Textbook of
PAEDIATRIC EMERGENCY MEDICINE

Second edition

EDITED BY

Peter Cameron MBBS MD FACEM
Professor of Emergency Medicine, The Alfred Hospital and Monash University, Melbourne, Australia

George Jelinek MD MBBS Dip DHM FACEM
Director, Emergency Practice Innovation Centre, St Vincents Hospital; Professorial Fellow, The University of Melbourne, Melbourne, Australia

Ian Everitt MBBS Dip Anat FRACP FACEM
Paediatric Emergency Physician, Princess Margaret Hospital for Children; General Paediatrician, Fremantle Hospital, Perth; General Paediatrician, Emergency Physician, Kimberley Health Service, Broome, Derby, Fitzroy Crossing, Australia

Gary Browne MD MBBS MSpMed FRACP FACEM
Professor of Emergency Medicine, The Children's Hospital at Westmead; Chair of Discipline of Emergency Medicine, The University of Sydney; Head of Academic Emergency Medicine, The Children's Hospital at Westmead, Sydney, Australia

Jeremy Raftos MBBS FRACP
Director of Paediatric Emergency Medicine, Women's and Children's Hospital, Children, Youth and Women's Health Service, Adelaide, Australia

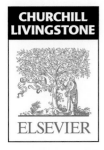

CHURCHILL
LIVINGSTONE

ELSEVIER

Edinburgh   London   New York   Oxford   Philadelphia   St Louis   Sydney   Toronto   2012

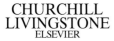

First edition 2006
Second edition 2012
   Reprinted 2012 (three times)

ISBN 9780702033681

British Library Cataloguing in Publication Data
A catalogue record for this book is available from the British Library

Library of Congress Cataloging in Publication Data
A catalog record for this book is available from the Library of Congress

your source for books,
journals and multimedia
in the health sciences

www.elsevierhealth.com

Working together to grow
libraries in developing countries

www.elsevier.com | www.bookaid.org | www.sabre.org

ELSEVIER   BOOK AID International   Sabre Foundation

The
Publisher's
policy is to use
**paper manufactured
from sustainable forests**

Printed in China

Textbook of
PAEDIATRIC EMERGENCY MEDICINE

Commissioning Editor: Timothy Horne/Jeremy Bowes
Development Editor: Helen Leng
Project Manager: Sukanthi Sukumar
Designer: Kirsteen Wright
Illustration Manager: Gillian Richards
Illustrator: Cactus

Preface to the second edition

Following the successful launch of the first edition as a companion to the *Adult Textbook of Emergency Medicine*, we have had considerable feedback on the content and layout from doctors, nurses and paramedics working in paediatric emergency practice from around the world. The feedback has been positive, particularly regarding the importance of a text with a standardised, easily accessible format. Despite major advances in computerisation, most clinicians studying detailed clinical material, still prefer a well-presented book with carefully edited text to on-line material. It is likely that further advances in technology will enable electronic versions of this text shortly and it is intended for this to occur after the printed version has been released.

In this edition we have reviewed each chapter and updated guidelines and management protocols where appropriate. Material has been reviewed by chapter authors and editors to ensure that it is consistent with best practice internationally. The structure has remained the same to enable easy access for readers.

Since the first edition, there has been consolidation of paediatric emergency medicine as a specialised domain of clinical expertise. Standards for paediatric patient care in emergency departments have been published in the United Kingdom and elsewhere and training programmes have been developed in many countries. There is a high degree of cooperation within the international emergency paediatric community and international networks for research (e.g. PERN – Paediatric Emergency Research Network) and other activities are being considered. Hopefully texts such as this can further consolidate the convergence of clinical knowledge and practice internationally.

This edition was developed over approximately 18 months with contributions from authors around the world including Australia, New Zealand, United Kingdom, Hong Kong, and the United States. The commitment and effort required to coordinate and cajole the many people involved, required dedication from all involved but we would particularly like to thank Helen Leng from Elsevier who remained focused throughout.

P. C.   2012
G. J.
I. E.
G. B.
J. R.

v

Preface to the first edition

For emergency physicians working in community hospitals, paediatric presentations are seen as the most challenging. There are very few critically ill children. However, the possibility of missing an early presentation of a potentially life-threatening illness is always present. Children are not always capable of communicating their problems verbally and the parents are inevitably anxious. There are numerous anecdotes of missed diagnoses resulting in catastrophic outcomes. With experience, emergency practitioners develop systematic approaches to overcome these problems. Unfortunately, this is often too late for trainees and clinicians rotating through low-paediatric-volume departments. The reality is that most emergency physicians, even when working in a specialised paediatric centre, will have limited exposure to critically ill children. Regular in-hospital training, courses such as the Advanced Paediatric Life Support (APLS) course, and access to simple reference material are all essential in overcoming this problem.

The purpose of this book is to provide a reference text for medical, nursing and paramedic staff involved in the provision of paediatric emergency care. The book provides a basic approach to the initial care of children with common emergencies whilst giving summary information on more complicated chronic presentations that may present to community hospitals as these conditions are increasingly treated outside the specialist centres. The contributors to the book have been deliberately selected from both specialist paediatric and emergency backgrounds, to ensure a broad perspective.

In Australasia, the United Kingdom, South-east Asia and many other regions, paediatric emergency medicine has fallen between specialist training groups with expertise from specialist paediatricians as well as emergency physicians. At times, this relationship has been strained with differing approaches to the management of emergency presentations and training of personnel working in paediatric departments. This is now being improved with joint training programmes and a more collaborative approach. Hopefully this book will help bridge some of the differences between the specialist groups.

This text should be seen as a companion to the *Textbook of Adult Emergency Medicine*, the second edition of which has been published and widely distributed in Australasia, South-east Asia and the United Kingdom. It is hoped that a simple straightforward approach to common emergencies will give the reader a method for managing likely emergency presentations. There are frequently many different approaches to managing common medical conditions. Where possible, we have tried to take an evidence-based approach. However, where limited evidence is available we have reverted to consensus amongst the experts in that area. As in most areas of medicine, most of our patient care is dependent on consensus rather than evidence.

For a textbook of this size, an incredible amount of work is necessary to ensure that content is correct and that the project finally comes together within a reasonable time frame. The individual contributors and publication staff at Elsevier should be congratulated. We would also like to thank Ms Mimi Morgan for her considerable patience in coordinating this project.

P. C.   2006
G. J.
I. E.
G. B.
J. R.

Contributors

Jason Acworth MBBS FRACP
Director, Paediatric Emergency Medicine, Children's Health Services, Queensland; Senior Lecturer, Paediatrics and Child Health, The University of Queensland, Brisbane, Australia

Navid Adib MBBS FRACP PhD
Paediatric Rheumatologist, Queensland Paediatric Rheumatology Services, Brisbane, Australia

Philip Aplin MBBS FACEM
Emergency Medicine, Flinders Medical Centre, Adelaide, Australia

Franz E Babl MD MPH FRACP FAAP FACEP
Paediatric Emergency Physician, Department of Emergency Medicine, Royal Children's Hospital; Associate Professor, Department of Paediatrics, The University of Melbourne; Research Fellow, Murdoch Children's Research Institute, Melbourne, Australia

Roger Barkin MD MPH FAAP FACEP
Emergency Medicine Physician, Aurora, Colorado, USA

Peter L J Barnett MBBS FRACP MSc FACEM MSpMed
Deputy Director, Department of Emergency Medicine, Royal Children's Hospital; Clinical Associate Professor, Department of Paediatrics, The University of Melbourne; Honorary Research Fellow, Emergency Research, Murdoch Children's Research Institute, Melbourne, Australia

Katherine Barton MBBS
Paediatric Emergency Senior Registrar, Department of Emergency Medicine, Princess Margaret Hospital for Children, Perth, Australia

Tom Beattie MB MSc FRCSE FRCPE FFSEM(RSPI) DCH
Consultant in Paediatric Emergency Medicine, Emergency Department, Royal Hospital for Sick Children, Edinburgh, UK

Andrew Berry AM FRACP
State Director, NETS (Newborn and paediatric Emergency Transport Service), NSW, Australia

Meredith Borland MBBS FRACGP FACEM
Deputy Director and Paediatric Emergency Physician, Emergency Department, Princess Margaret Hospital for Children, Perth; Joint Clinical Senior Lecturer, School of Paediatrics and Child Health and School of Primary, Aboriginal and Rural Health Care, University of Western Australia, Australia

Robyn Brady MBBS DCH MRCPI FRACP FACEM
Staff Specialist Paediatric Emergency Physician; Director of Emergency Medicine Training, Paediatric Emergency Department, Mater Children's Hospital, Brisbane, Australia

Drago Bratkovic MBBS FRACP HGSA
Unit Head, Metabolic Clinic, SA Pathology, Adelaide, Australia

Lindsay Bridgford CSM MBBS DCH DRANZCOG FACEM
Director of Emergency Medicine Training, Maroondah Hospital, Davey Drive, Australia

Andrew Bullock MBBS FRACP
Children's Cardiac Centre, Princess Margaret Hospital for Children, Perth, Australia

Danny Cass MBBS
Head of Academic Surgery and Director of Trauma, The Children's Hospital at Westmead, Sydney, Australia

Gervase Chaney MBBS FRACP
Paediatrician and Director, Postgraduate Medical Education, Princess Margaret Hospital for Children, Perth, Australia

Nicholas Cheng MBBS BSc(Med) DCH FRACP
Paediatric Emergency Physician, Emergency Department, The Children's Hospital at Westmead, Sydney, Australia

Raymond Chin MBBS DCH FRACP
Clinical Associate Lecturer, Paediatrics and Child Health, The Children's Hospital at Westmead and The University of Sydney, Sydney, Australia

Robin Choong MBBS FRACP FCICM
Senior Staff Specialist, Paediatric Intensive Care Unit, The Children's Hospital at Westmead, Sydney, Australia

Simon Chu MBBS DCH FACEM MMEd
General and Paediatric Emergency Physician, Emergency Department, Lyell McEwin Health Service, Adelaide, Australia

Pat Clements BSc BSocWk
Social Worker, Department of Emergency Medicine and Paediatric Intensive Care Unit, Royal Children's Hospital, Brisbane, Australia

Jane Cocks MBBS FRACP FACEM FCICM
Clinical Director, Neonatal and Paediatric Retrievals, MedSTAR Emergency Medical Retrieval, SA Health; Paediatric Emergency Physician, Paediatric Emergency Department, The Women's and Children's Hospital, Adelaide, Australia

David G Cooksley MBChB FACEM DIMC RCSE DRACOG ACCAM PGCertAME
Director, Trauma Service, The Townsville Hospital, Townsville, Australia

Elizabeth M Cotterell MBBS DipPaed FRACP MPH
Associate Professor, Paediatrics, School of Rural Medicine, The University of New England, Armidale, Australia

Lisa Coutts BNurs
Clinical Nurse, Department of Cardiology, Hollywood Private Hospital, Nedlands; Emergency Nurse, Emergency Department, Joondalup Health Campus, Joondalup, Perth, WA

Paul Craven BSc MBBS MRCP FRACP
Deputy Director and Senior Staff Specialist, Neonatal Intensive Care Unit, John Hunter Children's Hospital, Newcastle, Australia

Maree Crawford MBBS FRACP
Paediatrician and Senior Staff Specialist, Child Advocacy Service, Royal Children's Hospital, Brisbane, Australia

Nigel W Crawford MBBS MPH
Clinical Research Fellow, Murdoch Children's Research Institute, Royal Children's Hospital, Melbourne, Australia

Sarah Dalton BMed FRACP MAppMgtHlth
Paediatric Emergency Physician, Emergency Department, The Children's Hospital at Westmead; Retrieval Consultant, NSW Newborn and Paediatric Emergency Transport Service, Sydney, Australia

Andrew J Davidson MBBS MD FANZCA
Senior Anaesthetist, Royal Children's Hospital; Associate Professor, Department of Paediatrics, The University of Melbourne; Director of Clinical Research, Murdoch Children's Research Institute, Melbourne, Australia

Conor Deasy FCEM FACEM DIMC DCH DipTox MB BAO BCH BMedSc
Emergency Physician, Emergency and Trauma Centre, Alfred Hospital; Research Scholar, Department of Epidemiology and Preventive Medicine, Melbourne, Australia

Ronald A Dieckmann MD MPH FAAP FACEP
Professor Emeritus of Emergency Medicine and Pediatrics, University of California, San Francisco

Evelyn Doyle MB Bch BAO MRCPCH FRACP
Paediatric Emergency Physician, Emergency Department, Children, Youth and Women's Health Service, Adelaide, Australia

Linda Durojaiye MBBS BMedSci MRCP FRACP
Paediatric Emergency Physician, Emergency Department, Sydney Children's Hospital, Sydney, Australia

Daryl Efron MBBS FRACP MD
Paediatrician, Royal Children's Hospital; Senior Lecturer, Department of Paediatrics, The University of Melbourne; Honorary Research Fellow, Murdoch Children's Research Institute, Melbourne, Australia

Ian Everitt MBBS FACEM FRACP
Paediatric Emergency Physician, Princess Margaret Hospital for Children; General Paediatrician, Fremantle Hospital, Perth; General Paediatrician, Emergency Physician, Kimberley Health Service, Broome, Derby, Fitzroy Crossing, Australia

Tom Everitt MBBS FRACGP
General Practitioner, Casey Medical Centre, Melbourne, Australia

Michael Fairley MBBS FRANZCP
Child and Adolescent Mental Health, Prince of Wales and Sydney Children's Hospitals, Sydney, Australia

Bruce Fasher MBBS DRCOG DCH FRCP FRACP
Staff Physician, Royal Alexandra Hospital for Children, Sydney, Australia

Toby Fogg BM MRCS FACEM FCEM
Staff Specialist, Emergency Department, Royal North Shore Hospital, Sydney; Retrieval Specialist, CareFlight, Sydney, Australia

Peter Francis MBBS FRACP
Paediatrician, Frankston Hospital; Paediatric Nuclear Medicine Physician, Royal Children's Hospital, Melbourne, Australia

Gary Geelhoed MBBS FRACP FACEM MD
Clinical Professor, Director, Emergency Department, Princess Margaret Hospital for Children, Perth, Australia

Padraic Grattan-Smith MBBS MRCP FRACP
Honorary Consultant in Movement Disorders, Department of Neurology, The Children's Hospital at Westmead, Sydney, Australia

Joanne Grindlay MBBS DA FRACGP FARGP FACEM EMDM
Emergency Physician, Emergency Department, Royal Children's Hospital; Murdoch Children's Research Institute, Melbourne, Australia

Sonia Grover MBBS FRANZCOG MD
Director, Department of Paediatric and Adolescent Gynaecology and Associate Professor, Department of Paediatrics, Royal Children's Hospital, The University of Melbourne; Consultant Gynaecologist, Department of Obstetrics and Gynaecology, Mercy Hospital for Women, Melbourne, Australia

Naren Gunja MBBS FACEM
Medical Director, NSW Poisons Information Centre; Clinical Toxicologist, The Children's Hospital at Westmead; Clinical Senior Lecturer, Discipline of Emergency Medicine, Sydney Medical School, Sydney, Australia

Anthony Harrington MBBS FRACGP DARCS FACEM
Senior Consultant, Department of Emergency Medicine, Nambour General Hospital, Nambour, Australia

Andrew Harris MBBS FRACGP DipSportsMed ACCAM
General Practitioner, Sandringham Medical Centre, Melbourne, Australia

Wayne Hazell MBBS DipObs FACEM
Emergency Physician, Head of Emergency Medicine Education and Research, Middlemore Hospital, Auckland, New Zealand

Robert Henning FRCA FJFICM
Staff Specialist in Intensive Care, Royal Children's Hospital, Melbourne, Australia

Malcolm Higgins BMBS FRACP
Staff Specialist, Paediatric Emergency Department, Women's and Children's Hospital, Adelaide, Australia

Andrew J A Holland BSc (Hons) MBBS PhD Grad Cert Ed Studies (Higher Ed) FRCS (Eng) FRACS (Paed) FACS

Professor of Paediatric Surgery, The Children's Hospital at Westmead, The University of Sydney, Australia

Jason Hort MBBS MCRP FRACP
Senior Staff Specialist, Emergency Department, The Children's Hospital at Westmead, Sydney, Australia

Andrew Jan MBBS FACEM BA FAMAC MPhil
Director of Emergency Medicine, St John of God Hospital Murdoch, Perth, Australia

Andrew Stewart Kemp MBBS PhD FRACP
Professor of Allergy and Clinical Immunology, The Children's Hospital at Westmead, Sydney, Australia

Colin S Kikiros MBBS FRACS
Consultant Paediatric Surgeon, Princess Margaret Hospital for Children, Perth, Australia

Barbara King MBBS FRACP
Paediatric Emergency Physician, Princess Margaret Hospital for Children; Clinical Senior Lecturer, School of Paediatrics and Child Health, The University of Western Australia, Perth, Australia

Judith Klein MD FACEP
Assistant Professor of Emergency Medicine, San Francisco General Hospital Medical Center, San Francisco, USA

David Krieser MBBS FRACP
Paediatric Emergency Physician, Sunshine Hospital; Clinical Senior Lecturer, Paediatrics, The University of Melbourne, Melbourne, Australia

Richard Lennon MBBS FRACP FACEM CCPU MBioeth
Director of Emergency Paediatrics, Royal North Shore Hospital, Sydney, Australia

Stuart Lewena BMedSci MBBS FRACP
Paediatric Emergency Physician, Royal Children's Hospital; Research Affiliate, Murdoch Children's Research Institute, Melbourne, Australia

Michelle Lin MD
Associate Professor of Clinical Emergency Medicine, Department of Emergency Medicine, UCSF-San Francisco General Hospital, San Francisco, USA

Kevin Mackway-Jones FRCP FRCS FCEM
Professor of Emergency Medicine, Royal Manchester Children's Hospital and Manchester Royal Infirmary, Manchester, UK

Elly Marillier MBBS DCH FACEM
Emergency Physician, Emergency Department, Joondalup Health Campus; Clinical Senior Lecturer, The University of Western Australia, Perth, Australia

Jennie Martin MBBS DipCH FACEM
Senior Staff Specialist, Department of Emergency Medicine, Royal North Shore Hospital, Sydney, Australia

Karen McCarthy MBBch BAO FRACP
Paediatric Emergency Physician, Emergency Department, Starship Children's Hospital, Auckland, New Zealand

Helen Mead MBBS FRACP FACEM
Emergency Consultant, Emergency Department, Princess Margaret Hospital for Children; Senior Clinical Lecturer, School of Paediatrics and Child Health, The University of Western Australia, Perth, Australia

Alastair D McR Meyer BSc BMedSci MBBS FACEM
Emergency Physician, Southern Health (Casey Hospital & Monash Medical Centre); Director, Emergency Medicine Research, Casey Hospital; General Practitioner, Melbourne, Australia

Alistair Murray FACEM FCEM FRCS(A&E) DipIMC
Consultant in Emergency Medicine, St Vincent's University Hospital, Dublin, Ireland

Yuresh Naidoo MBChB FACEM
Director of Clinical Training, Emergency Department, Joondalup Health Campus, Perth, Australia

Murali Narayanan FRACP DNB DCH
Head of Department, Paediatrics, Kalgoorlie Regional Hospital, Kalgoorlie, Australia

Kenneth Nunn MBBS (Hons) FRANZCP FRCPsych PhD
Senior Consultant Child Psychiatrist, Acuity Reduction Team, The Children's Hospital,

Westmead; Department of Psychiatry, Faculty of Medicine, University of New South Wales, Sydney, Australia

Matthew O'Meara MBBS FRACP
Director of Emergency Medicine, Sydney Children's Hospital; Conjoint Senior Lecturer, School of Medicine, The University of New South Wales, Sydney, Australia

Ed Oakley MBBS
Director of Paediatric Emergency Medicine, Southern Health, Monash Medical Centre, Melbourne, Australia

Kim Lian Ong MBBS FRCS FHKCEM FHKAM FAMS
Consultant, Accident and Emergency, Pok Oi Hospital, Yuen Long, New Territories, Hong Kong

David Orchard MBBS FACD
Paediatric Dermatologist, Department of Dermatology, Royal Children's Hospital, Melbourne, Australia

Colin Parker MBChB DCH MRCPCH FACEM
Emergency Physician, Director of Emergency Medicine Training, Joondalup Health Campus; Emergency Physician, Princess Margaret Hospital for Children; Clinical Senior Lecturer, The University of Western Australia, Perth, Australia

Jacqueline E L Parkinson BPharm (Hons)
Senior Clinical Pharmacist, Pharmacy Department, Southern Health, Melbourne, Australia

Donald Payne MD FRACP FRCPCH
Associate Professor, Paediatric and Adolescent Medicine, Princess Margaret Hospital for Children; Associate Professor, School of Paediatrics and Child Health, The University of Western Australia, Perth, Australia

Scott Pearson MBChB FACEM
Emergency Physician, Emergency Medicine, Christchurch Hospital, Christchurch, New Zealand

Natalie Phillips MBBS MPhil FRACP
Department of Emergency Medicine, Royal Children's Hospital, Brisbane, Australia

Roderic Phillips MBBS FRACP PhD
Paediatric Skin Specialist, Royal Children's Hospital, Melbourne, Australia

Susan Phin MBBS FRACP
Paediatric Emergency Physician, The Children's Hospital at Westmead, Sydney, Australia

Colin V E Powell MBChB DCH MRCP FRACP FRCPCH MD
Senior Lecturer in Child Health, Department of Paediatrics, Cardiff University; Consultant Paediatrician, Department of Paediatrics, University Hospital of Wales, Cardiff, UK

Stephen Priestley MBBS FACEM
District Director and Senior Staff Specialist in Emergency Medicine, Sunshine Coast Health Service District, Nambour Hospital, Queensland, Australia

Michael Ragg MBBS FACEM DipO&G GradCertEBP
Emergency Physician, Emergency Medicine, Barwon Health, Geelong; Associate Clinical Professor, Deakin University School of Medicine, Melbourne, Australia

Pamela Rosengarten MBBS FACEM
Associate Professor of Emergency Medicine, Southern Clinical School, Faculty of Medicine, Nursing and Health Sciences, Monash University; Director of Education and Research in Emergency Medicine, Peninsula Health, Melbourne, Australia

John Ryan FCEM FRCSEd(A&E) FFSEM DCH DipSportsMed
Consultant in Emergency Medicine, University College Dublin; Associate Clinical Professor, St Vincent's University Hospital, Dublin, Ireland

Matt Ryan MBBS DRANZCOG MFM FACLM FFFLM(RCPUK) FACEM
Emergency Physician, Emergency Department, Werribee Mercy Hospital, Werribee, Australia

Kam Sinn MBBS FRACP
Emergency Paediatrician and Senior Specialist, Emergency Department, The Canberra Hospital, Canberra, Australia

Mike Starr MBBS FRACP
Paediatrician, Infectious Diseases Physician, Consultant in Emergency Medicine, Director of Paediatric Physician Training, Royal Children's Hospital, Melbourne, Australia

Greg Stevens BHB MBChB FACEM
Head of Emergency Medicine, Taranaki District Health Board, New Plymouth, New Zealand

Paul Tait MBBS FRACP
Senior Staff Specialist and Consultant Paediatrician, Child Protection Unit, The Children's Hospital at Westmead, Sydney, Australia

James Tibballs BMedSc MBBS MEd MBA MD MHlth&MedLaw DALF PGDipArts(Fr) FANZCA FACLM FCICM
Associate Professor, Intensive Care Physician and Resuscitation Officer, Royal Children's Hospital; Associate Professor, Australian Venom Research Unit, Department of Pharmacology, The University of Melbourne, Melbourne, Australia

James Tilleard MBBS FACEM
Emergency Physician, Nambour Hospital, QLD, Australia

Joseph Ting MBBS BMedSci MSc(Lond) PGDipEpi(LSHTM) FACEM
Senior Staff Specialist, Department of Emergency Medicine, Mater Public Hospitals; Clinical Senior Lecturer, Division of Anaesthesiology and Critical Care, School of Medicine, The University of Queensland; Retrieval and Clinical Coordination Physician, Careflight Medical Services Queensland, Brisbane, Australia

John Walsh MBChB MCHOrth FRCS FRACS
Director, Paediatric Orthopaedics Department, Mater Children's Hospital, Brisbane, Australia

Christopher Webber MBBS DipRACOG FRACP
Paediatric Emergency Physician, Emergency Department, Sydney Children's Hospital;

Deputy Medical Director, Newborn and paediatric Emergency Transport Service (NETS), NSW, Sydney, Australia

Julian White MBBS MD
Professor and Director, Toxinology Department, Women's and Children's Hospital, Adelaide, Australia

Richard P Widmer BDSc MDSc FRACDS
Clinical Associate Professor, Paediatrics and Child Health, The Children's Hospital at Westmead, Sydney, Australia

Barry Wilkins MD MA BChir
Senior Intensive Care Physician, Paediatric Intensive Care, The Children's Hospital at Westmead, Sydney, Australia

Gary Williams MBBS FRACP FJFICM
Staff Specialist in Intensive Care, Sydney Children's Hospital, Sydney, Australia

Frank Willis MBBS DCCH DCH GradDipHealthAdmin FRACP FRCPCH
Consultant, Emergency Department, Princess Margaret Hospital for Children; Clinical Senior Lecturer, School of Paediatrics and Child Health and School of Medicine, The University of Western Australia and The University of Notre Dame (Australia); Head of Paediatrics, Fremantle Hospital, Perth, Australia; Locum Consultant, Renal Unit, Royal Hospital for Sick Children, Glasgow, UK

Simon Wood MBBS DipPaed FACEM
Director of Emergency Medicine, Joondalup Health Campus, Perth, Australia

Simon Young MBBS DipCrim FACEM
Director, Department of Emergency Medicine, Royal Children's Hospital; Clinical Associate Professor, Department of Paediatrics, The University of Melbourne; Research Fellow, Murdoch Children's Research Institute, Melbourne, Australia

Contents

CONTENTS

CONTENTS

APPROACH TO THE PAEDIATRIC PATIENT

Section editor *Ian Everitt*

Discovery Library

Tel: 01752 439111

1.1 Approach to the paediatric patient

Ian Everitt • Andrew Jan • Andrew Harris • Tom Everitt • Lisa Coutts

ESSENTIALS

1 Gaining rapport with the child and the confidence of the parents is the key to assessing children.

2 A child needs to be approached according to chronological and developmental age.

3 Observation is a vital diagnostic tool, which is vastly more important in children than in adult patients.

4 The need for investigations is a balance between an invasive stress on a child and the potential gain of information to aid decision making.

5 Always back up discharge with a concrete action plan and definitive follow up.

6 It is often more important to exclude serious illnesses than make a definitive diagnosis.

7 Addressing parental concerns is an important part of the therapeutic process.

8 Emergency physicians should stay within their comfort zone and when in doubt, consult.

9 A febrile child should be considered as potentially sick until one can confidently conclude that he/she is well following a thorough assessment.

10 Always reflect on the potential fears of the child and parents.

Introduction

Who sees paediatric emergencies?

It is essential that all doctors are familiar with the recognition and management of the seriously ill child. The majority of children presenting to emergency departments are either taken to tertiary paediatric centres or mixed departments that see both adults and children. A small number will arrive, due to close proximity in an emergency, at adult departments where staff may be less familiar with the management of children. Likewise, paediatric emergencies occur remote from emergency departments and may require stabilisation by general practitioners, paramedical staff or laypersons prior to subsequent referral. It is an important role of emergency departments to be an available resource to support the community in the management of paediatric emergencies. This function may occur through advisory, liaison and educative processes.

Some critically ill children will arrive in a more predictable fashion via ambulance and some preparation can occur to plan for their initial treatment. On the other hand, a child in extremis may well be rushed in from a family car, without any prior warning of their arrival. Systems of preparedness for these situations are critical for the immediate assessment and optimal early management of children by emergency department staff (see Chapter 2).

Evolution of paediatric emergency medicine

In Australia and New Zealand there are currently only nine stand-alone tertiary paediatric emergency departments. Hence, the majority of paediatric patients present initially to mixed departments where approximately 10–30% of attendances are paediatric. This is similar to the UK, Canada and USA. Some of these children will require subsequent referral to a paediatric tertiary centre for ongoing specialist care. The role and functioning of emergency departments has changed dramatically over the past three decades. Paediatric emergency medicine (PEM) has now developed as a speciality of paediatrics and emergency medicine. The initial assessment and stabilisation of paediatric patients, which in the past was often deferred to intensive care or anaesthetic colleagues, is now an important role of emergency physicians. In Australasia, the development of PEM as a subspecialty of the College of Paediatrics has seen the establishment of a supervised training scheme by the Paediatric Emergency Medicine Special Interest Group for advanced paediatric trainees. A joint training programme overseen by both the Australasian College for Emergency Medicine and the Royal Australian College of Physicians oversees the training qualifications of paediatric emergency physicians. It is paramount that physicians and trainees in both specialist and general emergency departments are well trained and the facilities are appropriate for the resuscitation of critically ill children. Hence, the education and training of emergency physicians in the management of common paediatric emergencies is an important role of both paediatric and emergency colleges. Whether a trainee is seeking a career in a paediatric or a mixed emergency department, experience gained in both environments with exposure to the teaching of both paediatricians and emergency physicians is advantageous. Likewise, a rotation in paediatric intensive care and paediatric anaesthesia provides additional skills in resuscitation, airway management, haemodynamic support and monitoring of critically ill children. The APLS (Advanced Paediatric Life Support) and ATLS (Advanced Trauma Life Support) or equivalent courses are invaluable additional resources and are requirements to satisfy fellowship qualifications in the training of physicians who will be managing paediatric emergencies.

Identifying the potentially sick child

Of the vast number of children attending emergency departments, approximately 2–5% are classified as immediate emergencies (Australasian Triage Scale (ATS) 1 and 2) that require urgent assessment and management.[1] Importantly, children can present with a less urgent triage category, but may rapidly deteriorate from evolving sepsis or airway compromise. The majority of paediatric presentations consist of less emergent problems involving a wide spectrum of injuries and illness. Of this group of paediatric patients there is a subset where the diagnosis is not immediately apparent. Thus, paediatric patients can generally be divided into three broad groups: the obviously well,

the obviously sick or the potentially sick child. One of the major tasks for the emergency physician is to identify the 'sick child' from a large undifferentiated group of children who may present as potentially sick. It is by a 'filtering process' via history, examination, observation, investigation and consultation that one identifies the *potentially* sick child (Fig. 1.1.1). This group of patients includes: those children who have progressed to a severe form of a usually benign illness; those with early, subtle signs of a serious disease; or those who on initial assessment appear unwell, but require investigation to help rule out serious disease. It is often through *observation* of a child, that one is able to more accurately

assess each of these possibilities.[2] With experience, the ability to appreciate a 'sick child' improves; however, a good rule, particularly in the younger child, is, if in doubt, investigate, admit for a longer period of observation or seek the second opinion of a colleague.

Children with fever

The concept of 'occult bacteraemia' (OB) highlights the difficulties in detecting significant illness in febrile young children. With the recent advent of widespread vaccination to the common agents of occult bacteraemia (Hib, pneumococcus) the prevalence of

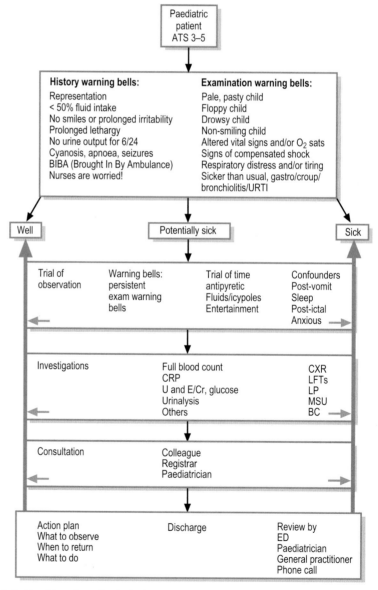

Fig. 1.1.1 Algorithm of paediatric decision making.

paediatric sepsis has diminished significantly and the clinical experience of managing septic children has been diluted in developed countries. Hence, one needs to have a planned approach to the assessment of febrile children at various ages. Bacteraemia can in its most manifest form present as a febrile, pale, pasty, mottled child, centrally warm but with cool peripheries. Some young children with bacteraemia, however, can appear completely well apart from fever. Investigations *may* help identify them with a high white cell count or c-reactive protein (CRP), but these inflammatory markers are unfortunately often non-discriminatory between benign and serious causes. The problem is not so much that children with OB are sick at that moment of time, but the possibility of the later development of serious bacterial sequelae necessitates timely treatment. Conversely, many bacteraemic children will spontaneously clear the organism without therapy. Therefore, these children remain in the potentially sick category of patients and are obligated to have either admission for observation or discharge with frequent planned reviews for sequelae and a definitive action plan for their parents should the condition change. The evidence for the use of prophylactic antibiotics in these children is controversial. The age of a patient and height of the temperature are useful risk factors to consider in the approach to individual patients. In children less than one month, any fever is significant, whereas older children are more at risk of serious illness with higher temperatures. Likewise, hypothermia can occur in overwhelming sepsis, particularly in neonates and infants.

Evolving illness in children

Due to differences in anatomy, physiology, development and psychology, children's diseases are age specific, with serious illness often taking time to evolve.[3] Many children present to an emergency department in the early stage of an illness and making a definitive diagnosis may require time. The clinical status of paediatric patients may also change rapidly. This can occur in response to prior trauma, evolving sepsis, toxin absorption or a seizure, and necessitate a change in the initial priority to receive

treatment. The younger the child, the greater the potential for rapid deterioration as the early manifestations of a serious illness may be subtle and non-specific. One must be vigilant for the early signs of compensated shock such as tachycardia, decreased capillary refill, mottled skin, cool peripheries, decreased urine output, or drowsiness. Early detection and fluid resuscitation at this point may prevent hypotension in a child with evolving sepsis. Children with severe and deteriorating respiratory illness will manifest fatigue. It is the early recognition of children with serious illness or the potential to deteriorate that is critical to the timely initiation of effective treatment.[2] An important principle in emergency paediatrics is to be proactive. One must be aware of the importance of regularly reviewing a child's response to a given therapy, escalate treatment if required and be vigilant for subtle signs of deterioration.

The environment

The physical environment of the emergency department needs to reflect a paediatric milieu with appropriately equipped cubicles for the reception of children accompanied by their carers. Despite the noise inherent in a busy department of sick children, the environment should be as calm and relaxed as possible. Wall or ceiling posters, mobiles, a selection of toys and books are useful to distract younger children from the distress and threat of an unfamiliar hospital environment. Posters of current popular characters such as 'Teletubbies', Blues Clues, Shrek, Wiggles or Harry Potter are useful. Not only do these characters make kids feel happy, but their active recognition provides a useful CNS diagnostic tool. A few initial moments gaining a child's confidence with a toy will usually reward the doctor with a more rapid and thorough assessment of the reluctant child. Supplies of stickers or bravery certificates are excellent rewards to have on hand for young frightened children who have undergone imaging or blood tests. If possible, in a mixed department, children should be completely separated from adult patients. Adult patients who are behaviourally disturbed will be distressing for a child and family to see or hear in a nearby cubicle.

Likewise if a child is to undergo a procedure during which he may become distressed, such as intravenous insertion or laceration repair, it is best performed in a closed dedicated procedure room. This will avoid visual or auditory distress to other children and parents. A mounted television/video monitor in this setting can be an excellent distraction during procedures, as an adjunct to analgesia and sedation. For neonates and small infants a radiant heater over the examination bed will aid temperature stability, examination and often the discovery of veins for cannulation.

The paediatric resuscitation area should include wall charts, which refer to emergency algorithms and drug dose guidelines, which can be rapidly referred to during the resuscitation of critically ill children. A white board is handy for pre-sizing and dosing for the imminent arrival of a sick child. Updated clinical guidelines in hard copy and electronic form in the management of common paediatric emergency conditions are a useful resource to be available within the department. Clinical pathways initiated in the emergency department can be useful in ensuring consistency of management from all levels of medical and nursing staff, as well as improving continuity of care in children who require admission to an inpatient unit.

Triage

Paediatric patients arriving in the emergency department should undergo triage according to standardised Australasian Triage Scale (ATS 1–5) so that they are seen in a prioritised fashion according to acuity. In mixed emergency departments where triage nurses may have had less paediatric experience, there has been a tendency to up-triage paediatric patients.[1] The use of scoring systems for specific conditions or a Triage Observation Tool may be helpful in improving the reliability of triage in young children, who may present with non-specific symptomatology.[4] A secondary nursing assessment should occur when the child is admitted to a cubicle, with further observations performed at the bedside, so that any change in condition can be detected early and acted on promptly. The senior doctor in the department should immediately be informed of children triaged as ATS 1 or 2 to direct timely management. In times of high workload, children with an ATS 3 may not be definitively assessed within 30 minutes and should have a senior doctor rapidly assess status and initiate therapy, if required. It may be necessary to modify normal triage systems when emergency department numbers are affected by surges in demand when significant influenza outbreaks or the like occur.

Fast tracking

Some initiation of treatment is appropriate during the triage process, such as the provision of analgesia for pain or an antipyretic in a child symptomatic of fever. It is important that children with pain are given early and appropriate analgesia or have injuries splinted when required. This will facilitate a more comfortable, reliable and expeditious assessment. The use of opiates, when required, will only enhance, rather than detract from the subsequent physician's physical examination.[5] The use of visual analogue scales such as the Wong–Baker faces may assist the assessment of a child's response to analgesia. A process of fast tracking appropriate children with single limb injuries for an X-ray prior to definitive medical review may improve efficiency through the department. Febrile children who present with a rash, not clearly due to a viral exanthema or benign phenomena, should be fast tracked to be seen by a senior doctor to consider the possibility of meningococcaemia. It is useful to have documented management plans for children who may recurrently present to the department. This includes conditions such as complex children, brittle asthma, cyclical vomiting or recalcitrant seizures where a clear plan of management can expedite care by ED staff.

The paediatric approach

The evaluation process of a child in the emergency department involves history, observation, examination and may include relevant investigations.

Each of these components needs to be considered in the formulation of a diagnosis and disposition plan. A child needs to be considered in the context of the family.

The assessment of children in the emergency department setting can be both challenging and very rewarding. It is a challenge to modify the clinical approach according to the chronological and developmental level of the individual child. Likewise, treating paediatric patients is a rewarding area of emergency medicine, as children will often respond rapidly to management within the time frame of the emergency department attendance.

Gaining rapport

Endeavouring to gain initial rapport with a child and the confidence of the parents is the key to assessing children in the emergency department setting. An unrushed, gentle and caring manner will rapidly settle the fears and anxieties of most children and their parents. This usually allows the examination to proceed in a non-threatening fashion and improves the reliability of clinical signs. It will take time, experience and the observation of colleagues' techniques for every emergency physician to develop their own individual approach to children. A thorough examination without causing distress to a child is very reassuring to a parent. Many children arrive at an emergency department miserable, in pain, fearful, or with some trepidation of what lies ahead. With a child-friendly approach by all staff, most will leave feeling much better and, hopefully, even having enjoyed the experience.

Age appropriate

The approach to any child in the emergency department is dictated by the child's age and developmental level. It is useful to have a modified approach to suit newborns, infants, toddlers, preschoolers, school children and adolescents. An understanding of the concept of 'the fourth trimester' is useful in dealing with crying phenomena in the first months of life, which will often precipitate emergency department visits (see Chapter 1.2). A preverbal or developmentally delayed child won't tell you of pain which has shifted to the right iliac fossa. An unwell 14-month-old clinging to mother may actively resist the initial attempts to be examined by a stranger. The absence of familiarity with a family or child that their family doctor may have may further impede the assessment of anxious children. When explaining procedures to children it is

important to be age appropriate and above all honest. Never tell a child 'you won't feel a thing!' prior to plunging a cannula through an EMLA anaesthetised cubital fossa. Rather, explain in age-appropriate terms what it may feel like and that it's OK to cry.

Maintaining a child's trust at all times is crucial and will positively influence any subsequent medical contacts the child may have. The demonstration of a procedure on a doll may decrease the anticipatory trepidation in a child.

The assessment of a child should always be carried out in the presence of the parent or carer, unless the child arrives by ambulance or other means without the parent/carer present, and the child's medical needs warrant immediate attention. Otherwise, it is prudent in the non-urgent situation to provide a staff member to support the child and defer the assessment until carers are present.

Development appropriate

Infants particularly benefit from the constant presence of their parent in their visual field in order to avoid stranger distress and are often best examined in the parent's arms. Neonates can be examined on the examination bed as long as they are kept warm. Toddlers, despite their evolving autonomy, will usually be less fretful if examined on a parent's lap. It is a useful sign of illness or other cause to note when young children do not exhibit these normal stranger anxieties. The preschooler who enjoys a sense of play and imagination can usually be relaxed during an examination or procedure by storytelling or engaging in play with a toy. An anxious early school-aged child may respond to participation in the examination or being asked about school or other more favoured activities. Adolescents, on the other hand, need to be approached in a more adult fashion and should be offered confidentiality and the opportunity to choose whether their parents are present (see Chapter 30.1).

In the event of an unatonable child resisting any examination, one may have to modify the approach to gain essential clinical findings in a gentle but firm manner. It is unusual, however, for a child to remain 'unexaminable' if appropriate analgesia is given and the child is left for a period of time undisturbed.

Parental involvement

In order to provide emotional support, parents should be encouraged to remain close to their child during any procedures. Parents who appear at risk of vagal syncope are best seated away from the 'viewing of action' but still in their child's earshot for verbal support. Children's behaviour often mirrors that of their parents, so gaining the confidence of the parent will often make an anxious child relax prior to procedures. The use of a confident, calm, caring approach will be rewarded by a child who will allow a more reliable examination. It is very reassuring to the parents to see that the doctor is experienced in dealing with children and anticipates the expected anxieties and reluctance to examination that a child may have when unwell.

History

The initial contact with the family should include an introduction of who you are. The parents should be addressed and the child greeted by name, in an age-appropriate manner. It is important to consider one's approach in terms of the needs of both the child's illness and the parental concerns. The history is generally elicited from the parent or caregiver but it is appropriate, in a verbal child, to augment this information by directly questioning the child.

Critically ill child

Sometimes the normal routine of history, followed by examination will need to be altered in a child who arrives critically ill. The management will need to be expeditious and occur simultaneously with the gathering of pertinent information from the parents. Parents should be given the opportunity to remain at the bedside of their critically ill child undergoing resuscitation, with a dedicated support person.

Parental issues

The clarity of the history given by parents can be affected by parental distress, anxiety or sleep deprivation. One should begin the history in a focused manner according to the presenting complaint. Later it may be useful to explore individual parental anxieties. One of the most important questions to a parent is, 'What is your biggest worry or fear?' Some parents may have specific concerns such as a fear their febrile child has meningococcal disease when community alertness to this condition is heightened. Addressing this concern may occupy most of the doctor's time. The parent of a child who has sustained an accidental scald or injury may be feeling distressed or guilty and sensitivity to this is required. Again, addressing guilt will involve much of the doctor's time.

Children-specific issues

In younger children, certain symptoms are less specific. The report of vomiting in an infant may be due to meningitis, pneumonia, tonsillitis or urinary sepsis rather than gastroenteritis. The assessment of wellness or otherwise in infants can be more challenging due to their limited psychomotor activities. Indeed, their spectrum of normal behaviours involves sleeping, waking to cry or demand a feed, followed by a return to sleep. Hence, it is important to enquire into their feeding status and sleep/activity pattern as an indicator of compromise due to illness. One needs to carefully clarify what their current intake is compared to their normal breast- or bottle-feeding. An infant who is feeding less than 50% of normal has significant compromise. It is important to note the report of a young febrile child who remains lethargic and fails to smile or interact with parents. In the otherwise well-looking infant, who appears mottled, clarify with parents whether this may be usual for their child (i.e. physiological cutis marmoratum versus sepsis). In assessing young children with trauma, a thorough history of the timing and mechanism of injury, noting the child's developmental capabilities, is paramount to detecting possible non-accidental injuries (see Chapter 18.2 on NAI).

Other useful information to cover in the paediatric patient history is shown in Tables 1.1.1 and 1.1.2.

Examination

Age appropriate

The examination technique used in paediatric patients depends on the age and developmental level of the child. The key is to gain the confidence and then the co-operation of the child. Older children are generally compliant, which allows them to be examined in a systematic fashion similar to adult patients. However, younger children usually need to be examined in a less formalised manner, whilst maintaining a high degree of vigilance. The order of the examination may need to be adapted according to the individual child's responses. In a reluctant examinee, clinical findings may be achieved by surreptitiously examining through play as the opportunity arises. Much can be ascertained in this situation by careful observation rather than a more threatening 'hands on approach'. Entertaining a young child in a professional manner during examination will generally allow the confounding influence of anxiety to diminish.

Table 1.1.1 History warning bells

- Child taking less than 50% of normal fluids
- The child with prolonged lethargy
- No urine output for six hours
- Prolonged irritability or inconsolability
- Report of cyanosis, pallor, seizures or significant apnoea
- The child who has not smiled over a period of hours
- Nursing staff feel the child is 'just not right'
- Unplanned re-presentations
- Parental concerns out of proportion to child's illness
- Brought in by ambulance
- History not compatible with injury/? non-accidental injury

Table 1.1.2 Important elements of the paediatric history

Presenting complaint
Pregnancy
Perinatal – delivery type, birth weight, need for resuscitation/special care nursery admission
Development – in a CNS problem, compatibility with injury mechanism
Immunisation status – need to clarify carefully
Previous illnesses/surgery/admissions/medications
Allergies
Infectious contacts/recent travel
Family history
Social history – family circumstances may influence a child's disposition
Fasting status if relevant
Feeds – normal bottle or breast feeds for comparison

Gentle, distraction, painful last

Children are usually reluctant to have any painful area disturbed. Confirming tenderness needs to be gentle and unhurried to minimise any distress, with appropriate prior analgesia. Many young children will respond to age-appropriate verbal banter during the examination, which distracts from the perceived threat of the examining hand. Alternatively, one may need to gently palpate a tender right iliac fossa, whilst using distraction such as the counting of the child's fingers. Sometimes a child may prefer their tender abdomen to be palpated with the examiner's hand 'through their own hand'. The examination needs to be adapted to the child's responses, deferring distressing phases until the final moment of examination. Time used initially to gain a child's confidence will make subsequent assessment more rewarding and the clinical signs more reliable. We have all experienced the frustration of trying to assess the abdomen of a screaming or fractious child who demonstrates the pseudo-rigid abdomen! Indeed, the most reliable method of excluding peritonism in a child does not involve any palpation of the abdomen. Asking a child to cough, walk, jump or climb the trolley are useful manoeuvres to help exclude peritoneal irritation.

The examination of ears and throat, tender abdomen or a painful injury, is best left till last in order not to upset a child and make the remaining routine examination difficult. If one detects that a child has an unfortunate fearful memory of a stethoscope or the like, a preliminary auscultation of a child's soft toy and warming the diaphragm will often allow this to subside. Distracters such as a soft toy placed in the hand may alleviate the examiner from the torture of the curious infant who yanks on the stethoscope tubing during auscultation.

Improvise

The examination of infants and young children is best done in the least threatening position. This is usually best whilst being held securely in the parent's arms or on the knee. If a young child is sleeping, the opportunity should be taken to perform auscultation, palpation of a fontanelle/abdomen, which will be altered in the crying state, prior to disturbing the child to wakefulness. A neonate examined supine needs to be kept warm with a blanket or a radiant heater. Hands should be warm. The crying fractious baby may be settled by offering a feed or a pacifier before the examination. The symmetry of normal infant reflexes is a useful screen for any focal motor problem or as a localiser of a painful limb that will modify normal symmetry of response.

Index of suspicion

The routine methods of examination for signs of meningism in children are unreliable. Asking the child to look upwards at an object or down to their umbilicus is a more useful screen to detect nuchal irritation. The presence of photophobia is sensitivity to ambient light as most children will be offended by a torch light in the eyes. In children less than two years old, the early signs of meningism are often absent and threshold for cerebrospinal fluid (CSF) examination adapted accordingly. Other significant but subtle features that may be missed on examination include persistent tachycardia or tachypnoea that is not clearly related to fever. One needs to be alert to the spectrum of stigmata of non-accidental injuries that may present to the emergency department (see Chapter 18.2 on NAI).

Respiratory examination

Noisy breathing in children can sometimes be difficult to determine if it is due to airway obstruction of intra- (lower airway) or extrathoracic (upper airway) origin. The localisation of airway obstruction to a particular segment of airway can often be aided by successive auscultation over the nares, mouth, larynx and peripheral airways. Remember, young children may manifest both upper and lower airway involvement ('crasthma, broup, cronchiolitis') with inflammatory involvement of both segments of the respiratory tract. Younger children are often easier to auscultate by listening through clothes (avoiding the 'stethoscope–cry reflex') from behind whilst being held by the parent. Detection of 'occult' asthma in a child with suggestive symptoms but no wheeze, may be aided by comparing the diminished volume and rate of airflow in expiration compared to inspiration, or alternatively re-auscultation after exercising the child in the ED. Young children with throat discomfort will be reluctant to volunteer a cough, but a gentle tickle of the axilla or palpating the anterior larynx will usually produce a bark to clarify suspicion of croup. Recognising the pattern of respiratory distress in a child from the end of the bed will often differentiate upper and lower airway obstruction, prior to any auscultation. Children with upper airway obstruction have slower inspiration, whereas gas-trapped wheezers will have diminished flow and speed of expiration on observation.

Abdominal examination

The abdominal examination needs to always conclude with the nappy area for otherwise occult torsions, hernias, skin problems and for stool examination, if present. The rectal examination in children is not routine and only performed with clear indication. One needs to be cognisant to maintain privacy and dignity, particularly when examining older children and adolescents. The examination of a child with possible sexual abuse is outlined in Chapter 18.1.

ENT last

In preschool age and younger children examination of the ears and throat is best deferred to last. A gentle, but rapid approach is necessary to achieve an accurate assessment of the oropharynx, followed by a cuddle from the parent. Despite the potential difficulty, the source of fever will often be overlooked if the throat is inadequately visualised in children. In infants, the throat is best examined with the child lying supine with both arms abducted alongside the head to prevent movement. A young child who is fearful of throat examination needs to be held as still as possible for a rapid, 'one gag, one look' approach. This is best performed after explanation, positioning the patient upright on a parent's knee, securing arms beside the trunk with the parent's dominant arm and holding the head straight-ahead with the other. 'Let's count your teeth' is a less threatening signal to most children to open the mouth, rather than mentioning 'the tonsil or throat' words, particularly if parents warn you that, 'Nobody has been able to get a look at his throat'. Some children require gently inserting the spatula between clenched teeth to touch the tongue to initiate a gag. Most

Table 1.1.3   Examination warning bells
The pale, pasty child
The floppy child
The child who appears drowsy
Alteration in vital signs, SaO_2
Early signs of compensated shock
The tiring child with respiratory distress
The child who never smiles despite appropriate prompting
The child who looks sicker than the usual child with gastroenteritis/croup/bronchiolitis/URTI
Other specific signs
Non-blanching rash – petechiae/purpura-sepsis
Bulging or full fontanelle – raised intracranial pressure
Bilious vomiting – bowel obstruction
High pitched cry – meningitis
Grunting – respiratory distress

older children, fortunately, will happily volunteer a view of the pharynx.

Following any distressing procedure it is important to acknowledge bravery in a frightened child. Likewise, giving a child an honest, developmentally appropriate explanation of what to expect prior to any procedure, such as an IV insertion, is to be encouraged. This is best done immediately prior to the procedure so that an anxious child's fears don't escalate in the intervening period (Table 1.1.3).

Observation

Observation is the distant examination of a child that begins prior to introducing oneself to the family, and continues after the examination, whilst one may be writing up notes or between seeing another patient. It also includes the noting of nursing remarks and vital signs recorded in order to obtain additional clues as to the sickness of a child. The trends of nursing observations over time are useful indicators to detect early signs of disease progression or the response to therapy. This 'ongoing triage', in effect, is particularly important to detect 'evolving illness' that may otherwise remain undetected.

LOOK, prior to examination

Before the 'laying on of hands', much can be gleaned by initially observing a child and parent in the cubicle, from a distance. One's first impressions of a child will often direct a subsequent approach. The child's state of activity and interaction with the environment and parents will often change when a strange doctor approaches. The process of evaluating a child differs from that of an adult by the greater importance of observation. It is important to emphasise the observation of a child to aid diagnosis in the emergency department setting. This is particularly important in evaluating children during their first three years of life. The 'end of bed' observations can be an important indicator for differentiating the potentially sick child.

Observational variables

The general appearance of a child should include noting level of alertness, eye contact, activity, quality of cry, posture, interaction with the environment, irritability, colour, hydration, perfusion, general growth and nutrition, respiratory distress and presence of any unusual smell (e.g. ketotic). The lack of normal resistance to examination or a procedure expected of a child is an important observation to note. The sick child may make none of the resistance expected to examination or venepuncture. Observational variables have been shown to be more predictive of serious disease than historical information in young children.[6] Likewise, clinical examination, considered alone, is a poor predictor of serious illness. Observation of a child needs to be performed as a separate process from the examination and may require a period of time for re-evaluation to detect disease progress. Researchers have used formalised scales such as the McCarthy Observation Scales to aid this assessment in febrile children.[7] In the ED setting, discussion of a child with a colleague can be a rewarding aid to decision making.

A child's posture, undisturbed, can be a useful clue to systemic illness, abnormal neuromuscular function or a painful limb or joint. Children with sepsis or meningitis may be floppy or flaccid. In other cases, the only sign of meningeal irritation may be a child who is holding his neck in a slightly extended position.

Observing breathing

When observing tachypnoea in a child, it is useful to determine whether a child has 'quiet tachypnoea' (breathing fast and quietly) with no evidence of increased work of breathing, such as may occur in conditions of fever, acidosis or cyanotic heart disease. Children with 'noisy tachypnoea' (breathing fast and hard) demonstrate increased work of breathing, due to conditions such as airway obstruction, pneumonia or heart failure.

Confounders

There are several observational confounders that can influence initial decision-making, when children can appear transiently sicker than they really are. There are many times when the initially sick-appearing child can pick up and appear well again over a short period of time. This situation usually occurs when the paediatric consultant is called and by the time he or she arrives the child is smiling and running around the department. The vomiting child will often look pale and 'pasty' for up to 20 minutes post vomiting. One-hour post antipyretic the symptomatic febrile child can look like a different child. Children initially emerging from a simple febrile convulsion can look well again in 20 to 30 minutes. A young child's physiological sleep can mimic septic drowsiness or somnolence resulting from head trauma. A fearful child, during examination, can escalate the examiner's perception of his illness.

Re-evaluate

This reinforces the power of observation. It allows time for a trial of fluids, reducing fever with an antipyretic, or seeing if a child responds to distraction. Subsequent re-evaluation of the child often allows one to differentiate whether a child is sick or well. The use of observation really allows one to identify the persistence of the initial abnormal examination findings. A child with intussusception may intermittently appear well and observation may be required to observe the clues to prompt the appropriate diagnostic investigation (Table 1.1.4).

When to investigate

One needs to be judicious with the use of investigations in children in the emergency department. Investigations serve more than

Table 1.1.4 Observation warning bells
Decreased level of alertness, activity, eye contact
Drowsiness or decreased interaction with the environment/parents
Abnormal posture
Abnormal quality of cry
Prolonged irritability or inconsolability
Ongoing pallor
Decreased peripheral perfusion or hydration appearance
Persistence of abnormal recorded vital signs
Respiratory distress/tachypnoea ('quiet' or 'noisy')
• Persistence of examination warning bells • Confounders – post vomit/seizure, high fever, normal sleep, anxiety

one purpose. They help confirm or refute clinical suspicions. Occasionally, parents appear to initially want more reassurance than simple clinical assessment and explanation.

Blood tests

Previous medical visits or advice may prompt a parent to feel that reassurance that their child is safe can only be confirmed by the 'magic of blood tests'. This may be especially so with a young-looking doctor. However, with clinical experience and clear explanation, parents can usually be counselled out of this option, when it is clearly not warranted clinically, by explaining that blood taking is not always straightforward in a chubby toddler and that sometimes two, three or occasionally more attempts are required. The potential psychological stress to the child is not worth the information that will be obtained in this instance. However, on the positive side, blood tests such as a full blood count (FBC) or a CRP may provide reassurance in some uncertain situations. At other times they are useless, for example to exclude meningitis in a child with clinical tonsillitis, as inflammatory markers are already raised.

Investigations may provide extra time for observation (by clinically reviewing the child!) and reassurance; however, if an investigation is performed and is abnormal, action must follow! The screening of urine in febrile young children is vital to detect occult urinary infection. In children less than 2 years old, dipstick analysis is inaccurate to exclude infection and microscopy must be performed to exclude pyuria. The appropriate techniques for obtaining urine are discussed in Chapter 16.4.

The parents

Parents who accompany their child to an emergency department are often anxious and fearful regarding the safety of their child. It is important to consider that the parents are entrusting the doctor with the well-being of their most cherished and precious possession. The management of the fears and the identification of the needs and expectations of the parents is an important role of the doctor attending to their child. Listening to and addressing the parents' concerns in a sympathetic and unhurried fashion is often the main therapeutic strategy to reassure an anxious parent that a child with a relatively minor illness is safe. Many parents may be sleep deprived due to attending to their sick child and this will influence their ability to convey a lucid history. The time spent at triage or in the waiting area in a busy emergency department can frustrate the most patient parent. This needs to be anticipated and acknowledged at the start of the consultation. Sensitivity to potential cultural issues is important in all interactions with carers.

Managing the parents

The emergency department visit may follow previous medical consultation(s) where their concerns may not have been addressed and it is important to explore these. Always acknowledge the parent's fears and anxieties; however, medical judgement should allow an objective decision about whether a child is sick or not. An exception to this is the parents of children with a chronic illness or special needs. They are usually correct when they judge that their child is sick. Aggressive and unreasonable carers will usually respond to a professional, polite and courteous senior doctor. There is usually a reason behind their behaviour that needs to be explored. Even the most anxious parent will usually respond to a thorough assessment of their child followed by an explanation of diagnosis and management. In unplanned second presentations where parents demand admission, it is usually best to admit.

Communication issues

Explanations to parents as a general rule should be appropriate to their level of understanding and education. Provision of handouts (with accompanying verbal explanation) or written instructions is useful to reinforce diagnosis and management. Reviewing a parent's understanding of instructions prior to discharge will allow clarification and avoid communication problems. Parents may have fears related to anecdotal advice from family/friends, misinterpretation of media reporting, or other sources, which need to be explored. Gaining the confidence of parents before they leave the department is an essential part of the therapeutic process and has a positive effect on compliance to therapy. It is useful to explain to parents the likely natural history of their child's illness and encourage review should significant deviations from this occur.

Management of paediatric patients

The urgency of management of children can be graded into the following categories:

- The critically ill child who requires immediate resuscitation and investigations and probable transfer to a tertiary centre.
- The sick child who needs immediate investigation and IV access.
- The child who warrants observation and a trial of fluids or antipyretics in the department. Consider the early placement of EMLA cream if further investigation may subsequently be necessary.
- The child that requires no investigation but whose parents need an explanation of the diagnosis and management.

The management of febrile young children is a large part of emergency paediatric practice. The current approach to those children without a clear focus is controversial and varies between institution and individuals. The two alternative approaches are risk- or test-minimising strategy (see Chapter 9). The current approach has been modified by the advent of pneumococcal vaccination. Certainly, it is reasonable, in a 3–36-month-old child, to be guided by clinical judgement alone with close planned review. If the child appears unwell, a sepsis screen is performed according to symptomatology. Neonates and small infants less than three months, where threshold for investigation is much lower, need to be approached according to departmental guidelines. Undifferentiated febrile children should be reviewed the next day and ongoing, until a definitive diagnosis is made or until the child returns to normal. Parents should be instructed to return to the department if their child deteriorates. The discharge action plan should give clear and understandable instructions on when to return. For example, in the febrile child, this should include: if child becomes more unwell, with decrease in intake to less than 50% normal, no urine output for six hours, or becoming drowsy beyond sleeping. Parents should be alerted to potential complications such as becoming limp, fitting or appearance of a rash, which warrant urgent review.

Turning the corner

Managing children is often about understanding the natural history of the illness and predicting when the child will 'turn the corner'. For example, one needs to be patient with a child who clearly has gastroenteritis who has been vomiting for two hours. Often a child will vomit hourly for eight hours, perhaps once or twice more and then improve. Advising the parents of the likely natural history of a condition and giving a clear action plan can be reassuring and prevent unnecessary re-presentation.

Decision making

Making decisions in paediatric emergency medicine is a balance of history, examination, intuition, knowing when to trust the parents and maintaining objectivity. If you feel uneasy with your diagnosis regarding a child, respect that feeling and gain support until you do feel comfortable with your decision. There are many strategies to do this:

❶ Consider early consultation with an emergency or paediatric consultant.
❷ Organise early follow up with a paediatrician or general practitioner.
❸ Have a colleague on the floor listen to the story or examine the child.

❹ Phone review the patient's family yourself, later that day or the next morning.
❺ Provide a concrete action discharge plan.
❻ Admit the patient for observation.

When to admit

The decision to admit or discharge a child from the emergency department is easily made when the child requires medical care that is only available in the hospital setting. The receiving ward will need to have appropriate resources for the ongoing management of the child, which should be clarified by discussion with the receiving inpatient unit/paediatrician. Some children may need to be discussed with, and transferred to a tertiary paediatric environment when they require, or have the potential to require, paediatric intensive care facilities or paediatric subspecialty management.

Factors influencing disposition

However, many other factors need to be considered in the disposition decision (Table 1.1.5). The threshold to admit a child is influenced by the child's age, availability of appropriate follow up, assessment of parent's ability to provide care and ongoing monitoring, the natural history of the illness and likelihood to deteriorate, social factors, comorbidity, distance from hospital, time of day, parental anxiety levels, availability of an early paediatric opinion, and the possibility that a child may be at risk. One needs to assess in a non-judgemental fashion the ability of the parents to carry out any ongoing treatment, and consider admission if

Table 1.1.5 Factors influencing admission threshold
Age of child
Availability of appropriate follow up/review
Parental ability to provide care and monitoring, social factors
Comorbidity
Distance from hospital
Time of presentation
Parental anxiety levels
To enable a paediatrician opinion
Possible child at risk outside hospital

there appears to be a need for ongoing support. When in doubt regarding whether or not to discharge a child, err on the side of caution. It may be prudent to consult, consider a period of observation in the emergency department, or admit the child to hospital.

Continuity of care

It is important for emergency department staff to liaise closely with the admitting paediatrician to provide continuity of care and to ensure ongoing care is expedited in the emergency department. Ongoing management and monitoring of the patient is an important role of medical and nursing staff after this decision has been made, particularly if there is a delay in the transfer process. Any significant change in a child's previous status or treatment needs to be communicated to the appropriate receiving team.

Observation ward

Significant compromise from many childhood illnesses is often transient and will often respond rapidly to interventions commenced in the emergency department followed by a period of observation. Parents can often be reassured during this period of observation in hospital that their child has remained well and will respond to management strategies that subsequently can be continued at home. Studies have shown that many children admitted to hospital only require a limited period of subsequent inpatient therapy and are discharged in less than 24 hours.[8] In a tertiary paediatric environment an effective way to manage these children is by admission to a short-stay observation ward. The emergency department needs to be appropriately resourced with staff to provide ongoing care and regular review of patients to expedite timely discharge. Conditions suitable for consideration of an observation ward admission will vary with local resources and may include asthma, croup, gastroenteritis, febrile convulsion, presumptive viral illnesses, non-surgical abdominal pain, minor trauma, post sedation recovery or ingestions.[9] In mixed departments, without the facility of a short-stay ward, it is often appropriate to use the paediatric ward to admit patients who would benefit from a period of observation (see Table 1.1.5).

Making a diagnosis

Not every child leaving the emergency department will do so with a specific diagnosis. The unwell febrile child needs to have serious diagnoses such as meningitis considered, before making a diagnosis of viral illness. Many children without a clear diagnosis can be managed expectantly and safely discharged home with organised review by a local doctor, paediatrician, or return to the department. Giving the parents clear instructions to return should the state of their child not follow an expected course is essential. Children are often seen early in the natural history of their illness and a diagnosis will only become clear with time. It is important to communicate clearly, verbally or in writing, with the doctor who will be following up the child. Close liaison with a local doctor who has referred a patient to the emergency department is essential. One should always respect the concerns raised by a referring local doctor who usually has the advantage of familiarity with the child and family.

THE ROLE OF THE GENERAL PRACTITIONER IN PAEDIATRIC EMERGENCY MANAGEMENT

Introduction

General practitioners (GPs) are the cornerstone and often the child's first contact within the Australian healthcare system. They are uniquely placed to have an intimate working knowledge of the biological, psychological and social dynamics that impact on a child's illness.

GPs are involved in the long-term care of family members, often for many years and in some cases several generations. It is this continuity of care and ongoing relationship with a family that is invaluable in assessing and triaging presenting medical conditions in children and their subsequent management. This is particularly important when caring for the health of children, who are often seen in the early prodromal phase of serious illnesses. It is the skill of the GP to differentiate the possibility of a serious illness in a child, particularly during the seasonal peaks of febrile presentations. This child may be non-specifically 'different' to similarly febrile children, but the experienced GP may just have a 'gut feeling' that a second opinion may be warranted and refer to ED.

There are two distinct areas where the general practitioner plays a vital role in paediatric emergency management:-

❶ Assessment, initial stabilisation and transfer of the child to the paediatric emergency department of the clearly 'unwell' or 'potentially unwell' child, and

❷ Ongoing management and follow up of the child after discharge from a hospital encounter.

Management prior to hospital care

The GP is more often than not the point of first contact for the potentially unwell child. The fundamental clinical medical tools of history taking and examination are used to make an initial assessment of whether the child can be treated in the community or requires referral to an emergency department for further opinion and management. This can be a challenging task as the GP is not afforded the luxury of observation over time, readily available ancillary testing such as pathology and imaging, nor an immediate further opinion from a specialist colleague. Particularly in the case of early or undifferentiated illness, the GP will need to make a judgement call on whether or not a child can be safely managed at home. Experienced GPs will not only use traditional methods of history and examination but will also listen to their 'gut feeling' when assessing children. This may involve attaching importance to red flag symptoms or signs or heeding the warning signs reported by an anxious, yet appropriately worried parent. This may depend not only on the medical status of the child but also the assessment of the social circumstances, education and competence of the parents/carers to detect their child is failing to 'turn the corner' or deteriorates. Often there is significant parental anxiety with an unwell child which cannot always be allayed by sound advice from an experienced GP when a child clearly has a self-limiting viral illness.

There may be parental demands for pathology testing to ensure 'nothing is missed' even though these may be deemed inappropriate by the family doctor. Parents may also report significant symptoms such as fever, an infant not feeding normally, cough or stridor which may no longer be present at the time of presentation to the GP. Some auscultatory chest findings are dynamic and therefore have a fluctuating presence, such as wheezing in bronchiolitis, so may vary greatly between the time of the GP and emergency department visit.

It is this complex interaction of both the medical and environmental factors which must be processed by the GP, often in the context of a 15-minute appointment. The outcome of this assessment may be the subsequent referral to hospital level care. Remember that the GP's decision is carefully considered with all the aforementioned factors coming into play.

Some of the more common reasons for referral to the ED may include the following;

- a serious time-critical illness which requires ambulance transfer, such as severe asthma, sepsis or meningitis;
- non-time critical illness which may not be responding to community based treatment and requires further investigation or parenteral antibiotics, such as evolving pneumonia;
- illness or injuries which are beyond the level of facilities available to the GP to manage, for example unstable limb fractures;
- parental concern and anxiety which cannot be sufficiently allayed by the GP; and
- social factors whereby the child cannot be adequately cared for or progress if monitored in the home setting due to lack of family resources.

It is imperative once the decision has been made to refer the child on to the emergency department, that the clinical assessment and concerns of the GP are adequately communicated to the physician who will be the next link in the management chain. This is best done with a phone call to the emergency department outlining the reasons for referral. In potentially serious illnesses the emergency department clinician can instruct the GP in any necessary treatment prior to transfer (for example, antibiotics and blood cultures in suspected meningitis or sepsis). A referral letter which contains the child's past medical history, allergies, immunisation status, list of current medications and any relevant investigations should accompany the child to the emergency department. This gives the treating doctor a head start in managing the child and avoids wasted time, effort and cost in repeating already established findings.

Management after hospital care

Once the child has been managed and discharged from the emergency department the circle of communication should include verbal and written feedback to the referring GP. This timely discharge communication contact has several benefits. First and foremost it ensures continuity of care for the child. If a treatment plan has been commenced by the hospital staff, the GP is then responsible for its implementation through continuing clinical assessment and adjustment of management according to progress. The natural history of illness and convalescence are dynamic processes which will vary from patient to patient and may require vigilant monitoring. This is most likely to be successful if the discharge plan is well communicated to the family doctor. It is vital that communication is not mislaid compromising patient care. The GP should receive information directly (fax or electronic) as well as via the patient or family as a back up if the usual communication systems fail.

Secondly, medical practitioners continue to accumulate knowledge and expertise throughout their careers so that reflective and sensitive feedback concerning outcomes of their referred patients is useful. This helps the GP to analyse and reflect upon their decision making processes and contribute to their evolving clinical acumen, which is a career long journey for all doctors. This is particularly so in the case of paediatrics as recognising the potentially unwell child can sometimes be as much art as science.

General practitioners can arrange further monitoring of the recovering child and is well placed to arrange further tests (for example chest X-ray following complicated pneumonia) or specialist follow-up if needed. Often the busy emergency department is not the easiest place, especially after hours, to arrange such important steps in the child's follow up care. The GP is also able to assess any psychological impact of the child's illness and offer ongoing support to the child and the family. These potential issues may not be evident at the time of the emergency department visit.

Integral to the communication process is a mutual respect between the GP and the emergency department physician with both having a respectful understanding and appreciation of the environment and challenges that each is working under. General practitioners have strong attachments to their patient and families and will appreciate a follow-up phone call and/or letter advising of the status of a referred child. The letter should be timely, with appropriate information including diagnosis, medication and results of investigations with an access phone number for any results pending. It should be presented in a clear concise form with a structured plan of management. Computer-generated letters are often more legible than hand written ones and reduce the chance of miscommunication in the discharge process. Some GP clinics now have secure email availability and may prefer to receive information this way.

If these strategies are implemented within a spirit of co-operation between GPs and emergency departments, this will ensure improved continuity of care and therefore better patient outcomes in the care of sick children.

Developmental milestones

It is important to have an understanding of the major developmental milestones throughout childhood for the provision of care to paediatric patients. These can be rapidly confirmed by examination or parental enquiry. This allows one to use an appropriate age-modified approach in the child's evaluation. Some specific behaviours, such as stranger anxiety in a 12-month-old,

Table 1.1.6 Normal milestones in first two years of life	
Neonate	Lift head, visually fix for period
6 weeks	Smile, follow past midline
4 months	Roll over
6 months	Sit, transfer toy between hands
9 months	Stand holding on, crawl, stranger anxiety
12 months	Walking, single words
18 months	Explorer (trauma/poisons), tantrums, several words
2 years	Combine words, run, jump

may challenge the assessment, so it is important to adapt the approach to these expected behaviours. Significant deviations from normal warrant consideration of paediatric referral. Useful early milestones are shown in the Table 1.1.6.

Growth

It is essential to measure a child's current weight on every emergency department visit in order to accurately dose any therapeutic drug and to quantify recent weight loss. Where a child is critically unwell and unable to be weighed, estimation can be made via Broselow or other charts. Between the age of one and ten years an estimation of weight is $2 \times (age + 4)$ kg. Standardised percentile growth charts are useful to confirm suspicion of failure to thrive or discrepancy in linear or cranial growth. The trend of growth plotted on a growth chart over time is more important than a single measurement. As a general rule, birth weight doubles by five months, and triples by one year. Newborns are often discharged from hospital in the first few days of life and may present in the first week to an emergency department. Following the expected initial weight loss, term babies should normally regain their birth weight by the end of the first week. Appropriate neonatal weight gain is an important index of wellness. Head circumference increases by 2 cm in the first three months, 1 cm in the next three months, followed by 0.5 cm per month thereafter (Table 1.1.7).

Table 1.1.7	Estimated normal growth		
Age	Weight (kg)	Height (cm)	Head circumference (cm)
Birth	3.5	50	35
1 year	10	75	47
2 years	13	88	49
>2 years	+2 kg yr^{-1}	+6 cm yr^{-1}	N/A

Table adapted from Fleischer and Ludwig, Textbook of Paediatric Emergency Medicine.[10]

Immunisation

It is not the role of the emergency department to provide routine immunisations to children. It is useful, however, to clarify a child's immunisation status with regard to the possibility of a particular infection such as epiglottitis, whooping cough or measles. Immunised children can, however, manifest a modified form of these infections. In children who are found to be incompletely or non-immunised, it is opportunistic to provide information regarding the normal vaccination schedule and refer to the local doctor or appropriate community facility for follow up (Table 1.1.8).

Vital Signs

It is necessary to interpret the vital signs according to the age of a particular child. A wall chart in the paediatric resuscitation area is a useful reference as a guide to these parameters. A good rule to remember is any child with a persistent respiratory rate >60 or heart rate >160 is definitely abnormal (Table 1.1.9).

Table 1.1.8	Australian standard vaccination schedule (0–5 years)*
Age	Vaccine
Birth	HepB
2 months	DTP, OPV, Hib-HepB,7vPCV
4 months	DTP, OPV, Hib-HepB, 7vPCV
6 months	DTP, OPV, 7vPCV
12 months	MMR, Hib-HepB, MenC
18 months	DTP
2–5 years	MenC
4 years	DTP, OPV, MMR

*This varies between states.

REFLECTION ON THE THOUGHTS OF CHILDREN AND PARENTS IN ED

The emergency doctor can gain much from the reflection of the insight of children and parents who have experienced the journey through the emergency department ... remember that every emergency department patient may reveal important lessons in our growth as care givers.

The thoughts of a child during the emergency department experience

"What comes to mind when I hear the word hospital? Huge needles, white every thing, people running around speaking doctors' language. Well, that's what I thought before I went, but I was proved quite wrong. For a start, the doctors and nurses actually spoke English (well most of the time) which made me feel more comfortable, being actually able to understand them. And they were all very friendly and smiling at you. In fact, the complete opposite to the stereotype storybook of needle brandishing doctors. I was so glad the corridors weren't thickly caked in white, but were dappled with different colours and pictures. Entering a place all white makes you feel quite nauseous, so I was glad for the variety. One thing I was a bit overwhelmed by was the size. To me, the ED was massive and I was amazed that it was only part of the hospital. I was so relieved that the ED had such a cheerful atmosphere that I wasn't really worried at all and I think that's what all hospitals should be like."

Thoughts on the emergency department through the eyes of a parent

"Anytime we have to take Aiden in to see the doctor we have to sedate him before we go ...
No white coats or uniforms...
It's so nice if the doctor takes time to talk to the parents first, not so clinical but to 'chew the fat' with the parents so the

Table 1.1.9	Normal vital signs			
Age	Weight (kg)	RR (per min)	HR (per min)	sBP (mmHg)
Birth	3.5	40–60	100–170	50
3 months	6	30–50	100–170	50
6 months	8	30–50	100–170	60
1 year	10	30–40	100–170	65
2 years	13	20–30	100–160	65
4 years	15	20	80–130	70
6 years	20	16	70–115	75
8 years	25	16	70–110	80
10 years	30	16	60–105	85
12 years	40	16	60–100	90
14 years	50	16	60–100	90

Adapted from RCH, Melbourne Clinical Guideline Site.[11]

child doesn't get scared when approached. . .

It's so much better if the doctor sits at the child's level so they don't feel like an adult is standing over them. . .

If the doctor is a nervous person, my child picks it up and this gets them nervous. . .

If the child says no during the examination, please don't push anything onto them. . .if they say no they mean no . . . give them some breathing space unless it's life threatening of course . . .

Don't have clinical stuff like needles, sharp containers visibly around or anything the child has a dislike for. . .

Perhaps a sedative prior to going to surgery again, as the next time he went for surgery he freaked out and it was so bad. He remembered everything when he entered the room and everyone was standing around him in scrubs, Dad had to hold him down whilst they gave him medication just to keep him on the bed. . .. Dad left crying. . .

Don't talk in the corridor about the child near the parents if possible. . .

The doctor/nurse talk can be insensitive to the child/parent even if the doctor/nurse don't realise it at the time. . .

It would be great if the staff have some sort of experience with a child with special needs before they see them in the hospital. . .

My child was unwell, miserable and clinging to me. The doctor was rough and tried to examine him instead of letting him settle and coming back later when he settled. . .

It's so frustrating when I tell doctors my child won't take oral medications and they just give oral medicines for us to struggle with at home, rather than considering a one-off injection which has helped in the past. . .

It gives us so much more confidence in the doctor if he explains what he's looking for during the examination, rather than just saying our child is fine when we're worried. . .

I like it when the doctor involves me during the examination of my child so I can distract their fear during the examination. . .

Some doctors only pretend to be hearing, but not listening to me when I tell them I'm worried about my child. . .

I'm so much more confident when the doctor is thorough but at the same time interacts playfully with my child. . .

I wish the doctor spoke to me separately about the scary operation details and then gave a non-fearful explanation to my child. I could have helped the doctor with how to explain things to my child without causing all that fear. . ."

References

1. Durojaiye L, O'Meara M. A study of triage of paediatric patients in Australia. *Emerg Med* 2002;**14**:67–76.
2. Luten RC. *Recognition of the sick child. Problems in paediatric emergency medicine.* New York: Churchill Livingstone; 1988. p. 1–12.
3. Browne GJ. Paediatric emergency departments: Old needs, new challenges and future opportunities. *Emerg Med* 2001;**13**:409–17.
4. Browne GL, Gaudry PL. A triage observation tool improves the reliability of the National Triage Scale in children. *Emerg Med* 1997;**9**:283–338.
5. Browne GJ, Chong RKC, Gaudry PL, et al. *Principles and practice of children's emergency care.* Sydney: McLennan and Petty; 1997. p. 1–5.
6. Waskerwitz S, Berkelhamer JE. Outpatient bacteraemia: Clinical findings in children under two years with initial temperatures of 39.5°C or higher. *J Paediatr* 1981;**99**(2): 231–3.
7. McCarthy PL, Sharpe MR, Spiesel SZ, et al. Predictive observation scales to identify serious illness in febrile children. *Paediatrics* 1982;**70**(5):802–9.
8. Browne G, Penna A. Short stay facilities. The future of efficient paediatric emergency services. *Arch Dis Child* 1996;**74**:309–13.
9. Scribano PV, Wiley JF, Platt K. Use of an observation unit by a paediatric emergency department for common paediatric illnesses. *Pediatr Emerg Care* 2001;**17**(5): 321–3.
10. Fleischer GR, Ludwig S. Understanding and meeting the unique needs of children. In: Fleischer GR, Ludwig S, editors. *Textbook of Paediatric Emergency Medicine.* 3rd ed Baltimore: Williams & Wilkins; 1993.
11. Royal Children's Hospital. *Clinical practice guidelines resuscitation: Emergency drug and fluid calculator.* Melbourne, Australia, 2003. [http://www.rch.org.au/clinicalguide/cpg.cfm?doc-id=5162].

1.2 The crying infant

Barbara King

ESSENTIALS

1 Define if this presentation is part of a recurrent stereotypical pattern in an otherwise well infant, or a single acute episode.

2 A careful history and examination will often lead to an appropriate diagnosis.

3 Screening tests, with the exception of urine culture, have little utility.

4 Review carefully carer's coping and supports.

5 Organise appropriate follow up.

Introduction

Crying is an important method of communication for infants.[1] Carers are usually able to identify and manage the cause (e.g. hunger, discomfort) and console the infant. Medical advice is sought if the crying is felt to be unusually intense or persistent or the infant is unable to be consoled by the usual methods.[2] 'Normal crying' was defined in Brazelton's 1962 study of 80 infants of American families selected to have minimal psychological stressors. There was a peak of crying to a median of $2\frac{3}{4}$ hours per day by 6 weeks, with a wide variation, and a decrease thereafter.[1] The classification of crying as normal or excessive is highly subjective and will vary according to infant, carer and situational factors. All three areas need to be assessed in this type of presentation.

Either a single episode of or recurrence of a pattern of excessive crying may precipitate emergency department (ED) presentation.[2]

Recurrent crying

Colic

Recurrent excessive crying in an otherwise healthy infant is often termed colic. This diagnosis can only be made if the pattern is recurrent and stereotypical[3] and a careful history, examination and period of follow up have ruled out important causes. The definition of colic varies but is frequently arbitrarily defined as a total of more than 3 hours per day of irritability, fussing and crying on at least 3 days a week for at least 3 weeks.[4] This pattern typically occurs in the afternoon or evening, ceasing by 3 to 4 months of age.[3]

Management

Current specific dietary, drug and behavioural strategies meet with limited success; however, cows' milk protein intolerance may have a role in a small proportion of infants.[4,5] The positive effects of changing from cows' milk based formula to casein hydrolysate formula have been noted to diminish with time, suggesting that colic is not related to allergy.[5] A trial of hydrolysate (e.g. Pepti-Junior, Alfare) may be appropriate in a formula-fed baby but its long-term use is likely to be unnecessary. It is notable that soy protein formulas may have similar adverse effects to those of cows' milk formulas.[5] Mothers of breastfed babies can exclude all dairy products (but ensure calcium supplementation) for 2 weeks as a trial.

Gastro-oesophageal reflux (GOR) is frequently cited as a possible cause of infant crying. Feeding difficulties and frequency of regurgitation ($>$ five times daily) are associated with pathological GOR as defined on oesophageal pH monitoring – there is a place for an empirical trial of proton pump inhibitors in this group.[6]

Anticolic medications should be avoided, as they have been shown to at best have no effect (simeticone) or risk serious adverse effects (anticholinergics).[4]

Behavioural interventions, including advice to reduce stimulation in combination with permission to leave the infant when the crying was no longer tolerable was effective when compared to a non-specific empathic interview.[4,7] Reduction of stimulation advice includes avoiding excessive patting, winding, lifting, vigorous jiggling and loud noises or toys. Carers were advised not to intervene in the early part of sleep when the infant may appear restless and also given an assurance that a certain amount of crying is normal.[4,7] It is important to remember that even if behavioural interventions do not change the infant's temperament, they may well alter the impact colic has on the carer and on carer–infant interactions.[8]

Carers very reasonably assume that there must be something wrong either with the child or their parenting for an infant to cry frequently and excessively. Much reassurance that the child is healthy can be gained from witnessing the conduct of a complete history and thorough examination. Similarly, an explanation that this is a common problem that does not reflect on their parenting, that some babies may be assisted by some simple behavioural techniques and that the carers will be supported by appropriate referral will also reduce anxiety considerably.

Acute crying

The causes of a single episode of excessive crying in an infant are vast. In an afebrile infant without a cause apparent to the carer, a careful history has been shown to provide clues to the final diagnosis in 20% of cases. Physical examination was revealing in more than 50% and a period of follow up often useful in patients where the diagnosis was still in question.[2]

Assessment

History includes the timing and amount of crying, duration of behaviour, measures taken to resolve the situation, specific carer concerns, the carer's response to crying, expectations and experience, specific social difficulties (including substance abuse), contact with child health nurse or other medical supports. A thoughtful review of the carer's supports and coping is essential.[9]

Also important are details of pregnancy, labour and neonatal difficulties, feeding activities including volumes of feed (considerations include under and overfeeding), dietary changes, past medical history, vomiting (gastrointestinal reflux, gastroenteritis, sepsis, meningitis). Consider changes in stools (constipation, gastroenteritis, bleeding anal fissure, intussusception), type of feeding (breast or bottle), type of milk, drug exposure, recent immunisation, fever, respiratory symptoms, rash, contacts with infectious illness and growth history.

Examination

A complete set of vital signs is essential, including oxygen saturation (tachypnoea with pneumonia, sepsis or metabolic acidosis, tachycardia with supraventricular tachycardia, sepsis or dehydration, desaturation with pneumonia or bronchiolitis). Examination should include tone and activity, alertness/conscious state (meningitis, encephalitis, sepsis, metabolic crisis, hypoglycaemia, electrolyte disturbance), perfusion, hydration, fontanelle (bulging with infection or trauma, sunken in poor feeding and dehydration), assessment of chest for respiratory distress, (pneumonia, bronchiolitis, metabolic acidosis, cardiac failure). An abdominal examination (herniae, testicular torsion, evidence of surgical abdomen), cardiovascular examination (murmurs, femoral pulses, cardiac ischaemia due to aberrant coronary vessels is a reported but extremely rare cause), ears (otitis media), oropharynx (herpes stomatitis, tonsillitis, upper respiratory tract infection).

Several additional manoeuvres may also assist:[2]

- fluorescein staining of cornea (corneal abrasion);
- palpation of long bones (fractures, osteomyelitis);
- inspection of skin beneath clothing (bruising);
- retinal examination (shaken baby syndrome);
- close attention to digits and genitalia (hair tourniquet).

Investigations

Investigations should be guided by initial clinical assessment. Screening investigations, with the exception of urine analysis and culture, have little utility.[2]

Disposition

The diagnosis of serious medical conditions during the initial clinical assessment will clearly indicate admission. Admission should also be considered in those cases where the clinical assessment is normal but the child continues to cry excessively in the ED beyond the time of the initial assessment. Persistent crying in these circumstances may be an indicator of serious illness.[2]

Occasionally it may be necessary to admit an infant with colic or minor medical problem to allow recovery of a sleep-deprived or poorly supported carer.[9] The involvement of social work services is appropriate under circumstances where the family or child is considered at risk. Serious injury to children by non-accidental shaking injury is preceded by other episodes of abuse or neglect in over 70% of cases.[10] Admission and social work assessment is always warranted if non-accidental injury or neglect is suspected.

Ensure appropriate follow up is organised for infants discharged from the ED – particularly where the diagnosis is not yet clear or where excessive crying is likely to be recurrent.

References

1. Brazelton TB. Crying in infancy. *Pediatrics* 1962; (April):579–88.
2. Poole SR. The infant with acute, unexplained, excessive crying. *Pediatrics* 1991;**88**(3):450–5.
3. Illingworth RS. Three month's colic. *Arch Dis Child* 1954;165–74.
4. Lucassen PLBJ, Assendelft WJJ, Gubbels JW, et al. Effectiveness of treatments for infantile colic: systemic review. *BMJ* 1998;**316**:1563–9.
5. Forsyth BWC. Colic and the effect of changing formulas: a double blind, multiple-crossover study. *J Pediatr* 1989;**115**:521–6.
6. Heine RG, Jordan B, Lubitz L, et al. Clinical predictors of pathological gastro-oesophageal reflux in infants with persistent distress. *J Paediatr Child Health* 2006;**42**:134–9.
7. McKenzie S. Troublesome crying in infants: effect of advice to reduce stimulation. *Arch Dis Child* 1991;**66**:1416–20.
8. Carey WB. The effectiveness of parent counselling in managing colic. *Pediatrics* 1994;**94**(3):333–4.
9. Singer JI, Rosenberg NM. A fatal case of colic. *Pediatr Emerg Care* 1992;**8**(3):171–2.
10. Alexander R, Crabbe L, Sato Y, et al. Serial abuse in children who are shaken. *AJDC* 1990;**144**:58–60.

APPROACH TO THE PAEDIATRIC PATIENT

2.1 Paediatric cardiopulmonary arrest (CPA)

Christopher Webber

ESSENTIALS

1 Prevention is the link in the Chain of Survival key to decreasing the incidence of death from Out-of-Hospital Cardiac Arrest (OHCA)[1]

2 Paediatric patients who sustain OHCA have similar survival to hospital discharge rates to adults who sustain OHCA.

3 CPA in children usually results from the development of progressive hypoxia and/or shock, which may be due to a myriad of causes.

4 The goal is to identify evolving hypoxia and shock early in seriously ill children and proactively instigate appropriate therapy to prevent the progression to cardiac arrest.

5 In contrast to adults, the most common arrest rhythm in children is non-VF/VT and is usually either asystole, pulseless electrical activity (PEA) or electromechanical dissociation (EMD).

6 Resuscitation organisations have developed guidelines for paediatric patients to include nuances of the newly-born, infant, young child and older child. Current recommendations simplify the differences in resuscitation approach between ages.

7 Allowing parents to be present and supported during the resuscitation of their child may be associated with a better long-term psychological outcome.

8 Unless CPA is associated with drug toxicity or some situations with profound hypothermia, neurologically intact survival is unlikely after 30 minutes of full CPR and several doses of adrenaline.

Epidemiology

Previous studies of paediatric Out-of-Hospital Cardiac Arrest (OHCA) have reported poor survival rates with severe neurological sequelae,[2,3] however more recent publications have challenged this reporting a similar rates of survival to hospital discharge as that of adults who sustain OHCA.[4,5]

The incidence of out-of-hospital arrest is reported as ranging from 2.6 to 19.7 per year per 100 000 paediatric population (age < 18 years), in the region of 30% achieving return of spontaneous circulation (ROSC), 24% surviving to hospital admission, and 12% surviving to discharge.[6]

Less than 10% of paediatric OHCA victims have a shockable rhythm on arrival of the prehospital care providers.[4,5]

Aetiology

The most common causes of cardiac arrest in children relate to the development of hypoxia and/or shock, the two pathways which, untreated, result in cardiopulmonary arrest. Shock is the clinical state of poor tissue perfusion. Thus, the primary organ systems involved are the respiratory and cardiovascular systems, and the central nervous system (CNS), which becomes compromised by hypoxia or decreased cerebral perfusion. Injury or diseases progressing to failure of these systems may then lead to cardiac arrest. CNS disorders, either with direct dysfunction or due to raised intracranial pressure, may cause respiratory arrest with the resulting hypoxia leading to cardiac arrest. The primary causes of cardiac arrest are heterogeneous and include trauma, sepsis, drug overdose, poisoning, immersion, critical respiratory illness and sudden infant death syndrome (SIDS). This list is by no means complete, and many other conditions may also progress to cardiac arrest.

Pathophysiology

Significant hypoxic and hypoperfusion insults to the myocardium are the common pathways that may progress to cardiac arrest in children. Hence, fluid or blood loss leading to shock, if left untreated, result in myocardial ischaemia and resultant cardiac arrest. Similarly, severe hypoxia also results in global myocardial dysfunction and subsequently cardiac arrest. Thus, preventive strategies must identify hypoxia and shock early and instigate appropriate management to improve oxygenation and organ perfusion, thereby preventing progress to cardiac arrest. Poisonings or ingestions may have a direct effect on the heart, causing an arrhythmia, coma, with subsequent respiratory arrest and hypoxia.

Outcome

Generally, the survival from respiratory arrest alone is much better than from cardiopulmonary arrest. Survival to discharge for children with respiratory arrest (pulse present) is around 75%, and of these up to 88% have a good neurological outcome. Reported survival rates from cardiac arrest in children have varied from 0% to 17%. Survival to discharge from hospital for paediatric OHCA is 7%[4,5] and 36% for in-hospital cardiac arrests.[7] 'Survival to discharge' is a very crude marker of 'success' as it does not include a measure of neurological function. Proactive early resuscitation of the pre-arrest child is important in order to have the most impact on outcome.

Unfortunately, the perception of the public, and even doctors and nurses, is that the expected survival rate is higher than this. Lay rescuers, physicians and nurses estimate the survival rate for cardiopulmonary arrest in children as being 63%, 45% and 41% respectively (compared to 53%, 30% and 24% for adult cardiopulmonary arrest).[8] Undoubtedly, fictional medical television programmes contribute to this bias, and even non-fictional medical programmes rarely show death as an outcome.

Differences compared to adults

When comparing children to adults in relation to cardiopulmonary arrest, there are several important differences. The aetiology of the event is usually different. Adults who collapse are more likely to have ventricular fibrillation or pulseless ventricular tachycardia, hence the time to defibrillation is the single greatest determinant of survival. Thus the *'phone first'* principle that applies to adults is not applicable to most infants and children, in whom the response should be *'phone fast'* (see Chapter 2.2 on Basic life support).

There are several anatomical and physical differences between children and adults. It is important to consider these differences in relation to the primary event leading to arrest and to the resuscitation techniques subsequently required (Table 2.1.1).

Development of resuscitation guidelines

In 1992 the American Heart Association guidelines for resuscitation were published. Subsequently representatives of seven resuscitation councils throughout the world,

Table 2.1.1 Important differences between children and adults	
Difference in children	*Implication*
AIRWAY	
Prominent occiput tends to cause neck flexion	Neck extension, into a neutral or sniffing position (slight extension), is required to optimise the airway for an infant or child respectively
Mandible is relatively smaller	More difficult intubation
Tongue is relatively larger	Tends to obstruct airway More difficult intubation
Larynx is more cephalad (located almost at base of tongue)	More difficult intubation - tendency for inexperienced operator to insert laryngoscope blade into oesophagus
Epiglottis is proportionally larger and more 'floppy'	Intubation may require straight-bladed laryngoscope to lift epiglottis forward to allow visualisation of vocal cords
Upper airways are more compliant (i.e. distensible)	Tend to collapse during increased work of breathing
BREATHING	
Chest wall more compliant (particularly the newborn infant and more so the preterm infant)	Less efficient ventilation, when increased work of breathing Earlier fatigue
Greater dependence on diaphragm to generate tidal volume	Distended stomach impairs ventilation Importance of venting stomach with gastric tube
CIRCULATION	
Maintains cardiac output and blood pressure by tachycardia initially	Diagnose and treat shock before hypotension develops Hypotension usually indicates late decompensation
GENERAL	
Head has proportionally greater component of body surface area	Loss of body heat during primary event or resuscitation Greater chance of head injury
Compliant chest wall allows transmission of energy to underlying organs, resulting in traumatic damage/rupture, rather than dissipation of energy	Pulmonary, hepatic and splenic injury may occur without overlying rib fractures
Development Language Motor development (fine and gross) Social and cognitive development (including abstract thinking)	Must be considered when interacting with the child and understanding injuries (accidental versus non-accidental)
Parental and staff considerations	Psychosocial issues Presence of family during resuscitation Staff pressure to continue resuscitation Impact on staff from death of child

including the Australian Resuscitation Council, formed the International Liaison Committee on Resuscitation (ILCOR). ILCOR advisory statements were produced. A subcommittee on paediatric resuscitation with representation from the American Heart Association and other paediatric representatives from ILCOR (Paediatric Working Group) further developed guidelines for paediatric patients. This group attempted to evaluate the level of evidence for resuscitation recommendations. It was important to attempt to avoid confusion between adult, paediatric and neonatal algorithms and ultimately the *International Guidelines 2000* were published. These were revised and published simultaneously in the journals *Resuscitation and Circulation* in 2005 and again in November 2010.[9] The Australian Resuscitation Council (ARC) and New Zealand Resuscitation Council (NZRC) released updated guidelines in December 2010. For the first time, both Councils published identical guidelines on-line, with both Councils' logos. Subsequently resuscitation courses, like the Advanced Paediatrics Life Support (APLS) course have been amended to be consistent with the international recommendations. APLS courses in Australia and New Zealand are consistent with ARC and NZRC recommendations.

Ethics of paediatric resuscitation

Presence of family

Over recent years, the benefit of allowing the family, mainly parents, into the resuscitation room during active resuscitation has become clearer. This practice has required a cultural change, and mandates appropriate and professional behaviour and language during resuscitation. Such practice should occur regardless of the presence of any 'outside' witnesses. It is a professional standard that all medical, nursing and other health professionals should aspire to and maintain. It is probably even more important that parents are offered the opportunity to witness the resuscitation, when the outcome is the death of their child.

In hindsight, parents who have witnessed the resuscitation of their child have valued this opportunity and despite the occasionally chaotic environment, common positive perceptions relate to the efforts made by staff. To achieve a positive (psychosocial) outcome, in relation to the presence of parents during resuscitation, the following issues should be considered:

- Parents being present during the resuscitation of their child should be regarded more as the norm than the exception.
- Parents should not be coerced into being present, but gentle encouragement and explanation by a senior member of staff is usually helpful.
- Senior members of staff engaged in resuscitation should not feel undue pressure as a result of the attendance of parents. Occasionally, however, it may be preferable for the parents to wait outside the immediate resuscitation area during challenging or visually disturbing procedures.
- Parents should have a dedicated support person, being a health professional, to remain with them throughout the resuscitation. The support person should obtain information from medical staff to keep the parents informed of their child's progress and explain procedures to the parents.
- Touching and talking to their child is often important for the parents where this is feasible.
- Parents need to have a quiet room to retreat to, if necessary. Discussion with family should not occur in a busy emergency department corridor as it will negatively affect the family's retention of information.
- Family requests and religious beliefs need to be respected.
- Obligations mandated by Coronial Law need to be explained with sensitivity.
- The emotional impact on all staff members when a child dies is considerable and this may be compounded by the distress of parents during and following the resuscitation.
- With any resuscitation, particularly those resulting in death, debriefing of staff is essential, as is organising the appropriate support and medical follow up of the parents.

Termination of resuscitative efforts

The decision to cease resuscitation efforts in a child in CPA is influenced by many factors. These include the total arrest time, clinical response to therapy, premorbid state of the child, potential for any reversible factors, likely neurological outcome, information from colleagues who care for a child with long-term medical problems and the parental wishes. In the initial stage of the arrested child arriving in the ED, these details should be rapidly established whilst resuscitation is continued in order to help guide subsequent management.

Termination of resuscitation in a newly born baby is likely to be appropriate if the baby remains in cardiorespiratory arrest at 15 minutes. Even after 10 minutes of documented asystole, survival without severe disability is unlikely.

For children in established cardiac arrest the overall outcome is poor. If the child requires adrenaline (epinephrine), and fails to respond to two doses, then survival is unlikely. Generally no longer than 30 minutes of advanced life support resuscitation is required to determine whether discontinuation of resuscitation is appropriate. Recurring/refractory VF or VT, toxic drug exposure or the presence of significant hypothermia in the setting of ice-cold immersion, are situations that may require more prolonged resuscitation efforts (see Chapter 22.2 on Drowning). Many children in cardiorespiratory arrest in Australia and New Zealand who are hypothermic, however, have lost body heat due to exposure, without spontaneous circulation after the arrest, and therefore this is unlikely to be neuroprotective.

Non-initiation of resuscitative efforts

Resuscitation should not be initiated if there are signs of prolonged death, like rigor mortis or post-mortem lividity. Children who are in a palliative phase of care should have an 'end of life care plan' that includes non-initiation of resuscitation should this have been previously determined by family and the child's coordinating specialist. Children with complex and disabling conditions will occasionally have life-threatening events occur. If prior discussions between parents (and child if appropriate) and physicians have not included limitations of interventions or medical support, then it is difficult to avoid commencing resuscitation. Early and urgent consultation with the child's primary physician is prudent in these situations. Physicians should not be coerced into undertaking care that they believe is morally wrong or fruitless.

There are specific situations in the newly born baby that may lead to the non-initiation of resuscitation, like extreme prematurity and congenital/chromosomal abnormalities not consistent with long-term survival. This issue is covered in Chapter 2.6 on neonatal resuscitation.

Consent

The philosophy of informed consent should be followed during any treatment, including resuscitation. The patient or the parents/guardian should have an explanation about the management (current and proposed), risks and potential outcomes. This may be limited during resuscitation but is the responsibility of the most senior physician involved with the child's care at the time. The decision to stop resuscitative efforts in the emergency department setting due to a lack of return of spontaneous circulation is a medical decision. It is not a choice that is offered to the parents. The circumstances are completely different to the discussion with parents about 'withdrawal of treatment', which usually occurs in an intensive care unit in a child who is ventilated but has a spontaneous circulation.

Non-accidental injury

It is important that all healthcare providers involved with children should be aware of their statutory obligations under state or federal law regarding notification of suspicion of non-accidental injury or neglect. Awareness of development of the child, feasibility or compatibility of the history with clinical signs and any delay in presentation should be considered when assessing this possibility. Regardless of the outcome of the resuscitation, if there is a suspicion of abuse or neglect, appropriate notification should be made.

Organ donation

Organ donation is usually a consideration for staff when a child is in an intensive care unit and generally not in the emergency department. The only situation where it may be contemplated in the ED is when post-mortem organs (like corneas, heart valves) may be retrieved for this purpose. In cases mandating notification of the coroner, then permission is required prior to any organ harvesting. Liaison with the appropriate local donor coordinator is essential. A senior member of staff should have this discussion with the parents and occasionally the parents themselves raise the issue.

If resuscitation has resulted in the return of spontaneous circulation but with likely brain death, subsequent organ donation may be feasible. The determination of brain death would usually occur in an intensive care unit, as a repeat examination for brain death, after a period of time, is required. Consultation with and consideration of transfer to a paediatric intensive care unit is required. The focus in the emergency department at this point is the ongoing care of the child and support of the family.

Death certificates, notification to the coroner and other legal issues

Death in the ED is, by itself, not an indication to notify the death to the coroner. Coroners' Acts vary from state to state and staff must be aware of their statutory obligations. Remember that if a death is to be notified to the coroner the body then becomes evidence and should be left intact at the termination of resuscitation. Common practices of taking hand/footprints, locks of hair, removing catheters and tubes must not occur or staff risk being held in contempt of court. Such mementos can be collected following the post-mortem examination. This usually requires liaison with staff in the forensic mortuary.

Some states have special processes in place for the management of sudden unexplained death in infancy (SUDI). Any sudden and unexplained death under 12 months of age warrants a detailed history as well as specific samples collected post-mortem to identify metabolic and genetic conditions. The Forensic Pathologist may need to have this drawn to their attention (e.g. see http://www.health.nsw.gov.au/policies/index.asp Search SUDI).

In the situation where a death does not require notification to the coroner, it must be clarified who can and will complete the death certificate, which includes the cause of death. Consultation with the primary physician involved with the long-term care of a child with chronic illness is obligatory. Medical staff need to be aware of other legal obligations, like the collection of blood alcohol specimens in pedestrian and vehicular accidents, but these would only be collected ante-mortem by hospital staff. These legal requirements vary between states.

References

1. Nolan J, Soar J, Eikeland H. The chain of survival. *Resuscitation* 2006;**71**(3):270–1.
2. Schindler MB, Bohn D, Cox PN, et al. Outcome of out-of-hospital cardiac or respiratory arrest in children. *N Engl J Med* 1996;**335**(20):1473–9.
3. Young KD, Gausche-Hill M, McClung CD, et al. A prospective, population-based study of the epidemiology and outcome of out-of-hospital pediatric cardiopulmonary arrest. *Pediatrics* 2004;**114**(1):157–64.
4. Atkins DL, Everson-Stewart S, Sears GK, et al. Epidemiology and outcomes from out-of-hospital cardiac arrest in children: the Resuscitation Outcomes Consortium Epistry-Cardiac Arrest. *Circulation* 2009;**119**(11):1484–91.
5. Deasy C, Bernard SA, Cameron P, et al. Epidemiology of paediatric out-of-hospital cardiac arrest in Melbourne, Australia. *Resuscitation* 2010;**81**(9):1095–100.
6. Donoghue AJ, Nadkarni VM, Elliott M, Durbin D. Effect of hospital characteristics on outcomes from pediatric cardiopulmonary resuscitation: a report from the national registry of cardiopulmonary resuscitation. *Pediatrics* 2006;**118**(3):995–1001.
7. Tibballs J, Kinney S. A prospective study of outcome of in-patient paediatric cardiopulmonary arrest. *Resuscitation* 2006;**71**(3):310–8.
8. Brown K, Bocock J. Update on paediatric resuscitation. *Emerg Med Clin North Am* 2002;**20**(1):1–26.
9. International Consensus on Cardiopulmonary Resuscitation and Emergency Cardiovascular Care Science. *Circulation* 2010;122:18 Supplement and *Resuscitation* 2010;81 Supplement.

2.2 Paediatric basic life support

Jane Cocks

ESSENTIALS

1 Paediatric cardiopulmonary resuscitation is different to adult resuscitation in many aspects, but the basic principles remain the same:

- Don't panic

- Get help

- Ensure both the patient and you are safe

- Initiate basic life support at the earliest possible moment: Airway, Breathing, Circulation.

2 Stabilise the cervical spine if the collapse follows any significant trauma.

3 DRSABC is a mnemonic to aid the sequence of events that should be followed when met with any collapsed patient. Check for **D**anger, **R**esponsiveness, **S**hout for help, Open the **A**irway, Check for **B**reathing and if patient is not breathing normally give 5 rescue breaths, if there are no signs of life commence **C**hest compressions.

4 Quality chest compressions involve compressing the chest to at least one third of the antero-posterior chest diameter at a rate of 100 compressions per minute with subsequent complete release to allow recoil of the chest wall.

5 Lone rescuers should use a 30:2 compression to ventilation ratio, while healthcare professionals performing two-rescuer CPR should use a 15:2 compression to ventilation ratio for all children, except in newly born where it is 3:1.

6 The rate of compressions is 100 per minute for all age groups, except in neonates where it is 120 per minute. The chest should be seen to fully recoil before the next compression is commenced.

Introduction

Basic life support (BLS) or basic cardiopulmonary resuscitation (CPR) is a process by which an individual's basic cardiac and respiratory functions can be restored and maintained through a combination of expired air resuscitation (EAR) and external cardiac compressions (ECC). The provision of BLS sustains the vital functions of the collapsed individual without the need for specialised equipment, minimising the potential hypoxic damage that may occur while advanced life support is being activated.

Paediatric versus adult basic life support

The aim of basic life support in all age groups is the same and the techniques utilised follow the same general principles, but paediatric BLS differs significantly from adult BLS in some very fundamental ways.

Aetiology of arrests

In adults the most common cause of cardiopulmonary arrest is a sudden, massive cardiac event with little preceding deterioration. Most adults requiring BLS measures are already in a state of full cardiopulmonary arrest, defined as a state of pulseless apnoea.

In children, the most common causes of cardiopulmonary arrest are hypoxic and, as a consequence, children generally undergo a period of deterioration with worsening bradycardia preceding the final arrested state. It is therefore important that paediatric BLS is commenced as soon as this bradycardic deterioration is noted and is not withheld until the patient becomes pulseless.

The currently accepted international recommendation for the commencement of external cardiac compressions (ECC) in children of all age groups who are unresponsive with no spontaneous breathing is a heart rate below 60 beats per minute (bpm).

Anatomy and physiology

The anatomy and physiology of the human body changes markedly with age, progressing from the immature neonatal form to the more adult form of the older child, and these changes are relevant to the provision of BLS at any particular age. The following differences from the adult form are of direct importance in the provision of BLS in children:

- *Airway*: Large head (particularly the occiput) and short neck leading to neck flexion; large tongue which is predominantly intra-oral; easily compressible oropharyngeal soft tissues; larynx lies more anteriorly and higher (C2–3); cricoid ring is the narrowest part of the airway; soft and short trachea.
- *Breathing*: Increased respiratory rate; more compliant chest wall; dependence on diaphragmatic breathing; reduced end expiratory lung volume.
- *Circulation*: Increased heart rate; more dependence on heart rate for delivery of adequate circulation; small absolute volume of circulating blood.
- *Metabolism*: Increased metabolic rate; increased body surface area (BSA).

BLS techniques and age

BLS techniques are modified depending on the child's age and size to ensure that they will be maximally effective. In view of this, children are arbitrarily divided into the following internationally accepted age groups:

- newborn/neonate: birth to 1 month old;
- infant: between 1 month and 1 year of age;
- small child: age between 1 and 8 years;
- large child: age older than 8 years.

Preparation and equipment

Basic CPR requires no extra equipment other than personnel trained in its administration. It is advantageous, however, to have available certain basic equipment to assist in the resuscitation process.

- Portable suction and suction catheters, for clearing secretions, improve the ability to achieve and maintain a patent airway.
- An oropharyngeal (Guedel) airway may assist in achieving a patent airway.
- A self-inflating bag and mask, suitable for the size of the patient, improves artificial ventilation and reduces the risk of cross infection.
- Oxygen for ventilation will further reduce the risk of hypoxic injury.

Basic life support sequence

A 'SAFE' approach

It is extremely important to ensure maximum rescuer and patient safety as a priority on first approaching the collapsed child. To this end, the Advanced Paediatric Life Support (APLS) course advocates a **'SAFE' approach** to collapsed patients. This acronym stands for:

- **S** = **S**hout for help. Call for assistance from surrounding people and request that an ambulance is called, do not leave the patient as immediate resuscitation may be required.
- **A** = **A**pproach with care. Ensure that you are not putting yourself at risk.
- **F** = **F**ree from danger. Remove the patient from immediate danger, if present.
- **E** = **E**valuate the ABCs (airway, breathing, circulation).

The activation of the Emergency Medical Services (EMS) should be performed as early as possible in the sequence of resuscitation, provided there are adequate numbers of bystanders to allow this to occur without delaying the commencement of BLS. Most paediatric arrests will have an underlying hypoxic cause and therefore any delay of BLS will significantly reduce its effectiveness. Commencement of BLS should therefore precede activation of EMS for a lone rescuer. In a witnessed sudden collapse of a child, the possibility of a sudden cardiac event is higher and activation of the EMS should occur immediately prior to commencement of BLS by a lone rescuer. These cases require rapid access to Advanced Cardiac Life Support measures, as is the case with most adult arrests.

Assess responsiveness

Assess the responsiveness of the patient by gently, but firmly, stimulating the patient and asking if they are OK. It is important to remember the possibility of cervical spinal injury and, if this is likely, stabilise the cervical spine by placing a hand on the patient's forehead prior to gently shaking their arm.

Airway

Open and maintain the airway

Position yourself at the patient's head, open the mouth and remove any obvious debris. Do not use a blind finger sweep in children as this may damage the delicate palatal tissues or move a foreign body further into the airway. Suction using a large-bore Yankeur catheter is useful for removing vomitus and secretions, preferably under direct vision.

Three manoeuvres will assist in opening and maintaining the airway (Figs 2.2.1, 2.2.2 and 2.2.3), which is most commonly obstructed by the child's tongue.

Head tilt

Place one hand on the patient's forehead and gently tilt the head back. In children the 'sniffing' position is desired, as in adult resuscitation. In an infant or neonate, a neutral position is required as they have a relatively large occiput and are naturally positioned in a sniffing position. A small towel placed under the infant's shoulders will eliminate the excessive neck flexion caused by the prominent occiput. If there is any possibility of cervical spine injury, the head tilt manoeuvre should be avoided.

Chin lift

Placing the fingers of the other hand on the jawbone, lift the chin, taking care not to compress the soft tissues of the floor of the mouth under the jaw.

Jaw thrust

Place two or three fingers under the angle of the mandible bilaterally, and lift the jaw upwards. This technique can be performed

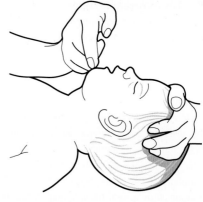

Fig. 2.2.1 Chin lift and head position in infants.

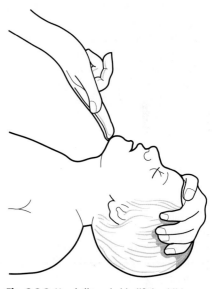

Fig. 2.2.2 Head tilt and chin lift in children.

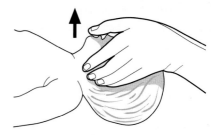

Fig. 2.2.3 Jaw thrust.

without head tilt and is indicated particularly if the possibility of cervical injury exists.

The patency of the airway can then be assessed by *looking* for chest movement, *listening* for breath sounds and *feeling* for exhaled breath. This assessment is best achieved from the patient's side, by placing an ear over the patient's mouth and nose, whilst watching the chest.

Oropharyngeal airway

Insertion of an oropharyngeal airway may assist in maintaining patency of the airway if the above manoeuvres are inadequate. An appropriately sized oropharyngeal airway should reach from the central incisors to the angle of the jaw. In infants and small children, the oropharyngeal airway should be inserted under direct vision 'the right way up'; that is, it should be inserted concave down in the position in which it will sit in the oropharynx. Gentle depression of the child's tongue with a spatula will help facilitate airway placement. In children older than 8 years, the usual adult oropharyngeal airway insertion technique may be used. This involves inserting the airway concave up and then rotating it through 180 degrees to sit snugly in the oropharynx. Oropharyngeal airways will not be tolerated in conscious or semi-conscious patients because of gagging. If this occurs, the airway should be removed. In this situation a nasopharyngeal airway may be a useful alternative in the patient who is not completely obtunded.

Cervical spine

Be aware of the risk of cervical spine injury if the collapse is following a motor vehicle accident (MVA) or other form of significant trauma. If this is likely, stabilise the cervical spine by placing one hand on either side of the head and maintaining the head in line with the body at all times. CPR in this case generally requires two operators to perform successfully. If a second operator is not available, attempt to immobilise the cervical spine between sandbags or in a hard cervical collar before proceeding.

Breathing

Once the airway is opened and patent, if the patient is not spontaneously breathing, deliver two to five slow rescue breaths via expired air resuscitation. Each breath is delivered slowly over 1 to 1.5 seconds' duration (inspiratory phase) and up to five may be required to ensure that two effective breaths are delivered.

Expired air resuscitation (EAR) is most commonly performed as 'mouth-to-mouth' but may also be delivered using 'mouth-to-mouth-and-nose' in the smaller child. In the 'mouth-to-mouth' technique, the rescuer

seals his or her mouth over the mouth of the patient, pinching off the nose with the free hand, whilst maintaining the patency of the airway with head tilt and chin lift. The 'mouth-to-mouth-and-nose' technique may be necessary for the infant or small child and in that case the rescuer's mouth should seal around the infant's mouth and nose. In the hospital setting the rescue breaths will be delivered utilising bag and mask ventilation (see Chapter 2.3 Paediatric advanced life support).

Ensure that the degree of chest excursion is frequently reassessed during the EAR. The chest must be seen to rise as if the child was taking a deep breath. Excessive tidal volumes or force may cause gastric dilatation and regurgitation. If there is no chest movement, the most likely cause is an obstructed airway due to poor positioning of the child's head. Reposition the patient using the above manoeuvres and retry. If there is still no chest movement, there may be a foreign body obstructing the airway, which can be removed with suction or forceps under direct vision (see below).

Circulation

Following the initial five rescue breaths, assess the circulation. Although the pulse check has always been considered the gold standard of circulation assessment, the International Liaison Committee on Resuscitation (ILCOR) recommendations suggest that for non-healthcare professionals, the assessment of pulse has both poor sensitivity and specificity and often delays the decision to commence ECC. The current recommendations, therefore, suggest that lay rescuers assess for 'signs of circulation', specifically the presence of normal breathing, coughing or movement in response to rescue breaths.

Healthcare professionals may check for a pulse as well as assessing for signs of circulation. The pulses that are easiest to feel are the carotid, brachial or femoral pulses and they should be palpated for no longer than a period of 10 seconds. The carotid pulse is difficult to feel in small children who have relatively short necks. If there is no pulse or severe bradycardia (heart rate <60 bpm) with signs of poor perfusion, then ECC on the lower half of the sternum should be commenced.

Chest compressions

The technique of providing ECC varies with the patient's age.

- Infants and neonates require compression with two fingers over the lower half of the sternum, avoiding the xiphisternum. An alternative technique involves the rescuer encircling the infant's chest with both hands and providing compressions with the thumbs at the same landmark site. This technique is felt to be more effective, but requires two rescuers to provide effective EAR and ECC (Figs 2.2.4 and 2.2.5).
- All other children require compressions with the heel of one or two hands over the lower half of the sternum, avoiding the xiphisternum (Figs 2.2.6 and 2.2.7).
- The emphasis in cardiac compressions is to minimise interruptions. The depth of compression is relative and should be one

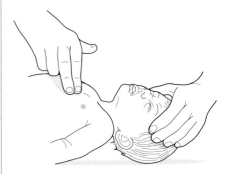

Fig. 2.2.4 Infant with two-finger technique of ECC.

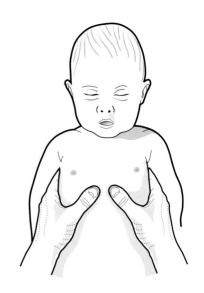

Fig. 2.2.5 Infant with two-thumb technique of ECC.

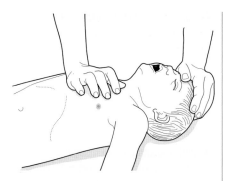

Fig. 2.2.6 Child with one-hand technique of ECC.

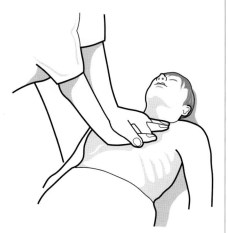

Fig. 2.2.7 Child with two-hand technique of ECC.

third to one half of the AP diameter of the chest in all age groups. The chest should be seen to fully recoil before the next compression is commenced. ECC should be performed on a firm flat surface.

• The rate of compressions is 100 per minute for all age groups, except in neonates, where it is 120 per minute (Table 2.2.1). Note that this is the rate or speed of compressions, not the actual number delivered per minute. The actual number of compressions delivered per minute will be less than 100 as there will be pauses for the delivery of EAR.

Compression to ventilation ratio

For a lone rescuer, external cardiac compressions should be combined with expired air resuscitation in a ratio of 30 compressions to 2 ventilations for all age groups (except neonates – see below). Healthcare providers performing two-rescuer BLS should use a ratio of 15 compressions to 2 ventilations

Table 2.2.1	Rate of ECC and ratio to EAR		
	Rate of ECC (per min)	Ratio of ECC:EAR	
		Single rescuer	Two rescuers
Newly born	120	3:1	3:1
Infant and small child	100	30:2	15:2
Large child and adults	100	30:2	30:2

for all infants and children (see Table 2.2.1). Note that the ratio of 30:2 is utilised in adults regardless of the number of rescuers.

Neonates require a combination of ECC:EAR at a ratio of 3 compressions to every 1 ventilation and a rate of 120 'events' per minute. This rate aims to achieve approximately 90 compressions and 30 breaths per minute.

It is important to check that the chest rises normally when the ventilation is provided to ensure that an effective breath is being delivered. When two rescuers are delivering BLS, the rescuer providing ECC should pause every 15th compression for the delivery of the breath. Once the airway is secured with intubation, this pause in ECC is no longer required.

Any interruption to basic life support measures should last no longer than 10 seconds, after which BLS should be promptly recommenced to optimise outcome.

Mechanical devices to provide chest compressions during ECC have been designed and tested only in adults and are not recommended for use in children.

Duration of BLS in the field

Continue BLS for a period of five cycles and then reassess the patient. If there is no return of spontaneous breathing or circulation and the rescuer is alone, he/she should seek help by activating emergency medical services. If the patient is small enough, the rescuer should take the patient with them and attempt to continue BLS whilst seeking help. If the patient is too large to be moved, the rescuer should position the patient on their side and leave to seek help. Once EMS has been activated, BLS should continue until EMS arrives or signs of life return.

Precautions and complications

Severe iatrogenic injuries are extremely uncommon in children who have undergone CPR, with an incidence of about 3%. The risk of infection to the rescuer from CPR is minimal, with the greatest risk being meningococcus from airway secretions. Standard antibiotic prophylaxis is recommended for any rescuer involved in the resuscitation of the airway of a patient with known or suspected meningococcal infection. There have been no reported cases of transmission of hepatitis B or HIV from mouth-to-mouth ventilation to date. Airway secretions, tears, sweat and vomitus are low-risk fluids, but extra precautions should be taken when contact with blood or other bodily fluids is likely.

Relief of foreign body airway obstruction

Presentation

Foreign body airway obstruction (FBAO) in both adults and children is commonly caused by the aspiration of food, but in children it may also occur during play with small objects. In both of these situations, it is likely that a parent or guardian will be present and the event may have been witnessed. Clinical signs will include the sudden onset of respiratory distress, associated with coughing, gagging and inspiratory stridor. These signs may also be caused by upper airway infections; however, the onset is slower and usually associated with other signs of infection, such as fever, lethargy, or coryza.

FBAO management in the responsive infant or child

In a child or infant who is responsive with good respiratory effort and forceful coughing, do not interfere with the child's spontaneous efforts. Any attempt to relieve the obstruction in this situation may dislodge the foreign body and worsen the situation by turning partial to complete airway obstruction. Call for help and get the child or infant urgently to an emergency facility.

Attempts to relieve FBAO should only be commenced when the cough becomes ineffective with increasing respiratory distress, or the child becomes unconscious or apnoeic.

FBAO management in the unresponsive patient

A combination of back blows and chest thrusts are utilised to relieve the obstruction. Abdominal thrusts are not recommended for any age group because of the risk of trauma to abdominal structures.

The sequence of response for an unresponsive, apnoeic patient with FBAO is as follows:

❶ Open the airway using chin lift or jaw thrust. Look inside the mouth and remove any visible foreign body. Do not perform a blind finger sweep because of the risk of damaging palatal tissues or pushing a foreign body further into the airway.

❷ Attempt up to five rescue breaths. If unsuccessful, reposition and try again.

❸ If rescue breaths are still unsuccessful, perform a sequence of five back blows and five chest thrusts.

- Deliver up to five back blows using the heel of the one hand between the shoulder blades, deliver five blows with sufficient force to dislodge a foreign body. Check after each back blow to see in the FB has been dislodged. Infants can be placed in a prone, head down position lying along the rescuer's forearm with the jaw supported by the rescuer's hand to deliver back blows (Fig. 2.2.8).

- If the obstruction is not relieved perform up to five chest thrusts utilising the same position and technique as for ECC but at a rate of one per second with sufficient force to expel the foreign object. Check after each chest thrust to see if the FB has been dislodged. Infants should be positioned supine lying along the rescuer's thigh, in a head down position (Fig. 2.2.9).

❹ If the obstruction is not relieved, continue the above sequence until the obstruction is relieved or for approximately one minute. If the patient remains unresponsive at one minute, seek help. If the patient is small enough, the rescuer should take the patient with them and attempt to continue FBAO

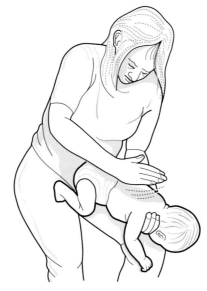

Fig. 2.2.8 Back blows in an infant.

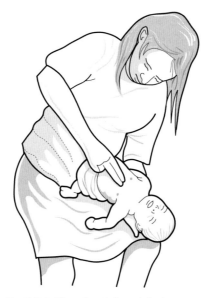

Fig. 2.2.9 Chest thrusts in an infant.

relief manoeuvres whilst seeking help. If the patient is too large to be moved, the rescuer should position the patient appropriately and leave to seek help.

For management in the emergency department setting see inhaled FB (Chapter 6.2).

FBAO management in the unresponsive child

A combination of abdominal thrusts, back blows and chest thrusts are utilised to relieve the obstruction. The sequence of response for an unresponsive, apnoeic child with FBAO is as for the infant except the rescuer should alternate between chest thrusts and abdominal thrusts with each cycle.

Abdominal thrusts (Heimlich manoeuvre) may be performed with the victim in the upright or supine position.

- With the child in the upright position (standing, sitting or kneeling), the rescuer stands behind the victim and places the fist of one hand on the child's abdomen above the umbilicus and below the xiphisternum. The rescuer's other hand covers the fist and both hands are thrust sharply inwards and upwards into the abdomen (Fig. 2.2.10).

- With the child in the supine position, the rescuer kneels at the child's feet or astride the child's hips. The heel of one hand is placed on the child's abdomen above the umbilicus and below the xiphisternum, the rescuer's other hand covers the first and both hands are thrust sharply inwards and upwards into the abdomen in the midline (Fig. 2.2.11).

- Abdominal thrusts should be repeated five times unless the foreign body is expelled before then.

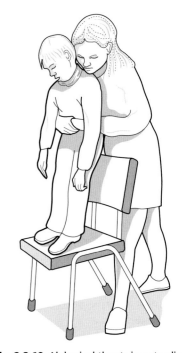

Fig. 2.2.10 Abdominal thrusts in a standing child.

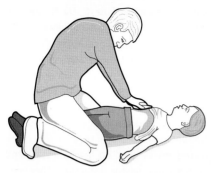

Fig. 2.2.11 Abdominal thrusts in a supine child.

- It is important to take care not to touch the xiphisternum or ribs during this manoeuvre due to the risk of internal damage.

Further reading

Advanced Life Support Group. *Advanced paediatric life support: The practical approach*, 4th rev. ed. London: BMJ Publishing Group; 2004.
Australian Resuscitation Council Guidelines, sections 12 and 13. http://www.resus.org.au/; December 2010.

Biarent D, Bingham R, Eich C, et al. European Resuscitation Council Guidelines for Resuscitation. Section 6: Paediatric life support. *Resuscitation* 2010;**81** (10):1364–88.
International Liaison Committee (ILCOR). Consensus on Science with Treatment Recommendations for Pediatric and Neonatal Patients: Pediatric Basic and Advanced Life Support. *Pediatrics* 2005;**117**(5).
Kleinman ME, de Caen AR, Chameides L, et al. Part 10: Pediatric basic and advanced life support: 2010 International Consensus on Cardiopulmonary Resuscitation and Emergency Cardiovascular Care Science With Treatment Recommendations. *Circulation* 2010;**16** (Suppl 2):S466–515.
Richmond S, Wyllie J. European Resuscitation Council Guidelines for Resuscitation. Section 7: Resuscitation of babies at birth. *Resuscitation* 2010;**81**(10):1389–99.

2.3 Paediatric advanced life support (PALS, APLS)

James Tibballs

ESSENTIALS

1 Diagnosis of cardiac arrest by pulse palpation alone is unreliable by healthcare personnel. If the patient is unresponsive, not breathing normally and a pulse cannot be identified within 10 seconds, give cardiopulmonary resuscitation (CPR) with external cardiac compression (rate 100/minute) and ventilation in a ratio of 15:2.

2 Ventilate initially with bag–mask ventilation. Avoid hypoxaemia during attempts at intubation which should be limited to 30 seconds.

3 The approximate *uncuffed* endotracheal tube size may be chosen for children over 1 year by the formula: size (mm) = age (years)/4 + 4. (*Cuffed* endotracheal tube: size (mm) = age (years)/4 + 3.5).

4 Confirm correct location of endotracheal tube in the trachea immediately after intubation by exhaled CO_2 detection and optimize cardiac compression and lung inflation by monitoring end-tidal CO_2.

5 Have a plan to cope with difficult and failed (impossible) intubation when bag-mask ventilation fails.

6 Obtain intraosseous access if a peripheral vein cannot be cannulated rapidly.

7 Administer lipid-soluble drugs (adrenaline [epinephrine], atropine, lignocaine and naloxone) via endotracheal tube if intravenous and intraosseous access is impossible.

8 Restore intravascular volume with a crystalloid solution (0.9% normal saline or Hartmann's solution) or a colloid in aliquots of 20 mL kg^{-1}.

9 Treat shockable rhythms (ventricular fibrillation, pulseless ventricular tachycardia) with a single direct current shock of 4 J kg^{-1} followed by immediate CPR for 2 minutes before re-analyzing the rhythm.

10 Institute therapeutic hypothermia (32–34°C) if the patient fails to resume consciousness after return of spontaneous circulation.

11 Base decisions to cease CPR on a number of factors including the duration of resuscitation, response to treatment, pre-arrest status of the patient, remediable factors, likely neurological outcome, opinions of personnel familiar with the patient and, whenever appropriate, the wishes of the parents.

Introduction

Definition of ALS

Advanced life support is cardiopulmonary resuscitation (CPR) with use of specific items of equipment available in the hospital or ambulance setting and the use of techniques and skills by specifically trained personnel. It includes the management of critically-ill infants and children in pre-cardiorespiratory arrest (CPA), during arrest and post-arrest.

The recommendations for advanced CPR given here are based on publications of the Australian Resuscitation Council,[1] the European Resuscitation Council,[2] the American Heart Association[3] and the International Liaison Committee on Resuscitation (ILCOR).[4] They are intended for use by medical and nursing personnel in hospital and by ambulance personnel in the field.

To add ability to knowledge, it is advisable to undertake a specialised paediatric cardiopulmonary resuscitation course such as the Advanced Paediatric Life Support (APLS) or Paediatric Advanced Life Support (PALS) courses.

Distinctions within the term 'paediatric' are based on combinations of physiology, physical size and age. Some aspects of CPR are different for 'the newly born', infant, small (younger) child and large (older) child. 'Newly-born' refers to the infant at birth or within several hours of birth. The management of the 'newly-born' infant is discussed in Chapter 26.1.

In this section, 'infant' refers to an infant outside the delivery room (the 'newly-born' infant) and includes the period starting from a few hours after birth up to the age of 12 months. Other terms such as newborn or neonate do not enable that distinction. 'Small/young child' refers to a child of pre-school and early primary school from the age of 1 to 8 years. 'Large/older child' refers to a child of late primary school from the age of 9 up to 14 years. Although ventricular fibrillation occurs in children, they are at less risk than adults. One guideline regards children of 8 years and over as adults specifically for use of semi-automated external defibrillators (sAED) out-of-hospital.

Diagnosing cardiac arrest

Healthcare personnel (doctors and nurses) have difficulty diagnosing cardiac arrest in infants and children if they rely on pulse palpation alone. Their accuracy is approximately 80% with a sensitivity of 0.85 and specificity of 0.65,[5] which means that in 15% of circumstances they would not give CPR when needed and would give it in 35% when not needed. While application of CPR is not harmful when there is a circulation, the withholding of CPR when there is none dooms the patient to die. The time taken to diagnose cardiac arrest is longer than hitherto realised[6] – as a group, healthcare personnel take an average of 15 seconds to exclude cardiac arrest by finding a pulse but 30 seconds to diagnose real cardiac arrest by the absence of a pulse. However, the accuracy and expediency of diagnosis are related to experience and training. Only experienced personnel who palpate pulses on a daily basis are able to detect a real pulse within 10 seconds but they, like inexperienced personnel, are unable to quickly diagnose cardiac arrest by the lack of a pulse and need on average about 25 seconds to confirm it. Clinical guidelines advise to spend no more than 10 seconds on pulse palpation and to combine whatever information is gained with observable signs of circulation such as responsiveness, movement and presence or absence of normal respiration. In short, if the patient is unresponsive and not breathing normally there is no point wasting time on pulse palpation (it is inaccurate and time consuming). Instead give CPR immediately.

Epidemiology

The causes of cardiopulmonary arrest in infants and children are many and include any cause of hypoxaemia or hypotension, or both. Common causes are trauma (motor vehicle accidents, near drowning, falls, burns, gunshots), drug overdose and poisoning, respiratory illness (asthma, upper airway obstruction, parenchymal diseases), post-operative (especially cardiac), septicaemia and sudden infant death syndrome.

Oxygen, ventilation and advanced airway support

Oxygen

Oxygen should be administered whenever hypoxaemia occurs but evidence from animal and newborn infant studies suggests that as soon as oxygenation is achieved the inspired oxygen (FiO_2) should be regulated to yield arterial oxygen partial-pressure in the normal range in order to limit oxygen-mediated cell damage. The only exception to administration of oxygen is when it may cause pulmonary vasodilation and thereby shunt blood to the lungs away from the systemic circulation, as may occur in an infant with a single ventricle which pumps blood to both circulations. Chronic hypoventilation is not an indication to withhold oxygen therapy during CPR for infants and children.

Numerous devices may be used to supply supplemental oxygen. The choice is dictated by the required inspired oxygen concentration (FiO_2), cost, avoidance of CO_2 rebreathing, imposed airway resistance and tolerance by the patient.

Oxygen catheters

These are easy to use, cheap, do not cause rebreathing and are well tolerated (permitting eating and drinking) but are limited to supply of up to 40% inspired O_2 because of restriction to gas flow (maximum 4 L min^{-1}) and limitation of gas reservoir (the nasopharynx). Sizes 6, 8 and 10 FG should be available and placed in the same nostril as the nasogastric tube, to limit airway resistance. Size 6 FG is suitable for infants, 8 FG for small children and 10 FG for older children. Excessive flow may desiccate mucosal membranes and cause gastric distension, which can embarrass respiration.

Oxygen is delivered by nasal cannulae (bi-pronged, 'nasal prongs'), which sit at the entrance to the nose or a few centimetres inside, need no humidification and do not cause gastric distension. They may become obstructed by mucus and may obstruct the nose. Flow rates for infants should be regulated by a low-flow meter, graduated 0–2.5 L min^{-1}. Rates of 0.24–4 L min^{-1} provide 40–70% O_2 to infants 1–10 kg body weight (BW). Improved oxygenation may be caused in part by positive end expiratory pressure (PEEP).

An oxygen catheter placed in the nasopharynx a distance equivalent to that from ala nasi to tragus provides a small amount of PEEP, and indeed may be used for that purpose. Oxygen concentrations of 30%, 40% and 50% approximately are provided by flows of 45, 80 and 150 mL kg^{-1} min^{-1} respectively. This technique to provide 'PEEP' may be useful to temporarily abort central apnoea in the young infant with RSV, whilst other treatment such as caffeine infusion is established.

Oxygen prongs

Non-humidified oxygen is subject to the same flow restriction as nasal catheters (up to 4 L min^{-1}). The use of 'high flow' (≥ 8 L min^{-1}) humidified oxygen as a means to provide CPAP and thereby prevent apnoea, although an attractive technique, has not yet proven to be advantageous in infants outside the premature age group.

Oxygen masks

Semi-rigid face masks of the Hudson type can supply approximately 35–70% O_2 at flow rates of 4–15 L min^{-1}. However, they may not be well tolerated by the infant or small child, and the distress they cause may consume energy in the tiring child. They may cause rebreathing or fail to deliver the desired FiO_2, especially when peak inspiratory flow rate (PIFR) is high, thus entraining excessive room air. Masks that incorporate a reservoir bag or a Venturi may deliver up to 80% O_2 but, likewise, may cause rebreathing if the flow rate does not match PIFR during respiratory distress.

Head boxes and incubators

A clear Perspex head box is the best way of administering a high concentration of oxygen to the unintubated infant. It allows a non-distressing delivery of oxygen and allows clear observation of the child. Precise oxygen therapy is possible but may be expensive and rebreathing, heat loss and desiccation are potential problems. To avoid rebreathing, a large flow rate $(10-12 \text{ L min}^{-1})$ of fresh gas with predetermined oxygen content should be introduced. The practice of introducing a low-flow rate of 100% oxygen into a head box (to gain a lesser concentration) may cause hypercarbia. If 100% oxygen is the only compressed gas available, lesser concentrations of oxygen may be attained without rebreathing by using a flow of 100% oxygen and a Venturi device. The relatively large capacity of an incubator precludes the attainment of a high concentration of oxygen, but limited oxygen therapy, up to a maximum of 60%, can be achieved at the cost of very high flow rates. The concentration of oxygen in the head box can be monitored with an analyser and help monitor the progress of the lung disease and oxygen requirements.

Ventilation

Bag–mask ventilation

As soon as practicable, mechanical ventilation with added oxygen should be commenced with either a bag–mask (bag–valve–mask) or via endotracheal intubation. Although intubation is preferred (see below), valuable time should not be wasted in numerous unsuccessful attempts. Initial effective bag–mask ventilation is a necessary prerequisite for successful paediatric CPR but it is a relatively difficult technique to learn and to perform well in emergency circumstances. Practice on mannequins or in an anaesthetic setting is invaluable in learning to perform this well for the infrequent paediatric resuscitation.

Bags of appropriate sizes should be available for infants, small children and large children. A bag of approximately 500 mL volume should be available for newborn infants and infants.

Insertion of an oropharyngeal (Guedel) airway may be necessary to facilitate bag-mask ventilation. Two types of resuscitation devices are available: flow-inflating and self-inflating bags. They can be attached to a mask, laryngeal mask airway (LMA), endotracheal tube or tracheostomy.

Flow-inflating bags

These are designed to give either positive pressure ventilation or to allow a patient to breathe spontaneously. They are exemplified by Jackson-Rees modified Ayre's T-piece. Gas flow must exceed $220 \text{ mL kg}^{-1} \text{ min}^{-1}$ for children and 3 L min^{-1} for infants, to prevent rebreathing during manual ventilation. It is possible to control precisely the concentration of inspired oxygen, which is an advantage, especially for the premature neonate at risk of oxygen-induced retrolental fibroplasia. However, considerable experience is necessary to provide adequate ventilation without barotrauma in the intubated infant. A pressure gauge and a relief valve should be incorporated in the circuit to help prevent barotrauma.

Self-inflating bags

These bags are designed only to give positive pressure ventilation. Rebreathing is prevented by one-way duck-bill valves, spring disk/ball valves or diaphragm/leaf valves. The Laerdal bag series (infant, child, adult) typifies these devices. A pressure-relief valve (infant and child size) opens at 35 cm H_2O (3.5 kPa). A pressure monitor can be incorporated in the circuit. Supplemental oxygen is added to the resuscitation bag, with or without attachment of a reservoir bag, whose movement may serve as a visual monitor of tidal volume during spontaneous ventilation when intubated. However, the valve may offer resistance for spontaneous ventilation and this is important to consider in the spontaneously breathing child just prior to the effect of relaxants of rapid sequence induction prior to intubation.

These bags should not be used to provide supplemental oxygen to a spontaneously breathing patient with a mask placed near or loosely over the face. With Laerdal and Partner bags, negligible amounts of oxygen $(0.1-0.3 \text{ L min}^{-1})$ issue from the patient valve when $5-15 \text{ L min}^{-1}$ of oxygen is introduced into bags unconnected to patients.[7] The patient valve is unlikely to open unless the mask is sealed well on the face. Although not recommended, if they are used in this way, it is vital to ensure that the patient valve opens or the reservoir bags deflates in unison with the chest movement.

The delivered oxygen concentration is dependent on the flow rate of oxygen, use of the reservoir bag, and the state of the pressure relief valve (whether open or closed). In the Laerdal series, with use of the reservoir bag and oxygen flow greater than the minute ventilation, 100% oxygen is delivered. Without the reservoir bag the delivered gas is only 50% oxygen, despite oxygen flow rate at twice minute ventilation. At an oxygen flow rate of 10 L min^{-1} to the infant resuscitator bag, the delivered gas is 85–100% oxygen without the use of the reservoir bag.

Rates and ratios of external cardiac compression and ventilation in ALS

The techniques of external cardiac compression and expired air resuscitation (mouth-to-mouth) or rescue breathing are described in Section 2.2. The recommended ratio of external cardiac compression to ventilation in basic life support by a single rescuer is $30:2^{1-4}$ which if able to be repeated 5 times in 2 minutes, with pauses for ventilations, would yield approximately 75 compressions and 5 breaths per minute.

In advanced life support the recommended ratio of compressions to ventilation by 2 rescuers is $15:2^{1-4}$ which, if repeated 5 times in 1 minute, with pauses for ventilation by bag–mask, would yield approximately 75 compressions and 10 ventilations per minute. When the patient is intubated, it is undesirable and not necessary to pause cardiac compressions to give ventilations because they can be delivered effectively during cardiac compressions and cardiac compressions can be given continuously without interruption. Every time cardiac compression is interrupted, cardiac stroke volume obviously falls to zero and then several successive compressions are required to re-establish the stroke volume achieved before interruption. Necessary interruptions to cardiac compressions should be minimized by co-ordinated planning, to for example, analyse the cardiac rhythm or to give DC shock. Effort must be directed towards minimizing "hands-off time" during requirement for cardiac compression.

Advanced airway support

Tracheal intubation

The trachea should be intubated as soon as practicable but it can be deferred if successful bag–mask ventilation can be given and should not be undertaken by inexperienced personnel out-of-hospital[8] because of complications and poorer outcomes compared with use of bag–mask ventilation. Nonetheless, intubation has numerous advantages, which include establishment and maintenance of the airway, facilitation of mechanical ventilation, titration of oxygen therapy, minimisation of the risk of pulmonary aspiration, enablement of tracheal suction, provision of a route for the administration of selected drugs and preferred for transport and long-term ventilation. Regurgitation of gastric contents is common during cardiac arrest.

Hypoxaemia should be avoided during attempts at intubation – which should be limited to 30 seconds. If difficulty is experienced, oxygenation should be re-established with bag–mask ventilation before a reattempt at intubation. Initial intubation should be via the oral route, not via the nasal route. The oral route is invariably quicker, is less likely to cause trauma and haemorrhage and the endotracheal tube is more easily exchanged if the first choice is inappropriate. On the other hand, a tube placed nasally can be better affixed to the face and so is less likely to enter a bronchus or be inadvertently dislodged during transport or other procedures. A nasal tube is preferred subsequently for long-term management. A nasogastric tube should be inserted after intubation to relieve possible gaseous distension of the stomach sustained during bag–mask ventilation.

Correct placement of the endotracheal tube in the trachea must be confirmed immediately. In the hurried conditions of emergency intubation at cardiopulmonary arrest, it is not difficult to mistakenly intubate the oesophagus or to intubate a bronchus. There is no substitute for visualising the passage of the tip of the endotracheal tube through the vocal cords, confirmation of bilateral pulmonary air entry by auscultation in the axillae, continuous observation of rise and fall of the chest on ventilation and maintenance of a pink complexion. In addition, it is recommended that correct placement of the endotracheal tube be

confirmed by capnography or CO_2 detection, with the realisation that CO_2 excretion can only occur with effective pulmonary blood flow. This implies that CO_2 detection cannot be expected unless spontaneous cardiac output returns or external cardiac compression is effective. Absent CO_2 detection mandates re-intubation or at least inspection that the tube is indeed passing through the vocal cords. High CO_2 indicates poor ventilation. Oxygenation should be confirmed with use of a pulse oximeter or measurement of arterial gas tension.

Endotracheal tube size

(Table 2.3.1)

Uncuffed sizes are 2.5 mm for a premature newborn <1 kg, 3.0 mm for infants 1–3.5 kg, 3.5 mm for infants >3.5 kg and up to age of six months, size 4 mm for infants seven months to one year (Table 2.3.1). The approximate size may be chosen for children over one year by the formula: size (mm) = age (years)/4 + 4. Tubes one size larger and smaller should be readily available. The correct size should allow a small leak on application of moderate pressure but also enable adequate pulmonary inflation. If the lungs are non-compliant, however, it may be necessary to insert a tube without a leak or insert a cuffed tube. Appropriate-sized **cuffed** tubes may be estimated by the formula: size (mm) = age (years)/4 + 3.5.

Depth of tube insertion

(Table 2.3.1)

The tube is inserted to a specific numerical depth to avoid accidental extubation or

endobronchial intubation. Assessment of the depth of insertion during laryngoscopy by noting passage through the vocal cords is not completely reliable since alteration of head position affects depth of tube insertion. The tube depth increases with neck flexion (goes in) and decreases (comes out) during extension. Since intubation is usually performed with the head extended, the tube depth increases when the laryngoscope is removed and the head assumes a position of neutrality or flexion. In a neutral head position, an appropriate depth of insertion measured from the centre of the lips for an **oral tube** is 9.5 cm for a term newborn, 11.5 cm for a 6-month-old infant, 12 cm for a 1-year-old. After 1 year the depth is given by the formula: depth (cm) = age (years)/2 + 12. An alternative formula for oral tube depth of insertion is: depth (cm) = size (mm) × 3 when an appropriate tube size for age is used. The appropriate depth of insertion for a **nasal tube** in this age group is: depth (cm) = age (years)/2 + 15. On a chest X-ray taken with the head in neutral position, the tip of the tube should be at the interclavicular line.

Laryngeal mask airway (LMA)

These have been used for resuscitation by medical, nursing and ambulance personnel trained in their selection and insertion. They may be used to maintain an airway and are a suitable alternative to the use of airway opening manoeuvres and use of oropharyngeal and nasopharyngeal airways. They are

Table 2.3.1 Endotracheal tube sizes (internal diameter) and orotracheal and nasotracheal depths for infants and children			
Age/body weight (kg)	Size (mm)	Oral depth (cm)	Nasal depth (cm)
Newly-born (3.5)	3.0	9.0	11.01–1.5
1–6 months	3.5	9.5–11	12–13
6–12 months	4.0	11.5–12	13–14
2–3 years	4.5	13–13.5	15–16
4–5 years	5.0	14–14.5	17–18
6–7 years	5.5	15–15.5	19
8–9 years	6.0	16–16.5	20
10–11 years	6.5	17–17.5	21
12–13 years	7.0	18–18.5	22
14–16 years	7.5	19	23

useful to establish an airway in the setting of airway obstruction or failed intubation.[9] An intubating LMA serves as a conduit for intubation.

However, the role of LMA in provision of mechanical ventilation remains uncertain. Like bag–mask ventilation, they do not protect the airway from aspiration, which occurs commonly during cardiopulmonary resuscitation. They are a suitable alternative to a face mask as a means to give ventilation before endotracheal intubation and when intubation is difficult. This is a better technique when the operator is unskilled in the use of LMA and intubation. Although insertion of an LMA is easier to learn than endotracheal intubation, training should not replace mastery of bag–mask ventilation. They should not be used in semiconscious patients or when the gag reflex is present and are not suitable for long-term use or use during transport when endotracheal intubation is far preferable. They are subject to dislodgment during movement and transport. Appropriate sizes according to body weight are given in Table 2.3.2.

Management of the difficult airway

Unfortunately, unanticipated difficulties with the airway and intubation or failures to follow a prepared plan to cope with difficult and failed intubation continue to cause deaths, irrespective of the degree of skill of the operator.

The airway can be difficult to maintain because of unusual anatomy, injury or ill-

Table 2.3.2 Laryngeal mask airways	
Sizes are available to suit body weight (kg) of newborns, infants and children	
Size	*Weight (kg)*
1	<5
1½	5–10
2	10–20
2½	20–30
3	30–50
4	50–70
5	70–100
6	>100

nesses or because of loss of natural maintenance after administration of drugs, which depress consciousness, muscle tone or activity. 'Airway difficulties' refer to maintenance of the airway, bag–mask ventilation and endotracheal intubation. Each situation may rapidly lead to hypoxaemic brain damage and death.

Resuscitators must be well-skilled in the management of the airway and provision of bag–mask ventilation. It is vital to possess good basic resuscitation techniques (see Chapter 2.2 on basic life support), to be familiar with equipment, to have skilled assistance and to have appropriate equipment ready-to-hand. They must also be familiar with manoeuvres to overcome difficulties with airway maintenance, bag–mask ventilation and intubation. Resuscitators must also have a pre-conceived plan to cope with difficult and failed (impossible) intubation, especially when bag–mask ventilation fails (Fig. 2.3.1).

An obstructed airway may be relieved by simple repositioning of the patient's head and neck, pharyngeal suction, use of an alternative airway-opening manoeuvre, insertion of an oropharyngeal or nasopharyngeal airway and help by an assistant. Persistent obstruction requires urgent endotracheal intubation.

Difficult intubation

With good technique, normally, intubation can be achieved via direct laryngoscopy with a direct line of sight to the glottis. Sometimes 'difficult intubation' is a consequence of anatomical abnormality, trauma or infection but sometimes it is simply the result of operator unpreparedness or incorrect choice or use of equipment or lack of knowledge of simple techniques to overcome difficulties.

Anatomical difficulties

Certain conditions imply that intubation will not be easy but it is prudent to inspect the facial and pharyngeal anatomy of every patient before giving sedation or anaesthesia. Common anatomical variants in many conditions, which will disallow a direct line of sight to the larynx are an 'anterior' larynx, prominent upper incisors, a large tongue or a small hypoplastic mandible. Thus Treacher Collins syndrome and Pierre–Robin syndrome (sequence) with mandibular hypoplasia and Beckwith–Wiedemann syndrome

with macroglossia are typical conditions in which difficult intubation should be anticipated.

Difficulty with intubation may be unanticipated, but may be predicted with three simple observations. One of these is the relative tongue/pharyngeal size ('Mallampati' test): if the faucial pillars, soft palate and uvula are obscured by the extended tongue on maximum mouth opening, intubation will be difficult. Another predictor is the extent of possible atlanto-occipital extension. If this is less than 35° intubation will be difficult. This corresponds to the angle between the occlusal surface of the upper teeth and horizontal plane when the head is maximally extended. The third predictor is the amount of mandibular space into which the tongue must be compressed to allow a line of sight to the glottis. This space can be judged by the distance from the thyroid cartilage or hyoid bone to the point of the mandible (thyromental, submental distances) or by the horizontal length of the mandible. In adult-sized patients a thyromental distance of greater than 6 cm and a mandibular length of greater than 9 cm predict easy intubation. Unfortunately, no such distances are known for children and infants.

Thus, the evaluation of intubation difficulty should include pharyngeal examination with extended tongue, inspection of mandibular size or submental space and examination of atlanto-occipital angle. These special measures should be in addition to routine history of airway management, as would have occurred in previous anaesthesia, inspection of nostrils and history and examination of cardiorespiratory function.

Equipment and technical difficulties

Although Magill's forceps are very useful for directing the tube into the larynx, the use of simple 'tricks' may facilitate intubation. For example, it is important that the patient's head and neck be correctly positioned in the so-called 'sniffing' position (neck flexed, head slightly extended) to offer the best line of sight to the larynx. In the neonate and infant, however, the head and neck should remain in the neutral position. The blade of a regular laryngoscope is designed to be introduced into the right side of the mouth (not the left)

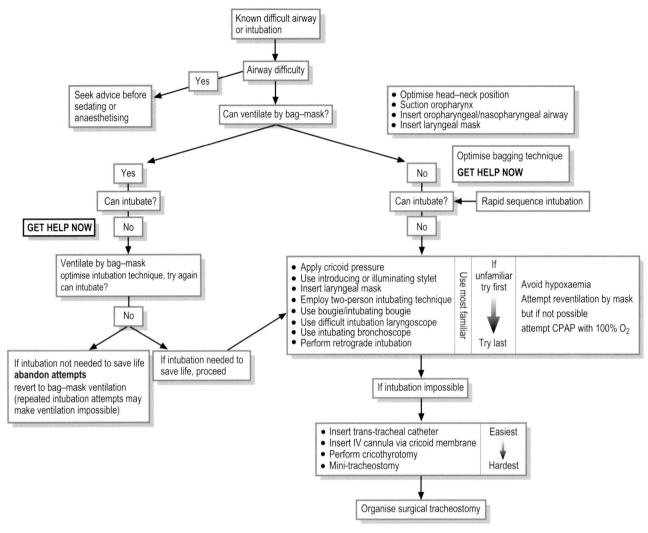

Fig. 2.3.1 Management of difficult and impossible intubation.

so that when the blade is subsequently centred the tongue is displaced to the left and an unimpeded view of the larynx and sufficient working space is afforded. The tip of a **curved**-bladed laryngoscope (Mackintosh type) is placed in the vallecula (space between base of tongue and epiglottis) whereas the tip of a **straight**-bladed laryngoscope is placed behind the epiglottis. The laryngoscope handle is then elevated upward and away from the operator to lift the tongue out of the line of sight to the glottis. The handle should not be elevated directly upwards or elevated back towards the operator – such actions may not displace the tongue sufficiently and fail to bring the glottis into view, and moreover may damage the upper teeth. The upper teeth should not be used as a leverage point.

The bevel of an endotracheal tube is angled so that it easily enters the trachea when introduced from the right side of the mouth. One should insert the tube keeping it oriented in a horizontal plane, rather than vertical, so that the presence of the tube does not impede the intubator's view of the larynx. This may be facilitated by an assistant pulling down on the corner of the mouth. When introduced from the left side, the tip of the bevel may stick at the laryngeal inlet – but this can be easily remedied by rotating the tube anticlockwise, thus changing the angle of approach and directing the tip more toward the centre of the laryngeal inlet rather than to its right side. If the tip of the upward curving tube sticks in the anterior larynx, flexion of the neck may direct the tube posteriorly and encourage it to enter the larynx. If the

larynx is anterior and difficult or impossible to see, use of an introducing stylet to create a more acute curve at the tube tip may achieve intubation and/or application of posterior cricoid pressure may bring the anterior larynx into view. A tube may be placed 'blindly' into the trachea with or without the use of a stylet or bougie over which a tube can be railroaded. Skilled anticipatory assistance and good suction by a dedicated airway nurse who anticipates the needs of the intubator are essential. Occasionally, a gentle finger of an assistant retracting the lip of the child may enlarge the oral opening to afford improved vision and field to place the endotracheal tube down the right side of the mouth.

Many other items of equipment are available to assist when intubation proves to be difficult. These include laryngoscopes that have a tip independent of the shaft of the blade, which is used to elevate the epiglottis (e.g. McCoy laryngoscope, Penlon), or which incorporate a prism to give a view of an anterior larynx (e.g. Belscope), illuminating stylets and intubating bronchoscopes. Illuminating stylets are malleable and give a 'Jack-o'-lantern' effect when correctly located in the trachea. All items of equipment are useless unless they are ready-to-hand and are familiar to the operator.

A two-person intubating technique may achieve intubation in difficult circumstances. In this, one person holds the laryngoscope with their left hand and applies cricoid pressure with their right to bring the larynx into view, while a second person applies suction, holds the lower lip out of the way and attempts to pass the endotracheal tube.

Another technique is retrograde intubation (translaryngeal-guided) in which a guide wire is threaded through a needle or intravenous catheter inserted cephalad through the cricothyroid membrane. The end of the wire is retrieved from the oral or nasal cavity, pulled taut and used as a 'tightrope' over which an endotracheal tube is railroaded into the trachea. Alternatively, a string can be tied to the end of the wire which is then drawn from the tracheal puncture. The proximal end of the string can be tied to the Murphy eye of a tube, which is then pulled from below into the trachea. A nasal endotracheal tube can be placed by joining a wire (or string) inserted into the oral cavity via the nasal route and joining it to the wire or string entering the oral cavity via the trachea. Retrograde intubation is a useful technique in cases such as facial trauma, trismus and upper airway masses.

Failed intubation

If endotracheal intubation is impossible when needed, the resuscitator must be able to oxygenate the patient while preparations are made for tracheostomy or until intubation can be somehow achieved.

Attempts at intubation should not be prolonged, so that hypoxaemia is not caused. Oxygenation should be restored with intermittent bag–mask ventilation. Likewise, intubation attempts should not be overly repetitive because the larynx will be traumatised and this may render bag–mask ventilation, previously possible, now impossible for

the more-skilled operator when they arrive. In situations where intubation is not absolutely needed (i.e. not life-saving) it is prudent to revert to bag–mask ventilation (if that is possible) rather than persist in intubation attempts, which could ultimately damage the larynx and render bag–mask ventilation impossible. If ventilation is not possible by mask, sometimes application of CPAP with 100% oxygen via an Ayre's T-piece will suffice to maintain oxygenation. Prolonged CPAP cannot be effectively applied with a mask using a self-inflating resuscitator bag.

If the airway is totally obstructed and neither bag–mask ventilation nor intubation can be performed, the situation is more desperate. Adequate oxygenation (but not normal ventilation) can be obtained by inserting a trans-tracheal catheter (Mallinck-rodt Medical Pty Ltd) otherwise intended for jet-ventilation, or a 14-gauge intravenous cannula percutaneously into the trachea caudad via the cricothyroid membrane (which lies immediately inferior to the thyroid cartilage). To do this, the patient should be lying straight, with the cannula in the midline and angled towards the feet. After removing the needle, the trans-tracheal catheter can be connected directly via its standard 22 mm connector to a bagging circuit. An intravenous cannula can be connected by various ways to a source of oxygen. One of these is direct connection to a resuscitator or a bagging circuit using a connector from a 3.0 mm endotracheal tube. Alternatively, the cannula can be connected to continuous oxygen supply via a three-way intravenous tap (to allow expiration) and a length of plastic tubing. Another option is use of plastic tubing alone that has a side hole cut or a Y-piece inserted, which is intermittently occluded to cause inspiration (1 second) and unoccluded (3 seconds) to allow expiration. With all these techniques care should be taken to allow expiration to avoid barotrauma. Expiration may need to be assisted by lateral chest compression as the arrested patient may not spontaneously expire much air. Ventilation is very difficult but oxygen can be supplied by sustained pressure.

A semipermanent solution for a totally obstructed airway is cricothyro(s)tomy. To do this the larynx is stabilised throughout the procedure with fingers of one hand

while skin over the thyroid–cricoid membrane (between the thyroid and cricoid cartilages) is incised with a scalpel held in the other. Then, bluntly dissect into the trachea with forceps in the midline or incise vertically with the scalpel. Insert a small tracheostomy, preferably bevelled, or a small endotracheal tube. Alternatively, perform percutaneous mini-tracheostomy. A formal tracheostomy should be organised while these measures are undertaken. An important part of a contingency plan to cope with unexpected difficulties is to have easily contactable more experienced operators.

Monitoring

Vital signs

Routine monitoring of heart rate, respiratory rate and blood pressure are essential for infants and children with critical illness. It is prudent to have ready access or to have displayed the normal age-related values visually available in the paediatric resuscitation area of the ED as an *aide-memoire*.

Oximetry

Transcutaneous oximetry (SpO_2) is essential monitoring in critically ill patients. It equates well to arterial haemoglobin oxygen saturation (SaO_2) but not when the SaO_2 is below 70%. Note that an SpO_2 of 90%, although only 10% below normal, represents a partial pressure of oxygen in arterial blood (PaO_2) of 60 mmHg, which is 40 mmHg below normal.

Expired CO$_2$ detection
Confirmation of endotracheal intubation

End-tidal CO_2 ($P_{et}CO_2$) is recommended after every tracheal intubation and during mechanical ventilation to guard against inadvertent oesophageal intubation and inadvertent extubation, particularly when the intubated patient undergoes transport to, within or between hospitals. Small movements of head and neck, as may occur for example on transfer from one trolley to another or to a bed, may dislodge an endotracheal tube. No CO_2 is excreted unless there is pulmonary blood flow so undetectable CO_2 after intubation basically represents non-tracheal intubation or absence of circulation, or both.

Regulation of cardiac compression and ventilation

To achieve optimum CO_2 excretion, cardiac output and pulmonary ventilation must be matched. A common error in advanced CPR is giving ventilation in excess of the limited cardiac output achievable by external cardiac compression, which is likely to be no more than a third of normal cardiac output. Ventilation can be safely reduced proportionately. Moreover, excessive ventilation not only interferes with performance of external cardiac compression but also increases intrathoracic pressure inhibiting venous return and cardiac output and may cause hypocarbia which causes cerebral ischaemia by vasoconstriction. On the other hand, inadequate ventilation contributes to hypercarbia, acidosis and cerebral vasodilation. After tracheal intubation, end-tidal CO_2 should be monitored by capnography. If end-tidal CO_2 is low, excessive ventilation and inadequate external cardiac compression (rate, depth of compression) should be excluded as causes.

Electrocardiograph (ECG)

The ECG should be displayed with either leads, pads or paddles. Drug therapy or immediate direct current shock is administered according to the existing rhythm. Electrolyte status, especially that of potassium and calcium, may be indicated by ECG patterns.

Vascular access

Peripheral venous cannulation

Access to the circulation via a peripheral vein should be attempted immediately on CPA. Any site is acceptable. Visible or palpable peripheral veins are to be found on the dorsum of the hand, wrist, forearm, cubital fossa, chest wall, foot and ankle. In infants, scalp veins are accessible and the umbilical vein can be used up to about a week after birth. The external jugulars are usually distended during CPR and easy to cannulate but this may be impeded by performance of intubation.

Intraosseous access

If peripheral intravenous access cannot be rapidly achieved, say within 60 seconds, intraosseous access should be obtained. This route has been used for patients of all ages.

It provides rapid, safe and reliable access to the circulation and serves as an adequate route for any parenteral drug and fluid administration. Syringing via a three-way tap is usually needed. The use of purpose-made intraosseous bone injection needles (e.g. Cook Aus Pty Ltd, 16g, 3 cm POWCH design) is preferable, although a short lumbar puncture type of needle with an inner trocar may suffice.

The handle of the device needle is held in the palm of the hand while the fingers grip the shaft about a centimetre from the tip. It is inserted perpendicular to the bone surface and a rotary action is used to traverse the cortex. Sudden loss of resistance signifies entry to bone marrow and the needle should stand unsupported. Correct positioning of the needle is confirmed by aspiration of bone marrow (which may be used for biochemical and haematological purposes) but that is not always possible. A bone marrow injection gun (Wais Med Ltd) which fires a needle a pre-set distance according to size of the patient or a bone marrow drill (EZ-IO, Vidacare) enables easy and rapid intraosseous infusion/injection for infants, children and adults. The latter device is preferred. Having an intraosseous drill available in the ED can provide extremely rapid access to the circulation in a child arriving in CPA.

Although many sites have been used for bone marrow injection, the easiest to identify is the anteromedial surface of the upper or lower tibia. The site of the latter is a few centimetres below the anterior tuberosity and the former a few centimetres above the medial malleolus. Care should be exercised to avoid complications, particularly cutaneous extravasation, compartment syndrome of the leg, and osteomyelitis. Contraindications include local trauma and infection.

Central venous cannulation

Cannulation of femoral, subclavian, or internal jugulars or external jugular veins are options. However, central cannulation is difficult in the setting of cardiorespiratory arrest and fraught with potential serious complications such as pneumothorax unless the operator is well practised. This technique is not recommended in the setting of an arrested child as the intraosseous route is more timely.

Endotracheal route

Drugs are absorbed into the circulation from the airways. Lipid-soluble drugs (adrenaline [epinephrine], atropine, lidocaine and naloxone) may be administered via the endotracheal tube if either intravenous or intraosseous access is non-existent. Although the optimal doses of these drugs by this route are not known, work in animal models suggests doses should be ten-times the intravenous doses. The drugs should be diluted in normal saline up to 2 mL for infants, 5 mL for small children and 10 mL for large children. It is acceptable and simplest to squirt the drugs from the syringe directly into the endotracheal tube and disperse them throughout the respiratory tree with bagging. Neither sodium bicarbonate nor calcium salts should be administered via the tracheal route because they injure the airways.

Other techniques

Surgical cutdown onto a long saphenous, saphenofemoral junction or basilic is a valuable skill sometimes required in traumatic exsanguination. Very occasionally, injection into the superior sagittal sinus of an infant[1] may be the only vascular access available. Any pre-existing functioning line can be used provided it does not contain any drug or electrolyte, which may have caused the CPA.

Fluid therapy

Circulatory hypovolaemia is expected in trauma, sepsis, dehydration and anaphylactic states. Restoration of intravascular volume should be with isotonic crystalloid solutions (0.9% normal saline or Hartmann's solution) or a colloidal solution such as 4% albumin. There is insufficient evidence to choose between these. Aliquots of 20 mL kg^{-1} intravenously or intraosseously are reasonable volumes to administer in shock states with titration against indices of vascular volume. It is reasonable to administer blood in traumatic haemorrhage if 40–60 mL kg^{-1} has not restored normal blood volume (70–80 mL kg^{-1}). The role of hypertonic solutions is not yet defined for children with hypovolaemic shock, but these solutions are in regular use for patients with severe head injury. Dextrose-containing solutions are inadvisable in acute resuscitation unless hypoglycaemia is proven since they may cause osmotic diuresis. Drugs should be flushed into the circulation with boluses of isotonic crystalloid solution.

Resuscitation drugs

Adenosine

This endogenous nucleoside is the drug of choice for treatment of supraventricular tachycardia (SVT) if circulation is adequate, otherwise DC shock is the preferred first treatment. It blocks AV node conduction and thus re-entry circuits, which are the usual causes of SVT in infants and children. It has a very short half-life (about 10 seconds) in the blood because it is deaminated and inactivated by adenosine deaminase on the surface of red blood cells. Hence, it must be delivered as a rapid bolus. The dose is 100–300 mcg kg^{-1} (commonly 100 mcg kg^{-1}) delivered rapidly intravenously (or intraosseously) and followed by a bolus of normal saline. If ineffective, the dose may be repeated and increased to the maximum recommended first and second doses as 6 and 12 mg.

Adrenaline (epinephrine)

Adrenaline is the most frequently used drug in paediatric advanced life support. Its α-adrenergic vasoconstrictive actions are considered the most important by increasing aortic diastolic pressure and coronary perfusion pressure. Its β-adrenergic actions enhance contractility and spontaneous contraction. The usual dose is 10 mcg kg^{-1} given intravenously or via the intraosseous route. It should be administered IV/IO every 3–5 minutes at the same dosage when indicated or run as an infusion of 0.05–0.3 mcg kg^{-1} min^{-1} (0.3 mg kg^{-1} adrenaline in 50 mL at 1 mL hr^{-1} = 0.1 mcg kg^{-1} min^{-1}). Higher bolus doses (up to 200 mcg kg^{-1}) or infusions may be administered in refractory asystole and bradyarrhythmic states but there is a risk of severe vasoconstriction, ischaemia, hypertension and onset of ectopy and tachyarrhythmias. If immediate access to the circulation is not available, it can be administered via the endotracheal route at a dosage of 100 mcg kg^{-1} but absorption is variable.

Amiodarone

This drug is used to treat a wide variety of atrial and ventricular dysrrhythmias including ectopic atrial tachycardia, junctional ectopic tachycardia (JET), ventricular tachycardia (VT) and DC-shock resistant ventricular fibrillation (VF). It inhibits α- and β-receptors, slows AV nodal conduction, and prolongs the QT interval and QRS duration. It thus may cause *torsade de pointes* VT. The loading dose is 5 mg kg^{-1} infused over several minutes to an hour depending on the dysrrhythmia being treated. Repeated doses to a maximum of 15 mg kg^{-1} may be given. Acute side effects are vasodilatation and hypotension and chronic effects are thyroid function disturbance, interstitial pneumonitis, corneal deposits and blue-grey skin discolouration.

Atropine

This parasympatholytic drug is used to treat bradycardia (<60 min^{-1}) caused by excessive vagal activity or a consequence of atrioventricular block (AV). If inadequate circulation or hypotension are present, severe bradycardia should be treated with adrenaline. Bradycardia caused by hypoxaemia should treated initially with ventilation and oxygen. The dose is 20 mcg kg^{-1} (minimum dose 100 mcg), which may be repeated after 5 minutes. Unresponsive bradycardia should be treated with adrenaline. Atropine should be given prior to RSI in young children to prevent the vagal stimulation of intubation that may cause bradycardia.

Calcium

Calcium should not be administered during acute resuscitation unless the cause of collapse is due to hypocalcaemia, hyperkalaemia, calcium channel blocker overdose or hypermagnesaemia. Although intimately involved in myocardial excitation-contraction coupling, it is not useful and possibly harmful, by causing cell death, in the regular treatment of asystole, electromechanical dissociation and ventricular fibrillation. Its use is associated with poor outcomes[10] and it should not be used without a definite indication. If it is indicated, the dose is 0.2 mL kg^{-1} of 10% calcium chloride or 0.7 mL kg^{-1} of 10% calcium gluconate and it may be repeated after 10 minutes according to the serum level if possible.

Glucose

Perturbations of glucose metabolism occur during critical illness. Infants are particularly at risk, as they have limited glycogen stores and may sustain hypoglycaemia, whereas the stress response may cause hyperglycaemia. Blood levels should be monitored regularly. Hypoglycaemia (<2.5 mmol kg^{-1}) should be treated with a dextrose infusion of approximately 6–8 mg kg^{-1}/min or equivalent. Bolus injection may be necessary (in situations such as seizure or coma due to hypoglycaemia) in which case an appropriate dose is 0.5 g kg^{-1} as provided, for example, by 5 mL kg^{-1} of 10% or 2 mL kg^{-1} of 25%. Such boluses, however, may cause hyperglycaemia and an acute rise in serum osmolality with osmotic diuresis and harmful rapid changes in brain osmolality. Hypoglycaemia and hyperglycaemia after brain injury should be avoided.

Lidocaine (Lignocaine)

This is a sodium channel blocker that decreases automaticity and suppresses ventricular arrhythmias. However, in infants and children it is considered ineffective unless dysrhythmia is associated with focal ischaemia. Although it has been traditionally used for shock-resistant VF and pulseless VT, it has no proven efficacy. If used, the recommended dose is 1 mg kg^{-1} (0.1 mL kg^{-1} of 1%) by rapid injection followed by an infusion of 20–50 mcg kg^{-1} min^{-1}. A low infusion dose is recommended if renal or hepatic dysfunction exists. Adverse side effects include myocardial depression with hypotension and central nervous system depression with depression of conscious state and convulsions.

Magnesium

Magnesium inhibits calcium channels and causes a reduction in intracellular calcium, thereby causing muscle relaxation, and is used as a bronchodilator in severe asthma. In resuscitation it is used to treat hypomagnesaemia and *torsade de pointes* VT (see earlier) – a dysrhythmia associated with prolonged QT interval, which may be congenital (e.g. Jervell–Lange–Nielson and Romano–Ward syndromes) or acquired. The causes of acquired prolonged QT interval are any cause of hypocalcaemia or hypomagnesaemia, drugs (notably tricyclics, phenothiazines, type IA antiarrhythmics such as quinidine and disopyramide, type III antiarrhythmics such as amiodarone and sotalol), central nervous system trauma and myocarditis/ischaemia. The dose of magnesium sulphate is 25–50 mg kg^{-1}

($0.1–0.2$ mmol kg^{-1}) by intravenous or intraosseous infusion over several minutes.

Sodium bicarbonate

Sodium bicarbonate may be used to counter measured metabolic acidosis in prolonged cardiac arrest but only after hypoventilation has been corrected and preferably only during hyperventilation. Although it can neutralise hydronium ions in the blood it may worsen intracellular acidosis. The product of bicarbonate and hydronium ions is carbonic acid, which freely dissociates to form water and carbon dioxide (CO_2) and, unless hyperventilation is given, the CO_2 may cross into cells, where it reforms carbonic acid and librates hydronium ions.

If indicated, an appropriate dose is 1 mmol kg^{-1}. Adverse effects include hypernatraemia and hyperosmolality, hypokalaemia, hypocalcaemia and metabolic alkalosis (which limits oxygen dissociation from haemoglobin). It should not be allowed to mix with catecholamines, which it inactivates, or with calcium salts, which it precipitates. The essential treatment of metabolic acidosis is treatment of the cause.

Vasopressin

The alternative to adrenaline as a vasopressor, vasopressin, has no better survival advantage for adult victims of in-hospital cardiac arrest,[11] and has not been adequately investigated for use during CPR for children.

Direct current shock

Unsynchronised DC shock is required as first treatment for VF and pulseless VT. If effective for VF it is called defibrillation. Synchronised DC shock may also be required for pulsatile VT and haemodynamically unstable supraventricular tachycardia (SVT).

Operators of defibrillators should be constantly alert to the possibility of inadvertent electrocution and cardiac arrest of themselves and others by misuse. Pads have advantages over paddles; they minimise risk of inadvertent shock to the operator and importantly, allow application of shock with minimal disruption to external cardiac compression. Paddles should be charged after placement on the patient, not before. Charged paddles should never be carried in one hand and never discharged in the air. If after charging, discharge is not needed, the paddles should be replaced in their storage holders before discharge. It is important that no-one is in contact with the patient or the bed or trolley at the time of discharge.

Defibrillators should have paediatric paddles of cross sectional area 12–20 cm^2 for use in children <10 kg. For others, adult-sized paddles (50–80 cm^2) are satisfactory provided the paddles do not contact each other. Selectable energy levels should enable delivery of doses 0.5–5 J kg^{-1}. Doses should be rounded up to the closest weight-based dose. For use in the anterolateral positions, one pad/paddle is placed over the mid-axilla opposite the xyphoid or nipple, the other to the right of the upper sternum below the clavicle. Conductive gel (confined to the area beneath the paddles) or gel pads and firm pressure are needed to deliver optimum energy to the heart without causing skin burns. An anteroposterior position of pads is the preferred positioning (one over cardiac apex or anterior chest, one over left scapula). Dextrocardia may be present with congenital heart disease and the position of the pads/paddles should be altered accordingly.

In the absence of a manual dose regulated defibrillator, semi-automated automatic external defibrillation (sAED) may be used for children but preferably should have an 'attenuated' adult dose. A dose of 50 J is appropriate for most infants and children. However, if a machine with such attenuated dosing is not available, the use of an adult sAED delivering 150–200 J is acceptable for infants and children[1–4] rather than leave untreated a shockable rhythm. The use of an sAED with adult doses of DC shock for children in hospital should not be considered unless a manual dose regulated defibrillator is not available or cannot be used or a body weight specific DC shock cannot be delivered within 3 minutes when indicated.

Management of pulseless arrhythmias (Fig. 2.3.2)

The following discussion assumes that mechanical ventilation with oxygen and external cardiac compression (ECC) have been commenced and continued if an adequate pulse rate is not detectable. The treatment of pulseless arrhythmias (ventricular fibrillation, ventricular tachycardia, asystole, electromechanical dissociation and pulseless electrical activity) are summarised in Fig. 2.3.2.

Specific causes of arrhythmias should be treated. For example, calcium channel blockade toxicity is treated with calcium IV or IO (chloride 10% 0.2 mL kg^{-1}, gluconate 10% 0.7 mL kg^{-1}); hyperkalaemia treated with calcium salt, sodium bicarbonate, hyperventilation, insulin and dextrose. All drugs should be flushed into the circulation with a small bolus of isotonic fluid. To prevent inactivation, drugs should not be mixed in the syringe or in infusion lines.

Asystole

Asystole should be treated with adrenaline (epinephrine) 10 mcg kg^{-1} IV or IO. If these routes are not available, adrenaline 100 μg kg^{-1} should be administered via endotracheal tube (ETT). Unresponsive asystole should be treated with similar doses (10 μg kg^{-1} IV, IO; 100 μg kg^{-1} ETT) every 3–5 minutes. Higher doses, up to 200 μg kg^{-1} IV or IO may be used, but have not altered outcome and predispose to complications (post-arrest myocardial dysfunction, hypertension, tachycardia). In newborn infants, the initial bolus dose is 10–30 mcg kg^{-1} (0.1–0.3 mL kg^{-1} of 1,10:000 solution). Persistent or recurrent bradyarrhythmia or asystole may require an infusion of adrenaline at 0.05–3 mcg kg^{-1} min^{-1}. Doses of <0.3 mcg kg^{-1} min^{-1} are predominantly β-adrenergic, doses >0.3 mcg kg^{-1} min^{-1} are predominantly α-adrenergic. Infuse into a secure large vein. If sinus rhythm cannot be restored, sodium bicarbonate 1 mmol kg^{-1} IV or IO may be helpful but do not allow mixing with adrenaline since catecholamines are inactivated in alkaline solution. Pacing is not helpful for asystole.

Pulseless electrical activity (PEA) and electromechanical dissociation (EMD)

A normal ECG complex without pulses is called electromechanical dissociation (EMD). If untreated, the ECG deteriorates to an abnormal but still recognisable state

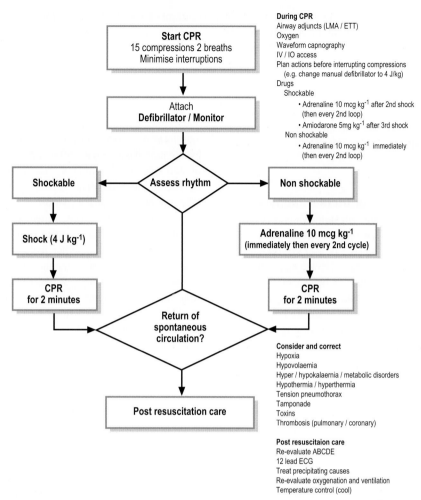

During CPR
Airway adjuncts (LMA / ETT)
Oxygen
Waveform capnography
IV / IO access
Plan actions before interrupting compressions
 (e.g. change manual defibrillator to 4 J/kg)
Drugs
 Shockable
   • Adrenaline 10 mcg kg⁻¹ after 2nd shock
    (then every 2nd loop)
   • Amiodarone 5mg kg⁻¹ after 3rd shock
 Non shockable
   • Adrenaline 10 mcg kg⁻¹ immediately
    (then every 2nd loop)

Consider and correct
Hypoxia
Hypovolaemia
Hyper / hypokalaernia / metabolic disorders
Hypothermia / hyperthermia
Tension pneumothorax
Tamponade
Toxins
Thrombosis (pulmonary / coronary)

Post resuscitaion care
Re-evaluate ABCDE
12 lead ECG
Treat precipitating causes
Re-evaluate oxygenation and ventilation
Temperature control (cool)

Fig. 2.3.2 Advanced cardiopulmonary resuscitation for infants and children. Adapted from resuscitation guidelines of the International Liaison Committee on Resuscitation, Australian Resuscitation Council, European Resuscitation Council and of the American Heart Association, December 2010. Australian Resuscitation Council. Key: CPR, cardiopulmonary resuscitation; ECG, electrocardiograph; IO, intraosseous; IV, intravenous; J, joules; kg, kilogram; mg, milligram; mcg, microgram.

when it is called pulseless electrical activity (PEA). Both conditions should be treated as for asystole and their causes ascertained and treated.

Ventricular fibrillation and pulseless ventricular tachycardia

In approximately 10% of paediatric cardiac arrests the initial identified rhythm is VF or pulseless VT. As soon as recognised, VF or pulseless VT should be treated with unsynchronized DC shock. If onset is witnessed in a monitored environment, a precordial thump may be given but its efficacy has not been proven.

Either monophasic or biphasic waveforms may be used. The optimum dose of external DC shock in terms of achieving first shock success with minimal damage to the myocardium is unknown. Some guidelines recommend a dose of 2–4 J kg⁻¹.[3,4] The dose of 2 J kg⁻¹ is considered too little by other guidelines[1,2] which advise 4 J kg⁻¹. This is supported by a recent study which showed that 2 J kg⁻¹ converted only about 50% of patients to a perfusing rhythm.[12] In contrast to previous recommendations, it is now recommended to give one shock followed immediately by uninterrupted CPR for 2 minutes without pausing to determine if another shock is required. Only in monitored

witnessed onset of VF and immediate availability of defibrillation (first dose within 30 seconds) is a stack of up to three shocks (each 4 J kg⁻¹)[1,2] without intervening CPR recommended. If ROSC has not occurred within 10 seconds of any of the 3 shocks CPR should be given. DC shock may be more successful if front and back placement of pads is used. Whatever position, use of pads rather than paddles enables minimal disruption to continuous external cardiac compression.

Failure of VF or pulseless VT to revert immediately to a perfusing rhythm with DC shock (4 J kg⁻¹) should be treated with another single DC shock (4 J kg⁻¹) after 2 minutes of CPR. Persistent VF or pulseless VT should be treated with adrenaline 10 mcg kg⁻¹ IV or IO or 100 mcg kg⁻¹ ETT followed by another single shock if necessary. Persistent (refractory) or recurrent VF or VT may be also treated with antiarrhythmics (amiodarone, magnesium) interspersed with single DC shocks followed by 2 minutes of CPR. Irrespective of other drug therapy, adrenaline should be administered every 3–5 minutes. Amiodarone is more efficacious than lignocaine for DC shock resistant VF and pulseless VT and is the preferred drug. The dose of amiodarone is 5 mg kg⁻¹ IV or IO over several to 60 minutes. It may be repeated to maximum of 15 mg kg⁻¹. If amiodarone is not available, lignocaine may be used in a dose of 1 mg kg⁻¹ IV or IO bolus followed by an infusion if successful at 20–50 mcg kg⁻¹ min⁻¹. Magnesium, 25–50 mg kg⁻¹ (0.10–0.20 mmol kg⁻¹) is indicated for polymorphic VT (torsade de pointes).

Management of pulsatile dysrhythmias

Bradysrhythmias

In all age groups, bradycardia is defined as a heart rate <60 min⁻¹ or rapidly declining rate with poor perfusion. Sinus bradycardia, sinus arrest with slow junctional or idioventricular rhythm and atrioventricular block are the most common preterminal arrhythmias in paediatric practice. Untreated, bradycardia will potentially progress to asystole. The treatment is reversal of the cause (hypoxaemia, hypotension, acidosis, hypothermia, intracranial hypertension) and, if unresponsive, adrenaline 10 mcg kg^{-1} IV or IO or 100 mcg kg^{-1} ETT. Bradycardia caused by vagal stimulation should be managed with cessation of the stimulus (e.g. oropharyngeal suctioning, laryngoscopy) and/or atropine 20 mcg kg^{-1} IV or IO (minimum dose 100 μg). Persistent vagal-mediated bradycardia should be treated with adrenaline 10 mcg kg^{-1} IV or IO. If facilities are available, pacing (oesophageal, trans-cutaneous, transvenous, epicardial) may be effective if sinus node dysfunction or heart block exist.

Tachydysrhythmias (Fig. 2.3.3)

Any heart rate above normal for age should be considered a tachydysrhythmia, particularly if associated with poor circulation and hypotension and if the patient has a history of cardiac disease, has had cardiac surgery or could have been poisoned with cardioactive drugs. Of course, such tachycardia may be the result, rather than the cause of poor circulation, i.e. sinus tachycardia (ST). It is important to determine the type and aetiology of the tachycardia, lest drug or other treatment exacerbate the situation. A history related to the tachycardia and a 12-lead ECG should be analysed carefully. If the diagnosis is not obvious, the rate and duration of the QRS are starting points to differentiate sinus tachycardia (ST), ventricular tachycardia (VT), supraventricular tachycardia (SVT) and wide QRS-complex SVT.

Pulsatile ventricular tachycardia

Haemodynamically stable VT may be treated with an antiarrhythmic agent such as amiodarone (5 mg kg^{-1} IV over 20–60 minutes) or procainamide (15 mg kg^{-1} IV over 30–60 minutes) or lidocaine (1 mg kg^{-1} IV over 2–4 minutes). Note that both amiodarone and procainamide prolong QT interval and should not be given together. If *torsade de pointes* (twisting of the peaks) is present, magnesium (25–50 mg kg^{-1}, 0.1–0.2 mmol kg^{-1} IV) may be used. If pulses are present but accompanied by hypotension and poor circulation, cardioversion is needed, in which case it should be synchronised at $\geq$2 J kg^{-1} under sedation/anaesthesia.

Supraventricular tachycardia

SVT is the most common spontaneous arrhythmia in childhood and infancy. Some infants may tolerate this rhythm for long periods; however, it may cause life-threatening hypotension. It is usually re-entrant with a rate of 220–300 min^{-1} in infants, usually less in children (approximately 180 min^{-1}). The QRS complex is usually narrow (<0.08 seconds), making it difficult sometimes to discern from sinus tachycardia. However, whereas ST is a part of other features of illness, SVT is a singular entity and whereas the rate in ST is variable with activity or stimulation, it is uniform in SVT and often of sudden onset and offset. In both rhythms, a P wave may be discernible.

If haemodynamically stable (adequate perfusion and blood pressure), initial treatment of SVT should be vagal stimulation. For infants and young children, application to the face of a plastic bag filled with iced-water is often effective, or alternatively

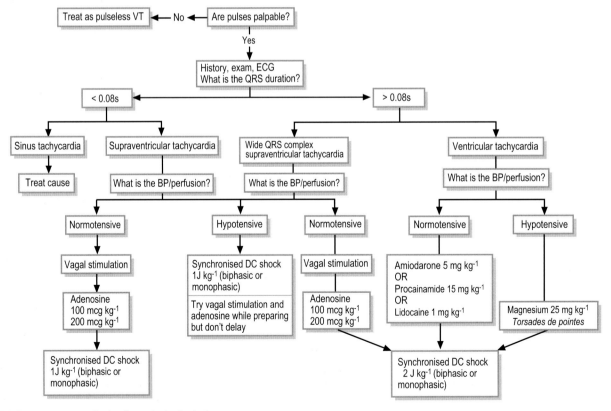

Fig. 2.3.3 Management of pulsatile tachydysrhythmias.

submersion of the face into a slurry of ice and water in a bowl. Older children may be treated with carotid sinus massage or asking them to perform a Valsalva manoeuvre – such as blowing through a narrow straw. If unsuccessful, give adenosine initially at 100 mcg kg^{-1} IV by rapid bolus (max dose 6 mg), increasing to 200 mcg kg^{-1} or 300 mcg kg^{-1}. In older children, it is important to describe the transient feeling of 'chest heaviness or breathing difficulty or fearfulness' that may accompany adenosine administration, and/or precede the adenosine with a small amnestic dose of midazolam. If unsuccessful, give synchronised DC shock (cardioversion)[13] initially at 0.5–1.0 J kg^{-1} but subsequently up to 2 J kg^{-1}. If at the outset SVT is accompanied by haemodynamic instability, proceed to cardioversion (synchronised 1.0 J kg^{-1}) immediately, although vagal stimulation or adenosine (IV or IO) may be used, provided they do not delay cardioversion. Verapamil should not be used to treat SVT in infants and should be avoided in children because it induces hypotension by vasodilation and negative inotropic effect.

Wide QRS complex supraventricular tachycardia

SVT with aberrant conduction may cause a wide-complex QRS (>0.08 seconds) and thus may resemble VT. If the blood pressure is low or circulation deemed inadequate, the rhythm should be regarded as VT and treated with synchronised DC shock at ≥2 J kg^{-1}. If pulses are absent, the rhythm should be regarded as pulseless VT and treated accordingly with DC shock.

Post-resuscitation management

Supportive therapy should be provided until there is recovery of function of vital organs. This may require provision of oxygen therapy, mechanical ventilation, inotropic/vasopressor infusion, renal support, parenteral nutrition and other therapy for several days or longer. Recovery of infants and children is usually slow because cardiorespiratory arrest is often secondary to prolonged global ischaemia or hypoxaemia, which implies that other organs sustain damage before

cardiorespiratory arrest. The cause of the CPA should be investigated and treated appropriately, e.g. sepsis or drug overdose. Particular care should be taken to ensure adequate cerebral perfusion with well-oxygenated blood. Hyperventilation to hypocarbic levels is contraindicated because of potential harmful cerebral vasoconstriction.

Survival and neurological outcome is better when deliberate hypothermia is used after cardiac arrest. ILCOR has recommended therapeutic hypothermia (32–34°C) for 12–24 hours for adults and children[1] who remain unconscious with spontaneous circulation after out-of-hospital cardiac arrest when the initial rhythm was ventricular fibrillation, and suggested that for any other rhythm, or cardiac arrest in hospital, such cooling may also be beneficial. The optimal duration of such requirement, however, is unknown but clinical studies among newborns suggest 72 hours.[14] Inadvertently hypothermic patients, provided temperature is above 32°C or greater should not be actively warmed and hyperthermia should be aggressively treated. If deliberate hypothermia is employed, shivering should be prevented with sedation and/or neuromuscular blockade. Seizures should be actively sought and treated with anticonvulsant.

Complications of CPR should be sought especially if secondary deterioration occurs. A chest X-ray should be obtained to check the position of the endotracheal tube, to exclude pneumothorax, lung collapse, contusion or aspiration and to check the cardiac silhouette. Invasive blood pressure measurement and periodic echocardiographic or bedside ultrasound examination are needed to specifically check contractility and to exclude a pericardial effusion. Measurement of haemoglobin, pH, gas tensions, electrolytes and glucose are important.

Cessation of CPR

Long-term outcome from paediatric CPR is poor, with approximately 5–10% of patients surviving out-of-hospital arrest[15] and 25–50% in-hospital cardiac arrest.[16,17] The decision to cease CPR should be based on a number of factors including the duration of resuscitation, its quality, response to treatment, pre-arrest status of the

patient, remediable factors, likely outcome if ultimately successful, opinions of personnel familiar with the patient and, whenever appropriate, the wishes of informed parents. In general, unless hypothermia or drug toxicity exists, survival to normality is most unlikely if there has been a failure to respond to full CPR after 30 minutes and several doses of adrenaline, unless environmental hypothermia was an important aetiological or consequential factor. In the newly-born infant, discontinuation of treatment is appropriate if CPR does not establish a spontaneous circulation within 15 minutes.[1] Family members should be kept informed, allowed to be present or asked if they want to be present during resuscitation (see Chapter 2.1).

Post-resuscitation staff management

Unfortunately, CPA occurring in hospital is often unexpected as when, for example, a moribund patient arrives unannounced in the emergency department, or a patient's condition deteriorates rapidly on the ward or when a mishap occurs under anaesthesia. These situations test the readiness, training, abilities and skills of individuals and the organisation of the institution. It is prudent to monitor performance with a view to improvement and not ignore the psychological impact that such events have on individuals. Sensitive debriefing sessions may be helpful to members of staff involved post resuscitation.

Prevention of cardiorespiratory arrest

Of course, hospital personnel should be well-trained and organised to treat unexpected cardiorespiratory arrest, but the far preferable course of action is prevention. Some paediatric hospitals have instituted 'Rapid Response Team' systems or 'Medical Emergency Team' systems, which can respond rapidly to deterioration in a patient's condition before cardiorespiratory arrest occurs, with consequent significant reductions in unexpected cardiac arrest (38%) mortality[18,19] (21%) and unplanned admission to intensive care.

References

1. *Australian Resuscitation Council Guidelines*. Melbourne. p. 12.1–12.7. http://www.resus.org.au.
2. Biarent D, Bimgham R, Eich C, et al. European Resuscitation Council Guidelines for Resuscitation 2010 Section 6. Paediatric life support. *Resuscitation* 2010;**81**:1364–88.
3. Kleinman ME, Chameides L, Schexnayder SM, et al. Part 14: Pediatric advanced life support: 2010 American Heart Association guidelines for cardiopulmonary resuscitation and emergency cardiovascular care. *Circulation* 2010;**122**: S876–S908.
4. de Caen AR, Kleinman ME, Chameides L, et al. Part 10: Paediatric basic and advanced life support: 2010 International Consensus on Cardiopulmonary Resuscitation and Emergency Cardiovascular Care Science with Treatment Recommendations. *Resuscitation* 2010;**81**:e213–e259.
5. Tibballs J, Russell P. Reliability of pulse palpation by healthcare personnel to diagnose paediatric cardiac arrest. *Resuscitation* 2009;**80**:61–4.
6. Tibballs J, Weeranatna C. The influence of time on the accuracy of healthcare personnel to diagnose paediatric cardiac arrest by pulse palpation. *Resuscitation* 2010;**81**(6):671–5.
7. Carter BG, Fairbank B, Tibballs J, et al. Oxygen delivery using self-inflating resuscitation bags. *Pediatr Crit Care Med* 2005;**6**:125–8.
8. Gausche M, Lewis RJ, Stratton SJ, et al. Effect of out-of-hospital pediatric endotracheal intubation on survival and neurological outcome: a controlled clinical trial. *JAMA* 2000;**283**:783–90.
9. Benumot JL. Laryngeal mask airway and the ASA difficult airway algorithm. *Anesthesiology* 1996;**84**:686–99.
10. Srinivasan M, Morris MC, Helfaer MA, et al. Calcium use during in-hospital pediatric cardiopulmonary resuscitation: a report from the National Registry of Cardiopulmonary Resuscitation. *Pediatrics* 2008;**121**: e114–e151.
11. Stiell IG, Hebert PC, Wells GA, et al. Vasopressin versus epinephrine for inhospital cardiac arrest: A randomised controlled trial. *Lancet* 2001;**358**:105–9.
12. Tibballs J, Carter B, Kiraly NJ, et al. External and internal biphasic DC shock doses for pediatric ventricular fibrillation and pulseless ventricular tachycardia. *Pediatr Crit Care Med* 2011;**12**:14–20.
13. Tibballs J, Carter B, Kiraly NJ, et al. Biphasic DC shock cardioverting doses for paediatric atrial dysrhythmias. *Resuscitation* 2010;**81**:1101–4.
14. Kochanek PM, Fink E, Bell MJ, et al. Therapeutic hypothermia: applications in pediatric cardiac arrest. *J Neurotrauma* 2009;**26**:421–7.
15. Deasy C, Bernard SA, Cameron P, et al. Epidemiology of paediatric out-of-hospital cardiac arrest in Melbourne, Australia. *Resuscitation* 2010;**81**:1095–100.
16. Tibballs J, Kinney S. A prospective study of out-of-patient paediatric cardiopulmonary arrest. *Resuscitation* 2006;**71**:310–8.
17. Meert KL, Donaldson A, Nadkarni V, et al. Multicenter cohort study of in-hospital pediatric cardiac arrest. *Pediatr Crit Care Med* 2009;**10**:544–53.
18. Chan PS, Jain R, Nallmothu BK, et al. Rapid response teams. A systematic review and meta-analysis. *Arch Intern Med* 2010;**170**:18–26.
19. Tibballs J, Brilli RJ. Pediatric RRSs. In: De Vita MA, Hillman K, Bellomo R, editors. *Textbook of Rapid Response Systems: Concepts and Implementation*. New York: Springer; 2011. p. 231–43.

2.4 Specific paediatric resuscitation

James Tibballs

Anaphylaxis

Persons receiving β-blocking drugs have a potentiated risk of anaphylaxis. In such patients, it is more resistant to therapy and lasts longer. Hypotension may be refractive to adrenaline. In such cases, glucagon (therapy for β-blocker toxicity) may be required along with infusions of adrenaline and dopamine. See Chapter 22.5 for the detailed account of the treatment of anaphylaxis.

Drowning

Victims of submersion incidents suffer global hypoxaemia and if arrested, global ischaemia. Associated injuries are aspiration pneumonitis and hypothermia. Aspiration of water and gastric contents is common (see Chapter 22.2). In addition, hypothermia (see Chapter 22.4) may be present, but unless the victim was subject to severe environmental hypothermia such as being submersed in ice-cold water (<5°C) or has profound afterdrop after removal from water, this reflects lack of perfusion and is a bad prognostic sign. Hypothermia should be treated but temperature not permitted to rise above 35°C if cardiac arrest has occurred (see Chapter 2.3).

The outcome is often determined by the extent of neurological injury. Bad prognostic indicators are prolonged duration of submersion, lack of bystander CPR, prolonged prehospital resuscitation, pulseless arrhythmia on arrival at hospital, fixed dilated pupils, severe acidosis and apnoea. Nonetheless, vigorous resuscitation should be instituted on arrival in hospital of the pulseless victim, if not already commenced by ambulance personnel, in order to clarify the clinical details whilst continuing resuscitation.

Intubation and mechanical ventilation with 100% oxygen should be instituted immediately. Regurgitation of stomach contents should be anticipated and a rapid sequence intubation technique with cricoid pressure should be used. Sedative drugs with cardiovascular depressive actions should not be used, or in minimally required doses only. The lung compliance is likely to be poor and it may be necessary to insert a larger-than-usual uncuffed or a cuffed endotracheal tube (preferred) to prevent a leak around the tube, to obtain adequate lung inflation in the setting of acute respiratory distress syndrome (ARDS) in order to achieve oxygenation. After restoration of cardiac rhythm myocardial contractility should be measured with echocardiography and optimised with inotropic agents.

During resuscitation, the goal is to provide maximum opportunity for cerebral recovery and this is achieved by restoring cerebral perfusion with well oxygenated blood and the avoidance of factors that decrease cerebral perfusion pressure. It is thus vital to restore cardiac output and blood pressure, to oxygenate blood and to avoid factors that would increase intracranial pressure, such as venous obstruction. Hypocapnia, hypercapnia, hypoglycaemia and hyperglycaemia should be avoided and convulsions treated.

Any pulseless arrhythmia may be encountered and should be managed along standard lines.

There are no important clinical differences between fresh and salt-water immersion. Altered levels of serum electrolytes, especially sodium and potassium, may be detected, but are uncommon and in any case do not influence acute resuscitation.

Toxicological emergencies

The standard resuscitation protocols may be inadequate in some toxicological emergencies, particularly when poisoning has occurred with cardioactive drugs.

Airway and ventilation management

Problems should not be created by treatment. Gastric lavage should not be undertaken unless the patient has ingested a significant toxin in significant amounts within the past hour. There are very few indications for gastric lavage. Gastric lavage should not be performed in the fully conscious or in the less-than-fully conscious patient, without prior securement of the airway with rapid sequence endotracheal intubation. Likewise, activated charcoal should not be administered by oro/nasogastric tube in a patient who is less-than-fully conscious, irrespective of the interval since ingestion. The risk of aspiration pneumonitis in these circumstances is significant. If activated charcoal is to given by naso/orogastruc tube, confirm it is in the stomach, not the lungs, prior to instilling the charcoal.

Drug-induced asystole

Infusions of KCl are hazardous. Molar solutions of KCl are in common use in intensive care units especially after cardiac surgery. They should not be available for regular ward use. An inadvertent IV bolus of potassium can cause asystole. Note that a 1 mL bolus of molar KCl (1 mmol) in a 10 kg child will theoretically raise the serum concentration by 2.5 mmol L^{-1} and cause immediate asystole.

Immediately acting treatment (within seconds) for hyperkalaemia is either 10% calcium chloride IV 0.2 mL kg^{-1} (or equivalent) or IV sodium bicarbonate 1 mmol kg^{-1} or both. Calcium antagonises the cardiac effects of potassium on the heart, while the bicarbonate lowers the serum concentration of potassium by a small amount. Better treatments of rapid onset (within minutes) are glucose 0.5 g kg^{-1} IV (e.g. 5 mL kg^{-1} of 10%) plus insulin 0.05 units kg^{-1} or salbutamol 0.25 mg kg^{-1} by aerosol or both. Slow treatment (within hours) is by resonium, oral or rectal, 0.5–1 g kg^{-1}.

Drug-induced bradycardia

Organophosphate and carbamate poisoning with bradycardia should be treated with atropine – repeated doses of 20–50 mcg kg^{-1} every 15 minutes or until secretions are dry and an acceptable heart rate is restored. In organophosphate poisoning (but not carbamate), pralidoxime can reactivate cholinesterase. The dose is 25 mg kg^{-1} IV over 15–30 minutes then 10–20 mg kg^{-1} per hour for 18 hours or more.

Bradycardia induced by β-blocker poisoning is treated with glucagon 7 mcg kg^{-1} IV then 2–7 mcg kg^{-1} min^{-1}. This is the preferred antidote because it stimulates non-catecholamine cAMP. Isoprenaline 0.05–3 mcg kg^{-1} min^{-1} by infusion may be used but it may cause β2-induced hypotension and should not be used if hypotension is pre-existing. Alternatively, an infusion of adrenalin (epinephrine) at 0.05–1 mcg kg^{-1} min^{-1} may be used.

Digoxin induced bradycardia may be treated with Digoxin Fab antibody in a dose of 10 vials per 25 of 0.25 mg tablets or per 5 mg elixir ingested. At steady state, the number of vials is calculated as serum digoxin (ng mL^{-1}) × (kg)/100.

Drug-induced tachyarrhythmias

The preferred treatment is a benzodiazepine such as diazepam or midazolam in doses that do not depress CNS function. Other treatments are the ultrashort-acting cardioselective β1 blocker esmolol IV 500 mcg kg^{-1} over 1 minute and then 25–200 mcg kg^{-1} min^{-1} by infusion. Treatments such as intravenous adenosine and DC shock are not likely to be effective because the toxic drug effect will be persistent. Calcium channel blockers such as verapamil may cause severe hypotension and should not be given.

Drug-induced hypertension

Hypertension may occur with poisoning by cocaine, amphetamine and similar substances, which cause vasoconstriction, tachycardia and arrhythmias. Benzodiazepines are the preferred treatment. Another alternative is a smooth muscle dilator such as sodium nitroprusside IV 0.5–2 mcg kg^{-1} min^{-1}, but its use mandates intra-arterial monitoring. Another choice is phentolamine IV 0.05–0.1 mg kg^{-1} and then an infusion of 5–50 mcg kg^{-1} min^{-1}. Propranolol, a non-selective β-blocker is contraindicated because it may paradoxically worsen hypertension when β2-adrenoreceptors are blocked.

Drug-induced ventricular tachycardia (VT) and fibrillation (VF)

Haemodynamically stable VT can be treated with anti-arrhythmic agents. Typical drug causes are tricyclic antidepressants, cocaine and amphetamines. These cause a monomorphic VT by increasing the QRS interval. Treatment should be sodium bicarbonate, especially in cases of tricyclic poisoning.

Both components of the sodium bicarbonate contribute to its antidotal effect – the sodium counters the sodium channel blockade effect of the drugs and the alkalosis reduces bioavailability. Induction of respiratory alkalosis is also beneficial. The preferred antidysrrhythmic agent is lidocaine. Phenytoin is no longer recommended. Polymorphic VT (*torsade de pointes*) of any cause should be treated with magnesium 25–50 mg kg^{-1} IV.

Pulseless VT or VF require DC shock. The use of adrenaline (epinephrine) in this situation should be limited to 10 mcg kg^{-1} boluses while higher doses which may cause recurrent VF or VT should be avoided. Propranolol is contraindicated.

Drug-induced shock

Shock may result from drugs that cause depression of myocardial contractility, vasodilatation or loss of intravascular volume, or combinations of these. An extreme rise in peripheral vascular resistance may also lead to myocardial failure. Whenever possible preload, contractility and afterload should be measured via a central venous line.

Preload deficiencies (hypovolaemia) are corrected with volume administration, titrated against blood pressure, right heart filling pressure and against pulmonary artery wedge pressure.

Infusion of dopamine is a suitable inotropic agent in doses of approximately 5–15 mcg kg^{-1} min^{-1}, although higher doses may be needed or other inotropic drugs added. If central access is not possible, infusion of dobutamine in a similar dose may be given via a peripheral venous access, at least in the short term. Other inotropic agents are infusions of calcium (0.03–0.1 mL kg^{-1} hr^{-1} of 10% $CaCl_2$, i.e. 3–10 mg kg^{-1} hr^{-1}), milrinone (50 mcg kg^{-1} loading dose then 0.375–0.75 mcg kg^{-1} min^{-1}) and glucagon. It is desirable to measure cardiac output or to assess contractility with echocardiography.

Vasodilatation is treated with an α-adrenergic agent such as noradrenaline (norepinephrine) infusion (0.05–1 mcg kg^{-1} min^{-1}) in the higher dose range. Other such agents are phenylephrine (1·5 μg kg^{-1} min^{-1}) and metaraminol (0.05–1 mcg kg^{-1} min^{-1}). Vasoconstriction is also obtained with vasopressin infusion (0.002–0.01 units kg^{-1} min^{-1}).

In selected circumstances, cardiac output can be supported with ventricular assist devices, extra-corporeal membrane oxygenation (ECMO) or intra-aortic balloon pumping, although the last named requires intrinsic cardiac rhythm. These techniques are sometimes used in toxicological emergencies in centres that use these techniques for cardiac surgery. They are only indicated when standard supportive measures are insufficient but the situation is recoverable, and organ damage, particularly brain damage, has not occurred. The principal risks with such techniques are haemorrhage, infection and mechanical failure.

Envenomation

The main principles of resuscitation, restoration of airway, breathing and circulation apply to victims of envenomation, but with additional special requirements related to the effects of venoms and the treatment of envenomation.[1]

Numerous venomous Australian terrestrial and marine creatures may threaten life (see Chapter 22.1). Snakes, spiders, ticks, jellyfish, octopuses and cone shells inject lethal venoms whereas the venoms of bees, ants and wasps cause anaphylaxis. The number of deaths due to envenomation in Australia is two to four per year. A similar number of deaths, one to three per year, are due to anaphylactic reactions to bee and wasp stings.

Death and critical illness is due to: (1) rapid onset neurotoxicity, with respiratory failure and airway obstruction by bulbar palsy; (2) haemorrhage and shock; and (3) renal failure secondary to rhabdomyolysis, disseminated intravascular coagulation (DIC; consumption coagulopathy, defibrination), haemorrhage or haemolysis. Rapid cardiovascular collapse within minutes after a snake bite may be due to anaphylaxis to venom, acute vasodilatation or to disseminated intravascular coagulation-provoked pulmonary hypertension and *cor pulmonale*.

Particular resuscitation problems encountered after envenomation include the following.

Respiratory failure and bulbar palsy

Many venoms contains neurotoxins. Respiratory and airway support may be required for a prolonged period. Although paralysis caused by some animals, e.g. blue-ringed octopuses, may be relatively brief, lasting perhaps several hours (if support is given), paralysis caused by some snake and funnel-web spider venoms may be lengthy. For example, a child considered to have been bitten by a Rough-scaled snake remained ventilator dependent for 10 weeks, although antivenom administration in that case was delayed.[2]

Coagulopathy and haemorrhage

Snake-bite-induced coagulopathy, and haemorrhage and shock, may be prolonged and may not respond readily to administration of antivenom and clotting factors. Antivenom alone does not *per se* restore normal coagulation. In the presence of haemorrhage, it is prudent to administer clotting factors if normal coagulation is not restored soon after antivenom administration, since serum levels of coagulation factors are not restored by liver function for approximately 6 hours after complete consumption of clotting factors during DIC. In the absence of any ability to measure the serum concentrations of venom components it is difficult to judge how much antivenom is required when the sole effect of venom is coagulopathy. Hitherto recommended neutralisation doses of antivenom have been found inadequate in canine and human plasma models of envenomation and coagulopathy.[3,4]

Rhabdomyolysis

Some envenomations cause rhabdomyolysis with implications for renal function, electrolyte disturbances (hyperkalaemia, hypocalcaemia) and muscle weakness. This is expected after envenomation by certain snakes (e.g. tiger snakes, black snakes, Beaked sea snake) and funnel-web spiders, particularly if antivenom therapy is inadequate or delayed. Myocardial muscle may be involved.

Cardiac dysrhythmias

Cardiac dysrhythmias have been observed after envenomation by some creatures. The venom of funnel-web spiders and that of the Irukandji jellyfish cause massive release of endogenous catecholamines, which may be responsible for tachydysrhythmia, stress-induced (Takotsubo) cardiomyopathy and ischaemia. The venom of the Box jellyfish

(*Chironex fleckeri*) can kill rapidly – the exact cause is still unknown but it may be related in part to dysrhythmia caused by hyperkalaemia secondary to haemolysis, or rapid onset of myocardial cytolysis caused by cell membrane pore-forming toxins.[5]

Hypertension

Severe hypertension may occur after bites from funnel-web spiders and after stings from jellyfish causing Irukandji syndrome. This is in part caused by release of endogenous catecholamines. Treatment could be with vasodilators, α-and β-adrenergic blockade. The infusion of magnesium may ameliorate the components of the Irukandji syndrome.[6]

Adverse reactions to antivenom

The treatment of some envenomations by antivenom may be complicated by reactions to antivenom. Adverse reactions to Australian snake antivenoms occur in approximately 8–13% of cases – which is relatively small compared to some overseas manufactured antivenoms, but not insignificant. It is thus prudent to prevent anaphylaxis by premedication with subcutaneous adrenaline (epinephrine) 0.25 mg for an adult, 5–10 µg kg^{-1} for a child. This recommendation stems from high-level scientific evidence: A prospective, double blind, randomised, placebo-controlled trial of 0.25 mg of subcutaneous adrenaline as premedication for snake antivenom in Sri Lanka found that subcutaneous adrenaline reduced the reaction rate from 43% to 11% ($p = 0.0002$) and reduced the severity of reactions.[7] Thus, although adrenaline has a potential to cause cerebral haemorrhage in a snake-venom induced coagulopathic state when given intravenously or intramuscularly, but not when given subcutaneously,[8] it should be administered. This controversial subject was subject to a systematic review,[9] which concluded: 'If clinicians believe local factors do not justify routine adrenaline, then they should test their belief in a randomised trial'. In contrast, more high-level evidence, a randomised, double blind, placebo-controlled trial of promethazine as a premedication for snake antivenom in Brazil[10] did not alter the reaction rate (25% placebo, 24% promethazine) and was thus not beneficial. Moreover, the effects of promethazine, hypotension and CNS obtundation might exacerbate the illness caused by envenomation. Promethazine is therefore contraindicated as a premedication.

Pressure-immobilisation bandage

Application of a pressure-immobilisation bandage is essential in the early management of selected envenomations. Elasticised bandages maintain pressure better than non-elasticised bandages. Delay in application or premature removal of a bandage may severely compromise resuscitation. Envenomations by snakes, funnel-web spiders, blue-ringed octopuses, and cone shells all warrant application of a bandage. The venoms of these creatures contain components that cause rapid onset of paralysis. The bandage serves to maintain venom at the bite or sting site[11] and hence prevents venom access to the general circulation and exerting systemic effects.

Unfortunately, application of a bandage is not always performed well or in a timely manner both before and after arrival of the victim at hospital. A critically ill victim should have a bandage applied in the Emergency Department, if one is not already in place on arrival and it should not be removed until antivenom, if indicated, has been administered.

References

1. Sutherland SK, Tibballs J. *Australian Animal Toxins.* Melbourne: Oxford University Press; 2001.
2. Patten BR, Pearn JH, DeBuse P, et al. Prolonged intensive therapy after snake bite. *Med J Aust* 1985;**142**:467–9.
3. Tibballs J, Sutherland SK. The efficacy of antivenom in prevention of cardiovascular depression and coagulopathy induced by brown snake (*Pseudonaja*) species. *Anaesth Intensive Care* 1991;**19**:530–4.
4. Sprivulis P, Jelinek GA, Marshall L. Efficacy and potency of antivenoms in neutralising the procoagulant effects of Australian snake venoms in dog and human plasma. *Anaesth Intensive Care* 1996;**24**:379–81.
5. Corkeron MA. Magnesium infusion to treat Irukandji syndrome. *Med J Aust* 2003;**178**:411.
6. Bailey PM, Bakker AJ, Seymour JE, Wilce JA. A functional comparison of the venom of three Australian jellyfish – *Chironex flekeri, Chiropsalmus* sp., and *Carybdea xaymacana* – on cytosolic Ca^{2+}, haemolysis and *Artemia* sp. Lethality. *Toxicon* 2005;**45**:233–42.
7. Premawardhena AP, de Silva CE, Fonseka MM, et al. Low dose subcutaneous adrenaline to prevent acute adverse reactions to antivenom serum in people bitten by snakes: Randomised, placebo-controlled trial. *Br Med J* 1999;**318**:1041–3.
8. Tibballs J. Premedication for snake antivenom. *Med J Aust* 1994;**160**:4–7.
9. Nuchpraryoon I, Garner P. Interventions for preventing reactions to snake antivenom. *Cochrane Database Syst Rev* 2003;**1**.
10. Fan HW, Marcopito LF, Cardoso JL, et al. Sequential randomised and double-blind trial of promethazine prophylaxis against early anaphylactic reactions to antivenom for bothrops snake bites. *Br Med J* 1999;**318**:1451–2.
11. Sutherland SK, Coulter AR, Harris RD. Rationalisation of first-aid measures for elapid snakebite. *Lancet* 1979; I:183–6.

2.5 Shock

Kevin Mackway-Jones

ESSENTIALS

1 Shock is a syndrome that arises because of acute failure of the circulation resulting in inadequate tissue perfusion. It may result from hypovolaemic, cardiogenic, distributive, obstructive or dissociative causes.

2 The normotensive child may have profound compensated shock.

3 As tachycardia may be a non-specific sign and hypotension occurs late, it is crucial to recognise the early features of shock in a child by assessing indices of peripheral perfusion and alterations of end organ function.

4 The initial management of shock should be volume expansion with a bolus of 20 mL kg^{-1} crystalloid. Further boluses are given according to clinical response. Occasionally, in the exsanguinating child, universal donor blood is indicated.

5 The ongoing management of the shocked child will depend on the specific cause and may include interventions such as: oxygenation, ventilation, glucose administration, cardioversion, broad-spectrum antibiotics, inotropic support, ductus arteriosus manipulation, adrenaline (epinephrine), atropine or surgical intervention.

Introduction

Shock, in the sense described in this chapter, is a syndrome that arises because of acute failure of the circulation. This acute circulatory failure results in inadequate tissue oxygenation and inability to remove the waste products of metabolism. Shock is a complex construct, having many causes and many expressions. The clinical diagnosis and management of shock is complicated by the fact that many organ systems become involved and because many of the 'signs of shock' actually arise because of the body's attempts at homeostasis rather than because of the underlying process.

The adequacy of circulation (and thereby the adequacy of tissue perfusion) requires proper functioning of the heart, vessels and blood. The heart must pump enough blood to meet peripheral oxygen demand; the vessels that deliver the blood to both the lungs and the other organs must be patent (that is not obstructed), be regulated appropriately at a macro level to ensure delivery of blood at an appropriate pressure to the organs requiring oxygen, and must function appropriately in the periphery so as to allow oxygen diffusion without fluid loss. The blood must have sufficient oxygen carrying capacity and must maintain the ability to allow oxygen exchange. Failure of any aspect of this complicated system will result in inadequate peripheral tissue perfusion and therefore shock.

Conventionally, shock is divided into the following five types:

- hypovolaemic
- cardiogenic
- distributive
- obstructive
- dissociative.

Hypovolaemic shock arises when there is circulatory volume inadequacy. This classically arises in trauma following haemorrhage or burns but it is also seen following gastrointestinal fluid losses such as diarrhoea and vomiting or third space losses such as in volvulus. Cardiogenic shock occurs when the heart fails to pump enough fluid. This can occur because the heart itself is failing secondary to infection, because the heart muscle has been injured (such as in cardiac contusion) or because of a problem with rhythm where the heart is beating too slow or too fast to achieve an adequate cardiac output. In distributive shock, peripheral vascular abnormalities result in failure to appropriately distribute pumped blood. This can be because of infection (as in the septic child), allergic reaction, spinal cord injury or drugs. Obstructive shock arises when there are abnormalities of flow. This can either be because particular vessels themselves are obstructed (such as in pulmonary embolus) or because of extra vascular abnormalities which obstruct the flow of blood (such as tension pneumothorax or cardiac tamponade). Finally, dissociative shock arises when the oxygen carrying capacity of the blood is too low (as in anaemia) or has been reduced, as in carbon monoxide poisoning.

Diagnosis and assessment

In all ill children the first need is to recognise the seriousness, or impending seriousness of the condition. This requires a systematic approach to assessment that involves looking at the airway, breathing, circulation, neurological status and exposing the child.

Airway

The ability to speak or cry without stridor indicates a patent airway. The presence of adequate breathing as assessed by looking at chest wall movement, listening and feeling for exhaled air also indicates an adequate airway.

Generally, shock affects the airway by reducing conscious level. In acute allergic reaction, airway obstruction (by swelling in the upper airway) and shock due to changes in vascular tone can both arise as part of the same process.

Breathing

The effort of breathing, efficacy of breathing and effects of inadequate respiration should be examined. Oxygen saturation and respiratory rate should be monitored.

Circulation

This is the crux of shock assessment since homeostatic mechanisms function particularly well in children and compensation for inadequate circulatory function is good. Consequently, in a child it can be difficult to detect circulatory failure until a late stage, hence one needs to be vigilant in detecting the earlier features of compensating shock.

Circulatory assessment should look at both circulatory status and also at the effects of inadequate circulation on other organ systems.

Heart rate and blood pressure are the classical measures of circulatory status but changes in skin perfusion (as shown by capillary refill and by skin pallor or temperature) can be more useful in detecting the early signs of compensated shock.

Heart rate

Tachycardia (relative to age norm) is a key sign of shock (see Chapter 1.1). This tachycardia is a homeostatic response to maintaining cardiac output. Bradycardia may occur pre-terminally in the child with overwhelming shock, and untreated will progress to asystole. The peripheral pulses may be weak, thready or absent.

Blood pressure

While it is true that a child with hypotension is shocked, it is not true to say that a child that is normotensive is not shocked. This is because maintenance of blood pressure is the key end point of the homeostatic response, and decompensation (and thereby hypotension) occurs late and may be precipitous. The accurate measurement of blood pressure in a distressed child can be a challenge in itself and a judgement as to whether a particular blood pressure is normal or abnormal in a particular age group in any particular circumstances is also challenging. Many widely quoted normal ranges by age are broad – furthermore many of these were derived in the resting outpatient child rather than in the seriously ill or injured child.

Capillary refill

The capillary refill time is measured by applying pressure to the nail bed or other area with visible circulation for some 5 seconds and then measuring the length of time it takes for the blanching to disappear. Central capillary refill such as over the sternum is more reliable than the peripheries, which can be influenced by vasoconstriction due to the ambient temperature effects. A capillary refill time of less than 2 seconds is normal. A capillary refill time of greater than 4 seconds is definitely abnormal. Capillary refill between 2 and 4 seconds should prompt further consideration of the presence of shock.

Changes in peripheral circulation (which are brought about by an increase in catecholamines) may also show as an increased core to periphery temperature difference (more than $2°C$ is a sign of poor perfusion) or as a noticeable centripetal temperature gradient. Reduced skin perfusion may result in a mottled, cyanosed, pale appearance and coolness on palpation. Some infants have physiological mottling (cutis marmoratum) in the first months of life due to 'immaturity' of the autonomic control of skin vessels, which commonly occurs with exposure. One must clarify with parents whether this mottled appearance is 'more than usual' in their child, as infants with cutis marmoratum will become more mottled if they have an accompanying illness causing shock.

Effects of circulatory inadequacy

Agitation and altered conscious level (that is response to voice or less) are important signs of circulatory inadequacy and the resultant cerebral hypoperfusion. In infants, the manifestations may be more subtle and increased 'irritability' or 'floppiness' or failure to recognise and make eye contact with parents may be the only obvious manifestation.

Increasing respiratory rate is an early sign of inadequate circulation. Latterly, as acidosis ensues, deep sighing respirations occur due to 'air hunger'.

Urine output will decrease with inadequate circulation. If a child has a urine collection device in place then a flow of some $2 \text{ mg kg}^{-1} \text{ hr}^{-1}$ in the child under one, and $1 \text{ mg kg}^{-1} \text{ hr}^{-1}$ in older children indicates adequate renal perfusion. If there is no urinary collection device then this can be difficult to assess, but the weight of wet nappies may be helpful.

Neurological status

As mentioned above, initially agitation and then subsequently depression in conscious level are associated with progressing shock. As in any other case of decreased conscious level a glucose stick test should be performed to exclude hypoglycaemia.

Initial management

The child with shock should be managed in the resuscitation area with monitoring of heart rate, blood pressure, respiratory rate, temperature and oxygen saturation. Urine output should also be monitored as an indicator of response to therapy. The airway and breathing should be managed as in any other case of the seriously ill child. Airway patency should be ensured and high-flow supplemental oxygen delivered. If ventilation is inadequate then this should be supported in the first instance with a bag-valve-mask device. Consideration should then be given to intubation and ventilation through an endotracheal tube if there is no improvement.

Circulation

Once airway and breathing have been managed, the next priority is to gain intravascular access. This should be obtained rapidly. An initial assessment to see whether there is a vein available to allow the placement of a short, relatively large, peripheral venous catheter is made. If it is likely that such a catheter can be placed, then up to two attempts can be allowed. If these attempts are unsuccessful (or if there is no possibility of placing a venous catheter) then intraosseous access should be gained. In most cases this is done over the medial aspect of the tibia just distal to the knee (see Chapter 23.1).

If neither peripheral venous access nor intraosseous access is possible or desirable, then a Seldinger (guide wire) approach to the femoral vein is probably the next route of choice.

As soon as intravascular access is obtained then blood should be drawn to be tested for haemoglobin, white cell count and platelets together with urea, electrolytes, acid base and lactate level. A blood culture should be taken and a glucose stick test performed to exclude hypoglycaemia.

An initial bolus of 20 mL kg^{-1} of fluid should be given. In most cases the initial fluid will be crystalloid but occasionally universal donor blood may be indicated. There is some controversy as to whether colloid should be administered in cases of sepsis, with proponents arguing that maintenance of oncotic pressure is important in this situation.

If a glucose stick test reveals significant hypoglycaemia then glucose should be administered (5 mL kg^{-1} of 10% dextrose). In such a case, hypoglycaemia may be the primary problem but it may also co-exist with other causes of serious illness and resuscitation must therefore be continued if immediate recovery does not ensue with correction of the blood glucose.

If a tachydysrhythmia is identified as a cause of established shock then cardioversion is indicated. This should be undertaken without delay. If the child is alert or otherwise responsive then sedation is usually indicated. If the tachydysrhythmia is supraventricular tachycardia then it may be quicker to give a single bolus of adenosine while preparing for cardioversion (see Chapter 5.9).

If no other cause of shock can be found then it is reasonable to give a broad-spectrum antibiotic as part of the initial treatment, as sepsis is the most common precipitant of shock in children. A third generation cephalosporin should therefore be given as soon as the blood culture has been taken, to children beyond the neonatal age, where amoxicillin and gentamicin are used as empirical sepsis cover.

Further management

Once the initial assessment and stabilisation is complete, then it is usually possible to take a more detailed history and undertake a comprehensive examination to try and establish the underlying condition.

The following specific conditions are dealt with in more detail below:

- hypovolaemia
- sepsis
- duct-dependent congenital heart disease
- heart failure
- acute severe allergic reaction (anaphylaxis)
- neurogenic shock.

Hypovolaemia

This diagnosis is usually made because of the presence of trauma, fluid loss from vomiting or diarrhoea or a surgical abdomen.

The further treatment depends on the response to initial fluid bolus. If there are still signs of shock then a second 20 mL kg^{-1} bolus should be given. At this stage a surgical opinion should be sought if an underlying surgical cause is suspected.

It would be most unusual for a child with gastroenteritis to require more than two boluses of crystalloid and, if this is the case, then an alternative diagnosis (such as an underlying intra-abdominal surgical problem or adrenal insufficiency) should be considered.

If the child shows no further signs of shock after two fluid boluses and the underlying diagnosis is gastroenteritis, then it will still be necessary to correct any underlying dehydration and this should be done in the normal manner (see Chapter 7.12).

Septic shock

Septic shock arises because of a complex combination of hypovolaemia (relative and absolute), cardiogenic shock (due to myocardial depression) and distributive shock. The underlying cause is, of course, the infection and this should be treated as a matter of urgency. As previously stated, any shocked child in whom there is not an obvious diagnosis should receive broad-spectrum antibiotics as part of the initial management. If a specific diagnosis of septicaemic shock is made and antibiotics have not been given then these broad-spectrum antibiotics (third generation cephalosporins) should be given immediately. Consideration should also be given for a specific prescription of anti-staphylococcal antibiotics such as flucloxacillin and vancomycin if there is evidence of cellulitis or a foreign body, or if the clinical picture is of toxic shock syndrome (high fever, confusion, scarlatina-form rash with desquamation and subcutaneous oedema).

In all cases a further bolus of 20 mL kg^{-1} of fluid should be given if there is not rapid restoration of normal circulation following the first bolus. A further fluid bolus should be administered (by IV push) if there is not a good response to the second. It is at this stage that urgent consideration to rapid sequence induction and elective intubation should be given. Many children will develop a degree of pulmonary oedema after the third fluid bolus and oxygenation can only be maintained by positive pressure ventilation (often with the addition of positive end-expiratory pressure).

Cardiogenic shock is also a feature of sepsis and this will require specific treatment. Dobutamine at a rate of 10 mcg kg^{-1} min^{-1} should be commenced and adjusted according to the response. Adrenaline (epinephrine) should be considered if there is no response to dobutamine.

Features of raised intracranial pressure due to meningitis can occur during treatment. This is usually presaged by a decrease in conscious level together with abnormal posturing or focal neurology. Early appropriate treatment should be commenced and this will include consideration of diuresis, intubation and ventilation and appropriate positioning of the patient. In this situation, a lumbar puncture is contraindicated.

Duct-dependent congenital heart disease

There are a number of congenital heart defects in which the presence of a patent ductus arteriosus is essential to the maintenance of pulmonary or systemic circulation. These conditions include pulmonary atresia, hypoplastic left heart syndrome, coarctation and critical aortic stenosis. The ductus usually closes functionally within 24 hours of birth – but may remain patent in the presence of cardiac abnormality.

Babies with critical pulmonary lesions will present within a few days of birth with tachypnoea and apparent breathlessness together with cyanosis, while those with systemic blood flow reduction will present with failure to feed, apparent breathlessness and collapse with poor peripheral circulation. The immediate impression, particularly in the latter group, may well be of severe sepsis and empirical antibiotics should be given until sepsis is excluded.

On examination, the babies are in heart failure (usually without a characteristic heart murmur), often with an enlarged liver and a gallop rhythm.

Immediate treatment is to maintain or increase ductus size with an infusion of alprostodil (0.05 mcg kg^{-1} min^{-1}). Immediate transfer to a cardiological centre is indicated.

It will usually be necessary to intubate and ventilate these children during transfer.

Heart failure

In babies, heart failure is usually due to structural heart disease, while in older children myocarditis and cardiomyopathy are the commonest underlying diagnoses.

Babies present with breathlessness, feeding problems and failure to thrive and restlessness. In older children more general complaints such as fatigue, anorexia, exercise intolerance and cough are common.

There are signs of increased effort of breathing with increased respiratory rate, recession and positioning. There is an increased heart rate with cool, pale peripheries together with hepatomegaly. On auscultation there may be a gallop rhythm and basal crepitations.

Oxygen should be given in all cases and broad-spectrum antibiotics administered if there is any suspicion of sepsis. As discussed earlier, alprostadil should be given if the lesion is potentially duct dependent. In other cases diuretics (furosemide 1–2 mg kg^{-1} day^{-1} in one to three divided doses initially) should be given urgently. A dobutamine infusion may be indicated to support the failing heart while urgent cardiological advice is sought.

Acute severe allergic reaction (anaphylaxis)

A diagnosis of acute allergic reaction will usually be made because of a history of a previous similar reaction, or because of the presence of typical early symptoms such as itching, facial swelling, urticarial rash, abdominal pain or wheeze.

The initial approach to shock is appropriate administration of fluid boluses. Anaphylactic circulatory shock will usually respond to adrenaline (epinephrine). The recommended dose is 10 mcg kg^{-1} given intramuscularly. Judicious use of 1:100 000 adrenaline solution given intravenously in small incremental boluses can also be effective. Over enthusiastic administration of adrenaline in the face of mild allergic reaction or, indeed, in the face of an anxiety attack has resulted in severe dysrhythmias. Caution should therefore be exercised (see Chapter 22.5).

If circulatory shock is resistant to the initial bolus of adrenaline then a further intravenous bolus of 20 mL kg^{-1} of fluid should be given. At this stage, if the diagnosis is clear, then an infusion of adrenaline at 0.1–5 mcg kg^{-1} min^{-1} should be commenced.

Neurogenic shock

A child with a spinal injury above T6 will have impaired sympathetic tone below this level once the initial catecholamine release that occurs at the time of injury has ceased to have an effect. The systemic vascular resistance will fall and the reflex tachycardia usually seen as a response to hypovolaemia will not occur. The overall outcome is generalised vasodilatation, bradycardia and loss of temperature control. Systolic blood pressure will fall below 90 mmHg but the skin will appear paradoxically warm and pink.

Initial management is with fluids and a single bolus of 20 mL kg^{-1} will usually achieve an acceptable blood pressure. Atropine (20 mcg kg^{-1}) can be given if heart rate falls below 50. Very careful handling is necessary as these children may suffer from postural hypotension if tipped or lifted suddenly. In the early stages fluid management is very important and this may require the insertion of arterial and pulmonary lines. Urinary catheterisation will be necessary as bladder control will be lost.

Concomitant absolute hypovolaemia due to trauma must always be considered, as neurogenic shock is invariably caused by trauma in children. Bleeding sources should be actively sought and managed in all children in whom hypotension persists, with early surgical consultation.

Further reading

Alderson P, Bunn F, Lefebvre C, et al. Human albumin solution for resuscitation and volume expansion in critically ill patients. *Cochrane Injuries Group Cochrane Database Syst Rev* 2003;**3**.

Alderson P, Schierhout G, Roberts I, Bunn F. Colloids versus crystalloids for fluid resuscitation in critically ill patients. *Cochrane Injuries Group Cochrane Database Syst Rev* 2003;**3**.

Bunn F, Alderson P, Hawkins V. Colloid solutions for fluid resuscitation. *Cochrane Injuries Group Cochrane Database Syst Rev* 2003;**3**.

Dark P, Woodford M, Vail A, et al. Systolic hypertension and the response to blunt trauma in infants and children. *Resuscitation* 2002;**54**(3):245–53.

Hartman ME, Angus DC, Clermont G, Kellum JA. Crystalloid solutions for fluid resuscitation in critically ill patients. *Cochrane Injuries Group Cochrane Database Syst Rev* 2003;**3**.

Kwan I, Bunn F, Roberts I. Timing and volume of fluid administration for patients with bleeding. *Cochrane Injuries Group Cochrane Database Syst Rev* 2003;**3**.

2.6 Neonatal resuscitation

Gary Williams

ESSENTIALS

1 Occasionally deliveries occur in the emergency department when labour cannot be delayed to enable transfer of the patient to a labour ward setting.

2 The emergency department should have available appropriate equipment and guidelines for the resuscitation of the newborn.

3 The unique physiological events at birth affect the resuscitative interventions in the newborn.

4 Ventilation is the main priority in the resuscitation of the newborn.

5 The heart rate is a reliable indicator of the newborn baby's degree of compromise and response to resuscitation. The easiest way to monitor newborn pulses is by palpation of the umbilicus.

6 Chest compressions are indicated if: (1) absent pulse; or (2) heart rate $<60\,\mathrm{min}^{-1}$ despite adequate assisted ventilations for 30 seconds.

7 Compressions and ventilations should be cycled at a ratio of 3 compressions to 1 ventilation to achieve approximately 120 events per minute.

8 The preferred site of the vascular access during neonatal resuscitation is the umbilical vein.

9 Drugs are rarely required in the resuscitation of the newly born.

10 Volume expansion should be with crystalloid $10\,\mathrm{mL\,kg}^{-1}$ boluses by slow push.

Introduction

Epidemiology

Between 5 and 10% of newborns require some assistance to begin breathing at birth and, in developed countries, approximately 1% need intensive resuscitative measures to restore cardiorespiratory function. It has been estimated that birth asphyxia significantly contributes to approximately 20% of the five million neonatal deaths that occur worldwide each year; outcome might therefore be improved for more than one million newborns per year through effective resuscitation at birth.

Neonatal resuscitation is unique in that it is required at a time when the newborn is undergoing a predetermined process of transition from a liquid filled intrauterine environment to spontaneous breathing of room air. There is an accompanying sequence of dramatic alterations in physiology, each of which may be altered and require correction.

There are two important caveats in this process. First, the achievement of lung expansion with an appropriate oxygen-containing gas leading to establishment of a functional residual capacity and adequate spontaneous ventilation is of primary importance. Second, the significance of a vital sign abnormality depends greatly on the time since birth and the time during which effective resuscitation measures have been administered. For instance, bradycardia immediately after birth prior to any resuscitative manoeuvres likely indicates an intrapartum stress. The same heart rate after 1 to 2 minutes of adequate ventilation suggests a different range of aetiologies and requires a different resuscitative response.

The majority of circumstances where newborn resuscitation is needed can be predicted, allowing opportunity for preparation of appropriate equipment and personnel. Factors placing the newborn at high risk for neonatal resuscitation include those listed in Table 2.6.1, due to maternal, fetal and intrapartum circumstances.

Aetiology and pathophysiology

The sequence of physiological changes in the newborn around birth includes:

- Cessation of alveolar fluid production and clearance of this fluid from the gas-exchanging part of the airway.

Table 2.6.1 Risk factors for need for neonatal resuscitation

Maternal	Fetal	Intrapartum
Premature or prolonged rupture of membranes	Multiple gestation	Fetal distress
Antepartum haemorrhage	Preterm (<35 weeks) or post-term	Abnormal presentation
Hypertension	(>42 weeks) gestation	Prolonged or precipitate labour
Diabetes mellitus	IUGR	Thick staining of amniotic fluid
Substance abuse	Polyhydramnios	Instrumental delivery or emergency caesarean section
Maternal infection or chronic illness	Congenital abnormalities	
Absence of antenatal care		

IUGR, intrauterine growth retardation.

- Spontaneous respirations and establishment of functional residual capacity (FRC).
- Fall in pulmonary vascular resistance (PVR) (lung expansion, oxygen).
- Rise in systemic vascular resistance (SVR) (umbilical artery constriction).
- Reversal of flow from left to right across foramen ovale and ductus arteriosus.
- Closure of the foramen ovale and ductus arteriosus.

This normal sequence may be interrupted at any point by:

- Inadequate clearance of endogenous lung liquid (precipitate, emergency or operative delivery) or excessive abnormal airway material (blood, mucus, meconium).
- Inadequate respiratory effort (maternal analgesics, central nervous system injury, sepsis) or excursion (congenital thoracic anomalies).
- Pulmonary disease preventing achievement and maintenance of adequate FRC (parenchymal disease, prematurity, space-occupying lesion) with secondary failure to lower PVR normally and possible intrapulmonary shunting.
- Compromised myocardial function (structural or functional cardiac abnormalities, hypoxia secondary to pulmonary dysfunction).

Interventions should occur in a defined sequence recognising the primary and crucial role of adequate ventilation and be guided by frequent reassessment of other vital signs.

Preparation

❶ Summon assistance: if it is anticipated that the infant is at high risk of requiring advanced life support resuscitative intervention, more than one experienced person should be mobilised.

❷ Communicate with colleagues to seek available antenatal and intrapartum data.

❸ In the case of extreme prematurity ($\leq$24 weeks' gestation) or known congenital anomalies, if time allows, the most senior care provider should seek to discuss with the family their beliefs and desires regarding the extent of resuscitation.[1]

❹ Prepare the environment: this includes a warm, draught-free area with adequate light, radiant heater, prewarmed blankets and a clock.

❺ Prepare required equipment (Table 2.6.2).

Assessment at birth

At birth the infant should be collected in a warm towel, dried and the umbilical cord clamped. Gentle stimulation may be provided (rubbing the back, flicking soles of feet if required) and an assessment of initial cry, respiratory effort, heart rate, colour and tone should be made virtually simultaneously (Table 2.6.3).

Ventilation

The initial assessment is an evaluation of the presence and quality of respirations.

- If respirations are adequate, the heart rate is evaluated.
- If respirations are shallow or slow, a brief period of stimulation may be provided.
- If the infant has not established adequate breathing by 30 seconds, face mask rescue breaths should be administered and if this is not successful with breathing established by 2 minutes, endotracheal intubation should be performed.
- There should be no delay in commencing rescue breaths if the infant is born with, or develops evidence of, asphyxia with signs of flaccidity, pallor and/or bradycardia (heart rate less than 60 min^{-1}).

Artificial ventilation

Various bag and mask systems are available for neonatal resuscitation. T-piece mechanical devices designed to regulate pressure, self-inflating bag or flow-inflating bag are all recognised as acceptable devices for ventilating newborn infants either via a face mask or endotracheal tube. Target inflation pressures, continuous positive airway pressure (CPAP) and long inspiratory times are achieved more consistently using T-piece devices than when using bags but the ability to achieve an increased inspiratory pressure when required in response to altered compliance (even for a few breaths) is greatest with the self-inflating bag. It is suggested in fact that the invariable success of rescue breathing at birth is because the FRC is established by an induced inspiratory effort via Head's paradoxical reflex (inspiratory effort induced by any lung inflation). The corollary is that face mask rescue breathing is unlikely to

Table 2.6.2 Equipment and drugs recommended for newborn resuscitation	
Equipment	**Drugs**
Stethoscope	Adrenaline (epinephrine) 1 in 1:10000 solution.
Suction catheters (6–12 French) and suction	Naloxone hydrochloride 1.0 or 0.4 mg mL^{-1}
8 French feeding tube and 20 mL syringe for gastric decompression	Dextrose 5% or 10%
Face masks	NaHCO$_3$ 4.2% solution
Oropharyngeal (Guedel's) airways	Volume expander (0.9% saline or 4% HSA)
Resuscitation system for PPV	
Laryngoscope with straight blade	
ET tubes 2.5 to 4 mm internal diameter	
ET stylets	
Tape for ETT and IV fixation	
Cannulae, syringes and UV catheterisation equipment	

HSA, human serum albumin; PPV, positive pressure ventilation.

Table 2.6.3 Apgar score			
Score	*0*	*1*	*2*
Heart rate	Absent	Less than 100	Greater than 100
Respiratory effort	Absent	Irregular	Crying
Muscle tone	Limp	Some flexion	Active motion
Reflex irritability	Absent	Grimace	Grimace and cough
Colour	Blue, pale	Acrocyanosis	Pink all over

be effective in the severely asphyxiated infant.

Regardless of these issues, it is generally accepted that higher inflation pressures (>30 cmH$_2$O) and longer inflation times (>1.5 seconds) may be required for the first several (≈5) breaths. Initial peak inflating pressures required are variable and unpredictable. In general, the minimum pressure required to achieve an increase in the heart rate should be used. Visible chest wall movement and an increase in the heart rate are the best indicators of adequate ventilation. Ventilations should be administered at a rate of 40–60 min^{-1} and after 30 seconds of effective ventilation, the heart rate should be evaluated.

Heart rate

Assessment of the heart rate can be done by palpating the umbilical stump, brachial or femoral pulse or auscultation of the apical heart sounds.

- The heart rate is a reliable indicator of the degree of compromise and response to resuscitation. It should be assessed at least every 30 seconds in the first 2 minutes if necessary, until the baby's required level of support is established.
- If the heart rate is less than 60 min^{-1} despite adequate assisted ventilation, compressions are required. When the heart rate is greater than 100 min^{-1}, only ventilation is continued. If the heart rate is between these two points, the level of intervention should be increased or decreased depending on the serial change in the heart rate.
- If the heart rate is not rising after 30 seconds of effective ventilation combined with chest compressions, then adrenaline (epinephrine) should be administered.

- Once a slow heart rate has increased above 60 min^{-1} and is rising, cardiac compressions may be discontinued.

Compression technique

If required, compressions should be instituted using the two-hand-encircling technique (preferred if greater than one rescuer) or two-finger technique (if only one rescuer or if access to the umbilicus is required). The lower third of the sternum (just below an imaginary intermammary line) should be depressed one third of the depth of the chest. These should be coordinated with ventilations (to avoid simultaneous delivery) in a ratio of 3:1 with about 90 compressions and 30 breaths each minute. The xiphoid portion of the sternum should not be compressed because such compression may damage the neonate's liver.

Colour

Once the heart rate has been evaluated, the infant's colour should be assessed by examining the trunk and mucosae.

- Peripheral cyanosis (acrocyanosis) is common in the first few minutes after birth and is not pathological.
- Central cyanosis reflects inadequate oxygenation and may be pulmonary or cardiac in origin. If present despite adequate ventilation and a heart rate greater than 100 beats per minute, supplementary oxygen should be administered until the cause of the cyanosis is known.[2]
- Using oximetry to guide oxygen administration may be valuable in these minutes to titrate oxygen and limit hyperoxia, especially in the premature. Remember that a SaO$_2$ of 70% is at the

lower end of the normal range at 5 minutes of age in a term baby.
- Pallor is suggestive of a decreased cardiac output and may be due to myocardial dysfunction, severe anaemia, hypovolaemia, hypothermia or acidosis.

Muscle tone and reflex irritability

These physical signs are valuable composite reflections of the adequacy of cerebral perfusion and oxygenation. As such, they constitute two of the five components of the Apgar score (see Table 2.6.3) used to assess a newborn's condition after birth.

Medications

Medications are rarely required during neonatal resuscitation. One study suggested medications were required in only 0.12% of all births, for severe fetal acidosis or ventilatory problems. This reaffirms the primary and critical importance of achieving optimal ventilation before resorting to medications in neonatal resuscitation.

Vascular access

Adrenaline (epinephrine) may be administered by intravenous (IV), intraosseous (IO) or endotracheal (ET) routes. If there is respiratory depression once heart rate and colour have been restored by adequate rescue ventilation, naloxone may be given via the intravenous (IV) or intramuscular (IM) route. The other drugs and volume expansion, detailed below, require emergency vascular access. Once vascular access is achieved, if the child remains in arrest, an adrenaline dose should be immediately administered via the IV route.

The preferred site of the vascular access during neonatal resuscitation is the umbilical vein, the larger thin walled single vessel (in comparison to the paired thicker walled arteries), which appears when the umbilical cord is trimmed 1 cm above the skin. A 3.5 or 5 French catheter flushed with saline (to remove any air in the tubing) should be inserted only until a good blood return is achieved (usually to a depth of 1 to 4 cm below the skin). Peripheral veins on extremities or scalp may be attempted or alternatively an intraosseous cannula may be placed on the medial aspect of the tibia just below the tibial tuberosity, if umbilical or other direct venous access is not readily obtainable.

Adrenaline (epinephrine)

Adrenaline is administered with the aim of producing α-adrenergic mediated vasoconstriction, an increase in coronary perfusion pressure and myocardial blood flow. Adrenaline is indicated if the heart rate remains less than 60 beats per minute after a minimum of 30 seconds of adequate ventilation and 30 seconds of combined ventilation and chest compressions. The recommended IV dose is 0.1–0.3 mL kg^{-1} of a 1:10000 solution (10–30 mcg kg^{-1}) repeated every 3 to 5 minutes as indicated. ET delivery, though of unproven efficacy, can be considered and requires a higher dose (up to 100 mcg kg^{-1}); it should be followed by 1 mL of normal saline and several good inflations to achieve optimal delivery to the pulmonary vascular bed. Most infant animal experimental dosing data supporting adrenaline's efficacy have been obtained in VF models and as such their value may not be directly applicable to the apparent preterminal bradyarrhythmia in an asphyxiated newborn with markedly elevated PCO_2.

Through the early 1990s some experimental and human data showed that higher intravenous doses of adrenaline (100 mcg kg^{-1}) were capable of achieving higher plasma adrenaline levels as well as greater myocardial and cerebral blood flow. However, several subsequent adult and paediatric studies showed no ultimate clinical benefit in survival or neurological outcome, with a significant risk of adverse effects from the higher dose (myocardial dysfunction or necrosis, hyperadrenergic states, reduced cerebral cortical blood flow). Specifically, there is an increase in potential risk of intraventricular haemorrhages (IVH) in preterm infants. For these reasons, the currently recommended initial IV dose remains 10 mcg kg^{-1} in neonates.

The ET route is likely to be the most accessible route for initial doses of adrenaline. Again, there is a paucity of both experimental and human data regarding dosage and efficacy of ET adrenaline in neonates. There are data to suggest a slower onset with a more prolonged and variable effect at higher dosages. For these reasons the dose recommended is 30–100 µg kg^{-1} every 3–5 minutes during arrest.

Bicarbonate

Although correcting acidosis during cardiac arrest to improve both myocardial function and adrenaline's effectiveness makes theoretic sense, there are few supportive experimental data. Most adult studies have found either no difference or that bicarbonate had deleterious effects on myocardial performance. There are no neonatal animal or human studies specifically examining this question. Bicarbonate administration has multiple possible adverse effects (metabolic alkalosis compromising peripheral tissue oxygen delivery, paradoxical intracellular hypercarbic acidosis). Pertinent to neonates are studies demonstrating large increases in plasma osmolality and reductions in cerebral blood flow, both of which may increase the risk of IVH in newborns. Therefore, bicarbonate administration is only recommended during prolonged arrests unresponsive to other therapy after establishment of adequate ventilation and perfusion. The dose is 1–2 mEq kg^{-1} of 4.2% solution by slow IV push over at least 2 minutes.

Naloxone

Naloxone is a narcotic antagonist, recommended for the neonate with respiratory depression secondary to narcotics given to the mother within 4 hours of delivery. Prompt institution of adequate ventilation is the first priority in such a situation and naloxone is not recommended for newborns whose mothers are suspected narcotic abusers as abrupt withdrawal may be precipitated. Following IV administration, onset of action occurs in 1–2 minutes and is variable in duration. The recommended IV dose is 0.1 mg kg^{-1}. Since the duration of action of narcotics may exceed that of naloxone, continued surveillance and repeat administration are often required. Naloxone may be administered IM, with some adult data suggesting slower onset and more prolonged duration of action via this route. There are no studies examining the ET route of administration in the neonate.

Dextrose

Hypoglycaemia is a potential problem for all stressed and asphyxiated babies and should be treated by using a slow bolus of 5 mL kg^{-1} of 10% dextrose IV, avoiding high blood sugar levels which have been shown to worsen CNS injury, at least in adults.

Volume expansion

If hypovolaemia is present because of known or suspected blood loss or loss of vascular tone following asphyxia, volume expansion may be appropriate. Isotonic non-dextrose containing crystalloid (normal saline or Ringer's lactate) 10 mL kg^{-1} intravenously over 5–10 minutes is recommended. Group O negative packed red cells may be indicated for replacement of large volume blood loss. Albumin-containing solutions are used less frequently because of limited availability, risk of infectious disease and an observed association with increased mortality. A recent randomised controlled comparison of albumin versus normal saline for hypotension in premature newborns showed that those who received albumin required significantly more volume expander to maintain normal blood pressure and had a higher mean percentage weight gain in the first 48 hours after birth.[3]

Specific resuscitation situations

Premature neonate

Preterm newborns have an increased likelihood of respiratory depression requiring assisted ventilation at birth. This occurs because of diminished lung compliance, weak respiratory muscles and immature respiratory drive and may make it difficult to establish and maintain an adequate FRC. For these reasons, infants born at or before 32 weeks gestation should receive face mask resuscitation by 30 seconds and be intubated at 60 seconds after birth if the onset of adequate spontaneous respirations is delayed. A recent study has shown that CPAP applied promptly to premature babies who breathe at birth may be effective in reducing need for ventilation. Also, because preterm infants often have low body fat and a high body surface area to mass ratio, they are more difficult to keep warm and therefore at increased risk of cold stress. For this reason babies <1500 g should be covered in food-grade heat-resistant plastic wrapping or placed in a polyethylene bag with the head excluded and a hat placed on the head. Rapid boluses of volume expander and use of hyperosmolar solutions may produce large fluctuations in blood pressure or osmolarity and therefore are not recommended.[3]

Meconium aspiration

Approximately one in 20 infants born through meconium-stained amniotic fluid (MSAF) develop meconium aspiration syndrome (MAS) due to aspiration into the distal airways either in utero or with the initial breaths following birth. However, of these, 25–50% require mechanical ventilation and 5% die. Although a long established practice, it is no longer recommended that infants delivered through MSAF undergo intrapartum suctioning of the oro- and nasopharynx once the head is delivered, prior to delivery of chest or shoulders. If the baby born through MSAF is not vigorous after delivery (depressed respirations, muscle tone or heart rate less than 100 min^{-1}) direct intratracheal suctioning (using continuous suction directly applied to the tracheal tube as it is withdrawn) should be performed. If meconium is recovered, the procedure should be repeated (if the heart rate is greater than 60 min^{-1}) before proceeding with resuscitation.

Congenital heart disease

Central cyanosis at birth apparently unresponsive to 100% oxygen particularly in a vigorous baby with adequate spontaneous respiratory effort and minimal respiratory distress may indicate duct-dependent cyanotic congenital heart disease (primarily right heart obstructive lesions, transposition of the great vessels and anomalous pulmonary venous return with complete atrial admixture). The major differential diagnoses are primary pulmonary hypertension or major pulmonary structural abnormalities (e.g. congenital diaphragmatic hernia). In such a circumstance ventilatory support requirement should be dictated by degree of respiratory distress with a target $PaCO_2$ of 35–40 mmHg.

Detailed cardiac auscultation should be attempted though there may be no abnormal murmurs audible; simultaneous pre- and postductal oximetry measurements should be performed. If a cyanotic cardiac abnormality is strongly suspected, documentation of preductal PaO_2 after breathing 100% oxygen for several minutes (hyperoxia test) will give the best indication of the presence and size of a significant intracardiac right to left shunt (see Chapter 5.1). An urgent bedside echocardiogram, if available, is indicated to delineate the cardiac anatomy. Where this is not available, one should consult with the local tertiary neonatal unit. If a diagnosis of a duct-dependent cyanotic cardiac lesion is confirmed on echocardiogram, IV alprostadil (PGE$_1$) 25–50 ng kg^{-1} min^{-1} restores and maintains ductal patency until definitive decisions regarding surgical correction can be made. The main side effects of this medication are flushing, fever and possibly apnoea if respiratory support is not already in place.

Alternatively, babies with duct-dependent systemic circulation usually due to some structural problem with left ventricular outflow (e.g. critical aortic stenosis, severe coarctation, hypoplastic left heart syndrome) may present in the first few days of life with heart failure and poor peripheral perfusion triggered by ductal closure. The most reliable physical signs of heart failure are tachycardia, tachypnoea and hepatomegaly. If shock is present (poor pulse volume, pallor, altered conscious state) respiratory support and fluid volume expansion may be required to restore the circulation. Subsequently, alprostadil or inotrope infusion and continuing judicious fluid administration may be required. The most important steps in restoring systemic circulation in this situation are artificial ventilation to normocapnia, together with re-establishing and maintaining ductal patency (see Chapter 5.5).

Post-resuscitation stabilisation

Post-resuscitation stabilisation should be directed towards preventing any ongoing or repeated primary insults (primarily to the brain) as well as limiting any secondary injury and organising a stable transfer to an appropriate neonatal unit.

- Artificial ventilation should be continued if required to maintain normocapnia (pCO$_2$ 35–40 mmHg).
- Oxygenation should be optimised (aiming for pO$_2$ 60–90 mmHg, although this target may be set higher in the face of documented pulmonary hypertension).
- ET tube migration or obstruction should be vigorously avoided.
- With regard to control of body temperature the primary goal is to achieve normothermia and avoid iatrogenic hyperthermia in infants who require resuscitation (see hypothermia in the Controversies section below).
- Blood pressure should be monitored meticulously and hypotension treated promptly with fluid resuscitation or inotropes as required.
- Close monitoring of body weight, fluid balance, electrolytes, calcium and magnesium is indicated.
- Evidence of hypoxic insult to major organs other than the brain should be sought (urinalysis, serum creatinine, liver function tests, serum troponin level, coagulation parameters).
- Both hyper- and hypoglycaemia may aggravate injury following hypoxic ischaemic insult and therefore normoglycaemia should be targeted.
- There is no evidence in neonatal post-resuscitation cerebral care for hypertonic or osmotic agents to treat or minimise cerebral oedema. The same applies to glucocorticoids and prophylactic anticonvulsant treatment. While the early use of barbiturates in the reduction of seizures, neuronal metabolic demands and excitatory amino acid production is theoretically sound, there are no solid data on which to support their use in this way following a perinatal insult.
- Liaison with and transfer to a neonatal intensive care unit (NICU) should be organised as soon as possible with clear documentation of the resuscitation interventions required and responses achieved.
- The parents should be kept well informed of the infant's condition and efforts made for them to have contact with the baby.

Prognosis

Predicting outcome at an early stage may be difficult but the most reliable early predictors of adverse outcome are abnormalities in the clinical examination (i.e. degree of encephalopathy) and electroencephalographic assessment. A sustained low-voltage EEG or discontinuous activity on EEG within 6 hours of birth are strongly predictive of death or significant adverse neurologic sequelae.

Controversies

❶ *Air or O$_2$ for newborn resuscitation.* Traditionally, 100% oxygen has been used for neonatal resuscitation, but recent animal studies and human trials have confirmed that ventilation with room air is equally successful in neonatal resuscitation. Use of air may have advantages (reduced oxidative stress, less delay in onset of spontaneous respirations). There may still be situations in which 100% oxygen is advantageous (pulmonary hypertension, diffusion abnormalities, alterations in cerebral blood flow). At present best evidence suggests that air should be used initially with supplementary oxygen if the infant's condition does not improve after effective ventilation. Data suggest that oxygen use in neonatal resuscitation should be individualised with the dose tailored to clinical response and monitored by oximetry.[2]

❷ *Hypothermia.* Traditionally, post-resuscitation care has involved heat-loss prevention or even external warming on the basis that this facilitates recovery from acidosis. However, recent animal studies have clearly shown that early modest cerebral hypothermia (32–34°C) can modulate hypoxic ischaemic injury.

Studies in human neonates are accumulating regarding the safety of induced hypothermia. At present cerebral hypothermia can not be routinely recommended. However, hyperthermia should definitely be avoided as there is strong evidence that this is deleterious.[4]

❸ *Ethics of resuscitation.* The decision to withdraw or withhold resuscitation from extremely premature newborns or those with severe congenital abnormalities requires clear communication with the family and accurate clinical data. Overall there is agreement that overly aggressive treatment is to be discouraged.[1]

❹ Recent studies demonstrate extremely poor survival rates for infants less than 23 weeks gestation (<1%) with a better but still poor rate for infants admitted to the NICU (5%). Mortality is less at 23, 24 and 25 completed weeks (11%, 26% and 44% survival in one large recent study). However, severe disability in childhood is present in 20 to 30% of survivors at these gestations and some disability can be expected in 50%.[5] Prognosis is probably better predicted by gestational age (if accurately known) rather than weight, though both factors have a role and gender is also important (lower mortality/morbidity in females).

❺ Non-initiation of resuscitation in the delivery room is appropriate for infants with confirmed gestation less than 23 weeks or birth weight less than 400 g,

anencephaly or confirmed trisomy 13 or 18. Options include a trial of resuscitation, non-initiation or discontinuation after further assessment. Initiation of resuscitation does not mandate continued support.

❻ International guidelines state that discontinuation of resuscitative efforts may be appropriate if resuscitation of an infant with cardiorespiratory arrest does not result in spontaneous circulation in 10 minutes.

References

1. Boyle RJ, Mcintosh N. Ethical considerations in neonatal resuscitation: clinical and research issues. *Semin Neonatol* 2001;**6**:261–9.
2. Richmond S, Goldsmith JP. Air or 100% oxygen in neonatal resuscitation? *Clin Perinatol* 2006;**33**:11–28.
3. So KW, Fok TF, Ng PC, et al. Randomised controlled trial of colloid or crystalloid in hypotensive preterm infants. *Arch Dis Child* 1997;**76**:F43–6.
4. Hoehn T, Hansmann G, Buhrer C, et al. Therapeutic hypothermia in neonates. Review of current clinical data, ILCOR recommendations and suggestions for implementation in neonatal intensive care units. *Resuscitation* 2008;**78**:7–12.
5. Wood NS, Marlow N, Costeloe K, et al. Neurologic and developmental disability after extremely preterm birth. *N Engl J Med* 2000;**343**(6):378–84.

Further reading

Escobedo M. Moving from experience to evidence: changes in US Neonatal Resuscitation Programme based on International Committee on Resuscitation Review. *J Perinatol* 2008;**28**:S35–40.
International Liaison Committee on Resuscitation. The International Liason Committee on Resuscitation (ILCOR) consensus on science with treatment recommendations for pediatric and neonatal patients: neonatal resuscitation. *Pediatrics* 2006;**117**(5): e978–88.
Richmond S. ILCOR and Neonatal Resuscitation 2005. *Arch Dis Child Fetal Neonatal Ed* 2007;**92**:F163–5.
Wu TJ, Carlo WA. Neonatal resuscitation guidelines 2000: framework for practice. *J Matern Fetal Neonatal Med* 2002;**11**:4–10.

TRAUMA IN CHILDREN

SECTION 3

Section editor *Ian Everitt*

3.1 Introduction to paediatric trauma

Danny Cass

ESSENTIALS

1 Trauma is the prime cause of death and serious injury throughout childhood, accounting for 60% of deaths.

2 Prevention strategies have resulted in most of the improvement in mortality during childhood.

3 The advent of trauma teams has led to great improvement in paediatric injury care.

4 Delayed management of airway obstruction and inadequate fluid management are the two most common contributors to preventable paediatric deaths in trauma.

5 The initial assessment of the seriously injured child should follow a structured approach so that life-threatening problems are rapidly identified and managed in rapid sequence.

6 It is important to provide early psychological support to other family members who arrive with the child with major injuries.

7 The team leader needs to co-ordinate the resuscitation of the child with multi-system trauma, so that patient care is at all times expeditious and tailored to the specific and prioritised needs of the child.

Prevalence

Overall, trauma is the number three cause of mortality (6%) and serious morbidity throughout life. However, trauma is the number one cause of death and disability between the ages of 1 and 44. Therefore it is the prime cause of death and serious injury throughout childhood – rendering it the most important health issue in children and adolescents. In most Western societies road trauma contributes about half (50%) of all serious injuries and deaths, with drowning incidents contributing up to 25%. The third major cause is burns and the remainder includes a range of miscellaneous causes. In most series, child abuse contributes less than 10% of all child deaths.

This chapter concentrates on those aspects of trauma management that are different in children. Overall, paediatric surgeons and paediatricians have taken a holistic view of trauma and have been heavily involved in aspects of prevention, immediate treatment and rehabilitation.

Prevention

Over the last decades, Australia has done well in reducing the death rate from approximately 11.5 deaths per hundred thousand to about 8.5 (World Health Organization).[1] However, while the death rate has been almost halved, it is still double that of some of the best OECD countries. Most developed countries have significantly reduced injury death rates. Unfortunately this is not the case in developing countries. While we have achieved much through prevention strategies, there is still more to be done.

Prevention has involved the work of legislators (seat belts, baby capsules, cycle helmets) through to educators and implementation groups such as 'Kidsafe'. Generally the community has been supportive of the minor inconveniences that accompany improvements in child safety.

Future progress will depend on campaigns refreshing the messages, as every few years there is a new generation of young parents and it cannot be assumed that a good campaign 3 to 5 years previously will suffice. There needs to be ongoing activity. We also need to be aware that we are promoting healthy, safe activities. This does not equate to safety above all other considerations. Our children should not be sitting in front of televisions and computer games and never going outside because that is perceived as being dangerous. Rather, through appropriate research we should further identify problem areas that are key factors in the causation of road trauma, drowning, house fires, serious falls and sporting injuries. Our children should be safely riding their cycles rather than believing that cycling is unsafe. This will require much more work by all levels of community as individuals, councils and governments. We do need to take account of children's needs for activity in homes, playgrounds, skateboard areas, walkways and cycle paths in order to plan prevention strategies.

Succinct treatment (salvage)

The advent of trauma teams and trauma systems in hospitals that receive paediatric patients has led to great improvements in paediatric injury care. It is estimated that there may have been a 20% decrease in mortality as a result of these systems. However, it is prevention that has resulted in most of the improvement in mortality.

Hospitals now have trauma teams ready to receive the child. This may occur by forward notification by the emergency management services. Trauma team activation should occur on notification when a child is at high risk of life-threatening injury according to prediction by pre-determined clinical and mechanism parameters (Table 3.1.1).

The trauma team should include a team leader, airway doctor, procedure doctor, and nursing staff from within the emergency department. Activation may involve alerting appropriate colleagues from radiology, anaesthetics, intensive care and surgical specialties according to local resources and protocols, in order to expedite emergent care. The activation process needs to be adapted to the varying local resources of the individual department, which vary between institutions.

Regular trauma meetings to review cases or videotape evaluation of resuscitation can provide education, with lessons learnt on 'how to do things better'. As major paediatric trauma is relatively uncommon, mock paediatric resuscitation scenarios can provide the emergency department staff with an opportunity to improve preparedness. There is now a good body of international literature available to keep the trauma team up to date with the optimal care of paediatric trauma patients. The use of a trauma proforma sheet may be useful for the documentation of the assessment and resuscitation of children with major injuries (see Table 3.1.1).

Clinicians often worry about managing children with major trauma and wonder how much they should treat them as adults and how much they should take note of their differences. In adults it is well established that the *A, B, C, D, E primary survey* approach is the correct paradigm. In managing paediatric trauma clinicians sometimes get confused. They have a vague memory that 'children are different'. They are not sure therefore whether to clearly follow the A, B, C, D, E or a different approach.

The best way to remember the acute management of trauma in children is to remember the a, b, c, d, e as lower case. That is, the sequence is exactly the same as in adults but there are additional nuances in children to optimise their care. However, more children suffer or die in the acute management of trauma by clinicians panicking and not following the A, B, C, D, E approach rather than doctors not being completely familiar with these nuances (see primary survey below). Delayed management of airway obstruction or inadequate fluid management are the two most common contributors to preventable paediatric deaths in trauma. Chapters 2.2 and 2.3 provide a detailed discussion of basic life support and advanced life support (ALS) techniques in children applicable in trauma.

The worst response is to panic and freeze. In this situation a child may be left un-intubated, whereas in an adult patient intubation would be performed as a reflex decision. A child with a Glasgow Coma Scale (GCS) of less than 8 should not be left with face mask oxygen; in an adult there would be rapid intubation. Similarly, intravenous lines can be difficult to insert in the shocked paediatric patient, and children may receive delayed fluid resuscitation if intraosseous access is not considered as an alternative where indicated. The supportive management of the child's family is a further important consideration in the emergency setting.

Primary survey

The initial assessment of the seriously injured child should follow a structured approach so that life-threatening problems are rapidly identified and managed in the appropriate rapid sequence. This approach is based on the prioritised principles as outlined in the teaching dictums of courses such as the Advanced Paediatric Life Support (APLS) and Advanced Trauma Life Support (ATLS) groups, which are invaluable for practitioners who deal with paediatric trauma.

The approach includes initially the **primary survey** with securing of (A) airway, (B) breathing and (C) circulation, and immediate management of threats to life. The stabilisation of the cervical spine occurs concurrently with airway management. Following this rapid initial stabilisation, a brief neurological assessment of the child should occur (D) with complete exposure for otherwise occult signs of injury and a prompt to consider environmental issues such as hypothermia (E).

In the team approach, the management should 'occur horizontally', with simultaneous attention to these priorities by designated members of the team, overseen by the team leader. The role of the primary survey is therefore to detect and treat abnormal physiology immediately in order to prevent potential secondary insults due to

---

Table 3.1.1 Major trauma predictors at high risk of life-threatening injury

Clinical parameters	Mechanism
Glasgow Coma Score <13 Systolic BP <90 Respiratory rate <10 or >30	High impact trauma Fall from significant height Crash speed >60 kph Ejection of child from MVA
Injury	Rollover MVA Death of same-car occupant
Penetrating injury to chest, abdomen, head, neck and groin Significant injury to two or more body areas Severe injury to head, neck or trunk Two or more proximal long bone fractures Burns of >15% or to face or airway	Pedestrian/cyclist struck at >30 kph

MVA, motor vehicle accident.
Source: Adapted from Cameron P. 2004. Textbook of Adult Emergency Medicine, 2nd edn.

hypoxia or hypovolaemia. A secondary survey follows with a head to toe, front and back examination of the child.

Paediatric differences

A. Airway and cervical spine control

In the setting of trauma, 'A' refers to securing of the child's airway with concurrent attention to the possibility of an unstable cervical injury. The cervical spine should be immobilised using an appropriate-sized hard collar, sandbags, tape and a spinal board where appropriate. It may be helpful in an infant to place a small towel under the space in the shoulder region caused by 'the elevation off the bed' by the prominent occiput at this age. As discussed in the ALS section in Chapter 2.3, the characteristics of the paediatric airway make it more vulnerable to obstruction. This can be exacerbated by the necessary supine positioning of the child on the resuscitation trolley. Due to comparatively higher oxygen demands and less reserve, a child manifests hypoxic decompensation earlier than adults. This reinforces the increased importance of airway management in achieving adequate ventilation. The initial airway-opening manoeuvre in trauma patients should be by the jaw thrust technique to maintain cervical spine immobilisation. Suctioning of any oropharyngeal soiling from blood, vomit, teeth or other foreign bodies may be necessary. Adjuncts such as the placement of an oropharyngeal airway may be required. In children, these should be placed into the oral cavity directly, using gentle depression of the tongue with a spatula to allow for atraumatic positioning. Nasopharyngeal airways are not recommended due to the potential presence of cribriform plate fractures, and trauma to the turbinates may cause bleeding that may further complicate airway patency.

The indications for intubation in children with major trauma are no different than those in adults. Thus, definitive airway intervention should occur in the child who is apnoeic (usually coma related), has persistent airway obstruction despite the above manoeuvres, is requiring bag–mask ventilation to achieve oxygenation, has respiratory insufficiency from major chest injury, has significant ongoing bleeding due to facial trauma compromising the airway or has high risk of subsequent compromise such as from an airway burn.

The technique of intubation should be rapid sequence with cricoid pressure. The control of the cervical spine during intubation should occur by manual immobilisation by a dedicated assistant. The patient should have continuous monitoring, pre-oxygenation and difficult airway adjuncts available, if required. The choice and dosage of the sedation agent (thiopentone, midazolam, propofol, or fentanyl, for example) may be individualised according to factors such as the level of coma, cardiovascular status of the child and the presence of other injuries. A rapidly and short acting muscle relaxant such as suxamethonium usually provides the most optimal intubation conditions, despite the potential for transient increase in intracranial and intraocular pressures with fasciculation. Children less than 2 years of age are prone to significant bradycardia on laryngoscopy, which may be blunted by the administration of atropine, prior to intubation. Confirmation of correct ETT placement should occur according to the methods described in Chapter 2.3. One needs to be prepared for the possibility of the difficult airway or failed intubation and have a planned algorithm to deal with this possibility. It is not the failed intubation that causes the problem, but the lack of a plan of action to alternatively oxygenate the patient in this situation, whilst summoning assistance.

B. Breathing and high-flow oxygen

All children with severe trauma should receive high-flow oxygen ($10–15 \text{ L min}^{-1}$) by a reservoir face mask, independent of the need determined by saturation monitoring. Inadequate spontaneous ventilation is supported by bag and mask assistance. If this need is ongoing, intubation is required. A rapid screen for life threats, such as a tension pneumothorax, should occur. This may require immediate decompression by needle aspiration for the child in extremis and a subsequent formal chest drain, as described in the section on chest trauma (see chapter 3.3). The possibility of developing tension due to a pneumothorax should be borne in mind as one of the potential precipitants of rapid deterioration following the initiation of positive pressure ventilation.

C. Circulation and stop haemorrhage

It is important to be aware that a child may be profoundly shocked from blood loss resulting from trauma well before the occurrence of hypotension. A child responds to hypovolaemia with tachycardia and increasing peripheral vascular resistance. Therefore, the assessment of circulation status needs to be focused on the heart rate, pulse volume and the parameters of skin perfusion such as capillary refill time, colour and temperature. Perfusion inadequacy should be proactively corrected with volume resuscitation, rather than waiting for hypotension as an indicator. Hypotension occurs late due to cardiac decompensation and indicates that a child is nearing collapse. Likewise, bradycardia is often a prelude to imminent arrest. The persistence of tachycardia in the child with trauma should prompt concern and evaluation for occult ongoing blood loss.

The child with major trauma requires urgent intravenous access with the largest practical cannulae into visible or palpable peripheral veins. In the shocked child, cephalic, femoral or great saphenous veins are usually the most accessible. Where vascular cannulation is unsuccessful, after 60–90 seconds, the child who requires immediate fluids or drugs to facilitate intubation, should have a rapid intraosseous needle placed as described in Chapter 23.11. This is clearly the second line method that should be used in children without hesitation, rather than cutdown techniques that may be applicable in adults. In certain circumstances, such as the small child backed over by a motor vehicle with obvious major abdominal, pelvic or lower limb trauma, it may be prudent to use additional alternative access into a vein that drains into the SVC (e.g. external jugular or subclavian). In this rare situation, lower limb intraosseous infused volume may not access the circulation effectively due to disruption of the normal continuity of the intraosseous and intravascular spaces.

Fluid resuscitation should initially be with crystalloid or colloid titrated to clinical response. Boluses of 20 mL kg^{-1} should be given using pressure infusion. In the hypotensive child who arrives in extremis the early use of uncross-matched O negative blood may be indicated. Otherwise, after two boluses of crystalloid or equivalent have been infused, ongoing hypovolaemia should be with crossmatched blood replacement. Whole blood or packed cells should be given in boluses of 20 and 10 mL kg^{-1} respectively. Fluids should be warmed in order to reduce the incidence of hypothermic stress complicating the resuscitation. The child with ongoing cardiovascular instability needs urgent surgical intervention.

Part of the circulation phase of management includes therapy to limit ongoing blood losses from external or fracture sites by direct pressure or splinting. This is of vital importance as a child's blood volume is only 80 mL kg^{-1} and small ongoing losses contribute to haemodynamic instability.

Although in major trauma the most likely cause of shock is blood loss, one needs to consider other possible contributors such as myocardial injury, pericardial tamponade, spinal shock or tension pneumothorax.

D. Disability

The most rapid way to assess a child's conscious level in the primary survey is by using the AVPU scale (see Table 3.2.2).

A child who scores a non-purposeful P or U correlates with a GCS of 8 or less and requires intubation and ventilation. The brief neurological assessment during the primary survey is completed by checking equality of pupil size and reactivity to light.

E. Exposure and environment

The child should be undressed fully to allow examination of the entire body in order to detect all external stigmata of injury. Once this is completed, the child should be covered by warm blankets. The potential for hypothermia can also be decreased by the use of radiant heaters and warm resuscitation fluids.

Other issues during initial stabilisation

Early analgesia

Children who have significant pain or distress need to have prompt provision of analgesia as soon as intravenous access is obtained. This is usually best achieved by titrating intravenous morphine in doses of 0.1–0.2 mg kg^{-1} to effect. Adequate analgesia allows a more rapid and reliable clinical assessment.

Continuous monitoring

This should include heart rate, blood pressure, respiratory rate, oxygen saturation and clinical assessment of perfusion.

Support of family members

It is important to provide early psychological support to other family members who arrive with the child with major injuries. This should occur via a senior member of the team assisted by a nurse or social worker who is dedicated to this role. Non-comatose children are often fearful and distressed and it is useful to have the parents available to provide comfort to them.

Secondary survey

The secondary survey follows when initial resuscitation has stabilised the child from immediate life threats. Continuous monitoring of vital signs and neurological status is paramount, as any deterioration should prompt immediate discontinuing of this phase of the assessment and return to the primary survey. The secondary survey should include:

❶ History – from ambulance staff, parents and child where possible.
A: Allergies
M: Medications
P: Past history
L: Last ate
E: Event – in order to clarify mechanism of trauma and potential for injury. The more detail in the history the more accurate the assessment of potential injuries.

❷ Head to toe, front and back examination – the child should have a methodical and thorough clinical examination to identify all injuries. The head, face, neck, chest, abdomen, pelvis, spine and extremities (see orthopaedic trauma below) need to be examined. A more formal neurological assessment should use a paediatric GCS. The spinal immobilisation needs to be maintained until clinical or radiological clearance, in cases where this is possible. During this phase, placement of an orogastric tube may occur if gastric decompression is indicated. A urinary catheter (with the standard precautions for a potential urethral injury) is indicated in the

unconscious child or where the accurate measurement of urine flow is required.

❸ Investigations – appropriate bloods should be sent on initial intravenous access, along with a bedside glucose measurement. In the multiply injured child, initial radiological films should potentially include a resuscitation room chest X-ray, lateral cervical spine and pelvis. A 12-lead ECG should be done where a child has sustained significant trauma to the chest.

Definitive care and disposition

After the secondary survey and reassessment of the child's physiological response to resuscitation, the next step is to prioritise injuries to determine the need and timing of further imaging or any surgical intervention. The general rule is if the child remains hypotensive despite a 1/2 blood volume resuscitation over the first 1 to 4 hours, the child needs surgery. Persistent fluid and blood resuscitation can quickly cause a coagulopathic state. It may be necessary to involve multiple surgical specialists depending on the child's injuries and the approach varies according to local resources. The team leader needs to coordinate these inputs so that patient care is at all times expeditious and tailored to the specific and prioritised needs of the child. In the non-paediatric tertiary environment, early liaison with appropriate colleagues from a trauma centre with the capacity for definitive care of a child with major injuries, will help determine the most appropriate means for the individual child optimally to reach definitive care. Transfer of a child to definitive care is discussed in Section 27.

Care in paediatric hospitals can result in lower rates of non-therapeutic laparotomies. The skill of the paediatric surgical trauma team is often in deciding when not to operate. Repeated examinations identify the child who is continuing to bleed and highlight the child who may have a hollow viscus injury. Patterns of injury, such as with seatbelt bruises, are often recognised and are able to be put in the context of the child's overall physiology. The optimal care of an injured child is in a paediatric institution where there is familiarity with children and a sufficient volume of work to maintain that. The care of the child throughout the hospital stay should include other important considerations such as early physiotherapy to stop limb contractures, early involvement of the rehabilitation team and schooling.

Orthopaedic trauma

A discussion of specific injuries and their management is dealt with in detail in Section 24.

Bony injuries are common in children who have multiple trauma. Once the child is stable, the secondary survey must include assessment of all limbs, clavicles, as well as ribs, pelvis and spine. The splinting of long-bone fractures before moving the patient from the resuscitation room is important, even in the face of other serious injuries. This avoids ongoing pain and blood loss as well as further soft tissue injury to the limb.

A careful tertiary survey the following day may reveal minor bony injuries, which were not detected during the initial resuscitation phase. These injuries need to be immobilised and, if necessary, a plan made for reduction as soon as the general condition of the child allows. Once the life-threatening injuries heal, a missed displaced bony injury is a major problem for the child in the longer term.

Isolated orthopaedic trauma is one of the most common types of trauma presenting to an Emergency Department. Review of history and mechanism of injury and an overall examination are needed to exclude concurrent injury. The possibility of a non-accidental injury must always be considered. The time of last oral intake should be documented and the child should receive nothing orally until the management plan is established.

In order to avoid causing further pain to a child, much of the examination of the fracture area can be done by observation.

- Lack of spontaneous movement gives a clue to the location of a painful injury.
- Deformity or angulation, swelling and bruising, or breach of the overlying skin suggests an open fracture.
- Gently eliciting localised areas of tenderness helps direct the most efficient use of radiology to identify the site of injury. It is best to exclude non-tender regions first. A co-operative child can point to the area of maximal tenderness, whereas in a younger child the parent may be able to indicate which areas cause the child to be apprehensive.
- The function and range of motion of surrounding joints should always be checked.
- Vascular complications can be assessed by colour, perfusion and pulses of the distal limb. As pain often limits motor function, neurological assessment to test sensory components is important.
- Compartment syndrome should be looked for when a displaced fracture has significant associated swelling. In children the volar surface of the forearm is frequently the site involved. Pain on passive stretch of involved muscles is the hallmark. Distal pulses may be preserved. Neurological dysfunction often develops.

Pain relief involves first immobilising the limb with a sling, a temporary backslab or seating the child in a wheelchair or bed. The need for medication for pain relief can then be assessed. Analgesia is required before radiological investigation, so that any limb movement necessary to take the appropriate films is less distressing for the child.

Plaster immobilisation in the Emergency Department should generally involve using a backslab technique, rather than a circumferential plaster because of the potential for early limb swelling. The slab should be of sufficient strength to keep the fracture stable. Plaster of Paris strips usually require 12 layers for the upper limb and 20 layers for the lower limb. For displaced fractures an initial temporary plaster slab can reduce movement and therefore pain at the fracture site during the X-ray. The soft padding can be used to line the plaster slab, rather than winding it around the limb to reduce movement on application.

The reduction of any displaced fractures should be done with appropriate analgesia, anaesthesia and sedation, which should be administered by a second doctor. Often this is best achieved with a general anaesthetic where there is significant need for manipulation or fracture instability. The reduction of any fracture in children should be done by a doctor with the appropriate training and experience, so that multiple attempts and further injury are avoided. Complicated fractures and those in which the reduction will be hard to maintain require additional expertise.

Appropriate orthopaedic follow up of even minor fractures in children is vital. Within 5–7 days the swelling subsides, and the back slab does not hold the fracture, which may lose position. At that stage a circumferential plaster can usually be used. Because the child frequently falls, a change in fracture position can easily occur. A repeat X-ray at review is necessary to determine if the fracture has maintained position.

Rehabilitation

Rehabilitation should start from the time of admission and there should be early involvement of the appropriate teams. There have been major improvements in the diagnosis and care of cervical spine injuries and management of severe head injuries. There needs to be continuing work on the outcome of minor head injuries and the debilitating long-term consequences of serious long bone fractures.

Finally, the child's social situation and propensity to partake in risky behaviour needs to be assessed, as there is some evidence that children with injuries tend to have further future injuries. Careful assessments of the child's social history may allow appropriate interventions. A full 'tertiary history' should include environmental factors (type of car / airbags / seatbelts / helmets / details of window falls / pool fence gates, etc.) so as to allow future prevention programs to be appropriately targeted.

Acknowledgement

The contribution of Mary McAskill as author in the first edition is hereby acknowledged.

Reference

1. *A League Table of Child Deaths by Injury in Rich Nations*. Innocenti Report Card Issue No. 2, United Nations Children's Fund; February 2001.

TRAUMA IN CHILDREN

3.2 Paediatric neurotrauma

David G. Cooksley

ESSENTIALS

1 Neurotrauma is the leading cause of morbidity and mortality in paediatric trauma.

2 The prevention of secondary brain injury is the primary focus of acute medical intervention in the emergency department.

3 A careful history and examination is important to assess the potential significance of the injury and determine the need for further investigation or admission for observation.

4 Clinicians should not attribute the cause of shock to head injury until other causes have been excluded. Infants may become hypovolaemic from the blood loss of an intracranial bleed. .

5 Any child with a GCS ≤14, clinical evidence of a skull fracture or penetrating skull injury should have an emergent cerebral CT scan.

6 The prime role of trauma resuscitation is to rapidly identify and correct hypoxia and hypotension in children with severe TBI, as they are significant contributors to secondary brain injury.

7 Rapid sequence oral intubation, with in-line stabilisation of the cervical spine, is the preferred technique for securing airway control in the head-injured child.

8 Children sent home from the emergency department following a head injury must be discharged to the care of a responsible adult who is given clear discharge instructions and a written head-injury sheet containing advice on when to seek review

9 The family of the child with a significant head injury requires appropriate support and explanation as an important facet of care whilst in the emergency department.

Introduction

Paediatric neurotrauma is a common presenting problem in emergency medicine practice. This chapter will deal principally with paediatric head injury or, more correctly, traumatic brain injury (TBI), and spinal cord injury. Spinal injury is also covered in Chapter 24.3.

Epidemiology

TBI covers a spectrum of injury from trivial to lethal. It is the leading cause of morbidity and mortality in paediatric trauma.[1] The number of children admitted to hospital in a recent study indicated an annual rate in Australia of 232 per 100 000 for those aged 0–4 years, 158 per 100 000 for those aged 5–9 years and 203 per 100 000 for those

aged 10–14 years.[2] These figures are higher than the overall, age standardised, annual rate of between 140 and 150 per 100 000 population.[2,3] It is important to remember that these figures only reflect hospital admissions and the true incidence of TBI in the community is much higher.[4]

In Australia the most common cause of TBI is falls, followed by motor vehicle related accidents.[2] A much smaller percentage result from being struck by objects, crushed, assaulted (non-accidental injury) and other miscellaneous causes. Males consistently outnumber females, with most studies reporting approximately a 2:1 ratio for all age groups. The overall incidence of spinal cord injury in Australia for children aged 0 to 14 years is unknown.[4,5] The age standardised incidence in the 15+-year-old population is 14 per million of population per year, with a male to female ratio

averaging 4:1, but peaking at 9:1 in the 15–24-year age group.[5]

Preventive strategies have made the most impact on the improved outcomes of paediatric trauma over the past two decades.

Pathophysiology

TBI, like spinal injury, can be divided into primary and secondary trauma. Primary trauma occurs during the initial impact to the head and only preventive measures such as using protective equipment (e.g. helmets and seatbelts), better engineering (e.g. safer roads), education and legislation can alter the extent of this primary injury. Secondary trauma or insult occurs when post-traumatic acute phase response and mediators, or subsequent physiological insults, such as hypoxia, hypotension and increased intracranial pressure, occur and cause further damage to the already traumatised tissues or structures. The prevention of secondary injury, particularly due to cerebral hypoxia and reduced cerebral perfusion, is the primary focus of acute medical intervention, which begins in the field via ambulance and continues in the ED setting.

Children have unique anatomical, physiological and developmental differences when compared to adults. They have a large head to body ratio, leading to a high centre of gravity (falls) and to the head being the primary 'target' for trauma. The skull is thinner and more plastic and thus transmits rather than attenuates impact.[6,7] Skull fractures are therefore more common in children and importantly, serious brain injury can occur without an associated skull fracture.[8–12]

In children, the dura is more closely adherent to the skull compared to adults, making extradural haematomas less common in children, particularly in infants.[7,13] Unfused sutures and an open fontanelle can expand to accommodate intracranial haemorrhage or cerebral oedema.[7] Some authors have thought children to be more prone to 'malignant cerebral swelling' that can cause rapid and sometimes fatal deterioration even after minor TBI.[9,14,15] However, this view has recently been questioned and swelling may be no more common in children than in adults.[16]

Physiologically, children have a lower systolic and mean arterial blood pressure, which implies a lower cerebral perfusion pressure (CPP). This, in turn, may cause problems with maintaining adequate cerebral perfusion if they have raised intracranial pressure. Infants and small children may become hypovolaemic with large intracranial bleeds. This is not seen in larger children or adults.[6]

Cerebral blood flow is often very low and may approach ischaemic levels following more severe TBI.[17] This may be related to a low brain metabolic rate in comatose patients, increased intracerebral pressure and vasospasm. Autoregulation of cerebral blood flow (CBF) may be lost following TBI, and in this setting CPP largely determines CBF. This underscores the importance of maintaining an adequate CPP in the head-injured patient, especially those with more severe injuries.

Head injury, as opposed to TBI, may be described as extra-axial or intra-axial. Extra-axial injury refers to pathology outside the brain parenchyma.[7,18] Extra-axial structures include the skull, structures between the skull and brain and the ventricular spaces within the brain. Common extra-axial lesions include skull fractures and extradural, subdural, subarachnoid and intraventricular haemorrhages. Extra-dural haemorrhage occurs, as its name implies, outside the dura. Medical literature often refers to this as 'epidural haemorrhage' but in Australasia the term 'epidural' is generally used only to describe lesions outside the dura of the spinal cord. Intra-axial injuries are true TBIs and include contusion, laceration, haemorrhage and diffuse axonal injury (DAI). DAI may result in considerable disability with little to see on radiological investigation.[7]

Classification

The generally accepted method of classifying severity of TBI is by using the Glasgow Coma Scale (GCS), although other measures such as duration of unconsciousness or amnesia are sometimes used. The GCS was first described for adults in 1974 and scores three variables: eye opening, verbal response and motor response (see 'examination' and Table 3.2.1).[19] It has proved to be a very useful tool in rating severity of TBI and prognosis.[7]

The problem with using the GCS on young children, particularly those aged less than 2 years, is that the best verbal response is limited by their language development. In an attempt to overcome this difficulty, modified GCSs have been proposed, including the so-called Child Coma Scale (CCS).[9,20] It is important to note that, unlike the GCS, the CCS has never been properly validated and many studies of head injury in children deliberately exclude those aged less than 2 years.

TBI is usually divided into three categories: mild, moderate and severe.

Mild TBI (GCS 14 to 15)

Mild TBI, sometimes termed 'minor' TBI, was originally defined as head trauma patients with a GCS from 13 to 15 (and/or varying periods of loss of consciousness (LOC) and amnesia).[21] The problem with this definition is that patients with GCS 13 have a significantly higher risk of intracranial injury, with subsequent risks for deterioration and neurosurgery, than patients with a GCS of 14 or 15. They more properly belong in the moderate head injury group.[15,22]

The original definition of GCS 13 to 15 continues to be used in international and Australasian literature but the recognised definition of mild TBI in Australasia is GCS of 14 or 15.[14] Some authors believe that even this is too liberal and the definition of mild TBI should be restricted to patients with a GCS of 15.[22,23]

Approximately 80% of children with TBI will fall into this category.[24] The reported incidence of intracranial haemorrhage (ICH) varies between 4 and 7% in children with GCS 15, and increases to approximately 10% in children with GCS 14.[10,15,25,26] The overall mortality in this group is reported to be as high as 2%.[15] These figures may be subject to significant selection bias.

The terms 'minimal' or 'trivial' TBI are sometimes used to describe a subgroup of mild TBI who meet the following criteria: GCS 15, normal neurological examination and no signs of a skull fracture.[23,25,27] Transient LOC or amnesia does not exclude patients from this subgroup.

Moderate TBI (GCS 9 to 13)

Approximately 18% of children with TBI fall into this category.[24] The incidence of ICH and overall mortality in this group of children is uncertain (almost all research focuses on either mild or severe TBI).

Severe TBI (GCS 8 or less)

Approximately 2% of children with TBI fall into this category.[24] Patients in this category are, by definition, comatose. Overall mortality in this group is between 30 and 40%.[28]

Table 3.2.1 Adult and child Glasgow Coma Scores (GCS)		
Score	Adult	Child
Eye opening		
4	Spontaneous	
3	To speech only	Same
2	To pain only	
1	No response	
Verbal		
5	Orientated in person, place and time	Happy/smiles/interacts normally
4	Confused	Crying but consolable
3	Inappropriate but intelligible speech	Inconsistently consolable
2	Incomprehensible sounds	Inconsolable and/or irritable
1	No response	No response
Motor		
6	Obeys commands	
5	Localises painful stimulus	
4	Withdraws to painful stimulus	Same
3	Flexor posturing to painful stimulus	
2	Extensor posturing to painful stimulus	
1	No response	

ASSESSMENT

History

Careful history and examination is important when assessing the significance of the injury and determining the need for further investigation or admission.

Initial assessment and treatment may need to occur simultaneously. Ensuring an adequate airway, breathing and circulation with resuscitation as required is the first priority. The best approach is to undertake a 'primary survey' with correction of life threats, followed by a 'detailed history plus secondary survey' as for any other trauma patient. Spinal precautions using immobilisation must be maintained until clinical and/or radiological clearance of the spine has been completed.

Assessment of the child may be extremely difficult, if not impossible, if the child is distressed with pain or is cerebrally irritated. The early use of a very small dose of parenteral narcotic such as morphine 0.05 mg kg^{-1} intravenously may make assessment and management much easier. Concern about masking changes in neurological function should not prevent the use of adequate analgesia for children who are distressed by pain.

The following historical information is relevant and should be ascertained if possible:

- time and mechanism of the injury;
- any loss of consciousness or period of altered level of consciousness and its duration;
- any post-trauma seizure-type activity;
- any post-injury vomiting;
- any headache or other neurological symptoms such as diplopia, weakness or altered sensation;
- any retro- or anterograde amnesia;
- progression of any symptoms and signs from the time of injury;
- details of pre-hospital care assessment and therapies.

The possibility of non-accidental injury (NAI) must always be considered in children with skull fractures or intracranial injuries. Be particularly vigilant with children aged <2 years, when a parent or carer has delayed seeking medical care or the stated mechanism is not in keeping with degree of injury observed.[12]

Past history that is particularly relevant in the context of neurotrauma is:

- previous head or spinal injury;
- congenital central nervous system (CNS) problems;
- CNS surgery (such as the insertion of a VP shunt);
- bleeding diatheses such as haemophilia or thrombocytopenia;
- psychomotor or developmental problems, such as autism, that make assessment particularly difficult.

It is important to remember:

- medications, and other ingestants that may influence assessment of a head injury including possible illicit drugs or medications and chemicals to which a young child may have gained access at home;
- allergies;
- immunisation status;
- last food or fluid intake.

Examination

Check vital signs, including bedside blood sugar level, to immediately exclude:

- hypoxia (SaO$_2$ ≤90% or PaO$_2$ ≤60 mmHg)
- hypotension (SBP ≤5th percentile for age or SBP <90 mmHg)
- hypoglycaemia (blood sugar level <3.0 mmol L^{-1}).

These reversible factors may be contributing to the child's altered level of consciousness and also cause secondary brain injury. Ascertain the child's weight, early, either by measurement or inference from the child's age, as it is necessary for calculating drug and fluid requirements.

Glasgow Coma Scale (GCS)

This should be used to define the child's level of consciousness and to monitor any change over time. Serial neurological observations should be performed regularly to monitor for deterioration or improvement in the child's conscious state. Once a child's GCS is normal and stable, the frequency of neurological observations can be decreased. It is important to note that the GCS is intended to score global function not focal deficit. When using the GCS to classify the severity of TBI, the best post-resuscitation score should be used.

If a painful stimulus is needed to test motor function, apply pressure to the supra-orbital margin to test for localisation of pain. This is superior to a 'sternal rub'. To test for withdrawal or abnormal flexion/extension, use a pen or pencil to apply pressure to finger-nail or toe-nail beds. Abnormal flexion is usually termed 'decorticate posturing' and abnormal extension termed 'decerebrate posturing' although this was discouraged in the original description of the GCS as it implied a specific physio-anatomic correlation.[19] The best score should be recorded after testing all four limbs and any discrepancy between limbs should be recorded separately.[5]

It should also be noted that it may not be possible to score verbal or motor function in some patients, for example those who are intubated (verbal score) or have a high-level spinal cord injury or limb injuries (motor score).

Table 3.2.1 allows comparison of the GCS and the CCS used by Hahn et al and others.[9,29] The CCS has never been properly validated and assessment of verbal response is somewhat subjective, particularly in children aged less than 6 months.[20]

A rapid assessment of a child's neurological disturbance can also be made using the **AVPU scale**, which denotes the child's response to stimuli (Table 3.2.2). The child who demonstrates a non-purposeful response to pain (withdrawal, flexor or extensor responses) has a level of consciousness consistent with a GCS of <9 and the unresponsive child, a GCS of 3.

Assess the child carefully for signs of trauma to the head, neck and thoracolumbar spine. A skull vault fracture may be

Table 3.2.2	AVPU scale	
A	Alert	
V	Responds to Voice	
P	Responds to Pain	Purposeful Non-purposeful
U	Unresponsive	

suggested by scalp haematoma, crepitus or palpable depression. A basilar skull fracture should be suspected in the presence of 'racoon eyes', Battle's sign (bruising around the mastoid process), haemotympanum or CSF rhinorrhoea/otorrhoea. Any sign of trauma above the clavicles increases the likelihood of intracranial pathology being detected on computerised tomography (CT) scanning.[30]

A careful examination of the cranial nerves and peripheral nervous system should follow to assess for any localising signs. If spinal cord injury is suspected the sensory level of injury (dermatome) should be defined, not forgetting to check for intact perianal sensation and normal anal tone. Hypotensive bradycardia, altered perspiration below the level of the lesion, priapism in boys and urinary retention all signify autonomic dysfunction, which may occur with spinal injury. Any sensory or motor function below the level of injury implies that the cord lesion is incomplete and denotes a better prognosis.

Pupil size, equality and reactivity, particularly in the unconscious child, should be checked and recorded. A dilated pupil is defined as >4 mm diameter, asymmetry as >1 mm difference between pupil size and non-reactivity as <1 mm movement when a bright light is used to test the reflex. The pupillary size and reaction may be also altered by direct trauma to the globe, so one needs to consider traumatic mydriasis when the overall features are not in keeping with an intracranial cause of unilateral pupillary dilatation. Whenever possible, neurological examination should include an assessment of gait.

Investigations

Bedside
Blood sugar level
This is better thought of as a 'vital sign' than a bedside investigation and should be measured at the same time as HR, BP, RR and SaO_2.

12-lead ECG
This should be performed in the child who has associated chest trauma and considered in any patient with moderate or severe head injury, as catecholamine release from TBI can cause myocardial effects.

Laboratory
In patients with mild TBI, laboratory investigations are not indicated unless there is known or suspected coexistent pathology such as haemophilia or thrombocytopenia.

In patients with moderate or severe TBI the following should be checked:

- Haemoglobin level and platelet count.
- Coagulation profile including fibrin degradation products (FDPs). Tissue thromboplastin released from the brain can cause coagulopathy and disseminated intravascular coagulation, the presence of which denotes a poor prognosis.[31,32]
- Electrolytes – these serve as baseline during fluid resuscitation and subsequent monitoring for hyponatraemia. Transient hypokalaemia is a well-recognised consequence of TBI and may occur even in mild cases. It usually resolves spontaneously after several hours and no treatment is required.
- Arterial blood gases should be considered, depending upon clinical situation. In ventilated patients arterial blood gases (ABGs) should be used to confirm that the end tidal CO_2 ($ETCO_2$) accurately reflects $PaCO_2$.

Radiological
Skull X-rays
Before the widespread availability of CT scanning, skull X-rays were often used to screen or help risk stratify which children should be observed in hospital or have a brain CT scan.[8,29] While it is acknowledged that children with a skull X-ray demonstrating a fracture have a higher incidence of ICH compared to those without a fracture, many children without fractures also have an ICH.[9–11,15,29] To compound this problem, the reported sensitivity and specificity of skull X-rays in detecting a fracture is reported to be as low as 21% and 53% respectively.[33] Emergency department staff need to be familiar with the interpretation of paediatric skull X-rays in order to minimise the misinterpretation of sutures or vascular markings as fractures and vice versa.

The role of plain films is very limited in seriously injured patients but may still have a role in helping to risk stratify very young children (age <2) with head trauma, who can be difficult to keep still for CT scanning

without sedation or general anaesthetic and in those in whom possible NAI is suspected.[34,35] Skull X-rays may also be useful in screening for depressed skull fractures or penetrating skull injury, particularly in environments where CT scanning is not readily available.

Cervical and thoracolumbar spine X-rays
These should be obtained for any child with suspected cervical or thoracolumbar trauma, or evidence of spinal cord injury, and those in whom the spine cannot be cleared clinically. Young children (age <10 years) are more prone to high cervical spine injuries whereas older children, like adults, are more prone to lower cervical spine injuries.[36] Spinal cord injury without radiological abnormality (SCIWORA) was thought to be principally a paediatric phenomenon but is in fact seen much more often in adults.[37]

A low threshold should be held for CT scanning the vertebral column in any child with high clinical suspicion of spinal injury or possible radiological abnormality on plain film.

CT scan
In cases of TBI, CT scan is the modality of choice for imaging the skull for fractures and brain for acute haemorrhage, oedema, mass effect, pneumocephalus and hydrocephalus.[7,38] It is rapid, inexpensive and can accommodate a wide range of life support and monitoring equipment. Any child with a persistent GCS ≤14, clinical evidence of a skull fracture or penetrating skull injury should have an emergent cerebral CT scan (Table 3.2.3; see also 'mild TBI'). The child needs to be accompanied by appropriate

Table 3.2.3   Indications for CT scan
- GCS <15 - Focal neurological deficit - Signs of skull fracture or penetrating skull injury
STRONGLY CONSIDER IF … - Persistent vomiting - History of LOC* - Post-traumatic seizure (delayed) - Post-traumatic amnesia - Moderate to severe headache - Underlying bleeding risk

*The duration LOC does not correlate well with the risk of intracranial pathology and anything greater than transient LOC (i.e. >1 min) should be considered significant.[12,23]

staff and monitoring equipment to the CT scan environment to continue optimal monitoring and rapidly manage any potential complications.

The CT is also used as the initial investigation of choice to further evaluate suspected spinal injury although it cannot exclude ligamentous injury and it provides limited information on injury to the spinal cord itself.[39,40]

Magnetic resonance imaging (MRI)

MRI is superior to CT scanning for detecting cerebral oedema, contusion and diffuse axonal injury in cases of TBI.[7] It is also superior to CT scanning for visualising the posterior fossa and brainstem regions. It is the investigation of choice for spinal cord injury and the actual patterns of haemorrhage and oedema within the cord carry prognostic significance.[39,41] MRI imaging of ligamentous tissues can be used to investigate possible spine instability. However, clinical correlation with MRI findings in 'mild' cases is still lacking.[40]

Management

Mild TBI (GCS 14, 15)

The management of mild TBI is controversial. The debate primarily focuses on the question of whether or not children in this group can be risk stratified and managed clinically without further investigation, or whether they need to have a cerebral CT scan regardless of clinical findings. Concern stems from the observation that even children with a GCS of 15 and a normal neurological examination can harbour clinically significant intracranial pathology with attendant risks for subsequent deterioration and death. One study of 429 children with mild TBI found that 16% of the children with GCS 15 and no LOC had significant IC injury.[42] Of these, 1.4% required neurosurgical intervention and 2% died.

On the other hand, CT scanning involves a significant radiation dose and concern has been expressed about the subsequent lifetime risk of radiation-induced malignancies which may be as high as 1 per 1500 scans in very young children.[43] Also, if very young, the child may require sedation or a general anaesthetic, with their attendant risks of apnoea, hypoxia, aspiration and prolonged

sedation.[12] In addition to the radiation risks, the cost of scanning all children with head trauma would be considerable.

The observation has been made that the greatest benefit in treating patients with TBI is not with aggressive management of the severely injured, but in preventing deterioration and complications in those with mild or moderate injuries who appear to be at low risk.[12]

Risk factors for IC injury or deterioration, such as LOC, amnesia, headache, vomiting, seizures and focal neurological deficit have been studied in an attempt to identify those children with mild TBI who do not require a CT scan.[11,15,18,26,30,35,42,44–47] The presence of any of these risk factors increases the likelihood of intracranial pathology and it is important to note that a child can have all of them and still have a GCS of 15. Prospective studies evaluating such clinical decision rules for imaging children with TBI are still to be completed.

The risk of developing clinically significant IC pathology following the initial trauma decreases over time. Although current Australasian guidelines for children suffering mild TBI suggest discharge after 4 hours of observation if the child has a GCS of 15 and is asymptomatic,[14] a large study of over 28 000 children admitted to hospital following head injury demonstrated that 6 hours of post-injury observation was required to identify all children who were likely to deteriorate.[48]

It has been estimated that a child with trivial head injury, who has no LOC and who is completely well (i.e. none of the above mentioned symptoms or signs) has a less than 1:5000 chance of significant IC pathology and can be discharged to the care of a responsible adult without further investigation.[23]

Based upon current knowledge, the management and disposition algorithm shown in Fig. 3.2.1 is suggested.

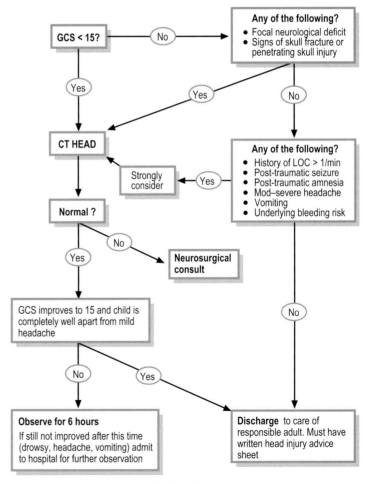

Fig. 3.2.1 Suggested management algorithm for mild TBI.

Moderate and Severe TBI

These groups will be considered together. It should be noted that the best GCS after resuscitation is used for classification of the TBI, and that a child with a GCS ≤ 8 is, by definition, comatose. The priorities of management include maintenance of the airway, oxygenation and cerebral perfusion.

Airway control, oxygenation and ventilation

It is important to rapidly identify and correct hypoxia as this is a significant contributor to secondary brain injury.[49–52] Supplemental oxygen should be applied in order to maximise oxygen delivery to any ischaemic tissue and the child's SaO_2 should be monitored.

Children who are not protecting their airway or maintaining adequate ventilation should be intubated and ventilated. In general, this would include any child with a GCS ≤ 8. In-line stabilisation of the cervical spine during rapid sequence oral intubation should occur to prevent potential secondary spinal injury. Rarely, the agitated or combative child with a higher GCS may require intubation in order to facilitate imaging or to stabilise a potentially at risk cervical spine until it can be cleared.

Pharmacological adjuncts to intubation should be used as required. However, care is required to avoid transient hypotension as this worsens neurological outcome (see below). The endotracheal tube should be securely fastened to the child's face with tape rather than using the standard 'tie around the neck'. This avoids the risk of impairing cerebral venous drainage and causing a consequent rise in intracranial pressure (ICP). Hard collars may also constrict the neck and therefore interfere with venous drainage, so need to be fitted correctly.

An orogastric tube should be passed to decompress the stomach. The nasogastric route should be avoided as inadvertent intracranial placement can occur if the child has a basal skull fracture.

SaO_2 and PaO_2 are not good indicators of adequate ventilation and continuous $ETCO_2$ monitoring should occur if the child is intubated. The child should be ventilated to maintain an $ETCO_2$ in the low–normal range (i.e. aiming for an $ETCO_2$ of 35 mmHg). Hypercarbia secondary to inadequate ventilation may result in cerebral vasodilation and secondary increase in ICP. Hypocarbia causes cerebral vasoconstriction and therefore decreases ICP, but increases the risk of causing or exacerbating cerebral hypoperfusion with secondary ischaemia.[53] Routine 'prophylactic hyperventilation' in adults has been shown to worsen outcome and presumably does so in children. Therefore hyperventilation to a $PaCO_2$ of 25 mmHg should be reserved for the child who is rapidly deteriorating with signs of increased intracranial pressure or cerebral herniation, such as new onset pupil asymmetry or rapidly decreasing GCS.

Circulation

Hypotension is the single most significant factor contributing to secondary brain insult.[49,51] Hypotension is defined as an SBP <90 mmHg in adults and a SBP <5th percentile for age in children.[49–52,54] One or more episodes of hypotension from time of injury through resuscitation at least doubles mortality and significantly increases morbidity.[49,51,54–56]

Despite studies focusing upon SBP, the true objective in the patient with TBI is to maintain an adequate CPP. This is the difference between mean arterial pressure (MAP) and intracranial pressure (ICP) [i.e. CPP = MAP – ICP]. The normal ICP is 0–10 mmHg and an ICP of 20 mmHg is generally regarded as the threshold for initiating specific therapy to reduce it. The optimal CPP is uncertain but consensus opinion recommends not less than 50 mmHg and not greater than 70 mmHg, as aggressive attempts to maintain CPP > 70 mmHg may also worsen outcomes.[57] In the pre-hospital and emergency department settings, the ICP is unknown so treatment is purely empirical. It is reasonable to aim for a MAP of between 70 and 90 mmHg that would maintain a CPP between 50 and 70 mmHg (i.e. allowing for ICPs up to 20 mmHg).

Initial resuscitation should be with dextrose-free isotonic solutions such as 0.9% saline or compound sodium lactate (Hartmann's) solution, although the use of hypertonic saline may be considered (see below). In the hypotensive patient, give a 20 mL kg^{-1} bolus (if using an isotonic crystalloid) and monitor the response. Repeat if the patient remains hypotensive. After a total of 40 mL kg^{-1} volume resuscitation, consideration should be given to the use of vasopressor support to maintain adequate MAP for cerebral perfusion. In the setting of hypovolaemia due to acute blood loss, ongoing resuscitation fluid will require blood product replacement.

Hypertonic saline

Hypertonic saline solutions have been used for initial resuscitation, as maintenance fluid and as specific treatment for raised ICP. In addition to rapidly restoring circulating volume, increasing blood pressure and reducing ICP, these solutions appear to have important and beneficial immuno-modulatory and neuro-chemical effects that may reduce secondary brain injury.[57,59]

A suggested regimen for the use of 3% saline for either initial resuscitation or to rapidly decrease ICP is to give a 5 mL kg^{-1} bolus, repeated if necessary according to patient response. It would appear that rapid changes in serum sodium concentration do not cause complications such as central pontine myelinolysis in humans, and most studies do not place an upper limit on serum sodium concentration.[59,60]

However, there have been no controlled trials demonstrating improved outcomes with hypertonic saline.

Mannitol

Mannitol has been used as both a resuscitation fluid (plasma expander) and as therapy for acute deterioration secondary to increasing ICP. Boluses of 0.25 g kg^{-1} to 1 g kg^{-1} body weight have been used successfully for short-term reduction of ICP.[61] Mannitol acts as an osmotic diuretic and can lead to subsequent problems with hypovolaemia and acute renal failure via acute tubular necrosis. A loop diuretic such as furosemide is sometimes used in addition to mannitol for treatment of acute rises in ICP. A urinary catheter is essential in any patient receiving mannitol or diuretics.

Positioning

The child's head should be kept in the midline to avoid jugular venous compression. Venous drainage is improved if the head of the bed is elevated 15–30 degrees, with resultant decrease in ICP. However, CPP is also reduced by this manoeuvre and there may be no net benefit unless ICP monitoring is in place and CCP adjusted as required.

Prophylactic anti-seizure therapy

Seizures that occur within seven days of a TBI are termed early post-traumatic seizures (EPTS) and those thereafter are late post-traumatic seizures (LPTS).[62] The overall incidence of seizures in children with TBI is probably between 5 and 15% but rises with increasing severity of TBI, occurring up to 40% of the time in those with a GCS ≤ 8.[51,62–64] Greater than 95% of PTS are early and approximately 80% of these occur within the first 24 hours.

Seizures may cause or exacerbate secondary brain injury by increasing cerebral metabolic demands, increasing intracerebral pressure and by causing or exacerbating cerebral hypoxia.[63,64]

The incidence of EPTS can be reduced by the use of prophylactic anticonvulsants such as phenytoin. Their use should be considered[65] in those with:

* GCS <10;
* seizure within 24 hours of injury;
* depressed skull fracture or penetrating head wound;
* subdural, extradural or intracerebral haematomas;
* cortical contusion.

It should be noted, however, that reduced EPTS does not translate into reduced mortality[65,66] and it remains to be seen whether or not an overall improved level of functioning occurs in those survivors given prophylactic anticonvulsant therapy. It should also be noted that prophylactic anticonvulsants do not alter the incidence of LPTS and their routine use after 7 days is not recommended.[65]

The management of active seizures should be with benzodiazepines and should follow the guidelines discussed in Chapter 8.3.

Antibiotics

Intravenous antibiotic prophylaxis with flucloxacillin 25–50 mg kg^{-1} 6-hourly should be given for compound skull fractures or fractures in communication with sinuses.

Steroids

Various steroids have been used in an attempt to improve outcome from TBI. To date no overall improvements have been identified and they may actually worsen outcome. Routine use is no longer recommended.[67–69]

Thermoregulation: prophylactic hypothermia and prevention of hyperthermia

Mild hypothermia (32–35°C) is known to decrease ICP and, in animal models, has been shown to be neuroprotective.[59,70,71] Outcomes in humans have not been consistently better and mild hypothermia may increase complications such as sepsis, pneumonia, bleeding and mortality in the TBI child.[59,72] Research is ongoing in this area and prophylactic hypothermia should be considered in consultation with local PICU intensivists regarding individual cases.

Hyperthermia is associated with a worse outcome in children with severe TBI.[72] It is not known if actively cooling the patient alters outcome and further research needs to be conducted in this area. In the meantime it would seem reasonable to attempt to cool a febrile brain-injured child.

Spinal cord injury

There is a great paucity of research into the optimal management of acute spinal cord injury in children. Therefore there are insufficient data to support diagnostic or treatment standards.[40] However, the principles of management of acute spinal cord injury are considered to be no different from TBI. The focus of therapy is to prevent secondary injury. Attention should be paid to the maintenance of strict spinal immobilisation, adequate oxygenation, ventilation, blood pressure and good supportive care as per moderate-severe TBI.

The use of high-dose steroids in acute spinal injury is controversial.[73,74] The issue is further complicated in the paediatric population by the fact that children <13 years were excluded from the major trials of steroids for spinal cord injury.[40] Routine use of high-dose steroids for spinal cord injury is no longer recommended by the Neurosurgical Society of Australasia.[14] If steroids are used, in consultation with local paediatric neurosurgical practice, they should be administered within 8 hours of injury. Practice currently varies between institutions.

The recommended dosing schedule is: methylprednisolone 30 mg kg^{-1} bolus over 15 minutes followed by a 45-minute break, then 5.4 mg kg^{-1} hr^{-1} continuous infusion for 23 hours.[14]

Supportive care

Immobilisation of children at risk of spinal injury is difficult when they are non-co-operative and needs to include the body as well as the head. Involvement of parents or carers and calming of the child are important adjuncts. Pressure area care should occur for all patients who are immobilised. Children who arrive in the emergency department on 'spinal boards' should be moved off them as soon as possible as pressure areas may develop rapidly.

Hard collars should be checked for correct fit and potential pressure areas. They should be changed to padded collars such as Aspen or Philadelphia collars if immobilisation is needed for an extended period.

A urinary catheter should be placed in children who require volume resuscitation, mannitol or diuretics, who are unable to communicate their need to micturate because of TBI, or who have a spinal cord injury.

The child's temperature should be monitored and inadvertent cooling avoided (see comments on thermoregulation above). The child's analgesic requirements should be regularly reviewed and analgesia titrated as required. Attention should be given to eye protection in children who are sedated or ventilated.

Family considerations

There are considerable immediate stresses during the initial stabilisation phases on the parents and family of the injured child. The family requires appropriate support and explanation whilst in the emergency department. If possible, it is useful to provide a dedicated staff member to be with them. The family should be kept well informed of the child's status and its proposed management by a designated senior medical member of the resuscitation team and consideration should be given to allowing parents into the resuscitation room to be with their child (see Chapter 2.1). Premature or vague conclusions of prognosis should be avoided until all relevant assessments and investigations have been made.

Disposition

The disposition for children with mild TBI has been outlined above. Children sent home from the emergency department following a head injury must be discharged to the care of a responsible adult who is given clear discharge instructions and a written head-injury sheet containing advice on when to seek review. Children who have had a significant concussive injury need to rest quietly for the next 24–48 hours – avoiding television, computers, music inputs, in order to minimise excessive visual-auditory stimulation in order for their symptoms to defervesce 'brain rest'. Returning to these activities too soon will often cause a recrudescence of their symptoms. Simple analgesics such as paracetamol can be used for mild headache, which should be expected to be short-lived. Any child with a suspected NAI should be admitted to hospital for safety and further evaluation.

All children with moderate or severe TBI or spinal cord injury should be transferred to a paediatric high dependency or intensive care unit for admission under the care of a neurosurgeon.

References

1. Martin C, Falcone R. Pediatric traumatic brain injury: an update of research to understand and improve outcomes. *Curr Opin Pediatr* 2008;**20**:294–9.
2. O'Connor P. *Hospitalisation due to traumatic brain injury, Australia 1997–98.* Australian Institute of Health and Welfare; 2002.
3. Khan F, Baguley I, Cameron D. Rehabilitation after traumatic brain injury. *Med J Aust* 2003;**178**(6):290–5.
4. Research Centre for Injury Studies. Spinal cord injury, Australia 1995/6. *Australian Injury Prevention Bulletin* 1998;**18**.
5. O'Connor. *December Spinal cord injury, Australia, 1999-00.* Australian Institute of Health and Welfare. 2001.
6. Anderson V, Catroppa C, Morse S, et al. Outcome from mild head injury in young children: A prospective study. *J Clin Exp Neuropsychol* 2001;**23**(6):705–17.
7. Poussaint T, Moeller K. Imaging of paediatric head trauma. *Neuroimaging Clin N Am* 2002;**12**:271–94.
8. Lazar L, Erez I, Gutermacher M, et al. Brain concussion produces transient hypokalemia in children. *J Pediatr Surg* 1997;**32**(1):88–90.
9. Hahn Y, McLone D. Risk factors in the outcome of children with minor head injury. *Pediatr Neurosurg* 1993;**19**:135–42.
10. Lloyd D, Carty H, Patterson M, et al. Predictive value of skull radiography for intracranial injury in children with blunt head injury. *Lancet* 1997;**349**:821–4.
11. Quayle K, Jaffe D, Kuppermann N, et al. Diagnostic testing for acute head injury in children: When are head computed tomography and skull X-rays indicated? *Pediatrics* 1997;**99**:e11.
12. Schutzman S, Greenes D. Paediatric minor head trauma. *Ann Emerg Med* 2001;**37**(1):65–74.
13. Moura dos Santos A, Plese J, Ciquini O, et al. Extradural hematomas in children. *Pediatr Neurosurg* 1994;**21**:50–4.
14. Neurological Society of Australasia and Royal Australasian College of Surgeons. *The Management of Acute Neurotrauma in Rural and Remote Locations.* 2nd ed. 2009.
15. Keskil I, Baykaner M, Ceviker N, et al. Assessment of mortality associated with mild head injury in the paediatric age group. *Childs Nerv Syst* 1995;**11**:467–73.
16. Lang D, Teasdale G, MacPherson P, et al. Diffuse brain swelling after head injury: More often malignant in adults than children? *J Neurosurg* 1994;**80**:675–80.
17. Bratton S, Chestnut R, Ghajar J, et al. Cerebral perfusion thresholds. *J Neurotrauma* 2007;**24**:S59–64.
18. Ratan S, Pandey R, Ratan J. Association among duration of unconsciousness, Glasgow Coma Scale, and cranial computed tomography abnormalities in head injured children. *Clin Pediatr* July, 2001;375–8.
19. Teasdale G, Jennett B. Assessment of coma and impaired consciousness. *Lancet* July 1974;81–3.
20. Simpson D, Reilly P. Paediatric Coma Scale. *Lancet* August 1982;450.
21. Mild Traumatic Brain Injury Committee of the Head Injury Interdisciplinary Special Interest Group of the American Congress of Rehabilitation Medicine. Definition of mild traumatic brain injury. *J Head Trauma Rehabil* 1993;**8**(3):86–7.
22. Culotta V, Sementilli M, Gerold K, et al. Clinicopathological heterogeneity in the classification of mild head injury. *Neurosurgery* 1996;**38**(2):245–50.
23. Committee on quality improvement, American Academy of Paediatrics. The management of minor closed head injury in children. *Paediatrics* 1999;**104**(6):1407–15.
24. Murgio A, Patrick P, Andrade F, et al. International study of emergency department care for paediatric traumatic brain injury and the role of CT scanning. *Childs Nerv Syst* 2001;**17**:257–62.
25. Davis R, Mullen N, Makela M, et al. Cranial computed tomography scans in children after minimal head injury with loss of consciousness. *Ann Emerg Med* 1994;**24**(4):640–5.
26. Schunk J, Rodgerson J, Woodward G. The utility of head computed tomographic scanning in paediatric patients with normal neurologic examination in the emergency department. *Pediatr Emerg Care* 1996;**12**(3):160–5.
27. Roddy S, Cohn S, Moller B, et al. Minimal head trauma in children revisited: Is routine hospitalisation required? *Pediatrics* 1998;**101**(4):575–7.
28. Johnson D, Krishnamurthy S. Severe paediatric head injury: Myth, magic, and actual fact. *Pediatr Neurosurg* 1998;**28**:167–72.
29. Hahn Y, Chyung C, Bartherl M, et al. Head injuries in children under 36 months of age. Demography and outcome. *Childs Nerv Syst* 1988;**4**:34–40.
30. Haydel M, Preston C, Mills T, et al. Indications for computed tomography in patients with minor head injury. *N Engl J Med* 2000;**343**(2):100–105.
31. Vavilala M, Dunbar P, Rivara F, et al. Coagulopathy predicts poor outcome following head injury in children less than 16 years of age. *Journal of Neurosurgical Anaesthetics* 2001;**13**(1):13–8.
32. Keller M, Fendya D, Weber T. Glasgow Coma Scale predicts coagulopathy in paediatric trauma patients. *Semin Pediatr Surg* 2001;**10**(1):12–6.
33. Homer C, Kleinman L. Technical report: Minor head injury in children. *Pediatrics* 1999;**104**(6):1380.
34. Gruskin K, Schutzman S. Head trauma in children younger than 2 years: Are there predictors for complications? *Arch Pediatr Adolesc Med* 1999;**153**(1):15–20.
35. Schutzman S, Barnes P, Duhaime A-C, et al. Evaluation and management of children younger than two years old
with apparently minor head trauma: proposed guidelines. *Pediatrics* 2001;**107**:983–93.
36. Eleraky M, Theordore N, Adams M, et al. Paediatric cervical spine injuries; Report of 102 cases and review of the literature. *J Neurosurg (Spine 1)* 2000;**92**:12–7.
37. Hendey G, Wolfson A, Mower W, et al. Spinal cord injury without radiographic abnormality; Results of the national emergency X-ray utilization study in blunt cervical trauma. *J Trauma* 2002;**53**(1):1–4.
38. Schwartz D, Reisdorff E. *Emergency Radiology.* USA: McGraw-Hill; 2000.
39. Sledge J, Dain A, Hyman J. Use of magnetic resonance imaging in evaluating injuries to the paediatric thoracolumbar spine. *J Pediatr Orthop* 2001;**21**(3):288–93.
40. Hadley M. Management of paediatric cervical spine and spinal cord injuries. *Neurosurgery* 2002;**50**(3): S85–99.
41. Frank J, Lim C, Flynn J, et al. The efficacy of magnetic resonance imaging in paediatric cervical spine clearance. *Spine* 2002;**27**(11):1176–9.
42. Simon B, Letourmeau P, Vitorino E, et al. Paediatric minor head trauma: Indications for computed tomographic scanning revisited. *J Trauma* 2001;**51**(2):231–8.
43. Brenner D, Hall E. Computed Tomography – An increasing source of radiation exposure. *N Engl J Med* 2007;**357**:2277–84.
44. Mandera M, Wencel T, Bazowski P, et al. How should we manage children after mild head injury? *Childs Nerv Syst* 2000;**16**:156–60.
45. Ng S, Toh E, Sherrington C. Clinical predictors of abnormal computed tomography scans in paediatric head injury. *J Paediatr Child Health* 2002;**38**:388–92.
46. Batchelor J, McGuiness A. A meta-analysis of GCS 15 head injured patients with loss of consciousness or post traumatic amnesia. *Emerg Med J* 2002;**19**:515–9.
47. Simon B, Letourneau P, Vitorino E, et al. Pediatric minor head trauma: Indications for computed tomographic scanning revisited. *J Trauma* 2001;**51**(2):231–8.
48. Sainsbury C, Sibert J. How long do we need to observe head injuries in hospital? *Arch Dis Child* 1984;**59**:856–9.
49. Philip S, Udomphorn Y, Kirham F, et al. Cerebrovascular Pathophysiology in Pediatric Trauma Brain Injury. *J Trauma* 2009;**67**(2):S128–34.
50. Chiaretti A, De Benedictis R, Della Corte F, et al. The impact of initial management on the outcome of children with severe head injury. *Childs Nerv Syst* 2002;**18**:54–60.
51. Chiaretti A, Piastra M, Pulitano S, et al. Prognostic factors and outcome of children with severe head injury: An 8 year experience. *Childs Nerv Syst* 2002;**18**:129–36.
52. Ong L, Selladurai B, Dhillon M, et al. The prognostic value of the Glasgow Coma Scale, hypoxia and computerised tomography in outcome prediction of paediatric head injury. *Pediatr Neurosurg* 1996;**24**:285–91.
53. Skippen P, Seear M, Poskitt K, et al. Effect of hyperventilation on regional cerebral blood flow in head-injured children. *Crit Care Med* 1997;**25**(8):1402–9.
54. Traumatic Brain Injury Guidelines Taskforce. Hypotension. *J Neurotrauma* 2000;**17**(6/7):591–5.
55. Winchell R, Simons R, Hoyt D. Transient systolic hypotension. A serious problem in the management of head injury. *Arch Surg* 1996;**131**:533–9.
56. Kokoska E, Smith G, Pittman T, et al. Early hypotension worsens neurological outcome in paediatric patients with moderately severe head trauma. *J Pediatr Surg* 1998;**33**(2):333–8.
57. Banks C, Furyk J. Review article: Hypertonic saline use in the emergency department. *Emerg Med Australas* 2008;**20**:294–305.
59. Walker P, Harting M, Baumgartner J, et al. Modern approaches to pediatric brain injury therapy. *J Trauma* 2009;**67**(2):S120–7.
60. Peterson B, Khanna S, Fisher B, et al. Prolonged hypernatremia controls elevated intracranial pressure in head-injured paediatric patients. *Crit Care Med* 2000;**28**(4):1136–43.
61. Bratton S, Chestnut R, Ghajar J, et al. Hyperosmolar therapy. *J Neurotrauma* 2007;**24**:S14–20.
62. Ong L, Dhillon M, Selladurai B, et al. Early post-traumatic seizures in children: Clinical and radiological aspects of injury. *J Paediatr Child Health* 1996;**32**:173–6.
63. Ratan S, Kulshreshtha R, Pandey R. Predictors of posttraumatic convulsions in head injured children. *Pediatr Neurosurg* 1999;**30**:127–31.

TRAUMA IN CHILDREN

3

64. Chiaretti A, Benedictis R, Polidori G, et al. Early post-traumatic seizures in children with head injury. *Childs Nerv Syst* 2000;**16**:862–6.

65. Bratton S, Chestnut R, Ghajar J, et al. Antiseizure prophylaxis. *J Neurotrauma* 2007;**24**:S83–6.

66. Haltiner A, Newell D, Temkin N, et al. Side effects and mortality associated with use of phenytoin for early posttraumatic seizure prophylaxis. *J Neurosurg* 1999;**91**:588–92.

67. Bratton S, Chestnut R, Ghajar J, et al. Steroids. *J Neurotrauma* 2007;**24**:S91–5.

68. Alderson P, Roberts I. Corticosteroids for acute traumatic brain injury (review). *Cochrane Database Syst Rev* 2009;(4).

69. Roberts I. Aminosteroids for acute traumatic brain injury. *Cochrane Database Syst Rev* 2009;(4).

70. Sydenham E, Roberts I, et al. Hypothermia for traumatic brain injury. *Cochrane Database of Systematic Reviews* 2009;(4).

71. Hutchison J, Ward R, Lacroix J. Hypothermia: Therapy after traumatic brain injury in children. *N Engl J Med* 2009;**358**:2447–56.

72. Natale J, Joseph J, Helfaer M, et al. Early hyperthermia after traumatic brain injury in children; Risk factors, influence on length of stay, and effect on short-term neurologic status. *Crit Care Med* 2000;**28**(7):2608–15.

73. Hurlbert R. The role of steroids in acute spinal cord injury; An evidence-based analysis. *Spine* 2001;**26**(24 Suppl.): S39–46.

74. Canadian Association of Emergency Physician Position Statement. *Steroids in acute spinal cord injury.* www .caep.ca; 2003 [Revised 22 January 2003].

Further reading

Beattie T. Minor head injury. *Arch Dis Child* 1997;**77**:82–5.

Bratton S, Chestnut R, Ghajar J, et al. Hyperventilation. *J Neurotrauma* 2007;**24**:S87–90.

Bratton S, Chestnut R, Ghajar J, et al. Blood pressure and oxygenation. *J Neurotrauma* 2007;**24**:S7–13.

Davis R, Hughes M, Gubler D, et al. The use of cranial CT scans in the triage of paediatric patients with mild head injury. *Paediatrics* 1995;**95**(3):345–9.

Mitchell K, Fallat M, Raque G, et al. Evaluation of minor head injury in children. *J Pediatr Surg* 1994;**29**(7):851–4.

Smally A. Management of minor closed head injury in children. *Paediatrics* 2001;**107**(5):1231.

Temkin N, Dikmen S, Anderson G, et al. Valproate therapy for prevention of posttraumatic seizures: A randomised trial. *J Neurosurg* 1999;**91**:593–600.

Traumatic Brain Injury Guidelines Taskforce. Glasgow Coma Scale score. *J Neurotrauma* 2000;**17**(6/7):563–70.

Traumatic Brain Injury Guidelines Taskforce. Pupillary diameter and light reflex. *J Neurotrauma* 2000;**17**(6/7):583–90.

3.3 Thoracic injuries in childhood

Philip Aplin

ESSENTIALS

1 Thoracic injuries in children are common, are usually due to blunt trauma and are often associated with other injuries.

2 The pathophysiological differences in children depend principally on their age and size. These must be appreciated in order to optimise outcome.

3 The most common injuries are pulmonary contusions, rib fractures, pneumothoraces and haemothoraces. These can usually be managed by a combination of adequate oxygenation, IV fluids, thoracostomy tube drainage and analgesia.

4 Injuries to the aorta and diaphragm may be clinically occult and CXR findings are often non-specifically abnormal. Further diagnostic evaluation is always indicated in suspect cases.

5 Surgical intervention is uncommonly required, but is indicated in cases of massive haemothorax, cardiac tamponade, major airway and oesophageal injury, as well as in aortic and diaphragmatic injuries.

6 ED thoracotomy is principally indicated in cases of penetrating chest trauma and an arrest or pre-arrest presentation.

Introduction[1-4]

Traumatic injury is the most common cause of morbidity and mortality in childhood and thoracic injuries are secondary to head injuries as a cause of mortality. Isolated chest injuries have a mortality of around 5% but this increases substantially when combined with head and/or abdominal injury to as high as 20%. Injuries to the great vessels, bronchi, lung lacerations and cardiac tamponade are the chest injuries most likely to cause early death. Small children provide a small target in blunt trauma, so multiple injuries should be expected.

A recent review of an Australian trauma registry database found multiple body region injury to be almost universal (99%) in cases of severe blunt chest trauma. The most frequent associated serious injuries were head (46%), lower extremity (32%) and abdominopelvic injury (30%). By far and away the commonest chest injuries were pulmonary contusion, haemopneumothorax and rib fractures.

The common mechanisms of injury vary with the age of the child. Overall, the majority (60–80%) are due to blunt trauma and involve a motor vehicle in over half. In infants and toddlers common mechanisms include being injured as passengers in motor vehicle collisions (MVC) or as pedestrians struck or run over by a vehicle (commonly in the driveway of the family home). Falls (from stairs, balconies, etc.) occur mainly in this age group. Child abuse also tends to predominate in this age group and should always be considered. In school age children motor vehicle and bicycle related trauma is common and sporting (± extreme sports) injuries increase in frequency with age. With adolescence the occurrence of penetrating trauma emerges, with an associated increased mortality risk; also, inexperienced teenage drivers have an increased incidence of MVC. Drug and alcohol intoxication is often associated with personal/interpersonal violence in this older age group.

There are a number of anatomical and physiological features of small children that must be appreciated when managing

Table 3.3.1 Important pathophysiological differences between children and adults in chest trauma

- Small target – multiple injuries common
- Narrow airway – prone to obstruction
- Anterior larynx – difficult intubation
- Increased surface area – increased risk of hypothermia
- Increased oxygen consumption, diaphragmatic breathing, low functional residual capacity – prone to hypoxia
- Increased pliability of ribs – decreased incidence of rib fractures
- Response to blood loss – hypotension is a late sign of shock
- Developmental considerations – paediatric coma scoring

Table 3.3.2 Indications for operative intervention in chest trauma

- Great vessel injury
- Pericardial tamponade
- Large haemothoraces
- Tracheobronchial injuries
- Oesophageal injury
- Diaphragmatic lacerations
- Open pneumothorax with major chest wall defect
- Penetrating chest trauma that crosses the mediastinum

Once stabilised, thoracic CT scan may be indicated to further delineate the extent of pulmonary injury, evaluate the great vessels and detect pneumothoraces. Analgesia should be initiated early in appropriate doses.

paediatric chest trauma. These are summarised in Table 3.3.1.

Initial approach in the ED[5]

Initial management follows the usual priorities. After ensuring airway patency, breathing should be assessed. High-flow oxygen should be applied. Signs of respiratory compromise and tension pneumothorax should be managed by needle decompression prior to chest X-ray (CXR) followed by chest tube insertion. A large haemothorax may compromise ventilation as well as circulation, requiring early chest tube placement and fluid resuscitation, whilst an orogastric tube (OGT) should be placed early to decompress the stomach, as gastric distension may compromise ventilation. Mechanical ventilation should be instituted for signs of ongoing respiratory distress/respiratory failure not relieved by optimisation of oxygen delivery, chest tube insertion, closure of open chest wounds and OGT placement. Ongoing signs of circulatory compromise without evidence of blood loss should raise the possibility of cardiac tamponade and myocardial contusion in a child with chest injuries. A portable CXR should be the first radiological test ordered. FAST (focused abdominal scan in trauma) scanning should occur early in the resuscitation of a child, where available, and imaging of the pericardium should always be included to detect haemopericardium. The vast majority of chest injuries in childhood can be managed non-operatively. Drainage of pericardial blood may occasionally be performed in the emergency department (ED) in an unstable patient if operative intervention

is not immediately available. Other indications for operative intervention are listed in Table 3.3.2. CT imaging of the chest should be used selectively. It is indicated in high impact trauma and when multiple injuries are present or suspected, particularly severe head injury where there is a high likelihood of associated severe chest injury.

Chest wall injury[6]

Rib fractures

The elasticity and flexibility of the younger child's chest wall leads to a lower incidence of rib fractures. Significant underlying intrathoracic injury can occur in the absence of rib fractures. In the 0- to 3-year age group rib fractures should raise the concern of abuse: in one study 2/3 of 0–3-year-olds with rib fractures were victims of abuse, and a careful assessment of all aspects of the clinical presentation is mandatory. Radiological findings suggestive of abuse include: multiple fractures, fractures of varying ages and bilateral fractures. A bone scan is a more sensitive test in the setting of potential abuse.

Rib fractures in children are a marker of potential severe associated injuries. Multiple rib fractures (>1) increase the risk of severe intrathoracic injury, multiple injuries and mortality. Fracture of the first rib requires significant force, mandating a high degree of suspicion of associated injuries to the great vessels and the trachea.

Flail chest injuries are rare in children and clearly indicate serious injury, with reduced ventilatory effectiveness and associated lung contusions contributing to the significant potential for respiratory failure.

Assisted ventilation is indicated for those with respiratory failure despite optimal non-invasive ventilation and analgesia or associated injuries, particularly to the head.

Management of rib fractures involves analgesia, treatment of associated injuries, ongoing assessment of the child's respiratory status and close observation for complications that may arise. Analgesic options in the ED include oral paracetamol (also available intravenously (IV)) and anti-inflammatories, intranasal fentanyl and titrated IV narcotics. Prevention of atelectasis and pneumonia is a priority.

Pulmonary injury[7,8]

Contusion

In children it is important to appreciate that significant lung injury can occur in the absence of rib fractures or other external signs of chest wall injury. Pulmonary contusion most commonly results from blunt injury and requires significant force. Pathological findings are intra-alveolar haemorrhage, consolidation and oedema causing V/Q mismatch, reduced lung compliance and subsequent hypoxaemia. CXR findings of increased pulmonary opacity may be present in the ED but may evolve over time. Computerised tomography (CT) scanning of the thorax may reveal contusion that is not evident on the initial plain films. Approximately half of the CXRs showing pulmonary contusion show other abnormalities, most commonly fractured ribs and pneumo/haemothoraces.

Management of pulmonary contusion involves:

- Maintenance of oxygenation. Supplemental O_2 is initially delivered by high flow mask (10–15 L min^{-1}). Persisting hypoxaemia requires non-invasive or invasive ventilatory support depending on severity and associated injuries.
- Pain relief should be provided as indicated.
- Excessive intravenous fluids should be avoided.
- Respiratory physiotherapy is useful.

Both acute respiratory distress syndrome and pneumonia may complicate pulmonary contusion.

Pneumothorax[4,9]

Traumatic pneumothoraces vary in their size and clinical significance. They occur in about 1/3 of children with significant thoracic trauma and associated injuries are common. All pneumothoraces should be considered as having the potential to cause cardiorespiratory compromise. The clinical signs of pneumothorax (PTX) vary from nothing to decreased air entry, hyperresonance and subcutaneous emphysema.

Small to medium sized pneumothoraces may not be visible on a portable supine CXR. Ultrasound of the chest may be incorporated into the FAST scan protocol to detect pneumothoraces and haemothoraces. The sensitivity of ultrasound in detecting these complications of chest trauma is superior to supine CXR but CT scanning remains the gold standard. Subtle signs on CXR include increased radiolucency on the ipsilateral side and a deep sulcus sign. Small pneumothoraces are commonly revealed on CT scan of the chest and/or abdomen. The significance and hence management of these small pneumothoraces is debated. A small uncomplicated PTX in a stable patient with isolated chest trauma, who is not likely to require positive pressure ventilation or prolonged transport (particularly aeromedical), can be considered for observation, high-flow O_2 and analgesia in a high-dependency unit setting. Most other traumatic pneumothoraces require the insertion of a formal chest drain.

Tension pneumothorax

This is a clinical condition resulting from increasing intrathoracic pressure, lung collapse and mediastinal shift with subsequent impaired gas exchange, decreased venous return and cardiovascular collapse. The diagnosis is clinical and treatment should precede radiology in clear-cut cases. Signs are of ↓ air entry, hyperresonance and hyperexpansion plus ↓ movement of the affected side. The signs of tracheal deviation and elevation of the jugular venous pressure (JVP) may be difficult to detect in children who have short necks. JVP elevation may also be absent if there is associated hypovolaemia. Patients are always tachypnoeic with respiratory distress and tachycardia, but hypotension is a late sign if solely due to a tension PTX. Immediate needle decompression with a 16G cannula inserted into the 2nd intercostal space in the mid clavicular line should occur whilst preparing for formal intercostal tube insertion via a lateral approach.

However, hypotension and/or hypoxaemia may have other causes in the traumatised child. The differential diagnosis of a tension PTX includes: haemorrhage; pericardial tamponade; haemothorax (which may cause tension); pulmonary contusion; and air embolism. Common, easily preventable/treatable causes that may occasionally be confused with a tension PTX are intubation of the right main-stem bronchus and gastric distension. Endotracheal tubes (ETT) must be inserted the appropriate distance (age/2 + 12 cm) and movement of the child's neck minimised. This is particularly so in small children where neck flexion (tube pulled out) or extension (tube down the [R] main bronchus) may result in the malposition of the ETT. An orogastric tube should be placed early.

Open pneumothoraces may occur with penetrating chest trauma. Respiratory compromise relates to the effects of the PTX, underlying lung injury and a 'sucking chest wound' if the defect is large enough. If the diameter of the chest wound is approximately 2/3 or greater than that of the trachea, air will preferentially be sucked into the chest on inspiration, leading to acute severe respiratory compromise. Management requires urgent wound coverage on three sides only with an occlusive dressing, to prevent the development of an iatrogenic tension PTX, and chest tube placement away from the wound. Once the chest drain is in place the wound can be sealed and arrangements made for definitive surgical care. Significant ongoing respiratory distress is an indication for mechanical ventilation.

Pulmonary lacerations[5]

Pulmonary lacerations are principally caused by penetrating injuries but can occur with blunt mechanisms especially associated with rib fractures. They usually result in a haemothorax (sometimes massive) or PTX and rarely can be complicated by air embolism. Air embolism typically occurs after the initiation of positive pressure ventilation and causes sudden haemodynamic deterioration with or without focal neurological signs. Development of a tension PTX, pericardial tamponade or massive haemothorax are the main other possibilities in the chest for such a sudden deterioration. Lung hyperinflation due to overly aggressive positive pressure ventilation may also cause cardiorespiratory compromise and risk barotrauma.

In the setting of deterioration after initiation of ventilation, by far the most likely cause is the development of tension PTX, which should be managed as above. In the rare event of air embolism, if suspected, management includes 100% oxygen, and reduction of the ventilation pressures. Emergency thoracotomy with clamping of the hilum on the affected side and aspiration of ventricular air has occasionally been life saving.

Haemothorax[9,10]

Clinically relevant haemothoraces occur in about 15% of cases of blunt chest trauma but are more common if the injury is penetrating. The source of bleeding is most commonly from lacerations to the lung, intercostal or internal mammary vessels or occasionally from mediastinal vessel injury (often fatal). Each hemithorax can hold up to 40% of a child's blood volume.

The clinical presentation is of varying degrees of hypovolaemia and respiratory compromise depending on the amount of blood lost into the chest, associated pneumothorax and the development of increased intrathoracic pressure. Chest examination reveals reduced air entry and dullness to percussion ± signs of tension. Management is with a chest drain. Drainage of massive haemothoraces may precipitate further bleeding as the tamponade effect is removed.

Blood loss from the chest tube, haemodynamic response to resuscitation, mechanism of injury (blunt vs. penetrating) and associated injuries (especially head) are used by cardiothoracic surgeons in determining the need for thoracotomy.

Indications for thoracotomy include:

- initial drainage exceeding >15 mL kg^{-1} of estimated blood volume;
- continued bleeding greater than 1–2 mL kg^{-1} hr^{-1};
- increasing bleeding;
- significant residual haemothorax post-tube drainage.

Management involves oxygenation and ventilatory support if indicated, urgent chest tube placement of the appropriate size via the lateral approach directed posteriorly and volume resuscitation. The concept of hypovolaemic resuscitation in uncontrolled traumatic haemorrhage has not been evaluated in children. However, it is important to consider early surgical intervention in any patient who is haemodynamically compromised due to haemorrhage or showing signs of ongoing bleeding.

Longer-term complications of haemothoraces include haematoma organisation with secondary lung entrapment and empyema formation. Prophylactic antibiotics are indicated when chest tubes are placed for penetrating trauma. The adult trauma literature suggests a reduced infection rate even in previously closed traumatic haemothoraces requiring drainage.

Tracheobronchial injuries[10]

These uncommon injuries may occur with penetrating or severe blunt trauma and have a high mortality if not recognised and treated rapidly. In blunt trauma intrathoracic airway injuries usually occur near the origin of the main stem bronchi. Typically they present with respiratory distress and signs of subcutaneous (SC) emphysema, pneumomediastinum and a tension PTX. Haemoptysis also occurs. In the case of PTX urgent chest tube placement is required and typically a large air leak will continue and there will be failure of lung expansion on CXR. At this point an airway injury is usually considered. A second chest tube should be placed and urgent cardiothoracic surgical consultation obtained. Once stabilised, a CT scan may be helpful in further injury delineation and assessing lung inflation, as massive SC emphysema can make CXR interpretation very difficult. Bronchoscopy is useful as a diagnostic modality in suspected tracheobronchial injury and operative intervention is often required.

Mediastinal injury[5,9,10]

Aortic transection

Aortic rupture is a rare event in young children but the incidence increases with

Table 3.3.3	CXR signs of aortic injury

- Widened mediastinum (mediastinum to chest ratio >0.25)
- Loss or abnormal contour of aortic knob
- Depression of left mainstem bronchus
- Deviation of the trachea to the right
- Deviation of the oesophagus (NG or OG tube) to the right
- Left pleural cap
- Left haemothorax
- Upper rib fractures

NG, nasogastric; OG, orogastric.

adolescents involved in high speed MVCs. About 80% occur at the aortic isthmus just distal to the origin of the left subclavian artery. Most are rapidly fatal at the scene. Diagnosis in hospital depends on clinical suspicion based on mechanism of injury, physical signs (often absent) and CXR findings. CXR in cases of aortic rupture is usually abnormal but findings are non-specific (Table 3.3.3) and the suspicion of aortic injury on clinical or radiological grounds requires further diagnostic imaging.

In young children the normal thymic contour may give the impression of a widened mediastinum. Further imaging usually involves CT angiography, aortogram or transoesophageal echocardiography depending on availability, expertise and local practices. The absence of signs of dissection and mediastinal haematoma on CT angiography is used to exclude aortic injury. Occasionally, formal aortography or transoesophageal echocardiography will be performed to exclude possible aortic injury.

Management in confirmed cases is surgical. β-blockers may be commenced pre-operatively in haemodynamically stable patients to reduce vessel wall stress.

Cardiac injuries[11]

As with aortic injury, clinically significant cardiac injury from blunt trauma in children is uncommon and is usually associated with other intrathoracic injuries. Pericardial tamponade can certainly occur with blunt trauma, though it is more common in penetrating injuries (see below). Myocardial contusion may manifest as an arrhythmia or otherwise unexplained tachycardia and/or hypotension. Valvular injury and septal defects are also reported. Diagnosis suffers from the lack of a gold standard and the questionable clinical relevance of test

results. Most of the evidence comes from adult trauma patients. A normal ECG has a high negative predictive value for the occurrence of clinically significant complications in suspected myocardial contusion. Evidence for the value of cardiac markers is lacking. Echocardiography is a very useful modality in assessing suspected clinically significant myocardial contusion such as the presence of unexplained hypotension, tachycardia or new murmurs.

In the absence of ECG abnormalities, hypotension or new murmurs, ongoing ECG monitoring is usually not required.

Commotio cordis[12,13]

The phenomenon of sudden cardiac arrest following a localised blow to the chest is well documented in children. In these cases autopsy fails to identify myocardial contusion, structural cardiac abnormality, conduction system or coronary artery pathology. The proposed theory is that a blow to the chest during the vulnerable phase of the electrical cycle induces ventricular fibrillation/ventricular tachycardia. Protective chest guards are recommended in at-risk sports.

Penetrating cardiac trauma[14]

In children this occurs predominantly in the adolescent age group. Cardiac lacerations may lead to rapid exsanguination or pericardial tamponade. Any penetrating chest or upper abdominal wound has the potential to injure the heart. Clinical signs of tamponade include tachycardia and elevation of the JVP (in the absence of hypovolaemia), with subsequent hypotension and cardiac arrest with pulseless electrical activity. The CXR is typically normal in the absence of associated mediastinal or lung injury. In trained hands and with satisfactory imaging conditions echocardiography has excellent accuracy in the detection of pericardial blood and can be done rapidly in the emergency department (ED). Management requires urgent cardiothoracic surgical involvement. A conscious patient with a perfusing blood pressure requires urgent surgery. A rapidly deteriorating patient in the ED requires needle pericardiocentesis if there is any surgical delay. Cardiac arrest with vital signs present at the scene and a short transit time to hospital or arrest in the ED is an indication for ED thoracotomy or pericardiocentesis depending on the skills of personnel available. Pericardiocentesis is performed using a long 16 or 18G over the needle cannula via the subxiphoid approach at a 35 degree angle to the skin and aiming at the left shoulder with ECG monitoring. Ultrasound control may assist where available. Aspiration of 10–20 mL may result in significant clinical improvements. The needle should be removed but the catheter should remain in place for repeat aspirations. Failure to aspirate blood does not exclude tamponade as the cannula may miss the pericardium or the pericardial blood may have clotted.

Diaphragmatic injury[9,10,15]

Diaphragmatic injury is another uncommon paediatric injury, but it is important nonetheless, as undiagnosed, complications eventually will arise, though this may take years. Left-sided injury is more common than right-sided in blunt trauma and associated intra-abdominal injury is common.

Upper abdominal penetrating trauma that injures intrathoracic structures (and vice versa) must also have caused diaphragmatic injury and requires repair. Diagnosis is difficult unless CXR reveals clear signs of herniated stomach or bowel or the nasogastric tube curling up into the thorax. More commonly the CXR is non-specifically abnormal with findings of an abnormal diaphragmatic contour with or without lower zone opacity. Often the diagnosis is made at laparotomy or laparoscopy for associated injuries. Barium studies are normal if bowel contents are not herniated. CT scanning may miss small tears. Magnetic resonance imaging may have a role in diagnosing these injuries. Suspected occult diaphragmatic lacerations in penetrating trauma

can be investigated by laparoscopy/thoracoscopy or open operation.

Oesophageal injury[5]

This is essentially only seen in penetrating trauma and in these cases a high index of suspicion is required, as missed injuries cause inevitable serious morbidity and mortality. On initial CXR a finding of mediastinal air is an early clue. Over subsequent hours an evolving sepsis with pleural effusions and mediastinitis ensues. Conscious patients able to verbalise complain of chest and epigastric pain but this is difficult to interpret in the setting of other chest injuries. Suspicion of an oesophageal injury must be followed by a Gastrografin study, oesophagoscopy or both. If positive, broad-spectrum antibiotics and urgent surgery are required.

ED thoracotomy[14]

The only definite indication for thoracotomy in the ED is in the scenario of penetrating chest trauma with loss of vital signs shortly before arrival in the ED or during ED resuscitation, with the purpose of pericardial drainage, repairing penetrating injury to the heart or controlling bleeding from the hilum or lung. Open cardiac massage can also be performed as well as cross-clamping of the aorta. The universally poor outcome of blunt trauma patients who arrive at the ED with no vital signs/signs of life argues strongly against performing ED thoracotomy in these patients. Blunt thoracic trauma patients who deteriorate in the ED despite full resuscitation may occasionally survive following ED thoracotomy but in general these very unstable patients should go to the operating theatre if possible.

Controversies

❶ The use of intercostal catheters in small traumatic pneumothoraces is debated – especially with positive pressure ventilation. The maximum size that can safely be treated conservatively is not defined.

❷ The role of ED thoracotomy, in low volume centres (which includes all Australasian paediatric centres), is not known.

References

1. Peclet MH, Newman KD, Eichelberger MR, et al. Thoracic trauma in children: An indicator of increased mortality. *J Pediatr Surg* 1990;**25**:961–5.
2. Black TL, Snyder CL, Miller JP, et al. Significance of chest trauma in children. *South Med J* 1996;**89**:494–6.
3. Nakayama DK, Ramenofsky ML, Rowe MI. Chest injuries in children. *Ann Surg* 1989;**210**:770–5.
4. Samarsekara S, Mikocka-Walus A, Butt W, Cameron P. Epidemiology of major paediatric chest trauma. *J Paediatr Child Health* 2009;**45**:676–80.
5. Fleisher GR, Ludwig S. *Textbook of paediatric emergency medicine.* 4th ed. Philadelphia: Lippincott Williams & Wilkins; 2000. p. 1341–60.
6. Garcia VF, Gotschall CS, Eichelberger MR, et al. Rib fractures in children: A marker of severe trauma. *J Trauma* 1990;**30**:695–700.
7. Bonadio WA, Hellmich T. Post-traumatic pulmonary contusion in children. *Ann Emerg Med* 1989;**18**:1050–2.
8. Allen GS, Cox CS, Moore FA, et al. Pulmonary contusion: Are children different? *J Am Coll Surg* 1997;**185**:229–33.
9. Bliss D, Silen M. Paediatric thoracic trauma. *Crit Care Med* 2002;**30**:1–13.
10. Wesson DE. Thoracic injuries. In: O'Neill JA, editor. *Paediatric surgery.* 5th ed. St Louis: Mosby; 1998. p. 245–60.
11. Dowd MD, Krug S. Pediatric blunt cardiac injury: Epidemiology, clinical features and diagnosis. *J Trauma* 1996;**40**:1–12.
12. Cantor RM, Leaming JM. Evaluation and management of pediatric major trauma. *Emerg Med Clin North Am* 1998;**16**:229–56.
13. Maron BJ. Blunt impact to the chest leading to sudden cardiac death from cardiac arrest during sports activities. *N Engl J Med* 1995;**333**:337–42.
14. Polhgeers A, Ruddy RM. An update on pediatric trauma. *Emerg Med Clin North Am* 1995;**12**:267–87.
15. Jackimczyk K. Blunt chest trauma. *Emerg Med Clin North Am* 1993;**11**:81–91.

3.4 Abdominal and pelvic trauma

Scott Pearson

ESSENTIALS

1 Children may have significant internal injury with little evidence of external trauma. The abdominal viscera are less well protected by the musculature and rib cage.

2 Meticulous assessment and reassessment will detect subtle abdominal injuries and a change in physiological status due to blood loss.

3 Persistent tachycardia may be the only clue of intra-abdominal haemorrhage in the child without other overt source of bleeding.

4 Unrecognised abdominal trauma is an important cause of preventable trauma deaths in children.

5 Selective non-operative management of solid visceral injuries is common but requires institutional support and may necessitate transfer of the child to a regional centre.

6 Pelvic fractures are a marker of severe injury, and there is a strong association with head, abdominal, and chest trauma.

7 The treatment of children with significant abdominal or pelvic trauma requires a planned team approach and early liaison with a paediatric surgeon and paediatric tertiary centre.

8 CT scan is the investigation of choice in stable children with abdominal trauma in consultation with a paediatric surgeon. Some patients will be safely managed by careful serial abdominal examinations without the need for CT scanning.

Introduction

Well over 90% of abdominal injuries in children are the result of blunt trauma. While penetrating injuries are increasing in incidence in the adolescent population, this remains an unusual phenomenon in most Australasian communities. Abdominal injuries resulting from blunt trauma commonly affect the solid organs, particularly the liver and spleen. Overall mortality is generally <5%, but obviously this depends on injury mechanism.[1] In children with multitrauma, the subtle early clinical findings of intra-abdominal injury may be masked by change in conscious state, and chest and limb injuries, and require repeated abdominal examination.

There are unique characteristics of children that predispose them to intra-abdominal injuries. The rib cage does not extend as far distally as in the adult, the ribs are more compliant, and the abdominal wall and musculature frequently thinner and less protective. The organs are closely packed together and there is less 'padding' soft tissue to absorb the kinetic energy transmitted by the impact.[2] The upper abdominal viscera are more at risk of injury, and relatively minor forces can be transmitted, resulting in a serious disrupting injury.[3]

The bladder is not as well protected by the bony pelvis as in the adult, increasing the risk of bladder injury in lower abdominal trauma. Gaseous distension of the stomach from air swallowing during crying or bag–valve–mask ventilation occurs rapidly and can impair ventilation. Likewise, acute gastric dilatation or a large bladder can seriously impede clinical assessment of the abdomen. The very compliant body of the child is capable of absorbing considerable amounts of kinetic energy without external signs, yet be associated with significant internal derangement.[3] Children are generally healthy, with few comorbidities and on few, if any, medications. In physiological terms, they are therefore able to compensate extremely well for blood loss.[2]

Early surgical involvement in treating children with abdominal injury is vital to care in the emergency department. The child with multiple injuries requires senior experienced clinicians involved in decision making during the resuscitation. Because such a patient invariably requires the involvement of several specialties, a trauma team approach, with clear leadership of the resuscitation, is imperative.

History

Obtaining details of the exact mechanism of injury cannot be over-emphasised. This often gives a clue to the potential injury pattern. Information can be obtained from witnesses, ambulance officers, family, friends, or care-givers. One member of the trauma team should be delegated to obtain this information, so that the primary survey can occur simultaneously.

Mechanisms of injury in children include pedestrians struck by motor vehicles, falls, occupants of motor vehicles involved in crashes, bicycle-related injuries, contact sports, assaults, and abuse. Falls are the most common mechanism. The events leading to the fall, and fall height and surface are all pertinent information that can usually be obtained rapidly. Information such as the aspect of the child when struck and likely speed of vehicles is useful in predicting injury patterns. Likewise, factors such as the use of restraint devices, type used, and wearing of a bicycle helmet, where appropriate, are helpful in defining the resulting injuries. Lap belts can be associated with rib and lumbar spine fractures, and upper abdominal organ injuries. Handlebar injuries may cause serious blunt intra-abdominal injuries. The resultant injuries to pancreas and duodenum can be subtle and delay the diagnosis. Hence the threshold for observation or imaging may need to be varied accordingly in children presenting with this mechanism of injury.

Small children are particularly at risk of being unsighted and backed over in driveways by reversing vehicles, and may sustain major internal injuries. The recognition of abuse as a causal mechanism in younger children and infants is important in patients with abdominal trauma. There may be minimal signs of external injury, and the reported history may suggest a minor incompatible mechanism or no history of injury at all. The emergency physician needs to maintain an index of suspicion in the infant who presents in shock or with an altered level of consciousness (see Chapter 3.2).

Other information, such as medications, allergies, and significant past history, should be obtained.

Examination

Primary survey focuses on the ABCs and may result in early interventions such as intubation or treatment of shock. The examination of the abdomen is usually delayed until the secondary survey. Where endotracheal intubation has already occurred, this invariably involves chemical sedation and paralysis. The information obtained by palpation of the abdomen in this situation is somewhat limited, and these children often require abdominal computerised tomography (CT) scanning, provided their vital signs are satisfactory and not deteriorating.

Vital signs are essential, particularly the respiratory rate, pulse rate, non-invasive blood pressure, and oxygen saturations. Attention should be given to the child's peripheral perfusion to detect early hypovolaemia and treat prior to the occurrence of hypotension. The blood pressure needs to be measured with an appropriately sized cuff for the child's habitus. Automated blood pressure machines, while useful in freeing staff to attend to other aspects of care, can be unreliable when hypotension exists and can result in delays in obtaining these recordings. Single vital sign recordings are of limited use, but it is the progression of recordings and the monitoring of perfusion that more accurately reflect volaemic state. In the critically ill child, pulse and blood pressure should be measured at 3–5-minute intervals.

The use of the terms *unstable* and *stable* is discouraged when conveying information regarding the child's status to colleagues. They are non-specific and are defined differently by individual practitioners. It is more useful, when relaying the circulatory status of a child, to convey the actual vital signs, progression over time, and response to fluid to indicate volaemic state. Other parameters, such as capillary refill time, have some limitations but can add to the assessment.

In children with less severe trauma, the technique of abdominal examination is important to reliably exclude significant intra-abdominal injury clinically. Where physical examination is to be relied on as the major indicator of abdominal injury, it should ideally be performed regularly by the same observer. With serial examination and vigilance to vital signs, changes are detected early and appropriate management implemented. The aim of the abdominal examination is to elicit physical signs, such as tenderness, rebound, guarding, or rigidity, which may require evaluation by CT scanning.

Pain from injuries and other distress all add to the difficulty of abdominal assessment. Judicious and early use of parenteral opiates is safe, decreases a child's distress, and allows a more accurate clinical assessment. Abdominal examination must be performed by gentle palpation with warm hands. There should be a brief but careful visual assessment of the abdominal wall for the distribution of any penetrating wounds, bruising, or marks (e.g. seat belt or handlebar). The presence of these warrants a prolonged observation period by admission, even for the child with no other positive findings.

Gastric dilatation may greatly impede examination as well as impair ventilation. Insertion of a nasogastric tube may facilitate examination by decompressing the stomach, while also reducing the risk of aspiration and improving diaphragmatic excursion. Aspiration of blood from the nasogastric tube usually signifies the presence of a significant intra-abdominal injury. A persistently distended abdomen after nasogastric tube insertion may signify intra-abdominal bleeding.

Information from clinical examination can usually be obtained by gentle palpation with occasional use of percussion tenderness. This technique is acceptable in children

with minor trauma who require careful re-examination. Auscultation of the abdomen has limited usefulness. Rectal and vaginal examinations are rarely indicated in the child with minor abdominal trauma.

In the child with only minor injuries, the way the child moves around the emergency trolley or walks can be a useful screening tool as to whether intra-abdominal injury exists.

Investigations

Laboratory

Blood should be taken for group and hold, full blood examination (FBE), liver function tests, amylase, and blood glucose. Urine should be obtained for examination. Some studies have demonstrated that elevated transaminases in combination with an abnormal physical examination are associated with intra-abdominal injury (although not a specific organ injury).[4,5] However, at present there are no laboratory studies that can be recommended as a screening tool for intra-abdominal injury.

In the context of pancreatic injury, serum amylase often rises, but the initial amylase may be normal, with increasing values over 3 days.[6]

Focused assessment by sonography for trauma (FAST)

Ultrasound has been promoted as a quick and effective initial screening tool in the evaluation of the abdomen in the traumatised child.[7–10] Ultrasound in this setting is aimed at the detection of free fluid in the peritoneal cavity. No attempt is made during this rapid assessment to identify solid visceral injury. This examination takes between 3 and 5 minutes, and can be achieved at the bedside in the resuscitation area. While there is much supportive literature for this modality,[7–9] there is also some cautionary research.[10] Detractors cite concerns of low sensitivities in the detection of free fluid; however, several studies have documented sensitivities from 89 to 100%. Providing the limitations of FAST are appreciated, it remains an invaluable tool, particularly in the assessment of the multiply injured child. Identification of free fluid in the stable child with normal vital signs should be followed by CT examination. The detection of free fluid in the child with deteriorating vital signs supports the decision for operative treatment. FAST ultrasound is operator-dependent and should be performed only by clinicians with appropriate training and credentialing.

CT scan

This is the investigation of choice in stable children with abdominal trauma in consultation with a paediatric surgeon. With the evolution and common acceptance of non-operative management of blunt abdominal injuries, diagnostic imaging is an essential component of the assessment process of the injured child. CT has emerged as the gold standard.[11] It identifies free intra-abdominal fluid, solid visceral injury and the injury configuration, and loops of bowel, and demonstrates free peritoneal gas. The retroperitoneum is well visualised. CT examination should be performed after the administration of intravenous contrast. This enables better visualisation, although in situations of renal hypoperfusion renal failure can be precipitated, and allergy to the contrast is a rare but potentially serious problem. The addition of oral contrast may increase diagnostic accuracy in detecting duodenal or pancreatic injury but this is controversial and institutional practice may vary.

CT scanning carries a radiation risk to the child. This needs to be considered when ordering such an investigation. CT scanning should be reserved for those patients in whom there is a high index of suspicion of intra-abdominal injury. Literature is now emerging that addresses the use of CT scanning in children.[12]

Formal ultrasound

A detailed upper and lower abdominal ultrasound examination takes longer to perform and is more observer-dependent than CT examination. Abdominal distension caused by ileus and luminal distension, and the presence of abdominal tenderness in the child, can make ultrasound examination more difficult. Hence there is little role for ultrasound in the definitive diagnosis of abdominal trauma, except when CT scan is unavailable.

General management

The assessment begins with primary survey and any life-saving interventions, while historical details are obtained simultaneously. Oxygen should be administered and vital signs monitored regularly. Vascular access is obtained early and appropriate blood samples for blood cross-matching, haematology, and biochemistry. Where there is delay in obtaining venous access, intraosseous access remains an effective method of resuscitation. Trauma series films of chest, pelvis, and lateral cervical spine should be obtained, when indicated, during the resuscitation. Views of thoracic and lumbar spine may also be required if indicated on mechanism or clinical findings. In the severely injured child, CT scanning may provide much of this information.

The abdominal examination is usually reserved until the secondary survey. Attention should be exercised to ensure that the child is warm to prevent the development of hypothermia during resuscitation.

Fluid therapy should begin with 20 mL kg^{-1} of warmed crystalloid (normal saline) and repeated if required. If further fluid therapy is required after two crystalloid boluses, blood should be used in volumes of 10 mL kg^{-1}. The rapidity of blood loss may rarely dictate the use of O-negative or group-specific blood rather than waiting for full cross-matched blood.

Early consideration of gastric decompression with a nasogastric tube assists abdominal assessment and aids ventilation. The insertion of a urinary catheter may be necessary, depending on the requirement to aid haemodynamic monitoring of fluid resuscitation and to detect haematuria. Perineal haematoma and blood at the external urethral meatus are contraindications to routine catheter insertion and mandate retrograde urethrogram or cystogram to assess the urethral integrity. In this situation, surgical opinion should be sought.

FAST ultrasound, when available, can be performed, often within the first 20 minutes of the patient's arrival, and may or may not show evidence of free fluid. Ongoing management is usually dictated by the haemodynamic response of the child to fluid resuscitation. CT examination is ideal but may not be possible in a very small number of exsanguinating children with deteriorating vital signs despite fluid resuscitation. In this situation, early surgical consultation regarding urgent laparotomy is required.

Surgical issues

Selective non-operative management of solid visceral injury in children is now well established. It is clear that bleeding from an injured spleen, liver, or kidney is generally self-limiting.[11] Success rates in excess of 90% with non-operative care mean that operative management is an exceptional event at many institutions. Pancreatic injuries, however, usually result in a higher incidence of operative intervention. Operative management is the rule for hollow viscus injuries. Some injuries, such as duodenal haematoma without evidence of perforation, may be managed without surgery. The decision about operative versus non-operative management is made by the surgeon who will have ongoing care of the child. This decision is strongly influenced by clear details regarding progression of vital signs, response to fluid therapy, and associated injuries. A non-operative approach must take place only in an institution with an available surgeon with a commitment to the injured child and dedicated paediatric intensive care or high-dependency facility.[13] This may necessitate the transfer of the child to a regional centre.

Penetrating trauma

Penetrating abdominal injury in a child usually requires exploration by laparoscopy or laparotomy. Because the abdominal wall is often thinner than in adults, penetration into the peritoneal cavity occurs more readily. A careful assessment, including a log roll for back examination, to exclude other injuries, is necessary. Gunshot wounds should be explored in theatre. The approach to initial resuscitation is identical to that for blunt trauma. An erect chest X-ray or lateral decubitus film helps to identify the presence of free air.

Pelvic fractures

A child who sustains a fractured pelvis has been exposed to severe trauma. These are uncommon injuries in children, occurring at half the frequency as in adults.[14] There are several major differences in the bony pelvis between the child and adolescent or the adult. There is greater elasticity in the sacro-iliac joints and pubic symphysis, and plasticity of the bone, in the paediatric pelvis, therefore greater amounts of kinetic energy must be involved to cause fracture. Avulsion fractures occur in children and adolescents because cartilage is weaker than bone. This occurs at the physis. Greater laxity of the joints in the paediatric pelvis means that single fractures occur more commonly, as opposed to the adult pelvis, where there is the double-break concept. Fractures occurring through epiphyseal and apophyseal growth centres may result in growth arrest, leg length discrepancy, and deformity. Children also have increased capacity for remodelling.[15]

The common mechanisms for pelvic fracture are motor vehicle accidents and motor vehicle-pedestrian collisions, followed by falls.[15]

There are several classification systems for pelvic fractures. None is ideal. Torode and Zeig described four groups of pelvic fracture but failed to include isolated acetabular fractures.[16] This has been modified by Silber et al,[15] whose classification by mechanism of injury and description is useful (Table 3.4.1).

Associated injuries increase in frequency with the increasing severity of fracture type. Other skeletal injuries are common, followed by head, abdominal, and pulmonary injuries. In one large series, 19% of the total group had visceral injures. Therefore, when a pelvic fracture is identified on initial X-ray, a thorough search for other injuries must be undertaken. The management of those other injuries usually takes priority over the pelvic fracture management.

Bladder injury, while more common than in the adult, is an infrequent association. In a review of 166 children with pelvic fractures, there was one urethral disruption and two bladder contusions.[15] There is a strong association of these injuries with straddle-type mechanism. Children commonly receive 'fall astride' injuries related to playground equipment or while riding bicycles.

In Silber's series, 97% of children were treated non-operatively.[15] The majority of these injuries (63%) were type 3 fractures. The remainder were type 2 (17%) and type 4 fractures (17%). In this series, six children died; all these deaths were due to associated injuries. The mortality rate from paediatric pelvic fractures is consistently less than 6% in recent studies.[14] In a study comparing paediatric and adult fractures, the mortality rate for children was 5.7% compared with 17.5 % in the adult group. Vascular injury and exsanguination in children is rare, in contrast to in adults. This is thought to be due to the greater skeletal flexibility and the greater ability of paediatric arteries to constrict after injury.

In those children in whom blood loss is significant, early involvement of an orthopaedic surgeon and interventional radiologist is essential to optimise management. External fixation and angiography have both been used successfully, particularly in adolescent children.

Disposition

Almost all children with significant abdominal or pelvic injury require admission from the emergency department. The nature and severity of the injuries and intended management determine the most appropriate location for this to occur. Surgical colleagues involved in the ongoing care of the child should have input into this decision.

Younger children who have experienced a significant mechanism of injury (e.g. fall from great height, high-velocity motor vehicle crashes, pedestrian hit, or run over by motor vehicle) but who are apparently injury-free or have only minor injuries should also be admitted for observation (for 12–24 hours). Abdominal injuries in young children may initially have minimal or subtle signs, which become more apparent after observation and serial examination. Because of the plasticity of the paediatric skeleton, significant internal derangement can occur without obvious external evidence of trauma.

Controversies

❶ The necessity to use double contrast for CT abdominal examinations. IV contrast is required, but the need for oral contrast is controversial.

❷ Defining the haemodynamically unstable child. When in doubt, discuss the child with an emergency or surgical colleague. Children can be profoundly hypovolaemic with normal vital signs or only tachycardia. Ongoing fluid requirements and indices of peripheral perfusion are important indicators of volaemic status.

❸ There is debate about which subset of blunt abdominal trauma patients can be safely managed with serial examination and without CT scanning.

In the older child, however, it may be appropriate to discharge the patient who is injury-free or has only minor injuries. This should occur after several assessments while in the emergency department and with arrangements for follow up with a medical practitioner within 24 hours. Parents should be instructed to return earlier should a

Table 3.4.1	Classification of paediatric pelvic fractures	
Type	Mechanism	Description
1	Avulsion	Separation through or adjacent to an apophysis
2	Lateral compression	Iliac wing fractures
3	Anteroposterior compression (usually)	Simple ring fractures: • isolated pubic rami fractures • disruption of the pubis symphysis without disruption of the sacroiliac joint • isolated acetabular fractures
4	Anteroposterior compression (usually)	Ring disruption fractures: • fracture (or diastasis) of both anterior and posterior structures • pelvic fracture with an acetabular fracture • straddle fracture: bilateral superior and inferior pubic rami fractures

Originally described by Torode and Zeig[16] and modified by Silber et al.[15]

child's symptoms change. In general, children with ongoing abdominal pain after trauma should not be discharged, regardless of negative imaging results.

References

1. Stafford PW, Blinman TA, Nance ML. Practical points in evaluation and resuscitation of the injured child. *Surg Clin North Am* 2002;**82**:273–301.
2. Gaines BA. Intra-abdominal solid organ injury in children: diagnosis and treatment. *J Trauma* 2009;**67**(2): S135–9.
3. Tepas JJ. Paediatric trauma. In: Moore EE, Mattox KL, Feliciano DV, editors. *Trauma*. 4th ed. New York: McGraw-Hill Education; 2003. p. 1075–98.
4. Holmes JF, Sokelove PE, Brant WE. Identification of children with intra-abdominal injuries after blunt trauma. *Ann Emerg Med* 2002;**39**:500–509.
5. Cotton BA, Liao JG, Burd RS. The utility of clinical and laboratory data for detecting intraabdominal injury among children. *J Trauma* 2004;**56**:1068–74.
6. Sjovall A, Hirsh K. Blunt abdominal trauma in children: Risks of nonoperative treatment. *J Pediatr Surg* 1997;**32**:1169–74.
7. Akgur FM, Aktug T, Olguner M, et al. Prospective study investigating routine usage of ultrasonography as the initial diagnostic modality for the evaluation of children sustaining blunt abdominal trauma. *J Trauma* 1997;**42**:626–8.
8. Thourani VH, Pettitt BJ, Schmidt JA, et al. Validation of surgeon-performed emergency abdominal ultrasonography in pediatric trauma patients. *J Pediatr Surg* 1998;**33**:322–8.
9. Corbett SW, Andrews HG, Baker EM, et al. ED evaluation of the pediatric trauma patient by ultrasonography. *Am J Emerg Med* 2000;**18**:244–9.
10. Coley BD, Mutabagani KH, Martin LC, et al. Focused abdominal sonography for trauma (FAST) in children with blunt trauma. *J Trauma* 2000;**48**:902–6.
11. Eppich WJ, Zonfrillo MR. Emergency department evaluation and management of blunt abdominal trauma in children. *Curr Opin Pediatr* 2007;**19**:265–9.
12. Rice HE, Frush DP, Farmer D, Waldhausen JH. APSA Education Committee. Review of radiation risks from computed tomography: essentials for the pediatric surgeon. *J Pediatr Surg* 2007;**42**:603–7.
13. Advanced Life Support Group. *Advanced Paediatric Life Support Manual*. 3rd ed. London: BMJ Books; 2001.
14. Ismail N, Bellemare JF, Mollitt DL, et al. Death from pelvic fracture: Children are different. *J Pediatr Surg* 1996;**31**:82–5.
15. Silber JS, Flynn JM, Koffler KM, et al. Analysis of the cause, classification and associated injuries of 166 consecutive pediatric pelvic fractures. *J Pediatr Surg* 2001;**21**:446–50.
16. Torode I, Zeig D. Pelvic fractures in children. *J Pediatr Surg* 1985;**5**:76–84.

3.5 Burns

Peter L.J. Barnett

ESSENTIALS

1 Burns are one of the leading causes of injury in children in Australia.

2 The definitive assessment of the 'depth' of the burn may be difficult early on, as the appearance can evolve during the first 24–48 hours.

3 The calculated amount of fluid (burn-deficient plus maintenance) to be replaced in 24 hours is only a guide and should be adjusted according to the child's haemodynamic response.

4 Children with major or complicated burns should be treated in a paediatric burns unit.

5 Consider non-accidental injury if the presentation is delayed or if the history given is inconsistent with the burn sustained.

6 Electrical injuries are more commonly seen in two age groups: toddlers within the home setting and male adolescents involved in risk-taking behaviour. High-voltage exposures have a more serious outcome, as they are more likely to be associated with injury to internal structures.

Introduction

Burns sustained by children are a common presentation to emergency departments and often cause significant distress to both the child and the parents. The mortality is increased in younger children. Deaths are generally related to flame burns, which may be complicated by inhalation of smoke and other toxic gases (e.g. in house fires). Early fatalities are related to respiratory complications, whereas late deaths are usually related to infection. The use of early debridement and skin grafting has led to an increased survival rate in patients who would previously have died because of infection.

Most burns are fortunately less serious, resulting mainly from scalds. These commonly occur in pre–school-aged children due to their inquisitive nature precipitating accidents in the home. Flame burns occur in older children often experimenting with inflammables. Chemical and electrical burns are uncommon. One must be alert to the possibility of burns presenting as a manifestation of non-accidental injury in a young child.

Several preventive strategies can help decrease the risk and degree of burns sustained, especially with thermal burns. Lowering the temperature of hot water heaters to a maximum of 50°C significantly increases the contact time needed to produce deep or full-thickness burns. Flame-resistant clothing and smoke detectors in homes have saved many lives. Spill-proof mugs, guards around wood fire stoves, and child-resistant taps have all been shown to prevent burns. Further prevention strategies will have a far bigger impact on burns than advances in burn management.

Pathophysiology

The skin is the largest organ in the body, and its functions include:

- preventing heat loss to the environment, thus regulating the body's temperature;
- preserving body fluids by preventing water loss from the body;
- acting as a barrier to infective organisms.

Therefore children with extensive burns have difficulty retaining fluid and regulating temperature, and are at risk of infection.

The skin is composed of two main layers.

❶ *Epidermis*: composed of stratified squamous epithelium, which is largely non-viable. It acts as the barrier to infectious agents as well as preventing fluid loss from the body.

❷ *Dermis*: contains the epithelial adnexal structures, e.g. hair follicles, sweat glands, and neural receptors for pain and pressure. It also contains blood vessels, which contribute to temperature regulation of the body via radiant heat loss.

After a burn, injury to the deeper specialised epithelial cells prompts a change into stratified squamous epithelium. These cells proliferate, gradually covering the burn with a non-epithelial barrier. Therefore, if the dermal structures are damaged, skin grafting is the only means to cover the skin. When these deeper layers are involved, scarring results and contractures may occur.

The depth of the burn will depend on the temperature of the substance in contact with the skin, the length of time the substance is in contact with the skin, and the extent of subsequent cooling of the burned skin area. Hypothermia due to cooling occurs quickly in children due to their higher surface area to weight ratio, compared to adults. Also, children have thinner skin, which leads to deeper burns for a given contact temperature and duration.

Classification

Burns are generally classified into superficial, partial thickness or full thickness. Previous nomenclature (first, second, and third degree) has been replaced to give a more accurate description of the burn. In the emergency department setting, the definitive assessment of the 'depth' of the burn may be difficult, as the appearance can evolve during the first 24–48 hours. Likewise, the burn is not generally uniform in depth, and it may take time to delineate between superficial and deeper areas. Superficial and partial-thickness burns are the most common burns seen in children.

Superficial

Superficial burns generally involve only the epidermal layer. These are commonly seen resulting from sunburn or minor scalds.

Blistering does not occur immediately but may over the next few days. The pain and swelling generally last only a few days. The skin is erythematous and blanches normally. The epidermis will often peel within 3–7 days and is completely healed by 7–10 days, without scarring.

Partial thickness

Partial-thickness burns occur when the whole epidermis is involved and part of the dermis. The more of the dermis that is involved, the increased scarring potential.

Superficial partial-thickness burns involve the papillary layer of the dermis and are characterised by erythema with blistering. The blisters may remain intact and later burst due to an external pressure. The skin underlying the blister has a pink or red colour and moist appearance. These burns are extremely painful, as the nerve endings are exposed. The deeper the burn, the slower the healing process. Generally, superficial partial-thickness burns heal in 2–3 weeks.

Deep partial-thickness burns involve the reticular layer of the dermis. They may be less painful than their more superficial counterpart, due to oedema lessening the exposure of the nerve endings. They are a paler colour with a speckled appearance due to thrombosed superficial vessels. The skin is non-blanching. It may initially be difficult to distinguish between full- and deep partial-thickness burns. Deep partial-thickness burns generally heal after 3–6 weeks. Scarring is common, and skin grafting is sometimes necessary.

Full thickness

Full-thickness burns generally occur after flame burns or after prolonged contact with a hot surface. Other causes include hot oil, prolonged immersion, or chemical burns. They involve the epidermis and all the dermis, including epidermal appendages. They have either a dry, hard, white, leathery appearance or may be black in colour. They usually have no sensation because the nerve endings have been destroyed, and pain is due to more superficial burns on the edge of the full-thickness burn. Full-thickness burns are able to heal only from skin regrowth from the edge of the burn, which causes scarring. Therefore most will require skin grafting.

All significant burns will become colonised with bacteria. Heat causes coagulation of tissue, which leads to oedema and non-viable skin. This will potentially become a rich source of nourishment for bacteria. Adequate debridement is required to reduce the risk of infection. Infection will increase the depth of skin damage and thus the degree of scarring.

The location of the burn is also important regarding potential scarring, contracture, and caring for the acute burn. Facial, hand, foot, and perineal burns may be difficult to dress. Hence the part of the body involved by the burn will influence whether inpatient or specialist care is required.

History

The history is generally obtained from the parent to clarify events. Ambulance officers may have important additional information. It is important to know the substance and estimated temperature of the substance that caused the burn (e.g. hot cup of tea, cooking oil, flame), and the duration of contact with skin (e.g. was the patient clothed at the time, in what, and for how long?).

With flame burns, was the patient trapped in an enclosed space, therefore at risk of inhalation problems, or was there any loss of consciousness? These features may suggest inhalation issues such as carbon monoxide poisoning. The historical information may determine the potential for associated injuries resulting from falls or explosions.

Non-accidental injury should be considered if the presentation is delayed or where the history given is inconsistent with the burn sustained or if the burn has distinctive distribution (e.g. glove and stocking). Past medical history and immunisation status, particularly for tetanus, should also be obtained (see Chapter 1.1).

Examination

Note that children who are distressed may require the provision of immediate appropriate analgesia at the outset to aid examination.

Primary survey

The initial assessment of the child should be directed to the presence of any features that suggest potential airway involvement. These include singed nasal hairs or eyebrow hairs, oral or facial burns, coughing up carbonaceous sputum, barking cough, altered voice, stridor, wheeze, or respiratory distress. Airway compromise (upper or lower) may have an insidious onset, so frequent re-examination of the child is vital during the first 12–24 hours. If stridor or hoarse voice is present, this indicates upper airway involvement, and early intubation is required prior to evolving oedema causing total airway obstruction. Delayed intubation in this setting can be increasingly hazardous due to distortion of the normal laryngeal anatomy. Scalds to the face rarely cause airway compromise, unless the child has ingested hot liquids.

The circulation status should be assessed next. Hypovolaemia resulting from third-space fluid loss will not occur for a few hours after a severe burn. Therefore, if early-onset cardiovascular instability is present, then an alternative explanation, such as bleeding, should be sought. The peripheral perfusion of limbs should be assessed where circumferential burns are apparent. Comparing the pulse wave forms of various digits on the limb using a saturation oximeter may assist this in questionable instances.

Evaluation of burn area

The extent and depth of the burn should be assessed after the patient has been stabilised. This is usually done from a body chart (Fig. 3.5.1), which can be useful to aid documentation of the burn. This chart is used because the surface area involved will alter depending on the age of the child and the parts of the body where the burn is located. A simple method, using the palmar surface of the child's hand and fingers, can also be used to estimate the area of burn. This correlates to approximately 1% of the child's total surface area. The adult formula using the 'rule of nines' can be used in adolescents older than 15 years.

Investigations

Patients who require intravenous resuscitation should have a baseline full blood count, electrolytes, creatinine and urea, and blood group and hold performed. In severe burns, replacement with blood, protein, and electrolyte may be necessary. Carboxyhaemoglobin levels should be obtained in patients with inhalation burns and extrapolated to the time of injury. A level of >15% on arrival in emergency suggests significant smoke inhalation. Urine output should be monitored in severe burns, both to guide adequacy of resuscitation and also to screen for presence of myoglobin.

Oxygen saturation monitoring and arterial blood gases (when indicated) aid clinical assessment of respiratory involvement. A chest X-ray should also be obtained if inhalation burns are suspected. Inhalation burns will evolve over time, and the initial film may be normal. The early appearance of X-ray changes generally indicates a more severe pulmonary injury.

Management

Prehospital

The main aims of prehospital care are stabilising ABCs, preventing ongoing burn injury, provision of analgesia, covering the area involved, and rapid transfer to an emergency department.

The first priority in any burn is to assess and stabilise the airway and breathing. Oxygen should be administered where there is suspected carbon monoxide poisoning with inhalation burns. Circulation is generally not a problem in the first hour after a major burn, and rapid transport to hospital should occur. If transfer time is greater than 1 hour, and the burn is greater than 20%, then intravenous fluid replacement should begin en route where possible.

The burns should be covered with water-soaked sterile cloth or the newer tea tree oil soaked pads. Excessive cooling of major burns causes hypothermia and worsens the patient's outcome. Recently sustained minor burns should be cooled under running water for at least 20 minutes. This acts to minimise the extent of the burn and also affords some pain relief.

Analgesia is generally required early, and a single dose of a narcotic (e.g. fentanyl 1.5–2 mcg kg^{-1} intranasally) is a good choice in burns less than 20%. Greater than 20%, then intravenous access should be obtained and analgesia titrated to responses as well as administering intravenous fluids.

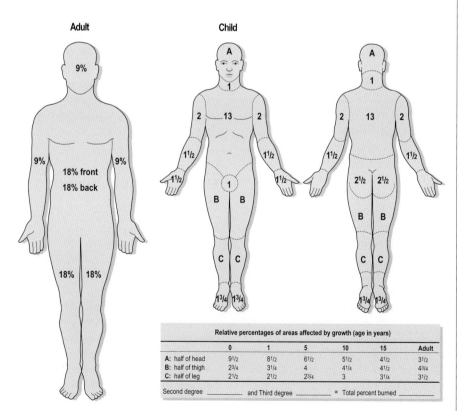

Fig. 3.5.1 Lund Browder chart for estimation of percentage size of burn.

Relative percentages of areas affected by growth (age in years)						
	0	1	5	10	15	Adult
A: half of head	9½	8½	6½	5½	4½	3½
B: half of thigh	2¾	3¼	4	4¼	4½	4¾
C: half of leg	2½	2½	2¾	3	3¼	3½
Second degree _____ and Third degree _____ = Total percent burned _____						

If electrical injury has been sustained, then cardiac monitoring should occur during transfer. Patients with chemical burns should undergo extensive washing of the affected area before transport.

Emergency department

The initial priority should focus on stabilisation of airway, breathing, and circulation, with concurrent provision of analgesia. If airway burns are suspected, then early intubation should be considered. Patients with obvious stridor due to upper airway compromise require urgent intubation. Supplemental oxygen should be instituted and oxygen saturation monitored.

Other potential indications for ventilation in major burns include:

- Extensive burns (>60–70%), to decrease the patient's work of breathing.
- Full-thickness circumferential chest burns, which may compromise chest expansion.
- Severe inhalational lung injury causing pulmonary oedema and hypoxaemia. Inhalation burns generally get worse in the first 12–24 hours, and ventilation may be needed during this time. Early consultation with paediatric intensive care colleagues in these instances is appropriate.

The fluid losses due to the burn itself do not cause early circulatory failure, and other contributing injuries should be sought in the patient with early shock. It is also important to note the time the patient is evaluated, relative to the time of the burn. Children who have delay (e.g. a few hours) in presentation may arrive with circulatory compromise from skin fluid losses.

Intravenous access should be placed in all children with burns body surface area (BSA) of >20%. Fluid resuscitation rates should be calculated using the time of the burn, not the time of presenting to the emergency department (see Fluid resuscitation, below). Peripheral venous access, preferably through non-burnt skin, is preferred over central venous access for the initial resuscitation. Monitoring of urinary output (via urinary catheter, weighing nappies) is important in determining the adequacy of fluid replacement. A nasogastric tube should also be inserted in children with severe burns, as gastric dilatation can occur, leading to respiratory compromise.

Analgesia should be given early, during the stabilisation of the A, B and C. Intranasal fentanyl (1.5–2 mcg kg^{-1}) is a good first up treatment. In severe burns, a morphine infusion should be started after adequate initial intravenous or intranasal analgesia has been given. Large doses of narcotics are sometimes needed in severe burns to control the pain. Intramuscular morphine is now obsolete given the use of intranasal fentanyl.

A careful secondary survey should then be undertaken, looking at the extent, depth, and anatomical relevance of the burns. It is important to determine if there are any circumferential burns to limbs and chest. In superficial or partial thickness burns, careful monitoring of circulation or ventilatory compromise is required. In full-thickness circumferential burns, an urgent escharotomy may be required to restore circulation to the limb or allow for adequate ventilation. A paediatric burn specialist should be consulted in this situation.

The secondary survey should also include careful examination for any other injuries requiring attention (e.g. head, neck, chest, limbs, pelvis, intra-abdominal). Burns to the face should also include fluorescein staining of the eyes to check for corneal involvement.

Fluid resuscitation

Fluid resuscitation should be calculated based on the weight of the child and the total surface area of the burn. Several formulas are used to calculate the resuscitation fluid requirement in the first 24 hours. The **Parkland formula** (BSA affected % × weight (kg) × 4) gives the number of millilitres of *resuscitation fluid* to be given over the first 24 hours. Half the fluid is given in the first 8 hours and the remainder in the subsequent 16 hours. The 24-hour period should begin from the time of the injury. Thus if a patient has received very little fluid in transfer, and it is 4 hours since initial burn, then the fluid calculated should be given over the next 20 hours, and half the calculated fluid given in the first 4 hours.

In addition, *maintenance fluid* for the 24-hour period should also be given. This is calculated as 100 mL kg^{-1} for 0–10 kg, 50 mL kg^{-1} for 11–20 kg, and 25 mL kg^{-1} for >20 kg. Thus a 30-kg child's maintenance = 1000 + 500 + 250 = 1750 mL over 24 hours. It is also important to monitor

ongoing losses (urinary output, respiratory loss, etc.).

The calculated amount of fluid (burn deficient plus maintenance) to be replaced in 24 hours is only a guide and should be adjusted according to the haemodynamic response. Patients need to be maintained in a positive fluid balance for the first 24–48 hours. The adequacy of fluid replacement is monitored by urine output and clinical parameters of perfusion. In children, 0.5–1 mL kg^{-1} per hour is the recommended urine output and should be monitored by a urinary catheter in severe burns. A central venous catheter is generally not required in the emergency department phase of management.

The type of fluid used varies between burn specialists, and it is best to be familiar with the preference of the local paediatric burns unit. In the shocked child, a 20 mL kg^{-1} bolus of normal saline should be given. This can be repeated if necessary to restore peripheral circulation. Ongoing replacement is generally with crystalloid in the first 24 hours, as colloid may leak through the burnt capillaries, causing worsening oedema. After 24 hours, colloid is used as part of the replacement fluids in the intensive care setting. When calculating the initial fluid requirements, it is important to subtract the bolus fluids given from this amount.

Additional fluids may be required in severe electrical burns causing muscle damage, as myoglobin may cause renal failure secondary to renal tubular deposition, and therefore maintaining adequate glomerular filtration is very important.

Management of burns
(Table 3.5.1)

Major burns

These patients should be treated in a specialised burns unit. Covering the burn with a sterile dressing is required prior to transfer. Specific dressing type is best decided after discussion with the receiving unit. Within the burn centre, patients are generally dressed with topical silver sulfadiazine (SSD) cream that should be changed each day. At each change, the wound should be cleaned with warm water and debrided to remove any avascular tissue (which may lead to infection). The burns are covered

Table 3.5.1 Admission criteria for paediatric burns unit

Require admission
- partial-thickness burns >20% BSA
- full-thickness burns >5–10% BSA
- smoke inhalation or airway burn is suspected
- child abuse suspected

Consider admission
- burn to hands, feet, face, perineum, or joints
- burns <20% BSA and other concerns e.g. age <12 months, parents not coping, etc.
- comorbidity
- other significant injuries

with a non-stick dressing over the SSD cream (e.g. Melolin), and then wrapped in crepe bandages to prevent contamination of the burn. The face and perineum are generally left open and covered with a water-based gel. SSD should not be used on the face, as the patient may spread it into the eyes. SSD is currently only recommended for inpatient care of patients with significant burns.

Minor burns

Patients with partial-thickness burns <20% or full-thickness burns <5–10% can often be managed on an outpatient basis and reviewed in a burns clinic.

There are several ways to dress wounds in the emergency department. Burns with intact blisters, unless over a joint surface or extremely large, should be left intact initially. The intact skin acts as a barrier to bacteria, and the skin underneath can heal. After 7–10 days, the intact blisters should be deroofed and the need for grafting assessed. If unclear at this stage, then they should be redressed and assessed in a further 7 days.

Superficial burns

Small superficial burns

With these small burns, a clear plastic dressing (e.g. Tegaderm) can be placed over the burn to provide protection and be left on until it also falls off. The disadvantage of this type of dressing is that fluid from the burn tends to collect under the dressing, is a rich source of 'food' for bacteria, and can lead to infection. Tegaderm is better applied after a few days, when the exudate from the burn has ceased. A more porous adherent dressing, such as Fixomul or Hyperfix is better when exudate is going to occur, as it allows some egress of fluid to occur. A covering dressing of gauze and crepe is needed for

the first few days. Removal of this type of dressing is problematic. Olive oil must be applied to the Fixomul several hours before the dressing can be removed, otherwise pulling the dressing off leads to removal of the new granulation tissue.

More extensive superficial burns

Most extensive superficial burns should be covered with Mepitel, Melolin and crepe bandage securing this with Hyperfix. Mepitel is a low adherent wound contact dressing made of silicone gel bound to a flexible polyamide net. The dressing is left intact until the patient is reviewed after 5–7 days. Repeat dressing may be required or the healing burn can be covered with Tegaderm or Hyperfix and be left on until it falls off.

Partial thickness/small full thickness burns

Use Acticoat, a silver impregnated barrier dressing, moistened with sterile water, covered with IntraSite Conformable, gladwrap, ± crepe bandage. Secure with Hyperfix. The exudate from the wound determines the number of dressing changes required. IntraSite Conformable is a soft hydrogel dressing that combines the advantage of IntraSite gel with a non-woven dressing. It creates a moist wound environment for the continued release of silver from the Acticoat. Patients should be reviewed between 3 and 7 days for a change of dressing and to assess if skin grafting is needed.

Superficial burns on the face should be managed non-dressed, and cleaned two or three times a day with warm water. Solugel or vaseline can be applied to the face or it can be left completely non-dressed. As a burn on the face starts to dry up, application of mild lanolin ointment/cream can be used to aid in healing by softening the skin. The burn should also be protected from the sun, as sunburn of an already burnt area causes increased pigmentation to the skin.

Superficial burns rarely become infected, but infection should be suspected if the patient: has unexplained fever, or has evolving pain, redness, and tenderness. Foul discharge from the burn does not always indicate that infection is present. In this case, the dressing should be changed earlier and the burn inspected, as antibiotics may not be indicated. As the skin heals under a

dressing, it becomes pruritic, which may require an antihistamine or cooling of the dressing (particularly in hot weather).

Tetanus prophylaxis is important in major burns or minor burns (which are contaminated). Antibiotics should be used only when a definite infection is present. Prophylactic use of antibiotics is not recommended.

Pain management for minor burns is generally achieved by the dressing itself. Covering the burn decreases the pain substantially. Generally, paracetamol with or without codeine should be sufficient during the first 24 hours.

Patients with burns involving hands, feet, or face should be referred to a burn specialist for ongoing management.

Electrical burns

Introduction

These are infrequent presentations to emergency departments but have unique problems. Electrical injuries are more commonly seen in two age groups: toddlers within the home setting and male adolescents involved in risk-taking behaviour.

Young children generally sustain electrical burns from low-voltage (<1000 V) or household currents (240 V). These may be due to frayed electrical cords or children inserting metal objects into power sockets. Mouth burns may occur when small children chew on power cords. In most states in Australia, safety switches are installed in all new houses, cutting the current when overloaded, thus preventing many severe electrical burns. These low-voltage exposures rarely result in significant internal injury, and most children are asymptomatic apart from distress from the cutaneous burn.

High-voltage (>1000 V) injuries are seen most often in adolescent males as a consequence of risk-taking behaviour (e.g. climbing electrical poles, train surfing). These high-voltage exposures have a more serious outcome, as they are more likely to be associated with injury to internal structures.

Clinical effects

Electrical currents preferentially flow along low-resistance tissues such as blood vessels, nerves, and muscles, rather than the skin, causing internal injury particularly if extremities are involved. There is generally an entrance and exit burn in non-water-related current injuries, with increased tissue damage at these sites. Wet or moist skin increases current flow dramatically by decreasing the tissue resistance.

Clinical manifestations vary according to the voltage exposure and may range from trivial to cardiac arrest, as follows.

Skin

- Entry and exit burns: well-demarcated pale areas with charred centre.
- Arc burns: heat produced can cause extensive tissue injury.
- Flame burns: due to ignition of clothing.

Cardiac
Arrhythmias:

- Low voltage: sinus tachycardia, atrial fibrillation, ventricular fibrillation. Myocardial injury is uncommon.
- High voltage: asystole.

Muscular

- Prolonged tetany of musculature: apnoea, fractures and dislocations.
- Muscle necrosis and rhabdomyolysis.

Neurological

- Acute: altered mental state; seizures; headache; speech, motor, or sensory disturbances.
- Delayed: spinal cord injury, memory and mood disturbance.

Renal

- Renal failure secondary to myoglobinuria.

Other

- Eyes: cataracts.
- Gastrointestinal tract: ulceration, perforation.
- Trauma following associated falls.

Management
Assessment of the child's A, B and C is the initial priority with electrical exposure, followed by examining for skin burns and potential internal injuries. A baseline 12-lead ECG should be done (unless a trivial exposure), and cardiac monitoring only continued if the initial ECG is abnormal or

the child is symptomatic (e.g. chest pain or impaired conscious state). A search for an entrance and exit wound should occur to determine the potential for deeper burns. Analgesia should be provided for the burn or muscle pain. Potential complications and associated injuries are treated on their merit.

Specific issues
Burns
All electrical burns warrant review by a burn specialist.

Fluids
Fluid requirements for significant electrical burns are underestimated using the Parkland formula, as most of the damage is internal. Therefore fluid requirements are significantly more than estimated, and one should aim to maintain a urine output of 2 mL kg^{-1} per hour.

Myoglobinuria
Muscle involvement leads to myoglobinuria, which may cause renal failure. Adequate fluid resuscitation and alkalinisation may help prevent renal failure.

Compartment injury
Compartment syndrome may also occur due to oedema and burn of the affected muscles. Fasciotomy may be necessary, with debridement of non-viable muscle.

Disposition
The following are general guidelines for admission and discharge after burns.

Admission
- Any high-voltage injury.
- Any child with evidence of cardiac or neurological abnormality.

Discharge
- Asymptomatic child with low-voltage injury with normal ECG.

Chemical burns

Many chemical agents can cause burns through accidental exposure. They are generally either acid or alkali. Acid burns cause

coagulation of the skin, which seems to limit the depth of penetration. Alkali burns cause liquefaction and thus result in a deeper injury. Caustic chemicals tend to give deeper burns than thermal injury, as there is generally a long duration of contact. Oedema tends to occur more quickly in chemical burns, which may cause a deeper burn to appear more superficial.

Treatment
Copious irrigation of the burn is the mainstay of treatment. Sufficient analgesia and topical anaesthesia is required to achieve this in a child. This can be done simply with water. Flushing of the burn should continue for at least 10–15 minutes and sometimes longer. Determination of wound pH via litmus paper may guide the duration of irrigation. If chemicals are introduced into the eye, then irrigation should continue until pH is neutral. This usually requires topical anaesthetic to the eye prior to flushing with saline. A Morgan lens is a good method of flushing eyes, as this requires less co-operation from the patient. Fluorescein staining of the eye should then determine the extent of the burn. Chemical burns to the eye require urgent ophthalmological referral. The treatment of a dermal chemical burn after decontamination should be the same as for any other burn.

Some chemicals may cause systemic toxicity from absorption through the burned skin, and these should be managed accordingly.

Further reading

Klein GL, Herndon DN. Burns. *Pediatr Rev* 2004;**25** (12):411–6.

Holland AJA. Pediatric burns: the forgotten trauma of childhood. *J Can Chir* 2006;**49**(4):272–7.

Sheridan R. Outpatient burn care in the emergency department. *Pediatr Emerg Care* 2005;**21** (7):449–56.

Hight DW, Bakalar HR, Lloyd JR. Inflicted burns in children: Recognition and treatment. *JAMA* 1979;**242**:517–20.

Dunn K, Edwards-Jones V. The role of Acticoat™ with nanocrystalline silver in the management of burns. *Burns* 2004;**30**(suppl 1):S1–S9.

Smith ML. Pediatric burns: Management of thermal, electrical, and chemical burns and burn-like dermatologic conditions. *Pediatr Ann* 2000;**29**(6):367–83.

Patel PP, Vasquez SA, Granick MS, Rhee ST. Topical antimicrobials in pediatric burn wound management. *J Craniofacial Surg* 2008;**19**(4):913–21.

Walker AR. Emergency department management of house fire burns and carbon monoxide poisoning in children. *Curr Opin Pediatr* 1996;**8**:239–42.

WOUND MANAGEMENT

Section editor Ian Everitt

4.1 Wound management

Ed Oakley

ESSENTIALS

1 The goals of wound management are to avoid infection, minimise discomfort, facilitate healing and minimise scar formation. The care of the patient as a whole should be the first management priority.

2 In children, management often requires sedation, adequate local anaesthesia and analgesia. Sedation should only be undertaken by personnel experienced in its use, and able to manage the complications of airway compromise, oxygen desaturation and respiratory depression.

3 The comprehension level and the co-operation gained from the child influence wound examination and the information gained. Distraction techniques, adequate topical anaesthesia and appropriate use of sedation can all aid in wound assessment in children. In the child less than 5 years old, observation of posture, symmetry and general movement is required.

4 Examination of function, sensation and circulation distal to the wound is best performed prior to exploration of the wound and prior to regional anaesthesia.

5 If presence of a foreign body is suspected, radiological investigation is advised.

6 Surgical debridement of non-viable tissue is vital to prevent wound infection or delayed wound healing.

7 Tissue adhesives are for external use only and should not be placed within wounds or used on mucous membranes.

8 In general, sutures are removed earlier in children than in adults.

9 Non-accidental injury should be considered, especially when the history and injury are inconsistent.

Introduction

Open wounds account for up to one third of paediatric emergency presentations; two thirds of open wounds occur in boys, and 40% involve a fall. The scalp and face account for more than 50% of all open wounds, and about 30% occur on the hands.[1-4] The goals of management of these wounds are to avoid infection, minimise discomfort, facilitate healing and minimise scar formation. Meticulous attention to wound care and repair should ensure the best possible outcome and functional result.

In children this often requires sedation in addition to adequate local anaesthesia and analgesia. Universal precautions should always be followed when assessing or managing any wound. Gloves (preferably sterile), drapes and eye protection are mandatory.

Anatomy of the skin

Skin is composed of two layers: dermis and epidermis. The epidermis acts as a protective layer for the dermis, preventing infection and desiccation. It is avascular and relies on diffusion of nutrients from the dermis. The dermis is rich in collagen and thus provides most of the tensile strength of the skin. It has a rich network of nutrient vessels and capillaries. The subcutaneous fat is composed of loose connective and adipose tissues.

Pathophysiology of wound healing

The stages of wound healing are coagulation, inflammation, proliferation and maturation. Wound healing is a sequential process that begins immediately after tissue injury. Coagulation is initiated by platelet aggregation then by fibrin clot formation. This supplies haemostasis and allows accumulation of neutrophils and monocytes, which herald the inflammatory phase. The inflammatory phase provides phagocytosis of bacteria, other foreign matter, and dead tissue in the wound. The macrophages release factors that stimulate proliferation of local fibroblasts in the dermis. These provide a collagen network and stimulate new vessel growth. This phase is characterised by pink granulation tissue and wound contraction. A warm moist environment that is supplied either by dressings or scab formation aids this process. Collagen synthesis reaches its peak towards the end of the first week of healing. Remodelling continues to occur for up to 12 months; thus the scar will usually fade and contract over the first 2 to 3 months and the final appearance may not be obvious for up to 6 months post injury.

A number of factors affect the healing of a wound. Adequate nutrition (including vitamins C and A, which are required for collagen formation) is essential. Corticosteroids and immunosuppressive drugs interfere with cellular proliferation and immunity, and anticoagulants inhibit clot formation and initial wound stabilisation. Infection interferes with collagen synthesis and will delay wound healing and cause an increase in scar tissue formation.

Tensile forces of the surrounding skin affect the healing and scar formation of a wound. The most cosmetically pleasing outcome occurs when the long axis of the wound is in the direction of maximum skin tension – along Langer's Lines of skin tension. Wounds that have long axis perpendicular to the lines of skin tension will heal with greater scarring, but there is significant inter-child variability. Dynamic skin tension caused by joint movement also impairs wound healing and causes increased scar formation, and immobilisation of joints while the laceration heals will minimise this effect.

Wound infection

Wound infection is relatively uncommon, occurring in about 5% of wounds presenting to emergency departments (EDs). In general, a wound in a child is less likely to become infected than a similar wound in an adult. Identified risk factors for infection include severe wound contamination, inadequate wound cleansing, inadequate debridement of dead tissue (especially in crush injuries), use of subcutaneous sutures, larger laceration (>5 cm) and site of injury. Specific sites identified as infection risks include axillae, perineum or groin, and feet. In general, limb wounds are at increased risk compared to head and neck wounds.[3,5,6]

Classification of wounds

Lacerations

Lacerations are the most common type of wound seen in the paediatric age group.[6] The edges are usually ragged. If the wound penetrates into the dermal capillaries it will bleed and if it extends into the subcutaneous tissue it will gape. Lacerations can be caused by tension on the skin (usually seen in areas with significant subcutaneous tissue) or by compression of the skin between an object and bone. There is always damage done to surrounding tissues and healing is therefore delayed. Compression injuries usually have more surrounding tissue damage and thus tend to heal more slowly.

Incised wounds

A sharp object such as a knife blade or glass shard makes an incised wound. The wound has margins that are clearly defined and there is little or no surrounding tissue damage. These wounds heal faster than lacerations and, in general, have a lower incidence of infection.

Abrasions

Abrasions are caused by sheering forces on the surface of the skin. The upper layers of the epidermis and sometimes dermis are scraped away. The depth of injury usually varies throughout the wound. If the epidermis alone is involved there is no bleeding, but a transudation of fluid. If the dermis is involved the wound will bleed and there is said to be an increased incidence of infection and foreign body retention.

Evaluation of the patient with a laceration

The care of the patient as a whole should be the first management priority. The airway, breathing and circulation should be assessed and treated as appropriate and a thorough secondary survey undertaken in most patients to exclude or allow management of serious injuries as well as detecting other minor injuries.

History

The mechanism of trauma (cut, crush, fall, bite, burn) and the time of injury are important as they may alter the management of the wound. Crush and bite injuries characteristically cause significantly more surrounding tissue damage and thus are more likely to have delayed healing or infection. When possible, determine the cleanliness of the inflicting object, the amount of blood loss, the presence of a foreign-body sensation, and the motor function and sensation distal to the affected area. The location of the wound should be noted and the possibility of injury to other structures explored.

The health status of the patient should be explored, especially with regard to chronic illnesses that may impact on wound healing – such as diabetes mellitus, obesity, malnutrition, chronic renal impairment, cyanotic congenital heart disease, chronic respiratory illness, tumours, and bleeding disorders.[3] Immunisation history should be obtained and further tetanus vaccination guided by the recommendations of the National Health and Medical Research Council (Table 4.1.1).[7] Current medications are important for both drug interactions with antibiotics that may be prescribed and for medications that may interfere with wound healing – such as immunosuppressive drugs and corticosteroids. A history of allergies must be determined prior to use of cleansing agents, dressings and tapes and prescription of medication. A history of latex allergy should be specifically sought. In wounds that require management under general anaesthesia or sedation a history of when the child last ate or drank is important. Non-accidental injury should be considered, especially when the history and injury are inconsistent.

Examination

Once assessment and management of more serious injuries has occurred, the patient should be assessed for the current severity of any chronic illness, and appropriate management initiated.

The co-operation able to be gained and comprehension level of the child influence wound examination and the information gained. Distraction techniques, adequate topical anaesthesia and appropriate use of sedation can all aid in wound assessment. A calm, unhurried, friendly approach, involving the parents, will maximise the chances of co-operation. Examination of the wound should be done with optimal lighting and with bleeding minimised. Examination of

Table 4.1.1 Tetanus prophylaxis in wound management

History of tetanus vaccination	Time since last dose	Type of wound	DTPa, DTPa-combinations, dT, dTpa, as appropriate	Tetanus immunoglobulin*
≥3 doses	<5 years	All wounds	NO	NO
≥3 doses	5–10 years	Clean, minor wounds	NO	NO
≥3 doses	5–10 years	All other wounds	YES	NO
≥3 doses	>10 years	All wounds	YES	NO
<3 doses or uncertain	–	Clean, minor wounds	YES	NO
<3 doses or uncertain	–	All other wounds	YES	YES

*Recommended dose for TIG is 250 IU to be given as soon as possible after the injury. If >24 hours has elapsed since the injury 500 IU should be given.
A combination vaccine should be used in order to boost community protection against pertussis:
< 8 years old DTPa-IPV (Infanrix-IPV)
> 8 years old dTpa (Boostrix)
Can use a diphtheria/tetanus toxoid vaccine (ADT) if pertussis vaccination is contraindicated.
Please note that CDT and tetanus toxoid vaccine are no longer available.
DTPa, acellular Diphtheria, Tetanus, Pertussis vaccine; dT = diphtheria tetanus; dTpa = booster diphtheria, Tetanus, pertussis vaccine.

function, sensation and circulation distal to the wound is best performed prior to exploration of the wound and prior to regional anaesthesia.[8–10]

Functional assessment requires the movement of all joints distal to the wound. In an older child each joint is examined individually on command and the strength documented. In the child less than 5 years old, observation of posture, symmetry and general movement is required. In wounds to the flexor tendons of the hand, close attention should be paid to the resting position of the fingers (partial flexion). The finding of extension of one finger at rest and the failure of the finger to flex at play or after application of a noxious stimulus confirms the tendon injury.

Injury to nerves is classically assessed with two-point discrimination and this should be possible in older children. Using a paperclip bent so that its ends are separated 4–8 mm is useful in this process. In upper limb injuries formal assessment of the median, ulna and radial nerves is required. In children less than 5 years old this approach needs to be modified. A noxious stimulus applied to the fingers will illicit sensation but risks losing patient confidence. Another method of determining intact innervation is to look for sweating of the fingers. Since autonomic response includes sweating, denervated fingers do not sweat. An ophthalmoscope can be used to examine for sweat beads or the cleaned body of a pen can be run over the fingers, with less resistance in the denervated, thus dry, segment. Arterial circulation is assessed by palpation of peripheral pulses, capillary return distal to the injury, and skin colour and temperature.

Assessment of the wound should include site, size, depth, nature of the edges, cleanliness, and presence of foreign bodies. The wound should be explored to determine the depth and involvement of any underlying tissues including vessels, nerves, tendons, ligaments, muscles, joints, bones and specialised tissues (especially ducts and glands). Bones adjacent to the wound should be palpated for deformity or crepitus and the wound searched for foreign bodies (including the sound of glass on the metal forceps). This assessment and exploration should take place after appropriate anaesthesia of the wound and any required sedation.

Investigation

If presence of a foreign body is expected radiological investigation is advised. In wounds caused by glass, all but superficial wounds should be investigated with plain soft tissue X-ray of the region to exclude a glass foreign body. Most glass foreign bodies more than 2–3 mm in size should be visible. If a radiolucent foreign body is suspected, ultrasound can be useful to both confirm the presence of the foreign body and provide a guide to its depth and location in the wound.[9–11] Other investigations should be determined by the findings of possible injuries to adjacent structures, such as bony X-rays for fractures.

Treatment of wounds

Wound anaesthesia

Analgesia and sedation are discussed in more detail in Section 20. Anaesthesia is required to adequately examine and then treat most wounds. Often, in children, analgesia and sedation will also be necessary, depending on the location of the wound, the involvement of underlying structures, and the age and anxiety of the child.

The options for anaesthesia include topical anaesthesia, local infiltration, regional anaesthesia, dissociative anaesthesia, or general anaesthesia.

Topical anaesthetics include ALA (adrenaline, lidocaine and amethocaine (tetracaine)) – commonly known as LET (lidocaine, epinephrine and tetracaine) in North America, or EMLA cream (eutectic mixture of local anaesthetics) – manufactured by AstraZeneca. ALA is highly effective on facial and head wounds but less so on limb wounds. It has replaced TAC (tetracaine, adrenaline and cocaine) in most institutions. Due to the vasoconstricting properties of adrenaline (epinephrine) these anaesthetics should not be used in areas of end arteries (finger tips, nose, lips, ears, genitalia). EMLA has been shown to be safe and effective when applied to limb wounds. Topical anaesthetics should be applied in the wound either as a liquid dripped onto a pledget of cotton wool placed into the wound or as a methylcellulose gel. The wound is then covered with an occlusive impermeable dressing and adequate anaesthesia is usually obtained within 30 minutes.[12–17]

Local infiltration is the classical method of anaesthetising a wound. The anaesthetic is injected into the wound margins. Pain of injection can be minimised by using warmed anaesthetic, buffering the drug with sodium bicarbonate (mix 10 mL of 1% lidocaine with 1 mL of 8.4% sodium bicarbonate), infiltrating slowly, using the lowest concentration possible, and using needles sized 25 gauge or smaller. The most commonly used local anaesthetic is lidocaine 1 or 2% with or without adrenaline (epinephrine) 1:100 000. The onset of action is rapid, with duration of action of 30 minutes to 1 hour. Addition of adrenaline (epinephrine) is useful to prolong the duration of action and help minimise bleeding; however, adrenaline (epinephrine) should be avoided in regions of end arteries (fingers, nose, lips, ears, genitalia), and its use may increase the risk of infection. The safe dose of plain lidocaine is 3 mg kg^{-1} or 6 mg kg^{-1} for lidocaine mixed with adrenaline (epinephrine).[3]

Regional anaesthesia is useful for facial, hand and foot lacerations, where nerves are readily accessible near bony landmarks. A regional nerve block involves anaesthetising the nerve or nerves that supply a specific anatomic region. Regional anaesthesia is especially useful for large lacerations and lacerations where local infiltration causes distortion of tissue anatomy. Regional anaesthesia is especially useful for anaesthetising digits. Lidocaine or bupivacaine hydrochloride 0.5%, which has duration of action of 3 to 6 hours, are the most commonly used agents. The safe dose of bupivacaine is 2 mg kg^{-1}.

Sedation is often required when treating lacerations in children. Options for sedation include benzodiazepines – such as midazolam or diazepam, fentanyl, nitrous oxide, ketamine, or propofol. Sedation should only be undertaken by personnel experienced in its use and able to manage the complications of airway compromise, oxygen desaturation and respiratory depression. Adequate equipment to deal with these complications should also be available. Some form of physical restraint may also be necessary to prevent excessive movement during repair; however, the aim must be to provide adequate analgesia and anxiolysis.[13,18]

Wound preparation and cleansing

Hair near the wound should only be removed if it interferes with the meticulous closure of the wound. If hair removal is desired the hair should be clipped, not shaved, as shaving disrupts hair follicles and increases the incidence of wound infection.[19] Eyebrow hair should not be removed because this may lead to abnormal or delayed regrowth.

The surrounding skin and wound edges should be thoroughly cleaned. This should be undertaken in a manner and with a substance that provides adequate antisepsis without tissue damage or impairing wound defence mechanisms. A solution such as aqueous povidone-iodine or aqueous chlorhexidene applied with gauze or cotton wool should be used. Care should be taken to minimise the amount of cleanser to penetrate the wound to minimise damage to wound defences increasing the risk of infection.

Surgical debridement of crushed or nonviable tissue is vital to prevent wound infection or delayed wound healing. However, as little tissue as possible should be debrided as possible. Manual removal with forceps of large particles of foreign material should also be meticulously undertaken. When a heavily contaminated wound contains specialised tissues such as tendons or nerves, consultation is recommended.

Once the wound is adequately anaesthetised it should be thoroughly cleaned. Irrigation is the method of choice for removing dirt and bacteria from wounds. In hospital, saline (0.9%) is the irrigation solution of choice, as it causes no tissue damage, but tap water can be used.[20] The ability of irrigation to decontaminate a wound is directly related to pressure of the irrigating stream, the size of the particles to be removed, and the volume of irrigant. At least 100–200 mL per 2 cm of laceration are required. The fluid should be injected from a 30–60 mL syringe via an 18 to 20 gauge cannula. Higher pressures should be avoided as they may cause tissue damage and increase the incidence of wound infection.[21,22] The volume and pressure of irrigation should be modified as necessary according to the location and cause of the wound. High-pressure irrigation does not enhance the dissemination of bacteria into soft tissue wounds, but excessive use can cause local tissue oedema enhancing risk of infection. Use of a device to minimise splashing of the irrigant is desirable and wearing of gloves, goggles and gown mandatory.[21, 22]

Antibiotic prophylaxis

The use of prophylactic antibiotics in wound care is controversial. Decontamination with appropriate irrigation techniques is more beneficial than the use of prophylactic antibiotics.[2,9,23,24] When indicated (Table 4.1.2), antibiotics should be given

Table 4.1.2 Indications for antibiotic prophylaxis in wounds
Wound characteristics
High risk anatomic site (hands, forefoot, groin, axilla)
Devitalised tissue
Extensive surrounding soft tissue injury
Stellate lacerations
Contaminated with body fluids or organic matter or dirt
Large lacerations (> 5 cm)
Closure delayed (> 12 hours)
High risk for endocarditis
Prosthetic heart valves
Patent ductus arteriosis
Structural heart disease
Tetralogy of Fallot
Ventricular septal defects
Coarctation of the aorta
Damaged heart valves
Immunocompromised children
Prior history of endocarditis
Intravenous drug use

as soon as possible. The initial dose should be given intravenously and be relatively large to provide rapid reliable high tissue concentrations. The first dose should be given before wound closure to ensure an effective concentration of antibiotic in the wound tissue fluid at the time of wound closure. When choosing an antibiotic the likely causative organisms should be borne in mind: the organisms contaminating the wound and the commensal organisms found in that region of the body. In general, bites and wounds in regions with high bacterial counts (hands, feet, groin) should be treated with antibiotics to cover *Staphylococcus epidermidis*, *S. aureus* and *Streptococcus* sp. The likelihood of anaerobic bacteria needs to be considered. Specific circumstances also need to be borne in mind. Patients at risk of endocarditis should have all wounds treated with antibiotics to cover *S. aureus* and *S. epidermidis*. Ampicillin/amoxicillin is the currently recommended drug in Australia. However, in communities where the incidence of penicillin resistance is high a cephalosporin and an aminoglycoside are recommended.

Wounds associated with fractures, tendon or muscle involvement should be considered for prophylaxis, as should large wounds, wounds with significant devitalised tissue such as crush injuries and stellate lacerations. Wounds contaminated with faeces should be treated with coverage of coliforms and anaerobic bacteria. Wounds in children with a compromised immune system should all be considered for treatment. Wounds with closure delayed more than 12 hours should also be considered high risk for infection. Treatment should be for 3 to 5 days with a penicillinase-resistant antibiotic such as a first generation cephalosporin or amoxicillin-clavulanic acid, with consideration to addition of metronidazole.[25]

Wound closure

The aim of wound closure is to reduce discomfort, aid healing and produce the best cosmetic result possible.[26] The technique chosen for wound closure depends on the type of wound. Most wounds in children can be managed with primary closure, as the risk of infection is relatively low. Infected, heavily contaminated wounds and wounds resulting from high-energy projectiles are best managed by delayed primary closure, with initial cleansing and packing then closure 3 to 5 days later, once the risk of infection has decreased. Wounds with delayed presentation (>24 hours), or those contaminated with saliva or faeces should also be considered for delayed closure. Some wounds, such as puncture wounds or contaminated wounds in areas of poor perfusion should not be closed but allowed to heal by secondary intention. Once it is decided to close the wound, a technique that allows apposition of the wound edges that is secure and accurate and holds the wound edges in apposition until the strength of the wound is sufficient should be chosen. With improved technology the options for wound closure are growing. Those presently available include sutures, staples, tissue adhesives and tapes.

Sutures

Suturing is the traditional method of wound closure. Sutures are divided into two classes on the basis of their degradation properties. Absorbable sutures degrade rapidly in vivo, and lose their tensile strength within 60 days. Sutures that degrade more slowly are classified as non-absorbable (Table 4.1.3 for individual suture material characteristics).

Absorbable sutures are made from either collagen or synthetic polymers. Gut sutures are manufactured from the submucosa of

Table 4.1.3 Characteristics of common suture materials

Suture material	Ease of handling	Tensile strength	Degradation (d)*	Tissue reactivity	Infection potential
Non-absorbable					
Nylon (Ethilon®, Dafilon®)	Average	Good	–	Low	Very low
Polypropylene (Prolene®)	Poor	Very good	–	Very low	Low
Silk	Good	Poor	–	High	High
Absorbable					
Surgical gut (fast absorbing	Poor	Average	4–7	High	High
Polyglactin (Vicryl Rapide®)	Average	Good	7–10	Low	Low
Chromic gut	Average	Average	10–14	High	High
Polyglactin (Vicryl®)	Average	Good	10–15	Low	Low
Polyglycolic acid (Dexon®)	Good	Good	25–30	Low	Low
Polydioxanone (PDS)	Average	Very good	25–30	Very low	Low

*Time to loss of 50% of tensile strength.

ovine or bovine intestines. The collagen is then treated to strengthen the material and increase resistance to tissue degradation (plain gut). Coating with chromium trioxide provides more resistance to absorption (chromic gut). These suture materials have a somewhat unpredictable absorption. Synthetic absorbable sutures have improved strength and delayed and more reliable absorption characteristics. Absorbable sutures are used for closing deep layers of a laceration and can be used for skin closure – especially where removing sutures in a young child may be difficult, or where procedural sedation is required to place sutures.

Non-absorbable sutures are made from either natural (silk, cotton, linen) or synthetic (nylon, Dacron®) fibres. They can also be classified according to their physical characteristics. Monofilament sutures are made from a single filament (nylon, Prolene®), and sutures containing multiple fibres are called multifilament (silk, cotton, nylon). Of these sutures, only nylon is available in both types of filament. Non-absorbable sutures are used to close fascial layers (where healing is slow) and for skin closure.[27,28]

Sutures come in varying sizes. The size of the suture to be used depends on the wound location and the tensile strength of the tissue to be sutured. Heavy sutures such as 4–0 should be used in the limbs and trunk, and should also be used on mucous

membranes and subcutaneous tissue. Heaviest sutures such as 3–0 should be used on thick skin (such as the sole of the foot) or over large joints. Small sutures such as 6–0 should be used on tissues with light tensions, such as facial skin and subcutaneous tissue.[27,28]

Needles

Needles come in varying sizes and shapes also. Needles are describes by the arc of curvature the needle possesses, and the shape of the needle itself. The most commonly used for skin closure is the circle (135°) needle or the ½ circle (180°) needle (Fig. 4.1.1). For closure of fascial layers ½ circumference needles are usually used. Needles that have two circumferences of curvature (compound needles) are able to be passed through the tissue with less rotation of the forearm. Needles come with different shapes as well as curvatures (see Fig. 4.1.1). A reverse cutting needle is the most common type used for skin closure. The needle cuts an inverted triangle and the suture sits on the base of the triangle, decreasing the likelihood of cutting out. A conventional cutting needle cuts a triangle into the skin and the suture sits in the apex of the triangle. For fascia a taper point needle is used. The cross-section of these needles is a circle that is tapered to a point. It does not cut but pushes the tissues aside, causing less tissue damage and reducing

Cross section

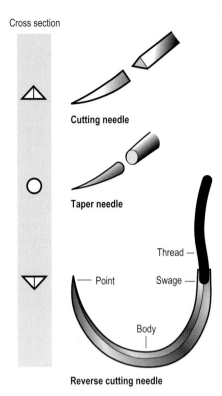

Fig. 4.1.1 Surgical needle characteristics and types. (From an original drawing by Elaine Wheildon.)

the chance of the stitch cutting out. For deep tissues that are stronger (such as tendon) a tapercut, or combination needle is used – it has a tapered body, but the point is a reverse cutting edge.[28]

Needles are grasped with a needle holder. The swage of the needle – the region where the needle is hollowed out to join with the suture – is the weakest point, and grasping the needle in this region should be avoided. The needle should be grasped in the body one half or two thirds of the distance from the tip of the needle.

Suturing techniques

For closure of a wound with sutures a number of instruments are needed to maintain a sterile field and to allow manipulation of the tissues and needle (Table 4.1.4). Finer instruments should be available for facial laceration repair.

Sutures should be placed to allow apposition of all injured layers of the skin. Proper suture placement should result in slight eversion of the wound edges, avoiding a depression of the scar when contraction takes place during wound healing. To ensure eversion of skin edges the skin suture must

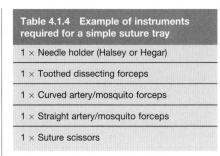

Table 4.1.4 Example of instruments required for a simple suture tray
1 × Needle holder (Halsey or Hegar)
1 × Toothed dissecting forceps
1 × Curved artery/mosquito forceps
1 × Straight artery/mosquito forceps
1 × Suture scissors

be placed so that an equal amount of tissue is included on each side of the wound, and so that the needle bite includes a broad base (Figs 4.1.2 and 4.1.3). This is accomplished by lifting the wound edge as the needle is passed through the skin on each side, maximising the deep tissues included in the suture.[28,29]

Most wounds sutured in the ED are closed with interrupted skin sutures. Synthetic non-absorbable sutures are most commonly used. However, rapidly absorbable sutures can be used to close the skin in children, avoiding the discomfort of suture removal. To place a simple interrupted suture the needle is held so the tip enters the skin at a right angle, and the hand rotated to ensure the needle remains at right angles to the skin throughout its passage, which aids in maximising the deep tissues captured in the bite. The stitch should be secured with an instrument tie and the knots secured to one side of the wound to minimise inflammation to the healing tissue. The initial throw should include two wraps of the suture material around the needle holder; subsequent throws should be wrapped once. The knot should be tied just tight enough to oppose the skin edges. Tying the knot too tightly will cause a reduction in the blood supply to the wound edges and increase the risk of infection and poor cosmetic outcome. Synthetic sutures with poor handling should have four or five throws per knot.[28–30]

The more sutures placed per centimetre, the finer the control over the wound edge. For facial lacerations, the skin sutures should be placed approximately 3 mm apart and enter the skin about 3 mm from the wound edge. For other areas of the body, sutures should be placed 4 to 5 mm apart and should pierce the skin about 5 mm from the wound edge. The number of sutures used to close a wound should be the minimal number that allows a desired cosmetic

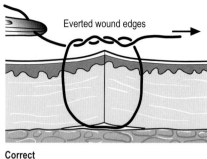

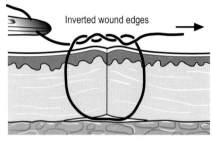

Fig. 4.1.2 Normal suture. Suturing technique for wound edge eversion.

outcome. In general, the better the blood supply, the closer together sutures can be placed.

There are generally two methods for closing a laceration, either suturing from one end to the other, or placing sutures that serially bisect the wound. A small linear wound is easily sutured from end to end, and long wounds without good landmarks on either side are most easily closed by placing the first stitch in the middle and then serially subdividing the wound. In wounds with definite landmarks, such as palmar skin creases or the vermillion border of the lip, the first suture should be placed to align these landmarks.[28,30]

Deep sutures should be placed where there are multiple layers of tissue involved and the skin sutures would be under tension. They are placed to reapproximate the dermal layers of the skin and remove skin tension, thus improving cosmetic outcome. Placing deep sutures inserts a foreign body into the wound and increases the risk of wound infection, so they should only be placed when necessary and the minimum number necessary used. For this reason, deep sutures should be avoided in the hands and feet. Deep sutures placed close to the skin are sometimes extruded through the wound. To place a deep suture, the needle is placed at the depth of the wound and removed at a more superficial level. The needle is then placed at the same superficial level on the opposite side of the wound and exits deeply so the knot is tied deeply in the wound (see Fig. 4.1.3).[28,30]

Special suturing techniques

A variety of special suturing techniques are available with the sole purpose of aiding the provision of skin apposition with everted wound edges. The vertical mattress suture is useful in regions with minimal subcutaneous tissue where the edges are difficult to maintain in eversion. The technique is begun the same way as a simple skin suture, but after the suture loop is made, the skin is re-entered 1 to 2 mm from the wound edge and then tied (Fig. 4.1.4). The horizontal mattress suture reinforces the subcutaneous tissue and relieves skin tension, but does not provide wound edge approximation as well as the vertical mattress suture (Fig. 4.1.5). The modified or half-buried horizontal mattress suture (or corner stitch) is the method of choice for closing a flap. It relieves tissue tension and avoids vascular compromise when approximating the tip of the flap (Fig. 4.1.6).[28,30]

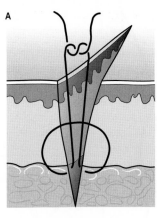

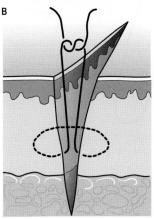

Fig. 4.1.3 Deep sutures. (A) The buried subcutaneous suture; (B) the horizontal dermal stitch.

A continuous suture can be used to close the laceration. It is faster to place than interrupted sutures, removal of sutures is easier and faster, and the tension is spread evenly along the wound. The continuous suture can be percutaneous or subcutaneous and made with absorbable or non-absorbable suture material. The disadvantages are that if one part of the suture breaks, the integrity of the whole wound is lost, and if the wound becomes infected, the whole wound needs to be opened to drain the pus. To place a percutaneous running stitch an interrupted suture is placed at one end of the wound and only the free end of the suture is cut. Suturing is continued along the wound in a coil pattern ensuring that the needle passes perpendicularly across the wound with each pass. The loop is tightened after each pass and the last stitch placed beyond the end of the laceration. The stitch is tied using the last loop as the tail.[28,30]

Correction of dog ears

A dog ear is the term given to a conical pucker of redundant skin that may develop at the ends of the wound during suturing. It is avoided by suturing the wound from the middle by sequentially bisecting the wound. Dog ears can be removed in many

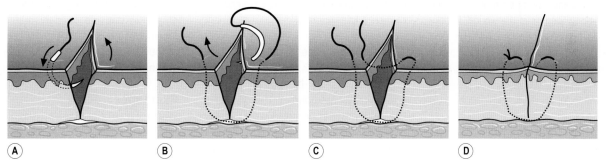

Fig. 4.1.4 The vertical mattress suture technique is useful to evert wound edges with a natural tendency to roll inwards despite correctly placed simple sutures. (From an original drawing by Elaine Wheildon.)

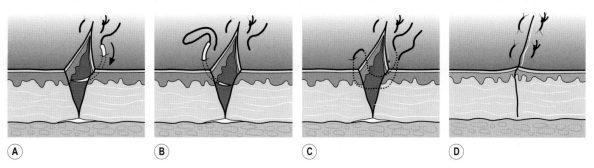

Fig. 4.1.5 The horizontal mattress suture redistributes tension and everts wound edges. (From an original drawing by Elaine Wheildon.)

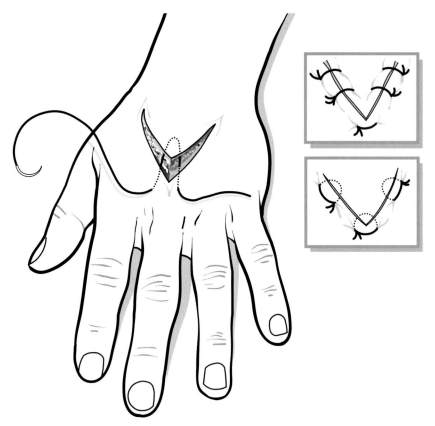

Fig. 4.1.6 Closure of a flap requires an initial suture of the apex, after which either simple or horizontal mattress sutures may be used. (From an original drawing by Elaine Wheildon.)

ways, the simplest of which is the overlap excision technique. The redundant skin is pulled across the wound from one side and excised along the line of the wound. Redundant skin from the opposite side is pulled across the wound and also excised along the line of the wound. The wound is then closed (Fig. 4.1.7).[28]

Staples

Stainless steel staples can be applied more rapidly than sutures, and they are associated with a lower rate of foreign body reaction and infection. Staples are generally considered especially useful for lacerations of the scalp, trunk, and limbs. However, they do not allow such meticulous wound apposition as sutures, and are slightly more painful to remove. They should not be used on the face or in any other wound where cosmetic outcome is a high priority.[31]

Tissue adhesives

Tissue adhesives have now been in use for several decades. The basis of the adhesive is a cyanoacrylate polymer. The cyanoacrylate polymerises in the presence of hydroxyl ions – found in water or blood – allowing them to bind to the skin. Tissue adhesives are for external use only and should not be placed within wounds or used on mucous membranes.

It is in the repair of lacerations to young children that tissue adhesives have become most popular. They are easy and relatively painless to apply and provide a cosmetic result that is as good as suturing, with no risk of causing suture marks. No removal is required, as they slough off in 7 to 10 days. They are, however, not suitable for use in all wounds. If the laceration cannot be approximated and the wound edges brought together with minimal tension, then tissue adhesive is not appropriate. Care should be taken not to apply too much tissue glue and to avoid placement over currently bleeding wounds, as the polymerisation is exothermic and the patient may notice a heat sensation. Also, contact with excess blood causes polymerisation above the skin, limiting the tensile strength of wound-edge closure.

The tissue glue is applied over the surface of the wound once its edges have been approximated by digital pressure. A number of thin layers of glue are applied across the wound and the wound held approximated for about 30 seconds. Care is taken not to allow glue to spill into eyes or orifices, and to avoid fixing forceps or gloves to the patient. The cyanoacrylates also act as their own dressing providing moist wound healing conditions under the glue, and have a degree of intrinsic antimicrobial activity. Careful attention to wound cleansing is still needed to avoid wound infections. In general, they are less expensive than sutures or staples and are strongly preferred by patients and families. A comparison of the various methods of wound closure is found in Table 4.1.5.[32–34]

Skin tapes

Skin tapes can be used to close small wounds with low tensile forces. They cannot be used over areas of motion such as over joints. Wound haemostasis is vital as the tapes will not stick to wet skin. Application of an adhesive agent to the skin adjacent to the wound is necessary to provide adequate adhesion of the tapes. These adhesive agents (e.g.

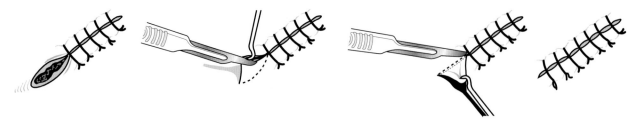

Fig. 4.1.7 Dog ear. Direct overlap excision technique. (From an original drawing by Elaine Wheildon.)

Table 4.1.5 Characteristics of wound closure techniques

Technique	Advantages	Disadvantages
Suture	Greatest tensile strength Meticulous closure	May require removal Painful/requires local anaesthesia ± sedation Slow application Costly Slow to apply Increased tissue reaction
Staples	Rapid application Low cost Low tissue reactivity	Less meticulous closure Painful/requires local anaesthesia ± sedation Requires removal
Tissue adhesives	Painless Rapid application No removal needed Low cost No risk of needle stick	Lower tensile strength Not for use over joints Slightly higher incidence of dehiscence
Surgical tapes	Least reactive Rapid application Patient comfort No risk of needle stick Low cost	Low tensile strength Difficulty maintaining adhesion May require use of toxic adjuncts to aid adhesion

Table 4.1.6 Timing of suture removal

Wound location	Time of removal (days)
Face	4
Scalp	5
Upper limbs, trunk	7–10
Lower limbs	8–10
Over joints	10–14

Tinc Benz®) are toxic to tissues and cause pain, so great care should be taken not to spill them into the wound. Tapes are not suitable for use in small children as they frequently pull them off. Tapes are a useful adjunct to wound closure, for example after suture removal or tissue adhesive application to decrease tension on the wound.

Post-wound-closure care

All patients should be provided with written information on care of their wound. Parents and children must understand the importance of ongoing wound care and be provided with instructions about follow up.

Dressing and suture removal

After the wound has been sutured it should be covered with a non-adherent occlusive or semiocclusive dressing to protect the wound from bacterial invasion and provide a moist healing environment and speed wound healing. Ideally, the dressing is left intact until suture removal. The dressing should only be removed if it becomes saturated or there is a risk of infection and inspection is warranted. If the wound is not covered with a waterproof dressing the dressing can be removed every few days for showering. Non-absorbable sutures should be removed at the appropriate time, depending on the

location of the injury. Removal of the sutures too early risks dehiscence; leaving sutures too long increases tissue reaction and the risk of cross-hatching and wound infection (Table 4.1.6). In general, sutures are removed earlier in children than in adults. Wounds closed with tissue adhesive should not be covered with an occlusive dressing, as the extra moisture will more rapidly decrease the ability of the glue to maintain wound edge apposition. The wound should be kept dry for 2–3 days, after which the patients may shower but should avoid bathing and swimming. Wounds closed with skin tapes should be kept dry to prevent premature removal.

Immobilisation and drains

Wounds that cross joints or are in areas of highly mobile skin should be immobilised. The joint should be splinted in the position of function for 7–10 days. Plaster of Paris can be used to make a cheap and easily applied splint, or a bulky dressing can be used to limit motion and prevent the child tampering with the wound.

In general, drains should not be used in wounds that have been closed as they promote wound infection. If a wound is considered at high risk for infection, delayed primary closure should be undertaken rather than closure and drainage.[9]

Treatment of selected injuries

Abrasions

In abrasions, the underlying tissues are relatively uninjured, providing a degree of protection against infection. Cleansing the abrasion is important to flush away bacteria and remove particulate matter, which should be removed to prevent infection or tattooing. Large abrasions or those heavily contaminated may need cleaning under general anaesthesia. After adequate cleansing and debridement the wound should be covered with a non-adherent occlusive or semi-occlusive dressing. A moist environment enhances healing, and the environment under a scab is ideal. However, wounds without extensive scab formation are more comfortable, so a dressing provides the moist environment. Children with large or deep abrasions should be reviewed in 2 to 3 days to check the wound. Ongoing review should be once or twice weekly.

Eyelid lacerations

A thorough eye examination needs to be performed for all eyelid lacerations. Attention should be given to the possibility of a ruptured globe (eccentric pupil) or trauma to the globe (hyphaema, dislocated lens or retinal detachment). Visual acuity should be measured and documented. Any wound that penetrates the tarsal plate or the inner canthus requires specialist attention, as do wounds involving the lid margins. Any wound that cannot be adequately assessed (e.g. in a young child) should be referred for evaluation under anaesthesia.[24]

Superficial wounds of the eyelid are relatively easily repaired with 6–0 fast absorbing gut, with sutures placed close to the wound edge. Care must be taken not to suture into the tarsal plate or other deep structures.[24]

Lip lacerations

Inspection of the teeth and oral mucosa is mandatory in all lip lacerations. Tooth injuries should be documented and referred for management where necessary; missing teeth warrant investigation to ensure they have not been inhaled or imbedded in the soft tissues of the mouth. Ideal anaesthesia is via nerve block of the mental or alveolar nerves for the lower lip or the infra-orbital nerve for the upper lip. Alternatives include sedation and direct infiltration, with or without application of methylene blue to the margins of the vermillion border.

Wounds that involve the vermillion border (the junction of the dry oral mucosa and the facial skin) must be exactly realigned to achieve acceptable cosmetic results. A 6–0 suture should be used, with the first suture placed to exactly reappose the vermillion border.[24] Further sutures should close the skin and the dry mucosal surface of the lip, with the wet mucosal surface only closed if it is gaping significantly.

Deep or through and through lacerations of the lip require deep sutures to repair the orbicularis oris muscle: if this is the case, an absorbable 6–0 suture should be used. The deep sutures should be placed after the initial suture is placed at the vermillion border and before tying that stitch.[24]

Tongue lacerations

Most tongue lacerations can be left to heal without intervention with good results. Large lacerations involving the free edge of the tongue should be repaired to avoid healing with a notch, interfering with the function of the tongue. Large flaps (that gap when the tongue is in the resting position) and lacerations that continue to bleed should also be repaired. Care should be taken when repairing these injuries because of the risk of airway compromise, especially considering moderate to deep sedation is likely to be necessary. General anaesthesia and repair in the operating theatre should be considered if there is doubt.

The tongue should be maintained in position by a gentle pull using a towel clip or 4–0 suture placed through the tip. Interrupted 4–0 absorbable sutures should be placed using full thickness bites to include both mucosal surfaces and the lingual muscle in each stitch. Multiple knots should

be used to secure the sutures and the parents warned that while the tongue is anaesthetised the child may bite through the stitch.[24]

Fingertip amputation

Young children tend to injure their fingertips in doors and windows. Most of the injuries in young children are contused lacerations or partial amputations, with complete amputation being less common. Older children are more prone to injury with knives or tools. Fractures are less common in the older age group. These wounds should be evaluated for tissue loss and with radiography for bony injury.

If the amputated fragment has been retained and involves any of the nailbed some surgeons reimplant as a graft, with approximately 50% chance of the graft taking. If the tissue is not retained or is small, and there is no bone on view, it is most appropriate to allow the wound to heal by secondary intention. Fingertips allowed to heal naturally have greater length and better sensory outcome than those treated with grafts. These wounds should be covered with a non-adherent occlusive or semiocclusive dressing to allow moist wound healing after thorough cleaning and debridement as needed. Follow up should be maintained until the wound is healed.

Injuries involving just the fingertip but not the nail heal very well. Injuries involving the nailbed or nail, but sparing bone, heal well. Those that involve the nailbed, nail and distal phalanx heal less well. Any injury with bone on view should be referred for specialist care.[23,24,35]

Nailbed lacerations

Trauma to the distal fingers is often associated with nailbed injury. An underlying fracture of the distal phalanx should be assessed with radiographs. Unrepaired nailbed lacerations can permanently disfigure the growth of the new nail from the matrix.

If the nail is lacerated, completely avulsed, or only loosely attached, the nailbed must be explored. This can be done under local anaesthesia with a ring block of the digital nerves or under general anaesthesia. The nail must be removed and the nailbed repaired with 5–0 or 6–0 absorbable suture material. The space between the nailbed and nailfold must be packed with

paraffin gauze or the nail replaced to prevent adhesions. If a fracture is present, antibiotics should be given. If the nail is partially avulsed only and is tightly adherent to the nailbed, it is reasonable to leave this intact as it will adequately splint and maintain apposition of any nailbed injury.[24]

Subungual haematoma

A subungual haematoma is a collection of blood between the nail and nailbed. It is most commonly seen with blunt fingertip injuries and may be associated with a fracture of the distal phalanx. Drainage of the haematoma usually provides symptomatic relief and should be undertaken whenever the haematoma is causing pain. Generally no local anaesthesia is required to drain the haematoma with cautery or needle burring using a 19-gauge needle. If there is an underlying fracture antibiotics should be administered. Nail removal for inspection of the nailbed should not be undertaken, regardless of the size of haematoma.[24]

Puncture wounds to the foot

Puncture wounds to the foot carry a high risk of infection and retained foreign body. All puncture wounds should be assessed for retained foreign body with radiography, and ultrasound for radiolucent foreign bodies. Anaesthesia with local infiltration or a posterior tibial nerve block is needed. The wound should be soaked to remove any scab on the surface, debrided and irrigated. The wound should be left open once any foreign material has been removed. The wound should be cleaned with an antibacterial solution (such as Betadine®) and dressed with a non-adherent dressing. Close review is important to detect infection early. Prophylactic antibiotics have not been shown to prevent infection and may predispose to *Pseudomonas* infection.

Bites

Animal bites

Animal bites are a common presenting problem for the ED. Dog and cat bites account for virtually all bites seen in the ED, with dog bites being about six times more common. Rodents and other animals account for less than 1 to 2% of bites.

Dog-bite injuries tend to be relatively large, relatively superficial crush injuries, which are seen most commonly on the face, neck and scalp in children. The overall infection rate for dog bites is about 10%, with facial wound infection rates of about 5%. Dog-bite wounds are infected with multiple organisms on all occasions, with both aerobic and anaerobic bacteria. It is reasonable to cleanse and close most dog bites, with antibiotic prophylaxis provided only to wounds that are high risk for infection (Tables 4.1.7 and 4.1.8). Amoxicillin with clavulanate is the most useful drug.

Cat bites, on the other hand, are typically puncture wounds with less surrounding tissue injury. They have bacteria inoculated deep into the wound, which is difficult to explore, irrigate or debride. The risk of infection is significantly higher than in dog bite – at least twice as likely – because of the puncture-type wound, the most common location of the bite being the hand, and the high incidence (about 80%) of *Pasteurella multocida* found in cats' mouths. *P. multocida* is a facultative, anaerobic Gram-negative rod that often results in rapidly progressive cellulitis. It is sensitive to the penicillins and variably sensitive to macrolides and first-generation cephalosporins. All these drugs have been documented as adequately treating infections of *P. multocida,* but treatment failures have been documented for erythromycin and first-generation cephalosporins. It is recommended that all cat bites receive prophylactic antibiotics (see Table 4.1.7).[36,37]

Human bites

Most human bites are probably at no more risk of infection than ordinary lacerations and they are not considered to carry a high risk of human immunodeficiency virus transmission. Prophylactic antibiotics have, however, been shown to reduce the risk of infection. Appropriate prophylactic antimicrobial choices for human bite injuries include amoxicillin with clavulanate.[36] However, the clenched-fist injury (or fight bite), which commonly causes a ragged laceration over the fourth or fifth metacarpophalangeal joint is at high risk of infection. These latter wounds should all receive prophylactic antibiotics, as should human bites (including self-inflicted bites) that have high-risk properties (see Tables 4.1.7 and 4.1.8).[36]

Controversies

❶ Subcutaneous sutures close deep wound dead space reducing fluid collection and infection, but deep sutures of themselves can cause infection by acting as a foreign body.

❷ Dressing practice for all wounds is changing to promote moist wound healing; this speeds rate of healing and improves wound comfort.

❸ A number of topical anaesthetic creams are being used in extremity wounds despite not being licensed for this use.

❹ Wound drains are not indicated in the management of wounds in the ED, and delayed primary closure is a preferred technique.

❺ Debridement should remove as little tissue as possible to maximise cosmetic outcome.

❻ Prophylactic antibiotics, while intended to prevent infection, have been shown in some wounds to increase the risk of infection with unusual organisms.

Table 4.1.7	Wound infection risk factors	
	High risk	**Low risk**
Biting species	Cat Human	Dog Rodent
Location of wound	Hand Over a joint Below knee Through and through oral	Face Scalp Mucosa
Wound type	Puncture Extensive crush Old	Large Superficial Recent

Table 4.1.8	Management of bite wounds	
Species	**Suturing**	**Antibiotics**
Dog	Yes	High-risk wound type only
Cat	Face only	All
Rodent	Yes	No
Human – hand bites	No	Yes
Human – other bites	Yes	Large wounds

References

1. Singer AJ, Thode Jr HC, Hollander JE. National trends in ED lacerations between 1992 and 2002. *Am J Emerg Med* 2006;24(2):183–8.
2. Young SJ, Barnett PL, Oakley EA. 10. Bruising, abrasions and lacerations: minor injuries in children I. *Med J Aust* 2005;182(11):588–92.
3. Hollander JE, Singer AJ. Laceration management. *Ann Emerg Med* 1999;34:356–67.
4. Capellan O, Hollander JE. Management of lacerations in the emergency department. *Emerg Med Clin North Am* 2003;21:205–31.
5. Hollander JE, Singer AJ, Valentine SM, Shofer FS. Risk factors for infection in patients with traumatic lacerations. *Acad Emerg Med* 2001;8:716–20.
6. Knapp JF. Updates in wound management for the paediatrician. *Pediatr Clin North Am* 1999;46: 1201–13.
7. NHMRC . *The Australian Immunisation Handbook.* 8th ed. Commonwealth of Australia; 2008.
8. Singer AJ, Hollander JE, Quinn J. Evaluation and management of traumatic lacerations. *N Engl J Med* 1997;337:1142–8.
9. Baruch J. Laceration repair. *J Gen Intern Med* 2005; 20(6):556–8.
10. Weinberger LN, Chen EH, Mills AM. Is screening radiography necessary to detect retained foreign bodies in adequately explored superficial glass-caused wounds? *Ann Emerg Med* 2008;51(5):666–7.
11. Anderson MA, Newmeyer WL, Kilgore ESJ. Diagnosis and treatment of retained foreign body in the hand. *Am J Surg* 1982;114:63.
12. Zempsky WT, Karasic RB. EMLA versus TAC for topical anesthesia of extremity wounds in children. *Ann Emerg Med* 1997;30:163–6.
13. Kennedy RM, Luhmann JD. Pharmacological management of pain and anxiety during emergency procedures in children. *Paediatr Drugs* 2001; 3(5):337–54.
14. Ernst AA, Marvez-Vails E, Nick TG, et al. LAT versus TAC for topical anesthesia in face and scalp lacerations. *Am J Emerg Med* 1995;13:151–4.
15. Blackburn PA, Butler KH, Hughes MJ, et al. Comparison of tetracaine–adrenaline–cocaine (TAC) with topical lidocaine–adrenaline (TLE): Efficacy and cost. *Am J Emerg Med* 1995;13:315–17.
16. Loryman B, Davies F, Chavada G, Coats T. Consigning "brutacaine" to history: a survey of pharmacological techniques to facilitate painful procedures in children in emergency departments in the UK. [see comment]. *Emerg Med J* 2006;23(11):838–40.
17. Priestley S, Kelly AM, Chow L, et al. Application of topical local anesthetic at triage reduces treatment time for children with lacerations: a randomized controlled trial.[see comment]. *Ann Emerg Med* 2003;42 (1):34–40.
18. Sectish TC. Use of sedation and local anesthesia to prepare children for procedures. *Am Fam Physician* 1997;55:909–16.
19. Seropian R, Reynolds B. Wound infection after preoperative depilatory versus razor preparation. *Am J Surg* 1971;121:251.
20. Moscati RM, Mayrose J, Reardon RF, Janicke DM, Jehle DV. A multicenter comparison of tap water versus sterile saline for wound irrigation.[see comment]. *Acad Emerg Med* 2007;14(5):404–9.
21. Stevenson TR, Thacker JG, Rodeheaver GT, et al. Cleansing the traumatic wound by high pressure syringe irrigation. *J Am Coll Emerg Physicians* 1976;5:17–21.
22. Wheeler CB, Rodeheaver GT, Thacker JG, et al. Side effects of high pressure irrigation. *Surg Gynecol Obstet* 1976;143:775–8.
23. Al-Nammari SS, Quyn AJ. Towards evidence based emergency medicine: best BETs from the Manchester Royal Infirmary. Conservative management or suturing for small, uncomplicated hand wounds. *Emerg Med J* 2007;24(3):217–8.
24. Brown DJ, Jaffe JE, Henson JK. Advanced laceration management. *Emerg Med Clin North Am* 2007;25 (1):83–99.

25. *Post traumatic wound infections. eTG complete (Internet).* Melbourne: Therapeutic Guidelines Ltd; 2009. *http://online.tg.org.au/ip/* [accessed 10.12.09].

26. Singer AJ, Mach C, Thode HCJ, et al. Patient priorities with traumatic lacerations. *Am J Emerg Med* 2000;**18**:683–6.

27. Lin K, Farinholt H, Reddy V, et al. The scientific basis for selecting surgical sutures. *J Long Term Eff Med Implants* 2001;**11**:29–40.

28. Ratner D, Nelson BR, Johnson TM. Basic suture materials and suturing techniques. *Semin Dermatol* 1994;**13**:20–6.

29. Sutures and Needles. *eMedicine* 2009; http://emedicine.medscape.com/article/884838-overview [accessed 15.11.09].

30. Suturing Techniques. *eMedicine* 2009; http://emedicine.medscape.com/article/1128240-overview [accessed 16.11.09].

31. Khan A, Dayan PS, Miller S, et al. Cosmetic outcome of scalp wound closure with staples in the pediatric emergency department: a prospective randomised trial. *Pediatr Emerg Care* 2002;**18**:171–3.

32. Holger JS, Wandersee SC, Hale DB. Cosmetic outcomes of facial lacerations repaired with tissue-adhesive, absorbable, and nonabsorbable sutures. *Am J Emerg Med* 2004;**22**(4):254–7.

33. Farion KJ, Osmond MH, Hartling L, et al. Tissue adhesives for traumatic lacerations: a systematic review of randomized controlled trials. *Acad Emerg Med* 2003;**10**(2):110–8.

34. Singer AJ, Thode Jr HC. A review of the literature on octylcyanoacrylate tissue adhesive. *Am J Surg* 2004;**187**(2):238–48.

35. Quinn J, Cummings S, Callaham M, Sellers K. Suturing versus conservative management of lacerations of the hand: randomised controlled trial. *BMJ* 2002;**325**:299–305.

36. Broom J, Woods M. Management of bite injuries. *Australian Prescriber* 2006;**29**:6–8.

37. Bites, Animal: Treatment & Medication. *eMedicine* 2009; http://emedicine.medscape.com/article/768875-overview [accessed 15.11.09].

CARDIOVASCULAR

Section editor *Ian Everitt*

5.1 Cyanotic heart disease and tetralogy of Fallot spells

Robin Choong

ESSENTIALS

1 Cyanosis is dependent on haematocrit and oxygen saturation.

2 Cyanosis is caused by arterial oxygen desaturation or increased capillary oxygen extraction.

3 The hyperoxia test helps differentiate cardiac from other causes of cyanosis:

- Measure SpO_2 in room air or low FiO_2;
- Remeasure SpO_2 in 100% O_2;
- If SpO_2 remains low consider a fixed intracardiac shunt (cyanotic congenital heart defect);
- If SpO_2 increases consider other causes, e.g. lung disease.

4 If a cardiac cause is suspected check the pulses, blood pressure, ECG, and chest X-ray. Consult with a neonatologist, paediatrician or cardiologist *early*.

5 Cyanosis may be due to a duct-dependent lesion. A prostaglandin infusion may be advised following consultation.

Tetralogy spells

1 Cyanosis is variable and depends on the amount of pulmonary blood flow and right-to-left shunting.

2 Hypercyanotic spells treatment:

- 'Knee-chest position' or over parent's shoulder with knees bent;
- Supplemental oxygen;
- Sedation: intravenous or subcutaneous morphine, 0.1 mg kg^{-1};
- Intravascular volume expansion.

3 In prolonged cyanosis consider a vasoconstrictor.

4 For prevention of spells, propranolol (0.5–1 mg kg^{-1} po qid).

5 A Blalock–Taussig shunt may be used for palliation before corrective surgery.

Introduction

Cyanosis is a bluish discolouration of skin and mucous membranes due to excessive concentration of reduced haemoglobin in the blood.[1] Cyanosis is evident when deoxygenated haemoglobin in the cutaneous veins reaches approximately 5 g dL^{-1}.[2] Deoxygenated haemoglobin may occur either from arterial blood desaturation or increased oxygen extraction by peripheral tissue. Central cyanosis is produced as a result of arterial desaturation, i.e. aortic blood carrying deoxygenated haemoglobin. Isolated peripheral cyanosis may result from excessive deoxy-haemoglobin caused by extensive oxygen extraction.[1] Haemoglobin level affects the presence of cyanosis. Cyanosis is detected at a higher oxygen saturation in children with polycythaemia and is more difficult to detect in children with severe anaemia. Causes of cyanosis are listed in Table 5.1.1.

Cyanotic congenital heart disease

Cyanotic congenital heart disease (CHD) generally presents in the neonatal period. In the newborn, mild cyanosis (mild hypoxia SaO$_2$ >85%) may be difficult to detect

---

Table 5.1.1 Causes of cyanosis[2–7]

Differential diagnosis

Arterial oxygen desaturation (central cyanosis [pO$_2$ <50 mmHg])
1. Airway
   - Airway obstruction
2. Breathing
   - Lung disease
   - Central nervous system depression (e.g. coma)
   - Respiratory muscle weakness
   - Reduced respiratory drive (e.g. morbid obesity)
3. Circulation
   - Intracardiac right-to-left shunt (e.g. cyanotic congenital heart disease, pulmonary hypertension)
   - Intrapulmonary shunt (e.g. pulmonary atrioventricular fistula)

Increased capillary oxygen extraction (peripheral cyanosis)

1. Circulatory shock, e.g. sepsis
2. Congestive heart failure
3. Environmental, e.g. cold
4. Acrocyanosis of the newborn (autonomic – may last 72 hours)

Abnormal haemoglobin (not related to level of oxygenation)

1. Methaemoglobinaemia (pO$_2$ >50 mmHg but low O$_2$ saturation)

---

clinically. Other confounding factors may be acrocyanosis (a normal finding, which may last 72 hours), polycythaemia (giving the appearance of cyanosis) and dark skin (cyanosis is more difficult to detect). Cyanosis is better appreciated in natural light than in artificial light.

Arterial oxygen saturation should always be assessed with pulse oximetry when considering cyanosis in the newborn. The hyperoxia test may help distinguish cyanosis caused by cyanotic heart defects from other defects.[2–4,8]

Hyperoxia test

- Measure SpO$_2$ in room air or low FiO$_2$.
- Remeasure SpO$_2$ after 15 minutes in 100% O$_2$.
- If SpO$_2$ remains low, consider fixed intracardiac shunt (cyanotic congenital heart defect). Most cyanotic CHDs have a PaO$_2$ <60 mmHg (8 kPa).
- If SpO$_2$ increases, consider other causes, e.g. lung disease. PaO$_2$ >150 mmHg (20 kPa) almost completely excludes cyanotic CHD.

Clinical features[2,7]

A comprehensive cardiac and respiratory examination is essential in any cyanosed child. The key features are:

- pulses – rate, rhythm, volume;
- blood pressure – all four limbs if the pulse volume is abnormal;
- precordial impulse – heaves, thrills;
- auscultation – abnormalities of P$_2$, murmurs;
- pre-and postductal oximetry (right arm versus left arm/legs) if there is differential cyanosis.

Investigations

Investigations are directed at likely causes, after history and clinical examination. They may include arterial blood gas, serum electrolytes, glucose levels, full blood count, haematocrit, and cultures.

The chest X-ray (CXR) can be very useful and should be examined carefully for heart size (normal cardiothoracic ratio in AP film is <0.6), oligaemic lung field with decreased pulmonary blood flow, e.g. tetralogy of Fallot, or pulmonary venous congestion with an obstructive lesion, e.g. totally anomalous pulmonary venous drainage (TAPVD), cor triatriatum.

Management

The presentation of cyanosis in an infant or child mandates urgent review by a neonatologist, paediatrician or paediatric cardiologist. Echocardiography may be necessary urgently. Early discussion with a neonatologist or cardiologist can help clarify possible diagnoses and initial management in the emergency department (ED) setting.

An important issue in the management of cyanosis in the newborn period is recognising the duct-dependent lesion. A duct-dependent lesion is one that results from the ductus arteriosus remaining patent so that blood flow is delivered to both the pulmonary and systemic circuits:

- Pulmonary atresia/critical pulmonary stenosis. The ductus shunts right-to-left to ensure adequate pulmonary blood flow.
- Coarctation of the aorta/critical aortic stenosis/interrupted aortic arch. The ductus shunts right-to-left to ensure adequate systemic blood flow.
- Transposition of the great arteries. Mixing is required usually at atrial, ductus and ventricular levels.

If a duct-dependent lesion is considered, consult a paediatric cardiologist or neonatologist before starting an intravenous infusion of prostaglandin E$_1$ (PGE$_1$, 5–25 ng^{-1} kg^{-1} min^{-1}). Important side effects are respiratory depression and fever. Avoid PGE$_1$ when a small heart accompanies cyanosis and pulmonary oedema, because these findings suggest TAPVD with obstructed veins (PGE$_1$ will worsen pulmonary oedema).

Chronic cyanosis stimulates a reactive polycythaemia that increases the oxygen-carrying capacity. When haematocrit reaches 65% or more, a large increase in blood viscosity occurs.

Hyperviscosity and coagulopathy often occur and in patients with a right-to-left intracardiac shunt may result in stroke and brain abscess.

TETRALOGY SPELLS

Introduction[2–10]

Hypercyanotic, hypoxic or cyanotic spells occur in young infants with tetralogy of Fallot. These occur most commonly under 6 months of age and may be precipitated by agitation from any cause. The cause is likely to be multifactorial, including a component of dynamic infundibular obstruction. The net result is an imbalance of pulmonary to systemic blood flow.

Tetralogy of Fallot consists of anterior deviation of the outlet septum leading to the characteristic morphological features of:

- subpulmonary infundibular stenosis ± pulmonary valve stenosis ± hypoplastic pulmonary arteries;
- subaortic perimembranous ventricular septal defect (VSD);
- aortic root overriding the crest of septum and VSD;
- secondary right ventricular hypertrophy;

Clinical features include:

- intense cyanosis;
- hyperpnoea and acidosis;
- quieter and shorter ejection murmur (compared to before the spell);
- irritability, lethargy, loss of consciousness, seizures, death.

Triggers include dehydration, exertion and emotional distress associated with crying (increases pulmonary vascular resistance and hence decreases pulmonary blood flow). The child may have a history of previous squatting. Spells are usually self-limiting though sequelae include hypoxic–ischaemic encephalopathy and death. Spells are less common since the advent of early systemic-pulmonary shunts or early corrective surgery.

Investigations

Investigations include laboratory testing and imaging as follows.

Laboratory

Blood gas analysis – usually shows acidosis with hypoxia.

ECG

The ECG in tetralogy of Fallot usually shows:

- right ventricular hypertrophy in the unipolar and standard leads;
- right axis deviation ($+120°$ to $+150°$);
- dominant R wave in the right and a dominant S in the left precordial leads;
- Right atrial hypertrophy;
- normal PR interval and QRS duration;
- tall, peaked T waves;
- reversal of the RS ratio.

Chest X-ray

The classic *coeur en sabot* or boot-shaped cardiac silhouette is caused by the elevation of the apex due to right ventricular hypertrophy, combined with a concavity in the area of the main pulmonary artery. A right-sided aorta is present in 25% of tetralogy patients.

Echocardiography

An echocardiogram will accurately confirm tetralogy of Fallot but is not useful in acute management of spells.

Treatment[2–6,8–13]

❶ If possible, the child should be in a quiet, calm environment. Being held in parents' arms often diminishes crying and helps pulmonary blood flow.

❷ The knee–chest or squatting position is preferred as it increases after-load, thus decreasing R to L shunting.

❸ Supplemental high-flow oxygen ($10–15$ L min^{-1} of 100% oxygen via mask) should be provided.

❹ Monitoring includes continuous ECG monitoring, pulse oximetry, and non-invasive BP.

❺ Morphine ($0.1–0.2$ mg kg^{-1} intravenously (IV) or subcutaneously (SC)) should be used to treat hyperpnoea and decrease systemic catecholamines, and often aborts crying, which perpetuates the spell.

❻ Consider a small fluid volume challenge ($5–10$ mL kg^{-1}) to increase preload and reduce dynamic outflow obstruction.

❼ Propranolol ($0.05–0.2$ mg kg^{-1} slow IV push over 10 minutes, repeat once every 15 minutes) can be used to block β-receptors in the infundibulum, thereby lessening RV outflow obstruction. Other β-blockers may be useful.

❽ Phenylephrine (phenylephrine, $5–10$ mcg kg^{-1} IV [maximum SC/IM dose $= 10$ mg]) increases afterload, thereby decreasing right-to-left shunt. Alternatives include metaraminol (0.01 mg kg^{-1} IV) or methoxamine (0.1 mg kg^{-1} IV).

❾ Consider NaHCO$_3$ ($1–2$ mmol kg^{-1} IV) for correction of acidosis.

❿ Check temperature and blood glucose. Correct hypoglycaemia and hypothermia.

Disposition

Organise hospital admission and paediatric cardiology consultation.

Failure to respond to the above treatment mandates intubation, ventilation and deep sedation or general anaesthesia and intensive care admission. Emergency surgery is rarely indicated.

References

1. Anderson DM. *Dorland's Illustrated Medical Dictionary.* Philadelphia: WB Saunders; 1994.
2. Park MK. Congestive heart failure. In: Park MY, editor. *Pediatric cardiology for practitioners.* 5th ed. Philadelphia: Mosby Elsevier; 2008.
3. Abelson WH, Garth Smith R. *Residents handbook of pediatrics.* 7th ed. Toronto: The Hospital for Sick Children, Toronto, Canada, BC Decker Inc; 1987.
4. Guzman MF, Hedley Brown A, Been M, et al. *Manual of cardiorespiratory critical care.* Sevenoaks, Kent: Butterworth; 1989.
5. Kilham H, Isaacs D. *The New Children's Hospital Handbook.* Westmead: RAHC; 1999.
6. Apitz C, Webb GD, Redington AN. Tetralogy of Fallot. *Lancet* 2009;**374**:1462–71.
7. Allen HD, Driscoll DJ, Shaddy RE, et al. *Moss and Adams' heart disease in infants. children and adolescents: Including the fetus and young adult.* 7th ed. Philadelphia: Lippincott Williams & Wilkins; 2007.
8. Nichols DG, Cameron DE. *Critical heart disease in infants and children.* 2nd ed. Philadelphia: Mosby Elsevier; 2006.
9. Siwik ES, Erenberg F, Zahka KG, Goldmuntz E. Tetralogy of Fallot. In: Allen HD, Driscoll DJ, Shaddy RE, et al., editors. *2007 Moss and Adams' Heart Disease in Infants, Children and Adolescents: Including the Fetus and Young Adult.* 7th ed. Philadelphia: Lippincott Williams & Wilkins; 2007.
10. Park MK. Tetralogy of Fallot. In: Park MY, editor. *Pediatric cardiology for practitioners.* 5th ed. Philadelphia: Mosby Elsevier; 2008.
11. van Roekens CN, Zuckerberg AL. Emergency management of hypercyanotic crises in tetralogy of Fallot. *Ann Emerg Med* 1995;**25**(2):256–8.
12. Baele PL, Rennotte MT, Veyckemans FA. External compression of the abdominal aorta reversing tetralogy of Fallot cyanotic crisis. *Anaesthesiology* 1991;**75** (1):146–9.
13. Nussbaum J, Zane EA, Thys DM. Esmolol for the treatment of hypercyanotic spells in infants with tetralogy of Fallot. *J Cardiothorac Anaesthesiol* 1989;**3** (2):200–2.

Further reading

Allen HD, Driscoll DJ, Shaddy RE, et al. *Moss and Adams' heart disease in infants, children and adolescents: Including the fetus and young adult.* 7th ed. Philadelphia: Lippincott Williams & Wilkins; 2007.
Apitz C, Webb GD, Redington AN. Tetralogy of Fallot. *Lancet* 2009;**374**:1462–71.
Breitbart RE, Fyler DC. Tetralogy of Fallot. In: Keane J, Fyler D, Lock J, editors. *Nadas paediatric cardiology.* 2nd ed. Philadelphia: Saunders Elsevier; 2006.
Nichols DG, Cameron DE. *Critical heart disease in infants and children.* 2nd ed. Philadelphia: Mosby Elsevier; 2006.
Park MK. Congestive heart failure. In: Park MY, editor. *Pediatric cardiology for practitioners.* 5th ed. Philadelphia: Mosby Elsevier; 2008.
van Roekens CN, Zuckerberg AL. Emergency management of hypercyanotic crises in tetralogy of Fallot. *Ann Emerg Med* 1995;**25**(2):256–8.

CARDIOVASCULAR

5

5.2 Heart failure

Robin Choong

ESSENTIALS

1 Congestive heart failure (CHF) is a clinical syndrome and may result from:

- excessive workload caused by increased pressure or volume, usually increased pulmonary blood flow, and/or

- normal workload faced by a damaged myocardium.

2 Clinical signs may include tachycardia, tachypnoea, increased work of breathing, sweatiness, cardiomegaly and hepatomegaly. In addition, infants may have failure to thrive, recurrent lower respiratory tract infections and respiratory distress.

3 In older children, new onset heart failure may be less overtly symptomatic. Malaise, decrease in the level of daily activity, abdominal pain, nausea, anorexia and weight loss may be present.

4 Current medications used in heart failure include diuretics, digoxin and angiotensin-converting enzyme inhibitors.

Causes of congestive heart failure[1-4]

Most cases of congestive heart failure in childhood result from congenital heart defects.

❶ Left-to-right shunts with increased pulmonary blood flow, e.g. ventricular septal defect (VSD), atrioventricular septal defect (AVSD), patent ductus arteriosus (PDA), atrioventricular septal defect, patent ductus arteriosus.

❷ Acute left heart obstruction, e.g. aortic stenosis, coarctation of the aorta, interrupted aortic arch, hypoplastic left heart syndrome.

A smaller number of cases may be from:

❸ Primary myocardial dysfunction, e.g. myocarditis, cardiomyopathy, anomalous left coronary artery.

❹ Other causes, e.g. anaemia, metabolic, toxic, dysrhythmia.

Age-based

The causes of congestive heart failure change with age. Congenital heart defects generally present in the first days or months of life. Acquired cardiac disease may occur at any age. The following lists the likely causes at particular ages.

First days of life
Asphyxia, left heart obstruction, metabolic, sepsis.

One day to one week of age
Left heart obstruction in duct-dependent lesions, e.g. aortic stenosis, coarctation of the aorta.

Large left-to-right shunt lesions, e.g. large VSD, AVSD, truncus arteriosus.

First month
Large left-to-right shunt, e.g. large VSD, AVSD, truncus arteriosus.

First three months
Large left-to-right shunt, e.g. large VSD, AVSD, truncus arteriosus.

Metabolic disease.

Acquired heart disease may occur at any age due to:

- inflammatory/infective, e.g. viral myocarditis, Kawasaki disease, pleuropericarditis, rheumatic fever;
- metabolic genetic, e.g. inherited cardiomyopathy;
- dysrhythmia, e.g. sustained SVT, ventricular tachycardia (VT);
- severe anaemia.

Clinical manifestations and investigations[1-4]

Presentation

Infants may present with problems related to feeding, such as sweating, tachypnoea, reduced volume of feeds leading to failure to thrive. Respiratory problems, such as cough, recurrent respiratory infections, tachypnoea and increased work of breathing are prominent. Lower respiratory tract infection may have features in common with congestive cardiac failure (CCF). Cardiac failure should be considered in atypical, persistent or recurrent cases of lower respiratory tract infection (LRTI), particularly in infants.

General features

- Tachycardia – due to fixed stroke volume.
- Tachypnoea – due to decreased compliance with increased lung water.
- Gallop rhythm, weak pulse.
- Failure to thrive – from decreased energy intake, increased energy expenditure.
- Cardiomegaly – may be due to left heart obstruction with left-to-right shunt or left ventricular dysfunction.
- Sweaty (cold sweat) – prominent with feeding.
- Fatigue/lethargy.
- Hepatomegaly – not specific to right heart failure unlike in adults, may occur with any aetiology.

Investigations
Routine

- Chest X-ray
  Cardiomegaly (in an AP film the normal cardiothoracic ratio is <0.6). Pulmonary plethora in left-to-right shunt. Pulmonary venous congestion in left heart obstruction/left ventricular dysfunction. Radiologic features include reticulogranular pattern, fluid in lung fissures, pleural effusions, pulmonary oedema.
- ECG
  Assess rhythm, myocarditis (voltages), ischaemia (ST-T wave).

Specialized
- Echocardiography.
- Cardiac catheterisation.
- Others: angiography (computerised tomography and magnetic resonance imaging), viral studies (blood, throat swab, faeces), chromosomal analysis, urine metabolic screen, myocardial tissue biopsy.

Referral
The diagnosis of cardiac failure in an infant or child mandates urgent review by a paediatrician or paediatric cardiologist.

Management[1-3,5-15]

Current medications used in heart failure include diuretics, digoxin and angiotensin-converting enzyme inhibitors.

Acute management
❶ Resuscitate with ventilatory support if required.
❷ If desaturated consider supplemental oxygen. Caveat: large left-to-right shunt lesions (e.g. truncus arteriosus) may worsen with high FiO_2. Consult early in these cases.
❸ Fluid restriction and diuretic therapy.
❹ Infants with left heart obstruction may present with cardiorespiratory failure when the ductus arteriosus closes. Prostaglandin infusion may reopen the ductus and assist systemic perfusion.

Diuretics
❶ Acutely: furosemide 1 mg kg^{-1} $dose^{-1}$ intramuscular (IM) or intravenous(IV) (anticipate hypokalaemia).
❷ Chronically: furosemide 1–3 mg kg^{-1} day^{-1} in divided doses, with spironolactone, 1 mg kg^{-1} $dose^{-1}$ po q12h. Beware potassium-sparing effect of angiotensin-converting enzyme inhibitors.

Digoxin
- Severe congestive heart failure treated with initial IV administration. Early failure in less distressed infants can be treated orally. All patients should have oral therapy as soon as possible. IV dosage is only 70–80% of amount used orally.
- The total digitalising dose (premature: 20 mcg kg^{-1}; infant: 30–40 mcg kg^{-1}; over 2 years: 30 mcg kg^{-1}) may be given as 1/2 stat, 1/4 in 6–12 hr, and 1/4 in another 12–18 hr.
- Maintenance dose (IV, oral) is 3 to 5 mcg kg^{-1} 12-hourly (maximum of 200 mcg (IV) to 250 mcg (oral)). If heart failure is not severe, then may start with a maintenance dose only.
- Digoxin is contraindicated in complete heart block, pericardial tamponade, hypertrophic cardiomyopathy and other outflow tract obstructions. Reduce dose in renal failure.
- Monitor with ECG and serum digoxin level (keep below 2.5 nmol L^{-1} [2.0 ng L^{-1}]).

Angiotensin-converting enzyme inhibitors
Angiotensin-converting enzyme inhibitors are used in heart failure due to large left-to-right shunts and heart failure caused by ventricular failure. Oral captopril (0.1–1 mg kg^{-1} $dose^{-1}$ 8-hourly) or lisinopril (0.1 mg kg^{-1} daily, increasing to 0.2–0.4 mg kg^{-1} daily over 4–6 weeks) may be used.

β-blockers
β-blockers have a role in paediatric heart failure though doses are extrapolated from adult data. However, their role in children with heart failure remains to be fully defined.

Levosimendan
Levosimendan is an IV calcium sensitiser used in acutely decompensated severe congestive cardiac failure. It has inotropic, vasodilatory and cardioprotective properties. In adults with severe cardiac failure, improvement in 31-day survival compared with dobutamine has been shown.

References

1. Park MK. Congestive heart failure. In: Park MY, editor. *Pediatric cardiology for practitioners*. 5th ed. Philadelphia: Mosby Elsevier; 2008.
2. Shaddy RE, Tani LY. Chronic Congestive Heart failure. In: Allen HD, Driscoll DJ, Shaddy RE, et al., editors. *2007 Moss and Adams' heart disease in infants, children and adolescents: Including the fetus and young adult*. 7th ed. Philadelphia: Lippincott Williams & Wilkins; 2007.
3. Abelson WH, Garth Smith R. *Residents handbook of pediatrics*. 7th ed. Toronto: The Hospital for Sick Children, Toronto, Canada, BC Decker Inc; 1987.
4. Guzman MF, Hedley Brown A, Been M, et al. *Manual of cardiorespiratory critical care*. Sevenoaks, Kent: Butterworth; 1989.
5. Chang AC, Hanley FL, Wernovsky G, Wessel DL. *Pediatric cardiac intensive care*. Baltimore, MD: Williams & Wilkins; 1998.
6. Shaddy RE. Optimizing treatment for chronic congestive heart failure in children. Crit Care Med 2001;29(Suppl): S237–40.
7. Schwartz SM, Duffy JY, Pearl JM, Nelson DP. Cellular and molecular aspects of myocardial dysfunction. Crit Care Med 2001;**29**(Suppl.):S214–19.
8. Clark IIIrd BJ. Treatment of heart failure in infants and children. Heart Dis 2000;2(5):354–61.
9. Buchhorn R, Hammersen A, Bartmus D, Bursch J. The pathogenesis of heart failure in infants with congenital heart disease. Cardiol Young 2001;11(5):498–504.
10. Kay JD, Colan SD, Graham Jr TP. Congestive heart failure in pediatric patients. Am Heart J 2001;**142**(5): 923–8.
11. Wernovsky G, Hoffman TM. Pediatric heart failure management: Solving the puzzle. Crit Care Med 2001; **29**(10 Suppl.):S212–13.
12. Shaddy RE. Beta-adrenergic receptor blockers as therapy in pediatric chronic heart failure. Minerva Pediatr 2001;**53**(4):297–304.
13. Shekerdemian L. Nonpharmacologic treatment of acute heart failure. Curr Opin Pediatr 2001;13(3):240–6.
14. De Luca L, Colucci WS, Nieminen HS, et al. Evidence-based use of levosimendan in different clinical settings. Eur Heart J 2006;**27**:1908–20.
15. Egan JR, Clarke AJB, Williams S, et al. Levosimendan for low cardiac output: A pediatric experience. J Intensive Care Med 2006;**21**(3):183–7.

Further reading

Allen HD, Driscoll DJ, Shaddy RE, et al. *Moss and Adams' heart disease in infants, children and adolescents*. 7th ed. Philadelphia: Lippincott Williams & Wilkins; 2007.
Archer N, Burch M. *Paediatric cardiology. An introduction*. London: Chapman & Hall Medical; 1998.
Park MK. Congestive heart failure. In: Park MY, editor. *Pediatric cardiology for practitioners*. 5th ed. Philadelphia: Mosby Elsevier; 2008.

CARDIOVASCULAR

5

5.3 Syncope

Linda Durojaiye • Andrew Bullock

ESSENTIALS

1 The most common cause of syncope in children is vasovagal.

2 A careful and detailed history will usually enable the diagnosis of vasovagal syncope to be established with confidence.

3 The main differential diagnoses of syncope in childhood include cardiovascular causes, seizures, migraines, hypoglycaemia, drugs, and psychogenic events.

4 A 12-lead ECG should be done for all children at the initial presentation with syncope.

5 Any child in whom a cardiac cause of syncope is either suspected or diagnosed should be referred to a cardiologist.

Introduction

Syncope is the term used to describe any event of sudden and transient loss of consciousness and postural tone.

The range of incidences of syncope occurring in childhood is described as being from 0.1–50%, with peak incidences occurring amongst toddlers and adolescents. The most common events seen in the paediatric setting are episodes of vasovagal syncope. Differentiating the common, benign vasovagal event from rare differential diagnoses is essential to the appropriate management of children who present with syncope.

By contrast, in the adult population syncope is the cause of 1–3% of all ED attendances, and malignant cardiac arrhythmias are commonly the underlying cause.

Aetiology

The final common pathway that leads to all episodes of syncope is a sudden decrease in delivery of metabolic substrates, namely oxygen and glucose, to the brain.

In childhood and adolescence the major cause of syncope is transient autonomic dysfunction.

In toddlers such episodes usually manifest as either blue breath-holding spells or 'reflex anoxic seizures' (also called 'pallid breath-holding spells'). The mechanism for the cyanosis in blue breath-holding spells is poorly understood. The precipitant for reflex anoxic seizures may be a noxious stimulus causing reflex asystole, which leads to an anoxic seizure.

In older children and in adolescents such episodes most commonly present as episodes of vasovagal syncope. A combination of hypotension and profound bradycardia, or either bradycardia or hypotension alone leads to cerebral hypoxia. Complete understanding of the underlying mechanisms is lacking. Other terms used to describe these episodes include neurocardiogenic syncope, vasodepressor syncope or neurally mediated syncope.

The differential diagnoses of syncope in childhood include cardiovascular causes, seizures, migraines, hypoglycaemia, drugs, and psychogenic events. These are listed in more detail in Table 5.3.1. It should be noted that situational syncope (syncope that occurs during micturition, swallowing cold liquids, defecation or coughing), and carotid sinus sensitivity are rare in the paediatric population. Mitral valve prolapse has not been conclusively proven to be a cause of syncope.

Clinical

History

A careful and detailed history will usually enable the correct diagnosis of the most common cause of childhood syncope, vasovagal syncope, to be established with confidence. Any unusual features of the history should raise suspicion of an alternate diagnosis.

A complete history should include the following:

- A description of the event by a witness, if possible. Ask specifically about duration of loss of consciousness, seizure activity, incontinence of urine, pallor or cyanosis, and post-ictal drowsiness or confusion.
- Any antecedent events such as sudden emotion or pain, anxiety, fasting, intercurrent illness, blood loss, or a hot environment.
- Activity and posture at the time of the event.
- Prodromal symptoms such as nausea, sweating, visual or auditory changes, an aura, perioral paraesthesia and carpopedal spasm, palpitations, dyspnoea or chest pain.
- Relevant medical history including previous episodes of syncope, cardiac disease, epilepsy, diabetes, drug use and past sexual activity.
- Family history of sudden collapse or death, cardiac disease, epilepsy, syncope and metabolic disease.

Vasovagal syncope

The typical history of vasovagal syncope is that the episode occurs whilst standing or sitting upright. There may or may not be a stressful antecedent event (this occurs less commonly in frequent recurrent vasovagal syncope). There is a **prodrome** of nausea, dizziness, visual disturbance and a sensation of warmth, followed by a period of loss of tone and consciousness. Witnesses will describe marked pallor. Seizure activity is unusual, but brief tonic–clonic activity or stiffening is possible, particularly if the patient fails to fall to a recumbent position. Urinary incontinence may also occur. Recovery to a normal level of consciousness is usually prompt once in the supine position. Children who recognise the prodrome may avoid a syncopal episode by assuming the lying position. The child may have a headache, or be fatigued for minutes to hours after the event.

Table 5.3.1 Causes of childhood syncope

Abnormality of circulation	Vasovagal syncope Reflex anoxic seizures Blue breath-holding attacks Cerebral syncope Acute volume depletion Chronic hypovolaemia Orthostatic hypotension Pregnancy

Cardiac causes	• Tachyarrythmias
	  Supraventricular tachyarrhythmias
	  Wolff–Parkinson–White syndrome
	  Ventricular tachycardia
	  Ventricular fibrillation
	
	• Conduction disturbances
	  Long QT interval
	  Atrioventricular block
	  Sinus node disease
	
	• Left ventricular outflow tract obstruction
	  Valvular aortic stenosis
	  Coarctation of the aorta
	  Idiopathic hypertrophic subaortic stenosis
	
	• Right ventricular outflow tract obstruction
	  Pulmonary stenosis
	  Tetralogy of Fallot
	  Primary pulmonary hypertension
	  Eisenmenger's syndrome
	  Large pulmonary embolism
	
	• Dilated cardiomyopathy
	  Myocarditis
	  Idiopathic
	  Coronary artery anomalies
	
	• Pericarditis with tamponade
	• Vertebrobasilar insufficiency

Central nervous system disorders	Seizure Migraine
Hypoglycaemia	
Hypoxia	
Drugs and poisons (no QT prolongation)	Antihypertensive drugs Antiarrhythmics Carbon monoxide poisoning Volatile nitrites Others
Psychogenic	Hyperventilation Hysteria Malingering Munchausen's by proxy Panic disorder

Cardiac syncope

A cardiac cause of syncope should be suspected in a patient with a history of congenital heart disease or with a family history of sudden unexplained death. Cardiac events are more likely to cause episodes of syncope that occur with no warning, with associated chest pain, during exercise, whilst sitting or supine, or in association with palpitations (though palpitations are frequently described by individuals with vasovagal syncope, and with hyperventilation).

Long QT syndrome is an ECG diagnosis that is associated with episodes of syncope or seizures caused by episodes of paroxysmal ventricular tachycardia (often *torsades de pointes*). It may result in sudden death. Syncopal episodes in patients with this diagnosis may be precipitated by exercise or a startle, or may be spontaneous. The condition may be congenital or acquired. The ECG in sinus rhythm reveals a prolonged QT interval. The QT prolongation may be minimal, and a high index of suspicion is needed to make the diagnosis. The QT interval is calculated with Bazett's formula:

$$QTc = \frac{QT}{\sqrt{RR}}$$

where QTc is the corrected QT interval (normal <0.44 seconds), QT is the QT interval in seconds, and RR is the RR interval in seconds.

Reflex anoxic seizures and blue breath-holding spells

Blue breath-holding spells are usually associated with a prolonged episode of crying after which the child has a prolonged forced expiration and apnoea, and becomes cyanosed. This may be followed by a brief period of loss of consciousness, with a rapid recovery to full normal activity. They occur in children between the ages of 1 and 5 years, with a peak incidence at the age of 2 years. They are more common than reflex anoxic seizures.

Reflex anoxic seizures occur when an infant is suddenly startled (for example by an injury). The infant is seen to give one or two cries, quietens and then becomes pale. There is then an abrupt loss of consciousness, during which the infant may have brief tonic posturing and upward eye deviation. Tonic–clonic movements may occur. Episodes usually last less than 1 minute, and are immediately followed by normal consciousness and posture.

Of these children, 85% have no further episodes after the age of 5 years, though 17% may get recurrence of syncopal episodes later in life. There is no increased tendency in these children to develop epilepsy, and there are no associated abnormalities found on electroencephalogram (EEG) testing.

Hypovolaemic states

There will usually be a history suggestive of fluid or blood loss and obvious signs of shock may be present. Orthostatic hypotension and tachycardia may be the only positive clinical signs. These tend to occur immediately, as distinct from the changes seen in vasovagal syncope, which occur after more prolonged orthostatic stress.

Seizures

It may be difficult to differentiate seizures from vasovagal episodes, as they may both be associated with brief convulsions as well as a loss of consciousness. A history of significant post-event disorientation is helpful in differentiating seizures from other causes of syncope. Seizures are also more likely to be associated with cyanosis, tongue biting, and a more prolonged period of loss of consciousness.

Hysterical syncope

Hysterical syncope is a diagnosis to be made once all other possible causes have been excluded, but clues strongly suggestive of the diagnosis are often witnessed during the event. The child will have no hypotension, bradycardia or pallor, and fluttering of half-closed eyelids may be seen.

Hyperventilation syncope

Syncope due to hyperventilation may be associated with a prodrome of lightheadedness and blurred vision. It is not as commonly seen as other symptoms associated with hyperventilation, such as feelings of anxiety, breathlessness and perioral paraesthesiae or carpopedal spasm.

Examination

A structured approach to the clinical examination of all children presenting with syncope is essential to ensure that all relevant findings are elucidated.

- The airway must be examined, and the work of breathing noted.
- The peripheral pulse rate, rhythm and character must be noted, and the orthostatic blood pressure recorded (this is abnormal if there is a decrease in systolic blood pressure of more than 20 mmHg between measurements taken in the supine and sitting or standing position). Cardiac auscultation and a 12-lead ECG should be performed on all patients.
- The level of consciousness, posture and mental state of the child should be noted, and pupils and fundi should be examined.
- The child's temperature should be recorded.
- The history and the initial assessment should direct further examination of the child. In addition to searching for clues to the cause of the syncope, it is important to examine the patient for any injuries sustained during the event.

Investigations

Clinical investigations within the emergency department

A 12-lead ECG should be done for all children at the initial presentation with syncope. The primary aim is the exclusion of a prolonged QT interval, and of any arrhythmia or other abnormality of conduction.

A blood sugar level is an appropriate investigation for the child with a history of fasting, or with a family history of metabolic disease.

A βHCG is indicated in fertile and sexually active adolescent females.

Other investigations are usually unnecessary, and if done should be appropriate to the clinical history and examination findings for the child.

Further investigations performed in the emergency department (ED) may include:

- cardiac monitoring and pulse oximetry for any child in whom the history is suggestive of an arrhythmia, or who remains unwell;
- blood haemoglobin concentration where a history suggestive of significant blood loss or anaemia is obtained;
- serum electrolytes, urea and creatinine, and urinary specific gravity where a diagnosis of dehydration is suspected;
- a chest X-ray where a structural cardiac abnormality is suspected;
- Urine drug screen for patients with a history or examination that suggests intoxication with a specific substance; this is not a useful investigation when done routinely.

Any abnormality found in these investigations should then direct further investigation and referral.

Outpatient investigations of syncope

Consider referral and further investigation for any child with an atypical history or abnormal examination, or with severe or frequent vasovagal syncope (Table 5.3.2).

Any child in whom a cardiac cause of syncope is either suspected or diagnosed must be referred to a cardiologist. It may be appropriate to arrange secondary investigations such as an echocardiogram or Holter monitoring prior to discharge from the ED after discussion with a paediatric

Table 5.3.2 Indications for referral and further investigation of a child with syncope

- Atypical history
- Abnormal cardiovascular or central nervous system examination
- Suspect cardiovascular cause
- Suspect seizure
- Recurrent and problematic vasovagal syncope

cardiologist. It should be noted that Holter monitoring is often unhelpful as symptoms rarely occur whilst the patient is monitored. Some children may go on to have electrophysiological studies, exercise stress tests or cardiac angiography.

Where a history obtained suggests that the child has had a seizure, an EEG should be arranged in consultation with the neurologist or paediatrician to whom they are referred.

Head-upright tilt-table testing may be done in children with frequent, recurrent syncope, and in those children in whom a cause for syncope is not certain. Protocols for the test vary, but the requirements are that the child has a period of supine rest before tilting and is then tilted at a defined angle for a period of time. The most common positive response seen is a combination of hypotension and bradycardia prior to syncope or near syncope. Other positive responses seen are either isolated hypotension or asystole prior to syncope.

Video surveillance with continuous ambulatory EEG and cardiac monitoring may be indicated where fictitious events are suspected.

Management of syncope within the ED

For most children the diagnosis of vasovagal syncope will be made, and the majority of these will be able to be discharged well from the ED. These patients must be given advice regarding the precipitants and management of vasovagal syncope. Avoidance of usual precipitating events is important. Children can also be taught to recognise the typical prodrome of the event, and to then attempt to prevent any loss of consciousness by sitting or lying with their feet elevated. They should be discharged into the care of a capable adult.

Carers of children with a diagnosis of either reflex anoxic seizures or blue breath-holding spells should be educated and reassured prior to discharge.

Children seen with hyperventilation syncope may require treatment by rebreathing. They should be encouraged to breathe slowly and regularly, with a paper bag held over their mouth and nose. Once their breathing is regular and their symptoms improved, they should be encouraged to be calm, and to sit or lie down for a time. Both the children and their carers should be taught the technique prior to discharge.

Management of all other children should be appropriate for their particular clinical condition.

Summary

The most common cause of childhood syncope is vasovagal syncope. Careful history and examination are essential in making the correct diagnosis. All children who present with their first episode of syncope should have a 12-lead ECG.

If there is an atypical history or if there are any abnormalities in the clinical examination the child must be investigated and referred appropriately.

For children in whom a diagnosis of vasovagal syncope is made, education and reassurance of both the child and their carers must be done prior to discharge from the ED.

Further reading

Braden DS, Gaymes CH. The diagnosis and management of syncope in children and adolescents. *Pediatr Ann* 1997;**26**:422–6.

Breningstall GN. Breath-holding spells. *Paediatr Neurol* 1996;**14**:91–7.

Fleisher GR, Ludwig S, editors. *Textbook of paediatric emergency medicine*. 4th ed. Philadelphia: Lippincott Williams & Wilkins; 2000.

Hannon DW, Knilans TK. Syncope in children and adolescents. *Curr Probl Paediatr* 1993;**23**:358–84.

Johnsrude CL. Current approach to paediatric syncope. *Paediatr Cardiol* 2000;**21**:522–31.

Lewis DA, Dahla A. Syncope in the paediatric patient. *Pediatr Clin N Am* 1999;**46**:205–19.

McLeod KA. Dysautomnia and neurocardiogenic syncope. *Curr Opin Cardiol* 2001;**16**:92–6.

McLeod KA. Syncope in childhood. *Arch Dis Child* 2003;**88**:350–3.

Narchi H. The child who passes out. *Paediatr Rev* 2000;**21**:384–8.

Prodinger RJ, Reisdorff EJ. Syncope in children. *Emerg Med Clin N Am* 1998;**16**:617–26.

Reuter D, Brownstein D. Common emergent paediatric neurological problems. *Paediatr Emerg Med* 2002;**20**:155–76.

Seifer CM, Kenny RA. Head-up tilt testing in children. *Eur Heart J* 2001;**22**:1968–70.

Strange GR, et al., editors. *Paediatric emergency medicine. A comprehensive study guide. American College of Emergency Physicians*. New York: McGraw-Hill; 1999.

5.4 Cardiovascular assessment and murmurs

Matthew O'Meara

ESSENTIALS

1 Cardiac problems are uncommon in children, but should be considered in an infant or child with respiratory distress, cyanosis, collapse or shock.

2 Key requirements on examination are palpation of the peripheral pulses and liver and auscultation of the heart.

3 Murmurs are commonly found on examination.

4 Children with murmurs should be referred if they have:

- Symptoms which may indicate cardiac disease (e.g. breathlessness, cyanosis, chest pain)

- Abnormalities of the heart sounds (e.g. fixed splitting of the second heart sound)

- A murmur that cannot be confidently identified as innocent

- A murmur with a thrill grade 4 intensity or greater.

5 Chest X-ray and ECG may help in suspected structural disease but are unlikely to be helpful in an asymptomatic child with a murmur.

Introduction

Approximately 1% of infants and children in developed countries have congenital cardiac problems. The majority are from congenital cardiac abnormalities (see Chapter 5.5). Acquired diseases include myocarditis, pericarditis, cardiomyopathies and coronary vascular disease such as Kawasaki disease (see Chapters 5.6–5.8).

History

The onset of the symptoms caused by a cardiac problem will depend on the severity of the haemodynamic disturbance. A child with congenital heart disease may present at birth with cyanosis, with symptoms related to cardiac failure at days to months of age or with a murmur heard incidentally during examination. A child with an acquired cardiac problem may present at any age.

The timing and onset of symptoms should be carefully noted. Babies with cardiac failure may present with breathlessness, feeding difficulties, inability to complete feeds and poor weight gain. If cyanosis is described, it is important to determine whether it is persistent or intermittent and its relationship to crying, feeding and activity. Normal infants may appear peripherally cyanosed when cold or febrile.

Details about the pregnancy are relevant for infants with cardiac problems. There are associations with maternal diabetes (structural heart disease, transient cardiomyopathy) and with maternal lupus (congenital heart block). Teratogenic drugs during pregnancy may cause heart disease, for instance alcohol (atrial septal defect (ASD), ventricular septal defect (VSD)), amphetamines (VSD, persistent ductus arteriosus (PDA), ASD, transposition of the great arteries (TGA)) lithium (Ebstein's abnormality), retinoic acid (conotruncal abnormalities) and valproic acid (ASD, VSD, aortic stenosis (AS), coarctation of the aorta (CoA)). Infections during pregnancy may also be implicated. Rubella is associated with PDA and peripheral pulmonary artery stenosis. Perinatal events such as fetal distress and asphyxia may cause an ischaemic insult and cardiomyopathy.

A family history of congenital heart disease or a sibling who died suddenly without clear cause found at post-mortem (e.g. undiagnosed QT syndrome), may be important. Most congenital cardiac defects are multifactorial and the risk of another sibling being affected is around 1–3%. Several diseases have an autosomal dominant pattern of inheritance, including hypertrophic obstructive cardiomyopathy (HOCM), supravalvular aortic stenosis, Marfan's syndrome, idiopathic mitral valve prolapse and some cases of ASD and long QT.

The onset of features of cardiac disease varies with the type of lesion. Most neonates with congenital heart disease are asymptomatic at birth. Infants with duct-dependent left-sided obstructive lesions usually present in the first 2 weeks of life as the ductus arteriosus closes. Cardiac output falls and shock develops. Infants with left-to-right shunting usually present after 4 weeks of age when pulmonary resistance has decreased and heart failure develops.

The pattern of breathing may provide clues. Increased work of breathing and grunting suggest left-sided obstructive lesions or respiratory illness. Effortless tachypnoea may be found with cyanotic heart disease (see Chapter 1.1).

Other features in history which suggest a cardiac cause, include recurrent respiratory infections, exercise tolerance, chest pain and episodes of palpitations or syncope.

Physical examination

Examining a child's cardiovascular system is similar to examining that of an adult, but particular attention should be paid to palpation of the peripheral pulses and careful auscultation of the heart. As with most paediatric examinations, tact and patience are often required to maintain co-operation and elicit the signs accurately. Infants and young children may be most settled in a parent's lap and occupied with a quiet toy or feeding. One may have to be flexible about the order of examination, taking the opportunity to auscultate during quieter moments.

A general assessment of the child comes first. Note whether the child appears well, has any dysmorphic features and assess whether growth is appropriate for age. Look at the tongue and mucous membranes for cyanosis. Central cyanosis is generalised; peripheral cyanosis occurs in areas of poor tissue perfusion, which are usually cold to touch. Examine the fingers for clubbing.

The peripheral pulses should be examined. Assess the rate, rhythm and character of the pulse. Compare the resting pulse rate to normal ranges for age (see Chapter 1.1). Variation of the heart rate with respiration (sinus arrhythmia) in children is more marked than in adults. The character of the pulse may change with a cardiac defect, surgical treatment or cardiac failure. Bounding pulses are often found in febrile children without heart disease but may be associated with patent ductus arteriosus or a systemic-pulmonary shunt for palliative treatment of cyanotic heart disease with decreased pulmonary blood flow. Reduced volume or delay of the femoral pulses compared with the right brachial pulse suggests coarctation of the aorta. Diffusely small pulses are associated with low-output cardiac failure or shock.

Blood pressure is a routine part of the cardiovascular examination in children. A cuff of the correct size should be wide enough to cover two-thirds of the length of the upper arm, be centred over the artery and have a bladder encircling at least two-thirds of the circumference of the upper arm. In general, fit the biggest cuff possible without covering the cubital fossa.

Chest examination starts with looking at the rate and work of breathing and comparing the respiratory rate to normal ranges. Evidence of previous surgery includes a sternotomy scar or less visible thoracotomy scar (from repair of coarctation, patent ductus arteriosus, pulmonary artery banding or insertion of systemic-pulmonary shunt).

The apex beat should be located and palpated for thrills. The presence of a thrill indicates that the murmur is pathological.

Auscultation of the heart starts with listening for the heart sounds, especially splitting of the second heart sound. In children, splitting is usually only audible during inspiration at the upper left border of the sternum. The absence of variation between inspiration and expiration (fixed splitting) occurs in atrial septal defects. Third heart sounds are heard in 20% of normal children. Listen for clicks in early systole (in aortic and pulmonary stenosis).

Murmurs should be assessed with regard to their:

- timing – systolic, diastolic or continuous;
- localisation – the point of maximum intensity;
- loudness – increasing loudness from grades 1 to 6;
- character – ejection, pansystolic, early/mid/late diastolic;
- radiation – audible in areas away from precordium.

Auscultation of the chest should note air entry and presence or absence of crackles.

Abdominal palpation should pay particular attention to the liver span, edge and presence of pulsation.

At the completion of the cardiovascular examination one should be able to determine whether the child is cyanosed or not and whether the child has cardiac failure. The pulses, blood pressure and precordial findings assist with the assessment of the type of cardiac problem, even if a specific diagnosis is not possible. A chest X-ray and electrocardiograph (ECG) may assist.

Chest X-ray

The chest X-ray is good at detecting volume overload, but less useful for hypertrophy without dilatation. Key features to assess on the chest X-ray are:

- patient name and date;
- cardiac position (dextrocardia, situs inversus);
- quality of the film – centring, penetration, degree of inspiration;
- cardiothoracic ratio (usually less than 50% but up to 60% in AP films in neonates);

- cardiac contour – especially size of pulmonary artery and position of the aorta;
- lung fields – vascularity.

In acyanotic heart disease with left-to-right shunting there may be increased pulmonary vascularity.

In cyanotic heart disease, increased pulmonary vascularity occurs in truncus arteriosus, totally anomalous pulmonary venous drainage (TAPVD) and TGA. Decreased pulmonary vascularity occurs with pulmonary atresia, tricuspid atresia, Ebstein's anomaly, tetralogy of Fallot and critical pulmonary stenosis.

Electrocardiography

The ECG is good at detecting hypertrophy and therefore conditions with pressure overload.

The rate, rhythm and axis should be assessed. Normal QRS axis varies with age. At birth, the range is from $+60°$ to $+180°$, at 1 year 1° to 100°, at 10 years 1° to 130°.

Systematically look at the P waves, PR interval, QRS complexes, ST interval and T waves.

Atrial enlargement

- Right atrial enlargement – peaked P wave with height of >2.5 mm (Fig. 5.4.1).
- Left atrial enlargement – P wave >0.08 s, may also be plateau or notched (Fig. 5.4.2).

Ventricular enlargement

Right ventricular hypertrophy (Fig. 5.4.3):

- R greater than S in V1 after 1 year;
- T wave upright in V1 after 1 week;

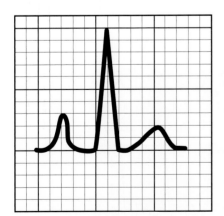

Fig. 5.4.1 Right atrial abnormality. Tall narrow P waves may indicate right atrial abnormality or overload (formerly referred to as *P pulmonale* pattern). From Goldberger: Clinical Electrocardiography: A Simplified Approach, 7th ed. 2006. Copyright © Mosby.

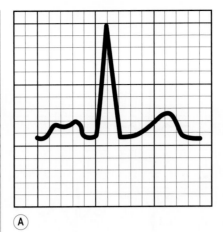

(A)

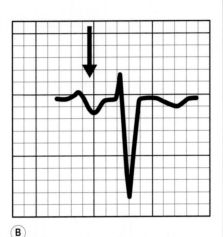

(B)

Fig. 5.4.2 Left atrial abnormality. Left atrial abnormality/enlargement may produce the following: **A**, wide, sometimes notched P waves in one or more limb leads (formerly referred to as *P mitrale* pattern); and/or **B**, wide biphasic P waves in lead V$_1$. From Goldberger: Clinical Electrocardiography: A Simplified Approach, 7th ed. 2006. Copyright © Mosby.

- SV6 greater than 15 mm at 1 week, 10 mm at 6 months, 5 mm at 1 year.

Left ventricular hypertrophy (Fig. 5.4.4).

- SV1 + rV6 greater than 30 mm to 1 year;
- SV1 + rV6 greater than 40 mm after 1 year.

The child with an asymptomatic murmur

Murmurs may be heard in around half of normal school-aged children and are heard even more frequently in infants. Many murmurs are innocent and can be recognised by their specific characteristics. Innocent murmurs occur when there is normal or increased blood flow through a normal heart and vessels.

Recognising common innocent murmurs enables exclusion of organic heart disease and the need for unnecessary investigation and referral.

There are four characteristic types of innocent murmurs

❶ Vibratory murmur.
❷ Pulmonary flow murmur.
❸ Carotid bruit.
❹ Venous hum.

The *vibratory murmur* (Still's murmur) is a short mid-systolic murmur best heard at the left sternal border or between the apex and the left sternal border. The murmur is of medium frequency and has a slight musical or vibratory character. It is often softer when the child stands or extends the neck and is louder when lying supine.

The *pulmonary flow murmur* is a soft blowing murmur maximal in intensity in the pulmonary area. Murmurs in this location are common in young children, but are often difficult to differentiate from an atrial septal defect or pulmonary stenosis, so may require assessment by a specialist.

A *carotid bruit* produces a rough ejection systolic murmur of medium frequency heard over the base of the neck, but is much softer below the clavicle.

A *venous hum* causes a high-pitched, blowing continuous murmur over the neck or sternoclavicular junction. It disappears when the child lies flat or when the neck veins are gently compressed.

Disposition

Referral for specialist consultation is indicated for a child with a murmur who has:

- symptoms that may indicate cardiac disease (e.g. breathlessness, cyanosis, chest pain);
- abnormalities of the heart sounds (e.g. fixed splitting of the second heart sound);
- a murmur that cannot be confidently identified as innocent;
- a murmur with an associated thrill (grade 4 intensity or greater).

Investigations

ECG and chest X-ray are readily available, but are poor screening tests for children with asymptomatic murmurs.

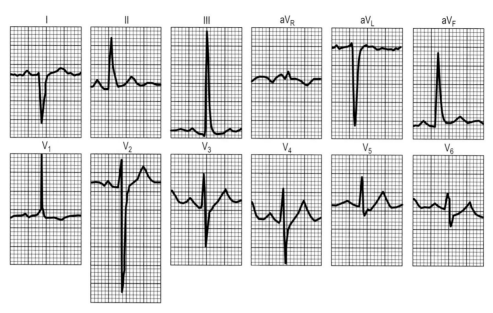

Fig. 5.4.3 Right ventricular hypertrophy. A tall R wave with an inverted T wave caused by right ventricular overload is seen in lead V₁ from a patient with tetralogy of Fallot. Marked right axis deviation is also present. (The R wave in lead III is taller than the R wave in lead II.) From Goldberger: Clinical Electrocardiography: A Simplified Approach, 7th ed. 2006. Copyright © Mosby.

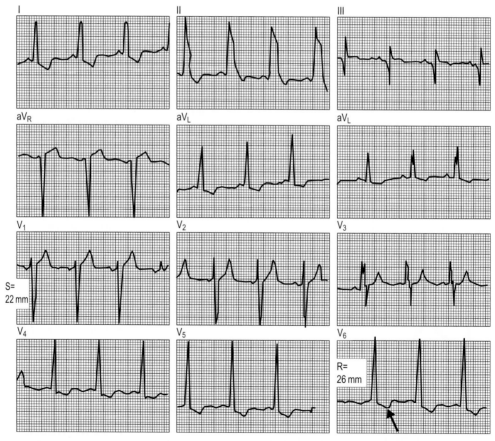

Fig. 5.4.4 Left ventricular hypertrophy. Tall voltages are seen in the chest leads and lead aV_L (R = 17 mm). A repolarization (ST-T) abnormality (*arrow*), formerly referred to as a "strain" pattern, is also present in these leads. In addition, enlargement of the left atrium is indicated by a biphasic P wave in lead V₁ and a broad, notched P wave in lead II. From Goldberger: Clinical Electrocardiography: A Simplified Approach, 7th ed. 2006. Copyright © Mosby.

The ECG is unlikely to disclose any unsuspected heart disease, but may assist in reaching the specific diagnosis when there is underlying pathology.

Similarly, screening asymptomatic children with a heart murmur chest X-ray is limited by poor sensitivity, specificity and reproducibility. Clinical assessment by a paediatrician or cardiologist correctly identifies almost all murmurs as innocent or needing further investigation. Echocardiography is not necessary in children identified by a specialist as having an innocent murmur

Further reading

Park MK. *Pediatric cardiology for Practitioners.* 5th ed. Philadelphia: Mosby; 2008.

5.5 Congenital heart disease

Matthew O'Meara

ESSENTIALS

1 Congenital cardiac disease is uncommon in children, but should be considered as a possible diagnosis in an infant or child with respiratory distress, cyanosis or shock.

2 The common congenital cardiac problems have characteristic clinical features that assist with clinical diagnosis and initial management.

3 The radiologic appearance of pulmonary blood flow and electrocardiographic features of axis deviation and ventricular hypertrophy assist the diagnostic evaluation.

Introduction

Incidence

Approximately 1% of infants and children in developed countries have congenital cardiac problems. Eight lesions account for 80% of all cases of congenital cardiac abnormalities: ventricular septal defect (VSD); patent ductus arteriosus (PDA); atrial septal defect (ASD); tetralogy of Fallot; pulmonary stenosis; coarctation of the aorta; aortic stenosis (AS); and transposition of the great arteries.

Common heart defects in infancy and childhood

Heart disease in children may present with the presence of an abnormal murmur, the development of symptoms or signs of congestive cardiac failure or central cyanosis. From an Emergency Department perspective, it is more important to identify the degree of cyanosis or cardiac failure, rather than identify the exact anatomic diagnosis. Clinical examination combined with the electrocardiograph

and chest radiograph will help the diagnostic process (Figs 5.5.1 and 5.5.2).

Clinical features

The age, severity of symptoms, and time of presentation of a child with congenital heart disease (CHD) vary depending on the specific defect, complexity and severity of the defect, and timing of the normal physiological changes that occur as the fetal circulation transitions to that of a neonate. The more severe or complex CHD lesions may not be clinically apparent immediately after birth. However, as the ductus arteriosus begins to close in the first few weeks of life, cardiac defects with obstructive lesions of the pulmonary or systemic circulations will be unmasked, and these infants will present clinically with acute cyanosis, shock, or both. Even the harsh systolic murmur of a large, isolated ventricular septal defect may not be heard until about the 4th to 6th week of life, when the left-to-right shunt across the ventricular septal defect increases due to the decrease in the pulmonary vascular

resistance. In general, the more severe the anatomic defect is (i.e., lack of pulmonary blood flow or lack of systemic blood flow), the earlier in life these conditions will manifest with cyanosis and shock.

The possibility of a congenital cardiac problem needs consideration in a child presenting with cyanosis, respiratory distress or shock. There are a number of general principles that may indicate a congenital cardiac problem.

- Is the child centrally cyanosed?
  - central cyanosis with normal breathing or only mild respiratory distress suggests a cardiac problem rather than a primary respiratory problem;
  - cyanosis that worsens with crying suggests a cardiac cause;
  - cyanosis that persists with oxygen suggests a cardiac cause.
- Does the heart sound normal?
  - Is there a murmur that cannot be confidently identified as innocent?
- Is the chest radiograph normal?
  - Is the heart shape abnormal?
  - Is the pulmonary vascularity increased or decreased?
- Is the electrocardiograph abnormal?
  - Is the axis abnormal?
  - Is there atrial or ventricular hypertrophy?

Acyanotic defects

These make up about 75% of all congenital heart defects. They include those associated with isolated left-to-right shunts such as VSD, ASD, PDA and those without shunting

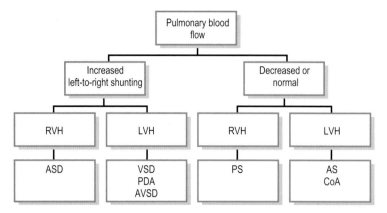

Fig. 5.5.1 Diagnostic approach to acyanotic congenital heart defects. AS, aortic stenosis; ASD, atrial septal defect; AVSD Atrioventricular septal defect; CoA, coarctation of the aorta; LVH, left ventricular hypertrophy; PDA, patent ductus arteriosus; PS, pulmonic stenosis; RVH, right ventricular hypertrophy; VSD, ventricular septal defect. Adapted from Marx: Rosen's Emergency Medicine, 7th ed. Copyright © 2009 Mosby.

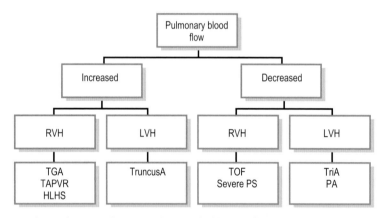

Fig. 5.5.2 Diagnostic approach to cyanotic congenital heart defects. BVH, biventricular hypertrophy; EA, Ebstein's anomaly; HLHS, hypoplastic left heart syndrome; LVH, left ventricular hypertrophy; PA, pulmonary atresia; PS, pulmonary stenosis; RVH, right ventricular hypertrophy; TAPVR, total anomalous pulmonary venous return; TGA, transposition of the great arteries; TOF, tetralogy of Fallot; TriA, tricuspid atresia; TruncusA, truncus arteriosus. Adapted from Marx: Rosen's Emergency Medicine, 7th ed. Copyright © 2009 Mosby.

such as AS pulmonary stenosis (PS) and coarctation of the aorta. See Fig. 5.5.1 for an approach to diagnosis based on radiological and electrocardiographic appearance.

Ventricular septal defect

VSDs make up 30% of all cardiac defects. The defect may be small or large and involve the membranous or muscular parts of the septum.

Clinical presentation depends on the amount of left-to-right shunting. A murmur may be noted incidentally on examination or congestive cardiac failure may develop in infants with larger defects and more shunting.

The characteristic clinical features of a VSD are a loud, harsh, high-pitched systolic murmur at the left sternal border, often associated with a thrill. The heart sounds are normal. Larger VSDs may cause a parasternal heave, a displaced apex beat, a softer systolic murmur and a diastolic murmur due to increased flow through the mitral valve. An infant with a large VSD will fail to thrive and become tachypnoeic, sweaty and tired with feeds.

The chest X-ray with small VSDs is normal. With larger defects there may be cardiomegaly and pulmonary plethora. The ECG often has features of biventricular hypertrophy.

Many small VSDs decrease in size or close spontaneously. In untreated cases complications of pulmonary hypertension and aortic valve prolapse may develop. Early surgical closure is indicated in cases where congestive cardiac failure develops in infancy or if pulmonary hypertension is present. Repair at a later age may be required if the defect fails to close or aortic valve prolapse develops.

Persistent ductus arteriosus

The ductus arteriosus, connecting the pulmonary trunk with the aorta, usually closes in the newborn period. It may remain open in premature infants or if the ductus is congenitally abnormal.

The clinical features depend on the size of the ductus. The only sign of a small ductus may be a continuous 'machinery' murmur at the upper left sternal edge. The diastolic component is often soft, creating the impression of a systolic murmur. With a large ductus the pulses may be bounding, the apex displaced and a mid-diastolic murmur audible due to increased flow across the mitral valve. An infant with a large PDA will fail to thrive, be tachypnoeic and may develop recurrent chest infections.

In small defects the ECG and chest X-ray are normal. Larger PDAs cause cardiomegaly, pulmonary plethora and left ventricular hypertrophy.

Premature infants with PDA may be successfully treated with indomethacin. Early closure is indicated in symptomatic term infants and premature infants following unsuccessful medical treatment of a PDA. Closure may be delayed in an asymptomatic infant with a small ductus. Closure with catheter may replace the traditional closure by ligation.

Atrial septal defect

ASDs are most commonly situated in the region of the fossa ovale and are called secundum ASDs.

Isolated ASDs cause an ejection systolic murmur in the pulmonary area, due to increased flow through the pulmonary valve. A soft mid-diastolic murmur may be heard at the lower sternum due to increased flow through the tricuspid valve. The pulmonary component of the second heart sound is delayed, causing wide fixed splitting.

Symptoms are mild. There may be mild effects on growth and exercise tolerance. Adults with unrecognised or unrepaired ASD may develop atrial arrhythmias and dyspnoea.

Chest X-ray shows increased cardiac size with pulmonary plethora. ECG shows partial right bundle branch block.

Closure is recommended for all cases with a significant shunt. Closure by catheter-delivered device is suitable in selected cases.

Atrioventricular septal defect

This group includes defects low on the atrial septum, abutting on the atrioventricular valves and may also involve the ventricular septum.

Defects involving the atrial septum and atrioventricular valves (AV) are known as ostium primum ASDs. The AV valves are usually abnormal, particularly the left AV (mitral) valve, which is cleft. Children with minor mitral regurgitation present with features like a secundum ASD. Infants with severe mitral regurgitation present with congestive cardiac failure.

When a significant ventricular defect coexists (complete atrioventricular septal defect), infants present with features similar to a large VSD with congestive cardiac failure in early months. This is the commonest cardiac defect associated with Down's syndrome.

The chest X-ray shows marked cardiomegaly and pulmonary plethora. ECG shows left axis deviation and partial right bundle branch block.

Surgical repair is required to repair the defects in the atrial and ventricular septa and AV.

Pulmonary stenosis

Pulmonary stenosis (PS) is the commonest obstructive malformation. The pulmonary valve is abnormal with thickened leaflets and partially fused commissures. The valve may be bicuspid.

The right ventricular outflow tract may be narrowed at other sites including infundibular stenosis, supravalvular stenosis and branch pulmonary stenosis.

Usually pulmonary stenosis is evident as an asymptomatic murmur. Moderate stenosis may lead to dyspnoea and angina with exercise and cardiac failure. More severe cases may present in infancy with cyanosis due to right-to-left shunting through a patent foramen ovale or ASD.

There is an ejection systolic murmur maximal in the pulmonary area, which radiates to the back. A thrill may be present. The pulmonary component of the second heart sound is soft. An ejection click in early systole can be heard at the left sternal border with valvular stenosis.

The chest X-ray may show a bump on the upper left heart border from poststenotic dilatation of the pulmonary artery. The ECG shows right ventricular hypertrophy in more severe cases.

Most cases can be treated with balloon dilatation.

Aortic stenosis

In aortic stenosis the aortic valve is abnormal with thickened leaflets and fused commissures. The valve is often bicuspid.

Left ventricular outflow tract obstruction may also occur due to hypertrophic subaortic stenosis and supravalvular aortic stenosis.

Most children present with an incidentally found murmur. Symptoms increase with age to include syncope, angina and dyspnoea on exertion and sudden death. Infants with critical aortic stenosis may present with severe cardiac failure.

The murmur is ejection systolic, maximal at the right sternal edge and radiates to the carotids. A thrill may be felt over the carotids, in the sternal notch or aortic area. An ejection click indicates valvular stenosis and is best heard at the apex. In more severe cases a forceful apical impulse may be present and the pulse pressure narrowed.

The ECG shows left ventricular hypertrophy in more severe cases.

Treatment options are open valvotomy or balloon aortic valvuloplasty but this may worsen aortic incompetence.

Coarctation of the aorta

There is a discrete narrowing of the aorta, near the site of the ductus arteriosus. There may be associated intracardiac anomalies including bicuspid aortic valve, AS, VSD and mitral valve abnormalities.

Coarctation may present in early weeks of life with cardiac failure or collapse with profound shock. Milder cases may only become evident with hypertension, a murmur or reduced femoral pulses in later years.

Physical findings are reduced volume femoral pulses. Delay of the femoral pulse compared to the brachial is evident only in later childhood after collateral vessels develop. The upper limb blood pressure may be elevated and a discrepancy occurs between upper and lower limb blood pressures of over 20 mmHg.

In infants with cardiac failure the chest X-ray will show cardiomegaly with pulmonary congestion. In later years the X-ray may show rib notching due to enlarged intercostal collateral vessels.

Infants with coarctation of the aorta develop cardiac failure from closure of the ductus arteriosus. In addition to supportive treatment, infusion of prostaglandin E1 may help maintain patency of the ductus in the collapsed shocked infant. Surgical repair is urgently required. Patients with milder degrees of coarctation require monitoring for development of hypertension.

Hypoplastic left heart

Some infants with severe aortic stenosis or coarctation of the aorta have associated gross hypoplasia of the left ventricle. Aortic and mitral valve atresia may also be present.

Infants with hypoplastic left heart present with shock in the first few days of life.

Resuscitation and infusion of prostaglandin E_1 (alprostadil) may help support. Treatment options include palliation and heart transplantation, although donors are rare.

Cyanotic cardiac defects

Cyanotic defects account for about one quarter of all congenital heart malformations.

There are three main types of defects – cyanotic defects with reduced pulmonary blood flow (e.g. tetralogy of Fallot), cyanotic defects with bidirectional shunting (e.g. truncus arteriosus) and cyanosis with separation of pulmonary and systemic circulations (e.g. transposition of the great arteries). See Fig. 5.5.2 for an approach to diagnosis based on radiographic and electrocardiographic features.

Tetralogy of Fallot

The four components of tetralogy of Fallot are PS, VSD, overriding aorta and right ventricular hypertrophy. The pulmonary stenosis is caused by infundibular muscular obstruction, often with valvular hypoplasia and commissural fusion, resulting in elevated right ventricular pressure. Although right and left ventricular pressures are similar, the resistance to ejection into the pulmonary circulation results in right-to-left shunting across the VSD into the aorta.

Cyanosis is often mild at birth and increases during infancy. Cyanosis is usually more obvious with crying or exertion. Hypercyanotic spells due to reduced pulmonary blood flow may occur and are characterised by marked pallor or cyanosis with respiratory distress, particularly after exercise (see Chapter 5.1). Children may have reduced exercise tolerance and squat on the ground. This manoeuvre increases systemic vascular resistance to reduce right-to-left shunting.

A systolic murmur due to infundibular stenosis is maximal at the left sternal edge and pulmonary area, radiating through to the back. The second heart sound is often loud and single as the sound of pulmonary valve closure is inaudible.

In untreated cases cyanosis gradually increases, resulting in decreased exercise tolerance, clubbing and growth retardation. Polycythaemia and thromboembolic complications may occur as well as endocarditis.

The chest X-ray shows a normal-sized heart with reduced pulmonary vascularity. The heart shape in severe cases has uptilting of the apex, resulting in a 'boot-shaped' heart. ECG shows right ventricular hypertrophy.

Total surgical repair may be possible in infancy if the pulmonary valve and vessels are suitable. If not, palliation to increase pulmonary blood flow can be achieved with a synthetic shunt between aorta and pulmonary artery (modified Blalock–Taussig shunt).

Persistent truncus arteriosus

In this rare defect, a single artery arises from the heart and branches into pulmonary artery and aorta. The truncal valve sits across a large VSD and receives blood from both ventricles.

Cyanosis is mild and congestive heart failure appears in the newborn. Systolic and diastolic murmurs are usually heard from flow through the truncal valve, which is often incompetent.

The chest X-ray shows cardiomegaly and pulmonary plethora. The ECG is often normal for age.

Surgical correction involves separating the pulmonary artery from the truncus, connecting it to the right ventricle with a valved conduit and closing the VSD.

Transposition of the great arteries

In this condition the aorta and pulmonary arteries arise from the incorrect ventricles. Deoxygenated systemic blood is directed through the right side of the heart and back into the aorta. Oxygenated blood from the pulmonary veins is directed through the left side of the heart and back into the pulmonary circulation. Survival is possible only if there are flows between each independent circuit through a foramen ovale, ductus arteriosus or septal defect.

Cyanosis is marked from birth. There may be a forceful right ventricular impulse but often no murmur. Metabolic acidosis may develop due to tissue hypoxia.

The chest X-ray shows a normal or slightly enlarged heart with increased pulmonary vascular markings. The abnormal arrangement of the great vessels gives the appearance of an 'egg on its side'. The ECG is normal or may show T-wave changes.

An urgent balloon atrial septostomy may be performed to increase interatrial shunting. Surgical correction with an 'arterial switch' operation is usually performed in early infancy. This also involves transferring the coronary arteries to the new aorta. An alternative is an intra-atrial patch ('atrial switch') to redirect blood flow at an atrial level (Mustard or Senning procedure).

Long-term complications of congenital heart disease

Bacterial endocarditis remains a risk with many congenital cardiac defects, especially palliated cyanotic congenital heart defects. Antibiotic prophylaxis should be carried out for procedures (see Chapter 5.7, Infective Endocarditis).

Arrhythmias may develop in children with congenital heart defects, particularly Ebstein's anomaly of the tricuspid valve, mitral valve prolapse, and after repair of transposition of the great arteries with atrial switch and repair of tetralogy of Fallot (see Chapter 5.9, Cardiac Arrhythmias).

Many patients who have undergone total corrective surgery for left-to-right shunts such as ASD, VSD or PDA will have few, if any, haemodynamic problems.

Children with repaired coarctation of the aorta may develop hypertension and restenosis. Late problems include coronary artery disease, congestive cardiac failure and ruptured aortic aneurysms.

Aortic stenosis often progresses with age. A gradient over 50 mmHg increases the risk of arrhythmias, syncope, sudden death, endocarditis and angina.

Patients with untreated VSD or atrioventricular septal defect may develop Eisenmenger syndrome with associated cyanosis and polycythaemia. Patients with palliated cyanotic congenital heart defects and patients with Eisenmenger syndrome should avoid situations in which dehydration may occur and lead to increased viscosity and risk of stroke. During illnesses such as gastroenteritis, diuretics may need to be decreased or temporarily discontinued in addition to ensuring adequate hydration status. High altitude, airline travel and sudden exposure to changes in environmental temperatures should also be avoided.

Further reading

Park MK. *Pediatric cardiology for Practitioners*. 5th ed. Philadelphia: Mosby; 2006.
Rosen's Emergency Medicine. *Concepts and Clinical Practice*. 7th ed. Mosby; 2009.

5.6 Acute rheumatic fever

Sarah Dalton

ESSENTIALS

1 Acute rheumatic fever (ARF) is a disease of connective tissue inflammation that may follow 2 to 4 weeks after a Group A streptococcal throat infection.

2 Diagnosis is based on the presence of carditis, arthritis, skin and neuropsychiatric sequelae.

3 The major complication of recurrent disease is progressive destruction of cardiac valves leading to rheumatic heart disease.

4 Treatment is comprised of eliminating streptococci, controlling joint pain and managing carditis, heart failure and chorea.

5 Antibiotic prophylaxis to prevent further attacks of ARF and episodes of infective endocarditis is mandatory.

Introduction

Acute rheumatic fever (ARF) is an acute inflammatory disease that may follow group A β-haemolytic streptococcal infection. It primarily affects connective tissue, causing carditis, arthritis and chorea and may follow a remitting and relapsing course for several years after the primary episode. Long-term complications of recurrent disease include progressive cardiac damage, which is associated with significant morbidity and mortality in the adult population.

Epidemiology

Rheumatic heart disease (RHD) is steadily decreasing in the developed world in association with improved standards of living and the availability of penicillin. Amongst developing countries prevalence is variable, with one of the highest prevalences worldwide found in the indigenous Australian communities. A family history of ARF is common, reflecting genetic predisposition as well as environmental influences.

Pathophysiology

The exact pathogenesis of ARF remains unclear. It is postulated that certain virulent strains of Gram-positive Group A β-haemolytic streptococci (*Streptococcus pyogenes*) invade the pharynx, leading to the production of anti-streptococcal antibodies, which cross-react with host connective tissue.

History

Acute rheumatic fever usually presents in school-age children but may present at any age. A history of pharyngitis several weeks previously is found in 70% of older children, but younger children are less likely to recall a sore throat. Typically, ARF presents with up to a week of high fevers, followed by several weeks of milder temperatures and the appearance of a rash (erythema marginatum). Specific symptoms include migratory joint pain, chorea, and neuropsychiatric manifestations such as abrupt personality change or poor attention span. There may be symptoms of congestive heart failure or non-specific symptoms such as weight loss, fatigue, pallor, headache and abdominal pain.

Examination

The diagnosis of ARF relies upon the identification of specific clinical features. The National Heart Foundation of Australia has developed diagnostic criteria which depend on the stratification of patient risk (Table 5.6.1). High-risk groups are those who live in communities with high rates of ARF or RHD such as Aboriginal and Torres Strait Islanders.

An initial episode of ARF may be diagnosed where two major or one major and two minor manifestations are present. The same criteria may be used to diagnose a recurrent episode, which otherwise requires the presence of three minor manifestations. All diagnoses require evidence of preceding Group A streptococcal (GAS) infection.

Carditis

A pancarditis, manifested as endocarditis, myocarditis or pericarditis, occurs in nearly 50% of cases of ARF. Clinical diagnosis begins with the identification of a new or changing murmur that must be distinguished from an innocent murmur in a febrile child. The mitral valve is most commonly affected, followed by the aortic valve. Myocarditis may be associated with a disproportionate sinus tachycardia or rhythm disturbance, such as first degree heart block. Signs of pericarditis or congestive heart failure may be present. Recurrent rheumatic fever leads to progressive valve damage and RHD.

Polyarthritis

The most common and earliest manifestation of ARF is polyarthritis or arthralgia. In up to one third of cases it may be the single presenting problem. Generally, large joints are involved, beginning in the lower extremities. The pain is often asymmetric, migratory and shows a marked response to aspirin. In most cases pain resolves within a week and virtually never results in permanent joint deformity.

Skin

Erythema marginatum

Erythema marginatum is a distinctive feature of rheumatic fever, but is only found in approximately 10% of patients. Lesions usually begin as small, pink, non-pruritic macules or papules on the trunk or limbs. The lesions gradually spread to develop a raised pink serpiginous edge with central clearing and remain late into the course of illness (Fig. 5.6.1).

Table 5.6.1 Diagnostic criteria for acute rheumatic fever

High-risk group	All other individuals
Major manifestations	
Carditis (including subclinical echocardiograph evidence)	Carditis (excluding subclinical echocardiograph evidence)
Polyarthritis, aseptic monoarthritis, or polyarthralgia	Polyarthritis
Erythema marginatum	Erythema marginatum
Subcutaneous nodules	Subcutaneous nodules
Chorea	Chorea
Minor manifestations	
Fever (documented >38°C)	Fever (documented >38°C)
ESR >30 mm hr^{-1} or CRP >30 mg L^{-1}	ESR >30 mm hr^{-1} or CRP >30 mg L^{-1}
Prolonged PR interval on ECG	Prolonged PR interval on ECG
	Polyarthralgia or aseptic monoarthritis

Amended from National Heart Foundation of Australia; Diagnosis and management of acute rheumatic fever and rheumatic heart disease in Australia – an evidence-based review. 2006.

Subcutaneous nodules

Subcutaneous nodules are an uncommon but highly specific manifestation of ARF. They are firm, non-tender nodules found over the extensor surface of the elbow, metacarpophalangeal joints, knees, and ankles. Up to three or four can appear in the first weeks of illness and may remain for up to a month.

Neuropsychiatric sequelae

Sydenham's chorea

Chorea occurs in up to 30% of patients with ARF, and is postulated to be due to cross-reactivity between anti-streptococcal antibodies and basal ganglia neurones. It presents with jerky, purposeless movement of limbs, speech impairment, involuntary grimacing or emotional lability, and may appear several months after the original GAS infection. Movements may be asymmetric and usually disappear during sleep. Generally symptoms improve in 1–2 weeks and resolve completely over 2–3 months, although the course can be variable. The presence of chorea is sufficient for the diagnosis of ARF without other manifestations, providing differential diagnoses have been excluded.

Investigations

Laboratory

Evidence of GAS infection

Preceding GAS infection should be demonstrated using a positive throat culture, rapid antigen detection test or elevated or rising anti-streptococcal antibody titre. Antibodies rise in the first month post-infection, plateau at 3–6 months, and normalise after 6–12 months (Table 5.6.2).

Acute phase reactants such as the erythrocyte sedimentation rate (ESR) and C-reactive protein (CRP) should be measured in all cases of possible ARF.

ECG

An ECG should be performed to identify pericarditis and first-degree heart block.

Imaging

To further evaluate ventricular and valvular morphology and function a chest X-ray and echocardiography are indicated. Echocardiography has an important role in the recognition of carditis, which may be clinically undetectable in up to one half of cases.

Differential diagnosis

Each clinical manifestation of ARF is associated with multiple alternative diagnoses, hence the need for strict diagnostic criteria. Sydenham's chorea is a diagnosis of exclusion after eliminating other causes of movement disorder such as drug toxicity, systemic lupus erythematosus (SLE), and Wilson's disease. Erythema marginatum is not specific for ARF, also being found in sepsis, glomerulonephritis and some drug reactions. Subcutaneous nodules are also seen in rheumatoid arthritis. Several systemic inflammatory conditions such as SLE and juvenile arthritis may fulfil all ARF diagnostic criteria and must be excluded.

Treatment

Acute management

Children who present with features of ARF should be admitted to hospital under a paediatrician for further evaluation and management. Management priorities are as follows:

1. Group A Streptococcus eradication

Following identification, GAS must be eliminated to prevent ongoing antibody formation. The National Heart Foundation of Australia recommends phenoxymethylpenicillin 10 mg kg^{-1} up to 500 mg po q12h for 10 days. Poorly compliant patients or those intolerant of oral therapy may receive single dose benzathine benzylpenicillin 450 mg intramuscular (IM) (<20 kg) or

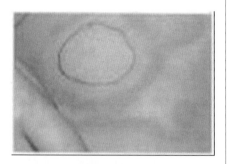

Fig. 5.6.1 Erythema marginatum. From Cohen & Powderly, Infectious Diseases, 2nd ed., Copyright © 2004 Mosby, An Imprint of Elsevier with permission.

Table 5.6.2 Upper limits of normal streptococcal serology

Age group	Anti-streptolysin titre (ASOT) (IU mL^{-1})	Anti-deoxyribonuclease B titre (Anti-DNase B) (IU mL^{-1})
4 to 5 years	120	100
6 to 9 years	480	400
10 to 14 years	320	380

Amended from National Heart Foundation of Australia; Diagnosis and management of acute rheumatic fever and rheumatic heart disease in Australia – an evidence-based review. 2006.

900 mg IM (>20 kg). Erythromycin may be substituted in cases of penicillin sensitivity.

2. Control of pain and inflammation

High-dose aspirin, 80–100 mg kg^{-1} day^{-1} in four divided doses, is indicated for control of pain and inflammation. It should not be commenced prior to definitive diagnosis, as discriminating clinical manifestations may be masked.

3. Treatment of carditis and control of heart failure

Prednisone may be indicated for severe carditis, but its use is controversial. Recommended dosage is 2 mg kg^{-1} day^{-1} continued for 1–3 weeks. Antifailure medication such as angiotensin-converting enzyme inhibitors or corrective valve surgery may be required, depending on the clinical situation.

4. Management of chorea

A variety of antipsychotics and anti-epileptics have been used to control Sydenham's chorea. Carbamazepine or valproic acid are commonly recommended, but their use is not universal and management should be undertaken with specialist consultation.

Prevention and prophylaxis

Continuous anti-streptococcal prophylaxis is recommended in all patients with a documented history of ARF to prevent recurrence with subsequent GAS infections. The National Heart Foundation of Australia recommends benzathine benzylpenicillin 450 mg IM (<20 kg) or 900 mg IM (>20 kg) every 4 weeks (or 3 weeks for selected high-risk groups). Oral phenoxymethylpenicillin 250 mg q12h may be used but is associated with poorer compliance and efficacy. In cases of penicillin sensitivity alternatives include oral erythromycin. Duration of therapy should be a minimum of 10 years after the most recent episode of ARF or until age 21 years. Prolonged therapy may be required for moderate to severe RHD and should be discussed with experts. Endocarditis prophylaxis is mandatory for those with residual valve disease (see Chapter 5.7 on Infective Endocarditis).

Prognosis

ARF resolves in most patients by 3 months. Complete spontaneous healing of valvulitis occurs in up to 80% of cases receiving prophylactic antibiotic therapy. Recurrent episodes of rheumatic fever are more common in younger patients and usually occur within 5 years. Prognostic indicators for chronic valve disease include total number of rheumatic fever episodes and time delay between onset of GAS and antibiotics in each instance. Of all patients with initial mitral valve insufficiency, up to 30% have evidence of RHD at follow up. This number increases substantially where aortic valve involvement, congestive heart failure or pericarditis was present at diagnosis.

Controversies

The role of echocardiography to diagnose ARF in the absence of a murmur is controversial. It can be difficult to distinguish the difference between echocardiographic features of pre-existing rheumatic heart disease and acute valvulitis. For this reason the National Heart Foundation of Australia excludes subclinical echocardiographic changes in diagnostic criteria unless the patient is from a high-risk group.

Further reading

Carapetis JR, Brown A, Wilson NJ, Edwards KN, Rheumatic Fever Guidelines Writing Group. An Australian guideline for rheumatic fever and rheumatic heart disease: an abridged outline. *Med J Aust* 2007;**186**(11):581–6.

Currie BJ, Brewster DR. Rheumatic fever in Aboriginal children. *J Paediatr Child Health* 2002;**38**(3):223–5.

National Heart Foundation of Australia (RF/RHD guideline development working group) and the Cardiac Society of Australia and New Zealand. *Diagnosis and management of acute rheumatic fever and rheumatic heart disease in Australia – an evidence-based review.* 2006.

Steer AC, Carapetis JR, Nolan TM, Shann F. Systematic review of rheumatic heart disease prevalence in children in developing countries: The role of environmental factors. *J Paediatr Child Health* 2002;**38**(3):229–34.

Stollerman GH. Rheumatic fever. Seminar. *Lancet* 1997;**349**(9056):935–42.

Therapeutic Guidelines: Rheumatology, version 1. Therapeutic Guidelines Limited; 2006.

Wilson NJ, Neutze JM. Echocardiographic diagnosis of subclinical carditis in acute rheumatic fever. *Int J Cardiol* 1995;**50**:1–6.

CARDIOVASCULAR

5

5.7 Infective endocarditis

Sarah Dalton

ESSENTIALS

1 Infective endocarditis is the microbial infection of cardiac endothelium.

2 Risk factors include congenital heart disease, central venous access, intravenous drug use and immunodeficiency.

3 Diagnosis is based on the presence of positive blood cultures with evidence of carditis, peripheral embolisation and immunological phenomena.

4 Acute management includes elimination of causative organisms and treatment of associated complications such as congestive heart failure.

5 Long-term chemoprophylaxis is recommended for procedures likely to result in bacteraemia in at-risk patients.

Introduction

Infective endocarditis (IE) is the microbial infection of the endothelial lining of the heart. Infection may be bacterial or fungal, and may arise in both structurally normal and abnormal hearts. Presentation can be acute or subacute and the long-term morbidity and mortality is high.

Epidemiology

Over the last decade the incidence of IE has increased owing to the improved survival of children with congenital heart disease and an increase in patients with central venous catheters. Up to 75% of children with bacterial endocarditis are known to have pre-existing cardiac abnormalities, most commonly ventricular septal defect and tetralogy of Fallot. Other risk factors include acquired valve disease, intravenous drug use, immunodeficiency and previous bacterial endocarditis.

Pathophysiology

Turbulent cardiac blood flow through a structurally abnormal heart can damage endothelium and lead to overlying thrombus formation. Transient bacteraemia may infect the thrombus and a vegetation is formed. The local effects of vegetations include valvular insufficiency, valvular obstruction, and perivalvular extension leading to intracardiac fistulae and conduction system abnormalities.

Extracardiac manifestations result from peripheral embolisation of thrombus material with subsequent infarction or infection of involved tissue. Mycotic aneurysms are secondary to bacterial embolisation causing infection and distension of the arterial wall and are most common in intracranial arteries.

Microbiology

Streptococcus viridans and *Staphylococcus aureus* are the most frequently encountered organisms in children with IE. Less common aetiological agents include enterococci, *Staphylococcus epidermidis* and Gram-negative HACEK bacilli – *Haemophilus*, *Actinobacillus*, *Cardiobacterium*, *Eikenella* and *Kingella* species. Fungal species such as *Candida* and *Aspergillus* may cause IE in neonates, immunocompromised patients and those with long-term central venous lines. Other agents such as *Coxiella*, *Pneumococcus* and *Listeria* are rare causes of endocarditis.

History

Patients with acute IE are often readily identified by systemic toxicity and high fever of short duration. The presentation of subacute endocarditis is more non-specific and usually includes fever, anorexia, malaise, cough, headache and arthralgia. A high degree of suspicion is required to identify these patients. Any presentation of unexplained prolonged fever, new neurological deficit or other embolic phenomena should be evaluated for endocarditis. Systemic embolisation occurs in up to 50% of patients with IE, and is most frequently seen in the first month post-diagnosis. Embolic events may cause infarction or abscess formation in the brain, lungs, kidneys, spleen, bone and extremities. Peripheral embolisation is often absent in acute endocarditis and right-sided heart disease, making their diagnosis more difficult. Endocarditis may also present with cardiac failure secondary to acute valvular dysfunction, fistulous tract formation or prosthetic dehiscence.

Examination

The physical signs of endocarditis may be subtle. A new or changing murmur may signify valvulitis, but can be difficult to distinguish from an innocent murmur or that of a pre-existing cardiac abnormality. Other findings include congestive heart failure or evidence of peripheral embolisation such as Osler nodes (tender, red nodules of finger pulps), Janeway lesions (non-painful, haemorrhagic areas of palms or soles) and splinter and subungual haemorrhages. These stigmata, which develop late in the course of disease, are unusual in children. Roth spots (retinal haemorrhages with a pale centre) are occasionally seen on funduscopy. Neurological deficit arises in 30–40% of patients from embolic infarcts, abscesses or intracerebral haemorrhage. Associated findings include splenomegaly in up to 30% of patients, and new onset clubbing may occur. Immune-mediated glomerulonephritis may result in haematuria, proteinuria and renal impairment.

Diagnosis is based on the modified Duke Criteria for Diagnosis of Infective Endocarditis (see below).

Modified Duke criteria

Major criteria

- Typical microorganisms from at least two separate blood cultures or a single positive blood culture for *Coxiella burnetii*.

- Mobile echodense intracardiac mass depicted on echocardiogram.
- Periannular abscess depicted on echocardiogram.
- New partial dehiscence of prosthetic valve depicted on echocardiogram.
- New valvular regurgitation depicted on echocardiogram.

Minor criteria

- Predisposing factor – history of intravenous (IV) drug use or congenital heart disease.
- Fever >38°C.
- Vascular phenomena – arterial emboli, pulmonary infarcts, mycotic aneurysm, intracranial haemorrhage, conjunctival haemorrhage, Janeway lesions.
- Immunological phenomena – glomerulonephritis, Osler nodes, Roth spots, positive rheumatoid factor.
- Positive blood cultures or serological evidence of infection not meeting above criteria.

These criteria determine three diagnostic categories: definite endocarditis, possible endocarditis and rejected cases. Definite diagnosis requires the presence of two major, one major with three minor, or five minor criteria. Possible endocarditis is defined by one major with one minor, or three minor criteria. Rejected cases are those where manifestations are explained by a clear alternate diagnosis or resolve after antibiotic therapy for 4 days or less.

Investigations

Laboratory

The most definitive test for IE is the identification of a known causative organism from more than one blood culture. In all cases of suspected endocarditis three sets of blood cultures should be collected from different peripheral sites prior to antibiotic administration. Up to 10% of all cases of IE remain culture negative, usually where organisms are highly fastidious, non-bacterial, or microbiological techniques are insufficient. Nonspecific inflammatory markers such as white cell count, C-reactive protein, erythrocyte sedimentation rate and rheumatoid factor may also be abnormal.

Imaging

The investigation of possible endocarditis should include an electrocardiogram (ECG) and chest X-ray (CXR) but findings are non-specific. A CXR may reveal evidence of cardiac or pulmonary complications but is not diagnostic of IE. Transthoracic echocardiography is the most definitive investigation and yields excellent images in most paediatric patients.

Accuracy can be increased using transoesophageal echocardiography (TOE), which should be considered in high-risk groups. Echocardiographic findings are also used to guide management such as surgical intervention.

Differential diagnosis

The presentation of IE is similar to many systemic inflammatory conditions. Positive blood cultures often distinguish the diagnosis, but in suggestive presentations where blood cultures remain negative, other diagnoses must be considered. Rheumatic fever, Kawasaki disease, systemic lupus erythematosus and leukaemia all have similar presentations, hence the need for rigorous diagnostic criteria.

Treatment

Medical

The medical management of IE includes eliminating causative microorganisms and treating complications such as congestive heart failure. The bacterial infection of vegetations is relatively protected and must be completely eradicated with prolonged parenteral therapy. As the aetiological agent is usually unknown at presentation, empiric antibiotic therapy should be commenced. Australian antibiotic guidelines recommend benzylpenicillin (45 mg kg^{-1}, max. 1.8 g) and flucloxacillin (50 mg kg^{-1}, max. 2 g) intravenously every 4 hours with daily IV gentamicin (4–6 mg kg^{-1}, max. 160 mg). Vancomycin should be added if there is a prosthetic valve, penicillin allergy, nosocomial infection or risk of methicillin-resistant *Staphylococcus aureus*. The duration of parenteral therapy is usually 4–6 weeks, modified by the aetiological agent and therapeutic response. Monitoring of drug levels

and consultation with microbiologists should be undertaken to optimise therapy.

Surgical

The need for surgical management of IE depends on the severity of complications and response to medical management. Perivalvular abscesses, obstructive vegetations, cardiac fistulae and prosthetic dehiscence often require surgery. Other indications include persistent bacteraemia, recurrent embolisation, and some cases of fungal endocarditis.

Prognosis

The overall mortality of IE remains approximately 25% and morbidity is also considerable, with up to 60% of confirmed cases developing significant complications. Poor prognosis is associated with *Staphylococcus aureus* infection and fungal disease. Severe cardiac failure, prolonged clinical symptoms and poor response to antibiotics are also associated with worse outcomes.

Prevention

Antibiotic prophylaxis for IE is recommended internationally but guidelines are based on expert consensus and vary across the world. Australian guidelines adopt recommendations from the American Heart Association and consider the underlying cardiac condition and risk of the proposed procedure.

Recommended conditions requiring prophylaxis:

- prosthetic cardiac valves;
- cardiac transplant with subsequent valvulopathy;
- rheumatic heart disease with valvular pathology;
- previous infective endocarditis;
- congenital heart disease if:
  - unrepaired cyanotic defect;
  - completely repaired defect with prosthetic material up to 6 months post procedure;
  - repaired defects with residual defect at prosthetic part.

Chemoprophylaxis depends on the procedure being performed. Australian guidelines suggest dental and upper respiratory tract procedures (e.g. reimplantation of avulsed tooth) receive amoxicillin (50 mg kg^{-1} orally) as a single dose 1 hour before the procedure. Cephalexin or clindamycin are alternatives for penicillin sensitivity. Genito-urinary and gastrointestinal procedures require ampicillin (50 mg kg^{-1} IV) just before the procedure, or vancomycin (25 mg kg^{-1} IV) if pencillin allergic. Endo-tracheal intubation and urinary catheterisation do not require antibiotic prophylaxis. Current therapeutic guidelines should be consulted to optimise management in each case.

Controversies

There is no published evidence to show that antibiotic prophylaxis prevents IE. Endocarditis is thought more likely to result from random bacteraemia than from that associated with dental, GI or GU procedures. The American Heart Association has recently revised guidelines to reduce the categories of patients for whom prophylaxis is recommended and Australian guidelines are in keeping with these recommendations.

Further reading

Baddour LM, Wilson WR, Bayer AR, et al. Infective Endocarditis; Diagnosis, Antimicrobial Therapy, and Management of Complications: A Statement for Healthcare Professionals. *Circulation* 2005;**111**:3167–84.

Fuster V. *The AHA Guidelines and Scientific Statements Handbook.* Wiley-Blackwell; 2009.

Milazzo AS, Li JS. Bacterial endocarditis in infants and children. *Paediatr Infect Dis J* 2001;**20**(8):799–801.

Prendergast BD. The changing face of infective endocarditis. *Heart* 2006;**92**:879–85.

Therapeutic Guidelines: Antibiotics, Version 13. Therapeutic Guidelines Limited; 2006.

Therapeutic Guidelines: Prevention of Endocarditis. Therapeutic Guidelines Limited; 2008.

Wilson W, Taubert KA, Gewitz M, et al. Prevention of Infective Endocarditis. *Circulation* 2007;**116**:1736–54.

5.8 Kawasaki disease

Daryl Efron

ESSENTIALS

1 Kawasaki disease is an uncommon ED presentation, but should be considered in any child with an unexplained prolonged fever, particularly in the presence of a rash and red eyes.

2 The diagnosis is *clinical* with presence of fever and four out of five other criteria.

3 Diagnostic criteria can appear sequentially and may not all be present at the same time, which can make early diagnosis difficult.

4 Patients with 'atypical Kawasaki disease' are being increasingly recognised, in whom full criteria are not met, but the patient has coronary artery abnormalities. These are often infants.

5 Any child with suspected Kawasaki disease should be treated immediately, regardless of the duration of symptoms.

6 Intravenous immunoglobulin (single dose of 2 g kg^{-1}) significantly reduces the risk of coronary artery abnormalities, especially if given in the first 10 days of illness.

Introduction

Kawasaki disease (KD) is an acute, self-limiting vasculitic illness predominantly affecting infants and young children. It is now a leading cause of acquired heart disease in children in Western countries. The diagnosis is made clinically, and effective treatment is available to reduce the likelihood of potentially fatal coronary vasculitis. KD was first described in 1967 as 'mucocutaneous lymph node syndrome' in a series of 50 Japanese children.[1] Although it is most common in Japanese and Korean children (annual incidence 90–150/100 000 children younger than 5 years), it occurs in all ethnic groups, with an annual incidence in the United States of approximately 10/100 000 children younger than 5 years old. The majority of cases (85%) occur in children aged less than 5 years of age. It is 1.5 times more common in boys than girls.[2]

Many features of KD suggest an infectious aetiology. These include: seasonal variation (peak in winter/spring); occasional outbreaks; 10-fold higher risk in siblings than in the general population; rarity in young infants (suggesting protection from mater-nally acquired antibody); low recurrence rate (4%, which suggests acquired immunity); as well as the resemblance of the clinical pre-sentation to other self-limiting infectious dis-eases, such as measles, adenovirus infection and staphylococcal toxic shock syndrome. However, despite much investigation of a variety of viral and bacterial pathogens, there is as yet no good evidence to implicate any known organism in KD. The ethnic vari-ation suggests a genetic predisposition.

There is debate as to whether the inflam-matory response in KD is initiated by a con-ventional antigen or a superantigen, and there are some immunological features to support both hypotheses. Unreplicated reports of increased expression of specific T-cell receptor V β-regions suggest toxin activation, whereas infiltration of paratra-cheal and vascular tissue with reactive clonal IgA plasma cells suggests entry of a conventional antigen via the respiratory route.[3]

Pathophysiology

The pathophysiology of KD involves vasculi-tis of medium-sized vessels including coro-nary, renal, hepatic and splanchnic arteries, beginning in both adventitial and intimal surfaces and proceeding toward the media. Coronary changes occur in approximately 20% of untreated patients.[4] Immune activa-tion involving cytokines and growth factors leads to inflammation and aneurysm forma-tion, with the risk of thrombosis. The process evolves for a long period after the acute illness. In the majority of patients with echocardiographically demonstrable coronary artery lesions, the vessels remodel and have a normal appearance within a year or so. However, there is evidence of subtle long-term changes in coronary artery function, the clinical significance of which remain unclear.[5] The risk of early adult coronary artery disease in these patients is unknown.

A diffuse inflammatory process of a variety of tissues has been found in autopsy specimens including lymph nodes, liver and gallbladder.[2] Endothelial changes are prominent, with hyperplasia, necrosis and thrombosis. Myocardial abnormalities include hypertrophy of myocytes and fibrosis.

Clinical features

KD should be considered in the differential diagnosis of all infants and young children with a fever, rash and red eyes, as well as those with a prolonged fever without an alternative explanation. The diagnostic criteria are outlined in Table 5.8.1.

The diagnosis can be made earlier than day 5 if other features are present. This is important, as there is evidence that earlier administration of intravenous immunoglobulin (IVIG) is associated with a shorter illness and reduced risk of coronary disease.[6]

The fever is often associated with irritability, which responds poorly to paracetamol. Over 90% of patients develop a rash, which can take any of a number of forms – scarlatiniform, morbilliform or maculopapular. It often has the appearance of a viral eruption or allergic reaction, but can appear urticarial. Petechiae are sometimes seen, as are micropustules. The red eyes demonstrate characteristic sparing of the avascular perilimbic region, giving the appearance of a

halo around the cornea. There is not usually an exudate. The changes may resolve rapidly, such that this important feature may be present only on history rather than being present when the child is examined. The cervical nodes are commonly unilateral and in the anterior chain. Generalised lymphadenopathy and splenomegaly are absent. The subacute phase occurs from 2–4 weeks, with resolution of fever. Desquamation (periungual) of fingers and toes may occur during this time.

KD is a multisystem disease with many and varied clinical manifestations. In addition to those in the diagnostic criteria, common features include marked irritability, diarrhoea, cough, arthralgia/arthritis, urethritis with sterile pyuria, otitis media, mild hepatic dysfunction, hydrops of the gallbladder and aseptic meningitis. Diagnosis is more likely to be delayed in older children, in whom less classical manifestations such as gastrointestinal and joint symptoms often predominate.[7]

Incomplete KD

Cases of incomplete or 'atypical KD' are being increasingly recognised, in which full criteria are not met, but the patient has coronary artery abnormalities. This is more common in young infants.[8] The incidence of coronary artery aneurysms is at least as high in incomplete KD as in classical cases. Given that infants under 6 months appear to be at increased risk of developing coronary abnormalities;[8] a lower threshold for treatment is probably indicated in this group. KD should be considered in all children with unexplained fever for 5 days and at least two major features of KD, and any infant with unexplained fever for over a week.[4]

Differential diagnosis

Depending on which features are present, a broad differential diagnosis needs to be considered in cases of possible KD. These include viral infections (e.g. measles, adenovirus, enterovirus), streptococcal and staphylococcal toxic-mediated illness (scarlet fever, toxic shock syndrome), drug allergy (including Stevens–Johnson syndrome), inflammatory

bowel disease, connective tissue disease, particularly Still's disease, and malignancy.

Complications

The major concern with KD is coronary artery disease. Younger children, especially under 12 months of age, are at highest risk. Changes seen include dilatation (ectasia) and discrete aneurysms. Aneurysms are classified according to the internal diameter into small (<3 mm), medium (3–6 mm), large (6–8 mm) and giant (>8 mm). Although aneurysms rarely form in the first 10 days of KD, echocardiographic signs of coronary arteritis may be seen, including perivascular brightness, ectasia and lack of tapering.[4] Other findings may include decreased left ventricular contractility, mitral regurgitation, and pericardial effusion.

Coronary artery occlusion is most likely to occur in giant aneurysms, through a combination of sluggish blood flow and fibrotic stenosis at proximal and/or distal ends of the aneurysm. Thrombosis of coronary aneurysms can cause myocardial infarction and sudden death. Mortality is increased over the background rate within the first two months. Rarely, myocarditis can occur, causing congestive cardiac failure or arrhythmias. Thrombosis of peripheral arteries can lead to ischaemia and gangrene.

Investigations

Any child who presents with possible features of KD should be discussed with a paediatrician.

There is **no definitive diagnostic test** for KD. Investigation is directed toward excluding alternative diagnoses, as well as gathering supporting evidence for the diagnosis of KD. At least one set of blood cultures should be taken, and cultures of urine, cerebrospinal fluid and other sites may be indicated. Serological testing for Group A *Streptococcus*, and for specific viruses such as measles may be helpful. In KD, the peripheral white cell count and inflammatory markers are generally significantly raised. The erythrocyte sedimentation rate may continue to rise as the child improves clinically. A marked thrombocytosis is commonly seen in the second to third week of the illness.

Table 5.8.1 Diagnostic criteria for Kawasaki disease

Fever (at least 5 days)
Plus four of the following five features:
- bilateral conjunctival injection
- enanthem – dry, cracked lips; oropharyngeal erythema; strawberry tongue
- exanthem – polymorphous
- peripheral changes – erythema (palms and soles), oedema (hands and feet), desquamation (2nd to 3rd week)
- cervical adenopathy

Pyuria, due to sterile urethritis, is often found on a voided sample (not on suprapubic aspirate (SPA) or catheter). Serum gamma glutamyl transferase is commonly elevated. Exclusion of markers for connective tissue disorders may be useful.

Echocardiography should be undertaken as soon as the diagnosis of KD is suspected. The American Heart Association guidelines suggest repeat echocardiograms at 2 weeks (time of maximal aneurysm formation), 6 weeks and 12 months (looking for late sequelae). If abnormalities are demonstrated on echocardiography, closer cardiological follow up may be required, depending on the lesion. A 12-lead ECG is most often normal but may show dysrhythmias, change in PR or QT intervals or non-specific ST changes.

Treatment

Treatment of KD is directed towards reducing the inflammation as rapidly as possible. The clinical markers of response to therapy are the temperature and patient's general well-being, supported by the white cell count and CRP.

IVIG therapy has been demonstrated to induce resolution of fever as well as significantly reduce the risk of coronary artery abnormalities (from around 20% to around 3–5%) if given within the first 10 days of the illness.[9] The precise mechanism of action of IVIG is unknown. Theories include saturation blockade of Fc receptors, direct antibody activity against bacterial superantigen, an unidentified causative pathogen or toxin, modulation of cytokine production or down-regulation of antibody synthesis. The optimal dose is 2 g kg^{-1} day^{-1} as a single infusion over 10–12 hours. There is some evidence that IVIG is also effective if given beyond 10 days;[10] however, treatment as early as possible is optimal.[6] IVIG should be given to patients with KD after the 10th day if they have persistent fever or other evidence of ongoing systemic inflammation.[4] The effect of IVIG in patients who have already developed coronary artery aneurysms is unknown, though there may be some benefit.[9] Different brands of IVIG may vary in their clinical effects, due to variation in sterilisation and other manufacturing procedures. As passive antibody acquisition

may interfere with immunogenicity, live vaccine administration (e.g. measles, varicella) should be postponed by 3 months in children who have been given IVIG.

In the 1980s, high-dose aspirin was shown to decrease the incidence of coronary artery involvement in KD.[11] The current role of aspirin in KD is difficult to determine as it has been used in combination with IVIG in the major trials. Many centres have used high-dose aspirin (80–100 mg kg^{-1} day^{-1} in 3–4 divided doses, for anti-inflammatory effect) initially, and then switched to low-dose (3–5 mg kg^{-1} day^{-1}, antiplatelet effect) after the patient's fever resolves. However, in patients treated with IVIG, concomitant use of high-dose aspirin initially does not appear to result in shorter duration of fever or hospitalisation than low-dose.[12] Furthermore, the incidence of coronary artery aneurysm appears to be independent of aspirin dose.[13] Therefore low-dose aspirin seems to be sufficient for initial treatment. Low-dose aspirin is continued for 6–8 weeks, and then stopped if there is no coronary involvement.

The role of corticosteroids in KD is a subject of continuing research. Studies of the addition of a single pulsed dose of steroids to IVIG as initial therapy have yielded conflicting results.[14,15] It is possible that a subset of patients at highest risk of developing coronary artery aneurysms may benefit; however, risk scores for stratification of patients have not been validated.

Refractory KD

Up to 15% of patients with KD treated with IVIG and aspirin have persistence or early recrudescence of fever, indicative of an ongoing vasculitic process.[16] This is a strong risk factor for the development of coronary artery aneurysms.[17] Children with ongoing or recurring fever beyond 36 hours after treatment with IVIG should be given a second dose of IVIG.[4]

Pulses of methylprednisolone (30 mg kg^{-1} daily for 1-3 days) have been used in cases unresponsive to two doses of IVIG.[18] Corticosteroids have been shown to reduce fever in patients with resistant KD; however, their effect on coronary artery abnormalities is uncertain.[4] A number of other treatments including plasma exchange, cyclophosphamide,

and tumour necrosis factor-α antagonists have been reported in children with refractory KD. The role of these therapies remains unclear.[4]

Prognosis

Mortality is less than 1%, being highest in those less than 12 months old. Recurrence is most likely to occur in children aged less than 3 years who had cardiac involvement initially, and usually within 12 months of the initial episode.[19] Patients with recurrent KD appear to be at increased risk for cardiac sequelae.

Children without demonstrable cardiac disease appear to have an excellent prognosis, with long-term follow-up studies demonstrating absence of clinical sequelae for up to 21 years.[20] It is possible, however, that individuals who have had KD are at risk of early atherosclerotic heart disease.

The prognosis for children who have had coronary artery aneurysms is less clear. Most small to medium-sized aneurysms resolve echocardiographically;[21] but healing involves fibrosis and calcification, with associated loss of vascular distensibility and reactivity. A proportion of coronary artery aneurysms progress to stenosis over time. Therefore children with KD who have had coronary artery aneurysms should have indefinite cardiology follow up. These patients will generally be treated with long-term antithrombotic therapy to prevent myocardial ischaemia. Children receiving long-term aspirin therapy should receive the influenza vaccine annually, to prevent Reye syndrome. New antiplatelet agents are under investigation.[22] There have been reports of the use of thrombolytic agents in patients with KD, with thrombus seen within coronary aneurysms.[23] Anticoagulation with warfarin is required for patients with 'giant' (≥8 mm) or multiple aneurysms, and surgical intervention (e.g. angioplasty, bypass grafting) is occasionally necessary.

Controversies

❶ The immunological mechanism of the inflammatory response in KD is the subject of continuing research – there is some evidence to support a conventional antigen, but other evidence suggests a superantigen.

❷ The optimal dose of aspirin in the acute febrile phase is uncertain.

❸ The role of steroids in KD is debated.

❹ The clinical significance of subtle long-term changes in coronary artery function in some patients who have had KD remains unknown.

References

1. Kawasaki T. Paediatric acute mucocutaneous lymph node syndrome: Clinical observation of 50 cases. *Arerugi* 1967;**16**:178–222 (in Japanese).
2. Burns JC. Kawasaki disease. *Adv Pediatr* 2001;**48**:157–77.
3. Meissner HC, Leung DYM. Superantigens, conventional antigens and the etiology of Kawasaki syndrome. *Pediatr Infect Dis J* 2000;**19**:91–4.
4. Newburger J, Takahashi M, Gerber M, et al. Diagnosis, Treatment, and Long-Term Management of Kawasaki Disease: A Statement for Health Professionals From the Committee on Rheumatic Fever, Endocarditis, and Kawasaki Disease, Council on Cardiovascular Disease in the Young, American Heart Association. *Pediatrics* 2004;**114**:1708–33.
5. Freeman AF, Shulman ST. Recent developments in Kawasaki disease. *Curr Opin Infect Dis* 2001;**14**:357–61.
6. Tse S, Silverman E, McCrindle B, Yeung R. Early treatment with intravenous immunoglobulin in patients with Kawasaki disease. *J Pediatr* 2002;**140**:450–5.
7. Stockneim JA, Innocentini N, Shulman ST. Kawasaki disease in older children and adolescents. *J Pediatr* 2000;**137**:250–2.
8. Rosenfeld EA, Corydon KE, Shulman ST. Kawasaki disease in infants less than one year of age. *J Pediatr* 1995;**126**:524–9.
9. Newburger JW, Takahashi M, Beiser AS, et al. A single intravenous infusion of gamma globulin as compared with four infusions in the treatment of acute Kawasaki syndrome. *N Engl J Med* 1991;**324**:1633–9.
10. Marasini M, Pongiglione G, Gazzolo D, et al. Late intravenous gamma globulin treatment in infants and children with Kawasaki disease and coronary artery abnormalities. *Am J Cardiol* 1991;**68**:796–7.
11. Koren G, Rose V, Lavi S, et al. Probable efficacy of high-dose salicylates in reducing coronary artery involvement in Kawasaki disease. *JAMA* 1985;**254**:767–9.
12. Hsieh K, Weng K, Lin C. Treatment of acute Kawasaki disease: Aspirin's role in the febrile stage revisited. *Pediatrics* 2004;**114**(6):e689–e693.
13. Terai M, Shulman ST. Prevalence of coronary artery abnormalities in Kawasaki disease is highly dependent on gamma globulin dose but independent of salicylate dose. *J Pediatr* 1997;**131**:888–93.
14. Wooditch A, Aronoff S. Effect of initial corticosteroid therapy on coronary artery aneurysm formation in Kawasaki disease: a meta-analysis of 862 children. *Pediatrics* 2005;**116**:989.
15. Newburger J, Sleeper L, McCrindle B, et al. Randomized trial of pulsed corticosteroid therapy for primary treatment of Kawasaki disease. *N Engl J Med* 2007;**356**:663.
16. Burns J, Glode M. Kawasaki syndrome. *Lancet* 2004;**364**:533.
17. Kim T, Choi W, Woo C, et al. Predictive risk factors for coronary artery abnormalities in Kawasaki disease. *Eur J Pediatr* 2007;**166**:421.
18. Wright DA, Newburger JW, Baker A, et al. Treatment of immune globulin-resistant Kawasaki disease with pulsed doses of corticosteroids. *J Pediatr* 1996;**128**:146–9.
19. Hirata S, Nakamura Y, Yanagawa H. Incident rate of recurrent Kawasaki disease and related risk factors: nationwide surveys of Kawasaki disease in Japan. *Acta Pediatr* 2001;**90**:40.
20. Kato H, Sugimura T, Akagi T, et al. Long-term consequences of Kawasaki disease: A 10- to 21-year follow-up study of 594 patients. *Circulation* 1996;**94**:1379.
21. Fukushige J, Takahashi N, Ueda K, et al. Long-term outcome of coronary abnormalities in patients after Kawasaki disease. *Pediatr Cardiol* 1996;**17**(2):71–6. Mar–Apr.
22. Williams RV, Minich LL, Tani LY. Pharmacological therapy for patients with Kawasaki disease. *Paediatr Drugs* 2001;**3**:649–60.
23. Tsubata S, Ichida F, Haramichi Y, et al. Successful thrombolytic therapy using tissue-type plasminogen activator in Kawasaki disease. *Pediatr Cardiol* 1995;**16**:186–9.

5.9 Cardiac arrhythmias

Gary Williams

ESSENTIALS

1 Focus initially on airway, breathing and circulation and then recognise and treat arrhythmias compromising cardiac output using the safest possible means.

2 If an arrhythmia is fast and regular try to assess the width of the QRS complex against age-based normal values.

3 Supraventricular tachycardia (SVT) accounts for 90% of all significant arrhythmias in children.

4 Any previous 12-lead electrocardiograph (ECG) may be of enormous value in diagnosing an arrhythmia.

5 Ventricular tachycardia (VT) has a wide range of potential aetiologies and treatment is based on an assessment of degree of compromise and morphology of the tachycardia.

6 Continuous recording of a single-lead ECG during acute resuscitation manoeuvres (adenosine administration, vagal manoeuvres, cardioversion) may yield very valuable information.

7 Any child with a significant arrhythmia should be discussed with a paediatric cardiologist at the earliest possible time.

Introduction

Identification and management of the child with a cardiac arrhythmia in the emergency department (ED) requires an initial focus on and, if required, attention to the patient's haemodynamic stability, followed by a team approach to diagnose and treat the arrhythmia if necessary. Although arrhythmias occur less frequently in acutely ill infants and children compared to adults, vigilance is required, as a correct acute assessment and management of the arrhythmia will have significant long-term consequences.

The primary aim of this initial assessment and resuscitation phase in an unstable patient is to recognise and treat arrhythmias that are compromising cardiac output using the safest means possible so that longer-term management decisions can be made in consultation with a paediatric cardiologist.

Normal conduction system

The normal heartbeat is initiated by an impulse which originates from the sinoatrial (SA) node located in the wall of the right atrium near the superior vena cava junction. The impulse is then propagated via conducting cells that form a specialised system throughout the heart. Initially the impulse travels across the atria and via transatrial internodal pathways that converge on the atrioventricular (AV) node. The impulse proceeds down the bundle of His to the right and left bundle branches; the impulse then finally spreads throughout the Purkinje fibres to depolarise the ventricular muscle. The conducting cells of this specialised system have a rapid conduction velocity to rapidly propagate the electrical impulse throughout the heart. The various parts of this conduction system are also capable of spontaneous depolarisation and impulse generation under abnormal conditions.

The SA node is normally the dominant (fastest) cardiac pacemaker but this can change if sinus node dysfunction occurs or if other parts of the conduction system develop increased automaticity. As stated above, the SA node is located near the junction of the superior vena cava (SVC) and the right atrium. The SA node is innervated by both sympathetic and parasympathetic nerve endings. Parasympathetic tone predominates during rest. Children are known to have relatively greater parasympathetic tone than adults and are also known to have developmental and age-dependent differences in action potential amplitude and conduction speed. Accordingly, there are age-dependent normal values for resting heart rate as well as PR interval and QRS duration, in addition to many other electrophysiology parameters (Table 5.9.1).

Depolarisation initiated in the SA node spreads rapidly through the internodal pathways to converge on the AV node. Usually, the atria and ventricles are electrically separated from one another by a ring of fibrous tissue at the atrioventricular junction (the annulus fibrosis). Accordingly, in usual circumstances, the impulse must pass to the His bundle via the AV node. The AV node is located in the inferomedial wall of the right atrium near the insertion of the septal leaflet of the tricuspid valve. Conduction through the AV node is slow to allow completion of atrial systole (and ventricular diastole). This delay (and therefore potentially the completeness of ventricular filling) can be reduced during sympathetic stimulation.

After leaving the AV node the impulse travels along the bundle of His for 1–2 cm along the posteroinferior margin of the membranous portion of the interventricular septum, before dividing into the right and left bundle branches. These extensions of the conducting system spread subendocardially across the ventricular chambers to the base of the papillary muscles. The left bundle separates into two distinct fascicles (anterior and posterior). From these specialised fibres the impulse spreads from endocardium to epicardium throughout the right and left ventricles.

Abnormally situated embryonic remnants of conducting tissue can persist as accessory tracts. These are most commonly found around the AV node and are capable of conducting electrical activity between the atria and ventricles thus bypassing the AV node. These remnants are the anatomical substrate for re-entrant tachyarrhythmias.

The cardiac action potential

The cardiac action potential is divided into five phases: 0, 1, 2, 3, 4.

Phase 0 is depolarisation due to voltage gated opening of sodium channels with sodium rushing into the cell. There is an intense entry of sodium for a brief period resulting in depolarisation of the entire cell as well as cell-to-cell propagation.

Phase 1 is a phase of partial repolarisation due to several factors but including chloride entry into and possibly potassium egress from the cell.

Phase 2 is the plateau phase thought to be important in coordinated and sustained ventricular contraction. During this phase there is slow inward calcium current and slow inward sodium current balanced by a gradually increasing outward potassium movement.

Phase 3 is repolarisation and it occurs by inactivation or closure of the slow calcium and sodium channels and then a voltage gated progressive opening of potassium channels leading to outward potassium ion movement and a progressively more negative membrane potential. Also during this phase, the fast sodium channels are reactivated and the cell is primed for further depolarisation.

During *phase 4*, an energy-dependent membrane Na–K ATPase removes the sodium and restores the potassium to the cell. Most myocardial cells maintain a constant level of depolarisation during this phase but Purkinje or conducting cells, by way of reduced outward potassium flow and some inward sodium flow, achieve slow depolarisation until the AP threshold is reached. These

Table 5.9.1 Normal resting heart rates, PR intervals and QRS durations in children				
Age	Heart rate mean (beats min^{-1})	Range	PR interval (ms)	QRS duration (ms)
<1 day	119	94–145	70–120	50–84
1–7 days	133	100–175	70–120	40–79
7–30 days	163	115–190	70–120	40–73
1–3 months	154	124–190	70–130	50–80
3–6 months	140	111–179	70–130	60–80
6–12 months	140	112–177	80–130	50–80
1–3 years	126	98–163	80–150	50–80
3–5 years	98	65–132	90–150	60–84
5–8 years	96	70–115	100–160	50–80
8–12 years	79	55–107	100–170	50–84
12–16 years	75	55–102	110–160	40–80

Source: Adapted from Liebman 1982.

conducting cells have a shorter duration action potential of lower amplitude, thought to be mediated more predominantly by slow calcium flux.

Vaughan Williams antiarrhythmia drug classification

Antiarrhythmic drugs are classified into five classes in the Vaughan Williams classification by the mechanism or channel that they most reliably affect during in vitro studies. There is, however, considerable overlap.

Class 1 drugs block the fast inward sodium channels and thereby increase the refractory period. This class is further subdivided into:

1a. Those that prolong action potential duration (e.g. quinidine);
1b. Do not change or shorten action potential duration (e.g. lignocaine); or
1c. Produce some mild action potential prolongation (e.g. flecainide).

It is fair to say that these are infrequently used in paediatrics, though lignocaine is still an option in the ventricular fibrillation protocol and flecainide may sometimes be used in supraventricular tachyarrhythmias.

Class 2 agents are β-blockers, which act by a combination of β-antagonism and a quinidine-like membrane stabilising effect. There is a slowing of conduction velocity, prolonging of action potential duration and a reduction of automaticity Their main clinical use is in treating supraventricular tachyarrhythmias (SVT, atrial fibrillation, atrial flutter) by increasing the refractory period of the AV node. Propranolol or atenolol may be used but in acute situations many clinicians favour esmolol, a very short-acting parenteral β-1-antagonist (half life 9 minutes), which can be useful in supraventricular tachycardia (SVT) and possibly ventricular tachycardia (VT).

Class 3 drugs act primarily as potassium channel blockers and basically prolong the phase 3 repolarisation phase, thereby causing a prolongation of the action potential and increase in the effective refractory period. This class of drug is particularly useful in ventricular tachyarrhythmias and includes amiodarone and sotalol.

Amiodarone is one of these antiarrhythmics with a plethora of effects, in that it is primarily class 3 (i.e. potassium channel blocker) but also has sodium channel blocking, β-antagonism and calcium channel blocking effects. Oral amiodarone has unusual pharmacokinetics, with clinical effect only apparent after several days of treatment and a half life of 3–15 weeks. Side effects are frequent and serious (corneal photosensitivity, hyper- or hypothyroidism, pulmonary fibrosis and pro-arrhythmia). Intravenous amiodarone is used in the acute management of post-operative tachyarrhythmias (usually junctional ectopic tachycardia, JET). In the adult ventricular fibrillation protocol, a randomised comparison between amiodarone and lignocaine found a greater chance of successful resuscitation (but not survival) with amiodarone. Therefore some authorities have recommended amiodarone as the agent of choice to help effect defibrillation after adrenaline (epinephrine). In haemodynamically stable VT the agent of choice is probably sotalol unless there is impaired ventricular function (EF <40%, signs of congestive heart failure) when amiodarone is recommended. In unstable or polymorphic VT the recommended agent depends a little on the initial trace. If it looks like *torsade de pointes* with the trace oscillating around the baseline (or in polymorphic VT with a normal QT interval), the clear recommendation is intravenous (IV) magnesium. If it is not *torsade-like* and the QT interval can be determined and is not prolonged, amiodarone is a second-line agent to β-blockers. If the QT interval is prolonged, then IV magnesium, followed if necessary by lignocaine, would be the recommended approach.

Sotalol is classified as a class 3 drug, although it is a non-selective β-blocker with additional class 3 properties. It therefore combines the β-blocking effect on the SA and AV nodes with prolongation of AP duration and lengthening of refractory period elsewhere in the heart. It is valuable acutely and long term in preventing SVT of all sorts and is the agent of choice in monomorphic stable VT with apparent normal ventricular function. Like amiodarone, it does increase the QT interval and is therefore pro-arrhythmic as well as having the other risks of hypotension and bradycardia, presumably resulting from its β-blocking effects.

Class 4 agents are calcium channel blockers and the prototype remains verapamil, which has wide-ranging effects on shortening the plateau phase and reducing contractility. Verapamil is primarily used in the adult setting because of its reduction of conduction velocity in the AV node, thereby controlling the ventricular response rate to SVT, atrial flutter or atrial fibrillation. Even in that situation it is still a second-line agent to adenosine for SVT termination in adults, provided there is good left ventricular (LV) function. However, because of serious bradycardia, hypotension and cardiac arrest in infants, it is not used in children. Instead, β-blockers are used in Wolff–Parkinson–White (WPW) syndrome and digoxin in non-WPW patients.

Finally, **Class 5** agents are a miscellaneous group and include adenosine and digoxin. Adenosine is an endogenous purine nucleoside with a very rapid half life (less than 5 seconds). It acts by depressing slow calcium channels and enhancing potassium conduction. Its main effects are to depress sinus node and AV node activity with a shortening of atrial refractoriness. Because of its effect in blocking AV nodal activity, adenosine is superbly suited to block re-entry phenomena, the most frequent cause of SVT in children. Series show that adenosine terminates 90–100% of SVTs but the arrhythmia re-initiates in approximately 25%. Other atrial tachycardias like multifocal atrial tachycardia, atrial flutter or atrial fibrillation are almost always resistant to adenosine. Adenosine is given in increasing doses from 50–200 mcg kg^{-1} every 2 minutes, using a two-syringe technique so that it can be flushed rapidly into the circulation. Side effects can be facial flushing, bronchospasm or sinus arrest. Adenosine is essentially very safe, although there is a single case report of VF occurring after a dose of adenosine in a neonate with a concealed WPW syndrome previously treated with digoxin.

Although adenosine is unlikely to be controlling in supraventricular tachycardias other than re-entrant SVT, the acute injection of adenosine may transiently slow AV nodal activity and allow the flutter wave or P wave morphology to be assessed. This may be very valuable in diagnosing the specific rhythm. In a haemodynamically stable wide complex tachycardia of uncertain origin, the differential diagnosis is primarily between VT and SVT with aberrant conduction. Adenosine administration might be discussed as a way of making this distinction (i.e. effective in the latter but not in the former). In the adult literature, unless SVT origin is strongly suspected, this practice is discouraged because of the potential for brief hypotension, and accelerated accessory pathway conduction following adenosine injection.

Digoxin is still very commonly used parenterally, acutely, and as a maintenance medication, primarily to slow AV conduction and decrease the ventricular response to atrial dysrhythmia like flutter or fibrillation. It provides rate control and sometimes converts supraventricular tachyarrhythmias. There is an important caveat with digoxin, that it may shorten accessory pathway refractoriness and increase the resulting ventricular response. Therefore, it should not be used in accessory pathway dysrhythmias like WPW syndrome. Virtually any arrhythmia can arise from intoxication with digoxin. This risk is greater with hypokalaemia and the acute treatment is intravenous Digitalis antibody.

Pathogenesis of arrhythmias

Bradyarrhythmias

Two mechanisms are responsible for bradyarrhythmias:

❶ Some form of sinus node dysfunction.
❷ Conduction system block.

Tachyarrhythmias

There are three fundamental mechanisms proposed for the generation of tachyarrhythmias:

❶ Re-entry.
❷ Enhanced automaticity.
❸ After depolarisations (triggered arrhythmias).

Re-entry

Re-entry exists when a closed loop of specialised conducting tissue allows an electrical impulse to travel in a circular fashion and permits atrial or ventricular electrical activation with each pass around the circuit. Re-entry may occur on a large (macro) or small (micro) scale. Atrial flutter and ventricular fibrillation are examples of micro re-entry; paroxysmal supraventricular tachycardia is an example of macro re-entry.

Macro re-entry usually involves the participation of an accessory conduction pathway. Accessory pathway conduction characteristics vary widely among patients. The accessory pathway in some patients conducts antegrade during sinus rhythm, whereas in others it conducts only retrograde during tachycardia. When anterograde conduction is possible down the accessory pathway the standard ECG will show pre-excitation with a short PR interval and wide QRS, including an initial delta wave resulting from the pre-excitation of the ventricle from the sinus impulse conducting through the accessory pathway before the impulse has passed through the normal conducting system. Patients with WPW usually manifest orthodromic tachycardia (forward excitation through AV node and rapid retrograde conduction via accessory pathway to create a circuit) but also (rarely) display antidromic tachycardia involving retrograde conduction up the usual atrioventricular route or via an alternative accessory connection.

Supraventricular tachycardia is the most common sustained tachyarrhythmia in children and almost always has a re-entry mechanism. Most commonly, particularly in children younger than 12 years of age, this re-entry is caused by an accessory atrioventricular connection (resulting in atrioventricular (or AV) re-entrant tachycardia). In adolescents, AV node re-entry is the mechanism in up to one third of patients. Previously we believed that this was due to a re-entry circuit within the compact AV node but a newer concept involves tissue, most likely atrial muscle, more than several millimetres outside the compact atrioventricular node.

The commonest mode of accessory connection-mediated re-entry tachycardia is orthodromic tachycardia, with the circular movement of the electrical impulse going antegrade through the atrioventricular node and then retrograde up the accessory connection.

Enhanced automaticity

The primary pacemaker cells of the SA and AV nodes usually demonstrate spontaneous depolarisation as well as having somewhat slower action potential propagation. The cells of the conduction system have more rapid action potential propagation but are also capable of spontaneous action potential generation if the opportunity arises. These cells are, however, normally overridden and kept refractory by the dominant (faster) pacemaker of the SA node. Under certain adverse physiological conditions (e.g. hypokalaemia, hypoxia) the threshold for spontaneous automaticity for these conducting cells may be altered. This potentially creates a situation of enhanced automaticity and secondary enhanced pacemakers. One example of a tachycardia due to enhanced automaticity is multifocal atrial tachycardia.

After depolarisations

After depolarisations are due to oscillations of the membrane potential during repolarisation that has reached the threshold membrane potential and triggered a second complete depolarisation. This process may become self-perpetuating. *Torsade-de-pointes* is the classic example of such a triggered arrhythmia.

General principles for arrhythmia management

❶ Direct primary attention to assessment and correction of ABCs.
❷ If patient has an acute arrhythmia with haemodynamic compromise (e.g. shock or loss of consciousness), assess whether the rhythm is fast and/or disorganised or slow and/or irregular. If the rhythm is fast or disorganised, cardioversion or defibrillation should take priority. If slow and/or irregular, cardiopulmonary resuscitation should commence.
❸ Obtain venous access and draw blood for biochemistry, specifically Na, K, Ca, Mg and blood sugar level.
❹ Record a 12-lead ECG as soon as possible.

Bradyarrhythmias

Normal heart rate varies as a function of age. Pathological bradyarrhythmia may present as fatigue, light-headedness or syncope in an otherwise well child or inappropriate absence of tachycardia in a critically unwell child under stress.

Sinus bradycardia

Sinus bradycardias can be caused in children by:

- parasympathetic stimulation (e.g. suctioning);

- metabolic disturbances (e.g. hypoxia, asphyxia, hypothermia);
- poisoning (e.g. β-blocker, calcium channel blocker);
- raised intracranial pressure;
- surgical injury to the sinoatrial node (e.g. following Mustard or Senning procedures for transposition, Fontan, closure of atrial septal defect or correction of total anomalous pulmonary venous drainage);
- cardiomyopathy.

Sinus node dysfunction

Sinus node dysfunction may manifest as sinus pauses (a transient interruption of normal sinus mechanism), or sinus exit block (abnormal propagation), either of which may occur with or without an associated escape rhythm and may evolve to sinus arrest.

Management

❶ Treatment is required if an adequate cardiac output is not being maintained.

❷ If possible, remove the cause (i.e. suction catheter).

❸ Ensure adequate ventilation.

❹ If life threatening, commence compressions and administer atropine 20 mcg kg^{-1} IV or EndoTracheal (ET) (minimum dose 100 mcg).

❺ If this is ineffective, or bradycardia recurs, use β-adrenergic agonist or adrenaline (epinephrine) bolus. Commence adrenaline (epinephrine) or isoproterenol by infusion while urgent preparations are made for temporary external or transvenous cardiac pacing.

Conduction disturbances: atrioventricular block

This involves delayed or incomplete conduction through the AV node. Causes include a congenital form (maternal systemic lupus erythematosus) and an acquired form. Acquired AV block occurs in poisoning, metabolic disturbances, myocarditis, rheumatic fever, Lyme disease, fibrosis in the area of the conduction system associated with previous cardiac surgery (particularly ventricular septal defect or atrioventricular septal defect closure, tetralogy repair or aortic valve replacement) and inferior myocardial infarction.

First degree AV block Is present when the PR interval is longer than usual for age (see Table 5.9.1) but normal sinus rhythm and 1:1 AV conduction is maintained. This is a normal feature of the ECG of endocardial cushion defects. It may occur in a normal heart during parasympathetic stimulation or digoxin treatment and usually does not require treatment.

Second degree Mobitz type I AV block (Wenckebach) Is characterised by progressive prolongation of the PR interval, culminating in a single non-conducted beat. This usually is a benign normal variant but may represent a temporary pathological prolongation of the atrioventricular node refractory period.

Second degree Mobitz type II AV block Manifests as a regular intermittent failure of P wave conduction while the PR interval remains constant. This is more likely attributable to a block within the His conduction system and as such has greater potential to progress to complete (3rd degree) atrioventricular block.

Third degree atrioventricular block (or complete heart block) Represents complete failure of atrial depolarisation to propagate to the ventricle. Anatomically the block may occur at atrioventricular node or at infranodal level. ECG will show complete dissociation of P waves and QRS complex. A narrow QRS junctional escape rhythm implies a nodal block whereas a widened slower QRS escape rhythm suggests an infranodal site for the block.

Clinical features Patient may be asymptomatic but will usually demonstrate an inadequate cardiac output, particularly in episodes of atrioventricular block associated with slower heart rate. In third degree AV block, cannon 'A' waves are visible in the neck and a slow cardiac rhythm with variable first heart sound is present on auscultation.

Management Emergency treatment is only required if cardiac output is inadequate. Optimise ventilation and initiate β-agonist by infusion while organising temporary external/transvenous cardiac pacing. This is definitely indicated in symptomatic children with Mobitz type II second degree AV block and 3rd degree AV block.

Bundle branch block

Bundle branch block patterns are unusual in paediatrics but occur when impaired conduction is present in the specialised intraventricular conduction tissue, resulting in delayed right or left ventricular depolarisation and a resulting broad aberrant QRS complex. Right bundle branch block (wide QRS with rSR pattern in right ventricular leads) may be a normal variant but also occurs in congenital heart disease (especially involving RVH), cor pulmonale and acute pulmonary embolism. Left bundle branch block (wide QRS with RR pattern in left chest leads) is associated with LV strain or hypertrophy or operated congenital heart disease.

Tachyarrhythmias

There is a wide range of tachyarrhythmias. Immediate diagnosis and management is best based on the width of the QRS complex when compared to age-based normal values.

Wide complex tachyarrhythmia

The differential diagnosis of a wide or broad complex tachycardia (i.e. QRS duration greater than normal for age, usually >0.08 seconds) is between:

❶ Ventricular tachycardia.

❷ SVT with intraventricular aberrant conduction (e.g. pre-existing bundle branch block).

❸ Atypical or antidromic SVT (where during the tachycardia antegrade conduction occurs down the fast accessory pathway and retrograde component goes via the atrioventricular node).

❹ Atrially originated arrhythmias conducted via an accessory connection to the ventricular muscle.

VT in children usually presents as a wide complex rhythm between 120 and 220 per minute. There is usually AV dissociation but retrograde VA conduction may occur. It may be mono- or polymorphic, sustained or non-sustained. Causes include metabolic abnormalities, poisoning, myocarditis, cardiomyopathy, ventriculotomy, ventricular tumours and congenital or acquired Long QT Syndrome.

Most children with VT are symptomatic with lethargy, symptoms of pulmonary congestion, poor circulation and possibly palpitations.

The other three differential diagnoses outlined above are unusual causes of a wide complex tachycardia in children. The most important differential to think about is SVT with aberrant conduction, because it should respond to vagal manoeuvres or adenosine administration. A previous electrocardiogram is of great value in determining the presence of an accessory pathway or a pre-existing bundle branch block in that these features point to SVT with aberrant conduction. Classically, VT is a wide complex tachycardia with a left access deviation and more frequently a left bundle branch block pattern, whereas a right bundle branch block pattern (with rSR in V_1) is more commonly seen in SVT. Again, the P wave morphology is crucial and if P waves can be distinguished, the loss of a one-to-one relationship between P wave and QRS complex is highly suggestive of VT. Sometimes, however, in VT there still may be a one-to-one ventriculoatrial relationship. The presence of fusion beats indicating an ectopic focus below the level of the AV node is also strongly suggestive of VT.

If there is strong evidence supporting a supraventricular origin and preserved LV function, vagal manoeuvres and/or adenosine administration can be tried. The caveat is that, in doing this, there is a small but important potential for hypotension and accelerated accessory pathway conduction from the adenosine administration that has been responsible for conversion of SVT to VT, or even worse on occasions.

If there are no pointers towards a supraventricular origin, or the above manoeuvres are unrewarding, the diagnosis is most likely VT.

If the patient is severely compromised, direct current cardioversion is clearly indicated. It is debated whether this is better synchronous or asynchronous, but most authorities recommend starting with synchronous cardioversion if there is a pulse, using a 1 J/kg shock from a biphasic defibrillator.

If the patient has reasonable perfusion, the recommended drug depends on the appearance of the VT. If the VT is monomorphic and the patient has preserved LV function, intravenous sotalol is the agent of choice, with amiodarone as a second-line agent. Amiodarone is definitely the drug of choice if LV function is impaired. If the rhythm is polymorphic, there should be some

further assessment of the trace. If the trace is *torsade*-like with complexes that vary in height and appear to twist around the baseline, intravenous magnesium is clearly recommended. If the QT interval is prolonged, IV magnesium followed probably by IV lignocaine is recommended. If the QT interval can be seen not to be prolonged, β-blockade is the primary approach, with amiodarone again the agent of choice if LV function is impaired.

Narrow complex tachyarrhythmia

A narrow complex tachycardia is defined as one with a QRS duration normal for age (approximately ≤ 0.08 seconds). The narrow QRS complex almost always indicates that these tachyarrhythmias are supraventricular.

SVT refers to a family of tachyarrhythmias requiring the atrium, AV node or both for their perpetuation. SVT accounts for 90% of all significant tachyarrhythmias in children. It is most useful to subclassify these tachyarrhythmias on the basis of site of origin and mechanism into primary atrial tachycardias (including MAT, atrial fibrillation and atrial flutter), atrioventricular reciprocating, AV nodal re-entry and junctional ectopic tachycardia. Primary atrial and junctional ectopic tachycardias will be dealt with later. Atrioventricular reciprocating and nodal re-entry tachycardias are the commonest forms of SVT in childhood.

Atrioventricular reciprocating tachycardia Occurs due to the presence of an accessory conduction pathway setting up a re-entry circuit. In the commonest variety (*orthodromic reciprocating*), the impulse travels antegrade via the AV node to the ventricles (as usual) and then retrograde via the accessory pathway back to the atria. If the accessory pathway is capable of conducting antegrade, *antidromic reciprocating* tachycardia can occur, with the impulse travelling in the opposite direction, i.e. forward down an accessory pathway, returning retrograde via the AV node.

AV nodal re-entrant tachycardia In this tachyarrhythmia the two conduction pathways are thought to be within or adjacent to the AV node. Beyond 5 years of age, this becomes the most common form of SVT. Classically, the P wave is buried within the QRS complex on ECG. In AV nodal re-entrant tachycardia, for long-term prophylaxis therapy digoxin is the preferred agent. However, β-blockers may be considered in resistant

cases, either alone or in combination with digoxin.

The crucial step in distinguishing between the above-mentioned atrial, atrioventricular or nodal tachycardias is an identification of the P wave and its relationship to the QRS complex. This is sometimes best done with a 12-lead ECG with the paper run at 50 mm s^{-1}. If epicardial leads are available (i.e. post-operatively), an 'atrial ECG' can be obtained by connecting the two atrial pacing leads to the right arm and right leg electrodes of a 12-lead ECG. Alternatively, a specialised transoesophageal pacing wire can be introduced, like a nasogastric tube approximately to the level of the nipple and then connected to lead V1 to display an oesophagoatrial ECG in lead V1, with the remainder of the leads showing a normal surface ECG. Because it is being recorded directly, the P wave will usually appear larger than the QRS complex in the surface ECG and by aligning simultaneously recorded surface and 'atrial' ECGs the position of the P relative to the QRS can be determined.

Atrially-driven tachycardias will have a P wave preceding each QRS. If the P wave is upright in inferior leads, the origin of the tachycardia is high in the atrium, whereas the P wave axis will be negative in inferior leads if there is AV nodal re-entry or a low atrial ectopic focus. The P wave is usually absent in junctional ectopic tachyarrhythmia or VT. An abnormal P wave morphology usually indicates an origin other than the sinus node and several morphologies will indicate multifocal atrial tachycardia (MAT). If the P wave follows the QRS complex, the differential diagnosis involves atrioventricular nodal re-entry tachyarrhythmia and ventricular tachycardia. If the P waves are dissociated from the QRS complexes, the diagnoses are most likely junctional ectopic tachycardia or VT.

Regardless of these diagnostic considerations, the approach is essentially the same. If the patient is acutely compromised, basic life support followed by attempted DC cardioversion with 0.5–1 J kg^{-1} of DC shock (under sedation if possible) and with continuous ECG monitoring is recommended. IV adenosine is an alternative if this is immediately available. If the patient has adequate perfusion, consider vagal manoeuvres/eliciting of diving reflex, administer adenosine in increasing doses as above.

The importance of a continuous 12-lead electrocardiogram during this process cannot be over emphasised. This is because just a few beats of sinus rhythm before reversion back to the tachyarrhythmia might well shed considerable light on the diagnosis. If the arrhythmia is resistant to adenosine, the next step is probably use of a β-blocker, with digoxin an alternative for maintenance (see below for caveats regarding digoxin in WPW).

Failure of adenosine to convert such a tachyarrhythmia makes unusual diagnoses more likely. For multiple atrial ectopic foci, sotalol is effective but probably only as a bridge to radiofrequency ablation. For JET the agent of choice is amiodarone. In atrial fibrillation/flutter, rate control can be achieved using digoxin but usually elective cardioversion is required to terminate the arrhythmia. In post-surgical cases recurrence is common and sotalol probably has the strongest demonstrated efficacy in reducing recurrences (and controlling ventricular rate) if they occur, though only as a bridge to possible cryoablation.

Wolff–Parkinson–White syndrome

WPW is present when the accessory atrio-ventricular connection allows ventricular pre-excitation by rapid antegrade conduction of the normal sinus impulse, thereby avoiding the normal delay in the AV node. This is present in 22–73% of cases of paediatric SVT and produces a shortened PR interval and slurred upstroke on the QRS complex (delta waves). It usually produces orthodromic reciprocating AV tachycardia but in a small proportion of cases (approximately 10%) an antidromic reciprocating tachycardia can occur.

If WPW is known to be present (by past history or presence of delta waves on a non-tachyarrhythmia ECG) β-blockers (propranolol or atenolol) are the agents of first choice (slow conduction through AV node with little, if any, effect on accessory pathways). Digoxin has traditionally been the drug of choice for prophylaxis against SVT in WPW but has pro-arrhythmia risks, particularly in antidromic reciprocating tachycardia (decreases accessory pathway refractory period, thereby facilitating accessory connection conductance of atrial arrhythmias), and should therefore be avoided. Sotalol combines β-blocker and

class-3 antiarrhythmic actions and is effective and safe in resistant SVT. There is also some evidence supporting a role for flecainide (class 1C agent) or amiodarone (class 3 agent) as maintenance treatments in resistant cases.

Atrial flutter

Atrial flutter is an atrial tachycardia that probably propagates via an intra-atrial re-entrant pathway. It is uncommon but can occur in infancy, when it is usually not associated with structural heart disease. Beyond infancy 95% of atrial flutter is associated with structural heart disease (Mustard/Senning operation for transposition of the great arteries, Fontan, repaired total anomalous pulmonary venous return).

Clinical features may include palpitations, cardiac failure or no symptoms, dependent on the rate of ventricular response. The ECG shows a characteristic saw-tooth flutter wave at 300 beats per minute, best seen in II, III and a VF with 2:1 or 3:1 AV block.

Infants without structural heart disease usually respond to low energy (0.5 J kg^{-1}) DC cardioversion, repeated after digoxin loading if initially unsuccessful. Atrial flutter is more resistant in the older patient who usually has associated structural cardiac disease. Amiodarone or class 1A agents have been shown to be effective. Radiofrequency catheter ablation may be valuable as a more definitive therapy.

Atrial fibrillation

Unlike in adults, atrial fibrillation (AF) is a relatively rare tachyarrhythmia in infants and children.

Clinical features may include irregular, rapid palpitations with cardiac failure if a rapid ventricular response is present. ECG reveals absence of discrete P waves with an irregularly irregular narrow, rapid ventricular complex.

Causes of AF may include atrial distension or scars, rheumatic heart disease, hyperthyroidism, hypocalcaemia, poisoning, or intra-thoracic pathology.

Management should focus on removing the cause if possible. Therapy is directed toward controlling the ventricular rate (primarily using digoxin or β-blockade to slow AV nodal conduction). Synchronised DC cardioversion is effective in conversion of atrial fibrillation to sinus rhythm but because of the embolic risk, the procedure

is avoided in children with long-standing atrial fibrillation, cardiac failure and/or enlarged atria.

Ventricular fibrillation

In confirmed ventricular fibrillation (VF), the first priority is rapid defibrillation. Basic life support should be initiated while a defibrillator is sought. There is increasing evidence that shock success is improved if effective chest compressions are provided for 1 to 3 minutes before defibrillation, especially if VF duration is longer than approximately 3 minutes before attempted defibrillation. Conducting pads or conductive gel should be placed on the chest in the left 5th intercostal space midaxillary line and second intercostal space to the right of the sternum, being careful that gel areas are not contiguous to avoid shorting of current. The paddles are applied, charged on the chest, 'stand clear' is called, and the operator verifies that this direction has been followed by other staff. Then 2 J kg^{-1} of current is discharged in asynchronous mode. CPR is resumed immediately after the first shock and continued for five cycles (about 2 minutes) before the next rhythm check. If VF persists, a second shock of 4 J kg^{-1} is administered and again CPR immediately resumed for five cycles. Early during these five cycles adrenaline (epinephrine) is administered and if VF persists on rhythm check a third shock of 4 J kg^{-1} is delivered. CPR is again immediately resumed and if the patient remains in VF, amiodarone 5 mg kg^{-1} by rapid IV bolus is the antiarrhythmic of choice. This is then followed by further attempts at defibrillation while CPR is continued. Lignocaine is a second choice agent, magnesium is recommended.

Controversies

❶ The appropriate energy dose for biphasic defibrillation in children is controversial.

❷ There is debate about the applicability and safety of automated external defibrillators for use in young children.

❸ Waveform analysis has the potential to reliably predict success of defibrillation and if so allow treatment alteration to improve outcome.

❹ Controversy exists around the requirement for ongoing prophylactic antiarrhythmic therapy for infants with paroxysmal supraventricular tachycardia when the natural history of this condition suggests fewer attacks with age beyond 12 months.

❺ The safety of amiodarone as antiarrhythmic agent of first choice in children with shock-resistant ventricular fibrillation has been questioned and its replacement by lignocaine suggested.

Further reading

Alexander ME, Berul CI. Ventricular arrhythmias: When to worry. *Pediatr Cardiol* 2000;21(6):532–41.

Anonymous. The International Liason Committee on Resuscitation (ILCOR) consensus on science with treatment recommendations for paediatric and neonatal patients: paediatric basic and advanced life support. *Pediatrics* 2006;117(5):e955–77.

Bink-Boelkens MTE. Pharmacologic management of arrhythmias. *Pediatr Cardiol* 2000;21(6):508–15.

Celiker A, Ayabakan C, Ozer S, et al. Sotalol in the treatment of pediatric cardiac arrhythmias. *Pediatr Int* 2001;43:624–30.

Chun TU, Van Hare GF. Advances in the approach to treatment of supraventricular tachycardia in the pediatric population. *Curr Cardiol Rep* 2004;6:322–6.

Kudenchuk PJ, Cobb LA, Copass MK, et al. Amiodarone for resuscitation after out-of-hospital cardiac arrest due to ventricular fibrillation. *N Engl J Med* 1999;341(12):871–8.

Liebman J. Tables of normal standards. In: Liebman J, Plonsey R, Gillette PC, editors. *Pediatric electrocardiography*. 1st ed. Baltimore: Williams & Wilkins; 1982. p. 82–133.

Luedtke SA, Kuhn RJ, McCaffrey FM. Pharmacologic management of supraventricular tachycardias in children. Part 1, WPW and AV nodal re-entry. *Ann Pharmacother* 1997;31:1227–43.

Luedtke SA, Kuhn RJ, McCaffrey FM. Pharmacologic management of supraventricular tachycardias in children. Part 2, Atrial flutter, atrial fibrillation and junctional and atrial ectopic tachycardia. *Ann Pharmacother* 1997;31:1347–59.

McKee MR. Amiodarone - an 'old' drug with new recommendations. *Curr Opin Pediatr* 2004;15:193–9.

Saul JP, Scott WA, Brown S, et al. Intravenous amiodarone for incessant tachyarrhythmias in children: a randomized, double-blind, antiarrhythmia drug trial. *Circulation* 2005;112:3470–7.

RESPIRATORY

Section editor *Ian Everitt*

6.1 Upper respiratory tract infections

Peter L.J. Barnett

ESSENTIALS

1 Over 95% of childhood URTIs are viral and do not require antibiotics.

2 Upper respiratory tract infections are common; children have between six and eight URTIs per year.

3 In the child with presumed URTI who has significant constitutional symptomatology one needs to consider alternative diagnoses.

4 Symptomatic nasal obstruction in infants should be treated with saline drops and gentle bulb aspiration. It is uncommon for simple URTIs to compromise feeding in infants; in this situation one needs to consider LRT involvement.

5 Stomatitis in children is usually caused by herpes simplex or coxsackie virus and symptomatic treatment to aid fluid intake is all that is required.

6 Tonsillitis in children under four years is usually viral in aetiology.

7 Tonsillitis is a feature of Epstein-Barr virus (EBV), thus always examine for node enlargement and organomegaly and features in the pharynx to suggest possible EBV.

Introduction

Infections involving the upper respiratory tract are the commonest infections seen in children and the most frequent reason for presenting to emergency departments (EDs). These infections may involve anatomical structures including the nasopharynx, mouth, ear and upper airway. Specific diagnosis needs to be made to decide whether antibiotic treatment is necessary. Most of these infections are mild and self-limiting, but complications can occur, leading to more serious disease.

Nasopharyngitis

Introduction

Nasopharyngitis or the common cold is a viral illness of the upper respiratory tract. This is commonly called an upper respiratory tract infection (URTI) even though it only affects part of the upper respiratory tract. An URTI is usually caused by rhino- and coronaviruses, but during the winter season, parainfluenza, respiratory syncytial virus (RSV) and metapneumovirus are also common. These later viruses may progress to croup, bronchiolitis or pneumonia. Other specific infections may begin with URTI symptoms and progress to involve the lower respiratory tract, e.g. influenza, *Bordetella pertussis*. If symptoms are persistent, an open mind regarding alternative diagnoses is required. In their first 6 years, children generally have between six and eight URTIs per year and children attending day care may have more. Not infrequently these may occur one after the other, leading to the impression of persistent symptoms rather than two to three separate infections. Breast feeding of babies may offer some protection, particularly in the first 6 months.

History

This illness is characterised by mild to moderate fever, blocked or runny nose, sneezing, mild cough (generally dry in the first few days) with an irritating sore throat if the child is able to verbalise this symptom. Infants may also become restless and irritable. Nasal congestion may interfere with feeding in infants under 6 months due to mechanical obstruction. Over the first few days the watery nasal discharge will become thicker and more mucopurulent. Nasal obstruction leads to mouth breathing and increased throat discomfort. The characteristic of the cough may change, becoming moist after a few days. Sputum production occurs but in small children is generally swallowed rather than expectorated and hence will not be reported by parents. The child is not particularly unwell. If a child has significant constitutional symptoms, one needs to consider alternative diagnoses such as lower respiratory infection or an influenza-like illness. Other family members may have or be recovering from cold symptoms. Symptoms usually peak around 1–3 days and disappear by 7–10 days although the cough may persist (up to 8 weeks – postviral cough). Bacterial complications are uncommon but should be considered if fever persist for longer than 3–5 days, ongoing mucopurulent nasal discharge for more than 2 weeks, child appears unwell or has lower respiratory tract signs (e.g. tachypnoea, grunting, wheeze, O_2 requirement).

Examination

The child appears well with nasal discharge, which may cause obstruction (particularly in babies). Mucopurulent discharge does not indicate a bacterial cause. The tympanic membranes may be slightly dull or pink in appearance with no evidence of fluid in the middle ear. The throat may be red but not associated with exudate or cervical lymphadenopathy. The chest is clear to auscultation, although there may be transmitted upper airway sounds, originating from the nasal passages. The cough may be dry or moist depending on the length of symptoms.

Investigations

There is no indication for investigations in a child with common cold.

Treatment

Therapy is supportive, with explanation and a management plan for parents. Parents need to ensure the child has adequate rest and fluids to maintain hydration. Nasal congestion/obstruction in infants may be improved with saline drops (one teaspoon salt in one cup boiled water and allowed to cool and kept in refrigerator for a few days only or commercial saline preparations) into the nares prior to feeds or sleeping. In addition, aspiration of mucus using a bulb

suction device is generally helpful. While feeding difficulty may occur due to nasal obstruction, infants with a presumed simple URTI who are unable to take normal feeds need to be carefully checked for features of lower respiratory tract (LRT) involvement.

The routine use of oral decongestants in infants is generally unhelpful and may cause side effects. In older children symptomatic of nasal obstruction, topical or oral decongestants may be used judiciously and topical decongestants never longer than 3 days, to avoid rebound nasal mucosal swelling.

There is no indication for antibiotics in this setting. Pharyngitis or tonsillitis associated with a URTI is viral in nature and will not respond to antibiotics. The inappropriate use of antibiotics in these patients may be a contributory factor to antibiotic resistance. Herbal remedies such as echinacea, vitamin C, or zinc have not been shown to benefit resolution of symptoms.

An explanation to parents of the expected natural history may decrease the likelihood of inappropriate seeking of antibiotics. Early review should be encouraged if their child's course deviates from that expected. Paracetamol is indicated if a child is symptomatic of fever or to diminish the discomfort of a sore throat.

Stomatitis

Introduction

Children with stomatitis often present to emergency due to difficulties in drinking. In children it is most commonly caused by herpes simplex virus (gingivostomatitis) or Coxsackie virus (e.g. hand, foot and mouth (HFM)). These viral infections cause vesicular lesions, which may involve the buccal mucosa, gingiva, tongue, palate and pharynx. Fungal infection with *Candida albicans* (thrush) may be seen in neonates or immunosuppressed children.

History

Primary herpes simplex produces a severe gingivostomatitis involving most of the mouth and characteristically has a few lesions on the outer lip area. Fever is prominent and can last for 7–10 days. The associated mouth pain can result in drooling, decreased oral intake and subsequent dehydration. Oral herpes can be spread to

the digits in patients who suck their fingers, leading to a herpetic whitlow. Coxsackie virus can produce ulcers involving the oral mucosa and skin areas (hands, feet and buttock areas). Thrush, generally seen in infants under 3 months, involves the tongue and buccal mucosa. It can cause feeding difficulties if severe but other issues need to be considered if mild.

Examination

Children may be distressed by mouth pain and have a high fever. Hydration should be assessed. Herpes causes multiple shallow ulcers of the oral mucosa and associated gingival inflammation. Hence, the oral features of herpes simplex virus infection tend to be more anterior on the gums, inner lips and tongue initially, and progress in a posterior direction. Coxsackie tends to cause fewer ulcers in the mouth, more on the palatal mucosa and is less likely to cause gingivitis. It is classically associated with vesicular lesions on the hands, feet and buttocks. Oral thrush presents with characteristic white plaques on the buccal mucosa and tongue. Clinical confusion may arise in the baby who has recently taken milk, which may give a similar appearance. Differentiation can be made by trying to scrape off the plaques, which either causes bleeding or they are unable to be removed.

Investigation

Diagnosis is clinical and usually requires no investigations. Immunofluorescence for herpes simplex may be required for isolation purposes or in the immunosuppressed.

Treatment

Viral stomatitis is self-limiting and symptomatic treatment to reduce pain and allow eating and drinking is the mainstay of therapy. Topical anaesthetic treatment such as Xylocaine viscous or gel 2% applied sparingly to the lesions, half an hour prior to drinking, may be beneficial. In addition, oral analgesics such as paracetamol ± codeine should also be used regularly. Icy poles (ice lollies), cool drinks or a soft diet may also be an effective way to achieve an adequate fluid intake. Frequent review is required to assess a patient's hydration status. The child with severe stomatitis, who is dehydrated, may require admission for intravenous fluids. Aciclovir has been used to hasten the resolution in immuno-compromised patients, but it has not been proven to be effective in normal patients admitted to hospital for hydration.

Treatment for oral thrush is either topical antifungal gel or oral drops four times a day for 10 to 14 days. Drops should be applied after a feed and inserted onto the buccal mucosa, not into the general oral cavity. Systemic antifungals are only indicated in immunocompromised patients.

Pharyngitis/tonsillitis

Introduction

Pharyngitis/tonsillitis is a common infection involving the throat, including the tonsils. In children, particularly in the first 4 years, a viral aetiology is most likely. Viruses that can cause pharyngitis include adenovirus, enterovirus, parainfluenza, or Epstein–Barr virus (EBV).

Group A *Streptococcus* is the most common bacterial infection of the throat, but only accounts for up to 20% of tonsillo-pharyngitis. The incidence is age related and is uncommon in children under 4 years of age. Twenty percent of children are colonised by Group A *Streptococcus,* hence, a positive throat swab may be incidental in a child with an acute viral infection. The clinical dilemma is distinguishing viral from acute bacterial infections.

History

Older children may complain of sore throat, headache, dysphagia or have referred abdominal pain. Younger children may present with less localising symptomatology with fever, decreased oral intake, drooling or clinging to parents. Patients presenting with associated coryzal symptoms (e.g. cough, nasal congestion, etc.) are unlikely to have a bacterial cause for their pharyngitis. In high-risk children (e.g. indigenous), one needs to consider the potential of post-streptococcal glomerulonephritis as a sequela.

Examination

Group A *Streptococcus* is most likely in the older child with fever, swollen tender cervical nodes, isolated sore throat and florid exudative tonsillopharyngitis. The presence of a scarlatiniform rash (red, sandpaper-textured skin) or a strawberry tongue is supportive of streptococcal infection. Enterovirus can cause, in infants/toddlers, an ulcerative or exudative pharyngitis associated with high fever, drooling and may be associated with vomiting/diarrhoea or a fine macular rash. EBV (infectious mononucleosis) is common in adolescents and can have a similar pharyngeal appearance to bacterial infection. The patient may have general swelling of the neck and face, due to marked cervical lymphadenopathy and enlargement of the spleen and liver (Table 6.1.1).

Investigations

The use of throat swabs in the ED remains controversial due to the *Streptococcus* A colonisation that occurs in up to 20% of children and since treatment with antibiotics only decreases symptoms by 1 day. A rapid strep test is very specific for *Streptococcus* A infection, but not very sensitive. If a rapid strep test is positive, this obviates the need for further testing. If one suspects EBV, a full blood examination (atypical lymphocytes) or monospot or EBV serology may be helpful, although the early monospot (within 1 week of onset of symptoms) can be falsely negative, particularly in younger children.

Treatment

Treatment of confirmed Group A streptococcal infection with antibiotics will decrease the length of symptoms approximately by 1 day (3 vs. 4 days) and decreases the likelihood of rheumatic fever. Oral penicillin is the drug of choice, either 250 mg bd (age <10 years) or 500 mg bd (age >10 years) given for 10 days. A long-acting parenteral penicillin (benzathine benzylpenicillin) is also effective in children who are refusing oral medication.

Most children with a sore throat have a viral infection and do not require antibiotics. Symptomatic relief using paracetamol or soluble aspirin/salt-water gargles may be helpful. Topical anaesthetic and oral steroids have been shown to decrease the throat pain. Ensuring adequate hydration improves the patient's general well-being. In those unable to drink and who are dehydrated, admission for intravenous fluids may be required. Children with severe tonsillomegaly and neck swelling from EBV can develop airway obstruction and may benefit from steroids. The threshold for antibiotic treatment needs to be lower in high-risk children (indigenous) who have an increased risk of glomerulonephritis.

Table 6.1.1 Features of viral and bacterial tonsillitis	
Viral	**Bacterial**
Age <4 years	Age >4 years
Associated cough, coryza, conjunctivitis, diarrhoea	Tender cervical lymphadenopathy
Lymphadenopathy, splenomegaly (e.g. EBV)	Scarlatiniform rash, oedematous tonsils or exudates
Oropharyngeal features of EBV	Absence of cough

Further reading

Dowell SF, Marcy SM, Phillips WR, et al. Principles of judicious use of antimicrobial agents for paediatric upper respiratory tract infections. *Paediatrics* 1998;**101**(1):163–5.

Dowell SF, Phillips WR, Schwartz B. Appropriate use of antibiotics for URIs in children: Part II. Cough pharyngitis and the common cold. *Am Fam Phys* 1998;**58**(6):1335–42.

Monto AS. Epidemiology of viral respiratory infections. *Am J Med* 2002;**112**(Suppl. 6A):4S–12S.

Heikkinen T, Jarvinen A. The common cold. *Lancet* 2003;**36** (9351):51–9.

Del Mar CB, Glasziou PP, Spinks AB. Antibiotics for sore throat. *Cochrane Database Syst Rev* 2006;(4):CD000023.

RESPIRATORY

6

6.2 Inhaled foreign body

Peter L.J. Barnett

ESSENTIALS

1 The presentation to an emergency department of a child with airway obstruction due to an inhaled foreign body can be life-threatening and requires rapid assessment.

2 One needs to have a prepared approach, which differentiates the situation of total from partial obstruction.

3 One needs to be cautious to avoid the potential to convert partial upper airway obstruction to complete obstruction by unnecessary interventions.

4 Many children who were initially symptomatic may be asymptomatic by the time they are seen in the emergency department and have minimal clinical findings.

5 The majority of objects are radiolucent and the radiological findings are those secondary to the physical presence in the airway.

6 Indication for bronchoscopy should be based on history, examination and radiological investigations. When in doubt, consult a paediatric respiratory physician.

Introduction

Foreign body (FB) aspiration usually occurs in children less than 3 years of age. Exceptions to this can exist, particularly in older children with developmental or neurological issues. Foreign bodies may lodge at any place along the airway from the hypopharynx to the segmental bronchus. Upper airway obstruction due to foreign bodies causes several deaths in Australia each year. The reason toddlers are more prone to aspiration is due to their general inquisitive nature, the presence of small food or non-food objects in the general home environment and their inability to efficiently grind food objects (due to lack of molar teeth).

The most common inhaled foreign bodies are food materials (e.g. peanuts, carrot or apple pieces) and small pieces of toys. Inhaled foreign bodies are rarely radio-opaque, therefore, often not visible on a plain X-ray. Foreign bodies in the upper airway account for only 5–10% of all inhaled objects, but have a higher mortality and morbidity due to their potential to cause high-grade obstruction of the airway proximal to the carina.

Upper airway foreign bodies

History

The presentation of a child with upper airway obstruction due to an inhaled foreign body can be life threatening and require a rapid careful assessment and management. These children present with acute onset of upper airway obstruction – which may be partial, total or fluctuating in severity. Oesophageal foreign bodies can cause upper airways obstruction due to adjacent airway compression, usually characterised by partial obstruction and significant drooling and saliva intolerance. There is generally no preceding history suggesting an infective cause such as croup or epiglottitis or allergic phenomena. Occasionally, the aspiration incident is witnessed as a choking episode, but often not, and a child is only discovered with breathing difficulty following an unwitnessed event.

Examination

A foreign body in the upper airway presents with acute signs of obstruction and respiratory distress. The signs reflect the degree of airway obstruction. In life-threatening cases there may be respiratory arrest with apnoea and cyanosis. Less urgent cases may have stridor, wheeze, cough and abnormal voice or cry. The child may be drooling.

Investigations

In a stable child with partial obstruction, a soft tissue X-ray may be useful to localise the foreign body, if radio-opaque. This is best performed portably in the emergency department (ED) so that the airway is clinically monitored, with ability to intervene if necessary.

Treatment

Total obstruction

Untreated, *total* airway obstruction will rapidly lead to hypoxia, loss of consciousness and subsequently cardiorespiratory arrest. In the child presenting with complete obstruction, basic life support should be commenced (see Chapter 2.4 on Resuscitation). The performance of back blows and chest thrusts to dislodge the foreign body should be followed by attempted ventilation with bag and mask. If these methods are unable to remove the foreign body and allow ventilation, then direct visualisation of the larynx and Magill forceps extraction of the foreign body should occur if possible. In the unlikely event of a foreign body visualised below the cords, suctioning may expedite its removal or, if not possible, advancing the object past the carina with an endotracheal tube or bougie may allow life-saving ventilation as a temporising measure.

Partial obstruction

The approach to the child with partial airway obstruction, but who is able to ventilate themselves to maintain adequate oxygenation, needs to be cautious. One needs to avoid the potential to convert the situation to one of complete obstruction by unnecessary interventions. It is best to leave the child undisturbed and as comfortable as possible. Small children are best kept in a parent's arms. Oxygen should be administered if required and tolerated. Causing distress and crying will usually worsen the degree of airway obstruction. The child needs to be carefully transferred from the ED to an appropriate environment where the object can be safely removed with anaesthetic, endoscopic and surgical facilities available. DO NOT attempt to remove the object by the methods mentioned above as this may convert the partial obstruction to complete obstruction.

Lower airway foreign body

History

The majority (70%) of patients presenting with an inhaled foreign body have a clear history to suggest an inhalation. However, up to 30% have a delayed presentation and/or no history of foreign body aspiration.

Patients generally present with sudden onset of coughing and choking, occasionally associated with a brief period of cyanosis. After the initial coughing episode, the child may have an audible wheeze and/or a persistent dry cough. However, many children who were initially symptomatic may be asymptomatic by the time they are seen in the ED. Depending on the size of the foreign body the symptoms may be mild. Foreign bodies tend to lodge in the right main stem bronchus more than the left, due to its less acute deviation from the lumen of the trachea. A patient may also suddenly deteriorate as the foreign body is coughed from one bronchus to the other causing increasing degree of lower airway obstruction. There may be a history of persistent cough or 'chestiness' after a remote choking event.

Examination

Examination usually reveals a well child with mild to moderate respiratory distress. The patient may have a cough. Auscultation may reveal diminished air entry on one side compared to the other ± unilateral wheeze.

There may be a fever and signs of collapse or consolidation if a foreign body has resulted in a segmental infection in delayed presentations. However, in some cases the inhaled object will be occult and the chest examination may be completely normal. A high index of suspicion is required, particularly if the history is suggestive.

Investigations

The initial investigation of the child with suspected inhaled foreign body should include a plain chest X-ray. The majority of objects are radiolucent and the radiological findings are those secondary to the physical presence in the airway. This may be normal or may show signs of unilateral hyperinflation.

Good quality inspiratory and expiratory X-rays are helpful. If there is air trapping, then the affected lung or part of the lung remains inflated in expiration. There may be segmental or lobar collapse distal to the foreign body particularly with delayed presentation. Fluoroscopy, if available, shows decreased movement of the diaphragm on the affected side.

Persistent changes on X-ray or recurrent pneumonia in the same place may signal an occult foreign body.

Treatment

Initially, the patient's airway and breathing should be assessed and oxygen given if required. Referral for bronchoscopy is the definitive treatment for confirmed or suspicious cases. Indications for bronchoscopy should be based on history, examination and radiological investigations '2 of 3 rule' (Table 6.2.1).

Patients should then be referred to an appropriate service, which can perform a rigid bronchoscopy to remove the foreign body. When in doubt, consult with a paediatric respiratory consultant.

Table 6.2.1 Indications for bronchoscopy
Two of the following
History • Coughing and choking episode and cyanosis or persistent cough after choking episode
Examination • Unilateral wheeze or unilateral decreased air entry
Investigations • Hyperinflation on expiration chest X-ray or subsegmental atelectasis or positive fluoroscopy

Children who have had a minor choking episode but no ongoing symptoms or signs and a normal X-ray can be discharged. Parents need to be instructed to return should any relevant symptoms evolve (wheeze, persistent dry cough, etc.).

If a child re-presents with ongoing symptoms after previous referral to a tertiary centre, clarify that an adequate assessment was made to rule out a foreign body at that review.

Prevention

Children under 3 years should be protected from access to toys with small parts or foods requiring molar function, as they are potential inhalation risks (e.g. peanuts).

Further reading

Digoy GP. Diagnosis and management of upper aerodigestive tract foreign bodies. *Otolaryngol Clin N Am* 2008;**41**: 485–96.

Heyer CM, Bollmeier ME, Rossler L, et al. Evaluation of clinical, radiologic, and laboratory prebronchoscopy findings in children with suspected foreign body aspiration. *J Ped Surg* 2006;**41**:1882–8.

Midulla F, Guidi R, Barbato A, et al. Foreign body aspiration in children. *Pediatr Int* 2005;**47**:663–8.

Malick MS, Khan AR, Al-Bassam A. Late presentation of tracheobronchial foreign body aspiration in children. *J Trop Pediatr* 2005;**51**(3):145–7.

6.3 Acute asthma

Colin V.E. Powell

ESSENTIALS

1 Acute asthma is one of the commonest paediatric presentations to an emergency department.

2 It is important to understand the patterns of asthma in children – infrequent episodic, frequent episodic, and persistent.

3 There are three major groups of factors contributing to 'high risk' asthma in children: previous severe asthma, management issues and psychological factors.

4 The most important parameters in the assessment of the severity of childhood asthma are the general appearance/mental state and work of breathing.

5 Life-threatening asthma is characterised by: silent chest, cyanosis, poor respiratory effort, exhaustion and altered mental state.

6 The main therapies for paediatric asthma include oxygen, inhaled bronchodilators and steroids modified according to severity.

7 Discharged patients should be given a clear asthma action plan and have appropriate follow up organised.

8 There are many areas of contention regarding the management of asthma in children and the recommended guidelines vary between countries. One should be familiar with the local paediatric guidelines.

Introduction

The National Asthma Campaign for Australia updated the 2002 guidelines in 2006[1] and this forms the basis of the chapter. However, there are other best practice guidelines[2,3] and national guidelines[4–7] and these are important resources for cross-reference and comparison to highlight the controversies.

Acute asthma is one of the commonest reasons for presentation to an emergency department and admission to a hospital. A recent review of admissions to nine paediatric emergency departments in Australia and New Zealand, examining over 300 000 presentations, demonstrated that acute asthma was the fourth most common presentation, accounting for 3.5% of the total number of presentations.[8] It is well recognised that in many cases admission to hospital may be preventable[9] if managed effectively by the family and medical team involved with a child's care. There are still great gaps between best practice guidelines and what actually happens in practice.[10–12]

Practice is highly variable, particularly for severe to critical acute asthma.[13]

History

Consider acute asthma when a child presents with signs of increase work of breathing, widespread wheezing and shortness of breath. There are other causes to consider such as mycoplasma pneumonia, aspiration, inhaled foreign body, and cardiac failure (Table 6.3.1). In the setting of a child with

Table 6.3.1 Differential diagnosis of asthma	
Acute	*Chronic*
Bronchiolitis, mycoplasma	Cystic fibrosis
Allergy	Cilial dyskinesia
Aspiration	Immune deficiency
Heart failure	Bronchiectasis
Foreign body	Airway abnormalities

a previous history of asthma or where asthma seems the most likely diagnosis, one can perform a primary assessment of severity and institute the initial treatment at the onset of history taking.

It is important to understand the patterns of asthma in children – infrequent episodic, frequent episodic, and persistent.[1] The pattern of asthma determines the need for preventive therapy. When a child is discharged from the emergency department (ED) or ward, consideration of the child's preventative treatment is essential.

Infrequent episodic asthma

Infrequent episodic asthma (IEA) is the most common pattern, accounting for 70 to 75% of children with asthma. In this pattern, children have isolated episodes of asthma lasting from 1 to 2 days up to 1 to 2 weeks, usually triggered by an upper respiratory tract infection (URTI) or an environmental allergen. The episodes are usually more than 6 to 8 weeks apart and these children are asymptomatic in the interval periods. They require management of the individual episode only and regular preventive therapy is unnecessary. Within this group there is a wide range of severity. Most are mild, but this group accounts for up to 60% of paediatric hospital admissions for asthma.[1]

Frequent episodic asthma

Frequent episodic asthma (FEA) accounts for approximately 20% of childhood asthma. This pattern is similar to IEA but the interval between episodes is shorter, less than 6 to 8 weeks, and the children have only minimal symptoms, such as exercise-induced wheeze, in the interval period. These children may benefit from regular preventive therapy such as low dose (not greater than 400 mcg per day) inhaled corticosteroids or leukotriene antagonist. Commonly, these children are troubled through the winter months only and may require preventive treatment for that part of the year.[1]

Persistent asthma

Persistent asthma (PA) accounts for 5–10% of childhood asthma. These children can have acute episodes like the categories above, but they also have symptoms on most days in the interval periods. These symptoms commonly include: sleep disturbance due to wheeze or cough, early morning chest tightness, exercise intolerance and spontaneous wheeze. Again, there is a wide range of severity in this group, ranging from those with mild symptoms 4 to 5 days per week readily controlled with low-dose corticosteroid preventive therapy, to those with frequent severe symptoms and abnormal lung function requiring intensive therapy.[1]

Acute episode

Mortality from acute asthma is fortunately rare – confidential enquiry into deaths from asthma suggests that there are three major factors contributing to the death.

- **The severity of the disease:** most children who have died from asthma have persistent asthma; however, a minority of children who have died have only mild to moderate disease.[4,14,15] Previous near fatal asthma, previous admission in the last year, previous admission to padiatric intensive care unit (PICU), heavy use of β_2 agonists, repeat attendances to the ED are all risk factors associated with risk of a severe attack, near fatal asthma or death.[4]
- **Medical management:** inadequate treatment steroids, heavy or increasing use of β_2 agonists, inadequate monitoring of the asthma and underuse of written asthma plans and delay in seeking help, have all been associated with deaths from asthma.[4,14,15]
- **Psychological factors:** non-adherence, poorly perceived symptoms, failure to attend clinics, conflict between child and parent or medical staff, family dysfunction are all risk factors associated with risk of death from asthma.[4,16]

A child should be considered as 'high risk' when attending the ED with an acute exacerbation of their asthma when there is a combination of features of previous severe asthma and one or more adverse psychological factors.

Examination

The most important parameters in the assessment of the severity of acute childhood asthma are general appearance/mental state and work of breathing (accessory muscle use, recession), as indicated in Table 6.3.2. Initial SaO$_2$ in air, heart rate and ability to talk are helpful but less reliable additional features. Wheeze intensity, pulsus paradoxus, and peak expiratory flow rate are not reliable.[2] Clinical signs of acute asthma correlate poorly with the severity of the asthma attack and none of the signs in isolation are predictive of severity.[4] Classification of an acute attack, using the NAC Australia guidelines[1] is as follows:

Investigations

Chest X-ray is not generally required in children with asthma, unless one has the suspicion of an alternative diagnosis or complication (air leak or atelectasis). Arterial blood gas and spirometry are rarely required in the assessment of acute asthma in children.

Differential diagnosis

During an acute episode of wheezing, asymmetry on auscultation is often found due to mucous plugging, but warrants consideration of foreign body. Consider other causes of wheeze (e.g. bronchiolitis, mycoplasma, aspiration, heart failure, or foreign body). Chronically wheezy children may have a diagnosis other than asthma, such as cystic fibrosis, cilial dyskinesia, immune dysfunction, developmental/congenital abnormality, upper airway problems or bronchiectasis. There may be clues in the family or perinatal history or symptoms and signs that may suggest an alternative diagnosis to asthma.[4]

Treatment

Treatment – mild

- Salbutamol by MDI/spacer (see below) – once and review after 20 minutes.
- Ensure device/technique appropriate.
- Good response – discharge on β_2 agonist as needed. Poor response – treat as moderate.
- Oral prednisolone (1 mg kg^{-1} daily for 1–3 days) if on prophylaxis or episode has persisted over several days.
- Provide written advice /action plan on what to do if symptoms worsen.

Table 6.3.2 Severity of asthma

Symptoms	Mild	Moderate	Severe and life-threatening*
Altered consciousness	No	No	Agitated *Confused/drowsy*
Accessory muscle use/ recession	No	*Minimal*	Moderate Severe
Oximetry on presentation (SaO$_2$)	>94%	94–90%	<90%
Talks in	Sentences	Phrases	Words *Unable to speak*
Pulsus paradoxus	Not palpable	May be palpable	Palpable
Pulse rate	<100	100–200	>200
Central cyanosis	Absent	Absent	Likely to be present
Wheeze intensity	Variable	Moderate–loud	Often quiet
Peak expiratory flow	>60%	40–60%	<40% *Unable to perform*
FEV$_1$ (% predicted)	>60%	40–60%	<40% *Unable to perform*
Arterial blood gases	Test not necessary	If initial response is poor	If initial response is poor *Yes*

*Life-threatening asthma is characterised by:[3]
- silent chest
- cyanosis
- poor respiratory effort
- hypotension
- exhaustion
- confusion
- coma

- Consider overall control and family's knowledge. Arrange follow up as appropriate (see discharge pack).

Treatment – moderate

- Give O_2 if O_2 saturation is <92%. Need for O_2 should be reassessed.
- Salbutamol by MDI/spacer (see below) – 3 doses, 20-minutely; review 10–20 minutes after 3rd dose and decide on admission or discharge.
- Oral prednisolone (1 mg kg^{-1} daily for 3 days).
- The few children of moderate severity who can go home must be discussed with a senior doctor and should not leave ED until at least 1 hour after their last spacer treatment.
- Arrange home treatment and follow up as above.

Treatment – severe

- Oxygen.
- Salbutamol by MDI/spacer (see below) or nebuliser – 3 doses 20-minutely; review ongoing requirements 10–20 minutes after 3rd dose – if improving reduce frequency, if no change continue 20-minutely, if deteriorating at any stage treat as life threatening.
- Ipratropium bromide (see below) by MDI/spacer or nebuliser. Three doses in the first hour every 20 minutes.
- Oral prednisolone (1 mg kg^{-1} daily); if vomiting give intravenous (IV) methylprednisolone 1 mg kg^{-1} or hydrocortisone 4 mg kg^{-1} 6-hourly.
- Involve senior staff.
- Arrange admission after initial assessment.

Treatment – life threatening

- Oxygen.
- Continuous nebulised salbutamol (0.5% undiluted).
- Nebulised ipratropium 250 mcg three times in 1st hr (20-minutely, added to salbutamol).
- Methylprednisolone 1 mg kg^{-1} or hydrocortisone 4 mg kg^{-1} 6-hourly.
- If deteriorating give IV salbutamol 15 mcg kg^{-1} over 10 minutes then 1–5 mcg kg^{-1} min^{-1}.
- If poor response to IV salbutamol, consider aminophylline 10 mg/kg IV (maximum dose 250 mg over 60 minutes). If currently taking oral theophylline, do not give IV aminophylline in ED – take serum level.

Following loading dose give continuous infusion (1–9 years: 1.1 mg kg^{-1} hr^{-1}, 10+ years: 0.7 mg kg^{-1} hr^{-1}; commence in ED if there will be >2 hours before transfer to ward).

- Magnesium sulfate 50% 0.1 mL kg^{-1} (50 mg kg^{-1}) IV over 20 minutes then 0.06 mL kg^{-1} hr^{-1} infusion with serum level 1.5–2.5 mmol L^{-1}.
- Involve senior staff, discuss with local PICU.
- Where intubation is indicated, ketamine is the induction agent of choice due to its bronchodilator action.

Disposition

Each child should have a written action plan on discharge from the ED. Observe the child's inhaler technique before discharge. Advise parents to seek further medical review should their child's condition deteriorate or if there is no significant improvement within 48 hours. At discharge all patients should have an outpatient appointment or appropriate follow up arranged with a paediatrician or local doctor as appropriate. Parents should be informed of other sources of information about asthma such as the Asthma Foundation. The concept of an asthma discharge pack is useful to ensure all aspects of discharge are considered. Adult data suggest that self-monitoring, regular review and written action plans can improve outcomes.[17] Two paediatric studies suggest that an intensive nurse-led discharge concentrating on education, written action plans and inhaler technique, appropriate follow up with discharge prescription for steroids can reduce readmissions and following morbidity.[18,19] A child should be ready for discharge when it is considered that they can be stable on 3–4-hour inhaled bronchodilators.[20] This is often a subjective decision.

Discharge pack

❶ Review need for preventative treatment.
   Consider preventative treatment if there are wheezing attacks less than 6 weeks apart, the attacks becoming more frequent and severe or there are increasing interval symptoms.
   Initial preventative treatment for frequent episodic asthma is inhaled steroids.
❷ Check inhaler technique.

Emergency attendance or admission should provide the patient and family with the opportunity to use an appropriate size space device and pMDI. Make sure the child and family can use the device adequately and know the importance of using it for all preventative therapy and treatment for significant exacerbations.
❸ Family education.
   On discharge from the ED or ward it is important that families understand the immediate management of their child's asthma. It is not appropriate to educate them on all aspects of asthma during an acute episode. This is best reserved for a visit to an outpatient clinic or local doctor at a time remote from the acute episode when a reasonable amount of time can be allocated and it is more likely that the information will be understood and retained.
❹ Prescription.
   A prescription for all medications should be provided at the time of discharge.
❺ Follow up.
   All patients should have a clear follow-up plan. For some it will be appropriate that they visit their local doctor for an early review, particularly if their condition deteriorates or fails to improve significantly with 48 hours. At discharge all patients should have an outpatient appointment or appropriate follow up arranged with a paediatrician within 4 to 6 weeks. This visit will be used for medical review and, most importantly, appropriate education about asthma management.
❻ Written action plan.
   All patients should have an individual written action plan and the discharging doctor should spend time going over the plan with the family.
❼ Communicate with the family doctor.
   For every emergency attendance or discharge, there should be communication with the patient's local doctor. The local doctor should receive a copy of the action plan.

Prognosis

Those with episodic asthma tend to improve throughout childhood, with asthma resolving by their adult years in approximately two-thirds. Those who continue to wheeze tend to have very mild asthma and maintain normal lung function. On the other hand, those with persistent asthma in childhood are more likely to continue to wheeze in their adult years (about two-thirds), with some impairment of lung function. Available evidence suggests that treatment does not influence the natural history of childhood asthma.[1]

Prevention

There are two areas of prevention to consider but the evidence is mostly inconclusive and confusing.[4]

Primary prophylaxis

These are interventions aimed at preventing the development of asthma and reduce its incidence. There is insufficient evidence to make recommendations about aeroallergen avoidance during pregnancy or early infancy, use of modified infant milk formulae, pre- and probiotic use, fish oil and other nutritional supplement use, immunotherapy and avoiding air pollutants. However, the only evidenced-based recommendations in this area are that:

- breast feeding should be encouraged as this will reduce the likelihood of developing asthma, particularly in families with an atopic history;[4]
- parents and parents-to-be should be advised not to smoke as, particularly maternal smoking antenatally and postnatally is associated with increased risk of infant wheeze.[4]

Secondary prophylaxis

These are interventions aimed at reducing the impact of the disease once developed. A number of non-pharmacological methods of secondary prophylaxis are debated: for example, allergen avoidance, house dust mite control measures, avoiding smoking and air pollution, antioxidant and mineral supplementation, fish oils and fatty acids use, breathing exercises, chemotherapy and immunotherapy. Recent evidence-based recommendations are that:

- In committed families, house dust mite avoidance by use of bed covers, removal of carpets and soft toys, dehumidification, high temperature washing of bed linen, and use of acaricides on soft furnishing may reduce morbidity from asthma.[4]

- Maternal smoking during pregnancy has an effect on lung development and infants whose mothers smoke are four times more likely to develop wheezy illness during the first year of life and thus environmental tobacco smoke should be avoided.[4]

If an organised discharge from hospital is completed as per recommendations (as above), then this is more likely to prevent readmission or re-presentation and reduce morbidity. A number of preventable factors associated with admission have been identified and these issues should be addressed at discharge: adherence issues, prophylactic treatment, action plan use and advice to prevent delay in seeking medical advice.[9]

Controversies

❶ Bronchodilator aerosol delivery

Pressurised metered dose inhalers (pMDI) and spacers are an effective way of delivering inhalation medication to treat mild to moderate and probably severe attacks of asthma.[21] Successful implementation[22,23] and sustained use of spacers after changeover from nebulisers has been demonstrated.[24] There are fewer side effects such as tachycardia, vomiting and hypoxia compared to when a drug is given via a nebuliser.[21] There is still debate as to cost in different countries and whether the pMDI/spacer combination use in adult acute asthma is as effective as nebulisers.[21] The pMDI/spacer combination is used less frequently in adult patients.[10] For mild and moderate asthma all of the eleven Clinical Practice Guidelines (CPG) in the PREDICT study recommended MDI and spacers; for severe asthma half of the CPG recommended spacer delivery and for critical asthma spacers were not recommended at all.[13] In the UK there has been a significant increase in the use of spacers in the hospital setting despite the asthma severity remaining stable over the last decade.[12] There are no data on the use of spacers in severe to life threatening asthma but clearly they are being used in the severe group.[13]

It probably doesn't make much difference what doses are given; if there is a response, cut down the dose, if there is no response, increase it! There are

similar dosing recommendations for nebulised bronchodilator; between 2.5 mg and 5 mg of salbutamol per nebuliser every 20 minutes[1-7] or frequent doses of 5–10 mg of nebulised teburtaline.[4] There is little evidence for any benefit for continuous nebulised (0.5% undiluted salbutamol) treatment compared to frequent intermittent doses of treatment[4] although many CPG recommend use in life-threatening exacerbations.[1-3] Indeed all the sites in the PREDICT study used continuous nebulised bronchodilator treatment in life-threatening asthma and 64% of sites recommended use in severe attacks.[13] There are some interesting data in the adult literature addressing the use of long acting β agonists in acute asthma, e.g. formoterol, which has a rapid onset of action and long duration of effect[6] (see Research/Future Directions section). Current BTS recommendation are, however, to stop long acting β_2 agonists if short acting β_2 agonists are required more than 4-hourly.[4]

❷ Ipratropium bromide

Repeated early doses of ipratropium bromide during the first 1–2 hours of presentation are associated with improved outcomes;[25] efficacy and safety have been demonstrated. It is recommended for children with severe and life-threatening attacks[1-7] but often overused in children with moderate and mild attacks'[10] with 37% of physicians reporting its use in moderate asthma exacerbations and 3% use in mild.[13] Although doses of inhaled ipratropium bromide are recommended for use with a metered dose inhaler and spacer[1-3,5] there are no data demonstrating that these doses are appropriate and this is a consensus statement recommendation. Different doses are recommended.

Standard doses of 250–500 mcg per dose for nebulised treatment seems universal.[1-7] Repeated doses of ipratropium bromide should be given early in children who are not responsive to β_2 agonists.[4] It is not clear whether there are any benefits from continued use after the attack has shown response to treatment. Once hospitalised, the addition of ipratropium to salbutamol and steroids appears to add no benefit.[26]

BTS recommend that the dose should be weaned down to 4–6-hourly or stopped once admitted.[4]

❸ Intravenous bronchodilators

The main problem with deciding which intravenous bronchodilator to use is that there are no good direct comparisons with the three intravenous treatments commonly used. There are certainly drug versus placebo studies but no head to head studies to endorse recommendations. Thus the referenced guidelines vary with recommendations.[1–7] The role of intravenous bronchodilators in addition to nebulised treatment remains unclear.[27]

Salbutamol – continuous intravenous infusions are recommended following on from a bolus or initial infusion, if the child does not respond, but different doses are recommended:[28]

The guidelines from the Global Initiative for Asthma (GINA) do not recommend intravenous β_2 agonists, stating there is no evidence for their benefit[25] and the AAP do not mention intravenous therapy.[7]

Aminophylline – there is no evidence that there is a role for aminophylline in children with mild to moderate exacerbations of their asthma. However, if a child is unresponsive to maximal inhaled therapy as above, then in the more severe and life-threatening attacks, aminophylline has been shown to have an effect on outcome (intubation).[29,30]

This is clearly a controversial area. There is no doubt that vomiting is a serious side effect from the higher doses of aminophylline and this may be the reason not to use it.[29]

Magnesium – **intravenous magnesium** relaxes smooth muscle and causes bronchodilation. Its exact place in the treatment of acute asthma in children has yet to be established. Doses of 40–100 mg kg^{-1} as a 20-minute infusion have been used with varying effects on lung function and asthma severity scores when compared to placebo.[31] NAC recommend using 50% 0.1 mL kg^{-1} (50 mg kg^{-1}) IV over 20 minutes for severe and life-threatening episodes, followed by an infusion of 0.06 ml kg^{-1} hr^{-1} (30 mg kg^{-1} hr^{-1}): target serum levels 1.5–2.5 mmol L^{-1}.[1] The use of intravenous magnesium sulfate in severe and critical exacerbations is discussed in the BTS guidelines but not fully endorsed[4] and GINA[5] does not recommend its use routinely in children but mentions it may be of benefit in severe asthma (no dose discussed). Magnesium is not mentioned in the other guidelines[2,3,6,7] for use in children. It is clearly being used in EDs in Australia and New Zealand in 50% of critical and 18% of severe exacerbations.[13]

Nebulised magnesium may have a role in adult asthma but there are few data on its role in children.[6] None of the guidelines recommend its use. A multicentre double blind RCT study of nebulised magnesium is currently under way in the UK.[32]

Adrenaline – this bronchodilator is not mentioned in the paediatric guidelines.[1–5] However, the GINA guidelines suggest it may be of use.[6] There is no doubt that some acute asthma may be anaphylaxis[33] and intramuscular adrenaline (epinephrine) may well have a role.[6] The dose suggested is 0.01 mg kg^{-1} up to 0.3–0.5 mg of 1:1000 adrenaline (epinephrine) every 20 minutes for three doses for acute asthma.[5] This treatment is very rarely used in acute asthma in a paediatric population.[10]

❹ Corticosteroids

There is no doubt that early use of steroids for an acute attack reduces not only the need for admission but also morbidity.[4,34] If a child can take a dose orally there is no benefit to administering it intravenously.[33,35] There are a number of different dosing regimens suggested: A 2-day course of dexamethasone has been shown to be as effective as a 5-day course of prednisolone and there may be some suggestions that this may help adherence.[36]

Inhaled steroids – there is insufficient evidence in children that inhaled steroids should replace oral or systemic steroids in acute exacerbations.[4] There are some adult data to suggest that high-dose inhaled steroids may have a value.[5]

❺ Leukotriene antagonists

Initiating oral leukotriene antagonists in primary care early at the onset of an exacerbation can result in reduced symptoms, time off school, healthcare resource utilisation and parental time off work in children with intermittent asthma.[37] There is no clear evidence that there is a role as intravenous therapy in acute asthma exacerbations; only adult data exist.[38] Current studies are reviewing the use of leukotriene antagonists in the management of acute asthma in children.

❻ Children less than 2 years of age

This age group can be difficult to assess and the different phenotypes of acute wheezing and indeed different labels used in different countries can cause problems when examining the literature on appropriate treatment.[4] In the recent update of the BTS guidelines where asthma is considered to be the likeliest diagnosis, β_2 agonists delivered by spacer and pMDI is the optimum delivery device; oral β_2 agonists are not recommended. There is little evidence that β_2 agonists or ipratropium bromide have an impact on wheezy children of this age in regard to their need for hospitalisation or length of stay.[4,39] Steroid therapy may have a role but this is still not clear.[4] There are problems differentiating between bronchiolitis and asthma in younger infants and this is outside the scope of this chapter.

❼ Intensive care management

The NAC and BTS recommendation is that once a child has severe enough asthma to require intravenous treatment they should be referred to a PICU or an PHDU even if they do not require intubation.[1,4] There are a number of indications for intensive care admission: deteriorating lung function, persisting or worsening hypoxia, hypercapnia, exhaustion, drowsiness, confusion, coma or respiratory arrest.[4] These features are clearly all part of a spectrum and the overall picture, plus lack of response to treatment, should indicate that the child should be admitted to a high dependency or intensive care area. They may not necessarily require ventilation. There are no absolute criteria and the decision needs to be made by an experienced physician/anaesthetist.[4,6] Non-invasive ventilation has had some success in adults but none of the paediatric guidelines recommend its use. Detailed discussion about ventilating a child with asthma is beyond the scope of this chapter. Helium and oxygen mixtures have been used in adults but again are not endorsed in the paediatric guidelines on current evidence.[6]

Future directions/research

The following list is a number of themes needing further development in acute asthma – it is by no means exhaustive.

Prevention of developing asthma and secondary prevention – can we reduce asthma morbidity?

Patient education and asthma care delivery – how best to deliver asthma care and how best to improve patients' and families' knowledge?

Gaps in practice and delivery of care – how best to audit asthma care and improve implementation of guidelines?

Improved assessment of acute asthma – what is the best predictor of asthma severity, need for treatment and hospital admission?

What should be the core outcomes measured for acute asthma research in children?

Are there different phenotypes of acute asthma with potentially different treatment modalities?

Do long-acting β_2 agonists have a role in treating acute asthma?

Pharmacogenomics – are there different genotypes with different responses to treatment?

Which is the most effective intravenous bronchodilator?

What is the best mode of delivery for aerosolised treatments?

Non-invasive ventilation – where does this have a role?

What is the role of inhaled magnesium, intravenous leukotriene antagonists and inhaled helium mixture?

References

1. National Asthma Council Australia Asthma Management Handbook. http://www.nationalasthma.org.au/; 2007.
2. Royal Children's Hospital, Melbourne. *clinical guidelines.* Available from http://www.rch.unimelb.edu.au/clinicalguide/; 2010 [accessed 13.10.10].
3. Sydney Children's Hospital Randwick NSW. Australia. Available from http://www.sch.edu.au; 2010 [accessed 13.10.10].
4. British Thoracic Society and Scottish Intercollegiate Guidelines Network updated. Available from http://www.sign.ac.uk/guidelines/published/; 2009 [accessed 13.10.10].
5. Canadian Association for Emergency Physicians. Available from http://www.cps.ca/; 2009 [accessed 13.10.10].
6. Global Strategy for Asthma Management and Prevention. Available from http://www.ginasthma.com; 2008 [accessed 13.10.10].
7. Hegenbarth MA. American Academy of Pediatrics Preparing for Pediatric Emergencies. *Pediatrics* 2008;**121**:433–43.
8. Acworth J, Babl F, Borland M, et al. Patterns of presentation to the Australian and New Zealand Pediatric Research Network. *Emerg Med Australas* 2009;**21**:59–66.
9. Ordonez GA, Phelan PD, Olinsky A, Robertson CF. Preventable factors in hospital admissions for asthma. *Arch Dis Child* 1998;**78**(2):143–7.
10. Kelly AM, Powell CVE, Kerr D. Snapshot of acute asthma: treatment and outcome of patients with acute asthma treated in Australian emergency departments. *Intern Med J* 2003;**33**:406–13.
11. Powell CV, Raftos J, Kerr D, et al. Asthma in emergency departments: combined adult versus paediatric only centres. *Paediatr Child Health* 2004;**40**:433–7.
12. Davies G, Payton JY, Beaton SJ, et al. Children admitted with acute wheeze/asthma during November 1998–2005: a national audit. *Arch Dis Child* 2008;**93**:952–8.
13. Babl FE, Sherriff N, Borland M, et al. Paediatric asthma management in Australia and New Zealand: practice patterns in the context of clinical guidelines. *Arch Dis Child* 2008;**93**:307–12.
14. Robertson CF, Rubinfield AR, Bowes G. Pediatric asthma deaths in Victoria: the mild are at risk. *Pediatr Pulmonol* 1992;**12**:95–100.
15. Martin AJ, Campbell DA, Gluyas PA, et al. Characteristics of near fatal asthma in children. *Pediatr Pulmonol* 1995;**20**:1–8.
16. Strunk RC, Mzrazek DA, Wolfson Fuhrmann GS, LaBrecque JF. Physiologic and psychological characteristics associated with deaths due to asthma in childhood. *JAMA* 1985;**254**:1193–8.
17. Gibson PG, Powell H, Wilson A, et al. Self-management education and regular practitioner review for adults with asthma. *Cochrane Database Syst Rev* 2002;(3). Art. No.: CD001117. doi:10.1002/14651858.CD001117.
18. Madge P, McColl J, Payton J. Impact of a nurse led home management training programme in children admitted to hospital with acute asthma. A randomized controlled study. *Thorax* 1997;**3**:223–8.
19. Wessldine LJ, McCarthy P, Silverman M. Structured discharge procedure for children admitted to hospital with acute asthma. A randomized controlled trail of nursing practice. *Arch Dis Child* 1999;**80**:110–4.
20. Storman MO, Mellis CM, Van Asperen PP, et al. Outcome evaluation of early discharge of asthmatic children from hospital: a randomized control trial. *J Qual Clin Pract* 1999;**19**:149–54.
21. Cates CJ, Crilly JA, Rowe BH. Holding chambers (spacers) versus nebulisers for beta-agonist treatment of acute asthma. *Cochrane Database Syst Rev* 2006;(2). Art. No.: CD000052. doi:10.1002/14651858.CD000052.pub2.
22. Powell CV, Maskell GR, Marks M, et al. Successful implementation of spacer treatment guidelines for acute asthma. *Arch Dis Child* 2001;**84**:142–6.
23. Gazarian M, Henry RL, Wales SR, et al. Evaluating the effectiveness of evidence-based guidelines for the use of spacer devices in children with acute asthma. *Med J Aust* 2001;**174**:394–7.
24. Cheng NG, Browne GJ, Lam LT, et al. Spacer compliance after discharge following a mild to moderate asthma attack. *Arch Dis Child* 2002;**87**(4):302–5.
25. Plotnick LH, Ducharme FM. Combined inhaled anticholinergic agents and beta-2 agonists for initial treatment of acute asthma in children (Cochrane Review). In: *The Cochrane Library.* Issue 3. Oxford: Update Software; 2001.
26. Goggin N, Macarthur C, Parkin PC. Randomized trial of the addition of ipratropium bromide to albuterol and corticosteroid therapy in children hospitalized because of an acute asthma exacerbation. *Arch Pediatr Adolesc Med* 2001;**155**:1329–34.
27. Travers AA, Jones AP, Kelly KD, et al. Intravenous beta2-agonists for acute asthma in the emergency department. *Cochrane Database Syst Rev* 2001;(1). Art. No.: CD002988. doi:10.1002/14651858.CD002988. *Cochrane Database Syst Rev* 2010 Issue 1, Copyright © 2010 The Cochrane Collaboration.
28. Browne GJ, Penna AS, Phung X, Soo M. Randomised trial of intravenous salbutamol in early management of acute severe asthma in children. *Lancet* 1997;**49**(9048):301–5.
29. Yung M, South M. Randomised controlled trial of aminophylline for severe asthma. *Arch Dis Child* 1998;**79**:405–10.
30. Ream RS, Loftus LL, Albers GM, et al. Efficacy of IV theophylline in children with severe status asthmaticus. *Chest* 2001;**119**:1480–8.
31. Rowe BH, Bretzlaff J, Bourdon C, et al. Magnesium sulfate for treating exacerbations of acute asthma in the emergency department. *Cochrane Database Syst Rev* 2000;(1). Art. No.: CD001490. doi:10.1002/14651858.CD001490. *Cochrane Database Syst Rev* 2010 Issue 1, Copyright © 2010 The Cochrane Collaboration.
32. Powell CVE. A randomised, placebo controlled study of nebulised magnesium in acute severe asthma in children. Available from http://www.controlled-trials.com/ISRCTN81456894 [accessed 13.10.10].
33. Rainbow J, Browne GJ. Fatal asthma or anaphylaxis? *Emerg Med J* 2002;**19**(5):415–7.
34. Smith M, Iqbal SMSI, Rowe BH, N'Diaye T. Corticosteroids for hospitalised children with acute asthma. *Cochrane Database Syst Rev* 2003;(1). Art. No.:CD002886. doi: 10.1002/14651858.CD002886. *Cochrane Database Syst Rev* 2010 Issue 1, Copyright © 2010 The Cochrane Collaboration.
35. Barnett P, Caputo GL, Baskin M, et al. Intravenous versus oral corticosteroids in acute pediatric asthma. *Ann Emerg Med* 1997;**29**:212–7.
36. Qureshi F, Zaritsky A, Poirier MP. Comparitive efficacy of oral dexamethasone versus oral prednisolone in acute pediatric asthma. *J Paediatr* 2001;**139**:20–6.
37. Robertson CF, Price D, Henry R, et al. Short course Montelukast for intermittent asthma in children: A randomize controlled trial. *Am J Respir Critical Med* 2007;**175**:323–9.
38. Camargo CA, Smithline HA, Marie-Pierre M, et al. A randomized controlled trial of intravenous montelukast in acute asthma. *Am J Respir Crit Care Med* 2003;**167**:528–33.
39. Everard M, Bara A, Kurian M, et al. Anticholinergic drugs for wheeze in children under the age of two years. *Cochrane Database Syst Rev* 2005;(3). Art. No.: CD001279. doi: 10.1002/14651858.CD001279.pub2.

6.4 Pertussis

Nigel W. Crawford • Colin V.E. Powell

ESSENTIALS

1 Pertussis infection is most common and severe in infants less than 6 months of age.

2 All children less than 6 months with pertussis should be admitted for a period of observation in order to assess the risk of significant apnoea.

3 Three stages of illness occur – catarrhal, paroxysmal and convalescent.

4 The mainstay of treatment is supportive. Admission allows for apnoea monitoring, oxygen and overcoming feeding difficulties.

5 Respiratory complications are the most common, with pneumonia the major cause of mortality (0.5–1%) in infants <6 months.

6 Treatment is with macrolide antibiotics (e.g. erythromycin for 2-week course), best if given early in the course of the illness.

7 Prevention is by universal immunisation with acellular pertussis vaccine in childhood, plus a booster in adolescence/adulthood.

Introduction

Pertussis or 'whooping cough' is a bacterial infection of the respiratory tract caused by the Gram-negative coccobacillus, *Bordetella pertussis*. The word pertussis itself means 'intensive cough' and was first described in 1578, when an epidemic occurred in Paris.[1] Pertussis is the preferred term because not all cases have the classical paroxysms of coughing, with an inspiratory 'whoop', which occur as a massive respiratory effort forces inhaled air against a narrow glottis.

Pathophysiology

Humans are the only reservoir and the incubation period is approximately 7–10 days. Transmission is primarily by direct contact with droplets via the airborne route. The organism is highly communicable early in the illness, with attack rates of 75–100% from symptomatic individuals to susceptible contacts. Pertussis is associated with a significant morbidity and mortality, particularly in young infants.

Epidemiology

With the advent of universal vaccination programmes in the 1940s the incidence of this disease decreased markedly. Due to concerns regarding immunisation, vaccination levels waned in the late 1970s and there was a resurgence in the number of cases. Worldwide there are approximately 250 000 deaths attributed to pertussis per year. There have been epidemics every 3–4 years in Australia, with epidemiological data showing an estimated incidence of 25 cases per 100 000 per year in 1996.[2,3]

History

The possibility of pertussis should be considered in a child presenting to the emergency department (ED) who has prominent coughing episodes. The diagnosis of pertussis is usually made on the basis of a suggestive clinical history, confirmed by isolation of the organism.

There are three characteristic stages of the illness and presentation is most commonly in the paroxysmal phase.

Stage 1: Catarrhal (1–2 weeks)

Upper respiratory tract infection symptoms, e.g. rhinorrhoea, conjunctivitis, malaise and low-grade fever.

Stage 2: Paroxysmal (2–6 weeks, can be longer)

Consists of paroxysms of coughing which may be followed by an inspiratory 'whoop'. Facial suffusion, with prominent eyes and protrusion of neck veins, may be seen during these paroxysms. The paroxysms can cause fatigue, which may impair an infant's ability to take feeds. Post-tussive vomiting commonly follows the coughing episode, but between times the child may appear quite well. It is important to note that young infants may present with apnoea as the only symptom. This can result in a presentation of sudden collapse (see Chapter 1.2).

Stage 3: Convalescent (1–2 weeks)

The paroxysms of coughing, whooping and vomiting decrease in number and severity. The cough may persist for a number of weeks/months and future episodes of upper respiratory tract infections may restimulate the coughing paroxysms.

Pertussis is most severe in infants younger than 6 months of age, particularly the non-immunised. It is these high-risk infants that particularly need to be identified and admitted for a period of observation to exclude significant apnoea events. In infants, the clinical manifestations can mimic those of bronchiolitis or other infective pneumonitis. In partially immune adults and adolescents, who have waning immunity, the presentation is less typical and can be that of a persistent cough.

Examination

The clinical findings depend on the stage of the illness when the child presents and one needs to look for potential complications. Some children will kindly display a typical coughing paroxysm in the ED and reinforce the description given by parents. This may include features of facial colour changes or a whoop that will suggest pertussis as the likely cause.

Other children may have little to find on examination, apart from mild coryza. In these, the diagnosis is based on a suggestive history and subsequent isolation of the organism. There may be visible mechanical sequelae, due to coughing and vomiting, such as petechiae or subconjunctival haemorrhages. Unless a secondary pneumonia or atelectasis due to plugging has occurred, the chest examination is generally unremarkable.

Investigations

The clinical diagnosis is traditionally confirmed by nasopharyngeal swab, with culture of the organism being the gold standard. The isolation rates for pertussis are best early in the course of the illness, prior to any antibiotic treatment. More recent investigations have focused on more rapid techniques, which may aid decision making in the ED. These include fluorescent antibody tests on post-nasal aspirate specimens, serology testing to anti-B. pertussis IgA, IgM or IgG, and polymerase chain reaction (PCR).[4]

The full blood examination, at the end of the catarrhal or early in the paroxysmal phase, can have a leucocytosis with a predominant lymphocytosis.

A chest X-ray may show perihilar infiltrates, interstitial emphysema or evidence of a secondary pneumonia.

Differential diagnosis

A 'pertussis-like syndrome' may be caused by other organisms, including: *Bordetella parapertussis*, adenoviral infections, *Mycoplasma pneumoniae* and *Chlamydia pneumoniae*. They often lead to a milder, shorter clinical course and can be isolated by a nasopharyngeal sample, or specific serology can be performed. In the first few months of life, viral bronchiolitis may cause a very similar clinical picture to that of pertussis and only be distinguished on the basis of the microbiology result.

Complications

Respiratory complications are frequent, with pneumonia the most common. It may be due to a secondary bacterial infection.

Occasionally, the pneumonia can be a severe necrotising form, which is the major cause of death. Atelectasis is common, resulting from mucous plugging and air leaks (pneumothoraces, interstitial emphysema or pneumomediastinum) may occur secondary to ruptured alveoli. Bronchiectasis is a rare late sequela.

Subconjunctival haemorrhages, rectal prolapse or inguinal hernia may occur due to increased intra-abdominal pressure. Cerebral anoxia with convulsions can occur in young children and encephalopathy is seen in approximately 1 in 10 000 cases.[3,5]

Treatment

All infants <6 months of age with suspected pertussis should be admitted with isolation, due to the risk of apnoea and other complications. This allows for a period of observation of coughing episodes and monitoring for apnoea and desaturations. Older children will require admission should they have significant apnoea/cyanosis or feeding problems. Treatment is mainly supportive via monitoring and the provision of oxygen and fluids.

Treatment with erythromycin is most effective if given early and has little effect in the paroxysmal phase. Recent studies have looked at the equivalence of the newer macrolides and a 5-day course of azithromycin or 7 days of clarithromycin may be as effective at eradicating the organism.[6] Co-trimoxazole is the drug of choice if macrolides are contraindicated. There is minimal chance of transmission after 5 days of treatment. Consider broader-spectrum antibiotics if there is evidence of superadded bacterial infection. The index case should be excluded from nursery/school until 5 days of treatment is completed.[6,7]

Chemoprophylaxis of contacts

Contact tracing is difficult, but the family and close household contacts should have a course of antibiotics regardless of immunisation status. There is poor placental transfer of *B. pertussis* antibodies, so pregnant women exposed around the time of delivery and their newborn infants should also receive chemoprophylaxis. The contacts should also have vaccination at the same time, particularly those under 8 years who

have not received their five DTPa vaccinations. There is no benefit from passive immunisation prophylaxis with human pertussis immunoglobulin.[3]

Prevention

Immunisation first commenced in the late 1940s with the triple vaccine, Diphtheria Tetanus Pertussis (DTP). This was initially a whole-cell vaccine but since the 1990s an acellular vaccine has been available. It has been shown to be as effective, preventing disease in 85% of cases with fewer side effects, and is now recommended.

Current immunisation schedule

DTPa: 2, 4, 6, and 4 years.

There are also multiple-combination vaccines available: e.g. DTPa-hepB. An adult-formulation pertussis-containing vaccine (dTpa) suitable for boosting adults and adolescents is recommended as a single dose at 15 to 17 years of age.[3] Complications of the vaccine may potentially present to ED and include: fever >38°C (uncommonly leads to a febrile convulsion), erythema at the injection site, persistent crying, drowsiness, vomiting, anorexia, systemic allergic reaction, and hypotonic–hyporesponsive episodes (rare, with no long-term sequelae).

Prognosis

The severity is directly related to age, with the illness normally milder in older children. Morbidity and mortality (0.5–1%) is still significant in infants under 6 months of age.

Controversies and future directions

❶ An encephalopathy has been controversially linked with the pertussis vaccination in the past, but the evidence is inconclusive, as the event is so rare and no causal link has been proven.[8] Pertussis vaccine does not cause infantile spasms, epilepsy or sudden infant death syndrome (SIDS).

❷ The drop in vaccination rates in the 1970s and the subsequent increase in the incidence of this preventable disease highlight the need for ongoing surveillance to monitor the uptake and efficacy of vaccinations, the frequency of adverse reactions and the incidence of epidemics. Further refinement and greater availability of the rapid diagnostic techniques will be helpful in making the diagnosis quickly and reliably. Progress in the sequencing of the genome of *B. pertussis* has also yielded a new field of research.[9] There is also a need for more studies on equivalence testing of different antibiotics for treatment of pertussis.

References

1. Cone TR. Whooping cough is first described as a disease sui generis by Balliou in 1640. *Paediatrics* 1970;**46**:522.
2. Andrews R, Herceg A, Roberts C. Pertussis notifications in Australia 1991 to 1997. *Commun Dis Intell* 1997;**21**(11):145–8.
3. National Health and Medical Research Council. *The Australian Immunisation Handbook 9th edn.* Canberra: Australian Government Publishing Service; 2008.
4. Heininger U, Schmidt-Schapfer G, Cherry J, Stehr K. Clinical validation of a polymerase chain reaction assay for the diagnosis of pertussis by comparison with serology, culture and symptoms during a large pertussis vaccine trial. *Paediatrics* 2000;**104**:312.
5. Miller D, Madge N, Diamond J. Pertussis immunisation and serious acute neurological illnesses in children. *Br Med J* 1993;**307**(6913):1171–5.
6. Lebel MH, Mehra S. Efficacy and safety of clarithromycin versus erythromycin for the treatment of pertussis: A prospective, randomized, single blind trial. *Pediatr Infect Dis J* 2001;**20**:1149–54.
7. Aoyama T, Sunakawa K, Iwata S, et al. Efficacy of short-term treatment of pertussis with clarithromycin and azithromycin. *J Paediatr* 1996;**129**(5):761–4.
8. Heininger U. Pertussis: An old disease that is still with us. *Curr Opin Infect Dis* 2001;**14**(3):329–35.
9. Girard DZ. Which strategy for pertussis vaccination today? *Paediatr Drugs* 2002;**4**(5):299–313.

Further reading

Cherry JD, Heininger U. Pertussis and other *Bordetella* infections. In: Feigin RD, Cherry JD, editors. *Textbook of Pediatric Infectious Diseases.* 4th ed., vol. 2. Philadelphia, PA: WB Saunders Co; 2004. p. 1588–608.

6.5 Community-acquired pneumonia

Mike Starr

ESSENTIALS

1 Viruses are the most common cause of pneumonia in children, although up to 40% of cases represent mixed infection.

2 *Streptococcus pneumoniae* is the most common bacterial cause.

3 X-ray findings do not correlate with aetiology.

4 Blood tests, including full blood count, inflammatory markers and blood culture are generally unhelpful.

5 Oral amoxicillin or intravenous benzylpenicillin are appropriate for empiric therapy of most children with pneumonia.

6 The addition of a macrolide antibiotic (e.g. roxithromycin) should be considered in children with atypical pneumonia.

7 The routine use of third-generation cephalosporins provides no additional benefit over the penicillins.

Introduction

Pneumonia is a common condition with significant morbidity and mortality. It is estimated to be responsible for approximately three million childhood deaths per year, most of which occur in developing countries.[1] Even in developed countries, pneumonia remains a major cause of acute morbidity and one of the most common reasons for paediatric hospital admissions.[2] The incidence of pneumonia is approximately 40 per 1000 children per year in those under 5 years of age, and 15 per 1000 children per year in 5–14-year-olds.[3–5]

In spite of how common it is, there is no single clinical or radiological definition that is widely accepted for pneumonia. It is investigated with a range of tests, the usefulness of which is known to be incomplete, and it is then often treated without knowledge of the aetiology. Fortunately, most children recover completely with empiric treatment.

Definition

There are various definitions that can be used for pneumonia. From a pathological point of view, it is defined as inflammation or infection of the lung parenchyma. In the clinical setting, the diagnosis is typically made on the basis of a constellation of clinical features, including fever, cough, tachypnoea and auscultatory findings, and confirmed by radiographic changes.

Aetiology

In the majority of cases of childhood pneumonia, the causative pathogen is not identified. Blood cultures are positive in under 5% of cases of pneumonia.[5,6] Transthoracic lung aspiration yields a cause in up to 69% of cases,[7,8] but is invasive. It is difficult to obtain adequate sputum for microscopy and culture in young children. Other indirect methods of identifying a cause, such as serology or immunofluorescence and culture of nasopharyngeal aspirates are neither sensitive nor specific.

Although an alveolar or lobar infiltrate on chest X-ray is considered by some to be suggestive of bacterial infection, chest X-ray changes cannot reliably predict aetiology.[9,10] Nor is any radiological pattern pathognomonic for viral or *Mycoplasma pneumoniae* infection.

Age is the best predictor of aetiology of pneumonia. In neonates, where bacterial causes predominate, Group B streptococci and *Escherichia coli* are the most common pathogens. Viruses, particularly respiratory syncytial virus (RSV), parainfluenza, influenza, metapneumovirus and adenovirus, are the most common cause overall, particularly in young children. The occurrence of recent local outbreaks and the clinical pattern may give a clue to the likely causative virus. These viruses appear to be responsible for approximately 40% of cases of community-acquired pneumonia in children who are hospitalised, particularly in those under 2 years of age, whereas *Streptococcus pneumoniae* is responsible for 27% to 44% of cases of community-acquired pneumonia.[11] Up to 40% of infections are mixed.[5] Infection with *Mycoplasma pneumoniae* and *Chlamydia pneumoniae* is usually considered to cause pneumonia in children of school age and in older patients, although more recent studies suggest that preschool-aged children have as many episodes of atypical bacterial pneumonia as older children.[11] Staphylococcal and Group A streptococcal pneumonia are uncommon, but should be considered in children who are severely unwell with invasive disease. These infections are more likely to be seen in indigenous and Pacific Islander children. More recently, infections with community-acquired multiresistant *Staphylococcus aureus* (CAMRSA) have emerged. CAMRSA results in a necrotising fulminant pneumonia with increased morbidity and mortality.

Gram-negative pneumonia is uncommon in children; non-typeable *Haemophilus influenzae* is mainly seen in children with underlying lung disease, such as cystic fibrosis and bronchiectasis.

The presence of a pleural effusion does not necessarily indicate more severe disease – *Strep. pneumoniae* remains the most common bacterial cause, with or without effusion.

Clinical findings

Pneumonia should be considered in any infant or child presenting with fever, cough, difficulty breathing, tachypnoea, increased work of breathing (nasal flaring, lower chest indrawing or recession), and auscultatory findings consistent with consolidation or effusion. However, the auscultatory findings may be unreliable in young children, particularly in those under 1 year. Infants may present with symptoms not obviously related to a lower respiratory tract infection, such as lethargy, vomiting, poor feeding, grunting, or poor perfusion. Children less than 3 months of age may present with apnoea. Tachypnoea is the most sensitive and specific sign[12] and may be the only clue in some children. Auscultatory findings, including asymmetrical breath sounds, crackles and bronchial breathing are less predictive. The presence of coryza or wheeze (particularly bilateral) suggests that bacterial pneumonia is unlikely.[6,13] Pneumonia located in the apex of the lung may present with neck pain and be confused with meningitis, whilst basal pneumonia may cause abdominal pain, suggestive of an acute abdomen. Conversely, an infant with grunting respirations may give the initial impression of an intra-abdominal problem.

The presentation of pneumococcal pneumonia is generally abrupt, whilst *M. pneumoniae* and viral infections more often present with a more indolent course, less fever, and other symptoms such as malaise, headache, arthralgia and rash.

Investigations

Posteroanterior chest X-rays are generally used to confirm pneumonia where there is clinical suspicion. However, they need not be performed routinely in older children with mild disease where the diagnosis may be made clinically. They are particularly important for confirming the diagnosis of pneumonia in children less than 5 years of age who present with fever and tachypnoea, unless classical features of bronchiolitis are present. Lateral X-rays do not confer much additional information in most cases.

Although, it is not possible to reliably predict aetiology or differentiate bacterial from viral pneumonia on chest X-ray, pneumococcal pneumonia typically presents with a lobar infiltrate or round pneumonia. Pneumatoceles, abscesses and cavities are associated most frequently with staphylococcal pneumonia but they are also seen in pneumonias caused by other bacteria. Bronchopneumonia is more typical of viral or other aetiology.

Large effusions may be difficult to differentiate from empyema. In some cases, ultrasound may be helpful in determining whether loculations are present.

Radiological changes lag behind clinical signs, and may persist for 4–6 weeks. Follow-up chest X-rays are unnecessary in most cases of uncomplicated pneumonia, but should be considered if symptoms and signs are persistent following treatment.

Most other investigations to determine microbiological aetiology are not particularly helpful in the emergency department setting to dictate immediate medical management. Rapid viral antigen tests, such as direct immunofluorescence assay for RSV and other respiratory viruses on nasopharyngeal aspirates, do not usually alter management. However, they may inform infection control strategies for young children admitted to hospital. Many respiratory pathogens may be identified using molecular methods, such as polymerase chain reaction (PCR) analysis of respiratory secretions.

Management

Patients should be stabilised as necessary with high-flow oxygen and fluid resuscitation. Many children will not require any specific treatment. Most children who are not too unwell and have lobar consolidation on chest X-ray can be managed as outpatients with oral amoxicillin 25 mg kg^{-1} (up to 1 g) three-times daily for 7 days. Children under 1 year of age, and those who are more unwell or hypoxic may require inpatient management (Table 6.5.1) and treatment with intravenous benzylpenicillin 50 mg kg^{-1} (up to 1.2 g) 6-hourly. Infants less than 3 months of age should also be given intravenous gentamicin 7.5 mg kg^{-1} daily.

Table 6.5.1 Possible indications for admission

Hypoxia, apnoea
Toxic appearance, poor feeding, dehydration
Age <1 year
Underlying lung disease or immunodeficiency
Extensive consolidation
Failed response to oral therapy

Antibiotic resistance among pneumococci is becoming more common. However, there is no difference in outcome between cases caused by susceptible and resistant strains, and amoxicillin or benzylpenicillin remains the treatment of choice.[14,15] The use of third-generation cephalosporins provides no additional benefit over these penicillins. They should be reserved for severe pneumonia where it may be important to cover beta-lactamase producers and Gram-negative bacteria.

Children presenting with coryza, wheeze, diffuse crackles and minimal chest X-ray changes may have viral pneumonitis. Admission may be necessary for supportive care, but antibiotics should be withheld. A trial of inhaled bronchodilator therapy may be useful in children who appear to have significant associated bronchospasm. A macrolide antibiotic, such as oral roxithromycin 4 mg kg^{-1} (up to 150 mg) twice daily for 7 days, should be considered for those with suspected *M. pneumoniae* infection.

Only children who are severely unwell require broader-spectrum antibiotics to include cover for *Staph. aureus* and Gram-negative bacteria: flucloxacillin 50 mg kg^{-1} intravenously (IV) (up to 2 g) 6-hourly plus cefotaxime 50 mg kg^{-1} IV 6-hourly. In settings or populations where CAMRSA is more prevalent, vancomycin 10–15 mg kg^{-1} per dose 6-hourly should be added.

A short course (3 days) of antibiotic therapy is as effective as a longer treatment (5 days) for non-severe pneumonia in children under 5 years of age.[16]

Complications

A child who remains very unwell and febrile after 48 hours of parenteral treatment should be reassessed for the possibility of empyema or, more rarely, lung abscess. In these cases, input from infectious diseases and respiratory specialists is advised.

Prevention

The introduction of conjugate *H. influenzae* type b (Hib) and *Strep. pneumoniae* vaccines into the routine immunisation schedule in many countries has led to a reduction in the burden of pneumonia caused by these two organisms.[17]

Conclusion

Pneumonia is a common illness in children. Viruses are the most common cause, and many children will not require any specific treatment. *Strep. pneumoniae* remains the most common bacterial cause, and amoxicillin remains the antibiotic treatment of choice.[18]

References

1. Campbell H. Acute respiratory infection: A global challenge. *Arch Dis Child* 1995;**73**(4):281–3 [Review: 38 refs].
2. Rudan I, Boschi-Pinto C, Biloglav Z, et al. Epidemiology and etiology of childhood pneumonia. *Bull World Health Organ* 2008;**86**(5):408–16.
3. Jokinen C, Heiskanen L, Juvonen H, et al. Incidence of community-acquired pneumonia in the population of four municipalities in eastern Finland. *Am J Epidemiol* 1993;**137**(9):977–88.
4. Murphy TF, Henderson FW, Clyde WA, et al. Pneumonia: An eleven-year study in a paediatric practice. *Am J Epidemiol* 1981;**113**(1):12–21.
5. Juven T, Mertsola J, Waris M, et al. Etiology of community-acquired pneumonia in 254 hospitalized children. *Pediatr Infect Dis J* 2000;**19**(4):293–8.
6. Durbin WJ, Stille C. Pneumonia. *Pediatr Rev* 2008;**29**(5):147–58.
7. Vuori-Holopainen E, Peltola H. Reappraisal of lung tap: Review of an old method for better etiologic diagnosis of childhood pneumonia. *Clin Infect Dis* 2001;**32**(5):715–26.
8. Vuori-Holopainen E, Salo E, Saxen H, et al. Etiological diagnosis of childhood pneumonia by use of transthoracic needle aspiration and modern microbiological methods. *Clin Infect Dis* 2002;**34**(5):583–90.
9. Bettenay FA, de Campo JF, McCrossin DB. Differentiating bacterial from viral pneumonias in children. *Pediatr Radiol* 1988;**18**(6):453–4.
10. Swingler GH. Radiologic differentiation between bacterial and viral lower respiratory infection in children: A systematic literature review. *Clin Pediatr* 2000;**39**(11):627–33.
11. Ranganathan SC, Sonnappa S. Pneumonia and other respiratory infections. *Pediatr Clin North Am* 2009;**56**(1):135–56.
12. Palafox M, Guiscafre H, Reyes H, et al. Diagnostic value of tachypnoea in pneumonia defined radiologically. *Arch Dis Child* 2000;**82**(1):41–5.
13. British Thoracic Society. Guidelines for the management of community acquired pneumonia in childhood 2002. *Thorax* 2002;**57**(Suppl. 1):11–24.
14. Friedland IR. Comparison of the response to antimicrobial therapy of penicillin-resistant and penicillin-susceptible pneumococcal disease. *Pediatr Infect Dis J* 1995;**14**(10):885–90.
15. Tan TQ, Mason Jr EO, Wald ER, et al. Clinical characteristics of children with complicated pneumonia caused by Streptococcus pneumoniae. *Paediatrics* 2002;**110**(1):1–6.
16. Haider B, Saeed M, Bhutta Z. Short-course versus long-course antibiotic therapy for non-severe community-acquired pneumonia in children aged 2 months to 59 months. *Cochrane Database Syst Rev* 2008;**16**(2): CD005976.
17. Theodoratou E, Johnson S, Jhass A, et al. The effect of Haemophilus influenzae type b and pneumococcal conjugate vaccines on childhood pneumonia incidence, severe morbidity and mortality. *Int J Epidemiol* 2010;**39**(Suppl. 1):i172–185.
18. Kabra SK, Lodha R, Pandey RM. Antibiotics for community-acquired pneumonia in children. *Cochrane Database Syst Rev* 2010;**17**(3) CD004874.

6.6 Bronchiolitis

Tom Beattie

ESSENTIALS

1 The diagnosis of bronchiolitis is clinical, based on history and examination.

2 Bronchiolitis typically affects children under the age of 12 months, but may occur in children up to 2 years of age.

3 As feeding by an infant is an important index of bronchiolitis severity, a careful history of a change in feeds is paramount.

4 High-risk patients include those with underlying chronic lung disease, congenital heart disease or corrected age less than 2 months of age.

5 In the very young infant, apnoea may be the predominant symptom with few respiratory signs. Likewise, in neonates a non-specific sepsis-like picture with collapse may occur.

6 Oxygen saturations fall with disease severity and SaO_2 levels below 94% indicate a need for admission.

7 The role of chest radiography is limited and only indicated if the diagnosis is unclear or in severe cases.

8 In patients being admitted, perform a rapid NPA or PNA to analyse for RSV or other respiratory viruses for isolation control.

9 Supportive care is the mainstay of treatment of bronchiolitis.

10 The decision to admit to hospital is based mainly on considerations of the child's need for oxygen, fluids or cardiorespiratory monitoring for apnoea.

Introduction

Epidemiology

Bronchiolitis is a common presentation to emergency departments, with a seasonal pattern. It typically affects children under the age of 12 months, but may occur in children up to 2 years of age. The peak age is between 2 and 8 months of age, with males more commonly affected. Approximately 1% of children will require admission for bronchiolitis, which is the leading cause of admission for children with lower respiratory tract disease in the Western world.[1] Epidemics of bronchiolitis occur during each winter, with the peaking of respiratory viruses. While respiratory syncytial virus (RSV) is the commonest organism responsible for bronchiolitis, others include parainfluenza virus, adenovirus, rhinovirus and influenza. Bronchiolitis may also complicate exanthems such as measles and varicella in young children. It is estimated that by the age of 2, 70% of children have been exposed to RSV. Despite the frequency, mortality is low at less than 1% of hospitalised babies. High-risk patients include those with underlying chronic lung disease, congenital heart disease, neuromuscular disorders or corrected age less than 2 months of age.[1]

Pathophysiology

Infection with RSV is associated with direct invasion of epithelial cells in the respiratory tract. Primary infection in young children and infants involves the lower respiratory tract. The bronchiolar epithelium is predominantly affected and an inflammatory response follows. Lymphocytes infiltrate the affected areas and oedema develops in the submucosa. Smooth muscle spasm ensues. The net result is that small airways become narrowed by the combination of oedema and muscle spasm, giving the typical clinical picture of bronchiolitis.

How this clinical picture emerges is still unclear. The role of pro-inflammatory regulators interleukin (IL)-6, IL-8, interferon-γ, and macrophage inflammatory protein-1β, as well as of the regulatory cytokine IL-10 in causing the disease as we know it, as opposed to facilitating healing and repair still remains to be elucidated.[2–4]

The incidence of concomitant or secondary bacterial infection is low, although otitis media may occur. In the very young infant, apnoea may be the predominant symptom, with few other respiratory signs. Likewise, in neonates a non-specific sepsis-like picture with collapse may occur. In reinfection with RSV or primary infection in older children, the symptoms are more limited to the upper respiratory tract, causing signs consistent with a severe common cold.

Clinical assessment

History

Bronchiolitis typically presents with a prodrome of upper respiratory tract infection over 1–2 days.

When the lower respiratory tract becomes involved, the hypersecretion of mucus causes the moist cough, onset of respiratory distress and resultant feeding difficulties. As ability to feed in an infant is an important index of bronchiolitis severity, a careful history of a change in feeds is paramount.

Examination

Examination of the child will reveal a combination of signs of upper respiratory tract infection (URTI), along with signs indicative of lower respiratory tract infection (LRTI), which may fluctuate between examinations. The fever is usually low grade. A moist cough is common and wheeze may be audible at the bedside.

Tachypnoea and tachycardia are usually in proportion to the illness severity. Infants who are estimated to be feeding less than 50% of normal feeds usually have oxygen saturations less than 94%. Cyanosis is seen in children with severe disease.

Chest examination may reveal hyperinflation and recessions of the chest wall due to increased work of breathing. Paradoxically, as an infant fatigues, the recessions will decrease. In this situation the diminishing air entry signifies progressive disease. Auscultation reveals wheezes that are generally symmetrical. There may be inspiratory crepitations. The auscultation findings are dynamic as coughing will move secretions to more proximal airways, with resultant temporary clearing of the wheeze. A short time later, as the fluid returns to the more peripheral airways, the wheeze returns. Hence, babies referred by a local doctor with 'marked wheeze' may initially appear to be wheeze free when seen in the emergency department (ED) a short time later. Re-examination later will confirm the presence of wheeze.[5]

Oxygen saturations fall with disease severity and SaO_2 levels below 94% indicate a need for admission.[4] McIntosh graded severity of bronchiolitis by simply documenting children as needing no oxygen, requiring oxygen and needing ventilation.[6] Certainly, increasing oxygen requirements will be associated with increasing severity of disease.

Assessment

In helping to assess an infant with bronchiolitis and the likely subsequent course, one needs to determine the onset of the respiratory distress or poor feeding phase of the illness. Most children have increasing work of breathing for 48–72 hours due to increasing secretions, before a plateau phase followed by resolution over 3–7 days.

The cough may persist for a further 7–10 days after resolution of the respiratory distress. In this way one can determine if a child is likely to deteriorate further, is probably stable at the peak of severity or improving at the time of the ED visit. It is the tiring consequence of the tachypnoea of bronchiolitis that impairs feeding ability, which is the important determinant of whether a child warrants interventions such as oxygen or intravenous fluids.

Assessment of the child with bronchiolitis requires several components to be considered. Several scoring systems for bronchiolitis

Table 6.6.1 Bronchiolitis severity and management

Severity	Signs	Management
Mild	Alert Feeding >50% normal Mild respiratory distress SaO_2 ≥94% NOT high-risk patient Age >6 weeks	Discharge home Smaller/frequent feeds Review in primary care
Moderate	Lethargic, tired Feeding <50% normal Marked respiratory distress Dehydrated SaO_2 <94% High-risk patient	Admit O_2 to SaO_2 >94% Minimise handling Consider NG or IV fluids Close observation
Severe	As above but with: Increasing O_2 requirement Fatigue Signs of CO_2 retention Apnoeic episode	Cardiorespiratory monitor Consider ABG Liaise with PICU

ABG, arterial blood gas; NG, nasogastric; PICU, paediatric intensive care unit.

have been developed to determine the severity of the disease. Table 6.6.1 shows the criteria used to help determine severity and management issues.

Differential diagnosis

The differential diagnosis of bronchiolitis includes cardiac failure, asthma and pneumonia (Table 6.6.2). Cardiac failure can present with many of the features of bronchiolitis – dyspnoea, tachypnoea, tachycardia, crepitations and palpable liver. Feeding may also be poor. However, infants with bronchiolitis will usually have the URTI prodrome and the onset of poor feeding is acute. The feeding difficulty in children with cardiac failure is less acute, leading to poor weight gains. Additional signs, such as a gallop rhythm or murmur, suggest an underlying cardiac abnormality. Recurrent episodes of wheeze associated with URTIs, particularly in older infants, can be difficult to differentiate from asthma. Pneumonia in infants can mimic bronchiolitis and the differentiation can be difficult. Some infants have persistent wheezing, which does not compromise activity or feeds and is unresponsive to inhaled bronchodilators ('fat happy wheezer').

Investigations

The diagnosis of bronchiolitis is clinical, based on history and examination. The role of chest radiography is limited and only

Table 6.6.2 Differential diagnosis of bronchiolitis

Asthma
Cardiac failure
Pneumonia
Neonatal sepsis – presenting as collapse
Happy wheezer – persistent wheezing in undistressed baby

indicated if the diagnosis is unclear or in severe cases. The typical radiological findings are hyperinflation of the lung fields, with bilateral increase in interstitial markings (particularly perihilar regions). There may be patchy atelectasis secondary to plugging or, in severe cases, collapse. Children with high fever, or a clinical impression of sepsis, may have superimposed bacterial infection, and a chest X-ray will aid exclusion of this diagnosis.[7]

Nosocomial infection and cross-infection can occur during bronchiolitis outbreaks. In patients being admitted to hospital, a nasopharyngeal aspirate (NPA) or posterior nasal aspirate (PNA) can be done to analyse for RSV or other respiratory viruses for isolation control. The development of near patient testing (NPT) kits for rapid diagnosis of RSV infection has aided infection control in some areas.[8] The rapid testing for RSV may be useful in cases of neonates to help with decision making where a child presents with fever, collapse or apnoea.

Other tests such as full blood examination are generally not useful in diagnosis. Severe cases may demonstrate CO_2 retention on arterial blood gases or electrolyte disturbance.

Treatment

Supportive care is the mainstay of treatment of bronchiolitis. The decision to admit to hospital is based mainly on considerations of the child's need for oxygen, fluids or cardiorespiratory monitoring for apnoea. Treatment options depend primarily on the severity of the disease.

Mild cases require an explanation to parents and advice regarding feeding to ensure adequate hydration. Smaller volume feeds offered more frequently to the child will usually ensure adequate hydration. Hence, the child who feeds 3–4 hourly normally, should be offered feeds every 1.5–2 hours. Parents should monitor urine output, and should be advised to seek review should feeding deteriorate or urine output fall significantly. Some parents become exhausted by the constant demands of infants with bronchiolitis, and an assessment of parental coping should form part of the clinical picture. If there are concerns about parental ability to provide the increased demands of feeding, admission should be considered.

Children with moderate bronchiolitis need to be admitted. The infant will need to be monitored clinically, with regular observation of heart rate, respiratory rate, ability to feed and level of fatigue. Oxygen saturation should be monitored and supplemental oxygen should be provided to maintain SaO_2 above 95% in those with saturations below 94% or unable to feed. Oxygen may be administered by head box, nasal prong or cannula, isolette, mask or tent. The choice of method of oxygen delivery needs to be tailored to the individual case. In small infants who are obligatory nose breathers, nasal prongs or cannulae may exacerbate the nasal obstruction in babies with copious secretions. Under 6 months of age a head box is usually the best, using an oxygen analyser to monitor the O_2 requirement. Older infants may tolerate an oxygen mask, but if distressed by this then using cot or tent oxygen may be necessary. In some infants who have self-limiting apnoeic episodes, continuous positive airway pressure may help buy time until the disease ameliorates. However, any persistence of apnoea or failure to maintain oxygenation would warrant consideration of ventilation using endotracheal intubation and admission to an Intensive Care setting. Clearly, the choice of treatment will depend on available expertise and equipment. In all situations an increase in O_2 requirement to maintain saturations indicates increasing severity and the need to escalate therapy accordingly.

Feeding can be continued orally initially in those with moderate bronchiolitis, with small frequent feeds as above. If the child cannot tolerate this, nasogastric feeds or intravenous fluids should be considered. Infants who do not have markedly increased work of breathing may come out of oxygen for feeds if tolerated.

There is no indication for antibiotic use for either mild or moderate bronchiolitis unless there is good evidence of secondary bacterial infection.

Children with severe disease need to be admitted to a facility where they can be continuously monitored by appropriate staff for ventilation should they deteriorate or have significant apnoea. Features of concern include the infant who is tiring, has escalating oxygen requirement or develops repeated and/or prolonged apnoeic episodes. Early discussion with the local paediatric intensive care unit staff will help to determine this need and organise appropriate transfer mechanism. Fluids should be given intravenously and adjusted according to volume status, urine output and electrolyte results. Children with underlying disease such as heart disease may need additional specific therapy.

Drug therapy

The role of various drug therapies in bronchiolitis is controversial and still undergoing research.

Two meta-analyses of the benefits of inhaled β agonists in bronchiolitis have proved inconclusive. A more recent Cochrane Review suggests some minimal benefit, while Patel has recently shown no benefit with albuterol (salbutamol).[9–12] Nebulised adrenaline (epinephrine) has similarly not been shown to provide benefit over a sustained timeframe. Isaacs suggested that if wheeze is the predominant sign then a trial of selective β agonist may help.[1]

Systemic or inhaled glucocorticoids are widely used in some parts of the world, but the evidence for their use is variable. A recent meta-analysis has shown some marginal benefit with systemic glucocorticoid use.[13] The role of ipratropium bromide is equally unclear and there is no clear-cut benefit to use.[14]

Nebulised adrenaline (epinephrine) and dexamethasone in combination have been shown in a multicentre trial in Canada to have some potential beneficial effect on the severity of the illness as determined by hospital admission.[15]

Ribavarin and antiviral immunoglobulins are not used in the ED setting, but may have a role in high-risk groups in intensive care. Ribavirin is expensive and has only marginal benefit when given aerolysed to high-risk patients with severe disease.[16] The role of immunisation against RSV is still under investigation.

Prognosis

The vast majority of children with bronchiolitis will recover over 7–10 days. The cough may persist for some weeks after the resolution of the respiratory distress. A small number may continue to wheeze and cough for several months and an indeterminate number will develop persistent wheeze and/or asthma. The exact relationship between these events is unclear. Further study is needed to elucidate the role of RSV in the development of subsequent reactive airway disease.

Prevention

The transmission of RSV occurs with contact with infected secretions. In the ED setting, attention to hand washing, stethoscope hygiene and cubicle use is important to prevent cross-infection between children.

Controversies

Treatment of bronchiolitis has changed little over the years, with the mainstay being supportive care. A considerable amount of research needs to be done on the classification of the severity of disease based on sound, objective data. Without this, the debate on treatment with β agonists, glucocorticoids, anticholinergic drugs and other therapies will persist, with anecdote continuing to supplant scientific data.

References

1. Isaacs D. Bronchiolitis. *Br Med J* 1995;**310**(6971):4–5.
2. Bont L, Heijnen CJ, Kavelaars A, et al. Peripheral blood cytokine responses and disease severity in respiratory syncytial virus bronchiolitis. *Eur Respir J* 1999;**14**(1):144–9.
3. Smyth RL, Mobbs KJ, O'Hea U, et al. Respiratory syncytial virus bronchiolitis: Disease severity, interleukin-8, and virus genotype. *Pediatr Pulmonol* 2002;**33**(5):339–46.
4. Bennett BL, Garafolo RP, Cron SG, et al. Immunopathogenesis of respiratory syncytial virus bronchiolitis. *J Infect Dis* 2007;**195**(10):1532–40.
5. Mulholland EK, Olinsky A, Shann FA. Clinical findings and severity of acute bronchiolitis. *Lancet* 1990;**335** (8700):1259–61.
6. McIntosh ED, De Silva LM, Oates RK. Clinical severity of respiratory syncytial virus group A and B infection in Sydney, Australia. *Pediatr Infect Dis J* 1993;**12**(10):815–9.
7. El-Radhi AS, Barry W, Patel S. Association of fever and severe clinical course in bronchiolitis. *Arch Dis Child* 1999;**81**(3):231–4.
8. Mackenzie A, Hallam N, Mitchell E, Beattie T. Near patient testing for respiratory syncytial virus in paediatric accident and emergency: Prospective pilot study. *Br Med J* 1999;**319**(7205):289–90.
9. Kellner JD, Ohlsson A, Gadomski AM, Wang EE. Efficacy of bronchodilator therapy in bronchiolitis. A meta-analysis. *Arch Pediatr Adolesc Med* 1996;**1150** (11):1166–72.
10. Flores G, Horwitz RI. Efficacy of β2-agonists in bronchiolitis: A reappraisal and meta-analysis. *Paediatrics* 1997;**100**(2 Pt 1):233–9.
11. Kellner JD, Ohlsson A, Gadomski AM, Wang EE. Bronchodilators for bronchiolitis. *Cochrane Database Syst Rev* 2000;**2**: CD001266.
12. Patel H, Platt RW, Pekeles GS, Ducharme FM. A randomized, controlled trial of the effectiveness of nebulized therapy with epinephrine compared with albuterol and saline in infants hospitalized for acute viral bronchiolitis. *J Pediatr* 2002;**141** (6):818–24.
13. Garrison MM, Christakis DA, Harvey E, et al. Systemic corticosteroids in infant bronchiolitis: A metaanalysis. *Pediatrics* 2000;**105**(4):E44.
14. Everard ML, Bara A, Kurian M, et al. Anticholinergic drugs for wheeze in children under the age of two years. *Cochrane Database Syst Rev* 2002;**1**: CD001279.
15. Plint A, Johnson D, Patel H, et al. Epinephrine and dexamethasone in children with bronchiolitis. *N Engl J Med* 2009;**360**(20):2079–89.
16. Everard ML, Swarbrick A, Rigby AS, Milner AD. The effect of ribavirin to treat previously healthy infants admitted with acute bronchiolitis on acute and chronic respiratory morbidity. *Respir Med* 2001;**95** (4):275–80.

6.7 Croup

Gary Geelhoed

ESSENTIALS

1 Croup is a common childhood problem with a peak incidence of 60 per 1000 child years in those aged between 1 and 2 years.

2 The loudness of stridor is variable and is not a reliable indicator of the severity of the airway obstruction.

3 All children who present to emergency departments with croup should be treated with steroids.

4 The steroids of choice are oral dexamethasone 0.15 mg kg^{-1} or prednisolone 1 mg kg^{-1}.

5 A compromised but functioning airway should never be made worse by upsetting the child.

6 Children who require adrenaline (epinephrine) may be sent home safely if they have also received steroids and have improved over a number of hours to have no stridor at rest.

Introduction

The term *croup* describes an acute clinical syndrome of hoarse voice, barking cough, and inspiratory stridor usually seen in young children. Croup results from swelling of the upper airway, in and around the larynx, usually as a result of a viral infection. Croup occurs seasonally, peaking in winter months due to the epidemics of upper respiratory viruses. Parainfluenza virus type 1 accounts for around half the cases during winter, with parainfluenza type 2, influenza type A, adenoviruses, respiratory syncytial virus, enteroviruses, and possibly *Mycoplasma pneumoniae* causing most of the other cases. Some of the viral exanthems, such as varicella, can cause concomitant croup by involvement of the upper airway in small children. Croup is a common childhood problem, with a peak incidence of 60 per 1000 child years in those aged between 1 and 2 years, although it may be seen up to the teen years. As such, it is by far the most common cause of acute upper airways obstruction likely to present to emergency departments.

The respiratory distress caused by obstruction tends to be most marked in younger children due to the small size of their larynx, the presence of loose submucous tissues, and the tight encirclement of the subglottic area by the cricoid cartilage. In children under 8 years of age, this is the narrowest region of the airway, hence any inflammatory swelling in this area results in a significant impingement of the airway. The younger child, who has a smaller diameter airway, requires an increased vigilance to assess the degree of airway compromise.

The lower airway involvement of laryngotracheobronchitis may also cause younger children to manifest wheeze due to concurrent inflammation producing mucus in the smaller peripheral airways. Likewise, occasionally, older children known to have asthma may exhibit signs of asthma in the setting of croup.[1]

Presentation

History

The typical presentation of croup is in a pre-school-aged child with a history of a recent onset of upper respiratory tract infection. The child subsequently develops a barking or seal-like cough, a hoarse voice and, if obstruction is severe enough, stridor. The stridor may initially be apparent only when a child is distressed, such as during crying. During crying or forced expiration the diameter of the upper airways physiologically narrows and, hence, stridor will manifest. Stridor, which is initially inspiratory, indicates obstruction at the laryngeal level or higher (i.e. upper airway). Expiratory stridor or biphasic stridor indicates more severe laryngeal obstruction or alternatively an obstruction occurring lower in the airway. The natural history of airway obstruction, when unmodified by steroids, is to increase slowly to peak over 24–48 hours. The airway compromise usually then resolves over a few days, although the laryngeal cough may persist longer.

Less common than infectious croup but usually more sudden in onset, older children may present with *recurrent or spasmodic croup* with no viral prodrome. This is thought to be allergic in origin. These children may have a history of atopy and suffer from asthma more than the general population. They should, however, be treated in the same manner as 'viral' croup. In the smaller child, particularly infants, problems with feeding, swallowing difficulties, and whether the child has been cyanosed should be ascertained.

It is important to enquire whether or not the child has had croup or other airway problems in the past and, specifically, whether the child has had any persistence of mild stridor in between acute attacks. This is important, as any child who has a pre-existing narrowing of the airway (infantile floppy larynx, laryngomalacia or other upper airway anatomical abnormalities) is more likely to proceed to severe obstruction with a superimposed acute obstruction. These children need to have a lower threshold for a period of observation as their obstruction may be more severe or persistent.

An immunisation history is important to check whether the child has had Hib vaccination if there is any suggestion that the condition could be epiglottitis; likewise, the very rare occurrence of diphtheria in the non-immunised.

Examination

Croup in children can generally be classified as mild, moderate, or severe (Table 6.7.1).

Most children with mild croup are not distressed and have only a barking cough with no stridor at rest or stridor audible only with physical activity, crying, or agitation. Crying causes physiological narrowing of the airway and will increase the respiratory distress. Hence the distressed, crying child's obstruction will often defervesce by allowing the child to be cuddled in the parent's arms. There may be signs due to viral illness, such as mild fever and nasal discharge. Children with mild cases can have their throats examined, but this should be deferred in more severe cases. A compromised but functioning airway should never be made worse by upsetting the child.

In more severe cases, the child may have a more pronounced stridor at rest. As airway obstruction progresses, increased work of breathing ensues and the child exhibits increasing substernal, intercostal, and subcostal retractions. Subtle signs of hypoxia causing altered consciousness may be reflected as anxiety or restlessness in a child. An obviously fatiguing child is a worrying sign. The child manifesting decreased air entry and respiratory effort, extreme pallor, and cyanosis requires immediate intervention.

The child's preferred position may also give clues as to severity of obstruction or to a diagnosis other than croup. Hyperextension or other abnormal positioning of the neck may suggest epiglottitis or a retropharyngeal abscess. It is unusual for the child with croup to be saliva intolerant or have any tenderness of the neck.

Table 6.7.1	Croup severity	
Sign or symptom	*Mild*	*Moderate or severe*
Stridor	None or only if agitated	Stridor at rest
Respiratory rate	Usually normal	May be decreased
Retractions	None	+ to +++
Air entry	Normal	Normal to decreased
Colour	Normal	May be pallor
Cyanosis	None	Late sign only
Conscious state	Normal	Restless or decreased

After Marks et al 2003.[2]

The use of a croup severity score may be helpful for less-experienced staff to assess children with croup and communicate findings with a colleague when seeking advice. As previously mentioned, some children may have concomitant wheeze in addition to the upper airway stridor and hence their pattern of breathing may be 'gas trapped' and cause hyperinflation of the chest with slow expiration phase, in contrast to those with pure croup alone.

Investigations

Croup is usually an easy 'spot diagnosis' and requires no diagnostic tests.

Oximetry is of limited value, as children may maintain near-normal oxygen saturations even when they have significant airway obstruction.[3] While it may have a role in cases of severe croup, this must be balanced with the distress caused by the monitoring probe in small children. In stable cases, where the diagnosis is unclear, a lateral soft tissue X-ray of the neck may be helpful to distinguish croup from epiglottitis or retropharyngeal abscess. However, the possible benefits of an X-ray need to be weighed against the risks of moving or disturbing the child when the obstruction is more than mild. A nasopharyngeal aspirate in croup is not necessary for diagnosis but may be useful for infection control for patients being admitted.

Differential diagnosis

It is important to establish that other, more sinister, causes of acute upper respiratory tract obstruction masquerading as croup are not present (Table 6.7.2). Especially in the younger child, one should enquire regarding longer-term symptoms preceding the present episode, such as low-grade stridor. This might suggest underlying congenital airway or vascular anomaly (e.g. tracheomalacia, subglottic

Table 6.7.2	Differential diagnoses of croup

- Epiglottitis
- Bacterial tracheitis
- Foreign body
- Congenital: laryngomalacia, subglottic stenosis, vascular ring, cord paresis
- Retropharyngeal abscess
- Allergic oedema
- Airway trauma

stenosis, bilateral cord paralysis, laryngeal web, or vascular ring compression of the trachea). One should also enquire as to possible airway trauma or toxic ingestion. Dysphagia and drooling may suggest epiglottitis, peritonsillar or retropharyngeal abscess, or foreign body in the airway or oesophagus.

Classic croup and epiglottitis are hard to confuse, as the latter usually presents as a pale, toxic, drooling child with a rapidly progressing course. Cough is generally not a prominent feature in epiglottitis. Children with epiglottitis may sit forwards, drooling saliva, and hold their neck in extension. In a child presenting with early epiglottitis, however, the distinction may be more difficult. Immunisation in developed countries, however, has made this distinction largely academic. Allergic angio-oedema may mimic croup after exposure to an allergen such as peanut. A child with 'severe croup' with a high fever, who does not respond to adrenaline (epinephrine) and steroids, may have tracheitis and will need consideration of a diagnostic laryngoscopy to provide a clear diagnosis. Likewise, the possibility of an inhaled foreign body should be kept in mind for children who don't respond to treatment or have a prolonged course. While usually parents will volunteer a history of an acute obstruction or a sudden coughing fit, the history of an inhaled object may not always have been observed and therefore reported. A definitive diagnosis may need to be made by directly viewing the upper airway, but this should be performed only by an experienced paediatric anaesthetist, intensivist, or emergency physician in an appropriate clinical setting (see below).

Treatment and disposition

Mild or moderate croup

All children who present to an emergency department with croup should be treated with steroids.[4] The mandatory use of steroids for croup in emergency departments results in a reduction in the relapse rate of those sent home,[5] the average length of stay in hospital falling, and the number of children needing intensive care and intubation dramatically reducing.[6,7] Prior to the regular use of steroids, a general rule of thumb was to admit children with stridor at rest (moderate) to hospital for observation, while

allowing those with occasional stridor and barking cough only (mild) to be managed at home. As many children will improve within a few hours of taking steroids, often they may be discharged home after a short stay in the emergency department or an observation ward. Factors such as the distance from medical care, the availability of transport, the time of day, the child's past history with regard to severe airway obstruction, and parental concern and attitude all need to be taken into account when making the decision to admit (Table 6.7.3).

Recommended steroid doses are oral dexamethasone in a one-off dose of 0.15 mg kg^{-1},[8] or an equivalent dose of prednisolone of 0.75 mg kg^{-1}. Most children with croup will require only one dose, but if the upper airway obstruction symptoms persist (as opposed to upper respiratory tract infection symptoms), a further dose may be given 18 to 24 hours later. It is often more convenient to use prednisolone (rounded off to 1 mg kg^{-1}) in the community, as it is more readily available. While one study[9] suggested that children treated with prednisolone may re-present more commonly than those treated with dexamethasone, Fifoot et al[10] did not confirm this finding. Steroids may be administered intramuscularly or intravenously in the child with severe obstruction, when there is concern that the child may aspirate or vomit, given their degree of respiratory difficulty.

Oral dexamethasone has been found to be as effective as inhaled steroids such as budesonide,[11] and to work as fast, at a fraction of the cost. A blinded randomised trial, submitted for publication, of dexamethasone 0.15 mg kg^{-1} compared to placebo that looked at croup scores at 10-minute intervals after administration showed a significant difference at

Table 6.7.3 Possible Indications for admission
• Upper airway obstruction at rest: fails to respond to steroids or adrenaline (epinephrine) and period of observation (4 hours)
• Severe croup or moderate croup that does not respond to treatment
• Infants <6 months
• Previous severe croup
• Underlying airway problem
• Inadequate social factors i.e. transport or lack of follow up
• Recurrent presentation

30 minutes.[12] Combining dexamethasone and budesonide is no more effective than dexamethasone alone.[11,13] There is no place for antibiotics in a typical case of croup. The use of 'steam' or humidified air is unproven,[14,15] despite its once common usage. The anecdotal report by parents of their child improving in the steam-filled bathroom at home is due to the defervescing of crying which occurs from cuddling in the room by the parent, rather than any steam effect.

Severe croup

Children with manifestations of severe obstruction should be given nebulised adrenaline (epinephrine). It is generally considered that adrenaline does not change the natural history of croup, such as length of stay in hospital or need to intubate, due to its short-lasting effects. It will, however, 'buy time' while waiting for the effect of steroids to occur. Rarely, in a worst-case scenario, adrenaline can be a useful temporising measure while organising the facilities and appropriate personnel for a child who may require intubation. The recommended dose (independent of age and weight) is 5 mL of 1:1000, nebulised with oxygen, which can be used for all children. This may be repeated after 10 minutes if needed and may help avoid the need for intubation in children who respond to steroids. 'Rebound' phenomenon may occur, where the upper airway obstruction may recur as the effect of the adrenaline wears off after 1–2 hours. While in the past it was recommended that any child who received adrenaline for croup should be admitted, a number of studies have now shown that children may be sent home safely if they have also received steroids and have improved to have no stridor at rest over a number of hours.[16,17] Children receiving nebulised adrenaline require close clinical monitoring of their response, particularly the change in air entry, in order to detect any deterioration.

Intubation needs to be considered in the child who has increasing upper airway obstruction, hypoxia, decreasing conscious state, or fatigue despite nebulised adrenaline. These children should be discussed early with a paediatric intensivist in order to optimise management. The ideal setting for this to occur is in theatre or a paediatric intensive care unit environment via gaseous induction, using an endotracheal tube 1.0-mm smaller than predicted by the child's size (see Chapter 2.3).

Prognosis

Most children with croup have mild symptoms, do not need hospitalisation, and will recover within a few days. Their symptoms will be shortened even further with the use of steroids. It should be pointed out to parents that steroids will have no effect on the duration of any underlying viral symptomatology. Despite the substantial impact of steroids, the occasional child will still follow a prolonged course of cough and marked stridor for many days. While other diagnoses, such as foreign body, need to be considered, most cases will settle with time.

Prevention

For most children, croup is a one-off episode and well tolerated, especially if steroids are used. Children who suffer repeated episodes of recurrent croup, as described above, may benefit from steroid use at home at the first sign of croup symptoms. Although no trials have evaluated this approach, anecdotal evidence suggests that this practice appears to have benefit.

Controversies and future research

❶ Although once controversial, steroids are now generally accepted for all children who present to emergency departments with croup.

❷ It is clear that both prednisolone and dexamethasone are effective in the treatment of croup; however, two direct comparisons have not resolved the question on whether the shorter half life of prednisolone results in more 'relapses' at home. While a once-only dose of dexamethasone is sufficient for the vast majority of children with croup, a second dose of prednisolone 24 hours later may be needed in some cases.

❸ Children with recurrent croup theoretically should benefit from early treatment at home, but no formal study to date has confirmed this.

References

1. Denny FW, Clyde WA. Acute lower respiratory tract infections in nonhospitalized children. *J Pediatr* 1986;**108**:635–45.
2. Marks M, Wilkinson D, Munro J. *Paediatric Handbook*. 6th ed Victoria: Blackwell Science; 2003.
3. Stoney PJ, Chakrabarti MK. Experience of pulse oximetry in children presenting with croup. *J Laryngol Otol* 1991;**105**:295–8.
4. Geelhoed GC. Croup. *Pediatr Pulmonol* 1997;**23** (5):370–4.
5. Geelhoed GC, Turner J, Macdonald WB. Efficacy of a small single dose of oral dexamethasone for outpatient croup: A double blind placebo controlled clinical trial. *Br Med J* 1996;**313**(7050):140–2.
6. Geelhoed GC. Sixteen years of croup in a Western Australian teaching hospital: The impact of routine steroid treatment. *Ann Emerg Med* 1996;**28**(6):621–6.
7. Dobrovoljac M, Geelhoed GC. 27 years of croup: an update highlighting the effectiveness of 0.15 mg/kg of dexamethasone. *Emerg Med Australas* 2009;**21**:309–14.
8. Geelhoed GC, Macdonald WGB. Oral dexamethasone in the treatment of croup: 0.15 mg/kg is as effective as 0.3 mg/kg or 0.6 mg/kg. *Pediatr Pulmonol* 1995;**20**:362–7.
9. Sparrow A, Geelhoed GC. Prednisolone versus dexamethasone in croup: A randomised equivalence trial. *Arch Dis Child* 2006;**91**:580–3.
10. Fifoot AA, Ting JYS. Comparison between single-dose oral prednisolone and oral dexamethasone in the treatment of croup: a randomized, double-blinded clinical trial. *Emerg Med Australasia* 2007;**19**:51–8.
11. Klassen TP, Craig WR, Moher D, et al. Nebulized budesonide and oral dexamethasone for treatment of croup: A randomized controlled trial. *JAMA* 1998;**279** (20):1629–32.
12. Dobrovoljac M. Geelhoed G.C. How fast does oral dexamethasone work in croup patients? A randomised double blinded clinical trial. *Emerg Med Australasia* 2009;**21**(4):309–14.
13. Geelhoed GC. Budesonide offers no advantage when added to oral dexamethasone in the treatment of croup. *Pediatr Emerg Care* 2005;**21**:359–62.
14. Neto GM, Kentab O, Klassen TP, et al. A randomized controlled trial of mist in the acute treatment of moderate croup. *Acad Emerg Med* 2002;**9**:873–9.
15. Bouchier D, Dawson KP, Fergusson DM. Humidification in viral croup: A controlled trial. *Aust Paediatr J* 1984;**20**:289–91.
16. Kelley PB, Simon JE. Racemic epinephrine use in croup and disposition. *Am J Emerg Med* 1992;**10**(3):181–3.
17. Prendergast M, Jones JS, Hartman D. Racemic epinephrine in the treatment of laryngotracheitis: Can we identify children for outpatient therapy? *Am J Emerg Med* 1994;**12**(6):613–6.

RESPIRATORY

6

GASTROENTEROLOGY AND HEPATOLOGY

Section editor **Ian Everitt**

7.1 Abdominal pain

Jason Hort

ESSENTIALS

1 Only a small percentage of children presenting with abdominal pain have an underlying surgical cause.

2 The age of the child with abdominal pain significantly influences the diagnostic possibilities.

3 The younger the child, the less reliable are the clinical signs of acute appendicitis.

4 The abdominal examination findings, rather than blood tests, are the most important contributor in assessing the need for surgical consultation.

5 Providing adequate analgesia to the distressed child and an unrushed gentle approach improve the reliability of physical findings and do not mask the detection of peritoneal findings.

6 Abdominal pain in children may have intra- or extra-abdominal causes.

7 Warning bells for a surgical problem include: pain that genuinely requires opiate analgesia, constant pain over a number of hours, inconsolability, a child who remains motionless despite severe pain (likely peritonism), associated pallor or shock, reproducible localised tenderness, guarding, rebound, abdominal distension, rigidity, bilious vomiting and representation.

8 Close observation with serial examination remains very useful in indeterminate cases.

9 It is not always possible to make a definitive diagnosis in the ED. A practical, systematic approach is required to exclude serious underlying possible causes. Discharged children in whom the diagnosis remains unclear need to have a clear action plan with early follow up organised.

Introduction

Abdominal pain is a common reason for children to attend an emergency department (ED), occurring in up to 5% of all presentations in some institutions.[1] Most commonly the underlying cause is non-surgical and surgery is required in only 1–7% of children who present with abdominal pain.[1,2] It is not possible to make a definitive diagnosis in all children with abdominal pain. In one study, as many as 15% of children presenting to emergency with abdominal pain did not have a specific diagnosis at their discharge. Some children arrive at the ED soon after the onset of symptoms and it may take time, expectant management and review before a diagnosis becomes clearer or the symptoms of a self-limiting cause resolve. It is important, however, to exclude causes of abdominal pain that may require early surgical consultation, observation or investigations within the ED.

The priorities in managing children presenting with abdominal pain are:

- triage and early appropriate analgesia;
- resuscitation with attention to ABCs as required;

- diagnosis formulation using history, examination and investigation;
- consideration of surgical review and management according to the likely diagnosis.

If a clear diagnosis cannot be reached in the ED, then exclusion of serious/life-threatening diagnoses is the priority. Subsequent disposition and follow up is dependent on various factors including: likelihood of a serious diagnosis; severity of the pain; availability of review; and psychosocial factors that may be contributory.

Pathophysiology

The sensation of abdominal pain is transmitted by either somatic or visceral afferent fibres.[3] Visceral pain from visceral peritoneum is poorly localised, whereas somatic pain arising from parietal peritoneum or the abdominal wall is more localised. Referred pain also occurs due to visceral and somatic pathways converging in the spinal column. Two examples of referred pain are diaphragmatic irritation leading to pain at the shoulder tip due to convergence of visceral and somatic pathways at C4, and somatic pain from pneumonia leading to T10–11 pain sensed in the lower abdomen.[3] Abdominal pain may occasionally be found to be psychosomatic in origin after a thorough assessment of alternative causes.

Aetiology

There is a broad range of causes of abdominal pain in children and one needs to initially keep an open mind regarding the diagnosis (Table 7.1.1). The age and sex of the child need to be considered, as well as features of the abdominal pain and associated symptoms, and examination findings to determine the diagnostic possibilities.

Assessment

Each child needs initial assessment and triage with attention to securing the ABCs and providing appropriate early analgesia. This will help achieve a more reliable

Table 7.1.1 Causes of acute abdominal pain in children

Inflammatory gastrointestinal
Appendicitis
Meckel's diverticulum
Mesenteric adenitis
Gastroenteritis
Food poisoning
Peritonitis
Peptic ulcer, gastritis
Hepatitis
Pancreatitis
Inflammatory bowel disease

Non-gastrointestinal
Tonsillitis, pharyngitis
Pneumonia (especially basal)
Pericarditis
Serositis
Pyelonephritis, cystitis
Pelvic inflammatory disease
Intra-abdominal abscess
Epididymitis

Generalised
Infectious mononucleosis
Acute rheumatic fever
Herpes zoster

Intestinal obstruction
Intussusception
Volvulus
Adhesions
Incarcerated hernia

Abdominal trauma
See Section 3

Gall bladder
Cholecystitis, cholelithiasis

Haematological
Leukaemia, lymphoma
Haemolytic crisis
Sickle cell disease
Neuroblastoma, Wilms' tumour

Endocrine
Diabetic ketoacidosis, hypoglycaemia
Adrenal insufficiency
Hyperparathyroidism

Vasculitic
Henoch–Schönlein purpura
Periarteritis nodosa
Kawasaki disease

Renal
Renal colic
Hydronephrosis
Nephrotic syndrome

Miscellaneous
Constipation
Colic
Toxic ingestion, e.g. lead
Torsion–testicular/ovarian
Ectopic pregnancy
Dysmenorrhea, Mittelschmerz pain
Mesenteric artery occlusion
Hypokalaemia
Acute intermittant porphyria
Familial Mediterranean fever
Abdominal migraine
Psychosomatic – including abuse

Source: Adapted from Rudolph 1996.

examination. A detailed history and thorough, gentle, and age-appropriate examination need to be performed.

History

In considering a child who has presented with abdominal pain with no history of trauma, five important questions have to be addressed:

1. The age of the child
The age of the child helps narrow the diagnostic possibilities. The most common diagnoses to consider according to age are:

Neonates and infants They usually present with a change in behaviour to signify pain.[4] This may be persistent crying, irritability, inability to be consoled, fussiness, sleeplessness, and poor feeding.[4] Serious or potentially life-threatening conditions not to miss in this age group are listed in Table 7.1.2.

The diagnoses of acute gastroenteritis or 'colic' need to be made after excluding more serious causes.

Preschool Common conditions include acute gastroenteritis, urinary infection, appendicitis, viral illness (mesenteric

Table 7.1.2 Serious conditions not to miss in neonates and infants

Surgical causes	Medical causes
Testicular torsion	Diabetic ketoacidosis
Appendicitis	Toxic, e.g. iron ingestion
Peritonitis	Sepsis
Necrotising enterocolitis	
Volvulus	Haemolytic uraemic syndrome
Intussusception	Urinary tract infection
Hirschsprung disease	
Incarcerated hernia	

adenitis), pneumonia, constipation and trauma-related abdominal pain.

School age Children of school age usually have acute gastroenteritis, urinary infection, trauma, appendicitis, constipation, viral-related, psychosomatic, inflammatory bowel or in older females consider gynaecological causes.

In the preschool and school-aged child, the commonest cause of abdominal pain is constipation. This is a diagnosis of exclusion after carefully considering alternative causes.[5]

Adolescents The causes of abdominal pain in adolescents expand to include various diagnoses of adulthood. In the female, pregnancy-related conditions must be considered, as well as other gynaecological conditions (see Chapter 15.1 on gynaecology).

2. Whether this is the first episode or recurrence of abdominal pain

A history of similar pain in a child may help to clarify the diagnosis. However, it is important to remember that children with chronic abdominal pain due to myriad causes may develop an acute abdomen and this needs to be considered at each presentation.

3. Whether there are other associated symptoms

Generally children with abdominal pain have other associated symptoms. A full symptom review is required, with particular reference to gastrointestinal symptoms. This includes vomiting, and whether it is bilious or blood stained, and the timing and quality of stool, including the presence of blood or mucus. The child with fever, voluminous diarrhoea and vomiting is likely to have gastroenteritis. However, particularly in young children, one must keep an open mind to other possibilities that can mimic or complicate gastroenteritis (see Chapter 7.8 pp. 172–175 on Diarrhoea and vomiting).

More general questions should assess the child's constitution – whether the child is febrile, lethargic, irritable, anorexic or has associated pallor. It is unusual for children with appendicitis to be hungry. The child with intussusception is often lethargic and pale. The presence of upper respiratory tract infection (URTI) or viral symptoms may suggest mesenteric adenitis. Dysuria or frequency may be reported in older children with a urinary tract infection. A typical rash or sore joints may indicate Henoch–Schönlein purpura as the cause of related vasculitic abdominal pain.

4. Whether there are any relevant pre-existing conditions

The child's past medical and surgical history should be fully explored. In older females an adolescent approach (see Chapter 30.1) and a menstrual and sexual activity history may be important. Family history and racial background may be relevant, along with a psychosocial history that may contribute if there is a suggestion of somatisation.

5. What are the characteristics of the pain?

These include location (generalised or localised), radiation, severity, quality (constant, episodic or of a colic nature), what improves and worsens the pain, along with the timing of the pain – gradual or sudden onset and whether the pain wakes the child. Direct questioning of the verbal child often augments the description of the characteristics of the pain as reported by a parent.

Pain that has a sudden onset may occur with perforated viscus, intussusception or torsion. The pain from appendicitis has a more insidious onset and usually increases over a period of hours. In both intussusception and mesenteric adenitis, the pain may cause episodic distress. Constant pain over a number of hours in a child usually suggests a significant underlying cause.

Examination

The abdominal examination of the young child with abdominal pain needs to be performed in an unhurried and gentle fashion. Toddlers may be better examined on the parent's lap. It is important to note the child's general appearance and any features of toxicity. Children with colicky pain often writhe around, whereas the child with peritoneal irritation usually remains still as movement exacerbates the abdominal pain. Providing adequate analgesia improves the reliability of physical findings and does not mask the clinical detection of peritoneal findings. It is best to very gently approach the painful quadrant of the abdomen last in distressed children, after pain subsides post analgesia, the child has relaxed and become accustomed to the examination.

One of the keys to the assessment is to determine the presence of focal tenderness or true peritoneal irritation. In children this can sometimes be difficult, as many voluntarily guard the abdomen when examined, irrespective of the cause of the abdominal pain. This is expected when a previous examination may have been distressing. Differentiating the presence of true peritoneal signs may be helped by distraction techniques, or by serial gentle examination over a period of time to determine true reproducibility of findings.

Eliciting rebound should begin with gentle palpation to avoid distress and resultant voluntary guarding. Signs consistent with peritonitis include refusing or being unable to walk, slow or stooped walking, or increased pain on coughing or movement, or the child lying motionless on the bed. Likewise, peritoneal irritation may be detected by asking if the child can expand or contract their abdominal wall by asking them to 'suck tummy in, then let it out'. The younger the child, the less likely they are to have reliable localising signs of appendicitis and the threshold for surgical review or observation needs to be adapted accordingly.

Important features of examination include the following:

- general appearance of the child;
- temperature and vital signs;
- jaundice;
- skin markings, e.g. abdominal bruising;
- abdominal distension;
- abdominal tenderness;
- guarding or rebound and/or rigidity;
- abdominal mass;
- bowel sounds;
- palpation of testes (in the male infant);
- presence of inguinal herniae;
- urinalysis.

Rectal examination in children, when rarely indicated, should be performed once, and ideally by the surgeon who may require the information. The interpretation of localised rectal tenderness is often difficult in children, as it is uncomfortable in all children and therefore does not often add to the assessment. The inguinoscrotal regions should always be checked for an otherwise occult hernia or torsion referring pain upwards to the abdomen. A sensitively performed, private, and chaperoned pelvic examination may be indicated in pubertal females.

The cause of abdominal pain in children may be extra-abdominal. The child with ileus may have intra- or extra-abdominal pathology including sepsis, urinary tract infection, pneumonia, or meningitis.

Important features in the examination of other systems that may present with abdominal pain include:

- respiratory - signs of basal pneumonia;
- ENT – URTI, tonsillitis or adenopathy;
- neurological – meningitis;
- endocrine – blood glucose level in diabetic ketoacidosis;
- haematological – pallor, lymphadenopathy;
- dermatological – rash, particularly purpura/petechiae of Henoch–Schönlein purpura, zoster;
- renal – oliguria, haematuria, hypertension in haemolytic uraemic syndrome.

Investigations

Many children have the diagnosis clarified by a physical examination alone. The need for investigations should be tailored to the individual case, where the diagnosis is unclear and the result of the test is likely to 'rule in or rule out' significant pathology.

Pathology

A full blood count may demonstrate leucocytosis, anaemia or film changes of haemolysis. However, the white cell count/differential is not particularly useful to determine if a child has acute appendicitis. Electrolytes, urea and creatinine assess changes resulting from fluid losses and impaired renal function. This may be indicated in the child who has had significant losses from diarrhoea or vomiting. Liver function tests are indicated in children with potential hepatic and gall bladder pathology. The possibility of pancreatitis can be assessed by serum amylase or lipase levels. A blood glucose level excludes diabetic ketoacidosis in the child presenting with abdominal pain who appears acidotic or has glucose and ketones in the urine.

Females of reproductive age should have a βhCG performed. Urinalysis, microscopy and culture are necessary to exclude renal pathology.

Imaging

The routine use of an abdominal X-ray is unhelpful to 'screen' children with abdominal pain. Specific situations where it may be helpful include: demonstrating the signs of bowel obstruction; free air, suggesting perforation; an ingested foreign body; calcification, including a faecolith in the appendix and Meckel's diverticulum; 'thumb-printing', suggesting gut ischaemia or a sentinel loop adjacent to inflammation; or a soft tissue mass. Calcification may also represent renal stones, neuroblastoma or teratoma.

An erect chest X-ray may be indicated to demonstrate gas under the diaphragm or evidence of a basal pneumonia.[3]

An ultrasound study can help evaluate liver, gall bladder and kidneys, as well as detect intussusception, features of appendicitis (if able to be visualised) or evaluate a palpable mass. An abdominal computerised tomography (CT) scan may be indicated in selected cases.

Management

The initial management of the child with severe abdominal pain should include assessment and securing of ABCs and administration of appropriate analgesia to relieve the child's distress. Children with similar pathophysiology can have markedly varied distress levels and analgesic requirements need to be individualised.[4] Concurrent anxiety may increase painful stimuli and this can be lessened by involving parents in comforting their child and using a child-friendly environment to distract and help calm the child. Using a visual analogue scale to evaluate severity of pain may be helpful to assess response to analgesia.

There is no contraindication to providing adequate analgesia for any child presenting in pain. It is much easier to perform a reliable examination on a child who is made comfortable. For severe distress, intravenous morphine titrated in increments controls most children's pain and will not mask the abdominal signs. Intra-nasal fentanyl is a useful alternative for rapid onset analgesia

(2–3 minutes) with the advantage of not requiring venous access, but its short duration of action (30–60 minutes) means longer-acting analgesia will be required if pain is ongoing.[6] Oral agents such as paracetamol, codeine or ibuprofen may be used in less severe pain. Serial examination of the child's abdomen and observation of vital signs over a period may be important to exclude significant pathology. Children with a potential surgical cause should be given nil by mouth, until surgical review.

Disposition

Children with significant abdominal findings need to have a surgical consultation. Not all children who present with abdominal pain will have a clear definitive diagnosis after their assessment has excluded a serious cause or the need for a surgical review. Some children with severe pain, but negative physical examination findings, where the diagnosis is not clear, will warrant admission for ongoing observation. Children who are discharged home need to have clear instructions given to parents regarding returning, should they deteriorate, and have a planned timely follow up by the local doctor.

ACUTE APPENDICITIS

Introduction

Appendicitis is the most common non-traumatic surgical emergency in children. It occurs slightly more commonly in males at any age, although it is uncommon in those under 2 years, and very rare in neonates. The peak incidence is at 9–12 years.

Clinical features

The clinical features of classic appendicitis are well known. Pain is felt initially in the periumbilical region due to visceral pain from obstruction of the appendix. There is often associated nausea, vomiting, anorexia and a low-grade fever. Later, there is migration of the pain to the region of the appendix. This more intense right lower quadrant pain results from irritation of the abdominal parietal lining. Up to 50% of adults have this progression of symptoms but it is less common in children.

Importantly, some children may have false localising diarrhoea or dysuria caused by irritation from an inflamed appendix. Fever is generally below 39.5°C, unless perforation has occurred. Asking the child to walk or hop to demonstrate pain with right leg movement may be useful in indeterminate cases to reveal the presence of true peritoneal irritation. Likewise, manoeuvres such as the iliopsoas, obturator or Rovsing's signs may help confirm suspicion of appendicitis. In children with clear signs of appendicitis, the rectal examination adds little value, is distressing for a child and does not alter management.[7]

Under the age of 2 years, vomiting (85–90%) and pain (35–77%) are the most common symptoms, with diarrhoea (18–46%) and fever (40–60%) less common. Sometimes grunting respirations (8–23%), cough or rhinitis (40%) and right hip symptoms (3–23%) may be misleading. Right lower abdominal tenderness is present in less than 50% so the diagnosis of appendicitis in this age group is often delayed, leading to perforation rates of 82–92%.

As children become older, right lower abdominal tenderness becomes more common (age 2–5 years, 58–85%), up to nearly all children in the school-age group, with some (15%) having generalised tenderness without perforation. In children 6–12 years, vomiting occurs in 68–95% of children, anorexia in 47–75%, diarrhoea in 9–16%, constipation in 5–28% and dysuria in 4–20%.

Differential diagnoses

These include mesenteric adenitis (less severe pain without peritoneal signs is usual and it is rare under 3 years of age), bacterial enterocolitis, pelvic inflammatory disease, urinary tract infection, Meckel's diverticulitis, intussusception and right lower lobe pneumonia.

Investigations

Children with a clear clinical diagnosis of acute appendicitis do not require investigations and delay of surgical consultation. In equivocal cases, imaging of the appendix may be helpful or demonstrate alternative causes of the pain.

No single test is diagnostic in appendicitis, with the white blood cell count insensitive and non-specific.[8] C reactive protein (CRP) levels >10 mg dL^{-1} have varying reported sensitivities (48–75%) and specificities (57–82%) in different studies on appendicitis. Normal CRP values do not exclude acute appendicitis in children.[8] On urine microscopy more than five white blood cells per high power field or the presence of red blood cells is found in 7–25% of children with appendicitis. Abdominal X-rays may show other pathology (e.g. right lower lobe pneumonia) and occasionally an appendiceal faecolith, but are also insensitive and non-specific for diagnosing appendicitis. Note the rare presence of an appendolith can give a more colicky nature to the pain.

Ultrasound Has reported sensitivity of 71–92% with specificity of 86–98% and is often used when there is initial diagnostic doubt. However, in one series patients undergoing sonography before appendicectomy had a longer delay before operation, a higher rate of misdiagnosis, and more postoperative complications. It is not uncommon for the appendix to be difficult to visualise (up to 10% of cases). High positive likelihood ratios and moderate negative likelihood ratios suggest that ultrasound can be used to confirm but not exclude a diagnosis of appendicitis.[8]

CT scan Abdominal helical CT scan in diagnosing appendicitis shows sensitivities from 87–100% and specificities 83–97% with signs of distension of the appendix, faecolith, focal caecal wall thickening and fluid collections in ruptured appendicitis. Some institutions have used a protocol incorporating ultrasound and subsequent CT scan with patients whose diagnosis is equivocal. They have shown this to be an accurate and cost-effective approach when compared with a negative appendicectomy rate of 23%. The American College of Radiology in general advocates the use of ultrasound over CT scan.

Magnetic resonance imaging (MRI) Recent studies suggest high sensitivity and specificity in adult patients with appendicitis.[9] However, several disadvantages including high cost, long duration of study, and limited availability mean MRI has a limited role at the moment. It appears potentially useful in pregnant patients with suspected appendicitis in whom ultrasound is inconclusive.[8]

Active observation Has also been used without investigation, with a positive predictive value of 97.9% in one series and a normal appendicectomy rate of 2.6%.

Management

The management of acute appendicitis is appendicectomy. Some children require intravenous rehydration, ongoing analgesia and antibiotics, if perforation is suspected.

The management of the child in whom the diagnosis is not clear, but may be possible early appendicitis, is more difficult and one needs to have a clear approach.

In some children it may be useful to perform imaging of the appendix such as ultrasound, particularly in older females who may have ovarian pathology as a cause of their pain. An expectant approach is appropriate in some children with a short history, with a clear plan of organised review over the next 6–12 hours. This may be achieved by actively observing the child in hospital or, if discharged, by arranging a definite early clinical review. Parents need clear instructions to return should their child's symptoms progress.

MECKEL'S DIVERTICULUM

Introduction

Meckel's diverticulum is a vestige of the omphalomesenteric duct, occurring in 2% of the population, with 2% of those with Meckel's diverticulum manifesting symptoms. The diverticulum is usually 60 cm proximal to the terminal ileum. Of symptomatic patients, 45% are under the age of 2, but it can present at any age. These findings are known as Meckel's rule of twos. The majority of Meckel's diverticuli contain gastric mucosa and may secrete acid.

Clinical features

The presenting features of a Meckel's diverticulum vary and may include abdominal pain, bowel obstruction, gastrointestinal haemorrhage, or perforation.

Meckel's diverticuli are the most common cause of significant lower gastrointestinal bleeding in children, usually from peptic ulceration within the diverticulum or adjacent ileum. It is classically painless bleeding, with stools either bright red or tarry, depending on the site and briskness of bleeding.

Diverticulitis causing crampy lower quadrant pain can occur in older children. A Meckel's diverticulum can be a lead point in intussusception, as well as causing intestinal obstruction by the formation of intraperitoneal bands, which can lead to the possibility of a volvulus or internal herniation.

Differential diagnoses

These include intestinal polyps, intussusception, anal fissures, midgut volvulus and bacterial enteritis.

Investigations

A Meckel's scan using [99m]technetium can be used, which is 75–85% sensitive and 95% specific[11] at demonstrating the ectopic gastric tissue, when bleeding is present.

Management

Management is intravenous fluid support with blood transfusion for massive bleeding. A Meckel's scan can be done in stable bleeding patients, but if unstable or with peritoneal signs, urgent surgical consultation must be obtained with a view to operative intervention. Definitive treatment is surgical excision, which may be done laparoscopically.

CHRONIC ABDOMINAL PAIN

Introduction

Chronic abdominal pain is defined as the presence of at least three discrete episodes of pain occurring over a period of 3 months or longer.[3] The reported prevalence of abdominal pain interfering with activities is 10–15% in children between 5 and 14 years. Causes of chronic abdominal pain are diverse and are listed in Table 7.1.3.

Signs and symptoms suggesting *organic disease* causing chronic abdominal pain in school-aged children include:

- persistent fever;
- poor weight gain or weight loss;
- child awakened from sleep;
- pain away from the umbilicus;
- radiation of pain to back, shoulder or lower extremities;
- persistent regurgitation, vomiting or dysphagia;
- bloody emesis or stools;
- associated altered bowel pattern;
- perianal disease;
- sleepiness following pain attacks;
- positive family history of peptic ulcer or inflammatory bowel disease.

Assessment

The assessment of the child with chronic abdominal pain involves a detailed history and examination. Blood pressure should be measured. The child who has no features to suggest an organic origin requires no testing, although some clinicians opt to perform a limited screen involving urinalysis, full blood count and erythrocyte sedimentation rate, and stool testing for ova and parasites and occult blood.

Diagnosis

The diagnosis of recurrent functional abdominal pain is based on history and a normal physical examination. Usually the patient has no worrying features (as listed above), has periumbilical or mid-epigastric pain, and rarely wakes at night from the pain. Psychosocial stressors may be evident. There may be secondary gain from the child's abdominal pain. Reassurance is the treatment of choice, although it is important to acknowledge that the child does experience pain. Cognitive–behavioural therapy may be useful for children who clearly have recurrent functional abdominal pain.[10]

Table 7.1.3   Causes of chronic abdominal pain

Gastrointestinal causes
Chronic recurrent functional abdominal pain
Peptic ulcer disease
Irritable bowel syndrome
Inflammatory bowel disease
Chronic or recurrent pancreatitis
Biliary colic
Appendiceal colic
Constipation
Partial bowel obstruction
Parasitic infection

Endocrine disease
Hyperparathyroidism
Addison's disease
Diabetes mellitus

Cardiovascular disease
Superior mesenteric artery syndrome
Coarctation of aorta

Neurological disease
Abdominal migraine
Migraine headaches
Familial dysautonomia

Haematological disease
Sickle cell disease
Porphyrias

Gynaecological disorders
Cystic teratoma of ovary
Endometriosis
Haematocolpos
Mittelschmerz

Musculoskeletal disorders
Discitis
Linea alba hernia
Painful rib syndrome
Muscle wall sprain

Other
Uteropelvic junction obstruction
Familial Mediterranean fever
Hereditary angioneurotic oedema

Source: Adapted from Rudolph 1996.[3]

Management

In the ED situation, the management of chronic abdominal pain depends on the possible diagnoses. Follow up should be ensured, particularly in the child with the suggestion of organic disease or the child missing a significant amount of school.

Controversies

❶ The best approach to investigations in appendicitis has not yet been settled.

❷ There is probably little need for a rectal examination in children with abdominal pain, but more research is needed before making definitive conclusions.

References

1. Scholer SJ, Pituch K, Orr DP, Ditttus RS. Clinical outcomes of children with acute abdominal pain. *Paediatrics* 1996;**98**:680–5.
2. Simpson ET, Smith A. The management of acute abdominal pain in children. *J Paediatr Child Health* 1996;**32**(2):110–2.
3. Rudolph A. *Rudolph's Textbook of Paediatrics.* 20th ed. USA: Appleton and Lange;1996.
4. D'Agostino J. Common abdominal emergencies in children. *Emerg Med Clin North Am* 2002;**20**:1.
5. Browne GJ, Choong RKC, Gaudry PL, Wilkins BH. *Principles and practice of children's emergency care.* Sydney: Maclennan and Petty;1997.
6. Borland ML, Jacobs I, Geelhoed G. Intranasal fentanyl reduces acute pain in children in the emergency department: a safety and efficacy study. *Emerg Med* 2002;**14**(3):275–80.
7. Dunning PG, Goldman MD. The incidence and value of rectal examination in children with suspected appendicitis. *Ann R Coll Surg Engl* 1991;**73**:233–4.
8. Kwok M, Kim M, Gorelick M. Evidence-based Approach to the diagnosis of appendicitis in children. *Pediatr Emerg Care* 2004;**20**(10):690–701.
9. Cobben L, Groot I, Kingma L, et al. A simple MRI protocol in patients with clinically suspected appendicitis: results in 138 patients and effect on outcome of appendectomy. *Eur Radiol* 2009;**19**(5):1175–83.
10. Banez G. Chronic abdominal pain in children: what to do following the medical evaluation. *Curr Opin Pediatr* 2008;**20**:571–5.
11. Behrman R, Kliegman R, Jenson H. *Nelson's Textbook of Paediatrics.* 16th ed. Philadelphia: WB Saunders; 2000.

Further reading

Bachoo P, Mahomed AA, Ninan GK, Youngson GG. Acute appendicitis: The continuing role for active observation. *Paediatr Surg Int* 2001;**17**(2–3):125–8.
Emil S, Mikhail P, Laberge JM, et al. Clinical versus sonographic evaluation of acute appendicitis in children: A comparison of patient characteristics and outcomes. *J Paediatr Surg* 2001;**36**(5):780–3.
Garcia-Pena BM, Taylor GA, Fishman SJ, et al. Costs and effectiveness of ultrasonagraphy and limited computed tomography for diagnosing appendicitis in children. *Paediatrics* 2000;**106**:672–6.

7.2 Gastrointestinal bleeding

Elizabeth M. Cotterell

ESSENTIALS

1 The causes of gastrointestinal (GI) bleeding in infants and children fall into age-specific diagnostic categories.

2 The majority of GI bleeding ceases spontaneously, requiring no treatment or treatment on the basis of a presumptive diagnosis.

3 A good history is important in determining the likely site of GI bleeding, the significance and acuity of the bleed and guides appropriate investigations.

4 Initial assessment is for signs of haemodynamic compromise due to the blood loss, followed by identification of underlying disease.

Introduction

Gastrointestinal (GI) bleeding in infants and children is an uncommon cause of presentations to an emergency department (ED) but nonetheless is an alarming symptom that concerns parents greatly. Fortunately, in the majority of infants and children, the cause is benign or relatively uncomplicated, and not associated with significant morbidity or mortality. There are, however, some less common conditions that occur in infancy and childhood that may be a cause of potentially life-threatening blood loss and require rapid assessment and resuscitation.

The epidemiology of GI bleeding in children is very limited. The reported incidence of GI bleeding of 6.4% in paediatric ICU patients[1] and the most frequent diagnoses confirmed endoscopically[2] (duodenal and gastric ulcers, oesophagitis, gastritis, and varices) represent selected populations and are not representative of the ambulatory paediatric population.

Definitions

Haematemesis is the vomiting of blood that may be either fresh (bright red) or altered by gastric acidity and described as 'coffee grounds'.

Melaena is the passage of black, tarry stool. This is caused by bacterial degradation of haemoglobin and implies that the bleeding has occurred over a period of hours.

Haematochezia is the passage of bright red blood per rectum. Haematemesis and melaena are usually indicative of an upper GI bleeding source. The passage of fresh blood per rectum usually indicates a source of blood from the lower GI tract. It can, however, derive from an upper GI source, especially in infants less than six months, due to rapid colonic transit times. Streaks of blood may be mixed with the stool, usually indicative of colitis, as compared to blood coating a hard or normal stool which may be due to an anal fissure.

Aetiology

The aetiology of GI bleeding is best considered within defined age groups, with some overlap between groups, and the likely location of the bleed, as guided by history and examination (Tables 7.2.1 and 7.2.2).

The term newborn infant who is breast fed and has GI bleeding is most likely to have ingested maternal blood either at the time

Table 7.2.1 Causes of upper GI bleeding (causes listed most common to rare)

Neonates (<1 month)	Infants (1 month to 1 year)	Toddlers and school age
Ingested maternal blood	Ingested blood	Ingested blood
Gastritis	Reflux oesophagitis	Reflux oesophagitis
Vascular malformations	Gastritis	Gastritis
Bleeding disorders	Mallory–Weiss tear	Mallory–Weiss tear
	Peptic ulceration	Oesophageal varices
	Vascular malformation	Peptic ulceration
	Bleeding disorders	Bleeding disorders

Table 7.2.2 Causes of lower GI bleeding

Neonates	Infants	Toddlers and school age
Ingested maternal blood	Anal fissure	Anal fissure
Necrotising enterocolitis	Protein sensitive enterocolitis	Juvenile colonic polyps
Protein-sensitive enterocolitis	Hirschsprung's enterocolitis	Infectious gastroenteritis
Hirschsprung's enterocolitis	Ischaemic enterocolitis	Meckel's diverticulum
Ischaemic enterocolitis	Infectious gastroenteritis	Intussusception
Infectious gastroenteritis	Meckel's diverticulum	Ischaemic enterocolitis
Congenital bleeding disorders	Intussusception	Haemolytic uraemic syndrome
	Haemolytic–uraemic syndrome	Henoch–Schönlein purpura
	Bleeding disorders	Inflammatory bowel disease
	Vascular malformation	Vascular malformation
	Inflammatory bowel disease	Bleeding disorders

Table 7.2.3 Chart for guided history taking for GI bleeding

Is it blood?
Consider haemoccult(r) test on stool samples and gastroccult(r) on vomit or NG aspirates
History of ingestion of food colouring or iron supplements

Is it from the GI tract?
Consider other sources for the blood
Ingestion of maternal blood at delivery or breast feeding
History of epistaxis, post ENT or oral surgery or pharyngitis

Where in the GI tract is it from?
Upper GI tract – haematemesis, melaena or haematochezia for profuse bleed
Lower GI tract – haematochezia, redcurrant jelly stools

Is it a significant amount?
Estimate acuity of bleed by history and assess clinical signs
Resuscitate immediately if haemodynamic compromise

Are there other concerning symptoms or signs?
Paroxysmal abdominal pain and/or lethargy – intussusception
Bilious vomiting – volvulus
History of chronic liver disease – oesophageal varices
Renal or haemotological abnormalities

of delivery or from breast feeding from cracked nipples. Premature infants are at an increased risk of necrotising enterocolitis, although it can occur in term neonates with birth asphyxia or cyanotic heart disease. Any sick newborn, compromised by hypoxia or hypotension is at risk of GI bleeding from stress ulcers. An infant who has not received parenteral vitamin K after birth, or has interference with vitamin K absorption, is at risk of haemorrhagic disease of the newborn. Formula fed infants may develop cow's milk protein intolerance within the first few weeks to months.

The bowel habit of the infant or child prior to onset of GI bleeding is important to note. Constipation associated with pain when straining at stool would make an anal fissure a probable diagnosis. The older infant or child with cerebral palsy may have severe gastro-oesophageal reflux and therefore most likely has an oesophagitis-related source of upper GI bleeding.

The key factor in identifying the cause of GI bleeding in toddlers and older children is the presence of associated symptoms. Crampy abdominal pain and diarrhoea with mucus and fresh blood may be caused by infectious gastroenteritis due to *Campylobacter, Shigella, Salmonella* and *Yersinia*. Intermittent colicky abdominal pain with episodes of lethargy occurring in intussusceptions may manifest with blood in the stools as a late sign.

Henoch–Schönlein purpura will manifest with the typical palpable purpura on extremities as well as abdominal pain. Certain diagnoses also have a recognised age pattern; juvenile polyps have a peak incidence of 1 to 6 years of age, intussusception peaks at 5 to 18 months, and inflammatory bowel disease more commonly presents in adolescence, although can occur at any age.

History

Details of the timing of the blood appearing in the vomitus or bowel motions, in relation to other events, may give a clue to alternative sources of the blood. For example, the ingestion of substances such as iron or food colourings, onset of epistaxis or recent oral or ENT surgery, indicate a source of bleeding other than from the GI tract (Table 7.2.3).

A history of recurrent retching or vomiting prior to the appearance of blood in the vomit suggests a Mallory–Weiss tear, but may occur in the absence of these symptoms. Symptoms of epigastric pain and nausea may be elicited with gastritis. Crampy abdominal pain with a passage of loose stools, with blood and mucus mixed throughout, suggest infectious or inflammatory colitis. Fresh blood coating the stool implies a lesion in the lower rectum or anus, such as a polyp or fissure.

A positive family history may be helpful, particularly with the less common causes, such as polyps, inflammatory bowel disease, coagulation disorders, haemorrhagic telangiectasia and Hirschsprung's disease. A medication history, including use of non-steroidal anti-inflammatory drugs (NSAIDs), salicylates and anticoagulants may provide further clues. Inadvertent ingestion of caustic agents and rodenticides containing warfarin-type agents should be considered in preschool-age children.

Examination

Initial assessment is for the presence or absence of any haemodynamic compromise due to the blood loss. This is uncommon in children but, if present, clinical assessment proceeds while resuscitation is commenced.

Specific findings in the physical examination of the GI tract may establish potential causes for the GI bleeding. The abdomen should be assessed for any localised tenderness or peritoneal signs. Children with minor bleeding in the setting of gastroenteritis will have a benign abdomen. The finding of hepatosplenomegaly with stigmata of chronic liver disease may suggest oesophageal varices as the cause. Palpation of a tender abdominal mass may support a diagnosis of intussusception. Visualisation of an anal fissure is important to confirm the source of blood on stools when the history is suggestive with the defect in the rectal mucosa usually superficial and posteriorly located. Consider *beta haemolytic streptococcal* infection if there is marked perianal erythema. Skin and mucus membrane examination may reveal signs of a bleeding tendency due to a coagulation or platelet disorder. Clinical signs of anaemia are more suggestive of a chronic picture of GI bleeding. Examination of the nose and throat may show a nasopharyngeal source for ingested blood.

In addition, parents may often provide evidence of the symptoms that they have reported, such as a cloth with blood-streaked vomitus or a nappy with bloody streaks in the faeces. In the event of a fresh sample of stool or vomit being provided, testing for occult blood will verify if GI bleeding has occurred.

Investigations

The appropriate investigation of GI bleeding needs to be tailored to the most likely cause on the basis of history and examination findings.

Blood tests

Blood tests for haemoglobin level and red cell indices may indicate a hypochromic microcytic anaemia and point to a chronic source of bleeding. Haematocrit changes in the acute setting are unreliable indicators of acute bleeding. Coagulation profile and platelet count should be checked if the history and examination findings suggest a bleeding diathesis or chronic liver disease.

If the GI bleeding has occurred in a breast-feeding infant, most commonly as streaks of fresh blood in the vomitus, then it may be possible to distinguish if the blood is maternal (ingested) rather than from the infant's gut by performing an Apt test. By diluting the blood from the sample with water (1:5), adding 1 mL of sodium hydroxide to the centrifuged mixture, foetal haemoglobin is resistant to denaturisation by alkali, as opposed to the brown–yellow colour that occurs in the presence of adult haemoglobin.

Stool testing

Stool samples for microscopy, looking for red and white cells, as well as for bacterial culture, should be sent if bacterial enterocolitis is suspected.

Endoscopy

The role of endoscopy for investigating GI bleeding in the acute setting in children is limited. It can, however, serve both a diagnostic and therapeutic role, especially in the case of oesophageal varices. Consultation with a paediatric gastroenterologist or surgeon is helpful in determining those patients most likely to benefit from this investigation.

Imaging

Nuclear medicine studies such as technetium pertechnetate scan for ectopic gastric mucosa in a Meckel's diverticulum may have a role in investigating the cause of GI bleeding. However, the Meckel scan has a relatively low negative predictive value and may not obviate the need for operative evaluation despite a negative scan, where clinical suspicion is high.[3] Other imaging techniques such as ultrasound and contrast air enema for intussusception should be considered in children under the age of 2 years with abdominal pain, GI bleeding and lethargy.

Treatment

Initial assessment and stabilisation

In the event of significant GI bleeding, the child or infant will develop signs of haemodynamic compromise. Cool peripheries, delayed capillary refill and tachycardia will be the first detectable signs. Hypotension occurs as a late sign of hypovolaemia in children.

Resuscitation should include the administration of high-flow oxygen, insertion of two large-bore cannulae and titrated 20 mL kg^{-1} fluid boluses with crystalloid. Children with significant GI bleeding require ongoing monitoring of heart rate, blood pressure, and urine output in the ED. These observations combined with frequent clinical assessment, help guide ongoing fluid therapy. Transfusion of cross-matched blood is indicated for ongoing or recurrent bleeding with haemodynamic instability unresponsive to initial fluid boluses. Correction of identified

coagulopathy with fresh frozen plasma, activated factor VII or platelet infusions may be needed to control the GI bleeding.

Pharmacological treatment

Studies addressing the use of H$_2$ antagonists and proton pump inhibitors (PPIs) for acute upper GI bleeding are restricted to the adult population. PPIs have been shown in systematic reviews to reduce the risk of further bleeding and need for surgery for peptic ulcers.[4] However, the routine use of H$_2$ antagonists or PPIs in children with acute GI bleeding cannot be recommended as bleeding gastric ulcers are very uncommon.

Intravenous somatostatin or octreotide have been shown to be effective for uncontrolled bleeding oesophageal varices by decreasing splanchnic blood flow; however, most variceal bleeding ceases spontaneously.

Bacterial enterocolitis is usually self limiting and does not require empiric antibiotic treatment.Children with gastroduodenal ulceration shown to be associated with *Helicobacter pylori* infection may benefit from antibiotic eradication treatment.

Infants with a presumptive diagnosis of cow's milk protein intolerance should be changed to a hydrolysed protein formula with expected improvement within days. Mothers of breastfed infants can be advised to eliminate all dairy products from their diet if this diagnosis is considered for their infant.[5]

Children with bleeding from an anal fissure may require laxatives to ensure regular soft stools so that the fissure will heal.

Surgery

Laparoscopy or laparotomy for investigation of lower GI bleeding may be both a diagnostic and therapeutic tool in children with GI bleeding of obscure origin. A study of 17 children with GI bleeding and no identifiable source after upper endoscopy and colonoscopy found that eight patients had Meckel's diverticulum at laparoscopy, five patients had other GI pathology that accounted for symptoms and four patients had normal findings.[6] Laparotomy may be necessary for acute abdominal emergencies such as intussusception unsuccessfully reduced at air enema, midgut volvulus or for management of continuous or recurrent active GI bleeding with haemodynamic compromise.

Endoscopic sclerotherapy

Injection sclerotherapy for oesophageal varices in children is well established with a reported efficacy of controlling active bleeding and eradication of varices exceeding 90%.[7] Complications can occur, including oesophageal ulceration leading to stricture formation. Variceal band ligation may be limited by size in infants and small children.

Dispositon

The decision to admit or discharge the infant or child with GI bleeding from the ED is very much influenced by the presumptive diagnosis. Given that the majority are self-limiting or respond readily to treatment, most patients can be managed on an out-patient basis. Those infants and children suitable for discharge will have no haemodynamic instability or significant co-morbidities at presentation to ED. High-risk patients with significant GI blood loss will need to be managed in an intensive care or high dependency unit. Children who present with recurrent GIT bleeding of unclear cause should be discussed with a paediatric gastroenterologist regarding the need for and timing of endoscopy.

Controversies

❶ The lack of evidence of benefit from the use of H₂ antagonists and PPIs for acute gastrointestinal bleeding in children has not prevented their frequent use.

❷ There is debate about the use of nasogastric aspiration as a diagnostic tool to establish an upper GI tract source of bleeding as it has low specificity for active bleeding.

References

1. Lacroix J, Nadeau D, Laberge S, et al. Frequency of upper gastrointestinal bleeding in a paediatric intensive care unit. *Crit Care Med* 1992;**20**:35–42.
2. Cox K, Ament ME. Upper gastrointestinal bleeding in children and adolescents. *Paediatrics* 1979;**63**:408–13.
3. Swaniker F, Soldes O, Hirschl RB. The utility of technetium-99m pertechnetate scintigraphy in the evaluation of patients with Meckel's diverticulum. *J Pediatr Surg* 1999;**34**:760–4.
4. Leontiadadis GI, Sreedharan A, Dorwrad S, et al. Systematic reviews of the clinical effectiveness and cost-effectiveness of proton pump inhibitors in acute upper gastrointestinal bleeding. *Health Technol Assess* 2007;**11**: iii–iiv, 1–164.
5. Maloney J, Nowak-Wegrzyn A. Educational clinical case series for pediatric allergy and immunology: Allergic proctocolitis, food protein-induced enterocolitis syndrome and allergic eosinophilic gastroenteritis with protein losing enteropathy as manifestations of non-IgE-mediated cow's mild allergy. *Pediatr Allergy Immunol* 2007;**18**:360–7.
6. Lee KH, Yeung CK, Tam YH, Ng WT, Yip KF. Laparoscopy for definitive diagnosis and treatment of gastrointestinal bleeding of obscure origin in children. *J Pediatr Surg* 2000;**35**:1291–3.
7. Fox VL. Gastrointestinal bleeding in infancy and childhood. *Gastroenterol Clin North Am* 2000;**29**:37–66.

Futher reading

Boyle JT. Gastrointestinal bleeding in infants and children. *Pediatr Rev* 2008;**29**:39–52. http://pedsreview .aappublications/org/cgi/content/full/29/2/3.

7.3 Gastro-oesophageal reflux

Daryl Efron

ESSENTIALS

1 The infant presenting with regurgitation/vomiting needs to have alternative causes considered, before concluding that the diagnosis is GOR.

2 GOR is a normal physiological phenomenon to which infants are particularly prone.

3 Infants with benign GOR appear healthy and thriving. If the child appears unwell, another cause should be considered.

4 Infants and children with uncomplicated GOR do not need any investigations.

5 Complications of GOR include failure to thrive, reflux oesophagitis, apnoea, aspiration pneumonia, and recurrent aspiration with chronic lung disease.

6 Antacids and antisecretory therapies can be helpful in reflux oesophagitis.

Introduction

Gastro-oesophageal reflux (GOR) is the regurgitation of gastric contents into the oesophagus. It is a normal physiological phenomenon at all ages. In most cases it is a benign self-limited condition which spontaneously resolves over a variable time period, usually in infancy. The refluxed gastric contents are generally rapidly cleared from the oesophagus without causing any significant clinical symptoms. Complications warranting medical intervention are uncommon. When complications do occur, it is referred to as GOR disease (GORD).

Pathophysiology

During periods of raised intra-abdominal pressure such as straining, there are a number of protective mechanisms which help to prevent GOR. These include contraction of the diaphragmatic crura around the lower oesophagus in the region of the lower oesophageal sphincter (LES), as well as compression of the intra-abdominal segment of the oesophagus. Many episodes of GOR are associated with transient relaxations of the LES.

In infants the LES is located above the diaphragm, rendering the above protective mechanisms ineffective. Therefore, infants are especially prone to GOR, particularly in the early months of life. However, with anatomical and physiological maturation, the natural history is of symptom resolution by late infancy in the vast majority. GOR is unusual in children older than 18 months.[1]

Some children are particularly predisposed to develop GORD. These include premature infants, children with neurological conditions, such as cerebral palsy or neurodegenerative disorders, and children with anatomical anomalies such as tracheo-oesophageal fistula. These children have poor oesophageal motility with reduced clearance of refluxed gastric contents.

History

The cardinal symptom of GOR is visible regurgitation of milk post-feeds. This is usually called vomiting, although in GOR the expulsion of gastric contents is generally by an effortless spill, whereas true vomiting involves forceful contraction of abdominal wall musculature. In GOR, the regurgitation is not particularly forceful and the milk usually soils the child's clothing. Likewise, the physiological 'posseting' of milk, which is common after feeding, usually just spills onto the child's chin region. This is in contrast to the more projectile vomiting of pyloric stenosis, where the milk often propels to a more distant location.

The history is crucial in considering potential differential diagnoses and in identifying complications. Careful questioning regarding the relationship of vomiting to feeds, the content of regurgitated material (e.g. is there blood or bile?), apparent associated distress, and feeding behaviour, is essential. Episodic irritability related to feeds may indicate GOR, although the association between irritability and GOR in infants is generally weak. Atopic features such as eczema and a family history raise the possibility of cows' milk protein allergy. A history of associated fever suggests an infective cause. Seizures and poor feeding raise the possibility of a metabolic or neurological disorder. Inquiry about associated symptoms such as poor weight gain and respiratory symptoms including apnoea, or wheezing is important to screen for potential complications. Onset of vomiting after 6 months of age is unusual in GOR and suggests an alternative cause.

Examination

Infants with benign GOR demonstrate a robust general condition. They appear well and are thriving. If the child appears unwell or lethargic another cause for the symptoms needs to be carefully considered. The presence of abdominal distension, abnormal tone, or hepatosplenomegaly suggests alternative diagnoses including anatomical anomalies, neurodevelopmental dysfunction or metabolic disorders. A pyloric tumour should be specifically palpated for in young infants. Note that occasionally, in a young infant with known GOR, a change in the character of the vomiting may indicate another evolving diagnosis on a background of GOR, such as pyloric stenosis or a urinary tract infection (UTI). Serial weight measurements should be plotted on the child's growth chart. Respiratory examination is important to identify signs of bronchospasm or recurrent aspiration, which may complicate GOR. Conjunctival pallor indicates anaemia, which may be secondary to reflux oesophagitis. The urine should be screened by microscopy and culture for an occult UTI causing vomiting.

Differential diagnosis

There are many causes of vomiting in children, and it is important to consider a number of alternative causes that may mimic GOR (see Chapter 7.8 on Diarrhoea and vomiting). These include: infection, e.g. urinary tract infection, gastroenteritis; surgical conditions, e.g. malrotation and volvulus, pyloric stenosis, intussusception; metabolic disorders, e.g. inborn errors, diabetes; food allergy and raised intracranial pressure, e.g. hydrocephalus, posterior fossa tumour, subdural haematoma (Table 7.3.1).

Complications

GOR may result in serious complications and is then referred to as GORD.

Table 7.3.1 Differential diagnosis of GOR
Urinary tract infection
Gastroenteritis
Surgical: volvulus, PS, intussusception
Food allergy
Neurological
Metabolic: inborn errors
Raised intracranial pressure

Failure to thrive

Some infants with GOR have poor weight gain, which may extend to failure to thrive (crossing two major centiles on a growth chart). This may result from reduced intake – either related to dysphagia or parental reduction of feed volumes offered, in an attempt to minimise regurgitation – or from inadequate absorption of ingested food due to excessive losses.

Respiratory

A number of respiratory complications may occur with GOR. Recurrent aspiration (often silent) results in chronic wheeze or cough, and alveolar disease may develop, with signs of tachypnoea and increased work of breathing. Exposure of the oesophageal mucosa to acid can trigger reflex bronchospasm, and persistent asthma symptoms may occasionally be related to GOR.[2] Intermittent (or even isolated) episodes of aspiration can cause pneumonia. Reflux of gastric contents into the upper airway can result in laryngospasm, presenting as an obstructive apnoea or apparent life-threatening event (ALTE).[3] However, it is unusual to be able to demonstrate an association between GOR and ALTE.

Oesophagitis

Reflux oesophagitis has become a popular clinical diagnosis given to infants presenting with excessive crying behaviour (so-called 'silent reflux'). There are many causes for infant distress, (including temperamental factors, food allergy) and peptic oesophagitis is only responsible for a minority of cases of infant distress.[4] These infants may have episodes of blood in the vomitus or develop iron deficiency anaemia due to the red cell loss. Rarely, an infant may develop feed aversion due to the distress of GOR.

Sandifer syndrome is abnormal trunk and neck posturing of infants in response to oesophageal pain due to refluxed gastric acid. These uncommon episodes can be quite stereotypic, such that they may be confused with seizures.

Investigations

In the majority of cases, a careful history and examination will clarify the likely diagnosis of GOR. Investigations may be required to exclude differential diagnoses, when the diagnosis is unclear.

Serum biochemistry including an acid base, to exclude the evolving metabolic hypokalaemic, hypochloraemic alkalosis of pyloric stenosis, and urine microscopy and culture to screen for a UTI, are relevant first-line tests in the vomiting infant. If the history or biochemistry is suggestive, a pyloric ultrasound should be performed to rule out pyloric stenosis.

Well and thriving infants and children with uncomplicated GOR should not be subjected to any investigations. There are a number of investigations that may be helpful in selected clinical situations. However, the interpretation of studies of oesophageal function and their clinical relevance is not straightforward.

Some children may require admission under a paediatrician for observation of feeding and the presence of regurgitation and consideration of further tests to clarify the diagnosis.

Barium meal and follow through is used to exclude anatomical problems such as malrotation of the small bowel. The observation of GOR merely demonstrates that the infant experienced an episode of reflux at the time of the study. The frequency of GOR episodes, their correlation with clinical symptoms, or the presence of complications cannot be determined from a barium study.

Oesophageal pH monitoring over 24 hours provides representative data about the pH at the lower oesophageal mucosa. A number of indices can be calculated from the monitoring: the frequency of GOR episodes; the length of episodes; and the reflux index – the proportion of time sampled that the oesophageal pH was less than 4 (exposure to gastric acid greater than 10% is usually considered abnormal). However, the association of GOR with oesophagitis is not strong. Infants often have abnormal oesophageal pH findings in the absence of histological features of oesophagitis and, conversely, infants with oesophagitis may have no evidence of significant GOR on pH study.[4] These infants presumably have an alternative cause for their oesophagitis, such as allergy. The precise role of oesophageal pH studies is contentious. It is a good test to confirm severe GOR prior to embarking on antireflux surgery, and there may be other clinical scenarios where it provides useful information, e.g. in conjunction with monitoring of respiratory rate, heart rate and oxygen saturations in investigation of apnoea or episodic hypoxaemia/bradycardia.

Oesophagoscopy and biopsy may be indicated for evaluating the presence and severity of oesophagitis, as well as to characterise the changes histologically, e.g. peptic, eosinophilic (allergic), Crohn's disease, Barrett's oesophagus.

Aspiration of gastric contents into the lungs can be identified by nuclear medicine study using radiolabelled milk (can detect aspiration events up to 24 hours following a feed). A chest X-ray $\pm$ computerised tomography scan of the chest can be used to evaluate for chronic lung disease.

Treatment

Children diagnosed with GOR need follow up organised with the local doctor, to ensure no alternative diagnosis is missed and to monitor for complications. Parents need an explanation of the symptoms and to be reassured that the natural history is for spontaneous resolution over months. It is unusual for GOR symptoms to persist beyond 12 to 15 months of age. If there is any doubt about the diagnosis, then a paediatric review should be arranged.

Simple measures

A number of conservative measures are commonly used to reduce the symptoms of GOR. These include posturing (elevation of cot ~30 degrees head up), thickening of feeds,[5] and changes to infant formulas. None of these have been demonstrated to modify clinical outcomes.[6] A trial of a partially hydrolysed formula may be indicated in GORD, e.g. GOR with failure to thrive. Prone sleeping position is best for reducing GOR[7] but is not generally recommended as it as associated with sudden infant death syndrome. Suggesting positioning a towel on the carer's shoulder may decrease the inconvenience of refluxed milk onto the parent during feeding.

Pharmacological

Pharmacological treatment of otherwise well, thriving infants with uncomplicated benign GOR is not indicated.[8]

In more severe cases, the pharmacological options include antacids, antisecretory therapies, and prokinetic agents. High-dose antacids can be effective in treating oesophagitis.[9] However, prolonged use can be associated with aluminium toxicity and is not recommended. H_2-receptor antagonists such as ranitidine have been shown to improve both histological changes and symptoms.[10] Proton pump inhibitors have well-demonstrated clinical efficacy in children with reflux oesophagitis[11,12] and appear to be safe. Prokinetic agents do not have clear evidence for symptom reduction;[13] however, a trial of domperidone or erythromycin may be worthwhile in GORD.

Surgical

Antireflux surgery has a limited role in cases of severe GORD, such as neurologically abnormal infants with recurrent aspiration pneumonia. The operation of choice is usually the Nissen fundoplication. Complications of the procedure include breakdown of the wrap, dysphagia, bloating and gagging. Some surgeons are now performing fundoplications laparoscopically.

Controversies

❶ The role of oesophageal pH studies in the evaluation for reflux oesophagitis is the subject of ongoing debate.

❷ Antireflux medications are not indicated for uncomplicated GOR, and are probably being overprescribed in infancy.

❸ Prokinetic agents have not been consistently demonstrated to reduce symptoms.

References

1. Campanozzi A, Boccia G, Pensabene L, et al. Prevalence and natural history of gastroesophageal reflux: pediatric prospective survey. *Pediatrics* 2009;**123**:779.
2. Balson BM, Kravitz EK, McGeady SJ. Diagnosis and treatment of gastroesophageal reflux in children and adolescents with severe asthma. *Ann Allergy Asthma Immunol* 1998;**81**:159–64.
3. Menon AP, Schefft GL, Thach BT. Apnea associated with regurgitation in infants. *J Pediatr* 1985;**106**:625–9.
4. Heine RG, Cameron DJS, Chow CW, et al. Esophagitis in distressed infants: Poor diagnostic agreement between esophageal pH monitoring and histopathologic findings. *J Pediatr* 2002;**140**:14–9.
5. Horvath A, Dziechciarz P, Szajewska H. The effect of thickened-feed interventions on gastroesophageal reflux in infants: systematic review and meta-analysis of randomized controlled trials. *Pediatrics* 2008;**122**:e1268.

6. Carroll AE, Garrison MM, Christakis DA. A systematic review of nonpharmacological and nonsurgical therapies for gastroesophageal reflux in infants. *Arch Pediatr Adolesc Med* 2002;**156**:109–13.
7. Meyers WF, Herbst JJ. Effectiveness of positioning therapy for gastroesophageal reflux. *Paediatrics* 1982;**69**: 768–82.
8. Khoshoo V, Edell D, Thompson A, Rubin M. Are we overprescribing antireflux medications for infants with regurgitation? *Pediatrics* 2007;**120**:946.

9. Cucchiara S, Staniano A, Romaniello G, et al. Antacids and cimetidine treatment for gastroesophageal reflux and peptic oesophagitis. *Arch Dis Child* 1984;**59**:842–7.
10. Simeone D, Caria MC, Miele E, et al. Treatment of childhood peptic oesophagitis: A double-blind placebo-controlled trial of nizatidine. *J Pediatr Gastroenterol Nutr* 1997;**25**:51–5.
11. Kato S, Ebina K, Fujii K, et al. Effect of omeprazole in the treatment of refractory acid-related diseases in childhood: Endoscopic healing and twenty-four hour intragastric acidity. *J Pediatr* 1996;**128**:415–21.
12. DeGiacomo C, Bawa P, Franceschi M, et al. Omeprazole for severe gastroesophageal reflux in children. *J Pediatr Gastroenterol Nutr* 1997;**24**:528–32.
13. Augood C, MacLennan S, Gilbert R, Logan S. Cisapride treatment for gastro-oesophageal reflux in children (Cochrane Review). In: *The Cochrane Library*. Issue 4. Chichester: John Wiley & Sons; 2002.

7.4 Pyloric stenosis

Kim Lian Ong

ESSENTIALS

1 Hypertrophic pyloric stenosis rarely occurs before the 1st week of life; it commonly presents at 2–8 weeks of age.

2 The main symptom is protracted vomiting; the infant is a hungry baby and metabolic derangements result from extensive and protracted vomiting.

3 The diagnosis is made by the characteristic clinical manifestations and the finding of a pathognomonic pyloric mass.

4 Ultrasonography is the diagnostic test of choice; in the absence of ultrasonography, barium upper gastrointestinal study is an effective means of diagnosis.

5 Treatment is directed at correction of derangements before definitive surgical repair by Ramstedt pyloromyotomy, a straightforward procedure with minimal complications.

Introduction

Hypertrophic pyloric stenosis (HPS) is a common gastrointestinal cause of gastric outlet obstruction in infants and is one of the most common surgical conditions of infancy.[1] It is caused by the idiopathic diffuse hypertrophy and hyperplasia of the circular muscle fibres of the pylorus with the proximal extension into the gastric antrum resulting in construction and obstruction of the gastric outlet. In response to outflow obstruction and vigorous peristalsis, stomach musculature becomes uniformly hypertrophied and dilated.

Epidemiology

Pyloric stenosis has an incidence of 2 to 4 per 1000 live births in Western populations[2] and it appears to be less common in infants in African and Asian populations. It is four to five times more common in males.[3] The cause of pyloric stenosis is unknown. Genetic, familial, gender and ethnic origin can influence the incidence rates of HPS. Offspring of parents with this condition have a higher risk of developing HPS and in many series first-born males are seen more frequently than the other siblings.[4]

Clinical presentation

Pyloric stenosis is not present at birth. In the early phase, there may just be regurgitation or occasional non-projectile vomiting. The onset rarely occurs before the first week of life and it commonly presents at 2–8 weeks of age; however, it is reported in premature babies prior to this corrected age. The peak usually occurs at 4 weeks and it is seldom delayed beyond the second to third month. Within a variable time after the onset of symptoms, the vomiting becomes more projectile and it generally occurs during or soon after feeding. However, at times, it may occur up to several hours later. The frequency of vomiting varies: in some infants vomiting occurs after each feed while in others it may be somewhat intermittent.

Shortly after vomiting, the infant is often hungry and will take another feed immediately. The vomitus is non-bilious but due to the frequency and force of vomiting, it may occasionally become blood tinged. The amount of stool may be very small and infrequent, depending on the amount of food that reaches the intestine. The degree of dehydration, lethargy and metabolic derangement depends on the time interval between the onset of symptoms and presentation. In some late presentations the infant may be severely malnourished, dehydrated or even collapsed.

It is important to note that it may take some time for the clinical features, metabolic disturbance and ultrasound findings to become established and one should not exclude HPS if symptoms persist / recrudesce after a relatively normal examination of an infant presenting very early. A planned review, should features evolve, is appropriate. Likewise, it is important to consider HPS in a previously benign 'posseting' or 'refluxy' baby whose regurgitation of milk has 'changed' in intensity or frequency rather than attributing this to 'posseting getting worse'. In this situation, the clue to the possibility of HPS is the change in the nature of the previous 'vomiting'.

Examination findings

With established HPS, the infant fails to thrive due to calorie losses, becomes dehydrated due to fluid losses and appears 'hungry' unless significant dehydration or alkalosis has started to affect the infant's activity level. The infant usually appears 'bright and active' unless significantly dehydrated, compared to the infant with a urinary tract infection who may be constitutionally unwell.

On physical examination, gastric distension or visible peristaltic waves may be seen moving from the left upper abdomen toward the epigastrium, and right side in some cases.[5] The palpable finding of a firm, mobile and non-tender ovoid mass ('olive') either to the right of the epigastrium or in the midline, deep to right rectus muscle and under the liver edge is diagnostic. This finding of a palpable mass requires much patience as the success of such a finding is dependent on an empty stomach and a relaxed anterior abdominal wall in a non-crying settled infant. If the stomach is significantly distended during palpation, aspiration of gastric contents using a nasogastric tube may be helpful to increase the likelihood of feeling the hypertrophied muscle. Also, palpation during a test feed may allow a previously non-palpable hypertrophied pylorus to be felt during peristaltic contractions. The best position for palpation is on the infant's left side. The inability to palpate an olive-shaped mass does not exclude the diagnosis of HPS and often an ultrasound is needed to clarify the diagnosis.[6]

With extensive and protracted vomiting, metabolic derangement will occur. Vomiting of gastric contents leads to depletion of sodium, potassium and hydrochloric acid, which results in the characteristic finding of hypokalaemic, hypochloraemic metabolic alkalosis.[7] The kidneys conserve sodium at the expense of hydrogen ions, resulting in a paradoxical aciduria. With the increasing degree of dehydration, renal potassium losses are accelerated in an attempt to retain sodium and fluid.

Imaging studies

Some clinicians believe that the palpation of an olive-shaped mass may obviate the need for a confirmatory imaging study, as a positive examination has high specificity.[8] Plain radiographs will often have been performed, given the history of vomiting, although they are of no diagnostic value. They may show gastric distension.

Ultrasonography is the now the diagnostic test of choice as it can be performed quickly and without radiation exposure. The accuracy is close to 100% when performed by experienced personnel,[9] having a sensitivity and specificity of 99.5% and 100% respectively.[10] The sonographic appearance of 'doughnuts' or 'bull's-eyes' on cross-section of the pyloric channel is most characteristic. A muscle thickness of the pylorus greater than 4 mm and a pyloric channel length of greater than 17 mm yield a positive predictive value of greater than 90%. For infants less than 30 days of age, these limits may be lower.[11]

In the absence of ultrasonography, barium upper gastrointestinal study is an effective means of diagnosing HPS. This study may be preferred over ultrasound as the cost-effective initial imaging study when the clinical presentation is atypical for HPS and favours other conditions more amenable to diagnosis by upper gastrointestinal study.[12] Positive findings include an elongated pylorus with antral indentation from the hypertrophied muscle. The pathognomonic finding is the appearance of a 'railroad track' sign caused by two thin parallel streams of barium traversing the pylorus. There is also a vigorously peristaltic stomach with delayed or no gastric emptying.

Upper GI endoscopy is performed on the very rare occasions when other imaging modalities are inconclusive and although it would demonstrate pyloric obstruction, it would be difficult to differentiate it from pyloric spasm.

Differential diagnosis

The diagnosis is made by the characteristic clinical manifestations of projectile non-bilious vomiting and the finding of a pathognomic pyloric mass. Other causes of vomiting, especially in early life, include achalasia of the oesophagus and a symptomatic hiatus hernia. Gastro-oesophageal reflux with or without hiatus hernia may have a similar presentation of persistent vomiting after feeding. Other non-pathological causes include feeding technique issues and overfeeding by an inexperienced enthusiastic carer.

Projectile vomiting may occur in some rare diagnoses such as pyloric membrane or pyloric duplication where a palpable mass may be felt.

Metabolic causes may mimic pyloric stenosis. Adrenal insufficiency results in profuse non-bilious vomiting but it is likely to result in metabolic acidosis rather than alkalosis as in pyloric stenosis. Unlike pyloric stenosis,

the serum potassium and urinary sodium concentration are elevated in adrenal insufficiency. Recurrent emesis with alkalosis or acidosis may be caused by some inborn errors of metabolism but usually there will be other associated clinical features, such as hypoglycaemia, coma or seizures to suggest a metabolic cause. Any vomiting infant needs to have a clean urine checked to exclude infection.

Management

The definitive treatment is surgical repair by a Ramstedt pyloromyotomy, which is the procedure of choice in which the pyloric mass is split, leaving the mucosal layer intact. This procedure is fairly straightforward, with minimal complications. The pylorus may be accessed by various incision techniques, including laparoscopic means. All methods are considered acceptable practice, with minimal differences in outcomes noted.[13]

The preoperative treatment is directed toward correction of fluid, electrolyte and acid–base imbalance which is important to achieve prior to anaesthesia. The amount of fluid resuscitation is based on the degree of dehydration. Correction of fluid and electrolyte imbalance can usually be achieved within 24-48 hours.

Resuscitation with a bolus dose of intravenous normal saline is required for moderate to severe dehydration and is given at $10-20 \text{ mL kg}^{-1}$. This is followed by rehydration with N/2 + 5% dextrose solution at 1.5 times maintenance rate over 24 hours.

Adequate amounts of both chloride and potassium are necessary to correct metabolic acidosis. The correction of potassium can be achieved by adding 10–20 mEq of KCl per 500 mL of intravenous fluid in patients with normal renal function. Chloride can be adequately replaced by normal saline or N/2 saline with 5% dextrose. During resuscitation urine output and electrolyte determinations should be performed regularly. In general, correction of chloride level to 90 mEq L^{-1} or greater is adequate for surgery to be performed.

Complications

Pyloromyotomy is associated with a low incidence of morbidity and mortality. A retrospective review of a large number of patients from two centres between 1969 and 1994 showed an overall 19% complication rate.[14] Therefore, complications are minimal when the pyloromyotomy is performed by experienced hands. The mortality associated with this procedure is less than 0.4% in most major centres.[15]

Controversies

❶ There is disagreement as to when vomiting becomes significant enough to warrant investigation as infants frequently regurgitate small amounts following a feed especially if they have caregivers with poor feeding technique. An important distinction may be the general appearance of the infant, as infants with regurgitation generally appear relatively well.

❷ It is not easy to palpate a pyloric mass as infants are irritable in the presence of protracted vomiting.

❸ The threshold for investigation with ultrasonography varies considerably.

References

1. Schwartz MZ. Hypertrophic pyloric stenosis. In: JA O'Neill, Rowe MI, Grosfeld JL, et al., Pediatric surgery. St Louis, USA: CV Mosby; 1998. p. 111–7.
2. To T, Wajja A, Wales PW, et al. Population demographic indicators associated with incidence of pyloric stenosis. Arch Pediatr Adolesc Med 2005;159:520–5.
3. Poon TS, Zhang AL, Cartmill T, Cass DT. Changing patterns of diagnosis and treatment of infantile hypertrophic pyloric stenosis: A clinical audit of 303 patients. J Pediatr Surg 1996;31:1611–5.
4. Murtagh K, Perry P, Corlett M, Fraser I. Infantile hypertrophic pyloric stenosis. Dig Dis 1992;10:190–8.
5. Spicer RD. Infantile hypertrophic pyloric stenosis: A review. Br J Surg 1982;69:128–35.
6. Forman HP, Leonidas JC, Kronfeld GD. A rational approach to the diagnosis of hypertrophic pyloric stenosis: Do the results match the claims? J Pediatr Surg 1990;25:262–6.
7. Rice HE, Caty MG, Glick PL. Fluid therapy for the pediatric surgical patient. Pediatr Clin North Am 1998;45:719–27.
8. Godbole P, Sprigg A, Dickson A, Lin PC. Ultrasound compared with clinical examination in infantile hypertrophic pyloric stenosis. Arch Dis Child 1996;75:335–7.
9. Hernanz-Schulman M, Sells LL, Ambrosino MM, et al. Hypertrophic pyloric stenosis in the infant without palpable olive: accuracy of sonographic diagnosis. Radiology 1994;193:771–6.
10. White MC, Langer JC, Don S, et al. Sensitivity and cost minimization analysis of radiology versus palpation for the diagnosis of hypertrophic pyloric stenosis. J Pediatr Surg 1998;33:913–7.
11. Lamki N, Athey PA, Round ME, et al. Hypertrophic pyloric stenosis in the neonate – diagnostic critical revisited. Can Assoc Radiol J 1993;44:21–4.
12. Olson AD, Hernanadez R, Hirschi RB. The role of ultrasonography in the diagnosis of pyloric stenosis: A decision analysis. J Pediatr Surg 1998;33:676–681.
13. Hingston G. Ramstedt's pyloromyotomy – what is the correct incision? N Z Med J 1996;109:276–8.
14. Hulka F, Harrison MW, Campbell TJ, et al. Complications of pyloromyotomy for infantile hypertrophic pyloric stenosis. Am J Surg 1997;173:450–2.
15. O' Neill JA, Grosfeld JL, Fonkalsrud EW, et al., editors. Principles of Pediatric Surgery. 2nd ed St. Louis, MO: Mosby; 2004. p. 467–79 [chapter 45].

7.5 Bilious vomiting

Andrew J.A. Holland

ESSENTIALS

1 Bilious vomiting generally indicates an intestinal obstruction due to surgical pathology.

2 Early referral to a paediatric surgeon is recommended.

3 Rarely, bile-stained vomiting may have a non-surgical medical aetiology.

4 Malrotation with volvulus usually presents in the first few weeks of life, but can occur at any age and is always a surgical emergency.

5 Small-bowel obstruction secondary to adhesions is less common in children than in adults and rarely settles with non-operative management.

Introduction

Any child presenting to the emergency department (ED) with bilious vomiting has a surgical cause of intestinal obstruction until proven otherwise. Bilious vomiting occurs when the vomitus contains bile. Typically, this is indicated by its bright green colour, although the discolouration may vary from a pale yellow to a dark greenish brown. Often the carer is aware of the importance of this sign and will have preserved a towel or item of clothing stained with the vomitus for inspection. For practical purposes, bilious vomiting indicates an intestinal obstruction. Some indication of the likely aetiology and level of the obstruction may be determined from the age of the child, the past medical history and length of illness prior to onset of vomiting. Rapid onset of bilious vomiting and a non-distended abdomen suggest a proximal obstruction, whereas late onset of bilious vomiting and abdominal distension, a distal obstruction. Immediate referral to a paediatric surgeon is indicated, as urgent surgical intervention may be required.

Causes

The possible causes of bilious vomiting are as shown in Table 7.5.1 and are discussed below:

Intestinal atresia

The term atresia implies maldevelopment of a lumen or opening that is normally patent. If there is just a narrowing of the lumen, this is termed a stenosis. Atresia of the intestinal tract can occur at any level, but in the context of bilious vomiting the level of obstruction is distal to the ampulla of Vater in the second part of the duodenum.

As the lesion is congenital, the child will present in the neonatal period, although increasingly, some of these infants are diagnosed on antenatal ultrasound scans.[1] Proximal lesions, such as duodenal or jejunal atresia, will usually present in the first 24 hours of life whereas more distal lesions, such as ileal or colonic atresias, can present later. Duodenal atresia may be associated with Down's syndrome and cardiac anomalies in up to 30% of cases.[2]

Table 7.5.1   Causes of bilious vomiting

Intestinal atresia

Anorectal anomalies

Meconium ileus

Hirschsprung's disease

Malrotation with volvulus

Irreducible inguinal hernia

Intussusception

Inflammatory

Meckel's diverticulum

Adhesions

Non-surgical

Anorectal anomalies

Typically the anus is imperforate and the rectum communicates with the urinary tract or perineum via a fistula. It may occur as part of the VACTERL association of anomalies (vertebral, anorectal, cardiac, tracheo-oesophageal, renal and limb).[3] The diagnosis should normally be made as part of the routine assessment of a neonate following delivery, but is occasionally missed, leading to a complete or partial distal obstruction and late onset bilious vomiting. Infrequently, the anomaly may present outside the neonatal period once the child commences solids.

Meconium ileus

This condition occurs in about 10–20% of neonates with cystic fibrosis (CF), although uncommonly it may occur in the absence of CF.[4] There may be a family history of CF. The condition results from the occlusion of the bowel lumen by abnormally viscous enteric secretions in the small bowel and may be complicated by an atresia.

Hirschsprung's disease

In this condition the enteric nervous system is abnormal, leading to a distal physiological obstruction. The condition is more common in males by a ratio of 4:1.[5] In 75% of cases, so called 'classical' Hirschsprung's disease (HD), a variable extent of the rectum and sigmoid colon is involved, leading to a distal colonic obstruction.[6] In the remaining 25% of cases, bowel proximal to the sigmoid colon will also be aganglionic. About 10% of children with HD will also have Down's

syndrome.[7] The cardinal feature of HD is the failure to first pass meconium within 24 hours of birth in a term infant, with the later development of bilious vomiting in the first few days of life.

Malrotation with volvulus

The mid-gut normally develops within a physiological hernia in utero. As this reduces towards the end of the first trimester, the mid-gut undergoes an anticlockwise rotation around the axis of the superior mesenteric vessels.[8] Failure of this process to occur results in malrotation. The onset of bilious vomiting usually indicates that the malrotated small bowel has obstructed as a result of twisting around its pedicle, although occasionally, this may occur as a result of associated congenital bands. There is a high risk of intestinal ischaemia, so urgent surgical intervention is required once the diagnosis has been confirmed.[9] Although malrotation most commonly presents in the first month of life, it can present at any time and even in adult life.[10]

Irreducible inguinal hernia

An irreducible inguinal hernia, particularly in a male, often contains bowel. The resultant obstruction of the bowel at the level of the external inguinal ring may produce bilious vomiting. Untreated, the irreducible hernia is at risk of producing intestinal ischaemia.

Intussusception

In intussusception the proximal bowel (the 'intussusceptum') invaginates or telescopes into the distal, receiving bowel (the 'intussuscipiens'). Initially this involves the ileum invaginating into itself, but then progresses to involve the colon. Most commonly, it presents in infants or toddlers with episodic colicky abdominal pain, which may be associated with vomiting or pallor. As the disease progresses, vomiting may become bilious, resulting from intestinal obstruction. The 'classical' redcurrant jelly stool of intussusception is a late phenomenon but occult blood can often be detected earlier.[11]

In older children above 3 years of age, intussusception is usually associated with a pathological lead point such as a Meckel's diverticulum (MD) or small bowel polyp.[12] It may also complicate CF and Henoch–Schönlein purpura.

Inflammatory

Complicated acute appendicitis, Meckel's diverticulitis or inflammatory bowel disease leading to the development of an inflammatory mass may result in intestinal obstruction. This presentation usually occurs when there has been a diagnostic delay of the primary pathology, often in children under 5 years of age.

Meckel's diverticulum

This represents a remnant of the omphalo-mesenteric duct and is present in about 2% of the population.[13] For reasons that are unclear, complications of a MD are more common in males.[13] MD may lead to a bowel obstruction either as a result of acting as the lead point for an intussusception, due to an associated band adhesion with volvulus or an internal hernia, or rarely an inflammatory mass due to Meckel's diverticulitis.

Adhesions

Bowel obstruction due to adhesions is uncommon in children following abdominal surgery.[9] This is fortunate as, unlike adults, the obstruction rarely settles with non-operative intervention.

Non-surgical

A wide variety of medical conditions may occasionally present with bilious vomiting, together with a variable degree of abdominal distension. Severe gastroenteritis with prolonged vomiting, sepsis, pyloric stenosis, hypothyroidism, meconium plug syndrome and the cyclical vomiting syndrome may all lead to a clinical picture similar to intestinal obstruction.[14] Any child presenting with bilious vomiting, however, requires paediatric surgical consultation to exclude a surgical cause.

Complications

The major complication of bilious vomiting due to intestinal obstruction is the potential for intestinal ischaemia if the diagnosis is delayed. Even short periods of ischaemia may lead to loss of the normal gut barrier function and a prolonged paralytic ileus. If there has been diagnostic delay with irreversible bowel ischaemia, perforation with peritoneal contamination can occur. In cases requiring extensive resection, short-bowel syndrome can result. In unrecognised cases, overwhelming septicaemia and even death can result.[9]

Investigations

A variety of investigations may be required in the child with bilious vomiting, but should not replace a focused history, clinical examination and surgical assessment.

Haematological and biochemical investigations are often normal unless the child is moderately to severely dehydrated. Acid–base derangement may occur secondary to the volume and content of the vomitus. If there is intestinal ischaemia, there is usually a marked leucocytosis. The blood glucose level should always be checked and the urine screened for sepsis.

The initial radiological investigations should be directed towards demonstrating obstruction and include plain films of the abdomen and chest. Free gas from a perforation can be seen on an erect chest, erect abdomen or decubitus abdominal views. Fluid levels consistent with intestinal obstruction may be seen on an erect or decubitus abdominal film, but can be normal and may occasionally occur in medical causes of bilious vomiting. Dilated small bowel is identified by the presence of the valvulae conniventes of Kirkring passing across the entire lumen, as opposed to the incomplete haustral markings in the colon. In neonates, these markings are usually not visible. There may be features to suggest intussusception (see Chapter 7.1 on Abdominal pain).

The use of further investigations will be directed by the likely pathology and surgical consultation. Contrast studies, either upper or lower, may be both diagnostic of the surgical cause and in the case of intussusception, potentially therapeutic, although now generally replaced by the safer air enema.[8,11] Ultrasound (US) has a limited role in the investigation of bilious vomiting, but may be useful as a screening tool in children with suspected intussusception and the detection of pathological lead points.[15] Whilst malrotation may be diagnostic of malrotation, it cannot be relied upon to exclude the diagnosis.[16]

Treatment

The treatment of intestinal obstruction in children involves analgesia, fluid and electrolyte resuscitation and definitive surgical management.

The child should be fasted. Neonates and infants require a warm environment to ensure temperature stability. Often large volumes of fluid have been lost from the intravascular space and 10–20 mL kg^{-1} fluid boluses of crystalloid solution may be required to treat shock. In addition, calculated maintenance and deficit fluid using half-strength normal saline with dextrose should be given. A gastric tube, at least 10 or 12F in size should be placed and regularly aspirated to decompress the stomach. Ongoing fluid losses should be charted and replaced on a mL for mL basis with intravenous normal saline. Hypokalaemia, if present, needs to be treated appropriately (see Chapter 10.5 on fluids and electrolytes). If required, intravenous analgesia should be given in the form of morphine 100 mcg kg^{-1} per dose and titrated to the response of the patient.

Most surgical causes of bilious vomiting will require operative treatment following further investigation.[9] Although adhesive obstruction may initially be treated non-operatively by a 24 to 48 hour period of gut rest, only rarely is this effective in children.

Controversies

❶ Radiological diagnosis of malrotation. False positives and negatives may occur with both contrast studies and US assessment.[17] Ultimately the clinician needs to make an assessment based on the patient's signs and symptoms in conjunction with information obtained from radiological studies.

❷ The role of laparoscopy in the assessment of small bowel obstruction in children.[18] There may be a role for laparoscopy as the first manoeuvre in the operative management of children with adhesive intestinal obstruction.

References

1. Dalla Vecchia LK, Grosfeld JL, West KW, et al. Intestinal atresia and stenosis: A 25-year experience with 277 cases. *Arch Surg* 1998;**133**:490–7.
2. Grosfeld JL, Rescorla FJ. Duodenal atresia and stenosis: Reassessment of treatment and outcome based on antenatal diagnosis, pathologic variance and long-term follow-up. *World J Surg* 1993;**17**:301–309.
3. Paidas CN, Pena A. Rectum and anus. In: Oldham KT, Colombani PM, Foglia RP, editors. *Surgery of infants and children: Scientific principles and practice.* Philideliphia: Lippincott-Raven Publishers; 1997. p. 1323–62.
4. Fakhoury K, Durie PR, Levison H, Canny GJ. Meconium ileus in the absence of cystic fibrosis. *Arch Dis Child* 1992;**67**:1204–1206.
5. Russell MB, Russell CA, Niebuhr E. An epidemiological study of Hirschsprung's disease and additional anomalies. *Acta Paediatr* 1994;**83**:68–71.
6. Kleinhaus S, Boley SJ, Sheran M, et al. Hirschsprung's disease: A survey of members of the surgical section of the American Academy of Paediatrics. *J Pediatr Surg* 1979;**14**:588–97.
7. Goldberg E. An epidemiological study of Hirschsprung's disease. *Int J Epidemiol* 1984;**13**:479–85.
8. Rowe MI, O'Neill JA, Grosfeld JL, et al. Rotational anomalies and volvulus. In: Rowe MI, O'Neill JA, Grosfeld JL, Fonkalsrud EW, Coran AG, editors. *Essentials of paediatric surgery.* St Louis: Mosby; 1995. p. 492–500.
9. Madonna MB, Boswell WC, Arensman RM. Outcomes. *Semin Pediatr Surg* 1997;**6**(2):105–11.
10. Powell DM, Otherson HB, Smith CD. Malrotation of the intestine in children: The effect of age in presentation and therapy. *J Pediatr Surg* 1989;**24**:777–80.
11. Losek JD, Fiete RL. Intussusception and the diagnostic value of testing stool for occult blood. *Am J Emerg Med* 1991;**9**:1–3.
12. Ong NT, Beasley SW. The leadpoint in intussusception. *J Pediatr Surg* 1990;**25**:640–3.
13. St-Vil D, Brandt ML, Panic S, et al. Meckel's diverticulum in children: A 20-year review. *J Paediatr Surg* 1991; **26**:1289–92.
14. Li BUK, Balint JP. Cyclic vomiting syndrome: Evolution in our understanding of a brain-gut disorder. *Adv Pediatr* 2000;**47**:117–60.
15. Bhisitkul DM, Listernick R, Shkolnik A, et al. Clinical application of ultrasonography in the diagnosis of intussusception. *J Pediatr* 1992;**121**:182–6.
16. Millar AJW, Rode H, Cywes S. Malrotation and volvulus in infancy and childhood. *Semin Pediatr Surg* 2003; **12**:229–36.
17. Dilley AV, Pereira J, Shi ECP, et al. The radiologist says malrotation: Does the surgeon operate? *Pediatr Surg Int* 2000;**16**:45–9.
18. Holcomb GW. Preface. *Semin Pediatr Surg* 2002;**11**:19.

7.6 Ingested foreign bodies

Scott Pearson

ESSENTIALS

1 Foreign bodies in the stomach or intestines are expected to pass spontaneously about 99% of the time if the child has normal anatomy.

2 Most complications occur when a foreign body is lodged in the oesophagus but a significant number of these will pass spontaneously.

3 Children who ingest a metallic foreign body and attend an ED should have X-ray localisation of the object. For coin ingestions, an alternative is localisation with a hand held metal detector.

4 Removal of disc batteries lodged in the oesophagus should occur urgently as mucosal injury can occur within a few hours.

Introduction

Ingestion of foreign (non-food) material is common in early childhood and often goes undetected whilst the child is playing and may not prompt a physician visit. The exact frequency of reported foreign body ingestions is uncertain. The literature in this field can be divided into three areas: descriptive studies of fairly large numbers of ingestion cases; studies primarily or exclusively about coin ingestion; and studies about disc batteries.[1] Common foreign bodies ingested that come to medical attention include coins, bones (fish, chicken), other metallic objects (pins, screws, keys, batteries), and plastic and rubber foreign bodies. In one large series of 1265 reported cases of foreign-body ingestions, age ranged from 7 months to 16 years with a mean of 5.2 years.[2] Most foreign bodies pass through the gastrointestinal tract without complications. The emergency physician should be aware of the few instances when emergent or semi-urgent intervention is indicated. Parents need to have clear guidelines regarding the treatment plan for children who are discharged to outpatient follow up.

History

In most instances, a thorough history can be obtained from parents or caregivers before a requirement for intervention. The nature of the ingested item is obviously imperative, as is the time of ingestion. The ingestion may have been witnessed or may have been reported (by an older child) or implied by the child's environment at the onset of symptomatology. It can be extremely useful if a replica of the foreign body can be easily obtained, especially in determining the type and size of disc batteries. Determining the immediate environment of the child at the time of ingestion can assist in revealing the possibility of any likely co-ingestants.

The symptoms experienced by the child since ingestion help determine the likely site of the foreign body but this has limitations. Many children are asymptomatic at presentation, which usually (but not always) suggests that the foreign body is lying in the stomach or more distal part of the gastrointestinal tract. Symptoms of vomiting, pain or discomfort on swallowing, drooling, irritability and refusal to take food or fluids may occur and suggest oesophageal foreign body. Several reports note that some children will be asymptomatic with foreign bodies lodged in the oesophagus, especially the distal oesophagus.[3,4] Even in the context of sharp fishbones, a prospective study found that symptoms were a poor predictor of the presence of fishbones, except for a sharp pricking sensation on swallowing.[5] Reports of abdominal pain or blood in the bowel motions should be noted. A history of previous oesophageal or other gastrointestinal disease is significant in determining a management plan and alerting one to potential complications. Significant developmental/

intellectual delay has been associated with major morbidity and mortality after foreign body ingestion.[2,6] This is often due to the vague symptomatology and delay in presentation.

Examination

For the majority of children the foreign body will have negotiated the oesophagus and general examination will be unremarkable. Vital signs should be recorded but once again are unlikely to be abnormal unless there is delayed presentation and the development of a complication.

Palpation of the abdomen will usually be normal. If the history alerts one to abdominal symptoms, the examiner may find localised tenderness or peritonism suggestive of intestinal perforation. This is rare.

Some children will have symptoms of proximal oesophageal or pharyngeal foreign body. In the older child or adolescent where this is due to bony ingestion (e.g. fish or chicken) there should be a careful examination of the oral cavity and pharynx by either indirect or direct laryngoscopy. Younger children are unlikely to co-operate with these procedures without sedation and an experienced examiner.

Investigations

All children with a history of ingestion of coins or batteries (or other radio-opaque foreign bodies) should have an X-ray performed to localise the foreign body. There is some controversy on this issue in relation to the need for X-rays in children who have ingested coins. Some authors (mainly hospital-based) note that even previously healthy children can be asymptomatic with an oesophageal coin and advocate early removal of oesophageal coins to prevent serious sequelae.[3,4] Other authors (notably in primary care) believe that routine X-rays in children having ingested a coin are unnecessary given that asymptomatic coin ingestion is rarely, if ever, associated with complications in otherwise healthy children.[7] It has been recognised that those patients presenting to an emergency department (ED) are a selected group and would be expected to have greater severity of symptoms and higher frequency of complications.[8] Hence the recommendation that all children with a history of coin ingestion *who attend* an ED, should have X-ray localisation of the coin performed. An alternative approach for coin ingestions is the use of a handheld metal detector for localisation of the coin. Several authors have confirmed the safety of this approach following a clear algorithm. Handheld metal detectors are not reliable at detecting metal foreign bodies other than coins.[9,10] If the ingestion is unwitnessed and the object looks like a coin on anteroposterior X-ray, be aware that a disc battery may have a similar appearance. In this situation, an additional lateral view will reveal an asymmetry, as the two sides of the disc battery have slightly different diameters. On the anteroposterior view one may also see the 'double ring' of both circumferences of the battery.

Treatment

Coins

Coins that reach the stomach almost always pass through the gastrointestinal tract without incident and further management is unnecessary unless symptoms arise. Coins that lodge in the oesophagus and have been unrecognised can cause complications such as oesophageal perforation, mediastinitis, acquired tracheo-oesophageal or aorto-oesophageal fistula formation – and death has been reported.[11] All children who are symptomatic should have a procedure to remove the coin. Asymptomatic children with proximal or middle-oesophageal coins should also have the coin removed as it is unlikely to pass spontaneously (20–30% in one series).[3] If there is a significant delay before the procedure (of more than a few hours) the X-ray should be repeated to ensure that spontaneous passage into the stomach has not occurred or a metal detector should be used to check if the position has clearly changed. Asymptomatic children with distal oesophageal coins can safely be observed as outpatients (depending on social circumstances) for 12–24 hours. The chance of spontaneous passage into the stomach has been reported to occur in 37–60% of patients.[3,4]

Glucagon has been found to be ineffective when studied prospectively in the management of oesophageal coins. Children should be referred to a specialist with expertise in paediatric endoscopy for endoscopic removal under appropriate sedation or anaesthesia. This may require transfer of the child to another institution, as local resources dictate. Other techniques have been described, such as oesophageal bougienage or Foley catheter extraction, but most emergency physicians will not manage sufficient children with this problem to develop expertise and appropriate safety of the procedure.

Disc batteries

Disc batteries are used for hearing aids, electronic devices and children's toys and cause tissue destruction due to their alkaline nature when in contact with moist membranes. Two deaths have been reported in the literature in situations of oesophageal batteries in children with delayed presentations.[12] Children with a history of possible ingestion of a disc battery should have an urgent X-ray performed. If the battery is lodged in the oesophagus, removal should be performed on an emergent basis because mucosal injury can occur in a few hours. Litovitz and Schmitz studied 2382 cases of battery ingestion over 7 years (97% were disc batteries) which were reported to a national registry.[13] There were only two major adverse outcomes, both occurring in children with oesophageal batteries. There were no deaths. There were 16 children with oesophageal disc batteries. In 88.3% the battery passed through the gastrointestinal tract with no symptoms or minor symptoms only. In 8.4% there were unrelated or unknown symptoms. As few as 3.1% of patients suffered moderate symptoms (defined as more pronounced or multiple episodes of nausea, vomiting, fever, bloody stools or emesis or changes in vital signs). Forty-four patients had arrested transit defined as identical non-oesophageal site on successive X-rays 48 hours apart: 17 in stomach; two in small intestine; 16 in the colon; and in nine at unidentified sites. Although more patients had minor or moderate symptoms in this group, none had major adverse effects. Outcome was more severe when there was arrested transit in the stomach. Battery transit time was known for 1366 patients. For the great majority (86.4%) the battery passed through the gastrointestinal tract in 96 hours.

Recommendations for ingested disc batteries are:

- All oesophageal batteries to be removed urgently by endoscopy.
- Asymptomatic children with subdiaphragmatic batteries can be observed at home with appropriate instructions to return if symptoms develop. It would seem reasonable to repeat an X-ray at 4 days and thereafter as required to detect the small group where arrested transit has occurred.
- Symptomatic children with subdiaphragmatic batteries should have surgical consultation to consider surgical or endoscopic removal of the battery, particularly if the battery case has split open or is not progressing along the gastrointestinal tract on sequential X-rays.[1]

Other metallic foreign bodies

Foreign bodies should be localised by X-ray and removed if lodged in the oesophagus. Other objects, including pins, needles and other sharp objects can be safely observed on an outpatient basis, with intervention occurring only if symptoms develop. In certain situations, where the object is lodged in the stomach, it may be appropriate to repeat an X-ray to ensure passage into the intestine. In many situations repeat X-rays are unnecessary unless symptoms develop. A more cautious approach is advisable when there is abnormal gastrointestinal anatomy.

Non-metallic foreign bodies

Sharp foreign material such as fish or chicken bones will usually impact in the pharynx or oral cavity and are considered elsewhere. X-rays may assist in localisation but many foreign bodies are not radio-opaque. Intervention is dictated by the presence or persistence of symptoms. The vast majority of other objects pass through uneventfully. Plastic bread-bag tags have been associated with small bowel obstruction and perforation. If there are symptoms of lodgement in the oesophagus the foreign body should be removed by gastroscopy, otherwise an observant approach is adequate, with the parents or caregiver receiving clear advice on when to return to the hospital.

Disposition

Most children will be managed in the ED and discharged. Some will be asked to return for further X-ray imaging but many will be advised to return only if symptoms or complications develop. Where admission is required this should be to a facility that is skilled in the endoscopic and surgical management of these children.

Prevention

Together with child-proofing the home to ensure that children are protected from access to potential poisons, this should extend to protection from small items that pre-school-age children can ingest. Great care should be exercised in relation to disc (button) batteries.

Controversies

Methods of removal of oesophageal coins/ batteries. There are some advocates of Foley catheter removal or oesophageal bougienage by emergency physicians or surgeons. Most centres utilise endoscopic removal by trained endoscopists.

References

1. Brown L, Dannenberg B. A literature-based approach to the identification and management of paediatric foreign bodies. *Pediatr Emerg Med Rep* 2002;**7**:19.
2. Cheng W, Tam PKH. Foreign body ingestion in children: experience with 1265 cases. *J Pediatr Surg* 1999;**34**:1472–6.
3. Soprano JV, Fleisher GR, Mandl KD. The spontaneous passage of esophageal coins in children. *Arch Pediatr Adolesc Med* 1999;**153**:1073–6.
4. Connors GP, Chamberlain JM, Ochsenschlager DW. Symptoms and spontaneous passage of esophageal coins. *Arch Pediatr Adolesc Med* 1995;**149**:36–9.
5. Ngan JH, Fok PJ, Lai EC, et al. A prospective study on fishbone ingestion. Experience of 358 patients. *Ann Surg* 1990;**211**:459–62.
6. Gilchrist BF, Valerie EP, Nguyen M, et al. Pearls and perils in the management of prolonged, peculiar penetrating esophageal foreign bodies in children. *J Pediatr Surg* 1977;**32**:1429–31.
7. Connors GP, Chamberlain JM, Weiner PR. Paediatric coin ingestion: a home based survey. *Am J Emerg Med* 1995;**13**:638–40.
8. Paul RI, Christoffel KK, Binns HJ, et al. Foreign body ingestions in children: risk of complication varies with site of initial health care contact. *Paediatrics* 1993;**91**:121–7.
9. Seikel K, Primm PA, Elizondo BJ, et al. Handheld metal detector localisation of ingested metallic foreign bodies. *Arch Pediatr Adolesc Med* 1999;**153**:853–7.
10. Lee JB, Ahmad S, Gale CP. Detection of coins ingested by children using a handheld metal detector: a systematic review. *Emerg Med J* 2005;**22**:839–44.
11. Byard RW, Moore L, Bourne AJ. Sudden and unexpected death: a late effect of occult intraesophageal foreign body. *Pediatr Pathol* 1990;**10**:837–41.
12. Blatnik DS, Toohill RJ, Lehman RH. Fatal complication from an alkaline battery foreign body in the esophagus. *Ann Otol Rhinol Laryngol* 1977;**86**:611–5.
13. Litovitz T, Schmitz BF. Ingestion of cylindrical and button batteries: an analysis of 2382 cases. *Paediatrics* 1992;**89**:747–57.

7.7 Hepatic failure

David Krieser

ESSENTIALS

1 Acute liver failure implies evidence of hepatocellular failure. Synthetic and metabolic processes may be affected.

2 Acute liver failure is a rare but serious problem in the paediatric population.

3 Many aetiologies require consideration: infectious, toxin-mediated, congenital (structural or metabolic) or infiltrative (malignancy, storage disease).

4 Infectious hepatitis is the most common cause worldwide, paracetamol toxicity the most common in the developed world.

5 Clinical information is vital to target appropriate investigation and treatment.

6 Management is largely supportive, and aims to maintain homeostasis until hepatic recovery or transplantation occurs.

7 Liaison with and transport to a paediatric liver transplantation centre is usually required. Consultation should occur early.

Introduction

Acute liver failure (ALF) is a rare but devastating presentation in children. The major functions of the liver include synthetic and metabolic functions. Synthetic functions include production of coagulation factors and albumin, while metabolic functions include: glucose metabolism, and waste product processing (e.g. bilirubin, nitrogenous compounds, drug elimination). ALF in children may be due to many causes (Table 7.7.1). The manifestations of coagulopathy, hypoglycaemia, jaundice, encephalopathy and hypoalbuminaemia reflect common disturbances of liver function.[1] ALF may be an immediate life-threatening process or a subacute process, with a spectrum of severity between those extremes. Medical management is multifaceted and focuses on supporting vital functions while hepatic recovery occurs or liver transplantation can be performed.

ALF has been defined in adults by clinical and laboratory criteria:

❶ Hepatocellular dysfunction (jaundice, coagulopathy, etc.) of rapid onset, and
❷ Encephalopathy within 8 weeks of jaundice.

The Pediatric Acute Liver Failure Study Group[2] has defined ALF in children as:

❶ Biochemical evidence of liver injury (usually less than 8 weeks' duration)
❷ No history of known chronic liver disease
❸ Coagulopathy not corrected with vitamin K
❹ International normalised ratio (INR) greater than 1.5 if accompanied by encephalopathy or INR greater than 2 if not accompanied by encephalopathy.

Table 7.7.1 Aetiology of liver failure

Neonates and infants		Older children	
Cholestasis	Biliary atresia	Infection: viral	Hepatitis A–D
	Choledochal cyst		Enteroviruses
	Intrahepatic bile duct paucity (Alagille's syndrome)		EBV
	Inspissated bile syndrome		Varicella
Idiopathic neonatal hepatitis			Adenovirus
Cystic fibrosis			CMV
Endocrine	Hypopituitarism		Herpes simplex
	Hypothyroidism		Rubella
Neonatal		Infection: bacterial	Listeria
haemochromatosis			Tuberculosis
Infection: viral	CMV		
	Herpes simplex	Infection: parasitic	Toxoplasma
	virus/HHV 6/VZV		
	EBV	Toxins and drugs	
	Parvovirus	Malignancy	Leukaemic infiltration
	Rubella		Lymphoma
	Reovirus type 3		Neuroblastomaa
	Adenovirus		Primary hepatic tumours
	Enterovirus		
		Wilson's disease	
Infection: bacterial	Bacterial sepsis	Hepatic venous occlusion	
	Urinary tract infection	Fatty liver	Obesity
	Tuberculosis		Pregnancy
	Syphilis	Hepatic hypoperfusion	Cardiogenic shock
Infection: parasitic	Toxoplasma		Hypovolaemic shock
Metabolic disease	Peroxisome function abnormality (Zellweger's)		Septic shock
	α_1-Antitrypsin deficiency		
	Bile acid metabolism		
	Urea cycle abnormalities		
	Amino acid metabolism abnormalities		
	Lipid metabolism abnormalities (Gaucher, Wolman, Niemann–Pick C)		
	Carbohydrate metabolism abnormalities (galactosaemia, fructosaemia, type IV glycogen storage disease)		
Toxins	Paracetamol		
	TPN		
	Hypervitaminosis A		
Tumour	Intra- and extra-hepatic		

HHV, human herpesvirus; VZV, varicella zoster virus.
Source: Modified from D'Agata ID, Balistreri WF 1999. Paediatrics in Review 20(11): 376–389.

This definition has been developed because the identification of encephalopathy, especially in infants and young children, can be very difficult. In addition, the onset of the illness may not be clear, particularly in metabolic disorders. For children with chronic liver disease who present with features of ALF, management principles are similar, although where specific therapy is available for an underlying disease then this should be considered as well.

ALF classification, using the time interval between the onset of jaundice and encephalopathy, has aetiological and prognostic importance (Table 7.7.2), despite the difficulties in identifying encephalopathy mentioned above. O'Grady et al[3,4] and Poddar et al[5] found that, in comparison with patients suffering acute or subacute liver

Table 7.7.2 Classification of ALF

Interval between onset of jaundice and encephalopathy	Classification
7 days or less	Hyperacute
8 to 28 days	Acute
5 to 12 weeks	Subacute

failure, those with hyperacute liver failure had a better prognosis.

Aetiology

Table 7.7.1 demonstrates the variety of diagnoses that may cause ALF in children. The aetiology can be grouped according to onset prior to or after the first year of life. In broad terms, infection, immune dysregulation, toxicity (including medication), infiltration, and inborn errors of metabolism are the causative pathways that may lead to ALF. Cases where the cause is not determined predominate in children under 3 years.

Neonates and infants

In the neonatal population, the estimated incidence of liver disease is approximately 1:2500. Biliary atresia and neonatal idiopathic hepatitis contribute 60% of all cases of cholestasis. In 80 infants under 12 months with ALF, inherited metabolic conditions were responsible for 42.5% of cases: neonatal haemochromatosis 16%, acute viral hepatitis 15%, and miscellaneous causes (toxins, autoimmune, malignancy) 10%. 16% of neonatal cases were undetermined.[6] Metabolic causes of liver failure include: disorders of the mitochondrial electron transport chain; disorders of protein, carbohydrate and lipid metabolism; and inherited causes of cholestasis.

Infectious hepatitis

Worldwide, infectious hepatitis is the greatest cause of ALF. Five RNA viruses (hepatitis A, C, D, E and G) and one DNA virus (hepatitis B) can infect the liver. Transmission of A and E is via the faecal-oral route. The remainder are transmitted via body fluids. Acute viral hepatitis is a clinical syndrome with systemic symptoms occurring after a virus-dependent incubation period. Jaundice ensues after hepatocyte necrosis reduces the liver's capacity to metabolise bilirubin. Fulminant hepatitis occurs in less than 1% of children with hepatitis A and in 1–2% of cases of hepatitis B. Fulminant disease occurs with hepatitis D in approximately 10% of cases and is more likely with super-infection. Hepatitis C can cause acute and chronic infection and rarely fulminant hepatitis. Severe acute hepatitis E infection is a leading cause of ALF in the tropics. Epstein–Barr virus (EBV), cytomegalovirus (CMV), herpes simplex virus, varicella zoster virus, human herpesvirus 6 and parvovirus B-19 are non-hepatotropic viruses that can rarely cause ALF. Consideration of, and investigation for, these viruses is important because specific therapy with antiviral medication is available for some of these pathogens.[7]

Toxins and medication

Paracetamol

Paracetamol toxicity is the most common cause of ALF in the developed world. Paracetamol is an analgesic and antipyretic freely available in many countries. It is metabolised by the hepatocyte and toxicity exhausts hepatic glutathione stores. Generation of toxic metabolites leads to centrilobular necrosis. Toxicity is unlikely with single doses under 150 mg kg^{-1}. Children are often given multiple doses of paracetamol and this can lead to toxicity if the cumulative daily dose is greater than 60 mg kg^{-1} day^{-1}. Factors predictive of hepatotoxicity include: age (lower incidence in children under 5), genetics (cytochrome isoenzyme polymorphisms are inherited), alcohol and tobacco use (relevant in adolescents), other medications and nutritional status.[8] Treatment of toxicity is discussed elsewhere in the text.

Anticonvulsants

Genetic predisposition has been purported for anticonvulsant induced hepatotoxicity.[2] Sodium valproate causes intracellular fat accumulation within the hepatocyte, and may be related to a primary defect of respiratory chain enzyme function.[2] Impaired metabolic functions within the cell may lead to necrosis. Children under 2 years and those on multiple medications are at highest risk. Carbamazepine may cause hepatitis and/or cholestasis during the first months of therapy. Clinically significant hepatotoxicity is rare.

Total parenteral nutrition

The aetiology of TPN-associated liver disease is largely unknown. The associations of sepsis, surgery, and other medications, which often co-exist, cannot be ignored as possible aetiological agents. This form of liver dysfunction will present in the intensive-care setting rather than the emergency department (ED).

Aspirin and Reye's syndrome

Mitochondrial dysfunction leading to acute encephalopathy, selective hepatic dysfunction and visceral fatty infiltration has been called Reye's syndrome.[9] Metabolic disorders have been later identified in some children initially diagnosed with Reye's syndrome. Mitochondrial oxidative phosphorylation and fatty acid β-oxidation are the metabolic pathways affected in Reye's syndrome. Preceding viral infection (classically varicella), immune mediators and aspirin (or its metabolites) all can limit normal functioning of these pathways. The association of aspirin with this disorder remains unclear despite a study by Forsyth et al,[10] which identified a dose–response relationship, and population studies that demonstrate that the decline in Reye's syndrome mirrors a decline in aspirin usage.[9,11]

Metabolic diseases associated with liver failure

Zellweger's syndrome (cerebrohepatorenal syndrome)

Autosomal recessive inheritance of this peroxisomal abnormality leads to abnormal bile acid synthesis, and abnormal fatty-acid oxidation. Multiorgan involvement (cardiac, pulmonary, neurological, renal) with failure to thrive and hypotonia are major early features. Jaundice occurs in 50% of cases. Therapy has not been shown to prolong life although histological improvement may occur on liver biopsy. Biopsy demonstrates abnormal mitochondria and absent peroxisomes. More information can be found at http://www.ncbi.nlm.nih.gov/omim/214100.

α$_1$-Antitrypsin deficiency

Approximately 1:4000 live births are affected by this autosomal recessive disorder. Cholestasis in the neonatal period, in the context of intrauterine growth retardation, hepatomegaly and failure to thrive is suggestive of this disease. Coagulopathy may occur in 2% of such infants and is usually responsive to vitamin K. Phenotyping of protease inhibitor (Pi) by isoelectric focus classifies children as: Pi ZZ (most commonly associated with liver disease), Pi SZ, Pi SS, Pi FZ and MZ (carrier state). Up to 50% of children with Pi ZZ will develop chronic hepatic failure leading to transplantation after development of cirrhosis. Bronchiectasis is rare in children. Liver transplantation will lead to functional restoration and phenotypic cure.

Tyrosinaemia

Linked to a gene on chromosome 15, tyrosinaemia is an autosomal recessive condition due to deficiency of fumarylacetoacetase which is the last enzyme in the processing of phenylalanine (pathway available at http://www.ncbi.nlm.nih.gov/omim/Images/tyrosine.html). This autosomal recessive disorder is characterised by progressive liver parenchymal damage and renal tubulopathy with generalised aminoaciduria. It is particularly common in parts of Quebec. Rapid progression may occur in infancy or an indolent course leading to hepatic cell carcinoma may occur in up to 37% of those over 2 years.

Galactosaemia

Occurring in approximately 1 in 40 000 live births, and inherited in an autosomal recessive fashion, this deficiency of galactose-1-phosphate uridyl-transferase leads to accumulation of galactose-1-phosphate in liver, brain and renal tubules. It is due to an abnormality on chromosome 9. Clinically these infants may present with progressive jaundice, hepatic failure, hypoglycaemia or cataracts. Multifactorial encephalopathy (hypoglycaemia, liver failure) may be present. These babies have an increased susceptibility to sepsis, especially due to Gram-negative organisms. This disorder is part of the routine newborn screening program and prenatal diagnosis is available via chorionic villus sampling. Treatment is via dietary control.

Wilson's disease

An autosomal recessive gene defect leads to this disorder of copper metabolism that occurs in 1:30 000 live births, linked to a gene locus on chromosome 13. Symptoms include: hepatic dysfunction (ALF, chronic active liver disease, insidious progression to cirrhosis), neuropsychiatric symptoms (behavioural disturbance, tremor, dysarthria, drooling and deteriorating school performance) renal tubulopathy, haemolysis and hormonal changes. Kayser–Fleischer rings are brown bands seen at the cornea–iris border. Low serum caeruloplasmin and high serum copper with high urinary copper characterise the laboratory abnormalities.

Alagille's syndrome

This autosomal dominant condition leads to intrahepatic biliary hypoplasia in association with cardiac, renal, ocular, facial and skeletal abnormalities. Alagille's syndrome has an incidence of 1:100 000 live births and is associated with abnormalities of chromosome 20. Peripheral pulmonary arterial stenosis, with or without pulmonary valvular stenosis, is the most common cardiac defect. Vertebral anomalies described as 'butterfly vertebrae' constitute the most common skeletal defect. Retinal pigmentation and posterior embryotoxon (requiring slit lamp examination) are present in the eye. The facies are 'triangular' with a broad forehead and a pointed mandible. Failure to thrive and jaundice are common presentations. Hepatic cirrhosis can develop in up to 50% of children.

Biliary atresia

Complete absence of all extrahepatic biliary structures is the usual malformation, leading to a clinical picture of jaundice, pale (acholic) stools and dark urine due to cholestasis.

A choledochal cyst may present in identical fashion and may co-exist with biliary atresia. Presentation is usually with prolonged neonatal jaundice or delayed onset of jaundice (age 2–3 weeks). This occurs in approximately 1:10 000 to 1:20 000 live births, with equal gender incidence. Following diagnostic testing (ultrasonography, nuclear medicine scan, occasionally liver biopsy), management is by surgical hepatoportoenterostomy (Kasai procedure) prior to 8 weeks of age, if possible, as earlier surgery improves outcomes.[12]

Mushrooms

Edible and inedible mushrooms can be difficult to distinguish. *Amanita phalloides* produces amatoxin, which is hepatotoxic. The toxin is a heat stable octapeptide. After a period of 6–48 hours the affected patient will start vomiting, complain of abdominal pain, develop diarrhoea, before neurological symptoms (coma, seizures) and hepatic failure commence, with a mortality of up to 30%. Cholinergic symptoms via muscarinic receptors may also occur and respond to atropine. Charcoal should be given to reduce absorption. Silibinin and high-dose penicillin G may assist in limiting hepatic damage.[13] Identification of the mushroom is important and may require referral to local botanists or mycologists.

Pathophysiology

Exposure to hepatotoxic agents such as: drugs, products of metabolism or infectious particles, in addition to immune responses, initiates hepatocyte injury that may progress to necrosis. Biopsy, when performed, reveals multilobular or bridging necrosis with reticulin framework collapse. Patterns related to aetiology can be seen, such as centrilobular necrosis in paracetamol toxicity or with circulatory shock. When normal regenerative processes do not occur, liver failure follows.[14] Astrocyte oedema may be seen and may be due to altered cell wall permeability, glutamate, ammonia, and neurotransmitter balance.[15]

Hepatic encephalopathy occurs through the interplay of three factors:

❶ Reduction in synthesis of substances essential for normal brain function;

❷ Production of substances that are neurotoxic; and

❸ Reduced elimination of neurotoxins.

Contributions from ammonia, inflammatory cytokines, benzodiazepine-like compounds and manganese[16] lead to neuronal dysfunction and altered interaction of astrocytes with neurons. This leads to the clinical manifestations of hepatic encephalopathy. The balance of inhibitory (e.g. GABA) versus excitatory (e.g. glutamate) neurotransmission is altered in hepatic encephalopathy.[9] Ammonia appears to augment inhibitory neurotransmission. In addition, the role of sepsis, either via systemic immune response[17] or via lipopolysaccharides directly,[18] hypoglycaemia and raised intracranial pressure is important in the development of encephalopathy.

Presentation

History

History and examination findings are significantly influenced by the age of the child. Neonates may present with jaundice and care must be taken to differentiate physiological jaundice or 'breast milk' jaundice from pathological jaundice. The presence of acholic (pale) stools is characteristic of cholestasis. Investigation (see below) will be directed at identifying the cause of cholestasis. Jaundice in the context of dysmorphic features, cardiac murmur and ocular abnormalities suggest Alagille's syndrome. The development of jaundice after a change in diet may suggest metabolic abnormalities of carbohydrate metabolism such as galactosaemia or hereditary fructose intolerance.

Infants and older children may present with a history of loss of appetite, vomiting, fevers, or abdominal pain, prior to the development of jaundice. Infectious hepatitis (e.g. hepatitis A, EBV or CMV) is the most likely cause in this situation. EBV infection may be suggested by a history of sore throat and lymphadenopathy. A dietary and travel history for hepatitis A may be relevant. Hepatitis B and C infection needs to be considered if a history of exposure is obtained. In adolescents, the use of illicit drugs and sexual activity must be explored confidentially. In areas where strict screening is performed, children who receive blood product transfusions (e.g. malignancy, renal failure, haemophilia, haemoglobinopathy) are at very low risk for the acquisition of hepatitis B and C. An infant presenting with encephalopathy and jaundice may have a metabolic disease (fatty acid oxidation, carbohydrate metabolism) and the possibility of consanguinity needs exploration. Previous surgery for a choledochal cyst or for biliary atresia is important in the context of a child presenting with jaundice and/or hepatic failure. Exposure to hepatotoxins such as paracetamol, anticonvulsants, aspirin or mushrooms must be identified, as specific treatments can be implemented. Pruritus with jaundice, dark urine and pale stools may be the presenting features of cholestasis in an older child.

Examination

Hepatomegaly and jaundice are the most frequent findings. The character of the liver edge may offer additional information: for example, a firm, nodular surface suggesting cirrhosis or fibrosis; tenderness suggesting acute hepatitis. Note that in cirrhosis liver span may be reduced. Splenomegaly suggests portal hypertension or infiltration (e.g. storage disease, extramedullary haematopoiesis, malignancy). Abdominal examination will also identify ascites if present.

As discussed above, specific diseases associated with liver failure will have other features. The phenotypes of galactosaemia, Alagille's syndrome, α_1-antitrypsin deficiency and Wilson's disease may be identified by careful clinical examination. Neurological evaluation is essential and the presence of asterixis important in a child with liver failure in order to assess for, and classify a stage of, hepatic encephalopathy, if present (Table 7.7.3). In young children

encephalopathy, which occurs late, is difficult to detect. Cutaneous features such as bruising, petechiae or bleeding may indicate an associated coagulopathy. In children with chronic liver disease there may be signs such as spider naevi, caput medusae or finger clubbing.

Investigations

Investigation of the child with hepatic failure focuses on identifying the extent of liver dysfunction and on identifying the cause. History and examination findings must guide investigation. ED screen should include a full blood examination, liver function tests including conjugated and unconjugated bilirubin, blood glucose, coagulation screen, renal function and arterial blood gases. Further potentially relevant investigations such as viral serology, copper and caeruloplasmin levels, Pi typing, lactate level, drug screens, urine metabolic screen, or imaging should be determined after discussion with a paediatric hepatologist. Note that the international normalised ratio for coagulation and the serum bilirubin concentration are not predictive of post-transplant survival, while renal dysfunction requiring dialysis is associated with a higher mortality.[14] Escudie et al[19] found a prothrombin index below 10% (INR approx 6) 4 days after *Amanita phalloides* ingestion was predictive of fatal outcome.

Management

The management of acute liver failure involves supportive care, complication management and specific treatment modalities

where they exist. Therapy needs to be initiated in the ED prior to transfer to a paediatric intensive-care environment. The initial management issues are listed in Table 7.7.4. Intubation and ventilation may be required due to coma or respiratory failure. Respiratory failure itself is multifactorial: altered cardiac output; capillary leak; possible oliguria; and significant fluid requirements contribute. Fluid management may be complex in the face of renal failure and electrolyte imbalances. Vitamin K, fresh frozen plasma or cryoprecipitate may be required to correct symptomatic coagulopathy. Intravenous fluids containing 10% dextrose or more are usually required to correct hypoglycaemia and then maintain normoglycaemia. Lactulose is given in hepatic encephalopathy to reduce absorption of nitrogenous wastes. Neomycin and/or metronidazole, given enterally, reduce the enteric bacterial load and the production of nitrogenous wastes. Proton pump inhibitors, H_2-receptor blockers and/or sucralfate are given to limit the risk of gastric ulceration in the context of coagulopathy. Sepsis is a common and serious complication, and will exacerbate liver failure and requires aggressive antimicrobial management. Raised intracranial pressure and, more specifically, reduced cerebral perfusion pressure are important complications of ALF. Both these effects may be improved by therapeutic cooling. Therapeutic cooling (32–33°C) reduces brain energy metabolism, normalises cerebral blood flow, reduces ammonia delivery, reduces oxidative pressure on astrocytes and reduces brain glutamate.[14]

A bridge to liver transplantation may be created via the use of liver support devices. These have not undergone extensive testing as yet. Artificial systems using filtration,

Table 7.7.3 Stages of hepatic encephalopathy		I	II	III	IV	
					IV a	IV b
Symptoms		Lethargy, euphoria, poor concentration	Drowsiness, erratic behaviour, disorientation	Stuporous but rousable, incoherent speech	Responsive to pain	No response
Signs		Reduced cognitive performance (drawing figures, memory)	Asterixis, incontinence, fetor hepaticus	Asterixis, hyper-reflexia, rigidity	No asterixis, areflexia, flaccidity	
EEG		Normal	Generalised slowing, theta waves	Markedly abnormal, triphasic waves	Markedly abnormal bilateral slowing, delta waves, cortical silence	

Source: Modified from Suchy FJ 2000. Fulminant hepatic failure. In Behrman RE (ed). Nelson Textbook of Pediatrics, 16 edn.

Table 7.7.4 Initial management tasks	
Management tasks	
Observation of:	Vital signs Pulse oximetry Level of consciousness Urine output (may need indwelling catheter)
Monitoring of:	ECG Blood glucose Acid/base status (blood gases) Coagulation Liver function tests Serum electrolytes
Insertion of:	Vascular access (peripheral, central, intraosseous) Nasogastric tube (for gastric drainage and administration of neomycin and lactulose)
Supplementation of:	Glucose Potassium Albumin Coagulation factors (vitamin K, frozen plasma, cryoprecipitate, platelets) Oxygen (may require endotracheal intubation) Intravascular volume if required
Identification of:	Treatable cause if present (toxic, infectious, metabolic) Evolving encephalopathy Raised intracranial pressure

Table 7.7.5   The King's College criteria
Features associated with a poor prognosis
• Unknown aetiology • Toxin associated (other than paracetamol) • Age under 10 years • Age over 40 years • Jaundice for more than 1 week prior to encephalopathy • Serum bilirubin over 300 μmol L^{-1} • INR over 3.5 • pH less than 7.3 • Serum creatinine over 300 μmol L^{-1}

Source: Data from O'Grady et al 1989.
Gastroenterology 97: 439–445.

dialysis or ion exchange or bioartificial systems (human or non-human hepatocytes within an artificial framework) are available. Anecdotal reports of these systems include reduction in serum copper in Wilson's disease-induced ALF that allowed stabilisation prior to transplantation.[20]

The development of liver transplantation has allowed children with irreversible liver failure to survive. The paucity of available donors and contraindications to transplantation limit the number of children able to receive liver transplants in the acute setting. Contraindications to transplantation include: uncontrolled systemic infection; extrahepatic metastasis in liver tumours, irreversible neurological injury; and multiorgan failure. Living donor transplantation has increased the number of liver transplants in children. Auxiliary partial orthotopic transplantation allows the transplanted liver segment to function while a diseased native liver recovers and regenerates. This technique also may allow for the discontinuity of antirejection medication once the native liver recovers.[21] Disease-specific treatment is available for paracetamol toxicity. Intravenous *N*-acetylcysteine (NAC) is given in addition to supportive measures. Herpesvirus-induced fulminant hepatitis may respond to aciclovir. Children with Wilson's disease may respond to chelation therapy pending transplantation. Certain metabolic diseases can be managed through dietary manipulation or metabolic pathway manipulation.

Disposition

Management of the child with ALF requires a multidisciplinary team of physicians, nursing staff and allied health personnel in an intensive-care environment. The invasive nature of monitoring and maintaining such patients will necessitate transport to a paediatric intensive-care unit. Transportation will require stabilisation and continued monitoring of the above parameters, with intervention occurring en route if necessary. Liver transplantation will require the involvement of surgeons and anaesthetists in addition to those already involved within the paediatric intensive care unit. The transplant service should be consulted early in such cases.

Prognosis

The mortality of ALF is approximately 60%. Of children with Stage 4 hepatic encephalopathy, 80% will die. Sepsis is the cause of death in approximately 10% of children with ALF. The King's College criteria (Table 7.7.5), based on multivariate analysis of 588 patients with fulminant hepatic failure, provide clinical and laboratory parameters predictive of mortality. A single adverse factor was associated with 80% mortality; three adverse factors were associated with 95% mortality. Paracetamol toxicity was associated with a better prognosis. If paracetamol toxicity was the reason for ALF then the presence of a single adverse risk factor places mortality risk at 55%. It is important to compare these figures with the 20–30% mortality rate of all children undergoing liver transplantation.

The United Network for Organ Sharing (UNOS) has developed the Model for End-Stage Liver Disease (MELD) for patients over 12 years. The Pediatric End-Stage Liver Disease score is for patients under 12. Both assess risks of death while waiting for transplantation in order to prioritise available organs. The PELD score uses: albumin, bilirubin, INR, growth failure and age at listing (for transplantation) while the MELD score uses creatinine, bilirubin and INR in predictive modelling (www.unos.org).

Prevention

Viral hepatitis requires public health and legislative intervention to be controlled. Immunisation against hepatitis A and B, improved hygiene, reduced overcrowding and the promotion of harm-minimisation through 'safe sex' and reduction in the sharing of needles among intravenous drug users may have impacts on the incidence of viral hepatitis. Vaccines for hepatitis A and B are available but expense and distribution problems act as barriers in the developing world.

The widespread availability of paracetamol contributes to its position as the leading cause of ALF in the developed world. Limiting packet size, 'child-proofed' containers and even reducing distribution to pharmacies alone may reduce the incidence of paracetamol poisoning.

Screening of embryos or parents after the identification of a metabolic disease will assist in reducing the incidence of such diseases, if parents consider termination of pregnancy an option. Genetic counselling is mandatory in such cases. Direct gene therapy for such diseases remains elusive.

Controversies and future directions

❶ Transplantation remains the gold standard therapy and case reports of auxiliary partial orthotopic liver transplantation demonstrated that a transplanted liver lobe functioned satisfactorily until native liver recovery occurred in a case of mushroom toxicity.[22]

❷ Cerebral cooling for management of raised intracranial pressure associated with ALF may offer some benefits and requires more research.

❸ Prognostic scores have been developed according to aetiology of ALF and need more prospective research: in paracetamol hepatotoxicity, arterial pH, serum lactate and prothrombin time and creatinine; in mushroom toxicity, prothrombin time and creatinine appear more predictive. A patient with Wilson's disease requires transplantation if encephalopathy is present, although serum bilirubin, INR, aspartate aminotransferase and white cell count are important predictors of the need for transplantation. In general, predictors of poor outcome include: poor renal function, a PELD score >25, and age under 24 months and onset of encephalopathy within 7 days of onset of jaundice.[4]

References

1. D'Agata I, Balistreri W. Evaluation of liver disease in the pediatric patient. *Pediatr Rev* 1999;**20**(11):376–89.
2. Bucuvalas J, Yazigi N, Squires RH. Acute liver failure in children. *Clin Liver Dis* 2006;**10**(1):149–68.
3. O'Grady J, Schalm S, Williams R. Acute liver failure: redefining the syndromes. *Lancet* 1993;**342**(8866):273–5.
4. O'Grady J. Modern management of acute liver failure. *Clin Liver Dis* 2007;**11**(2):291–303.
5. Poddar U, Thapa B, Prasad A, et al. Natural history and risk factors in fulminant hepatic failure. *Arch Dis Child* 2002;**87**(1):54–6.
6. Durand P, Debray D, Mandel R, et al. Acute liver failure in infancy: a 14 year experience of a pediatric liver transplantation center. *J Pediatr* 2001;**139**(6):871–6.
7. Fontana R. Acute liver failure including acetaminophen overdose. *Med Clin North Am* 2008;**92**(4):761–94.
8. Larsen AM. Acetaminophen hepatotoxicity. *Clin Liver Dis* 2007;**11**(3):525–48.
9. Glasgow J, Middleton B. Reye syndrome - insights on causation and prognosis. *Arch Dis Child* 2001;**85**:351–3.
10. Forsyth BW, Horwitz RI, Acampora D, et al. New epidemiologic evidence confirming that bias does not explain the aspirin/Reye's syndrome association. *JAMA* 1989;**261**(17):2517–24.
11. Belay E, Bresee J, Holman R, et al. Reye's syndrome in the United States from 1981 through 1997. *N Engl J Med* 1999;**340**(18):1377–82.
12. Serinet M, Wildhaber B, Broue P, et al. Impact of age at Kasai operation on its results in late childhood and adolescence: a rational basis for biliary atresia screening. *Pediatrics* 2009;**123**(5):1280–6.
13. Schilsky ML, Honiden S, Arnott L, Emre S. ICU management of acute liver failure. *Clin Chest Med* 2009;**30**(1):71–87.
14. Suchy FJ. Fulminant hepatic failure. In: Kliegman R, Rudolf M, editors. *Nelson Textbook of Pediatrics*. 18th ed. Saunders; 2007.
15. Sundaram V, Shaikh O. Hepatic encephalopathy: pathophysiology and emerging therapies. *Med Clin North Am* 2009;**93**:819–36.
16. Munoz SJ. Hepatic encephalopathy. *Med Clin North Am* 2008;**92**(8):795–812.
17. Shawcross DL, Davies NA, Williams R. Systemic inflammatory response exacerbates the neuropsychological effects of induced hyperammonemia in cirrhosis. *J Hepatol* 2004;**40**:247–54.
18. Pedersen HR, Ring-Larsen H, Olsen NV. Hyperammonemia acts synergistically with lipopolysaccharide in inducing changes in cerebral hemodynamics in rats anaesthetised with pentobarbital. *J Hepatol* 2007;**47**:245–52.
19. Escudie L, Francoz C, Vinel J-P, et al. Amanita phalloides poisoning: Reasessment of prognostic factors and indications for emergency liver transplantation. *J Hepatol* 2007;**46**(3): 466–73.
20. Sen S, Felldin M, Steiner C, et al. Albumin dialysis and Molecular Adsorbents Recirculating System (MARS) for acute Wilson's disease. *Liver Transpl* 2002;**8**(10):962–7.
21. Kerkar N, Emre S. Issues unique to pediatric liver transplantation. *Clin Liver Dis* 2007;**11**(2):323–35.
22. Rosenthal P, Roberts J, Ascher N, Emond J. Auxiliary liver transplant in fulminant failure. *Paediatrics* 1997; **100**(2):E10.

GASTROENTEROLOGY AND HEPATOLOGY

7.8 Diarrhoea and vomiting

Christopher Webber

ESSENTIALS

1 'ABC fluids in and out' is a useful tool in taking a history.

2 Not all diarrhoea and vomiting is gastroenteritis.

3 Vomiting may be a non-specific symptom of a more serious medical problem.

4 The differential diagnoses are extensive.

5 Young infants with diarrhoea must be managed with caution.

Introduction

Common symptoms

Vomiting and diarrhoea are common symptoms that affect infants and children. These symptoms may occur separately or in combination. Clinicians must exercise caution when evaluating infants presenting with fever and vomiting who do not have diarrhoea, as the list of differential diagnoses is extensive, including some conditions with significant morbidity and mortality.

Frequency of presentation

By far the commonest condition causing vomiting and diarrhoea in children is gastroenteritis. A urinary-tract infection (UTI) must be considered in all infants with vomiting, with or without fever. The presence of diarrhoea makes a urine infection much less likely, and in this situation the diagnosis is more likely to be gastroenteritis.

Definitions

Vomiting is an active process involving muscular contraction expelling the stomach contents orally. In comparison, gastro-oesophageal *reflux* is the passive regurgitation of gastric contents, most commonly liquid. In the newborn and young infant gastro-oesophageal reflux is common and may be considered normal if it is not associated with consequences like pain or failure to thrive.

Diarrhoea refers to the frequency and consistency of stool being frequent, loose or liquid. The stool may also contain blood and mucous, both of which are abnormal.

Fever is present when the body's temperature is elevated above normal. Actual definitions of fever vary, but a core temperature of about 36.5–37.2°C is normal. The site used to make the measurement also affects measured temperature. Generally aural (tympanic) temperatures are less accurate. Per-axilla temperatures are lower than rectal temperatures by about 0.5–1°C. Although rectal temperatures more closely reflect the body's core temperature, per-axilla temperatures are more convenient to measure and socially acceptable to the patient. Needless to say, an infant with cardiovascular compromise and peripherally 'shutdown' should have a rectal temperature checked, as a per-axilla temperature may not accurately reflect core temperature and falsely reassure the physician.

Clinical evaluation

History
Presenting complaint and past history

Always listen to the parents or carers of the child. Generally, they know the infant or child best and physicians are unwise to ignore their concerns. Explore the symptoms further and in more detail, if necessary. Is there blood in the vomitus, or blood or mucus in the stool? Sometimes important associated symptoms are not volunteered by parents, and are only alluded to when directed by a focused history. Specific information regarding the nature and content of the vomiting and diarrhoea needs clarification. In the child with a possible infectious condition, it may be important to clarify whether there have been infectious contacts or recent overseas travel. Review of the past history should include any significant medical or surgical problems and whether the child is thriving.

ABC – fluids in and out

This schema provides a simple structure for obtaining the history, and may be used to advise parents about concerning symptoms that may develop subsequently. Alertness and activity (**A**) provides information about the neurological state of the child. Lethargy and poor interactivity are concerning symptoms in a young child. The behaviour of the baby whilst feeding is also important. Parents may note poor suck and sleepiness during feeding; and the breastfeeding mother may comment more precisely about the quality of the infant's suck. Breathing (**B**), specifically rapid or laboured breathing, and poor circulation (**C**), as indicated by mottling and coolness of the peripheries, are also worrying signs.

The child's fluid intake and urine output as a percentage of usual or normal provide very important markers of the unwell infant or child. The number and 'wetness' of the nappies is used as the indicator of urine output. Thus, using an evaluation of 'fluids in and out', one should be concerned when these are less than 50% of normal for the child.

Examination

General observation

In the absence of a life-threatening emergency it is always worthwhile to make a careful observation of the child, either whilst talking with the carer or to the child. This general observation phase is invaluable in the paediatric assessment, particularly in young children. During this observation look and listen for the following:

❶ Airway noises (stridor, sturtor, grunt or wheeze).

❷ Tachypnoea (measure the respiratory rate).

❸ Colour (centrally and peripherally, look for cyanosis and mottling).

❹ Alertness and activity (or inter-activity, particularly with child's carer[s]).

Note that the ABCD approach (airway, breathing, circulation, disability) is utilised.

Assessment of the state of hydration is critical. It is well recognised that clinicians tend to overestimate the degree of dehydration, consequently excessive amounts of intravenous fluid may be administered. Accurate premorbid and current weight may aid this assessment. The following is a revised guide for the assessment of dehydration:

- < 3% – no clinical signs; reduced urine output;
- 3% – mild dehydration; mild tachycardia, dry mucous membranes;
- 5% – moderate dehydration; lethargy, tachycardia, reduced skin turgor, sunken eyes/fontanelle;
- 10% – severe dehydration; clinical signs of shock (tachycardia, thready pulses, reduced perfusion, particularly centrally).

Always check carefully for a rash, as petechiae and purpura may be inconspicuous or subtle. Examination of the ears, nose and throat, is frequently left until the end of the examination, to avoid potential distress impairing the remainder of the examination.

Cardiovascular and respiratory status

It is important to evaluate the cardiovascular and respiratory systems in the infant with vomiting for the following reasons:

- shock may be present due to either septicaemia or fluid loss from vomiting and/or diarrhoea;
- septicaemia may be the cause of the symptoms;
- pneumonia or other respiratory infections may cause vomiting;
- effortless tachypnoea may indicate a metabolic acidosis.

The pulse rate and pulse volume may identify a rapid thready pulse indicating poor perfusion. Capillary refill is often thought to be a poor indicator of circulatory status, as the peripheral perfusion (hands and feet) may be affected by environmental temperature. The comparison of central (anterior

chest) and peripheral capillary refill, with other data like heart rate, pulse volume and consciousness state, allows an assessment of the adequacy of the circulation. The presence of shock indicates inadequate tissue perfusion. It is present when there is a rapid, thready pulse, delayed capillary refill, especially if central (>2 seconds), and abnormal neurological status including agitation, lethargy, or coma. The diagnosis of shock is not reliant on the presence of hypotension, particularly in children. Delay in identifying shock until the child is hypotensive risks severe compromise and potential progress to cardiac arrest.

Septicaemia, with or without meningitis, may cause fever, vomiting and diarrhoea. Some bacterial pathogens that cause gastroenteritis may also cause septicaemia, such as *Salmonella* and *Shigella*.

Respiratory examination of the infant with fever, cough and vomiting may identify tachypnoea and grunt that alert the clinician to the possibility of pneumonia. Grunting is an expiratory noise, usually intermittent, and generates PEEP (positive end expiratory pressure) by partially closing the glottis during expiration. Percussion note for dullness may be more valuable than auscultation for crackles or bronchial breathing. Be aware of the child with abdominal pain and grunt as they may have a lower lobe pneumonia.

Abdominal examination

The abdomen is examined for distension, tenderness and guarding. Take note of the child's resting posture and how they move spontaneously or on request, both in the bed or walking. A gentle, unrushed examination provides more information.

Presence of guarding and rebound can be elicited with gentle flexion/relaxation of the fingers of the examining hand (at the metacarpophalangeal joint). Evaluate for organomegaly – liver, spleen and kidneys. Are there any masses? The pale, vomiting child may have intussusception. Examine for anal fissures and other perianal abnormality that may indicate inflammatory bowel disease.

Neurological examination

The child may have impaired consciousness either due to systemic illness, shock or a primary neurological problem. The unwell

infant who is vomiting may have meningitis. Likewise, raised intracranial pressure (ICP) may cause vomiting. Cushing's triad includes bradycardia, hypertension and abnormal respiration, but is generally associated with a marked elevation of the ICP. On neurological examination, check for any asymmetry of movement, tone and reflexes, as a cerebral abscess may cause fever and vomiting. Focal seizures generally indicate focal pathology and should be considered the same as a focal abnormality on examination.

Temperature

Always measure the temperature of the vomiting child. If the child's circulation is compromised then consider continually monitoring the temperature with a rectal probe. The body's temperature varies over time, and in the unwell patient it is crucial to continue to monitor for fever over a period of time. Remember that some modes of measurement underestimate the core temperature or are an inaccurate reflection of the core temperature (see above). The child with overwhelming sepsis may not mount a fever and, indeed, may be hypothermic.

Differential diagnoses

This list is extensive and varies depending upon the combination of symptoms, vomiting and/or fever and/or diarrhoea, as well as the examination findings:

- gastro-oesophageal reflux;
- viral illness;
  - gastritis/enteritis;
  - non-specific, generalised viral illnesses;
- gastroenteritis – viral, bacterial;
- otitis media/URTI/tonsillitis/ pharyngitis/stomatitis;
- urinary tract infection (UTI);
- septicaemia;
- meningitis/encephalitis;
- pneumonia;
- appendicitis;
- metabolic/endocrine problems;
- intestinal obstruction including malrotation (± volvulus);
- cyclical vomiting;
- malabsorption including cows' milk protein enteropathy;
- colitis (including Crohn's disease, ulcerative colitis, pseudomembranous colitis).

The child with recurrent vomiting warrants particular attention, with consideration of diagnoses like malrotation, UTIs and cyclical vomiting. An abdominal X-ray may be helpful, but after surgical consultation an upper gastrointestinal contrast study may be required. A child thought to have cyclical vomiting should be referred to a paediatrician for follow up. Beware of children with a pre-existing condition (or 'label') such as cyclical vomiting as they may develop other acute conditions. These children require careful reconsideration at each presentation before concluding 'another vomiting episode'.

Investigations

Remember, only order tests that aid the decision making and management of the patient. Reference ranges are frequently based on the standard deviation in a population, so a result outside the range may not necessarily indicate abnormality or pathology. This may inadvertently lead the clinician to order more unnecessary tests.

Not every child who is medically assessed requires investigations. The tests required depend on the possible differential diagnoses and the severity of illness (Table 7.8.1). Don't forget simple bedside tests like urine analysis (UA) and blood

---

Table 7.8.1 Tests that may be useful in the child with vomiting or diarrhoea

Common tests:
- Urine analysis
- Urine culture
- Stool
  Microscopy, culture
  Rotavirus antigen
  Giardia (often tested by RIA, avoiding the need for multiple samples for ova and parasites)
- Biochemistry – electrolytes, urea/creatinine, blood glucose
- Full blood count

Less common tests:
- Liver function tests
- Blood gas (venous or arterial)
- Blood culture
- Amylase
- Insulin, growth hormone, cortisol (if hypoglycaemic)
- Lactate
- Urine metabolic screen
- CXR to exclude pneumonia
- AXR to exclude intestinal obstruction

AXR, abdominal X-ray; CXR, chest X-ray; RIA, radioimmunoassay.

---

glucose. This information can be invaluable in assessing the child with diarrhoea and vomiting. In this context, check the specific gravity and for ketones. Glycosuria may indicate diabetic ketoacidosis. If the UA is positive for nitrites or leucocytes, then an appropriately collected urine specimen should be cultured. The specimen to be cultured should be collected attempting to minimise contamination, even if re-collection is required.

Generally urine culture is unnecessary where acute gastroenteritis is likely (i.e. when there is diarrhoea) but is mandatory in the infant or baby with acute vomiting and fever. Urinary symptoms like dysuria and frequency can be expected in children from about 4 or 5 years of age, allowing a more selective approach to those who require urine culture. 'Bag urines' (collected in an adhesive, sterile plastic bag) have a high contamination rate and are best avoided when performing a urine culture, but are satisfactory for a simple UA. Although more difficult to collect, a 'clean catch urine' provides a sample less likely to be contaminated. This is collected with an open nappy, a poised parent, with an open sterile container, waiting patiently to 'catch' the spontaneously voided urine. Those babies and infants deemed to be at higher risk of a UTI or who are more seriously unwell may require more rapid testing by either a suprapubic aspirate ('bladder tap') or an in–out catheter urine collection. Any child who is toilet trained and requires a urine culture should have mid-stream urine collected.

The child who is previously well and thriving who presents with vomiting and hypoglycaemia, if ketotic, is likely to be hypoglycaemic from starvation. In the absence of ketonuria, metabolic and endocrine abnormalities need to be considered. It may be necessary to assay growth hormone, insulin and cortisol, as well as performing a urine metabolic screen. Collecting appropriate specimens when hypoglycaemic is important. Blood samples collected in a lithium heparin tube (plasma) and plain tube (serum) should allow blood glucose to be measured concurrently with hormone levels. Other samples may also be needed. Consultation with a paediatrician or paediatric endocrinologist may be prudent.

In a young, breastfed infant with blood in vomitus or stool it is important to distinguish swallowed maternal blood from infant's blood. An Apt test distinguishes between the two due to presence of HbF. To perform the test, add the bloody stool/vomitus to a test tube with about 5 mL of tap water. This lyses the red blood cells. After allowing to settle, the "supernatant" should be pink to continue. If so, add 1 mL of 1% sodium hydroxide. Remaining pink indicates infant's blood (HbF) whereas changing to a yellow-brown colour over 2 minutes indicates maternal (adult) blood.

The microscopy of the diarrhoeal stool may be important. The presence of stool white cells, without a viral or bacterial pathogen, in the young infant, may indicate cows' milk protein intolerance.

Management

Intravenous fluids
- Bolus.
- Rehydration.
- Glucose.

The management will depend on the need for immediate resuscitation and subsequently, the provisional diagnosis. A fluid bolus is used to restore circulating volume and is therefore warranted when signs of shock are present. This must not be confused with strategies of 'rapid rehydration' in dehydrated children. Intravenous fluids containing dextrose must not be used as volume expanders. The choice of crystalloid fluid for a bolus is either normal saline (0.9%) or Hartmann's solution. If these crystalloids are not available, and a bolus is required, then a colloid should be used (e.g. 4% NSA or Gelofusine).

In dehydrated, but not cardiovascular compromised children, it is safer to commence initial intravenous rehydration with fluids that contain at least 75 mmol L^{-1} sodium, i.e. 0.45–0.9% NaCl solution. Commonly available fluids include 0.45% NaCl + 5% glucose, 0.9% NaCl (normal saline) and Hartmann's solution. Normal saline (0.9% NaCl) with 5% glucose is also currently available. Hypoglycaemia is not infrequent, both at presentation or subsequently, thus dextrose-containing fluids are appropriate in all children, particularly in the young infant or those who have had insufficient caloric intake and are ketotic. Intravenous fluids are commonly manufactured as 'isotonic' with plasma, by varying the glucose concentration to balance the sodium chloride (e.g. 0.45% NaCl + 5% glucose). The addition of dextrose to many commercially available solutions (such as normal saline) makes them 'hypertonic' compared to plasma. However, due to rapid equilibration of the dextrose with extravascular space this is not clinically significant. In this context, 0.9% NaCl + 5% glucose is an appropriate intravenous fluid to use (may be made by adding 50 mL of 50% glucose to 450 mL of 0.9% NaCl).

Be aware of the potential of SIADH in unwell children. The rate of fluid administration may need to be altered depending upon the initial biochemistry, the diagnosis and the clinical progress of the child. Monitoring fluid balance is essential in the unwell infant or child.

Nasogastric rehydration is commonly used in dehydrated infants with gastroenteritis. See Chapter 7.12.

Antibiotics

Any specific management like administration of antibiotics depends on the provisional diagnosis, and the severity of illness. Most acute diarrhoeal illnesses are viral and self-limiting and therefore do not require antibiotics. Clearly it is preferable that appropriate cultures be taken prior to administration of antibiotics, although in the severely unwell, febrile patient broad-spectrum antibiotics should not be delayed whilst awaiting collection of all cultures. It would be preferable, but not essential, that a blood culture be undertaken prior to such administration.

Consultation

Consultation with more experienced staff, either emergency physicians or paediatricians should be encouraged, especially for complex or severely ill infants or children. Assistance may be required for clinical evaluation and technical procedures in critically ill children.

Transfer

Local experienced senior clinical consultation and review should occur prior to transfer. The child who requires transfer to a facility that provides a higher level of care needs an experienced evaluation regarding the level of escort, urgency and mode of transport required to safely achieve the transfer.

Conclusions

Differential diagnostic possibilities

For each patient the differential diagnoses vary depending on the constellation of symptoms (fever, vomiting, diarrhoea or others). Keep an open mind and always re-evaluate clinical data. Don't be distracted by a child's previous diagnoses or labels.

General approach

'ABC fluids in and out' is a useful tool in taking a history. Caution must be exercised in the infant who has fever and vomiting, as differential diagnoses include serious illnesses, like meningitis. The younger the infant, the more challenging the evaluation and the less reliable the clinical examination. If in doubt, seek consultation from a colleague. The telephone is a useful and powerful tool for clinicians and the value of consultation should not be underestimated.

Further reading

Craig JV, Lancaster GA, Taylor S, et al. Infrared ear thermometry compared with rectal thermometry in children: a systematic review. *Lancet* 2002;**360** (9333):603–9 [Review; 48 refs].

Craver RD, Abermanis JG. Dipstick only urinalysis screen for the pediatric emergency room. *Paediatr Nephrol* 1998;**11** (3):331–333 [1998 erratum appears in Paediatr Nephrol 12(5): 426].

Gorelick MH, Shaw KN. Screening tests for urinary tract infection in children: a meta-analysis. *Pediatrics* 1999;**104** (5):54.

Gorelick MH, Shaw KN, Baker MD. Effect of ambient temperature on capillary refill in healthy children. *Paediatrics* 1993;**92**(5):699–702.

Hewson PH, Gollan RA. A simple hospital triaging system for infants with acute illness. *J Paediatr Child Health* 1995;**31** (1):29–32.

Neville KA, Verge CF, O'Meara MW, Walker JL. High antidiuretic hormone levels and hyponatremia in children with gastroenteritis. *Pediatrics* 2005;**116**(6):1401–7.

Neville KA, Verge CF, Rosenberg AR, et al. Isotonic is better than hypotonic saline for intravenous rehydration of children with gastroenteritis: a prospective randomised study. *Arch Dis Child* 2006;**91**(3):226–32.

Shaw KN, McGowan KL, Gorelick MH, Schwartz JS. Screening for urinary tract infection in infants in the ED: which test is best? *Paediatrics* 1998;**101**(6):E1.

GASTROENTEROLOGY AND HEPATOLOGY

7.9 Hepatitis

Franz E. Babl

ESSENTIALS

1 Hepatitis A, B and C are the main viral agents of acute hepatitis in children in Australia.

2 Aboriginal children in certain areas of Australia are at higher risk of hepatitis A than non-Aboriginal children.

3 Acute hepatitis due to the various hepatotropic viruses is clinically indistinguishable.

4 The younger the child the more likely viral hepatitis will be asymptomatic or only mildly symptomatic without jaundice.

5 Severe hepatitis, especially with synthetic dysfunction, should be urgently referred to a paediatric gastroenterologist.

6 Hepatitis A and B are vaccine preventable and post-exposure prophylaxis is available for both.

7 In addition to toxin- and drug-related hepatitis, a variety of metabolic and systemic illnesses can present with the clinical picture of acute or chronic hepatitis in children.

Introduction[1–5]

Hepatitis is defined as inflammation of the liver due to a number of possible causes. Jaundice or icterus implies a yellow discolouration of skin, sclera and mucous membranes due to hyperbilirubinaemia which may or may not be caused by hepatitis.

In children, the presentation of hepatitis includes a diverse number of viral and non-viral causes. Viral hepatitis continues to be a major health problem in developing and developed countries and can present as an acute or chronic illness.

Aetiology

- Infection
  - hepatotropic viruses, e.g. hepatitis A, B, C, D, E;
  - other viruses with hepatic involvement, e.g. Epstein–Barr virus (EBV), cytomegalovirus (CMV);
  - bacterial infections with hepatic involvement, e.g. leptospirosis, brucellosis, Q fever, cat-scratch disease, gonococcal perihepatitis (Fitz–Hugh–Curtis syndrome), syphilis, typhoid fever or associated with septicaemia;
  - amoebic.
- Drug and toxin related liver injury (Table 7.9.1).
- Chronic hepatitis.
- Persistent viral infection (hepatitis B, C, D).
- Autoimmune hepatitis.
- Sclerosing cholangitis.
- Metabolic diseases, e.g. Wilson's disease, α_1-antitrypsin deficiency, cystic fibrosis.
- Systemic illnesses, e.g. inflammatory bowel disease, cardiac disease, total parenteral nutrition.

Viral hepatitis in children can present with various manifestations, ranging from asymptomatic seroconversions especially in infants, mildly symptomatic and anicteric presentations with symptoms of a flu-like or gastroenteritis-like illness, to fulminant hepatic failure as well as chronic hepatitis leading to cirrhosis and hepatocellular carcinoma. In adults, chronic hepatitis is defined as biochemical or histological changes that persist for more than 6 months. This definition in children would inappropriately delay the diagnosis of several childhood causes of non-viral chronic hepatitis which respond to specific medical therapy. Persistence of abnormal serum aminotransferase tests beyond 3 months warrants aggressive evaluation to define the aetiology of the liver injury. A child with clinical evidence of chronic liver disease should be referred to a paediatric gastroenterologist for further evaluation without the 3 month observation period.

History

Acute symptomatic viral hepatitis classically presents with a 1-week prodromal phase with non-specific symptoms of nausea, vomiting, malaise, anorexia and low-grade fever, followed by an icteric phase with dark urine followed by jaundice and pale stools. Prodromal symptoms fade with the onset of jaundice but anorexia and malaise may persist, and localised hepatic pain or tenderness and pruritus may develop. Important historical clues indicating an infectious aetiology are attendance of child care and possible disease among peers and childcare workers, exposure to highly endemic communities in Australia (e.g. remote Aboriginal communities) or overseas, attendance of schools and residential facilities for the

Table 7.9.1 Patterns of hepatic drug injury	
Centrilobar necrosis	Paracetamol Halothane
Microvesicular steatosis	Valproic acid
Acute hepatitis	Isoniacid
General hypersensitivity	Sulfonamide Phenytoin
Fibrosis	Methotrexate
Cholestasis	Chlorpromazine Erythromycin Oestrogens
Veno-occlusive disease	Cyclophosphamide
Portal and hepatic vein thrombosis	Oestrogens Androgens
Biliary sludge	Ceftriaxone
Hepatic adenoma or carcinoma	Oral contraceptives Anabolic steroids

disabled, exposure to blood products, injection drug use and high risk sexual activity (men who have sex with men). A history of acute drug or toxin ingestion or ongoing therapeutic use of potentially hepatotoxic agents should be elicited. The history should also explore the possibility of acute or chronic presentations of metabolic and systemic illnesses associated with liver disease e.g. neurological complaints in Wilson's disease, respiratory difficulties in cystic fibrosis, or a history of cardiac disease.

Examination

Although jaundice is the hallmark of hepatitis, many children will present anicteric. Carotenaemia, which also causes a yellow-orange tinge of the skin due to high intake of carotenoids in carrots and other vegetables, can be differentiated from jaundice by the lack of scleral involvement. In addition to jaundice, physical examination in acute hepatitis may show tender hepatomegaly and mild splenomegaly. Arthralgias or arthritis and rashes can occur with hepatitis B. Signs of chronic liver disease should be specifically looked for including clubbing, leukonychia, palmar erythema, spider naevi, bruising, scratch marks, asterixis, ascites, prominent abdominal veins, oedema and signs of fat-soluble vitamin deficiency.

Investigations

Laboratory tests for hepatitis can be expensive and many may not be clinically useful in the emergency setting. Initial studies should include a full blood count, total and fractionated serum bilirubins, aspartate aminotransferase (AST), alanine aminotransferase (ALT), gamma glutamyl transferase (GGT) and prothrombin time (PT). A serum alkaline phosphatase level may be difficult to interpret in growing children because levels increase with bone growth. Serum AST, ALT and GGT are indicative of hepatocellular damage rather than 'liver function tests'. Slight elevations of AST and ALT do not always predict mild disease and both can fall with end-stage liver disease. PT is the most useful indicator of synthetic function. If the aetiology of the hepatitis is unknown, anti-hepatitis A immunoglobulin M (IgM), hepatitis B surface antigen (HBsAg), IgM anti-hepatitis B core (HBc) and anti-hepatitis C virus (HCV) antibody should be obtained. If these tests are negative, other viral causes such as EBV and CMV should be considered. If no viral cause can be identified, metabolic and systemic causes of acute and chronic hepatitis should be excluded. Wilson's disease can be detected by measuring serum coeruloplasmin levels and 24-hour urinary copper excretion, cystic fibrosis by measuring sweat electrolytes, α-antitrypsin deficiency by measuring serum α_1-antitrypsin levels.

Viral hepatitis[1-4]

Over the past decades the knowledge about the viruses that cause hepatitis has increased and is still evolving. The agents identified to cause hepatitis as their primary disease manifestation include hepatitis A virus (HAV), hepatitis B virus (HBV), hepatitis D virus (HDV) and formerly non-A, non-B designated viruses, hepatitis C (parenteral transmission) and hepatitis E (enteral transmission). HBV is a DNA virus whereas the other hepatotropic agents are RNA viruses. HAV and HEV are not known to cause chronic disease whereas the others can develop chronic infection. All five viruses can cause fulminant hepatitis with acute liver failure. A child with evidence of synthetic dysfunction (prolonged prothrombin time, hypoglycaemia, hyperammonaemia, lactic acidosis) with or without positive viral serology should be urgently referred to a paediatric gastroenterologist. Patients with severe hepatitis should be transferred early before intensive care therapy is required.

There are a number of other hepatotropic viruses which play a less well defined role in the pathogenesis of acute and chronic liver disease such as hepatitis G virus and TT virus. It is virtually impossible to clinically distinguish an acute infection due to one agent from another. Diagnosis is therefore dependent on the use of serologic and nucleic acid based assays. Many other viruses can cause hepatitis as part of their clinical spectrum, such as EBV and CMV.

Hepatitis A[1-3,6-9]
Aetiology
HAV is an RNA virus classified as a member of the picorna virus group.

Epidemiology
The most common mode of transmission is person to person by the faecal–oral route. In developing countries, and also in certain Aboriginal communities, where infection is endemic, most persons are infected in the first decade of life. In developed countries, including much of Australia, infection may occur at an older age when susceptible adults travel to endemic areas. In Australia, the main patterns of hepatitis A are large, slowly evolving community outbreaks involving childcare centres, residential facilities, communities of intravenous drug users and male homosexuals, sporadic cases due to travel to endemic areas and point source outbreaks from contaminated food, water or an infected food handler. Faecal–oral transmission from asymptomatic infections, particularly in young children, likely accounts for many of the approximately 50% cases where the source cannot be determined.

The incubation period is 15–50 days (mean 30 days). The highest titres of HAV in stool occur during 1 to 2 weeks before the onset of illness, when patients are most likely to transmit HAV.

Clinical course
Hepatitis A is an acute self limited illness associated with fever, malaise, jaundice, anorexia and nausea. In children under 6 years of age symptomatic hepatitis occurs in only 30% and few will have jaundice. In older children and adults infection is usually symptomatic, typically lasting several weeks, and 70% will have jaundice. Prolonged or relapsing disease can occur though no chronic infection occurs. Fulminant hepatitis is rare but is more frequent with underlying liver disease.

Laboratory tests
HAV specific IgM and IgG antibody tests are available. IgM is invariably present by the time the patient presents and indicates current or recent infection and usually persists for 3 to 6 months. Anti-HAV IgG is detectable shortly after the appearance of IgM. The presence of anti-HAV IgG indicates past infection (or possibly immunisation) and immunity.

Management

There is no specific treatment for hepatitis A. Most patients can be managed at home. Hepatotoxic agents should be avoided. No specific dietary restrictions are required. Pruritus associated with cholestasis, which develops in 5–10%, may be treated with cholestyramine, an H_1-receptor blocker or local therapy.

Children and adults with acute HAV infection who are food handlers or work in child-care settings should be excluded for 1 week after the onset of illness. Hospitalised patients require contact precautions for 1 week after the onset of illness if they are incontinent or in nappies. Patients should be admitted if warning signs of acute liver failure develop (repeated vomiting, deepening jaundice and increasing prothrombin time), and transfer to a liver transplant centre is indicated at the onset of acute liver failure (increased prothrombin time and clouding of consciousness).

Immunisations and post-exposure prophylaxis

Hepatitis A vaccines are highly immunogenic in both children and adults, with very high efficacy in preventing hepatitis A, approaching 100%. The duration of immunity is not known but there is no current evidence that booster doses are required. There are a number of different vaccines available, also in combination with other vaccines, with variable age, dose and vaccination schedules. Vaccination is recommended for susceptible persons travelling to countries and areas with high endemic rates of HAV infection, Aboriginal and Torres Strait Islander children residing in parts of Australia, those whose occupation or life style may put them at risk of acquiring hepatitis A, people with intellectual disabilities and people with chronic liver disease of any aetiology including those with hepatitis B or C. Hepatitis A vaccination of children in Aboriginal communities has been shown to lead to rapid decline in hepatitis cases in both indigenous and non-indigenous people.

Post-exposure prophylaxis with normal human immunoglobulin (NHIG) is indicated for household and sexual contacts within 2 weeks of exposure and for unimmunised children and employees in outbreaks in the day care setting and in well-defined or closed communities. There are insufficient data for the use of hepatitis A vaccine alone for post-exposure prophylaxis.

Hepatitis B[1–3,6,10–12]

Aetiology

HBV is a DNA-containing hepadnavirus. Important components include hepatitis B surface antigen (HBsAg), hepatitis B core antigen (HBcAg) and hepatitis B e antigen (HBeAg).

Epidemiology

HBV is transmitted through blood or body fluids such as semen, cervical secretions, wound exudates, and saliva of HBsAg positive persons, in particular if they are chronically infected. Modes of transmission are through blood and blood products (now rare due to screening), sharing of needles, percutaneous or mucous membrane exposure to infective body fluids and homosexual and heterosexual activity. Perinatal transmission usually occurs during delivery rather than intra-uterine. Non-sexual transmission occurs in household settings primarily from child to child, and young children are at highest risk. Although the exact mechanism is unknown, it is likely due to frequent interpersonal contact of non-intact skin or mucous membranes with secretions or saliva or the sharing of inanimate objects, as HBV can survive at ambient temperatures for 1 week or longer. HBV is not transmitted by the faecal–oral route. Prevalence of HBV infection varies markedly from country to country, with low rates in Australia, the US, Canada and Western Europe and high endemic rates in South-East Asia, China, the Pacific Islands and other developing countries as well as some Australian Aboriginal communities. First generation immigrants usually retain the carrier rate of their country of origin, but subsequent generations show a decline in carrier rate irrespective of vaccination.

The incubation period is 45 to 160 days with an average of 90 days.

Clinical course

HBV virus infection causes a wide spectrum of diseases ranging from asymptomatic seroconversion, subacute illness with non-specific symptoms or extrahepatic symptoms and clinical hepatitis with jaundice to fulminant fatal hepatitis. Asymptomatic infection is most common in young children. Symptomatic illness is indistinguishable from other forms of hepatitis. Some patients will show extrahepatic manifestations early in the disease including arthralgias, arthritis, macular rash and papular acrodermatitis (Gianotti–Crosti syndrome). The rate of chronic HBV infection is age dependent. It occurs in up to 90% of infants infected by perinatal infection, 25–50% of children 1 to 5 years of age, and 2–6% of older children and adults with HBV. Chronic HBV infection can lead to chronic liver disease and cirrhosis and primary hepatocellular carcinoma later in life, though it can occasionally occur in children. The risk of death from HBV related cirrhosis or liver cancer is approximately 25% for persons who become chronically infected in early childhood.

Laboratory tests

Antigen and antibody tests for HBV are available to detect acute infection, resolved infection, immunity after immunisation and persons at high risk of transmission. HBsAg is detectable during acute infection. If the infection is self limited it disappears before serum anti-HBs can be detected (the 'window phase'). IgM anti-HBc allows the detection of acute or recent infections, including those in HBsAg negative patients during the 'window phase'. Persons with chronic HBV infection are positive for HBsAg as well as anti-HBc antibody. Both anti-HBs and anti-HBc antibodies are detected in persons with resolved infection, whereas anti-HBs alone is detected after hepatitis B vaccination. The presence of HBeAg and HBV viral DNA by polymerase chain reaction (PCR) indicates ongoing viral replication, increased disease activity and infectivity.

Management

For acute hepatitis B there is no specific therapy and management is otherwise similar to hepatitis A. Follow-up laboratory studies are important to assess the development of carrier state and chronic liver disease. Interferon-α, lamivudine and other antiviral agents are being used to treat chronic hepatitis B infection with long-term remission and reduced complications. Children with chronic HBV infection should be managed with the involvement of a paediatric gastroenterologist and screened periodically for disease activity and by abdominal ultrasound for hepatic complications. Liver transplantation is a possible therapy in end-stage chronic hepatitis.

Immunisations and post-exposure prophylaxis

Hepatitis B vaccines are produced by recombinant DNA technology. They are highly efficacious, safe and provide long-term protection. The vaccines are part of universal childhood immunisations in many Western countries, including Australia, and should be used for other persons at high risk of exposure such as healthcare personnel, haemodialysis and human immunodeficiency virus (HIV) patients, patients receiving blood products, and those with chronic liver disease. Hepatitis A and B combination vaccines are available.

The vaccine is also used for post-exposure prophylaxis in unimmunised household and sexual contacts of persons with acute HBV infection, newborns of HBsAg positive mothers (the baby injection site should be washed prior to injection to decrease needle inoculation contamination), and after accidental occupational percutaneous exposure to blood that contains or might contain HBsAg. To provide immediate protection, the latter two groups should also receive hepatitis B immunoglobulin. All patients with hepatitis B infection should also be immunised with hepatitis A vaccine.

Hepatitis C[2,3,13,14]
Aetiology

HCV is a small single-stranded RNA virus with multiple genotypes. HCV is a member of the flavivirus family.

Epidemiology

Infection is spread primarily by parenteral exposure to blood and blood products. Screening of blood donors and blood products and inactivation procedures for HCV have virtually eliminated the risk of post-transfusion hepatitis due to this agent.

At increased risk are injection drug users, haemophilia patients who received untreated clotting products in the past, haemodialysis patients and persons with high-risk sexual behaviours. The risk of maternal to infant (vertical) transmission, which is the most likely source of HCV infection in developed countries, is 5–10%. In Australia there are an estimated 125–250 children infected vertically each year. Incubation time is 2 weeks to 6 months, with an average of 6 to 7 weeks.

Clinical course

The signs and symptoms of HCV infection are usually indistinguishable from HAV and HBV infection. Acute disease tends to be mild and insidious in onset and in children most infections are asymptomatic. Only 15% of patients develop symptomatic acute hepatitis. Persistent HCV infection occurs in the majority of infected children even in the absence of biochemical evidence of liver disease. Most children with chronic HCV infection are asymptomatic. Chronic liver disease and cirrhosis can follow and primary hepatocellular carcinoma can occur in these patients in later life.

Laboratory tests

HCV infection can be detected using total anti-HCV antibody assays and HCV RNA by PCR. However, the diagnosis of HCV is difficult as antibody assays may be negative early in the course of the acute illness.

Management

All patients with HCV infection should be considered infectious and refrain from donating blood products and sharing tooth brushes or razors. They should be counselled on avoiding hepatotoxic agents including medications and alcohol. Susceptible children should be immunised against hepatitis A and B. Infected children do not need to be excluded from day care. HCV is not a contraindication to breastfeeding.

Interferon-α, ribavirin and other antiviral agents, usually in combination, have been used for treatment of HCV infection in children and adults, with combination therapy showing better outcome than single drug therapy. Liver transplantation is indicated in end-stage liver disease. HCV infected children require ongoing care by a paediatric gastroenterologist.

There is no hepatitis C vaccine and immunoglobulin has not shown efficacy for post-exposure prophylaxis.

Hepatitis D[2,3]
Aetiology

HDV is a particle consisting of an RNA genome and a delta protein antigen (HDAg), both of which are coated with hepatitis B surface antigen (HBsAg).

Epidemiology

HDV causes infection only in persons with acute or chronic HBV infection. HDV requires HBV as a helper virus and cannot produce infection in the absence of HBV. It can cause infection at the same time as the initial HBV infection (co-infection) or infect a person already chronically infected (superinfection). Acquisition of HDV is similar to HBV, i.e. by parenteral, percutaneous or mucous membrane inoculation. High prevalence areas include southern Italy, parts of Eastern Europe, South America and the Middle East. HDV infection is rare in Australia.

Incubation period for HDV superinfection is 2–8 weeks; in co-infection with HBV the incubation period is similar to hepatitis B (45–160 days; average 90 days).

Clinical course

The importance of HDV infection lies in its ability to convert an asymptomatic or mild chronic HBV infection into a fulminant or rapidly progressive disease. Acute co-infection with HBV and HDV usually causes an acute illness indistinguishable from acute HBV infection alone, except that the likelihood of fulminant hepatitis can be as high as 5%.

Laboratory tests

Diagnosis can be made by detecting IGM-specific anti-HDV antibody and HDAg. If markers for HDV infection exist, HBV co-infection can be differentiated from superinfection in an established HBsAg carrier by testing for IgM hepatitis B core antibody. Absence of this core antibody suggests that the person is an HBsAg carrier.

Immunisations

Because HDV cannot be transmitted in the absence of HBV infection, hepatitis B immunisation protects against HDV infection.

Hepatitis E[2,3]
Aetiology

The HEV is an RNA virus and is the only known agent of enterically transmitted non-A non-B hepatitis.

Epidemiology

Transmission of HEV is by the faecal–oral route. It is more common in adults than children and has a high case-fatality rate in pregnant women. Cases have been reported in epidemics and sporadically in developing countries. HEV in Australia has been reported in returning travellers from endemic regions and in the Northern Territory. Outbreaks have been associated with contaminated water. Chronic infection does not seem to occur.

Clinical course

HEV causes a self-limited acute illness with jaundice, malaise, anorexia, fever, abdominal pain and arthralgia. Subclinical infection also occurs.

Laboratory tests

Diagnosis can be made by detecting IgM anti-HEV in serum or by detecting HEV RNA by PCR in serum or faeces.

Viral hepatitis due to other viruses

EBV, CMV, HIV, herpesvirus, varicella zoster, rubella, adenoviruses and enteroviruses, as well as yellow fever and dengue fever in tropical and subtropical areas, are also known agents causing acute hepatitis in children. EBV and CMV are ubiquitous and most persons are infected by the time they reach young adulthood. If tests for hepatitis A, B and C are negative, EBV and CMV are among the most likely additional agents to consider. However, hepatic involvement with these viruses is usually only one component of a multisystem disease.

Drug and toxin-induced liver injury[3,15]

The liver is the main site of drug metabolism and is particularly susceptible to structural and functional injury from drugs and toxins. The clinical spectrum varies from asymptomatic biochemical abnormalities to fulminant liver failure. Children may be more or less susceptible than adults to hepatotoxic reactions. For example, liver injury after halothane is rare in children and paracetamol toxicity is unusual in infants compared with adolescents, whereas most cases of fatal hepatotoxicity associated with sodium valproate use have been reported in children. Excess or prolonged therapeutic administration of paracetamol combined with reduction in caloric intake may produce hepatotoxicity in children. When considering adverse reactions to medications with liver involvement clinicians need to consider all drugs taken in the previous months including prescription medications, over the counter medications and complementary medicines. In Australia the most commonly reported alternative and complementary medicines associated with hepatotoxicity according to the Adverse Drug Reactions Advisory Council (ADRAC) are kombucha tea, echinacea, evening primrose tea and valerian.

Hepatotoxicity can be predictable or idiosyncratic. Predictable hepatotoxicity implies a high incidence in exposed persons with dose dependence. Examples are paracetamol or antimetabolites such as methotrexate. Idiosyncratic hepatotoxicity is infrequent and unpredictable. It is not dose dependent, may occur at any time during exposure to the agent and may be immunologically mediated as a result of prior sensitisation.

The pathological spectrum of drug induced liver disease varies widely and is rarely specific (see table). The laboratory features also vary widely. After exclusion of other causes of liver disease, the cessation of a temporally related offending medication with normalisation of liver function tests is usually sufficient to establish a diagnosis. Treatment is mainly supportive. *N*-acetylcysteine is used as a specific antidote in preventing paracetamol toxicity. The prognosis of drug or toxin induced liver injury depends on its type and severity. Injury is usually completely reversible with the withdrawal of the offending agent. The mortality of submassive hepatic necrosis with fulminant liver injury may, however, exceed 50%.

Chronic hepatitis

Overview

Chronic hepatitis can be caused by persistent viral infection (hepatitis B, C and D), autoimmune hepatitis, sclerosing cholangitis, metabolic diseases such as Wilson's disease, α_1-antitrypsin deficiency, cystic fibrosis, Indian childhood cirrhosis and other inborn errors of metabolism and systemic illnesses such as inflammatory bowel disease, cardiac disease and liver disease associated with parenteral nutrition. In addition, drugs and toxins can produce chronic hepatitis.

Autoimmune hepatitis

Autoimmune hepatitis (AH) is characterised by progressive destruction of hepatocytes in association with circulating auto-antibodies, but in the absence of other known causes of chronic liver disease. AH type I occurs mainly in females and presents with lethargy, jaundice and the typical findings of chronic liver disease. Antinuclear antibodies (ANA) are found in the majority. AH II is clinically similar but ANA is negative and anti-liver–kidney microsomal antibodies are present. Liver biopsy shows piecemeal necrosis without involvement of the biliary tract. Both forms of AH can be associated with other autoimmune manifestations such as thyroiditis, glomerulonephritis, haemolytic anaemia and erythema nodosum. AH generally responds to corticosteroid therapy.

Sclerosing cholangitis

Sclerosing cholangitis (SC) is characterised by chronic inflammation of the intra- or extrahepatic biliary tree. Primary SC is associated with inflammatory bowel disease or immune deficiency, secondary SC results from an obstructive process in the biliary system such as stones or post-operative stricture. Primary SC can occasionally be associated with antibodies such as ANA. Although histology includes periductal inflammation, differentiation from other causes of chronic hepatitis often requires cholangiography demonstrating typical biliary abnormalities. Supportive therapy does not prevent disease progression to cirrhosis.

Metabolic causes of chronic hepatitis

Wilson's disease is an autosomal recessive disorder caused by a defect in biliary copper excretion. Excessive intrahepatic accumulation of copper causes liver cell damage followed by fibrosis and cirrhosis. Extrahepatic accumulation of copper in brain, cornea and kidney accounts for extrahepatic manifestations of neurological abnormalities and Kayser–Fleisher rings. Initial presentation of Wilson's disease may resemble acute viral, fulminant or chronic hepatitis with variable extrahepatic findings. The importance in considering Wilson's disease, though uncommon, lies in the ability to treat patients and other family members with penicillamine, a chelating agent.

α_1-Antitrypsin deficiency is caused by a deficiency of the major serum protease inhibitor, α_1-antitrypisin. Various allele combinations account for α_1-antitrypsin deficiency, of which some are more prone to cause chronic liver disease than others. The course of liver disease is highly variable. Liver transplantation is curative. There is no other effective therapy.

Cystic fibrosis can be associated with biliary cirrhosis and chronic liver disease. In addition, cholelithiasis may occur in the second decade of life.

Systemic disorders causing chronic liver disease

Hepatobiliary disease may complicate ulcerative colitis and Crohn's disease. Fatty liver, cholangitis, chronic hepatitis, cirrhosis, portal vein thrombosis, sclerosing cholangitis and cholelithiasis have been associated with inflammatory bowel disease. Hepatic congestion and injury may occur as a complication of severe chronic or acute congestive heart failure or cyanotic heart disease. Hepatic dysfunction is due to hypoxaemia, systemic venous congestion and low cardiac output.

Liver dysfunction is the most common metabolic complication of total parenteral nutrition (TPN). Cholestasis associated with TPN is potentially fatal and is the major factor limiting long-term TPN use. Pathogenesis is multifactorial. In general, with administration of oral feedings a gradual resolution of the liver disease occurs.

Future directions

❶ Improved public health measures to minimise transmission of viral hepatitis including universal immunisations for children and targeted immunisations for high-risk groups.

❷ The development of a vaccine against HCV infection is a priority but remains elusive.

❸ The optimal monitoring, indications for therapy and the role of antiviral agents in chronic hepatitis B and C in children remain to be defined.

References

1. Australian Government. Department of Health and Aging. National Health and Medical Research Council. *Hepatitis A and B. The Australian Immunisation Handbook.* 9th ed. Available from http://www.health.gov.au/internet/immunise/publishing.nsf/Content/Handbook-home; 2008 [accessed 15.10.10].
2. American Academy of Pediatrics. *Hepatitis A–E. 2006 Red Book: Report of the Committee on Infectious Diseases.* 27th ed. Elk Grove Village, IL: American Academy of Pediatrics; 2006. p. 326–61.
3. Balistreri WF. Part XVII The digestive system. Section 6. The liver and biliary system. In: Kliegman RM, Behrman RE, Jenson HB, Stanton B, editors. *Nelson's Textbook of Pediatrics.* 18th ed. Philadelphia: Saunders Elsevier; 2007. p. 1657–713.
4. Denson LA. Other viral infections. In: Kleinman RE, Goulet O-J, Mieli-Vergani G, et al., editors. *Walker's Pediatric Gatrointestinal Disease.* Ontario, Canada: BC Decker, Hamilton; 2008. p. 859–64.
5. Harris W. Chapter 8. Gastroenterology. *Examination Paediatrics.* 4th ed. Chatswood, NSW: Elsevier Australia; p. 190–252.
6. Australian Government. Department of Health and Aging. National Health and Medical Research Council. *National Immunisation Program Schedule.* Available from http://www.immunise.health.gov.au/internet/immunise/publishing.nsf/Content/E875BA5436C6DF9BCA2575BD001C80BF/$File/nip-schedule-card-july07.pdf [accessed 15.10.10].
7. Koff RS. Hepatitis A. *Lancet* 1998;**351**:1643–91.
8. Hanna JN, Hills SL, Humphreys JL. Impact of hepatitis A vaccination of Indigenous children on notifications of hepatitis A in north Queensland. *Med J Aust* 2004;**181**:482–5.
9. Van Damme P, Banatvala J, Fay O, et al. Hepatitis A booster vaccination: is there a need? *Lancet* 2003;**362**:1065–71.
10. Mast E, Mahoney F, Kane MA, Margolis HS. Hepatitis B vaccine. In: Plotkin SA, Orenstein WA, editors. *Vaccines.* 4th ed. Philadelphia, PA: Saunders; 2004.
11. Gill JS, Bucens M, Hatton M, et al. Markers of hepatitis B virus infection in schoolchildren in the Kimberley, Western Australia. *Med J Aust* 1990;**153**: 34–7.
12. Aggarwal R, Ranjan P. Preventing and treating hepatitis B infection. *Br Med J* 2004;**329**(7474):1080–6 Review.
13. Maheshwari A, Ray S, Thuluvath PJ. Acute hepatitis C. *Lancet* 2008;**372**(9635):321–32. Review.
14. Kesson AM. Diagnosis and management of paediatric hepatitis C virus infection. *J Paediatr Child Health* 2002;213–8.
15. Ryan M, Desmond P. Liver toxicity: could this be a drug reaction. *Aust Fam Physician* 2001;**30**:427–31.

Further reading

Australian Government. Department of Health and Aging. National Health and Medical Research Council. *The Australian Immunisation Handbook.* 9th ed. Available from http://www.health.gov.au/internet/immunise/publishing.nsf/Content/Handbook-home; (accessed 15.10.10).

American Academy of Pediatrics. *Red Book: Report of the Committee on Infectious Diseases.* 27th ed, Elk Grove Village, IL: American Academy of Pediatrics; 2006.

Kleinman RE, Goulet O-J, Mieli-Vergani G, et al, editors. *Walker's Pediatric Gatrointestinal Disease.* Ontario, Canada: BC Decker, Hamilton; 2008.

7.10 Intussusception

Kim Lian Ong • Ian Everitt

ESSENTIALS

1 A high index of suspicion is needed to make an early diagnosis.

2 Most cases are idiopathic.

3 Intussusception is the most common cause of bowel obstruction in children between 3 months and 3 years of age.

4 Paroxysmal colicky abdominal pain/distress is the most common symptom.

5 Profound lethargy may be the presenting feature in 10% of cases.

6 Bilious vomiting and redcurrant stools present LATE.

7 Morbidity and morbidity is increased by a delayed diagnosis.

Introduction

Intussusception is a common cause of paediatric bowel obstruction, particularly in children less than 2 years of age. Intussusception occurs when a bowel segment (usually the small intestine) invaginates into the lumen of a more distal lumen of bowel. The invaginated segment, known as the intussusceptum, is carried distally by peristalsis while the mesentery and vessels are squeezed within the engulfing segment (intussuscipiens). The resulting venous congestion is the cause of the blood and mucous in the stool, the classic 'redcurrant jelly' stool that may result in some cases. Intussusception occurs most commonly at the terminal ileum when the terminal ileum is carried through the ileocaecal valve into the colon (ileocolic ∼90%) and in some instances the telescoping small bowel may even reach the rectum.

Aetiology

Most cases of intussusceptions are *idiopathic* without any mass lesion acting as a lead point or an apex of the intussusceptum. In *non-idiopathic intussusception*, the following may act as lead points:

❶ Meckel's diverticulum or polyp related.
❷ Haemolytic–uraemic syndrome.
❸ Cystic fibrosis with inspissated bowel content.
❹ Henoch–Schönlein purpura (HSP) with intramural haemorrhage.
❺ Lymphoma and leukaemia involving the bowel wall.

Epidemiology

Most of the children are younger than 1 year of age, and the peak incidence occurs in infants between 5 and 10 months of age. Intussusception is the most common cause of intestinal obstruction in patients between 3 months and 3 years. Patients under 3 years of age with intussusception usually do not have a mass lesion as the lead point, the telescoping is idiopathic and they are usually responsive to non-operative reduction. Older children may have a surgical lead point to the intussusception and require operative reduction.

The estimated incidence is 1 to 4 per 1000 live births. There is an overall male preponderance, with a male-to-female ratio of approximately 3 to 1. Mortality with treatment is rare. Morbidity is increased by a delay in diagnosis and is likely to be due to bowel wall necrosis and perforation. Delay will cause prolonged intestinal obstruction with persistent vomiting, causing resultant dehydration and electrolyte imbalance.

Clinical

Clinically, the **four classic symptoms** and signs of vomiting, abdominal pain, abdominal mass and bloody stool described in patients with intussusception are present in less than one half of patients with the disease.[1,2] Intestinal obstruction is often the presenting sign.

The patient is usually in the infant age group and is previously healthy and well nourished, with acute onset of symptoms. The presentation is one of sudden onset of intermittent colicky abdominal pain, manifesting as episodic bouts (1–10 minutes) of crying. One of the descriptions sometimes given by the caregivers is the drawing up of the legs to the child's abdomen and then kicking the legs in the air. The child is often inconsolable during an episode of distress. Often the child will appear **pale** due to increased vagal tone caused by the telescoping bowel. Between the episodes, the child may be flat, lethargic or fall asleep exhausted, whereas some children will resume normal activity until another bout of distress occurs.

There is poor feeding, vomiting, and there may be passage of loose or watery stools. The child may have one or more episodes of loose stool which may be followed by blood or mucus per rectum within 12–24 hours. The mixture of mucus and shed blood described as 'redcurrant jelly' is a **late sign**. The diarrhoea, which occurs early, may lead to a misdiagnosis of gastroenteritis, so intussusception should be considered in any young child having episodic distress in the setting of a diarrhoeal illness. Initially the vomiting is non-bilious but it becomes bilious when intestinal obstruction occurs. There may be a preceding upper respiratory tract infection, which can sometimes distract from the true cause of the child's distress. This condition is unusual in children who are malnourished. The child usually appears chubby and in good health. The child when observed will be seen to have paroxysmal crying spells which represent episodes of abdominal pain between periods of lethargy. In late presentations, the child may be floridly shocked and minimally reactive from collapse.

One must be mindful of the small subset of 'encephalopathic' intussusceptions that present without symptoms to suggest a gastrointestinal problem ('painless presentation'). These children will present with lethargy, sweating and pallor which may be episodic.

Most children appear pale, but with pink conjunctivae. On examination, a right hypochondrium or mid-abdominal sausage-shaped mass may be palpated and this is best felt when the child is quiet between spasms of colic. Abdominal palpation may be soft and appear non-tender in some cases, whereas some children will elicit non-specific guarding. If obstruction has occurred distension and tenderness will be present. The nappy should be checked for any blood, and in suspicious cases a gentle rectal swab may reveal otherwise occult blood. Rarely, the bowel can progress to present rectally and prolapse. The presence of fever and leukocytosis are late signs and may indicate transmural gangrene and infarction. The occurrence of intestinal gangrene and infarction can be suggested by the presence of peritonitis, with the physical signs of rigidity and involuntary guarding.

Often patients with intussusception do not present with classic signs and symptoms, which may lead to an unfortunate delay in diagnosis, with disastrous consequences. Therefore it is essential to maintain a high index of suspicion for intussusception when evaluating a child presenting with abdominal pain, especially those less than 5 years of age or those who have HSP and episodic severe pain.

Investigations

All children should be resuscitated and stabilised prior to any imaging.

Abdominal X-ray

A plain abdominal radiograph may be performed, as a screen or if a reliable ultrasound is not readily available. Early in the course of the disease it may be normal, or it may show an absence of air in the right upper quadrant and a right-sided soft tissue shadow giving an impression of an intracolonic mass. There may be dilated small bowel and an absence of intraluminal gas in the region of the caecum. The presence of stool and air fluid levels in the caecum makes the diagnosis of intussusception less likely.[3,4] The accuracy of plain radiography in diagnosis or exclusion of intussusception ranges from 40 to 90%. In cases of established bowel obstruction, distended bowel loops and air-fluid levels will be present. The presence of any free air indicates perforation and precludes non-operative intervention.

Traditionally, the diagnosis of intussusception is made by the use of an enema, either using air or barium. Contrast enema is a quick and reliable investigation and is often also therapeutic. Barium has traditionally been the contrast material used but perforation can result in barium and faecal peritonitis.[5-7] The availability of near-isotonic water media and the use of air as a contrast medium[8,9] have changed the traditional therapeutic approach. The advantages of air reduction are its rapidity and safety compared with barium. In the case of perforation during the procedure, air enema has been shown to result in a smaller tear than hydrostatic enema with markedly less spillage of faeces.[10] In addition, air has no deleterious consequences within the abdominal cavity.[11,12]

Findings on contrast examination include the classical 'coiled spring sign', which is caused by the contrast material tracking around the lumen of the oedematous intestine and the 'meniscus sign' is produced by rounded apex of the intussusceptum protruding into the column of contrast material.[13]

Ultrasound

This is the imaging of choice to demonstrate intussusception. There are some recent studies to suggest that ultrasound is highly sensitive and specific for the diagnosis of intussusception. Some authors reported the sensitivity to be close to 100% in identification of intussusception, even in relatively inexperienced hands.[14-16]

The classical ultrasonographic sign on a longitudinal plane is the 'pseudokidney sign', which is an oval or tubular structure with a hyperechoic centre surrounded by hypoechoic periphery. The hyperechoic areas represent mesenteric fat pulled with the vessels and lymph nodes into the intussuscipiens while the hypoechoic border is the oedematous wall of the intussuscepted intestinal head. On the transverse plane, a 'target sign' is classic and appears as a circular mass with a hyperechoic centre surrounded by a hypoechoic outer rim.[17]

Management

The treatment in the emergency department is to initially provide stabilisation depending on the child's clinical condition and consult with a paediatric surgeon. Intravenous fluids should be started for resuscitation (normal saline bolus) and subsequent rehydration as required. The stomach should be decompressed by use of a nasogastric tube, if there is a bowel obstruction.

Non-operative reduction by air enema (hydrostatic reduction) is now generally accepted as the modality of treatment for most patients. Absolute contraindications include peritonitis, perforation or profound shock.[18]

Outcome

Various authors have reported reduction rates of between 80 and 90% using air enema.[19-20,26-28] The perforation rate is quoted to be less than 1%.[18,19] Factors that are associated with lower reduction and higher perforation rate, especially if more than one of the following are present: (a) patient's age: younger than 3 months or older than 5 years; (b) long duration of symptoms, especially if more than 48 hours; (c) passage of blood per rectum; (d) significant dehydration; (e) small bowel obstruction and (f) the presence of dissection sign on contrast study.[20-25]

Surgical reduction is now performed after failure to achieve reduction or when it is contraindicated to perform non-operative reduction.

The overall mortality rate of intussusception is less than 1%.[18] Mortality rates observed among children in industrialised countries are lower than those in developing countries.[1,28-33] Some of these deaths are preventable and may be related to reduced access to or delays in seeking health care, factors known to be associated with mortality in children with intussusception.[31-33] Therefore, early diagnosis and management play an important role in the reduction of mortality.

References

1. Simon RA, Hugh TJ, Curtin AM. Childhood intussusception in a regional hospital. *Aust N Z J Surg* 1994;**64**:699–702.

2. Kim YS, Rhu JH. Intussusception in infancy and childhood: analysis of 385 cases. *Int Surg* 1989;**74**:114–8.

3. Heller RM, Hernanz-Schulman M. Applications of new imaging modalities to the evaluation of common pediatric conditions. *J Pediatr* 1999;**135**(5):632–9.

4. Sargent MA, Babyn P, Alton DJ. Plain abdominal radiography in suspected intussusception: a reassessment. *Pediatr Radiol* 1994;**24**:17–20.

5. Grobmyer A, Kerlan R, Peterson C, Dragstedt L. Barium peritonitis. *Am Surg* 1984;**50**:116–20.

6. Mahvoubi S, Sherman N, Ziegler M. Barium peritonitis following attempted reduction of intussusception. *Clin Pediatr* 1983;**23**:36–8.

7. Yamamura M, Nishi M, Furubayashi H, et al. Barium peritonitis. Report of a case and review of the literature. *Dis Colon Rectum* 1985;**28**:347–52.

8. de Campo JF, Phelan E. Gas reduction of intussusception. *Pediatr Radiol* 1989;**19**:297–8.

9. Shiels WE 2d, Maves CK, Hedlund GL, Kirks DR. Air enema for diagnosis and reduction of intussusception: clinical experience and pressure correlates. *Radiology* 1991;**181**:169–72.

10. Shiels WE 2d, Kirks DR, Keller GL, et al. John Caffey Award. Colonic perforation by air and liquid enemas: comparison study in young pigs. *AJR Am J Roentgenol* 1993;**160**:931–5.

11. Hernanz-Schulman M, Foster C, Maxa R, et al. *Fecal peritonitis and contrast media: experimental protocol to assess synergistic effects and to compare relative safety of barium sulfate, water-soluble ionic media, saline and air.* Presented at the 35th Annual Meeting of The Society for Pediatric Radiology. Orlando, Florida; 1992 May 14–17.

12. Hernanz-Schulman M, Vanholder R, Schulman G. Inhibition of neutrophil phagocytosis by barium sulfate. Presented at the 37th Annual Meeting of The Society for Pediatric Radiology. Colorado Springs, Colorado; 1994 Apr 28–May 1.

13. del-Pozo G, Albillos J, Tejedor D, et al. Intussusception in Children: Current concepts in diagnosis and enema reduction. *Radiographics* 1999;**19**:299–319.

14. Bhisitkul DM, Listernick R, Shkolnik A, et al. Clinical application of ultrasonography in the diagnosis of intussusception. *J Pediatr* 1992;**121**:182–6.

15. Bowerman R, Silver T, Jaffe M. Real-time ultrasound diagnosis of intussusception. *Radiology* 1982;**143**:527–9.

16. del-Pozo G, Albillos J, Tejedor D. Intussusception: US findings with pathologic correlation – the crescent-in doughnut sign. *Radiology* 1996;**199**:688–92.

17. Pendergast LA, Wilson M. Intussusception: a sonographer's perspective. *J Diagn Med Sonogr* 2003;**19** (4):231–8.

18. DiFore JW. Intussusception. *Semin Pediatr Surg* 1999;**8**:214–20.

19. Hadidi AT, El Shal N. Childhood intussusception: a comparative study of nonsurgical management. *J Pediatr Surg* 1999;**34**:304–7.

20. Katz M, Phelan E, Carlin JB, Beasley SW. Gas enema for the reduction of intussusception: relationship between clinical signs and symptoms and outcome. *AJR* 1993;**160**:363–6.

21. den Hollander D, Burge DM. Exclusion criteria and outcome in pressure reduction of intussusception. *Arch Dis Child* 1993;**68**:79–81.

22. Reijnen JAM, Festen C, van Roosmalen RP. Intussusception: factors related to treatment. *Arch Dis Child* 1990;**65**:871–3.

23. Barr LL, Stansberry SD, Swischuk LE. Significance of age, duration, obstruction, and the dissection sign in intussusception. *Pediatr Radiol* 1990;**20**:454–6.

24. Stephenson CA, Seibert JJ, Strain JD, et al. Intussusception: clinical and radiographic factors influencing reducibility. *Pediatr Radiol* 1989;**20**: 57–60.

25. Fishman MC, Borden S, Cooper A. The dissection sign of nonreducible ileocolic intussusception. *AJR* 1984;**143**:5–8.

26. Gorenstein A, Raucher A, Serour F, et al. Intussusception in children: Reduction with repeated delayed air enema. *Radiology* 1998;**206**:721–4.

27. Ein SH, Alton D, Padler SB, et al. Intussusception in the 1990's: Has 25 years made a difference? *Pediatr Surg Int* 1997;**12**:402–5.

28. Ein SH, Alton D, Palder SB, et al. Intussusception in the 1990s: has 25 years made a difference? *Pediatr Surg Int* 1997;**12**:374–6.

29. van Heek NT, Aronson DC, Halimun EM, et al. Intussusception in a tropical country: comparison among patient populations in Jakarta, Jogyakarta, and Amsterdam. *J Pediatr Gastroenterol Nutr* 1999;**29**:402–5.

30. Meier DE, Coln CD, Rescorla FJ, et al. Intussusception in children: international perspective. *World J Surg* 1996;**20**:1035–9.

31. Stringer MD, Pledger G, Drake DP. Childhood deaths from intussusception in England and Wales, 1984-9. *Br Med J* 1992;**304**:737–9.

32. Adejuyigbe O, Jeje EA, Owa JA. Childhood intussusception in Ile-Ife, Nigeria. *Ann Trop Paediatr* 1991;**11**:123–7.

33. Mangete ED, Allison AB. Intussusception in infancy and childhood: an analysis of 69 cases. *West Afr J Med* 1994;**13**:87–90.

7.11 Herniae

Andrew J.A. Holland

ESSENTIALS

1 The key diagnostic steps are detailed history from the carer and a careful clinical examination.

2 Radiological investigations have little, if any, role in the management of inguinal herniae in children.

3 A hernia that is not reducible may be associated with ischaemia and an urgent surgical opinion should always be sought.

4 In children, unlike in adults, it is the gonad rather than the bowel structures that is most at risk from an inguinal hernia.

Introduction

A hernia is defined as the protrusion of a viscus or part of a viscus into an abnormal location. The most common herniae occurring in children are inguinal and umbilical – femoral herniae are rare. A variety of descriptive terms is applied to herniae in these locations, often incorrectly. This may lead to diagnostic confusion and inappropriate delays in referral.

Herniae are usually classified based on two characteristics: anatomical location and whether or not the hernia is reducible. An irreducible hernia may result in ischaemia of either the contents of the hernia or adjacent structures. Treatment of an irreducible hernia is thus a surgical emergency. The use of the terms incarceration (irreducible) and strangulation (arrest of circulation) should be avoided, as all irreducible herniae may be associated with ischaemia.

Types of herniae

Inguinal

The incidence of inguinal herniae in children has been reported to be between 0.8% and 4.4%,[1] rising to 18.9% to 30% of preterm infants.[2,3] Inguinal herniae are six times more common in boys and are more common in twins.[1,4] Around 1 in 10 inguinal hernias are non-reducible at presentation, although a careful history from the parents will often elucidate earlier signs and symptoms. In this group, over two-thirds are under 1 year of age.

In children, inguinal herniae are almost always indirect.[5] The hernia exits the peritoneal cavity via the internal inguinal ring to enter the inguinal canal, leaving the canal via the external inguinal ring. The sac is intimately related to the contents of the spermatic cord. It is compression of the testicular vessels by hernial contents that may render the testis ischaemic. In contrast, in females the risk of ischaemia to the ovary and adnexae usually occurs as a result of torsion of these structures within the hernial sac.

Rarely, direct inguinal herniae may occur, with some series reporting an incidence of up to 5%.[6] Typically, these children have either had previous inguinal surgery, a connective tissue disorder or were delivered at less than 30 weeks' gestation. The clinical management and surgical approach remains similar to indirect inguinal herniae.

Inguinal herniae usually present as a swelling in the inguinal region first noticed by the carer when changing or bathing the child, especially if crying or straining.[7] The swelling may extend into the scrotum in boys or the labia majora in girls. Persistent tachycardia, overlying erythema and marked tenderness suggest an irreducible hernia complicated by ischaemia.[8] Occasionally, an irreducible hernia may present with vomiting and abdominal distension as a result of intestinal obstruction.

A hernia can be differentiated from a hydrocele as the latter transilluminates and does not usually extend into the inguinal region. In neonates, these differences may be less obvious and a hernia may appear to transilluminate. Encysted hydroceles of the cord and, rarely, testicular torsion may also cause diagnostic confusion. Where there is any doubt regarding the diagnosis, a paediatric surgeon should be consulted.

Femoral

Femoral herniae are rare in children, accounting for between 0.4 and 1.1% of all groin herniae.[1,9] They are often not diagnosed prior to surgery and are one cause of recurrent 'inguinal' herniae in children. Typically, most present between 4 and 10 years of age and there is an equal sex incidence. Clinically, the hernia presents as a swelling that is inferior and lateral to the pubic tubercle. As in adults, femoral herniae are associated with a high incidence of complications, so prompt surgical intervention is required.

Umbilical and paraumbilical herniae

A true umbilical hernia occurs through the umbilical ring as opposed to a paraumbilical hernia that results from a defect *adjacent* to the umbilical ring.

Umbilical herniae are very common, occurring in up to 18.5% of infants under 6 months of age.[5] They are more common in Afro-Caribbean children and in premature infants, when the incidence rises to between 41.6 and 75%.[10,11] The vast majority of umbilical defects appear to close spontaneously with increasing age, largely irrespective of the size of the defect. Given the very low risk of the hernia becoming non-reducible, surgical repair is only indicated for those herniae that persist beyond 3 and 5 years of age, or in the very few that present with symptoms.[12]

Paraumbilical defects do not close with increasing age and should be referred for elective repair on diagnosis.

Epigastric herniae

These herniae occur as a result of a defect, often only a few millimetres in size, in the linea alba between the umbilicus and the xiphisternum. The child presents with a small swelling in this region that may be associated with pain, usually due to entrapment of extraperitoneal fat. Once diagnosed, elective surgical repair is required.

Complications

Complications of an irreducible hernia are more likely to occur if the child presents late or there is diagnostic delay. The most common adverse sequelae include gonadal ischaemia and bowel obstruction. Enteric ischaemia, perhaps leading to perforation, remains rare.

Treatment

All inguinal hernias require surgery due to the risk of bowel ischaemia and compression of adjacent gonadal structures. If the hernia is reducible, the patient should be discussed with a paediatric surgeon regarding the timing of follow up. Neonates and infants should be assessed within 1 week of presentation and scheduled for early elective surgery because of the high risk of the hernia becoming irreducible in this age group. Carers should be advised to re-present urgently if signs and symptoms of an irreducible hernia develop.

Indirect inguinal hernias have traditionally been treated by a herniotomy, with removal of the hernial sac following its ligation at the internal ring. This procedure has a high success rate with a low incidence of important complications such as injury to the vas and subsequent testicular atrophy.[6] Laparoscopic correction involves suture ligation of the hernial sac from within the abdominal cavity and appears to have a slightly higher recurrence rate than open surgery.[13] Direct hernias are generally repaired primarily without the use of mesh.[6]

If the hernia does not spontaneously reduce, a paediatric surgeon should be contacted urgently. In the absence of signs or symptoms suggestive of ischaemia, manual reduction by an experienced clinician may be attempted. The child should be given appropriate analgesia. A two-handed technique is required: one hand from above disengages the hernia from the external ring and the other from below reduces the hernia by gentle direct pressure. If there are signs suggestive of ischaemia, emergency surgery is required.

Controversies

❶ The role of routine contralateral inguinal exploration in children with a unilateral inguinal hernia remains controversial. A recent systematic review suggested that, as the overall risk of developing a metachronous hernia in childhood was 7.2%, routine contralateral exploration was not warranted.[14]

❷ The use of intraoperative laparoscopy for the assessment of the presence of a contralateral inguinal hernia has been advocated but even if positive may not necessarily correlate with subsequent development of a symptomatic hernia on that side.

References

1. Bronsther B, Abrahams MW, Elboim C. Inguinal hernia in children – a study of 1000 cases and review of the literature. *J Am Med Women's Ass* 1992;**27**:522–5.
2. Darlow BA, Dawson KP, Mogridge N. Inguinal hernia and low birth weight. *N Z Med J* 1987;**100**:492–4.
3. Harper RG, Garcia A, Sia C. Inguinal hernia: A common problem of premature infants weighing 1000 grams or less at birth. *Paediatrics* 1975;**56**:112–5.
4. Bawkin H. Indirect inguinal hernia in twins. *J Pediatr Surg* 1971;**6**:165–8.
5. Rescorla FJ. Hernias and umbilicus. In: Oldham KT, Colombani PM, Foglia RP, editors. *Surgery of infants and children*. Philadelphia: Lippincott-Raven; 1997. p. 1069–81.
6. Brandt ML. Pediatric hernias. *Surg Clin North Am* 2008;**88**:27–43.

7. Johnstone JMS. Hernia in the neonate. In: Freeman NV, Burge DM, Griffiths M, Malone PSJ, editors. *Surgery of the newborn*. Edinburgh: Churchill Livingstone; 1994. p. 321–30.
8. Kapur P, Caty MG, Glick PL. Paediatric hernias and hydroceles. *Pediatr Clin North Am* 1998;**45**:773–89.
9. Radcliffe G, Stringer MD. Reappraisal of femoral hernia in children. *Br J Surg* 1997;**84**:58–60.
10. Crump EP. Umbilical hernia: Occurrence of the infantile type in Negro infants and children. *J Pediatr* 1952;**40**:214–23.
11. Vohr BR, Rosenfeld AG, Oh W. Umbilical hernia in low birth weight infants (less than 1500 grams). *J Pediatr* 1977;**90**:807–8.
12. Meier DE, OlaOlorun DA, Omodele RA, et al. Tarpley JL. Incidence of umbilical hernia in African children: Redefinition of 'normal' and re-evaluation of indications for repair. *World J Surg* 2001;**25**:645–8.
13. Zitsman JL. Pediatric minimal-access surgery: update 2006. *Pediatrics* 2006;**118**:304–8.
14. Ron O, Eaton S, Pierro A. Systematic review of the risk of developing a metachronous contralateral inguinal hernia in children. *Br J Surg* 2007;**94**:804–11.

7.12 Gastroenteritis

Susan Phin

ESSENTIALS

1 Most children with gastroenteritis and mild-moderate dehydration can be successfully rehydrated with oral rehydration solutions either by mouth or nasogastric tube.

2 Oral rehydration solutions (ORS) should be used for oral rehydration, not fruit juices, soft drinks or sports drinks.

3 It is important to use appropriate intravenous fluids for bolus or maintenance phases of rehydration.

4 Careful instruction to parents in how to give oral fluids appropriately is vital.

5 Antidiarrhoeal and most antiemetic medications should not be used in children.

6 Early refeeding with age-appropriate foods should be encouraged.

7 Timely reassessment is vital and, if the child does not progress as anticipated, other diagnoses and complications should be considered.

8 Other diagnoses should be considered, especially in the presence of:

- An infant less than 6 months of age
- High-grade fever
- Bilious vomiting
- Significant abdominal pain
- No diarrhoea
- Blood in vomitus or stool
- Drowsiness/reduced level of consciousness.

Introduction

Acute gastroenteritis is an inflammation of the gastrointestinal tract. It is one of the commonest reasons for children to present to an emergency department (ED). Most children under 5 years of age have experienced an episode of gastroenteritis and most can be successfully managed without admission to hospital. Worldwide, however, gastroenteritis still remains a significant cause of morbidity and mortality.[1]

Aetiology

Gastroenteritis is caused by a wide range of pathogens including viruses, bacteria and parasites (as shown in Table 7.12.1). In developed countries, the majority of episodes are due to viruses, with rotavirus being by far the most common pathogen. The most common bacterial causes are *Salmonella* and *Campylobacter*. *Shigella*, *Yersinia* and *Escherichia coli* are less common, while *Vibrio cholerae* is seen in developing countries. Parasites such as *Giardia* and *Cryptosporidium* are sometimes the infective agent.

In general a bacterium is more likely to be the causative agent if:

❶ There is blood or mucus in the stool.
❷ There is significant abdominal pain.
❸ There is a high-grade fever.

These infective agents cause gastroenteritis by one or more mechanisms. Some directly invade the bowel wall, e.g. *Salmonella* or *Shigella*, some produce toxins prior to ingestion, e.g. *Staphylococcus aureus*, and some multiply and produce toxins within the gastrointestinal tract, e.g. *Shigella*.

In an uncomplicated acute bout of gastroenteritis, determining the causative pathogen is usually unnecessary, as this usually does not alter the management.

History

Most children with acute gastroenteritis present with a history of diarrhoea and vomiting. Abdominal pain and fever are sometimes accompanying symptoms. It is important to ask for specific details about these symptoms, to increase the certainty of the diagnosis of gastroenteritis and also to help assess the risk of dehydration in the child.

Diarrhoea refers to loose or liquid stools. The frequency, volume (small to voluminous) and consistency (semisolid to watery) and

Table 7.12.1   Common causes of acute gastroenteritis

Viruses	Bacteria	Parasites
Rotavirus	Salmonella	Cryptosporidium
Norwalk virus	Campylobacter jejuni	Giardia lamblia
Enteric adenovirus	Shigella	Entamoeba histolytica
	Escherichia coli	
	Yersinia enterocolitica	
	Vibrio cholerae	

Table 7.12.2   Standard assessment scale for severity of dehydration

Variable	Mild	Moderate	Severe
Thirst	+	++	+++
Dry mucous membranes	+	++	+++
Reduced urine output	+	++	+++
Lethargy	−	+	+++
Sunken eyes	−	+	++
Reduced skin turgor	−	+	++
Tachycardia	−	+	++
Poor perfusion	−	+	++
Tachypnoea	−	−	+
Hypotension	−	−	+

the presence of blood or mucus are all important. Similarly, the frequency and nature (bilious or non-bilious) of the vomiting are also important. The words 'my child is vomiting everything he tries to drink' can be used by parents to describe a child who has had either two or 20 vomits in the last 24 hours. It is important, therefore, to be specific in questioning.

The abdominal pain that can be associated with gastroenteritis is crampy in nature and commonly more pronounced in bacterial gastroenteritis. It is not accompanied by focal or significant findings on abdominal examination. If fever is a symptom, the height of the fever can be helpful. Although children with rotaviral gastroenteritis are often febrile, it is not usually high-grade. Such fevers are more likely in bacterial gastroenteritis or in other diagnoses altogether.

Specific details about the amount of fluid tolerated by the child are vital in assessing the risk of dehydration. Parents are usually able to estimate whether, over a 24-hour period, the child has taken one-quarter, one-half or three-quarters of normal intake. Intake that is consistently less than half of normal is of concern.

Specific questions about urine output (i.e. heaviness and frequency of wet nappies) are also important. Fewer than four wet nappies in 24 hours is of concern when assessing hydration status.

Questions about the level of alertness and activity of the child are also important. Lethargy may simply be an indication of significant dehydration in a child. However, more severe lethargy and drowsiness (particularly if out of proportion to that expected for the dehydration) may indicate another more serious diagnosis as the cause of the child's symptoms, such as enteroviral meningitis.

Examination

The aim of the clinical examination is to exclude signs of an alternative cause of the symptoms, other than gastroenteritis (see Chapter 7.8) and to assess the degree of dehydration.

Occasionally pathogens causing gastroenteritis can cause extraintestinal disease. This can occur particularly with *Shigella* and *Salmonella*. *Shigella* can cause central nervous system irritation, which can manifest as encephalopathy or seizures. This may occur prior to the onset of diarrhoea. *Salmonella can* cause a bacteraemia, which can lead to focal infections including osteomyelitis and meningitis. The infant under 6 months of age is particularly at risk.

Assessment of dehydration

The accurate assessment of dehydration is difficult. Studies have shown that medical personnel tend to overestimate the degree of dehydration.[2] The gold standard in assessment of dehydration is a loss of weight compared with a recent pre-illness weight. For example, a 1-year-old weighing 10 kg a week ago who presents with gastroenteritis for 3 days and now weighs 9.5 kg, is approximately 5% dehydrated. However, a recent weight is rarely available in the ED. Therefore, tables such as Table 7.12.2 use a combination of clinical symptoms and signs to estimate the degree of dehydration.

It is important to remember that some of the signs and symptoms of dehydration can be affected by other factors. Mouth breathers have dry mucous membranes. Watery diarrhoea can make it difficult to assess if the child has a wet nappy from urine output. Crying can cause a sunken fontanelle to appear full. Tachycardia may be caused by a crying, anxious or febrile child; therefore it is the context and trend of the pulse that is important.

Various studies have attempted to validate combinations of these signs and symptoms with varying degrees of standardisation and scientific validity.[2–5] Difficulties arise as some of the signs are subjective and gold standards differ.

Gorelick et al[5] performed a good study in Philadelphia in 1997, which looked at the 10 clinical signs shown in Table 7.12.3. Using a gold standard of serial weight gain, they found that <3 signs correlated with <5% dehydration, 3–6 signs correlated with 5–9% dehydration and >7 signs correlated with >10% dehydration.

Laboratory investigations in the assessment of dehydration

There are few data to support the usefulness of laboratory tests in the assessment of dehydration due to gastroenteritis. Dehydration is thought to typically cause a metabolic acidosis. It is true that vomiting can cause a metabolic acidosis by several mechanisms including volume depletion, lactic acidosis and starvation ketosis. However, isolated vomiting can also cause a metabolic

Table 7.12.3   Ten clinical signs of dehydration

1. Decreased skin elasticity
2. Capillary refill >2 seconds
3. General appearance (ill-appearing, irritable, apathetic)
4. Absent tears
5. Abnormal respirations
6. Dry mucous membranes
7. Sunken eyes
8. Abnormal radial pulse
9. Tachycardia (HR >150)
10. Decreased urine output

Source: Gorelick et al.[5]

GASTROENTEROLOGY AND HEPATOLOGY

7

alkalosis through loss of gastric acid. In addition, isolated diarrhoea can cause a metabolic acidosis through loss of bicarbonate in the stool, but the child who can increase oral intake to keep pace with the diarrhoeal losses may not actually be dehydrated. Despite these confounding factors, it has been shown that serum bicarbonate is significantly lower in children with moderate or severe dehydration (mean 14.5 mEq L^{-1} and 10.3 mEq L^{-1}) than in children with mild dehydration (mean 18.9 mEq L^{-1}).[3] Raised serum urea levels have also been thought to reflect dehydration, but with even less evidence.

From a practical point of view, it is not vital to put a specific percentage on the degree of dehydration, particularly when the accuracy of such a specific percentage is questionable. What is important is to allocate the child into a broad category of dehydration, for example, mild, moderate or severe, which determines what treatment should be commenced, and then to reassess the child and the degree of dehydration within a specific timeframe.

Differential diagnosis

Many other conditions can masquerade as gastroenteritis by presenting with a combination of vomiting, diarrhoea, fever, or abdominal pain. These include:

- other infections, e.g. urinary tract infection, meningitis;
- surgical diseases, e.g. intussusception, bowel obstruction, appendicitis;
- raised intracranial pressure, e.g. blocked ventriculoperitoneal shunt;
- metabolic diseases, e.g. diabetic ketoacidosis, inborn errors of metabolism.

Features of concern to suggest the possibility of other cause include:

- age less than 6 months;
- high-grade fever;
- bilious vomiting;
- significant abdominal pain;
- no diarrhoea;
- blood in vomitus or stool;
- drowsiness/reduced level of consciousness.

See Chapter 7.8 on diarrhoea and vomiting, for more details on differential diagnosis.

Investigations

In uncomplicated acute gastroenteritis, it is usually not necessary to perform any investigations, as they will not alter management. Indications to consider performing investigations include:

- uncertainty about diagnosis;
- severe dehydration;
- the child's clinical course not progressing as anticipated;
- commencement of intravenous rehydration.

Stool cultures do not change management in simple gastroenteritis; therefore they are not usually warranted. If bacterial gastroenteritis is suspected a stool sample may be performed, although this will not change management in the majority of cases. A stool sample may be taken for public-health reasons, or to reassure the doctor that there is not another cause for the blood and mucus in the stool.

Urine culture is usually unnecessary when the diagnosis of gastroenteritis is clear. However, if there is little diarrhoea, particularly if the child is under 6 months of age, it may be necessary to exclude a urinary tract infection. It is important that a *clean* specimen is collected to avoid contamination by stool contents.

Electrolytes, urea and creatinine are usually unnecessary in children with gastroenteritis who are mild to moderately dehydrated and who are to receive oral fluids, as they will not usually alter management. If, however, the child does not improve as expected, or deteriorates despite rehydration, or the child was initially severely dehydrated, these tests along with a blood glucose level and perhaps other investigations, will be required.

A full blood count and blood culture are unnecessary in acute gastroenteritis. However, if the diagnosis is uncertain it may be reasonable to perform these tests. In the younger infant, particularly the under 3 month age group, if bacterial gastroenteritis is likely, the possibility of systemic *Salmonella* infection should be considered and blood culture and intravenous antibiotics considered.

If significant abdominal pain is present and surgical pathology such as intussusception or bowel obstruction seems more likely than simple gastroenteritis, other investigations such as abdominal X-rays, ultrasound or air enemas may be required.

Treatment

Mildly dehydrated

Children in developed countries presenting to EDs with gastroenteritis are often only mildly dehydrated or not dehydrated at all. Most can be managed as outpatients with oral fluids alone. Educating the parents in how to give fluids, and observing them giving a trial of fluids to the child, are important to empower the parents to provide ongoing oral rehydration at home.

The essential things to ensure are:

- the parent knows the appropriate oral fluids to give;
- the parent knows how, and is able, to give the oral fluids correctly to optimise success;
- the parent will have the child reviewed by the local doctor within 48 hours;
- the parent knows what worrying signs and symptoms to look for that would require representation.

If the above criteria cannot be satisfied, the child may need to be admitted. This is particularly so in the younger infant or those with profuse gastrointestinal losses, as they have a higher risk of becoming dehydrated. See 'moderately dehydrated' for further treatment options in those patients.

Appropriate oral fluids

Oral rehydration solutions (ORSs) are the appropriate fluids to rehydrate children with gastroenteritis. These are specifically designed fluids that contain the correct amounts of sodium, glucose and other electrolytes and are of the appropriate osmolality to maximise water absorption from the gut. They use the principle of glucose-facilitated sodium transport, whereby glucose enhances sodium and secondarily water transport across the mucosa of the upper intestine. The sodium and glucose concentrations and the osmolality are of vital importance.

The WHO ORS has a sodium concentration of 90 mmol L^{-1}. In developed countries with non-cholera diarrhoea, it is generally thought that 90 mmol L^{-1} is a little high, as non-cholera gastroenteritis does not result in the same sodium losses that are seen in cholera. Many different ORSs with varying sodium concentrations have been developed. It has been shown[6] that water absorption across the lumen of the human intestine is maximal using solutions with a sodium concentration of 60 mmol L^{-1} and this is the concentration recommended by the European Society of Paediatric Gastroenterology and Nutrition.[7] Studies have also shown that hypo-osmolar solutions are most effective at promoting water absorption.[8–10]

Studies have also examined rice-based ORSs and their effect on stool output and duration of diarrhoea when compared with glucose-based ORSs. Rice-based ORSs appear to have benefits in cholera diarrhoea but not in non-cholera diarrhoea.[11]

The composition of various ORSs and other fluids is shown in Tables 7.12.4 and 7.12.5. Fruit juices and soft drinks are inappropriate because of the minimal sodium content and the excessive glucose content and hence excessive osmolality. Diluting these solutions will not address the grossly inadequate sodium content, nor will it result in an optimal glucose concentration or osmolality. Sports drinks are also inappropriate, with too low sodium levels and too high glucose levels and osmolalities.

Method of giving oral fluids

The important message is to give small amounts of fluid frequently, for example 0.5 mL kg^{-1} every 5 minutes. The fluid can be measured in a syringe and given to the child either by syringe, teaspoon or cup. The child is far more likely to tolerate these small amounts of fluid than a whole bottle at once. If the child tolerates this fluid the parent can gradually increase the volume and decrease the frequency of the fluid offered. Success can be optimised in the ED setting by giving the parents a documentation chart to fill in, which shows the fluid given and any vomits or diarrhoea or urine passed.

It is important to educate the parents that seeing a doctor will not cure the vomiting and diarrhoea. Small, frequent amounts of fluid will hopefully minimise the vomiting, but will not reduce the diarrhoea. The aim is for the input to exceed the output enough to rehydrate and then maintain hydration. Parents will know if they are succeeding by observing their child for the following symptoms and signs.

Indications for re-presentation

Parents should be given some indication of symptoms and signs that will prompt re-presentation. These need to be relatively easy for a parent to detect. They will be related to two things:

❶ The child is, or is at risk of becoming, more dehydrated
  - persistent vomiting despite small amounts of oral fluids frequently; or
  - no wet nappy for 8 hours; or
  - increasing lethargy.
❷ Gastroenteritis may not be the correct diagnosis
  - bilious vomiting; or
  - significant abdominal pain; or
  - drowsiness.

Refeeding

- Breast-fed infants – breast-feeding should continue throughout the episode of gastroenteritis, including the rehydration phase.
- Formula-fed infants – full-strength normal formula should be started as soon as the infant is rehydrated. This can be supplemented with an ORS for ongoing losses, for example offer 10 mL kg^{-1} after each diarrhoea. However, children with no dehydration and mild gastroenteritis are the least likely to take an ORS because of the salty taste. In this instance increased amounts of normal fluids in conjunction with age-appropriate feeding may be sufficient.
- Early refeeding – studies have shown that early refeeding does not worsen or prolong the duration of diarrhoea, nor increase vomiting or lactose intolerance, and leads to a significantly higher weight gain after rehydration.[12] Early reintroduction of age-appropriate foods is now recommended.

Moderately dehydrated

Some children who present to EDs with gastroenteritis are moderately dehydrated. These children can be rehydrated in several ways. Some are successfully rehydrated with oral fluids alone, as previously described. Some fail this and require additional intervention. Increasing numbers of hospitals in developed countries are using oral rehydration therapy (ORT) via continuous nasogastric infusion.[13,14] This is where an ORS is infused continuously down a nasogastric tube with a pump such as a Kangaroo pump. Nasogastric infusions should not be used

Table 7.12.4	Composition of oral rehydration solutions				
ORSs	Na (mm L^{-1})	Carbohydrate			Osmolality (mOsm L^{-1})
			(mm L^{-1})	(%)	
WHO	90	G	111	2	331
Gastrolyte	60	G	90	2	240
Gastrolyte-R	60	RSS	6 (g L^{-1})	2.5	226
Hydralyte (solution or iceblock)	45	G	90	2.5	240

G, glucose; RSS, ice syrup solids.

Table 7.12.5	Composition of oral fluids		
Oral fluids	Na (mm L^{-1})	Carbohydrate (mm L^{-1})	Osmolality (mOsm L^{-1})
Apple juice	3	690	730
Sports drinks	20	255	330
Soft drinks	2	700	750

when the child has an ileus or is comatose. Oral rehydration therapy has been the method of choice in developing countries since the 1970s. However, it has taken longer to become accepted in developed countries. This is despite numerous studies that show that it is as effective as intravenous rehydration but less expensive[13-21] and reduces lengths of hospital stay.[13]

Different regimens are used for continuous nasogastric rehydration. The European Society of Paediatric Gastroenterology and Nutrition recommends calculating the fluid deficit and replacing that over 4 hours.[22] The American Academy of Pediatrics recommends that mildly dehydrated children receive 50 mL kg^{-1} over 4 hours and moderately dehydrated children receive 100 mL kg^{-1} over 4 hours.[23] Other regimes recommend a fixed volume, for example 40 mL kg^{-1} over 4 hours for all mild to moderately dehydrated children followed by a reassessment and retrial of oral fluids.[24] This takes into account the tendency for medical officers to overestimate the degree of dehydration[2] and the desire to avoid subsequent over-hydration. The important thing to remember is that, whatever regimen is used to rehydrate the child, fluid status should be regularly reassessed.

Intravenous rehydration

Intravenous rehydration should be used to rehydrate children with gastroenteritis who fail nasogastric therapy or deteriorate.

The volume (mL) of replacement fluids is calculated using the formula: weight (kg) × dehydration (%) × 10. Maintenance fluids are then calculated, with one method being to give 100 mL kg^{-1} for the first 10 kg, 50 mL kg^{-1} for the second 10 kg and 20 mL kg^{-1} for each subsequent kilogram. The volumes for rehydration and maintenance are then added together and divided by 24 to calculate the hourly rate.

The recommended fluid used to rehydrate children with gastroenteritis has changed over recent years. It is now recommended that for children, excluding neonates and infants <3 months of age, 0.9% (150 mmol L^{-1}) saline + 2.5% (or 5%) glucose should be used.[25,26] Studies have shown that children with gastroenteritis have inappropriately high levels of antidiuretic hormone and increased incidence and risk of hyponatraemia[27] and that low

sodium solutions cause hyponatraemia while solutions with a sodium content of 130–154 mmol L^{-1} are protective.[28] As in nasogastric rehydration, it is important to regularly reassess the child's fluid status. If the child remains on intravenous fluids for >24 hours, it is important to recheck the electrolytes.

If the child is significantly hypernatraemic the rate of infusion needs to be reduced to rehydrate the child over 48–72 hours. The aim is to avoid a rapid fall in the serum sodium level as this can precipitate cerebral oedema. It is still reasonable to start with 0.9% (150 mmol L^{-1}) saline + 2.5% (or 5%) glucose to prevent a rapid initial fall in serum sodium, but this may need to be changed to 0.45% (75 mmol L^{-1}) saline + 2.5% (or 5%) glucose, depending on progress of the electrolytes, which need to be rechecked frequently. If the child is hyponatraemic, 0.9% (150 mmol L^{-1}) saline + 2.5% (or 5%) glucose should be used. Senior paediatric advice should be sought if the serum sodium level is significantly abnormal.

Rapid intravenous rehydration: Interest in rapid intravenous rehydration for children with gastroenteritis has emerged in recent years in developed countries. It has long been used in developing countries.[29,30] There have been a number of studies in developed countries over the last several years that have looked at this issue[24,28,31-33] and shown that this seems to be a safe and effective way to rehydrate children with gastroenteritis who require intravenous therapy. An example of this type of regime is giving 0.9% (150 mmol L^{-1}) saline + 2.5% glucose at 10 mL kg^{-1} hr^{-1} for 4 hours.[34] It is important that lower sodium-containing fluids are **not** used.

Severely dehydrated

Although this is a relatively rare occurrence in developed countries, it is vital to diagnose and institute immediate treatment, as this is a medical emergency. The child is usually shocked and needs immediate intravenous access and resuscitation with a 20 mL kg^{-1} bolus of normal saline or Hartmann's solution. If the child remains shocked the bolus should be repeated. Senior advice should be sought about any child presenting in this condition. During insertion of the cannula, blood should be taken for electrolytes, urea, creatinine, glucose, full blood count and

venous blood gas. Blood cultures can also be taken at the same time if indicated.

Glucose-containing fluids such as 0.45% (75 mmol L^{-1}) saline + 2.5% glucose or 0.225% (37.5 mmol L^{-1}) saline + 3.75% glucose *should never be used for resuscitation boluses*. Although these solutions are technically isotonic, the glucose is rapidly metabolised, so effectively it is as if a hypotonic solution has been given, with the resultant risk of rapid fluid shifts and cerebral oedema. It is important to differentiate these resuscitation boluses from rapid rehydration therapy. The resuscitation boluses are given over several minutes and *do not* contain glucose. The rapid rehydration fluids are given over several hours and *do* contain glucose.

After the initial resuscitation, replacement plus maintenance fluids are given as per above. It is important to reassess the child's hydration status regularly and look for any indication that another diagnosis is the cause of the child's condition. Electrolytes, urea and creatinine need to be regularly repeated while the child remains significantly unwell.

Other treatments
Antibiotics

Antibiotics are rarely indicated in gastroenteritis. They are of proven benefit for treatment of only the following situations:

- *Shigella*
  Intravenous ampicillin in severe disease
  Oral ampicillin or trimethoprim-sulfamethoxazole in milder disease
  Shortens illness duration, eradicates organism.
- Invasive *Salmonella* infections – e.g. septicaemia, osteomyelitis, meningitis
  Intravenous cefotaxime or ceftriaxone
  Antibiotics prolong excretion in gastroenteritis.
- Traveller's diarrhoea – trimethoprim-sulfamethoxazole.
- *Campylobacter* septicaemia – erythromycin or gentamicin. Not indicated in uncomplicated gastroenteritis.

Anti-diarrhoeal and anti-emetic medications

Anti-diarrhoeal medications are *not indicated* in children with gastroenteritis. Most anti-emetic medications are also *not indicated*. There is little evidence of efficacy and a high incidence of side effects such as dystonic reactions and sedation in infants and young children. There have been some recent studies[35–37] that show that ondansetron may have some clinical benefit in this setting by reducing vomiting, but they do not decrease the length of illness and may prolong the diarrhoea.[37] Experienced clinicians who wish to use this medication in this setting should generally limit its use to a single dose.

Disposition

In the past, many children were admitted to hospital with gastroenteritis when perhaps they did not need to be.[38] With the emergence of 'Short Stay Wards' or 'Emergency Observation Units', where patients can be admitted to a special area within the ED for a finite time of less than 24 hours, hospital inpatient admission rates for children with gastroenteritis have fallen.[24] In these units children can be rehydrated (orally or via rapid nasogastric or intravenous infusion) over a period of a few hours and then sent home after appropriate education and advice. This is provided that the medical officer is confident about the diagnosis of gastroenteritis and that the criteria set out in the 'mildly dehydrated' section are fulfilled. Care needs to be taken especially with young infants, as they become dehydrated more rapidly than older children and are more likely to have another diagnosis.

Paediatric staff in non-children's hospitals can potentially be utilised to help manage these patients in conjunction with ED staff. An admission to, and discharge from, these 'Short Stay Wards' causes much less disruption to the child and family and allows hospital resources to be used for other patients requiring inpatient admissions. Some children, however, still require an inpatient admission for successful management.

Prognosis

Gastroenteritis in children is generally a benign, self-limiting disease, with dehydration being the major potential complication. If this is recognised early and the child is rehydrated appropriately, the child should recover completely with no adverse sequelae.

Controversies and future directions

❶ Interest has arisen in the use of probiotics such as *Lactobacillus* GG in the treatment of acute gastroenteritis. Early studies seem to suggest that it may shorten the diarrhoeal illness.[39] Further research is necessary.

❷ The use of anti-emetics such as ondansetron in children may decrease the vomiting frequency in gastroenteritis, but does not decrease the length of illness and may prolong the diarrhoea.[35–37] Further research is necessary.

References

1. World Health Organization. *The treatment of diarrhoea: A manual for physicians and other senior health workers.* Geneva: WHO; 1995 (WHO/CDR/95.3 Rev 3 10/95).
2. Mackenzie A, Barnes G, Shann F. Clinical signs of dehydration in children. *Lancet* 1989;2(8663):605–7.
3. Vega RM, Avner JR. A prospective study of the usefulness of clinical and laboratory parameters for predicting percentage of dehydration in children. *Pediatr Emerg Care* 1997;13:179–82.
4. Duggan C, Refat M, Hashem M, et al. How valid are clinical signs of dehydration in infants. *J Pediatr Gastroenterol Nutr* 1996;22:56–61.
5. Gorelick MH, Shaw KN, Murphy KO. Validity and reliability of clinical signs in the diagnosis of dehydration in children. *Paediatrics* 1997;99(5):E6.
6. Hunt JB, Elliott EJ, Fairclough PD, et al. Water and solute absorption from hypotonic glucose-electrolyte solutions in human jejunum. *Gut* 1992;33:479–83.
7. Booth I, Ferreira R, Desjeux JF, et al. Recommendation for composition of oral rehydration solutions for the children of Europe. Report of an ESPGAN working group. *J Pediatr Gastroenterol Nutr* 1992;14:113–5.
8. Ferreira RMCC, Elliott EJ, Watson AJM, et al. Dominant role for osmolality in the efficacy of glucose and glycine-containing oral rehydration solutions: Studies in a rat model of secretory diarrhoea. *Acta Paediatr* 1991;81:46–50.
9. Hunt JB, Thillainayagam AV, Salim AFM, et al. Water and solute absorption from a new hypotonic oral rehydration solution: Evaluation in human and animal perfusion models. *Gut* 1992;33:1652–9.
10. International Study Group on Reduced-osmolarity ORS Solutions. Multicentre evaluation of reduced-osmolarity oral rehydration salts solution. *Lancet* 1995;345:282–5.
11. Gore SM, Fontaine O, Pierce NF. Impact of rice based oral rehydration solution on stool output and duration of diarrhoea: Meta-analysis of 13 clinical trials. *Br Med J* 1992;304:287–91.
12. Walker-Smith JA, Sandhu BK, Isolauri E, et al. Recommendations for feeding in childhood gastroenteritis. *J Pediatr Gastroenterol Nutr* 1997;24:619–20.
13. Gremse DA. Effectiveness of nasogastric rehydration in hospitalised children with acute diarrhoea. *J Pediatr Gastroenterol Nutr* 1995;21:145–8.
14. Mackenzie A, Barnes G. Randomised controlled trial comparing oral and intravenous rehydration therapy in children with diarrhoea. *Br Med J* 1991;303:393–6.
15. Sharifi J, Ghavami F, Nowrouzi Z, et al. Oral versus intravenous rehydration therapy in severe gastroenteritis. *Arch Dis Child* 1985;60:856–60.
16. Issenman RM, Leung AK. Oral and intravenous rehydration of children. *Can Fam Physician* 1993;39:2129–36.
17. Vesikari T, Isolauri E, Baer M. A comparative trial of rapid oral and intravenous rehydration in acute diarrhoea. *Acta Paediatr Scand* 1987;76:300–305.
18. Santosham M, Daum RS, Dillman L, et al. Oral rehydration therapy of infantile diarrhoea. *N Engl J Med* 1982;306:1070–6.
19. Tamer AM, Friedman LB, Maxwell SRW, et al. Oral rehydration of infants in a large US urban medical center. *J Pediatr* 1985;107:14–9.
20. Listernick R, Zieserl E, Davis AT. Out-patient oral rehydration in the United States. *Am J Dis Child* 1986;140:211–5.
21. Nager AL, Wang VJ. Comparison of nasogastric and intravenous methods of rehydration in pediatric patients with acute dehydration. *Paediatrics* 2002;109 (4):566–72.
22. Sandhu BK, Isolauri E, Walker-Smith JA, et al. Early feeding in gastroenteritis. *J Pediatr Gastroenterol Nutr* 1997;24:522–7.
23. American Academy of Pediatrics, Provisional Committee on Quality Improvement, Subcommittee on Acute Gastroenteritis. Practice parameter: The management of acute gastroenteritis in young children. *Paediatrics* 1996;97:424–35.
24. Phin SJ, McCaskill ME, Browne GJ, Lam LT. Clinical pathway using rapid rehydration in children with gastroenteritis. *J Paediatr Child Health* 2003;39:343–8.
25. Children's Hospital Australasia working party. *Interim recommendations: Intravenous fluid types for children and adolescents.* 2010.
26. National Patient Safety Agency. *Reducing the risk of hyponatraemia when administering intravenous fluids to children.* 2007. Available from http://www.npsa.nhs.uk/nrls/alerts-and-directives/alerts/intravenous-infusions/ [accessed 15.10.10].
27. Neville KA, Verge CF, O'Meara MW, Walker JL. High antidiuretic hormone levels and hyponatraemia in children with gastroenteritis. *Pediatrics* 2005;116 (6):1401–7.
28. Neville KA, Verge CF, Rosenberg AR, et al. Isotonic is better than hypotonic saline for intravenous rehydration of children with gastroenteritis: a prospective randomised study. *Arch Dis Child* 2006;91 (3):226–32.
29. Slone D, Levin SE. Hypertonic dehydration and summer diarrhoea. *S Afr Med J* 1969;34:209–13.
30. Rahman O, Bennish ML, Adam AN, et al. Rapid intravenous rehydration by means of a single polyelectrolyte solution with or without dextrose. *J Pediatr* 1988;113:654–60.
31. Reid SR, Bonadio WA. Outpatient rapid intravenous rehydration to correct dehydration and resolve vomiting in children with acute gastroenteritis. *Pediatrics* 1996;28 (3):318–23.
32. Moineau G, Newman J. Rapid intravenous rehydration in the pediatric ED. *Pediatr Emerg Care* 1990;6 (3):186–8.
33. Brewster DR. Dehydration in acute gastroenteritis. *J Paediatr Child Health* 2002;38:219–22.
34. NSW Department of Health. *Infants and Children: Acute Management of Gastroenteritis – Clinical practice guideline.* 3rd ed. 2010.
35. Freedman SB, Adler M, Seshadri R, et al. Oral ondansetron for gastroenteritis in a pediatric emergency department. *N Engl J Med* 2006;354(16):1698–705.
36. Reeves JJ, Shannon MW, Fleisher GR. Ondansetron decreases vomiting associated with acute gastroenteritis: a randomized, controlled trial. *Pediatrics* 2002;109(4): e62.
37. Chubeddu LX, Trujillo LM, Talmaciu I, et al. Antiemetic activity of ondansetron in acute gastroenteritis. *Aliment Pharmacol Ther* 1997;11(1):185–91.
38. Elliott EJ, Backhouse JA, Leach JW, et al. Pre-admission management of acute gastroenteritis. *J Paediatr Child Health* 1996;32:18–21.
39. Guandalini S, Pensabene L, Zikri MA, et al. Lactobacillus GG administered in oral rehydration solution to children with acute diarrhoea: A multicentre European trial. *J Pediatr Gastroenterol Nutr* 2000;30:54–60.

7.13 Constipation

Bruce Fasher

ESSENTIALS

1 It is important to understand the physiology and development of gut transit to recognise the normal (often regarded as abnormal).

2 Constipation is a common reason for children to present to EDs with abdominal pain.

3 Management depends on the child's age and whether the problem is acute or chronic.

4 The patient's and parents' real concerns need to be acknowledged.

5 Issues to be addressed include:

- natural history;

- the aims of treatment (empty the bowel and establish pharmacological rhythm and then wean to biological rhythm);

- the likely duration of treatment;

- the anticipated setbacks;

- the need for a coordinator clinician (normally unavailable in an ED).

6 Treat from the top, once at night and titrate the dose according to the response. Avoid treatment per rectum if at all possible, to draw attention away from any anal obsession to achieve bowel actions.

7 Be able to refer to a resource who is known to be interested in managing the condition and to ensure appropriate ongoing review and support.

Introduction

Constipation in childhood engenders in clinicians unwarranted anxieties about management. Defining terms and understanding normal physiology and its variants, the frequent blurring in paediatric medicine between physical and emotional factors and their impact on normal development along with evidence-based data can provide the clinician with an algorithm for management.

Management varies according to age and whether constipation is acute or chronic. The emergency department (ED) is a difficult place from which to manage constipation, especially chronic constipation, for success requires ongoing maintenance therapy and contact with a committed and interested clinician. This is best achieved through the child's local doctor, with input from a sympathetic paediatrician in difficult cases if deemed appropriate.[1,2]

Definitions

❶ *Constipation* is delay or difficulty in defecation, sufficient to cause significant distress.

❷ *Encopresis* is the passage of a normal stool in an abnormal place.

❸ *Soiling* is the frequent involuntary passage of loose or semi-loose stools in clothing. This is usually overflow incontinence as the liquid stool escapes around an impacted rectal faecolith.

Pathophysiology

The rectum and anal canal have two tasks, to store faeces temporarily and to evacuate at a socially convenient time. The distending rectum evokes a wave of contraction with inhibition of the smooth muscle tone of the internal anal sphincter, resulting in a sensation of the urge to defecate. An urgent desire to defecate occurs as the stool stretches the sensitive zone of the upper anal canal. This urge is overcome by the voluntary contraction of the external sphincter and the levator ani muscles. Eventually the rectum habituates to the stimulus of the enlarging faecal mass and the urge to defecate subsides. With time this retentive pattern can become automatic.

It is understandable, therefore, that the child who is afraid to use the non-private, wet, smelly school lavatory, and allows his rectum occasionally to overcome the external sphincter, as he is relieved to arrive home, albeit with 'poo in the pants' – is really a normal variant rather than true encopresis.

There is a wide variation of physiology and normal development as can be seen in the age range of successful potty training. To produce a stool at will is one of the child's first major achievements and most gain satisfaction from framing their success in a pot. If too much persuasion is provided, especially if full control has never been attained, the child's profound disappointments are compounded by disapproval and hostility from the parents. Like most adults, most children seek solitude to defecate.

Management basics

❶ Be interested. The patient has often been pushed from pillar to post, with a quick fix, and reviewed in 3 months. Recognise that the parents and the patient have a concern, which can be the cause of major family dysfunction.

❷ Endeavour to treat from the top, orally, rather than continue to direct attention to the rectum and anus with suppositories and enemas. The exception is when a fissure needs managing with ointment or Xylocaine ointment if defecation can be anticipated.

❸ Develop a pharmacological armamentarium of stool softeners or osmotic aperients. Stimulants (e.g. senna) may cause abdominal discomfort with colic in infants.

❹ Be aware that ongoing management by a single interested clinician is desirable as the constipation will often relapse, and gains are often small (three steps forward, two steps back).

❺ This makes constipation difficult to manage in EDs. Such departments need to have appropriate and willing referral resources. Outpatient appointments rarely work for the same reasons – difficulties with continuity of care and the ability to be seen relatively urgently (albeit that encouragement with management, behavioural modification and aperient dose titration is often all that is necessary and can often be done by phone by the interested clinician).

❻ The significant risk of relapse dictates that a period of maintenance therapy is necessary before weaning off medications. It might be appropriate to let the patient and family know that if it has taken 2 years to arrive at this stage it is highly likely it will take 2 years or so to regain the rectum's natural motility and sensitivity.

Constipation in babies

Never again in life will the stooling pattern, and indeed the stools, be so closely examined as in the period of nappies being changed prior to toilet training. Straining at stool is often marked and then misconstrued as constipation whereas it is a simple reflection of the urge to defecate sensation. Plantar flexion of the toes is a similarly objective sign (at all ages).

Breast-fed infants may pass a stool after each feed or as infrequently as once every few weeks. As long as the stool is of normal quality (often referred to as scrambled eggs) and of great volume there is no reason for concern. For a couple of days prior to defecation the infant may be, not unreasonably, somewhat unsettled.

Just weaned, bottle-fed infants may produce dry, hard stools with difficulty and sometimes traces of fresh blood. Attention to water intake, perhaps addition of extra

sugar (brown sugar is better) or sorbitol ($1-3$ mL kg^{-1} noct.) will help soften the stool. Formula switching is usually unproductive, although it is recognised that some forms of cows' milk intolerance may present with persistent constipation.

Should constipation persist and the clinician is confident that mother's description is of constipation, red flags should alert other considerations.

Fever, vomiting, bloody diarrhoea, failure to thrive, anal stenosis, abdominal distension, history of delayed passage of meconium, polydipsia or polyuria should prompt a search for physical causes.

Conditions to consider are listed in Table 7.13.1.

Acute constipation

Acute constipation often occurs after febrile illnesses, change in diet or environment, especially when intake has been low (e.g. low post-operatively). A fissure in ano, usually from the passage of a hard faecolith, may cause pain, sphincter spasm, withholding and the start of a vicious cycle leading to chronic constipation with megacolon and overflow incontinence. Also consider the management of a fissure-in-ano which may be hiding in the anal skin folds.

Most acute constipation resolves spontaneously but given the risk of chronic constipation, especially if there has been a previous tendency to constipation, it may be prudent to commence gentle oral therapy early.

Table 7.13.1 Conditions possibly causing persistent constipation

- Anal anomalies (stenosis, stricter, malposition)
- Spinal anomalies (spinal dysraphism, sacral agenesis)
- Hirschprung's disease
- Hypothyroidism
- Metabolic – hypercalcaemia, hypokalaemia
- Coeliac disease
- Cows' milk intolerance
- Lead poisoning
- Intellectual impairment
- Child abuse
- Cystic fibrosis
- Dietary – inadequate roughage, excessive cows' milk intake
- Psychogenic – parent-child and environment issues
- Drug related – anticholinergic, sympathomimetics, codeine

Chronic constipation

Chronic constipation is defined as persistent delay and difficulty in defecation often associated with soiling (overflow incontinence). Symptoms may be temporarily relieved by laxatives but relapse rapidly. This is why the ED is not the ideal place for long-term management, but may offer acute intervention for immediate relieve of unpleasant symptoms and to gain the family's confidence by explaining management and natural history.

These children usually present in the school-age group. There may be a history of fissure, pain and withholding then ongoing constipation for months or years. The colon, rectum and upper anal canal become loaded with faeces, insensitive and hypotonic. Soiling develops with loose faeces escaping around an inspissated hard faecolith. Faeces are often palpable per abdomen. Social rejection in the class, due to the malodorous state, is often the first impetus for the patient themselves to seek cure. This, with loss of ability to defecate at will, takes a toll on the child's emotional stability. They have often undergone multiple management regimens from dietary manipulation to manual disimpaction, delivered by a variety of healthcare workers.

Investigations

When there is doubt regarding the diagnosis, a plain abdominal X-ray is useful to demonstrate faecal loading. Demonstration of the X-ray findings to the parents may be additionally useful to aid adherence to prolonged therapeutic strategies.

Management

The management of acute versus chronic constipation varies mainly in nuance and the extent and duration of treatment.

The aim of treatment is that in gaining the family's confidence the clinician recognises that there is a very real concern, and a plan can be instituted to:

❶ Exclude physical treatable causes with careful history, examination and investigations as warranted.

❷ Empty the rectum, preferably 'from the top' i.e. through *oral agents* rather than per rectum.

❸ Establish a pharmacological bowel rhythm and pattern, which may need support for several years.

❹ Allow the enlarged rectum/colon to re-establish its own inherent physiological bowel pattern and tone and to regain its normal sensation.

❺ Continue maintenance for some time before considering slowly weaning off pharmaceuticals.

This will involve:

- Enthusiasm on part of managing clinicians.
- Non-punitive behaviour on part of the parents.
- Adjunctive behavioural modification interventions with achievable goals.
- Acknowledging the need for patience, determination and resolution as the most chronic cases will take years to resolve.
- Stool lubricants, paraffin oil, the taste of which has been well masked in Australia by Parachoc, using a nocturnal dose starting at 10 mL and titrating dose according to response (not recommended less than 1 year old due to possible aspiration pneumonia).
- Osmotic laxative, lactulose or sorbitol, initially 3 mL kg^{-1} noct. as a 70% solution, titrating dose according to response.
- Stimulants, senna starting at 2.5 mL noct. titrating dose according to response (side effects are possible colic, and if used in combination with a lubricant it may just make the faecolith spin around).
- Good results have been achieved using sachets (according to the directions) of

Macrogol 3350 which is available in several palatable commercial presentations. The Macrogol 3350 induces a laxative effect by osmosis, is virtually unchanged and unabsorbed in the gut and has no known pharmacological activity. Electrolytes are present in the formulation, realising virtually no net loss of sodium, potassium or water.

Only should oral therapy be inadequate *or* if a large impacted stool in rectum is causing significant acute distress: treatment from below may be necessary.

- Suppositories of glycerin may be helpful, especially in acute constipation.
- Microlax enemas are also helpful in the acute situation.
- Phosphate enemas (these should be avoided in children less than 2 years old; persistent use may cause hyperphosphataemia, hypocalcaemia and tetany).
- Enemas, soap and water (tap water and magnesium have potential toxicity).

Disimpaction of an obstinate rectal faecolith may require:

- Polyethylene glycol – electrolyte solution lavage, 25 mL kg^{-1} hr^{-1} (to 1000 mL hr^{-1} by nasogastric tube); causing nausea, bloating, cramps, aspiration pneumonia. This will require the child to be admitted to hospital.
- Manual disimpaction under general anaesthesia.
- There is no evidence-based medicine to suggest the success or otherwise of anal dilatation (Lord's procedure), and some consider permanent external sphincter damage may occur.

Maintenance therapy

Focuses on the prevention of recurrence and should be instituted straight after successful disimpaction or for the child presenting without disimpaction. This involves, as above, dietary interventions, behavioural modification, laxatives, patience and enthusiasm.

Dietary changes

Those commonly advised include increased fluid intake, absorbable and non-absorbable carbohydrate, (sorbitol is found in prune, pear and apple juice). No randomised control study confirms the benefit of this. Forceful implementation would then seem undesirable.

Controversies and future directions

The role of serotonin type 4 receptors in the neurochemical basis of peristalsis may provide a more logical pharmaceutical approach to the future management of constipation.

References

1. Clayden GS. *Constipation and soiling in childhood. Problems of childhood.* London: BMA; 1976.
2. Baker SS. Constipation in infants and children: Evaluation and treatment. *J Pediatr Gastroenterol Nutr* 1999;**29** (5):612–26.

Further reading

Liptak GS. Constipation. In: Meyer, et al., editors. *Evidence-based paediatrics and child health.* London: British Medical Journal Books; 2000.

NEUROLOGY

Section editor *Ian Everitt*

8.1 CSF shunt complications

Richard Lennon

ESSENTIALS

1 Emergency physicians should consider the possibility of a shunt complication in any child with a cerebrospinal fluid (CSF) shunt presenting to an ED because symptoms and signs of malfunction may be non-specific, subtle and of gradual onset.

2 The most common shunt complications are malfunction (undershunting and overshunting) and infection.

3 Shunt infection is much more likely to occur in the 6 months following insertion or revision.

4 CT scan and plain X-rays of shunt hardware ('Shunt Series') are the preferred imaging methods for detecting shunt malfunction; however, these tests are not 100% sensitive and patients should be referred to the neurosurgical service if clinical suspicion persists.

5 Before performing any procedure on a shunt, it is best to consult with the treating neurosurgeon.

Introduction

The intervention of cerebrospinal fluid (CSF) shunting for CSF accumulations has brought about long-term survival and avoidance of disabilities in children suffering from hydrocephalus. Unfortunately, the insertion of inert non-growing hardware in infants and children who are usually very active and can expect to grow 20 to 30 times their birth weight leads to a high rate of shunt complications. Some studies find that 60% or more shunts need revising after several years. The task of the Emergency Physician is to diagnose those complications, commence time critical treatments and refer to a neurosurgical service when appropriate.

Types of shunt

Many types of CSF shunt may be encountered in paediatric emergency practice. There are also many different types of shunt hardware; however, most have the same basic structure, which comprises a proximal tube that takes CSF, usually from the lateral ventricle, to the outer surface of the skull. At this point there is usually a subcutaneous one-way valve and possibly a pumping device. There may also be an antisiphoning device. The distal tubing is tunnelled under the skin to the drainage site, which is most commonly the peritoneal cavity. The distal catheter usually contains valves that prevent back flow. Variations on the positioning of the proximal tubing include placement in the subdural or subarachnoid space and placement in cystic malformations such as the Dandy Walker syndrome and also in the spinal canal as in lumbo-peritoneal shunts. Variations in the placement of the distal catheter include the right atrium, the pleural cavity and the gall bladder. By far the most common is the peritoneal cavity, with these alternatives only being used if the peritoneal site is contraindicated.

Shunt problems that may present to an emergency department (ED) are listed in Table 8.1.1.

Clinical presentation

The developmental stage of the child with a CSF shunt can cause considerable variation in the clinical presentation of shunt complications. The most obvious is the presence of an open anterior fontanelle in infants up to the age of approximately 9 to 18 months. Simply looking and feeling the fontanelle allows an estimation of intracranial pressure. A bulging fontanelle is a highly specific but not very sensitive sign of under-shunting;

Table 8.1.1 Complications of CSF shunts

- Infection
- Malfunction
  Blocked proximal catheter
  Blocked distal catheter
  Loculation of lateral ventricle
  Valve dysfunction
  Overshunting/slit ventricle syndrome
  Disconnection
- Abdominal pseudocyst
- Migration of distal catheter
- Invasion of abdominal organs (VP shunt)
- Peritonitis, ascites (VP shunt)
- Pulmonary emboli (VA shunt)
- Glomerulonephritis (VA shunts)
- Brain tumour metastases
- CSF ascites
- Pleural effusion (pleural shunts)

Table 8.1.2 Signs and symptoms that on their own warrant immediate referral to neurosurgical service

Bulging fontanelle
Decreased level of consciousness
Fluid tracking around shunt tubing
Loss of upward gaze (sunset eyes)
Signs of local infection (usually <6 m post op)
  Erythema of site
  Erosion/ulceration
  CSF leak
  Purulent drainage
Meningismus
Peritonitis

a sunken fontanelle can be a sign of overshunting.

The cranial sutures in children are not fused and can undergo diastasis due to raised intracranial pressure. The older a child is, the longer and higher the intracranial pressure has to be to cause diastasis. This also means that the head circumference will rapidly increase when there is inadequate shunting. Therefore it is important to measure the occipitofrontal circumference and compare it with previous records if available and plot it on growth centile charts. A head circumference that is rapidly crossing centiles in an upward fashion or a head circumference that is in the very high centile range especially when the other parameters, weight and length, are not, is an indicator of undershunting. Another implication of unfused cranial sutures is that because this allows an increase in cranial volume it retards the rise in intracranial pressure. This may be the reason that small infants present with more non-specific signs and symptoms than older children.

The most common question an emergency physician will have to answer when confronted with a child who has a CSF shunt is 'Should I refer this patient to the neurosurgical service?' A recent study by Piatt et al[1] attempted to quantify the power of various symptoms and sign to predict shunt malfunction or infection. Table 8.1.2 shows the strongly predictive signs and symptoms that allow referral to be made on the basis of that single finding. This may be done even before computerised tomography (CT) scanning, as the neurosurgeon may prefer to have the scan done locally to allow for easier

comparison with previous scans (see discussion of CT scanning below). Table 8.1.3 shows the signs and symptoms with strong positive predictive power but not strong enough to warrant immediate referral if just one feature is present on its own. Thus in a patient with a ventriculoperitoneal shunt (VPS) who presents with fever alone, an initial general work up for a cause of the fever is warranted and then consideration for referral to neurosurgery made if no definite cause for the fever is found. However, fever with another feature listed in Table 8.1.3, such as headache, warrants early neurosurgical referral. The question of whether to send the child home is more difficult. The absence of any of the symptoms and signs listed in Tables 8.1.2 and 8.1.3 does not rule out shunt malfunction or infection. If concerned about shunt infection, this is much less likely if the patient is more than 6 months from the last shunt insertion or revision. However, this does not exclude shunt malfunction. Where a symptom or sign that is not of high predictive power is adequately explained by another diagnosis (e.g. vomiting with diarrhoea and

Table 8.1.3 Symptoms and signs may warrant neurosurgical consultation (see text)

Abdominal pain
Fever
Nausea/vomiting
Irritability
Headache
Abnormal shunt pump test
Accelerated head growth

recent contact with a case of gastroenteritis) CSF shunt complication is very unlikely. For cases where CSF shunt complications are neither ruled in or out on historical and examination findings, one must resort to investigations and/or observation and/or neurosurgical consultation.

History

Parents may present very early, reporting vague and non-specific symptoms, particularly if the child has had a similar presentation of shunt malfunction previously.

The most common presentation of children with shunt obstruction is headache, vomiting and/or drowsiness. It is notable that seizures occur on neither of the above lists. This is because many children with shunts also have epilepsy, therefore seizure alone has a poor correlation with shunt complication. It is important to remember that distal shunt problems may present with abdominal symptomatology such as pain and distension.

Symptoms suggesting possible infection include fever, lethargy, irritability, or features of meningism. There may be concurrent symptoms of shunt obstruction.

Examination

For examination features of raised intracranial pressure see Chapter 8.2. Features of infection e.g. fever, rigors, lethargy, localised redness, swelling and peritonism (ventriculo-peritoneal shunt) or pleurisy (ventriculo-pleural shunt) should be sought.

Shunt evaluation

The extent of the shunt course itself should be examined thoroughly. The older child is usually the best at finding the shunt hardware under his/her hair. This should be palpated and, if possible, inspected for inflammation of the skin along the shunt route. Many have a silicon-pumping bulb, which is used both for checking the patency of the shunt and for access to sample CSF.

Most reservoirs can be compressed easily and rapidly refill in a few seconds. Incompressibility of the bulb is usually due to obstruction of the distal catheter. This is the less common site of obstruction. If the bulb compresses easily but does not refill, then the proximal catheter is blocked. This is the 'shunt pump test'. An abnormality of the test did not perform well enough to warrant immediate referral in Piatt's study.[1] This is because it can be difficult to tell if a test is abnormal or not. The return of the chamber after depression can take a number of minutes and may take longer if the choroid plexus is drawn into the catheter causing partial or complete obstruction. This is the reason why shunt pump tests should be kept to a minimum as multiple tests can not only cause blockage with choroid but also other debris and the ventricular wall, and can cause low pressure headache.

CSF tracking around the proximal catheter can form a fluctuant swelling around the burr hole in the skull where the shunt enters. This indicates a blocked proximal catheter or disconnection and the child requires neurosurgical consultation.

The entire subcutaneous catheter should be carefully inspected and palpated for continuity and the abdomen examined for evidence of peritonitis or pseudocyst formation.

Investigations

On rare occasions, insertion of a needle into a shunt pumping chamber may be useful for both diagnostic and therapeutic reasons but should generally be performed by neurosurgical colleagues. The exception is in the rapidly deteriorating child, where contact with the neurosurgeon is delayed or where in remote locations after discussion with the treating neurosurgeon it is considered important to get some information to help with a decision to transport. In the case of a moribund child, an emergency physician may relieve the raised intracranial pressure by inserting a 25-gauge butterfly needle into the bulb/pumping chamber at 45 degrees to the skin under strict aseptic technique.[2] It is important not to advance too deeply as the needle can damage valve mechanisms so badly that replacement is necessary. The pressure can be measured with a similar technique to that used in a lumbar puncture and then CSF drained off until the pressure is 10 cmH$_2$O.

In the stable child, an X-ray of the entire shunt may demonstrate a disconnection or kinking causing blockage. The CT scan is the usual preferred method of imaging, because it provides clear images in a short space of time. However, difficulties associated with obtaining a CT scan need to be considered. One difficulty is keeping the child still long enough to obtain adequate images even with rapid CT scanners. In infants, firm wrapping and sucrose on a dummy or pacifier may be sufficient to keep them still. When these fail procedural sedation or general anaesthesia are required. This is less desirable because of anaesthetic risk, longer delays, use of resources, and the potential to temporarily obscure one of the important signs of raised intracranial pressure (ICP), decreased level of consciousness. Another consideration is the harmful effects of the radiation exposure. A protocol designed to minimise radiation exposure in children should be used and the head angulated to avoid radiation exposure to the eyes. This reduces the risk of premature cataract formation. These precautions may not be routine at institutions that do not frequently scan children and the clinician may have to ensure that these things are done. Some studies have examined magnetic resonance imaging (MRI) as an alternative to CT scanning; however, the scan takes longer, makes it difficult to access the child, often requires the child to be sedated or anaesthetised and often does not provide images as clear as a CT.

Enlarged ventricles on scanning may indicate undershunting due to obstruction. However, this may be chronic and comparison with previous CT scans is necessary for accurate interpretation. Obliteration of the perimesencephalic cistern is a particularly worrying sign and mandates urgent neurosurgical consultation. The scan may also show the reason for malfunction (e.g. catheter tip embedded in brain tissue) or it may show a ventriculitis when the lining of the ventricles enhances with contrast. Alternatively, neuroimaging may reveal small 'slit-like' ventricles. These are thought to be due to overshunting and may be non-compliant. This leads to sharp fluctuations in ICP, with very little change in CT appearance. The management of this complication is a neurosurgical challenge. The emergency physician needs to be aware that small ventricles do not mean a normal ICP. Nuclear medicine shunt function studies are also used in some centres for diagnosing shunt blockage. An abdominal ultrasound may be useful to identify a CSF pseudocyst.

Aspects of some CSF shunt complications

Infection

The diagnosis of shunt infection is not always straightforward. In a retrospective case series[3] the presenting symptoms were as listed in Table 8.1.4.

The positive predictive value of these symptoms was even greater in the first 9 months following insertion of the shunt because 80% of all shunt infections occur in this time. There is also an increase in VP shunt infections after laparotomy. Case reports also mention other symptoms such as rigors whenever a ventriculoatrial shunt is manipulated. The most useful investigation is initially the CSF white cell count, which is elevated in approximately 70% of cases. The blood white cell count is elevated in only 30% of cases. A positive CSF culture is the gold standard, although this may be negative in those children who have been on antibiotics. Bacterial antigen detection and polymerase chain reaction testing may be helpful in this situation.

Staphylococcus epidermidis is the most common bacterium isolated, followed by other coagulase negative staphylococci and *Staph. aureus*. Less commonly Gram-negative bacteria, such as *Propionobacter* and *Streptococcus pneumoniae* and *Candida* infections, have been reported.

Table 8.1.4 Shunt infection presenting symptoms[2]	
Symptom	*Percentage of cases of infection with symptom*
Shunt malfunction	33%
Fever	26%
Localised wound or shunt tract inflammation	22%
Abdominal pain or pseudocyst	19%

Initial antibiotic therapy can be tailored to findings on Gram stain from a CSF tap and/or cultures from previous infections. If the patient has no contraindications flucloxacillin or dicloxacillin should be in all empirical regimens with Gram-negative cover considered after consultation with neurosurgeons and an infectious-disease specialist. In the majority of cases the shunt will have to be removed and replaced at a later date, with some temporary measure in the meantime.

Early post-operative complications

Wound dehiscence and purulent discharge are much more likely in the first few weeks after shunt insertion. If there is early overshunting this can lead to such a degree of brain shrinkage that the subdural bridging veins are broken and subdural haematomas form. Also, the presence of blood or fibrin in the CSF increases the risk of proximal blockage. At the other end of the shunt peritonitis and wound infection is more likely in the early post-operative period.

Migration and penetration of shunts

In various cases the distal end of VP shunts have migrated into the thorax, liver, bowel lumen and even out of the anus and mouth.

Several liver abscesses have been reported. Treatment involves removing the distal part the tube, possibly repairing damaged organs and often a temporary alternative shunting method.

Glomerulonephritis

This is a complication of ventriculoatrial shunts, which are rarely used today. This is usually a gradually progressive illness which requires a high level of suspicion for diagnosis. Treatment is usually to remove the shunt and replace it with an alternative.

Trauma in children with a CSF shunt

In a child who has a CSF shunt in place and is subject to trauma the emergency physician should seek to answer the following questions:

Was there a direct impact upon the shunt hardware? Relatively minor trauma to the shunt may cause breakage and malfunction which may not become manifest until some days or weeks following the trauma; also, a direct blow may cause shunt movement and damage to tissues surrounding the shunt. Intracranial haemorrhage following moderate impact in sporting events has been reported. Impacts on distal tubing may cause shunt penetration of abdominal viscera.

Is there an open wound that may communicate with the shunt or the CSF? This would increase the risk of infection. Thus a scalp wound near the entry point of the tubing into the cranial cavity may cause a pneumocephalus and may lead to meningitis. At the other end, a bowel perforation may cause a distal shunt infection.

In addition to these questions there is the possibility that the presence of the shunt and/or the underlying pathology may make the child more likely to have some complication of trauma. The most common example of this is subdural haematoma from rupture of bridging veins that have been stretched by brain shrinkage after shunt placement.

References

1. Piatt JH, Garton HJ. Clinical diagnosis of ventriculoperitoneal shunt failure among children with hydrocephalus. *Pediatr Emerg Care* 2008;**24**(4):201–10.
2. Roberts JR. *Clinical Procedures in Emergency Medicine.* 5th ed. Philadelphia, PA: WB Saunders Company; 2009.
3. Williams DG, Hayes J, McCool S. Shunt infection in children: presentation and management. *J Neurosci Nurs* 1996;**28**(3):155–62.

8.2 Raised intracranial pressure

Richard Lennon

ESSENTIALS

1 A rapidly expanding head circumference in an infant prior to suture fusion, is an important sign of raised ICP.

2 The open anterior fontanelle allows direct palpation of ICP in children up to 9–18 months of age.

3 In rare circumstances an emergency procedure, such as a subdural or a ventricular tap, can be performed through the anterior fontanelle in infants.

4 A brain CT scan or MRI can rule out many causes of raised ICP, but does not exclude raised ICP itself and thus should not be the sole basis for deciding whether or not it is safe to perform a lumbar puncture.

5 Acute severe elevation of ICP is a true emergency often requiring intubation and ventilation, infusion of mannitol 1 g kg^{-1} and early consultation with neurosurgeons.

Introduction

Normal physiology

Normal intracranial pressure (ICP) is 6–18 cmH$_2$O. It is the product of the intracranial contents mainly blood, brain and cerebrospinal fluid (CSF) and the resistance of the cranial vault. Normal ICP has a diurnal cycle that is higher in the early hours of the morning when one is normally supine during sleep. Therefore the symptoms of raised ICP, such as headache and vomiting, are usually worse in the morning. Intracranial pressure may be raised by anything that can cause an increase in the volume of its contents or a decrease in the size of the cranial cavity (Table 8.2.1). This section will not cover the diagnosis and management of raised intracranial pressure associated with trauma. Those issues are covered in Chapter 3.2.

Most CSF is made by the choroid plexus in the lateral third and fourth ventricles. A normal child makes approximately 20 mL hr^{-1} and the total volume is 50 mL in an infant, rising to 150 mL in an adult. It flows through the foramen of Monro into the third ventricle, then down the aqueduct of Sylvius, which is usually only 2 mm wide, and 3 mm long in a child. This leads into the fourth ventricle and from there via the foramina of Luschka and Magendie to the basal cisterns. From there the CSF flows over the surface of the cerebellar and cerebral hemispheres to be reabsorbed through the arachnoid villi on the superior sagittal sinus. CSF can also be reabsorbed through several other channels, including a small amount through the choroid plexus and via lymphatics. Intracranial pressure will be raised whenever there is obstruction to the flow or reabsorption of CSF or in the rare circumstance where CSF production is increased.

Table 8.2.1 Causes of raised intracranial pressure

A. Increased CSF (hydrocephalus)
1. Decreased absorption
   - Obstructive
   - Communicating
2. Increased production

B. Swollen contents
1. Meningitis
2. Encephalitis
3. Cerebral oedema
   - Hypo/hypernatraemia
   - Post-ischaemic
   - Post-traumatic/diffuse axonal injury

C. Space-occupying lesion (SOL)
1. Tumours
   - Primary
   - Secondary
2. Haematomas
   - Extradural
   - Subdural
   - Intracerebral/intraventricular
3. Abscesses/cysts
4. Arteriovenous malformation
5. Congenital cysts

D. Decreased or fixed intracranial volume
1. Depressed skull fracture
2. Premature fusion of cranial sutures (craniosynostosis)

E. Pseudotumour cerebri (benign intracranial hypertension)

Measurement of ICP

Intracranial pressure is usually estimated from lumbar puncture (LP) manometry, when performed on a child lying in the lateral decubitus position in a relaxed posture. Measuring CSF pressure in a screaming child is likely to be inaccurate because of the temporary rise caused by high venous pressure. Similarly, the person holding the child in the fetal position for the LP should relax their grasp and allow the child to stretch out temporarily while the pressure is being measured. If the LP is being done under a general anaesthetic, attempts should be made to normalise the pCO$_2$, so that the pressure reflects awake ICP. If a lumbar puncture is performed on a child in a sitting posture measurement of hydrostatic pressure is likely to be elevated compared to ICP. Adjustment of the sitting posture LP pressure to reflect intracranial pressure is difficult because multiple factors affect the relationship, including; the height of the child, their posture and their emotional state. Nevertheless, if the child is very co-operative, pressure measurement can still be attempted by carefully laying the child on their side straight after the needle has entered the subarachnoid space.

Particular issues in children

Infants

An infant's inability to communicate and smaller repertoire of behaviours makes raised intracranial pressure more difficult to diagnose and one needs to have a high index of suspicion as the presentation may be subtle.

The infant does not have a rigid cranial vault until fusion of the cranial sutures. This is a gradual process occurring throughout childhood; therefore ICP can cause diastasis of the cranial sutures in children, however, this is rare in children over the age of 7 years and even rarer now that computerised tomography (CT) scans and magnetic resonance imaging (MRI) allow for earlier diagnosis. Because of this flexibility, increasing intracranial contents in the infant will cause a lesser increase in the ICP and a greater increase in the head circumference than it would in older children or adults. This is one of the reasons why acute increases in ICP in infants are often not easily detected by the infant's subtle change in behaviour patterns.

The measurement of head circumference (occipitofrontal) is a useful means of detecting intracranial pathology. The head circumference should be plotted on centile charts, using prior measurements, if available, to determine if there has been a trend to cross percentiles. The child's length and weight should be plotted concurrently, to evaluate if the head is disproportionately large or small. When the cranial sutures separate due to expansion, percussion of the skull makes a sound similar to that of a 'cracked pot'. This is known as Macewen's sign.

Conversely, the open anterior fontanelle allows direct palpation of intracranial pressure up to the age of 9 to 18 months. It is highly recommended that one closely observes the fontanelles of normal infants, to help one identify abnormalities in clinical practice. The normal fontanelle will bulge slightly when the infant is lying down. It will become depressed when the child is sat up. It will bulge more prominently when the infant is crying or straining. The normal fontanelle will have an arterial pulsation more apparent when the infant is upright.

The fontanelle also provides access for emergency procedures such as the draining of a traumatic subdural or a ventricular tap. Fortunately the need for these procedures in the emergency department (ED) rarely arises. When it does, however, it should be done by a neurosurgical specialist (or trainee if sufficiently experienced). In centres where such help is not rapidly available, over-the-phone advice from a neurosurgeon may help with both the decision to do the procedure and the technique.

Clinical features of raised intracranial pressure

The symptoms and signs that lead to a diagnosis of raised ICP (RICP) will vary with the age, severity and rate of development. In slower onset conditions such as brain tumours the most common scenario in infants is the gradually progressive onset of drowsiness/lethargy, morning irritability and vomiting, with an expanding head circumference. In older children there are progressive early morning headaches, but no dramatic increase in head circumference.

Brain tumours may also present with focal neurological signs before there is a significant rise in ICP due to direct invasion of neural pathways. Other symptoms may include a head tilt, which is due to unilateral 4th cranial nerve palsy causing a vertical strabismus. The child will compensate for this by tilting the head. This often occurs with posterior fossa tumours. However, there are other causes of head tilt such as sternomastoid 'tumour' in the newborn and benign torticollis. In obstructive hydrocephalus, paralysis of upward gaze is common due to third nerve dysfunction. This leads to the classic picture in the infant of a big head and 'sunset' eyes. Some infants will become irritable on watching TV or looking at books because of diplopia. Parents may notice strabismus and older children will complain of diplopia.

Often there will be regression in motor milestones due to ataxia and/or weakness. Personality changes may occur.

As pressure increases, the pressure itself may cause focal neurological symptoms and signs. These may be due to several mechanisms, which include:

- impingement on, or disruption of, a cranial nerve, cranial nerve nucleus or higher centre;
- impingement on a blood vessel supplying any of the above;
- in hydrocephalus, stretching of corticospinal tract fibres around enlarging ventricles causes upper motor neuron signs in the legs;
- focal seizures may accompany raised ICP and leave an infant with a Todd's paresis.

In the more rapid onset conditions, such as intracranial haemorrhage, rapid onset of drowsiness and vomiting, with or without focal neurology, is the rule. When there is a large intracerebral pressure differential across a fixed structure, such as the tentorium, the brain will herniate. There are several herniation syndromes.

The central herniation syndrome

Generalised midline or bilateral swelling above the tentorium cerebelli causes the midbrain to herniate through the tentorium. This leads to dysfunction of the midbrain and higher centres due to compression, causing:

- drowsiness;
- initially *small* reactive pupils;
- decorticate posturing;
- as the process worsens pupils become midrange;
- posture becomes decerebrate;
- bilateral 6th cranial nerve palsies may become apparent when attempting the doll's-eye reflex;
- these are accompanied by Cushing's triad, i.e. hypertension, bradycardia and abnormal breathing patterns (alternating tachypnoea/bradypnoea and fluctuating depth of respiration).

The lateral mass herniation syndrome

A unilateral supratentorial swelling will give rise to a pattern of events formerly known as the uncal herniation syndrome. Imaging studies now show that herniation of the uncus happens very late in the process and is not responsible for most of the signs. Features in approximate sequence are:

- contralateral hemiplegia;
- drowsiness;
- ipsilateral pupillary dilatation (partial 3rd nerve palsy);
- complete 3rd nerve palsy as pressure increases (can be bilateral);
- ipsilateral hemiplegia (midbrain being pushed against edge of tentorium);
- Cushing's triad.

Cerebellar tonsillar herniation syndrome

A wide variety of signs and symptoms arise from posterior fossa masses. However, sometimes as the cerebellar tonsils are pushed through the foramen magnum and the medulla with its respiratory control centres is compressed, the following sequence occurs:

- patient complains of a stiff neck;
- drowsiness;
- nystagmoid eye movements;
- apnoea.

Other examination findings in raised ICP

General observation

In the unco-operative irritable child, general observation from a distance is a vital part of the examination. It may reveal a large and/ or an asymmetric head, evidence of trauma, gait, speech or visual disturbance. Watching a playful child from a distance will yield a lot more useful neurological information than an attempted formal examination of a screaming unhappy one.

Fundi

Although often difficult to visualise in children, fundal examination is of vital importance. Using a parent as a visual distraction will often help. With patience, the disc can usually be visualised through an undilated pupil. One may be able to visualise retinal venous pulsations. The implication of these pulsations is that intracranial pressure is less than peak venous pressure. Papilloedema is less common in infants with raised ICP due to the 'decompressing' presence of an open anterior fontanelle. Examination of the fundi is less useful in acute severe raised ICP, as papilloedema takes days to evolve. Other retinal findings associated with raised ICP include retinal haemorrhages, which have a strong association with non-accidental injury, aneurysms and arteriovenous malformation that may be associated with similar intracranial lesions, and subhyaloid haemorrhages which may be seen in patients with subarachnoid haemorrhages. In some instances it may be useful to ask an ophthalmologist to examine the child through dilated pupils.

Peripheral neurological signs

The development of 'handedness' is not apparent in normal infants under 1 year of age. If handedness is apparent in infancy, it is usually due to a neurological or musculoskeletal lesion, some of which are associated with raised ICP. Hydrocephalus may produce lower limb signs with gait disturbance in the ambulant child. In infants, this may be apparent when the child is held up by hands around the chest with the legs suspended in midair. Spasm of the adductors will cause scissoring of the lower limbs.

Investigations

Imaging the brain will often reveal the underlying pathology in children with raised intracranial pressure. However, there are several drawbacks that must be borne in mind when deciding to obtain a scan.

One must be sure that it is safe to move the child to the scanner room where facilities for resuscitation and access to the patient are less than ideal. CT or MRI scans may be falsely reassuring, especially in the case of pseudotumour cerebri (PTC or benign intracranial hypertension) or meningitis, where the appearance may be normal even when the pressure is dangerously high. To keep an unco-operative child still may require a general anaesthetic, with its concomitant risks. However, as scanning technology improves, the time required for a scan is getting dramatically shorter. Many infants can often be successfully scanned with the use of a 'dummy' (comforter) dipped in a sucrose solution and firm wrapping. Likewise, in older children, the presence of a parent in the scanner room may permit the avoidance of anaesthesia. Otherwise the decision to use general anaesthesia or procedural sedation depends on the clinical situation, local policy and skill mix, with safety always being the first consideration.

An MRI scan is more likely to require anaesthesia in younger children, as they usually take longer and patient access is more difficult. Finally, when obtaining CT scans, one must consider the risks of radiation causing cancer, which in a CT scan of the head in a child is estimated to be 1:1000–1:10 000 over the lifetime of the child.[1] Head ultrasound is an option for initial imaging in infants. This is good at imaging the lateral ventricles and surrounding structures but dependent on operator experience. However, ultrasound is less able to image the subdural space around the vertex and the posterior fossa region which may need to be considered in the adequacy of the clinical scenario.

Management of raised ICP

Acute severe increases in ICP are a true emergency and children with features of the herniation syndromes should be treated in the resuscitation area of the ED or the neurosurgical operating theatre. A neurosurgeon should be consulted as early as possible.

In this situation efforts should be directed towards maintaining cerebral oxygenation and perfusion by supporting the child's ventilation and circulation, if necessary using rapid sequence intubation (RSI) and mechanical ventilation. Some drugs used in RSI and the manipulation of the airway itself may cause a further transient rise in intracranial pressure. Several strategies have been used to avoid this transient rise including administering an IV dose of lignocaine just prior to RSI and giving a 'defasciculating' dose of a non depolarising neuromuscular blocking agent just before the Succinylcholine. There are no studies looking at what effect the use of these strategies has on patient outcome. This author's opinion is that it is more important to avoid hypotension and hypoxia during RSI because there is strong evidence that these are harmful. Therefore this author does not use these strategies because it is a change in the usual practice of the department which more likely lead to errors and delays in the RSI process. (See the end of the chapter for further reading on this issue). Intracranial pressure can be reduced by giving intravenous mannitol $1 \, g \, kg^{-1}$ and nursing the patient in a 30° head up position. Mannitol should not be given if the patient has circulatory failure (i.e. hypotension or hypoperfusion) as the osmotic diuresis that it causes could exacerbate the hypoperfusion. Just as in trauma so in medical illnesses C (circulation) comes before D (disability) meaning that a perfusing blood pressure must be maintained if there is to be any cerebral perfusion pressure. There is strong evidence against prolonged hyperventilation because vasoconstriction impairs cerebral perfusion despite the reduction in intracranial pressure. pCO_2 should be kept between 35 and 40 mmHg unless the above measures have been unsuccessful or herniation is progressing, in which case the pCO_2 can be taken down to 25 mmHg for a brief period while further measures are commenced. Whilst these measures are taking effect consideration and management of the underlying cause should be undertaken. This will be aided by a concise history and some rapid bedside testing such as blood gas, which may reveal conditions such as hyponatraemia or any infusions containing free water. If an infant in this situation does not respond to these measures, a neurosurgeon should be urgently consulted regarding a ventricular or subdural tap via the open fontanelle. In older children who do not respond adequately, the options depend on the clinical situation and the underlying cause. Therapeutic options include: consulting neurosurgeons and getting an urgent CT scan; palliating or treating an underlying cause urgently (e.g. high-dose dexamethasone for vasogenic oedema or hypertonic saline for hyponatraemia); or maintaining cerebral perfusion pressure by maintaining mean arterial blood pressure at above normal levels with fluids and inotropes and reducing cerebral metabolic demand with drugs such as thiopentone. Other neurosurgical interventions include: craniotomy; insertion of external ventricular drain; and insertion of a CSF reservoir or a complete CSF shunt. Where a shunt is already present this may be tapped (see Chapter 8.1 on shunt complications). Consideration should also be given to prophylactic anticonvulsants because seizure will cause a further acute rise in ICP. Once initial stabilisation is underway and neurosurgeons are involved referral to a paediatric ICU is mandatory.

Children with less severely raised ICP usually need investigation and treatment of the cause, usually under the care of paediatric neurosurgeon whilst avoiding interventions that may increase ICP. One should avoid the infusion of hypotonic fluids for a vomiting child or the administration of certain drugs. Children with hydrocephalus will usually require admission for consideration of a shunt, or 3rd ventriculostomy.

Some particular causes of raised ICP

Iatrogenic

Any child receiving intravenous fluids, especially for treatment of diabetic ketoacidosis (DKA), who develops headache and/or drowsiness and/or seizures during therapy should be considered to have raised ICP until proven otherwise. A thorough assessment should be made and electrolytes checked for disturbances that may lead to cerebral oedema. Imaging should be considered. If cerebral oedema is confirmed or not excluded then the child should be treated as above and observed in a paediatric intensive care unit.

Pseudotumour cerebri (PTC or benign intracranial pressure)

This condition is characterised by sustained raised ICP causing symptoms similar to a cerebral tumour but with no anatomical abnormality on neuroimaging. It is usually due to decreased CSF re-absorption. PTC has many causes (Table 8.2.2). It is more prone to occur in overweight pubescent girls, in whom no cause is found. The presentation is usually with headaches and vomiting, which are worse in the morning. Some patients may complain of transient visual obscuration with blurring or darkening of vision that lasts less than 30 seconds. Later there may be unilateral or bilateral 6th nerve palsies causing diplopia on lateral gaze. Papilloedema is often the only positive physical finding. The most significant complication of PTC is loss of vision. This begins with an enlargement of the blindspot associated with papilloedema,

Table 8.2.2   Causes of pseudotumour cerebri

1. Idiopathic
2. Venous obstruction
3. Metabolic
   - Hypervitaminosis A
   - Hypoparathyroidism
   - Addison's disease
   - Obesity
   - Pregnancy
   - Galactosaemia
4. Drugs
   - Oral contraceptive pill
   - Glucocorticoids
   - Tetracyclines
   - Isotretinoin
   - Nalidixic acid
   - Nitrofurantoin
5. Haematologic
   - Anaemia
   - Polycythaemia
6. Infections
   - Roseola infantum
   - Chronic complicated otitis media
7. Others
   - Guillain–Barré A syndrome

and later progresses with erosion of the peripheral visual fields. Left untreated the patient with persistent PTC will eventually develop optic atrophy and blindness.

Investigations include CT scan or MRI, followed by lumbar puncture to measure opening pressure. Lumbar puncture may be both diagnostic and therapeutic. The CSF has a high pressure, but analysis reveals normal protein, glucose, cell count and no microorganisms.

Therapeutic CSF taps should aim to decrease the ICP by 50% under the guidance of a paediatric neurologist. This may be curative. However, in most cases repeat lumbar punctures and/or acetazolamide are required. It is believed that acetazolamide works by reducing CSF production. In severe cases a lumboperitoneal shunt or optic nerve sheath fenestration may be required. One needs to exclude any treatable underlying cause. Anticoagulants should be given for venous thrombosis and drugs such as glucocorticoids should be ceased or weaned if possible. Referral to a paediatric neurologist is mandatory.

Reference

1. Brenner DJ, Elliston CD, Hall J, et al. Estimated risks of radiation-induced fatal cancer from pediatric CT. *AJR* 2001;**175**(2):289–96.

Further reading

Behrman RE, Kliegman R, Jenson HB, editors. *Nelson Textbook of Pediatrics*. 16th ed. Philadelphia: WB Saunders; 2000.

Bisan Salhi, et al. In defense of the use of lidocaine in rapid sequence intubation. *Annals Emerg Med* 2007;**49**(1):85–6.

Clancy M, Halford S, Walls R, Murphy M. In patients with head injuries who undergo rapid sequence intubation using succinylcholine, does pretreatment with a competitive neuromuscular blocking agent improve outcome? A literature review. *Emerg Med J* 2001;**18**:373–5.

Roberts JR. *Clinical Procedures in Emergency Medicine*. 3rd ed. Philadelphia: WB Saunders.

Robinson N, Clancy M. In patients with head injury undergoing rapid sequence intubation, does pretreatment with intravenous lignocaine/lidocaine lead to an improved neurological outcome? A review of the literature. *Emerg Med J* 2001;**18**:453–7.

Vaillancourt Christian, et al. Opposition to the use of lidocaine in rapid sequence intubation. *Annals Emerg Med* 2007;**49**(1):86–7.

8.3 Seizures and non-epileptic events

Padraic Grattan-Smith

ESSENTIALS

1 Seizures are the most common life threatening emergency presentation to EDs requiring immediate management.

2 The diagnosis of a seizure is based on a careful history.

3 There are many paroxysmal events or 'funny turns' in children, which can mimic seizures.

4 A bedside dextrostix should be performed on the child who is having a seizure. First-ever seizures should have blood sent for formal glucose, electrolytes, calcium, magnesium and phosphate levels.

5 The acute management of the child having a seizure involves supporting airway and breathing and the graduated use of antiepileptic drugs to terminate the seizure.

6 Parental reassurance and education regarding seizures, BLS and safety issues are an important facet of management in the child presenting with a first convulsion.

Introduction

An epileptic seizure can be defined as a disturbance in neurological function, resulting from uncontrolled excessive neuronal activity in the central nervous system.

The subject of seizures and their differential diagnosis is large. This chapter provides essential information that may be useful in formulating diagnosis and treatment in the emergency department (ED). There is insufficient space for a detailed discussion of the role of the electroencephalogram (EEG) and other investigations.

General comments

There are a number of conditions that must always be considered in children experiencing 'unusual events'. Hypoglycaemia can cause both partial and generalised seizures. It may also 'illogically' produce focal neurological signs. Abnormalities of electrolytes, calcium, magnesium and phosphate can present in a similar fashion. Cardiac arrhythmias associated with prolonged QT interval may cause epileptic seizures that seem to follow the arrhythmia. Sudden loss of consciousness during, or immediately after, intense exercise or associated with strong emotion, raises the possibility of an underlying cardiac cause.

A family history of premature unexplained sudden death in a young relative should also raise this possibility.

Some variants of migraine may be difficult to distinguish from seizures. Acute confusional migraine often follows minor head trauma. The episodes may last for a number of hours. The child is 'concussed', confused and often vomiting. Basilar artery migraine is associated with confusion or loss of consciousness and brainstem symptoms and signs. Neither diagnosis should be made at the first presentation and without further investigation. On the other hand, occipital epilepsy can cause vomiting, visual loss and severe headache. The presence of tonic eye deviation early in the event is a strong clue that this is a seizure rather than migraine.

Pseudoepileptic seizures and Munchausen's syndrome by proxy always need to be considered in the differential diagnosis of atypical epileptic seizures. However, the diagnosis is often difficult and the ED is usually not an appropriate setting to make a confident diagnosis of either of these conditions.

Classification of seizures

Seizures are conceptually divided into *generalised seizures* where the onset is from all brain regions simultaneously and *partial seizures*, where the seizure arises from one area in the brain. In *simple partial seizures* there is no alteration of consciousness. With *complex partial seizures*, alteration of consciousness occurs. Partial seizures may spread and become secondarily generalised.

Status epilepticus is said to occur where a seizure lasts more than 30 minutes or there is incomplete recovery between seizures over this time period. **In practical terms, any child who arrives in the ED still fitting, should be regarded as a medical emergency.** Status epilepticus can occur in both convulsive and non-convulsive forms.

Febrile seizures

Febrile convulsions are not regarded as a form of epilepsy but are discussed because of their frequent presentation to EDs. Typically they occur in children between 6 months and 6 years of age. They are common, affecting around 3% of children. Most children who have febrile convulsions have only one, but 25–30% will have a recurrence. The risk of recurrence is greater in infants less than 12 months, *where it may be as high as 50%.*

Febrile convulsions most commonly occur in the setting of viral illnesses such as an upper repiratory tract infection, pharyngitis, gastroenteritis, or an exanthem such as roseola infantum. Much less commonly, pneumonia or a urinary tract infection may be the underlying cause. Febrile seizures typically occur relatively early in the course of an infectious illness and sometimes the convulsion is the first sign that the child is unwell.

Most febrile seizures are generalised and brief, lasting less than a few minutes. The child returns to normal after a short (usually less than 30 minutes) postictal period. The seizures may be clonic, tonic–clonic or atonic where the child may simply seem to stop breathing. Examination should confirm the presence of a fever, identify the source of the fever, and exclude signs of central nervous system (CNS) infection or of a focal neurological process. Most children with an uncomplicated febrile seizure who have completely recovered and have a clear source of infection require no blood tests or other investigations.

Prolonged (lasting >10 minutes) and complicated (focal, multiple) febrile seizures can occur. Underlying meningitis/encephalitis must always be considered in the child who fails to return to normal, has multiple or prolonged seizures or has residual neurological signs. The threshold to perform a cerebrospinal fluid (CSF) examination is lower when the child is less than 12 months of age or has been on antibiotics, which may mask the usual signs of meningism. However, lumbar puncture can be dangerous in the child with focal signs such as a hemiparesis or if there has been a rapid deterioration in conscious level or an abnormality of respiratory rhythm. Consultation with senior colleagues is advised if there is doubt about the safety to perform a lumbar puncture.

Children with seizures are seen in the ED in two broad settings:

❶ The child who is seen after an event. Was this a seizure?
❷ The child who is still fitting.

THE CHILD SEEN AFTER THE EVENT

History

The diagnosis of seizures is based almost entirely on the history.

The parents or any witnesses of the event should be taken through the episode systematically. An exact description of what took place is crucial in making a correct diagnosis. What was the child doing when it started? What was the very first sign of a problem, and what followed? If abnormal movements were present, did they principally involve one side of the body? How long did the event last? What was the child like afterwards? How long before the child was back to normal? Was there any faecal or urinary incontinence or tongue biting? Was there any apnoea or colour change?

Witnessing a sudden loss of consciousness in a child is an extremely upsetting event for any observer, particularly the parents. Many parents report that they thought their child had 'stopped breathing' and commenced various resuscitation techniques. There are

obvious limitations to the history, but it remains the single piece of information most likely to provide a diagnosis. It is also worth talking to the verbal child about what happened. Even young children can sometimes give very helpful accounts if spoken to soon after the event.

It is important to establish whether there may have been provocative factors, such as sleep deprivation, a febrile illness, head trauma or potential exposure to epileptogenic medications. A past history of similar events should be sought. It is also important to ask about a family history of seizures or unusual turns and to review the child's developmental milestones.

Examination

The physical examination is often normal, but it must be carefully performed, looking for fever, evidence of intercurrent illness and abnormal neurological signs. Other important diagnostic clues include a Todd's paralysis, skin lesions of tuberous sclerosis or morphological features of a chromosomal disorder or other underlying neurological abnormality associated with a seizure disorder. The finding of lateral tongue trauma or incontinence supports a suspicion of seizure when the diagnosis is unclear. The febrile child needs to have an underlying meningitis or encephalitis excluded.

In infants, the sudden onset of frequent seizures and failure to regain consciousness is a common presentation of child abuse and a careful retinal examination must be performed, looking for retinal haemorrhages.

Differential diagnosis

Tonic–clonic seizures, myoclonic seizures and clonic seizures, in general, can occur at any age. They are well described in standard textbooks and will not be discussed here except to discourage the tendency to loosely label any event with loss of consciousness as a 'tonic–clonic' seizure.

Although there is overlap, it is helpful to approach the problem in terms of age of presentation. For neonatal seizures refer to Chapter 2.6.

Infancy
Seizure types
Infantile spasms Typically take the form of 'salaam' seizures. There is characteristic sudden flexion of the arms, head and trunk in a brief spasm. Asymmetrical or extensor spasms can occur. The characteristic feature of established infantile spasms is that the episodes occur in *runs* (clusters) which can continue for 10 minutes or more. In the early phases, the spasms may be mild and relatively infrequent, making diagnosis difficult.

Lennox–Gastaut syndrome In this syndrome there are multiple seizure types, including atypical absences, myoclonic seizures, drop attacks, nocturnal tonic seizures and generalised tonic–clonic seizures. In the early phases, which can be seen in late infancy, the child may present with atypical absences. These have somewhat slower onset than typical absences and there may be obscuration rather than complete loss of consciousness. Great caution should be taken with any child presenting in the first 2 years of life with 'absences', as this may be an early manifestation of Lennox–Gastaut syndrome.

Complex partial seizures in infancy
May present as episodes of altered consciousness, with autonomic symptoms and also with apnoea. An underlying tumour (most often in the temporal lobe) may cause this type of seizure.

Non-epileptic events of infancy
The following events can mimic seizures in young children and are usually distinguished by a careful history.

Breath-holding spells
These are always provoked by an unpleasant stimulus. This is usually minor trauma, e.g. a bump on the head, but the child being scolded or frustrated may provoke them. Somewhat arbitrarily, breath-holding attacks are divided into:

❶ *Pallid breath-holding* attacks, where after a short cry, the infant loses consciousness, becomes pale and there may be tonic stiffening.
❷ *Cyanotic breath-holding* attacks, where after vigorous crying, there is breath-holding in expiration and loss of consciousness.

As in syncopal episodes there may be brief clonic jerking after an episode. The story of provocation is usually clear, but at times there can be diagnostic confusion, for example, when a child who is playing happily is found unconscious on the floor and no precipitating event was observed.

Benign neonatal sleep myoclonus

This is characterised by myoclonic jerks, which can be quite violent and asymmetric, but are confined to sleep. The infant is otherwise normal.

Benign paroxysmal vertigo

Sudden episodes of acute unsteadiness occur without alteration of consciousness. The child typically clutches onto whatever is nearby. The episodes are usually brief, lasting seconds to minutes. The parents may notice nystagmus during an episode. There may be multiple episodes per day.

Shuddering attacks

The infant's body 'shivers' as though cold water had been poured on its back.

Self-stimulatory episodes ('infantile masturbation')

These are seen in girls. The thighs are generally clenched tight, with the legs crossed at the ankles. There are pelvic undulatory movements. The infant may look extremely flushed and upset and may be sleepy afterwards.

Stereotypies

There are hand-flapping or other repetitive limb movements. These are usually repeated in exactly the same way each time. Although common in children with autism, they also occur in children who are otherwise normal.

Day-dreaming

Is common at all ages in childhood. The child may stare straight ahead and at times not respond to being called.

In daydreaming, stereotypic behaviours and self-stimulatory episodes, the event can usually be immediately stopped by physical interaction with the child, e.g. by tickling them.

Childhood
Seizure types

Absence seizures Are usually brief staring spells characterised by a sudden loss of consciousness and an abrupt end to the seizure. There is no post-ictal period. With longer absences, automatisms may occur. The events usually last less than 10 seconds, and multiple episodes may occur per day.

Complex partial seizures There may be an aura (actually a partial seizure), a more prolonged episode of altered consciousness in which the child may be partially responsive and a post-ictal period characterised by drowsiness and a desire to sleep.

Benign focal epilepsy of childhood In its typical form, presents with the child awaking from sleep at around 2–4 a.m. making a 'glugging' or 'clucking' noise. This is followed by a clonic seizure involving one side of the body, including the face. The child may be awake during the seizure and find it very frightening. Not uncommonly, this seizure becomes secondarily generalised.

Nocturnal frontal lobe seizures Are rare but may be mistaken for night terrors and 'pseudoseizures'. Seizures should be considered if there are multiple stereotyped events occurring in the one night, if the episodes are very brief or if they occur only in the second half of the night.

Non-epileptic events of childhood:

Night terrors Usually occur within the first few hours of the child going to sleep. Typically the child screams and is found sitting up in bed with widely dilated pupils and appears to be extremely fearful. This may last for half an hour or more. The child is eventually comforted and goes off to sleep. The next morning the child has no memory of the event.

Nightmares In contrast, these usually occur in the second half of the night. The child goes into the parent's bedroom afraid because of a 'bad dream'. The child usually has a good memory of the dream, although he/she may not want to discuss it.

Paroxysmal kinesigenic dyskinesia Brief episodes of dystonic or choreoathetoid movements involving the limbs are provoked by sudden bursts of exercise. There is no alteration of consciousness.

Late childhood and adolescence
Seizure types

Juvenile myoclonic epilepsy This usually develops in the early teenage years. Typically there are myoclonic jerks in the morning soon after awakening. These may not be mentioned to the parents. The first presentation is often with an early morning generalised tonic–clonic seizure. A history of early morning myoclonus should always be sought in this situation.

Non-epileptic events

Syncope Is usually a vasovagal response provoked by a stressful situation, such as seeing blood or standing for a prolonged period in hot weather. There is a feeling of light-headedness, nausea and then a progressive fading out of vision. As mentioned above, there may be brief stiffening and clonic jerks in the course of syncopal episodes. Unusual forms of syncope in adolescence include 'stretch syncope' provoked by neck hyperextension and shoulder abduction while stretching and 'hair grooming syncope', which seems to be provoked by strong pulling of the hair while combing or brushing. Children with intellectual handicap may repeatedly provoke episodes of loss of consciousness by hyperventilating and then performing the Valsalva manoeuvre.

Rage attacks These consist of sudden episodes of directed anger, usually provoked by being thwarted in some way. A careful history will usually differentiate a rage attack from non-directed aggression, which can occur in the post-ictal state. This usually occurs when a patient in a confused post-ictal state is restrained or surrounded by a crowd of people.

THE CHILD WHO IS STILL FITTING

The child with convulsive status epilepticus

When a child is fitting on arrival at the ED, the seizure is likely to have continued for at least 15 minutes. There is a risk of brain damage or death if the seizure is not rapidly controlled and respiration appropriately supported. There needs to be a clear plan for the immediate management of the convulsing child. The child should be taken directly to the paediatric resuscitation area with ready access to anaesthetic and airway resuscitation facilities.

Airway, breathing and circulation need to be assessed and simultaneously managed. The child should receive high-flow oxygen via mask or assisted by bag and mask, if ventilation is inadequate. Basic airway manoeuvres and suctioning may be required. Oxygen saturation should be monitored continuously. Intravenous access should be gained and a Dextrostix checked immediately to exclude hypoglycaemia. Blood should be taken for glucose, electrolytes, calcium, magnesium and phosphate and full blood count. Children on maintenance anticonvulsants should have their drug level taken.

At the same time, a history should be rapidly obtained regarding:

- the duration of the seizure;
- previous episodes (and if there is a particular drug most likely to be effective);
- precipitating events;
- medications the child is taking;
- whether drugs have already been given for the seizure;
- the presence of underlying neurological problems.

Drug therapy

If the child has received no treatment for the seizure prior to arrival, the following approach is suggested.

First line

Initial treatment is with benzodiazepines, which are rapidly acting, using intravenous (IV) diazepam 0.25 mg kg^{-1} or IV midazolam 0.15 mg kg^{-1}. If the seizure has not stopped within 5 minutes the dose can be repeated. The potential side effects of respiratory depression or apnoea need to be anticipated.

Second line

If after another 5 minutes the fit continues, IV phenytoin 20 mg kg^{-1} as an infusion over 30 minutes or IV phenobarbital 10–15 mg kg^{-1} as an infusion over 30 minutes should be given. These 'second-line' agents need to be given *slowly* by intravenous infusion, and therefore will take time to control the seizure. If continued seizure activity is causing *respiratory compromise* or it is felt their severity may result in brain injury, it may be necessary to use further benzodiazepines and be prepared to support respiration or to proceed to use barbiturates, which require intubation.

Third line

If there has been no response after a further 5 minutes, thiopental 5 mg kg^{-1} and intubation using rapid sequence induction, is the next step. The decision to intubate to control a seizure needs to involve consideration not only of the length and severity of the seizure but also the degree of respiratory embarrassment to the child. Mild seizure activity that is not compromising a child can be tolerated longer than a major convulsion that is impairing oxygenation. These children will need to be subsequently managed in a paediatric intensive care unit.

There are almost endless variables in this situation. If intravenous access is a problem, midazolam 0.15 mg kg^{-1} may be given intramuscularly, or into the nose or buccal space, or diazepam 0.5 mg kg^{-1} may be given rectally. Intraosseous injection can be used. If the child has already received a benzodiazepine beforehand, a second dose may be given on arrival, followed by phenytoin as it is less likely to cause respiratory depression than the combination of phenobarbitone and a benzodiazepine.

In a severely handicapped child who has frequent bouts of status epilepticus where there is a desire to avoid intubation, paraldehyde 0.4 mL kg^{-1} rectally may be tried if there has been no response to benzodiazepines, phenytoin or phenobarbital.

Absence, atypical absence and complex partial status are much less common than convulsive status but should be considered in children who are obtunded or have bizarre behaviour without obvious cause. If there is doubt an EEG should be performed. If an EEG is unavailable and CNS infection and metabolic causes have been excluded, 'waking up' soon after an IV dose of a benzodiazepine is a useful diagnostic clue of 'non-convulsive' status.

Investigations

These depend on the clinical setting but some general rules apply.

Blood tests

All children having a seizure should have a bedside Dextrostix followed by a formal blood glucose to exclude hypoglycaemia. At the same time full blood count, electrolytes, calcium, magnesium and phosphate levels should be checked in order to exclude a metabolic cause. These are exceedingly rare beyond the infant age group in the child who has returned to normal and the yield is negligible, unless there are other clues to promote an electrolyte disturbance.

Neuroimaging

As a general rule, patients with focal seizure or examination findings, features suggesting raised intracranial pressure or seizures in the setting of trauma, should have urgent neuroimaging. The computerised tomography scan of the brain has the advantage of relative ease of access but it should be remembered that the magnetic resonance scan is a better test in almost all instances except traumatic brain injury.

EEG

An urgent EEG is very useful in cases where convulsive status epilepticus has been treated but the patient remains unconscious and there is a suspicion of continuing non-convulsive status. It is also very helpful in the child presenting with an altered state of consciousness and absence or complex partial status is suspected. In the child who has recovered from a brief seizure an EEG done soon after presentation may be useful, e.g. showing focal changes that suggest a secondarily generalised seizure. There is no reason to delay getting an EEG soon after a fit but this will be limited by the resources that are available.

Disposition

Children who have prolonged or multiple seizures, focal seizures, or abnormal neurological examination, or where the diagnosis is unclear, should be admitted for observation and paediatric or neurological review. Children who are having increased frequency of seizures or are known to have prolonged, or clusters of seizures warrant admission and observation until stabilised.

Not all children presenting with an uncomplicated first seizure need to be admitted to hospital. Those who have a first generalised seizure, with normal neurological examination and metabolic work up, can be followed up on an outpatient basis. This is usually best achieved by discussion with a general paediatrician or neurologist colleague to determine the timing of imaging and an EEG and formal review. Other influences on the decision to admit may include the age of the child, parental anxiety and any intercurrent illness issues.

If the event has clearly been a brief seizure, it is important to discuss the nature of this with the parents and provide some reassurance that it has not caused brain damage. First-aid measures should be discussed with the parents so that they have a clear plan should their child have a further seizure at home. The parents should be warned that further seizures can occur. It is important to take care that the child is not in a potentially dangerous situation should this happen. A particular risk is swimming without careful adult supervision. This advice should be reviewed at the organised follow up. Children who are discharged after a febrile convulsion should be reviewed by their local doctor within 24 hours to follow progress and reinforce the safety issues.

Controversies and future directions

❶ Unlike in other countries, the intravenous form of sodium valproate has not been used widely (if at all) in Australia.

❷ In the future, newer intravenous agents such as levetiracetam may come to be increasingly used in the acute management of seizures.

❸ Given the efficacy and safety of midazolam by the IM or IN route, many clinicians argue that there is no place for rectal diazepam, given its impracticality and unpredictable absorption by this route.

Further reading

Chin RF, Neville BG, Scott RC. Meningitis is a common cause of convulsive status epilepticus with fever. *Arch Dis Childhood* 2005;**90**:66–9.

Maytal J, Shinnar S, Moshe SL, Alvarez LA. Low morbidity and mortality of status epilepticus in children. *Paediatrics* 1989;**83**:323–31.

Mitchell W. Status epilepticus and acute repetitive seizures in children, adolescents and young adults: Etiology, outcome, and treatment. *Epilepsia* 1996;**37**(Suppl 1):S74–80.

Sofou K, Kristjansdottir R, Papachatzakis NE, et al. Management of prolonged seizures and status epilepticus in childhood: a systemic at review. *J Child Neurol* 2009;**24**:918–26.

The Status Epilepticus Working Party. The treatment of convulsive status epilepticus in children. *Arch Dis Child* 2000;**83**:415–9.

Verity CM, Ross EM, Golding J. Outcome of childhood status epilepticus and lengthy febrile convulsions: Findings of national cohort study. *Br Med J* 1993;**307**:225–8.

8.4 Acute weakness

Richard Lennon

ESSENTIALS

1 The fact that a child has acute weakness may be obscured by an inability to communicate and a smaller repertoire of activities. The possibility of a neuromuscular problem must be consciously considered by the clinician.

2 Conversely, a small child may not move a limb because of pain rather than weakness. A history and examination for evidence of trauma should be performed and appropriate diagnostic imaging considered.

3 Respiratory insufficiency due to weakness may occur with surprising rapidity and may be compounded by aspiration. Careful assessment and close monitoring for this complication must be made.

4 Abnormal reflexes are important in localising the cause of acute weakness. If some are *absent*, especially distally, it suggests a lower motor neuron dysfunction. If all are *present* it suggests muscle dysfunction and if they are *increased* it suggests an upper motor neuron weakness.

5 The presence of a sensory level indicates a spinal cord lesion. One should consider investigating this with an urgent MRI to determine whether or not urgent surgery is needed.

Introduction

The acutely weak child is challenging to the emergency physician because she/he can present in many different ways with many different diagnoses. In particular, the preverbal child may present with only regression in motor milestones or bruising on the face from increased frequency of falls. The diagnosis in such children can range from a tick bite to Duchenne pseudohypertrophic muscular dystrophy.

Presentation

In infants of less than 3 months, parents are usually quite sensitive to abnormalities of the infant's behaviour. They may bring a baby in complaining of poor feeding, decreased activity or being 'floppy'. The older infant may be noted to lose milestones such as ceasing to crawl or walk. 'Ataxia' may be the predominant feature in preschool and school-age children. Sometimes children may present with an associated feature of illness, such as the rash of dermatomyositis or an obvious engorged tick. In general, the older the child is, the more typical the presentation. However, even in this group, as in adults, there is a wide range of presentations, e.g. cranial nerve palsies in the Miller–Fisher variant of Guillain–Barré syndrome.

Trauma masquerading as weakness

Trauma is dealt with in detail in other chapters of the book. However, it should noted that non-accidental injury (NAI) can present as 'acute weakness' in the infant and young child. Shaken baby syndrome may present as a lethargic irritable child with little or no bruising. The apparent focal weakness may be due to an underlying fracture. Likewise, emotional and nutritional neglect may also lead to weakness. Hence, NAI must be considered in the differential diagnosis of the acutely weak child (see Chapter 18.2).

Primary survey approach

General inspection

This is done by looking for both cause and effect of the weakness. An abnormality of the primary survey severe enough to cause generalised weakness (e.g. respiratory distress) is usually the obvious presenting problem. Hypoglycaemia in a child can, in rare circumstances, present with focal weakness. It is important in the 'weak', floppy infant to consider the possibility of intussusception or other intra-abdominal pathology. In an infant with intussusception, prostration mimicking severe 'weakness' and lethargy may be the only presenting sign. When one comes to exposure in the primary survey of the weak child a thorough search has to take place for ticks (don't forget to look in deep skin folds), possible venomous bites and stings, and rashes, such as those caused by enteroviruses. Enteroviral rashes are usually scattered maculopapular but may be petechial. A close inspection should be made for bruises and other suggestive signs of NAI. A quick assessment of the child's nutritional state and the appropriateness of weight for age should be estimated. The size of the child's head and its proportion to the body should be noted and centiles should be plotted later in the detailed examination phase.

ABC

The effects of weakness may include airway compromise from bulbar palsy (e.g. hoarse voice, stridor, and aspiration of secretions). Severely impaired ventilation will be clinically apparent. However, mild or moderate impairment can be subtle and can rapidly progress to cause respiratory embarrassment. Therefore, if possible, respiratory function tests should be serially performed on all children presenting with neuromuscular weakness. Arterial or venous blood gases should also be considered in this assessment. (Table 8.4.1 for predictors of needing intubation and mechanical ventilation.) Circulatory defects may arise from disturbance of the autonomic nervous system. This is characterised by labile blood pressure, heart rate and postural hypotension.

Disability

The neurological part of the primary survey can give early hints as to the site of the lesion(s) involved. The classic description of peripheral neuromuscular weakness is an alert, but anxious looking, child that has a paucity of limb movements. If respiratory failure or facial weakness have intervened this appearance will not be present. Conversely, intracranial causes of weakness are usually associated with some degree of obtundation.

The weak infant classically lies in a frog leg posture with all limbs lying on the bed, abducted at the hips and flexed at the knees. Asymmetry may be apparent in those with a focal weakness. With central causes of weakness (e.g. acute hydrocephalus) hypertonic posturing may be seen, with scissoring

Table 8.4.1 Predictors of the necessity for ICU/HDU admission
Bulbar palsy
Vital capacity <20 mL kg^{-1}
>30% reduction in vital capacity from baseline
Flaccid quadriparesis
Rapidly progressive weakness
Autonomic cardiovascular instability

adduction of lower limbs. Autonomic dysfunction may lead to associated fever or hypothermia. In any child with weakness one needs to consider whether the findings could be caused by a toxidrome (e.g. organophosphate poisoning).

Once the primary survey has been completed, and any abnormalities corrected, then a detailed history and examination should be performed.

History

If, on questioning, the weakness has been chronic then the list of possible diagnoses is extensive and is beyond the scope of this text. Such children should be stabilised and referred to the appropriate paediatric service for diagnosis. However, it is possible that a child with chronic weakness could undergo an acute deterioration, such as influenza in a child with a Duchenne muscular dystrophy. In infants the distinction between acute and chronic weakness is less relevant. In those children with conditions covered by this chapter, the history needs to focus initially on finding treatable causes. Detailed enquiry should be made about any possible tick bites or other venomous bites or stings. Enquiry should also be made about the availability of various medications and poisons around the house.

A precise time course for the illness should be obtained, along with the pattern of evolution of the weakness. Whether it is *ascending* from lower limbs up, whether it is *lateralised* and whether it has *progressed* or not. A sudden onset may suggest a vascular or epileptic event. Rapid onset weakness may follow an intoxication or envenomation. Other causes are more subacute and may have progressed over weeks. The family history should be reviewed, and whether there is consanguinity. A history of recent infectious illnesses may be relevant. Immunisation history regarding polio vaccination is important and diphtheria is still a common cause of weakness in third world countries. Any overseas travel should be noted.

Examination

A detailed but focused examination is then performed, that attempts to establish the level and the nature of the lesion.

The following lists the important distinguishing features of the different levels of the neuromuscular system which may present with weakness.

❶ Muscular:
- usually proximal more than distal weakness;
- reflexes preserved until very late;
- may have tender muscles;
- these children often have a positive Gower's sign (see below).

❷ Neuromuscular junction:
- fatigability;
- reflexes are preserved if the muscle is not fatigued or the disease is not severe.

❸ Lower motor neuron weakness:
- more peripheral than proximal weakness;
- reflexes are lost early in the illness.

❹ Upper motor neuron weakness:
- apart from an initial flaccid phase, tone and reflexes are usually increased;
- spinal cord lesions are usually associated with a sensory level;
- intracranial problems are associated with features of encephalopathy, decreased level of consciousness, speech dysfunction, ataxia, and bulbar dysfunction.

It may be difficult to perform a formal neurological examination in an unco-operative infant or small child. Often in these situations, one can get a lot of information just by watching the child play. Another useful test is known as Gower's sign. The child is laid on their back on a firm surface and encouraged to stand. A child with proximal muscle weakness will not be able to sit up but will have to roll on to its abdomen get up on all fours and then 'climb up its legs' using its hands. Although reflexes are a good guide they are by no means foolproof. Upper motor lesions will usually have increased reflexes with increased tone. However, immediately after a spinal cord insult there may be a flaccid paralysis below the level of the lesion with absence of reflexes. Also, in transverse myelitis, there may be patchy combinations of upper and lower motor neuron signs. Early in Guillain–Barré syndrome the reflexes may be preserved and, likewise, very late in myopathic weakness, distal reflexes may be lost. Acute myositis is usually associated with tender muscles.

Investigations

Laboratory
Tests that may be useful in the acutely weak child include:

- *a full blood count*, which may reveal anaemia, nutritional disorders, leukaemia, or signs of infection;
- abnormalities of electrolytes especially potassium, calcium, phosphate, sodium may cause weakness;
- urea and creatinine – renal failure may present as generalised weakness, but more likely cause an abnormality of electrolytes;
- creatine kinase is often raised in muscular causes of acute weakness;
- endocrine function tests – especially thyroid and adrenal (see below);
- lumbar puncture (see below)
- electrophysiological studies (electromyogram (EMG), electroneurogram (ENG)).

Imaging
- *Urgent magnetic resonance imaging (MRI)* of spine (where progressive spinal cord lesion is suspected);
- Computerised tomography (CT) or MRI of brain (where central cause is suspected);
- Chest X-ray (e.g. for suspected aspiration).

SPECIFIC CONDITIONS CAUSING ACUTE WEAKNESS

Though not exhaustive, the following sections give some detail on the more common causes of acute weakness seen in children and also the rarer ones that must be diagnosed and treated in emergency.

Guillain–Barré syndrome

Introduction
Guillain–Barré syndrome (GBS) is an acute polyradiculopathy. It is now considered a group of diseases with two main pathological mechanisms; demyelination and axonal degeneration. In the paediatric population it is more common in late childhood (4–9 years of age) and in males (1.5 times higher risk). It is uncommon, estimated at less than 1/100 000 person years in people less than 17 years of age. It is primarily a lower motor neuron disease affecting the myelin sheath with variable damage to axons. It is an immune-mediated reaction, usually to a recent infection. Antibodies to various gangliosides are found in the serum of patients with GBS and matching antigens are often found in the preceding infectious agent. Infections known to be associated with GBS include *Campylobacter*, *Mycoplasma*, Epstein–Barr virus, Coxsackie viruses, influenza viruses, echoviruses and cytomegalovirus. The greater the axonal damage, the longer and the less complete is the recovery.

History and examination
Children usually present with weakness, falls, regression of motor milestones or ataxia. They also complain of muscle pain in the early part of the illness. Cranial nerves are involved in 40–50% of cases, with the facial nerve most commonly involved. The Miller–Fisher variant presents with oculomotor palsies, ataxia and areflexia.

On questioning, the parents often give a history of a generalised viral, respiratory or gastroenteritis illness in the preceding 2 weeks. In the early part of the illness the child may have paraesthesiae. Classically, the paralysis is ascending and symmetrical. The majority present with mostly distal weakness; however, about 15% have extensive proximal muscular involvement.

Papilloedema is rare, but may occur in GBS and is associated with raised intracranial pressure. Paralysis of the respiratory muscles is common and must be monitored carefully. Sympathetic nervous system involvement can produce profuse sweating, hypertension, postural hypotension and disturbances of sphincter function. Fatal cardiac arrhythmias have been reported in association with these signs. Although primarily a motor problem, sensory disturbance does occur, especially impairment of position sense. As mentioned above, reflexes are usually absent though increased reflexes and extensor plantar responses are occasionally found in the early phase of the illness.

The weakness may evolve rapidly within hours. However, it usually takes 1–2 weeks to reach the maximal weakness. Then, in the 2nd to 4th week of the illness, recovery is apparent and most children have recovered by 2 months, although some take as long as 18 months. Rarely, GBS will present in the newborn and is known as congenital GBS. They present as floppy babies that are areflexic and have elevated cerebrospinal fluid (CSF) protein.

Laboratory findings

An isolated elevation in CSF protein is the characteristic clinical finding of GBS. The CSF cell count is usually normal, although 5% of children may have a pleocystosis of 100 or so cells. Approximately 10% of children will have a normal CSF protein. The protein may be raised if a lumbar puncture is done later in the illness as it rises to a maximum after 4–5 weeks. The ENG characteristically shows conduction block, although this may not become apparent until weeks into the illness.

Differential diagnosis

As laboratory tests may be normal in early GBS and signs may be variable, it is important to exclude other causes of acute weakness (Table 8.4.2).

Treatment

The main role of the emergency physician in the treatment of GBS is in monitoring, prevention and treatment of cardiovascular and respiratory complications. In addition to

Table 8.4.3 Predictors of the necessity for intubation and ventilation in GBS

Vital capacity $\leq$20 mL kg^{-1}
Maximum inspiratory pressure $\leq$30 cmH$_2$O
Maximum expiratory pressure $\leq$40 cmH$_2$O
Tidal volume <5 mL kg^{-1}
A sustained increase of pCO$_2$ to $\geq$50 mmHg
An increasing respiratory rate
Increasing oxygen requirement
An increased use of accessory muscles and paradoxical diaphragm movements; these reflect restrictive lung-chest wall movement and low lung volumes

monitoring of vital signs and cardiac rhythm, frequent examinations and (if possible) lung function tests should be performed. As noted above, progression to respiratory failure can be surprisingly rapid and the indicators for intubation listed in Table 8.4.3 should be actively sought to avoid respiratory arrest. The other less emergent treatments of GBS are either intravenous immunoglobulin or plasma exchange. This is indicated if the child can not walk unaided, has bulbar palsy, has rapidly progressive weakness, or worsening respiratory status. The immunoglobulin dose

is usually 2 g kg^{-1} given in divided doses with variable regimes.

Prognosis

Prognosis is usually good in those treated and supported appropriately. Most children reach maximum weakness in 2 to 4 weeks then remain stable for 1–3 weeks and then recover fully over a period of time that varies from 6 weeks to many months. Approximately 85% of children recover completely. Mortality is 2 to 4% and is due to cardiovascular and respiratory complications.

Disposition

Children with suspected GBS should be admitted and closely observed for the evolution of severe weakness that can occur. The findings outlined in Table 8.4.1 will assist in deciding who should go to an intensive care unit (ICU)/high dependency unit and who should go to the general ward. Children with any one of these features should be monitored in a paediatric ICU.

Tick paralysis

Ticks that can cause paralysis are found throughout the world. In Australia *Ixodes holocyclus* is the main paralysing tick; it is found on the east coast. Other ticks have been known to cause paralysis, but they are rare. The toxin previously called holocyclotoxin is now thought to be several toxins. The toxins inhibit the release of acetylcholine from motor end plates. The paralysis usually occurs 5 to 7 days after the tick attaches. The paralysis can resemble GBS in the form of an ascending paralysis and is an important differential diagnosis because removal of the tick is necessary for recovery. The envenomation most frequently presents with cranial nerve palsies. Although the tick is often located in the vicinity of the palsy, this is not always the case and in all cases a thorough examination should be made for multiple ticks. The paralysis can be severe and require ventilation. Australian tick paralysis may get worse in the 48 hours following tick removal, and children should be monitored carefully during this time. Conversely, with children presenting with paralysis one should ask if a tick was removed in the last 48 hours. Deaths have usually been due to respiratory paralysis; however, there have been reports

Table 8.4.2 Differential diagnosis of GBS

Diagnosis	Features/action to exclude
Puffer fish, Shell fish and Blue ringed octopus poisoning, Ciguatera	History of ingestion or bite often a descending paralysis
Tick paralysis	Thorough examination of hair/skin creases
Snake envenomation	History; check for bite site; coagulation screen, creatine kinase
Spinal cord lesion	Look for upper motor neuron/mixed features and a sensory level; if suspected perform MRI
Periodic paralysis	Usually a sudden or very rapid onset, reflexes are diminished but preserved; check family history; measure serum potassium; do ECG
Infant botulism	Almost exclusively in infants; ask for history of eating honey; culture stools for *Clostridium botulinum* and test for botulinum toxin
Poisoning (e.g. organophosphate, lead)	History of exposure; toxidrome; check levels where suspected
Myasthenia gravis	Often cranial nerves involved; fatigability; look for antibodies; perform Tensilon test
Vasculitis (e.g. polyarteritis nodosa)	Check urinalysis; look for autoantibodies if suspected
Myositis (e.g. dermatomyositis)	Reflexes preserved; no ophthalmoplegia; look for characteristic rash; check creatine kinase; EMG
Poliomyelitis, diphtheria, other enteroviruses	Usually has fever and sore throat in diphtheria; ask about immunisations; no sensory changes

of myocarditis and autonomic effects on the heart. Treatment includes supportive therapy then careful removal of the tick(s) ensuring that the mouthparts are removed along with the body. This can be made easier by applying a pyrethrum spray, which suffocates the creature and makes it loosen its grip. Squeezing the tick is not recommended as this may inject more toxin. Human Tick Antivenom is no longer available. The treatment of tick paralysis is supportive; this may well include intubation and ventilation for several days after tick removal.

Other envenomations

Snake and spider bites are discussed in detail elsewhere in the text (see Chapter 22.1). Usually the history and accompanying symptoms will give the diagnosis. Death adder envenomation is usually a purely neurological presentation so in the weak non-verbal child a thorough look for a bite site is indicated.

Botulism

Poisoning with botulinum toxin can present in three ways:

❶ Infant botulism;
❷ Food-borne botulism; and
❸ Wound botulism.

Infant botulism

Although rare, several cases of infant botulism have been reported in Australia in the last few years. Infant botulism is caused by release of botulinum toxin into the bloodstream from *Clostridium botulinum* bacteria colonising the intestines. Part of the toxin enters the terminal bouton of cholinergic motor nerves and enzymatically disables the mechanism by which acetylcholine-containing vesicles attach to the cell membrane. This process is irreversible and recovery occurs by sprouting new unmyelinated motor neurons. Risk factors for babies contracting this disease include exposure to honey in the first six months (honey is not recommended for babies under 1 year), decreased frequency of stooling and lack of breast-feeding.

Diagnosis of this condition is characterised by:

- age group – the infants are almost always less than 6 months; however, there are reports in infants up to 1 year and older children with abnormal bowel anatomy;

- nature of onset – the infants always start with bulbar palsies because that is where the blood supply is greatest; this is a descending paralysis;
- fatigability, but lack of reversibility with edrophonium or neostigmine;
- absence of fever;
- absence of an altered mental status;
- absence of sensory defects;
- normal CSF.

Clostridium botulinum may be cultured from the stools and the toxin may be found in stools or serum through polymerase chain reaction or enzyme-linked immunosorbent assay tests. Mouse bioassay is also available where sterilised stools are injected into a mouse to see if it becomes paralysed. If suspicion is high, foods in the child's residence can be tested for *C. botulinum*. The EMG is characteristic.

The difficulty is in early diagnosis. A weak suck is often put down to generalised illness and it is often only the mother who notices the lack of expression on the infant's face. A high index of suspicion needs to be maintained.

Treatment is by supportive care and administration of botulinum antitoxin. Antibiotics are not recommended unless there is secondary infection (e.g. pneumonia). This is because they may increase toxin release when the bacteria lyse and divulge their contents. Tube feeding is recommended as it restores peristalsis, which is essential for clearing *C. botulinum* from the gut. If antibiotics are used, aminoglycosides should be avoided because these worsen the paralysis. About half of the patients end up needing intubation and ventilation. Hospital stay is an average of 1 month but varies widely. Infants seem to recover completely.

There are two antitoxins available. Equine-derived antitoxin, a small amount of which is held in the Commonwealth Serum Laboratories, and botulism immune globulin (BIG), a human-derived hyperimmune globulin, which in a recent randomised controlled trial reduced hospital stay from 6.6 weeks to 2.6 weeks. It is not available outside the United States.

Food-borne botulism

This is due to consumption of food in which there is preformed toxin. It is associated with home-canned foods. It differs from infant botulism in that it can occur in any age group and

one third of cases have gastroenteritis-like symptoms. The illness usually begins about 18 to 36 hours after ingestion, but onset can range from 2 hours to 8 days. Presentation is similar to infant botulism but more obvious because of the patients' greater age. The treatment is similar.

Wound botulism

This is perhaps the rarest form. The differences from the other forms are the presence of a wound, which may be obviously infected, and the presence of fever. The incubation period is 4–14 days. This requires aggressive treatment with antibiotics and antitoxin.

Spinal cord lesions

These are usually distinguished from peripheral nerve disease by upper motor neuron signs. However, in many cases initially the reflexes and tone are diminished (e.g. 'spinal shock' after trauma). In other cases, there may be patchy upper and lower motor neuron involvement such as in transverse myelitis. Therefore spinal cord lesions need to be considered in the differential diagnosis of the weak child. The key to spinal cord lesions is the presence of a sensory level. However, in transverse myelitis and in a preverbal child this may be difficult to establish. If a spinal cord lesion is suspected, the investigation of choice is an urgent MRI. This is time-critical as a space-occupying lesion in the narrow canal can rapidly cause permanent damage to the surrounding cord.

Transverse myelitis (TM)

The aetiology of this acute spinal cord inflammation is still uncertain. Hypotheses include microbial antigen cross-reaction with neural elements, bacterial superantigen inflammation and direct microbial invasion. Rarely, it is associated with systemic diseases such as systemic lupus erythematosus and multiple sclerosis. It is likely that TM will be found to be several diseases and perhaps treatment will need to be tailored to the specific aetiology.

This disease usually has a rapid onset of predominantly lower limb weakness and altered sensation. Neck stiffness and fever are present early in most cases along with low back pain or abdominal pain. The sensory level is usually around the mid-thoracic region below which pain, light touch and temperature sensation are impaired. However, joint position and vibration sense are more preserved. Bladder and bowel disturbance is common, although this may be difficult to determine in a child in nappies. Tone is usually flaccid early in the illness with decreased reflexes, followed by increased tone and hyperreflexia as the disease progresses to its peak over the next 2–3 days. Sixty percent of patients recover fully over weeks to months.

Urgent MRI usually shows fusiform oedema around the site of the sensory level. CSF shows a moderate lymphocytosis and mildly raised protein.

Treatment is controversial, with case-control studies indicating a benefit with glucocorticoids, whereas prospective trials show no benefit. Treatment decisions should be made in consultation with a paediatric neurologist.

Spinal cord trauma

This is discussed in Section 3.

Spinal cord space-occupying lesions

These include epidural abscess, tumours, syringomyelia and arteriovenous malformations. Since syringomyelia is almost always a chronic condition it will not be dealt with here.

Tumours

These may be intramedullary (e.g. low-grade astrocytoma), extramedullary intradural (e.g. meningioma) and extradural (e.g. lymphoma). They usually have a more gradual onset than the other diseases mentioned in this chapter but the early signs may be missed and the child may present when signs are rapidly evolving due to high intramedullary pressures. Progressive gait and bladder disturbance with back pain and absence of fever are characteristic signs. Recent onset of scoliosis may be a feature. There may be a mixture of signs with upper motor neuron signs in the lower limbs and lower motor neuron signs in the upper limbs.

Urgent MRI is the investigation of choice, followed by consultation with surgeons and/or radiation oncologists. If MRI is unavailable, CT or plain X-ray may show abnormalities. However, these should only be done if they do not delay transfer to an MRI capable centre.

Arteriovenous malformations

These are usually in the thoracic region. They may cause symptoms as a space-occupying

lesion causing compression or by stealing circulation from the nearby cord. The history is usually subacute, unless a haemorrhage or ischaemia has intervened. Clues to the diagnosis on examination include a cutaneous angioma over the region and a bruit on auscultation. MRI/MR angiogram will give the diagnosis but angiography is usually required to define the lesion fully and to decide on whether to treat with surgery or embolisation.

Epidural abscess

This is a rare disease in children, who usually present with back pain and rigidity, fever, leucocytosis and a raised erythrocyte sedimentation rate. These symptoms may be followed by spinal neurological signs. MRI is the investigation of choice, but there is controversy over whether treatment should be by surgery or antibiotics alone.

Tethered cord/diastematomyelia

These are two conditions that tend to fix the cord of the child, which has to 'move up' the canal as the child grows. They rarely present with acute weakness, although there may be sudden exacerbations on flexion and extension. Examination over the spine may reveal sentinel lesions such as a tuft of hair, a sacral pit, a lipoma, or a cutaneous haemangioma.

Myasthenia gravis (MG)

This condition, which is usually due to acetylcholine receptor autoantibodies, leads to easy and rapid fatigability of muscles. This may occur in children in three forms.

Transient myasthenia of newborns

This occurs where the mother has myasthenia. Maternal antibodies to the acetylcholine receptor (AChR) cross the placenta and the baby is born with fatigable muscle weakness. These babies may show very little motor activity for days after birth. Alternatively, they may just have feeding difficulty that worsens during the day. This illness improves within weeks as the maternal antibody levels diminish in the child's blood. The only treatment is supportive by tube feeding and intubation and ventilation, if severe. The babies recover completely and have no increased risk of MG.

Congenital myasthenia

This is a lasting condition due to a genetic disorder. It is not due to antibodies to the AChR.

Acquired myasthenia

The incidence of this is low, though not insignificant. In an Italian study the annual incidence was 3.3 per million children <15 years; about 1% of total MG cases. The presentation is usually with ptosis, ophthalmoplegia or bulbar weakness. The clue on history is the worsening of symptoms as the day progresses due to fatigue. Peripheral muscles, especially limb girdle and hand muscles, are also involved. Reflexes are preserved but diminished. Clinical tests for fatigability such as getting the child to look up for 60–90 seconds and watching for ptosis, or to flap one arm 'like a bird' for a minute and then comparing its strength with the other arm are very useful.

Diagnosis can be made with three tests. First, an anticholinergic drug may be given. Edrophonium, the usual drug used in adults may cause cardiac arrhythmias in small children, so neostigmine is preferred. Atropine is given beforehand to block the muscarinic effects. These drugs should abolish the fatigability. Second, the EMG is characteristic and usually obviates the need for muscle biopsy. Third, AChR antibodies can be measured in the blood. Early diagnosis is important because, if untreated, this disease will often progress to life-threatening severity.

Associations with MG commonly found in adults, such as thymoma, are rare in children. Differential diagnosis includes botulism, chronic low-grade organophosphate toxicity and tick paralysis.

In the ED the child may present as an initial episode or because of a crisis of weakness. These crises may be myasthenic, due to exacerbation of the underlying condition or cholinergic due to excessive anticholinesterase treatment, which leads to over stimulation and exhaustion of receptors. Classically, a cholinergic crisis has the cholinergic toxidrome features of hypersalivation, pulmonary oedema and muscle fasciculation. However, in someone with myasthenia the cholinergic crisis may only be manifest by weakness. Distinguishing between a myasthenic and cholinergic crisis may be difficult. History may give a clue if medications have been missed or an overdose of pyridostigmine has been taken. A therapeutic trial of edrophonium may help, but should not be undertaken if there is significant risk of a cholinergic crisis. In the latter case supportive treatment and measurement of blood cholinesterase activity may be the only option.

Long-term treatment of MG comprises anticholinesterases and a variety of immunosuppression, IgG infusion or thymectomy. In MG:

- Do not give neuromuscular blocking agents (e.g. suxamethonium, vecuronium) as these may paralyse the MG patient for days or even weeks.
- Do not give aminoglycoside antibiotics as these exacerbate the weakness.

Poliomyelitis and other enteroviral infections

Poliomyelitis is now exceedingly rare; however, one should always ask about immunisation status in the acutely weak child. If the child is not immunised one should ask about contact with infants recently immunised with Sabin (oral weakened live poliovirus) vaccine. Infants excrete the virus after the immunisation and this is where most recent cases of poliomyelitis have come from. The other source of infection is in developing nations, where immunisation rates are low. The illness itself usually presents with symptoms related to the virus's portal of entry through the gut and upper respiratory tract. Patients have fever, sore throat, anorexia, nausea, vomiting, generalised non-specific abdominal pain, malaise and headache. The great majority of poliovirus infections end here or are asymptomatic. In those patients who progress there is often an asymptomatic period of 1–2 days followed by symptoms of aseptic meningitis with neck and often entire spine stiffness. There may be mild transient neurological deficits such as bladder paralysis and loss of abdominal and anal reflexes. Those who progress to paralytic polio will usually do so 8–12 hours after the superficial reflexes are lost. Poliovirus can infect and destroy neurons from the motor cortex down to the anterior horn cells. However, most commonly the paralytic form presents with patchy asymmetrical lower motor neuron weakness. Bulbar weakness is also a frequent presentation and often the picture is mixed. Rarely there are also encephalitic and ataxic presentations.

Diagnosis is based on the immunisation history, the clinical picture and a lumbar puncture showing a moderate pleocytosis, initially of neutrophils but then changing to monocytes. Serology and culture of stool, throat swab and rarely CSF will often reveal the organism. Treatment is supportive only. Infection control authorities need to be informed.

Bell's palsy

A sudden or rapid onset of a unilateral lower motor neuron palsy is not a rare occurrence in children. Estimated annual incidence varies from 3 to 10 per 100 000 children per year. Its aetiology is uncertain. The disease commonly begins 2 weeks after an infectious illness, which suggests a post-infectious autoimmune or allergic aetiology. Lyme disease has been associated and serology should be done if the patient has been in an endemic area. Epstein–Barr, mumps and herpes simplex viruses have also been associated with this disease. An association with hypertension has suggested another aetiology related to pressure necrosis of the nerve due to swelling in the narrow facial canal.

The patient often presents with pain around the ipsilateral ear and may also complain of abnormal hearing. About half have loss of taste sensation to the anterior two-thirds of the tongue and there may be hemifacial 'dysaesthesia' due to the proprioceptive fibres to the facial muscles in the facial nerve.

The differential is extensive but the diagnosis can be determined by a thorough history and clinical examination. One should look for evidence of trauma (be aware of non-accidental injury), central nervous system dysfunction, aural lesions (e.g. the Ramsay Hunt syndrome), other cranial nerve dysfunctions, hypertension and GBS. Acute lymphoblastic leukaemia and even sarcoidosis have been reported.

Treatment is controversial, as the prognosis in children is better than in adults. Complete recovery occurs in 60 to 80% of patients, with near complete recovery in the remainder. In one study average time to recovery was about 7 weeks with a range of 9 days to 7 months. Uncontrolled studies have claimed a benefit for early corticosteroid therapy. However, controlled studies in adults have shown a benefit for oral glucocorticoids in Bell's palsy. This and the less reliable evidence in children prompt this author

to recommend glucocorticoids in all but the mildest cases of Bell's palsy. There is even less evidence for antiviral agents in the absence of apparent viral infection (e.g. the Ramsay Hunt syndrome). If the eyelid does not completely close steps should be taken to protect the cornea from exposure keratopathy, i.e. artificial tears and eyeglasses during the daytime, ointment and a protective eye chamber at night.

Toxic neuropathies

A long list of substances can cause acute weakness. Some of the more common ones are listed here.

Anticholinesterases

The organophosphates and carbamates are commonly used insecticides, which can cause poisoning through skin, oral or pulmonary exposure. They inhibit cholinesterases, allowing acetylcholine to persistently stimulate the nicotinic and muscarinic receptors, which then can become refractory and thus cause weakness. This weakness is usually accompanied by the cholinergic toxidrome (see Chapter 21.2 on toxicology) and, indeed, it is usually the respiratory and cardiac features that predominate. However, there is an *intermediate syndrome* where 12 hours to 7 days after the initial poisoning, one finds proximal limb weakness that is unresponsive to atropine or pralidoxime. There may also be respiratory and bulbar paralysis. Recovery from this is usually complete. *Late neurotoxicity* arises 4–21 days after the acute exposure, causing a mixed sensory motor deficit, which may take weeks or months to recover, or may be permanent. Diagnosis is by identification of the poison at source or in urine or serum drug screens and also by measuring serum cholinesterase activity level. Treatment is supportive and with antidotes atropine and pralidoxime. Muscle relaxants will have a prolonged effect and should be avoided if possible.

Lead and other heavy metals

Lead, mercury and arsenic are all known to cause neuropathies, often taking the form of mononeuritis multiplex. It is uncommon for these to present as acute weakness. Nevertheless, a history of exposure should be sought and appropriate specimens taken if the cause of the acute weakness is unclear.

Chemotherapeutic agents

Vincristine, vinblastine and cisplatin are known to cause a peripheral neuropathy. Any child who is on, or has recently had, chemotherapy needs to have this ruled out as a possible cause.

Hereditary neuropathy

Rarely, a patient with an undiagnosed hereditary neuropathy presents with an acute exacerbation. A thorough history will reveal the chronicity of the problem. Such patients should be referred to an appropriate paediatric neurology service.

Muscular disorders

Juvenile dermatomyositis

Juvenile dermatomyositis is a systemic vasculitis thought to be triggered by infection. Both enteroviruses and Group A *Streptococcus* have been implicated. This is the most common myositis of childhood. Its peak age of incidence is 6 years. Because of its gradual onset this uncommonly presents as acute weakness. The child may well present with the rash before weakness has become apparent.

The rash appears on sun-exposed areas, especially the malar region of the face and a purple discolouration of the eyelids is apparent (heliotrope rash). The rash may also be found on the extensor surfaces of the arms and legs, thorax, ankles and buttocks. The fingers develop thickening of the skin over joints, called Gottron's papules. The weakness comes on about 2 months after the rash and is usually very slow in onset. Small children may be noted to become gradually inactive and older children have increasing difficulty with sport. Proximal muscle activities, such as climbing up stairs, reveal the weakness first. The vasculopathy can affect any muscle group and children may present with aspiration dysphagia or hoarse voice due to pharyngeal muscle weakness. The affected muscles are often tender and sometimes swollen.

The vasculitis can affect any organ system. Subclinical myocarditis and conduction defects are often found at diagnosis. Less common effects include renal dysfunction, hepatosplenomegaly, retinitis, iritis, seizures, depression, bowel dysfunction and pulmonary disease.

Diagnosis is made on the clinical picture associated with a raised serum creatine kinase. There are typical changes on muscle biopsy and electromyogram. There may also be elevated autoantibodies, liver function tests and abnormalities on MRI.

Complications include calcinosis of muscles, subcutaneous fat and fascia. These are more likely if the illness is prolonged and are decreased by aggressive treatment. Calcinosis lesions may become infected and lead to septicaemia.

These children may require judicious use of pain relief and require referral to a specialist paediatric unit. Treatment options range from sunscreen for the rash through to immunosuppression with glucocorticoids and chemotherapeutic agents, depending on the severity of the disease. Prognosis is generally good in children, with approximately 80% making a good recovery.

Infectious myositis

Viral infections such as influenza can uncommonly cause a myositis that may in its severest form lead to rhabdomyolysis and myoglobinuria. Various bacteria including *Streptococcus and Mycoplasma* species have been reported to cause a focal myositis with tender muscles. These usually present with the other features of the infection and myalgia, rather than acute weakness. The weakness is only found on close examination, if the myalgia permits. The creatine kinase is raised. The prognosis is generally good although permanent muscle damage may ensue, especially in focal bacterial myositis.

Metabolic/endocrine myopathies

Most endocrinopathies can produce weakness by several mechanisms. Often this is just myalgia and fatigue, but true myopathies can develop. This weakness usually responds to the treatment of the underlying endocrine disorder. Endocrinopathies can be associated with electrolyte disturbances that lead to weakness (e.g. hypokalaemia in Conn's syndrome) or with primary muscle diseases, such as hypokalaemic periodic paralysis with thyrotoxicosis.

The periodic paralyses are a series of genetic ion channel disorders that lead to acute episodes of weakness lasting from 1 hour up to more than a day. They often come on after rest, during sleep or following exercise, but never during exercise. Diagnosis is by measurement of electrolytes during an attack or response to a metabolic challenge or by gene mutation identification. Hypokalaemic periodic paralysis usually occurs in adolescence. The patient will have low potassium during attacks. Conversely, hyperkalaemic periodic paralysis usually comes on in early childhood. The attacks are more frequent, occurring up to several times a day and are associated with an elevated or normal potassium. The identification of these diseases is important, as they are treatable.

Somatisation disorders/malingering

Occasionally, children may present with a psychogenic cause of weakness. The findings of a careful neurological examination will demonstrate inconsistencies and the child will be able to perform manoeuvres that require more strength than normal walking (e.g. knees giving way but not falling). Reflexes will be normal. Usually, no laboratory tests or imaging are necessary. However, if there is any doubt, consultation and investigation should be undertaken.

Once you have made the diagnosis it is best to take the parent or carer aside and discuss the diagnosis with them. Confrontation of the child is rarely helpful and it is often best to reassure the child that this is not serious and that they will get better. This gives the child an exit from the medical review with dignity intact. An effort should be made to find the underlying psychological reason for the presentation, which may be anything from school avoidance to sexual abuse. Consultation with social work or psychiatry may be indicated for ongoing counselling.

Further reading

Behrman RE, Kliegman R, Jenson HB, editors. *Nelson Textbook of Pediatrics.* 16th ed. Philadelphia: WB Saunders; 2000.

Emilia-Romagna Study Group on Clinical and Epidemiological Problems in Neurology. Incidence of myasthenia gravis in the Emilia-Romagna region: A prospective multicenter study. *Neurology* 1998;**51**(1):255–8 [brief communications].

Lawn ND, Fletcher DD, Henderson RD, et al. Anticipating mechanical ventilation in Guillain–Barré syndrome. *Arch Neurol* 2001;**58**:893–8.

Odaka M, Yuki N, Hirata K. Anti-GQ1b IgG antibody syndrome: Clinical and immunological range. *J Neurol, Neurosurg Psychiatry* 2001;**70**:50–5.

Tang T, Noble-Jamieson C. A painful hip as a presentation of Guillain-Barré syndrome in children. *Br Med J* 2001;**322**:149–150.

8.5 Acute ataxia

Joanne Grindlay

ESSENTIALS

1 The most common causes of acute cerebellar ataxia in children are post-infectious (acute cerebellar ataxia), drug intoxication and posterior fossa tumours.

2 Clinical features suggestive of a brain tumour and hence warranting further investigation include headache, vomiting, papilloedema, cranial nerve dysfunction or behavioural changes.

3 Ataxia is not uncommonly a presenting symptom of poisoning or excessive therapeutic drug levels, particularly anticonvulsants.

4 A number of neurological conditions may present with an unsteady gait (pseudo-ataxia) due to acute weakness.

5 Investigations in the child with ataxia are directed by the history and clinical features detected on examination.

6 While ataxia may be seen in post-concussion syndrome, conditions requiring acute intervention should be sought by CT scan.

7 Most children with significant ataxia require admission for investigation and observation.

Introduction

Ataxia is an uncommon, but important paediatric presentation to the emergency department (ED). Ataxia is a disorder of movement manifest by the loss of coordination, most apparent as a disturbance of gait, with intact muscle strength. It may be associated with a disturbance of balance. Ataxia is most often caused by a loss of function of the cerebellum, which controls the coordination of movement. Disease of the peripheral sensory nerves or the spinal column, particularly affecting proprioception, may also lead to ataxia as a result of abnormal inputs into the cerebellum. Cortical ataxia results from cerebral cortical dysfunction, particularly of the frontal lobe, while vestibular ataxia results from disease of the inner ear. Rarely, psychiatric causes of 'ataxia' may also be seen as a manifestation of conversion reaction. The most common diagnosis of acute ataxia in children is a post-infectious ataxia called acute cerebellar ataxia (see below). This is a diagnosis of exclusion, made after consideration of other causes (Table 8.5.1). These include poisoning, metabolic disorders and organic brain lesion.

There are numerous hereditary conditions causing chronic ataxia that may present in childhood. These include: Friedreich's ataxia, hereditary cerebellar ataxia, spinocerebellar ataxia and ataxia telangiectasia. The progressive nature of these conditions and their associated signs differentiate these from the acute ataxias.

Pathophysiology

Cerebellum

The cerebellum consists of two lateral hemispheres, divided into anterior and posterior lobes by the primary fissure. The hemispheres are joined by the vermis in the midline. The cerebellum connects to the cerebral cortex and brainstem via three paired sets of peduncles, the superior, middle and inferior cerebellar peduncles.

Cerebral hemispheres and vermis

There are three functional parts of the cerebellum. These are the archaecerebellum, the palaeocerebellum and the neocerebellum. The archaecerebellum is formed by the flocculus, nodule and lingula of the vermis. It has only vestibular connections, which travel in the inferior cerebellar peduncle. The archaecerebellum controls balance. Dysfunction leads to truncal ataxia characterised by a drunken gait, with swaying of the trunk and titubation when sitting, standing or walking. Typically there is neither alteration in fine movements nor nystagmus. Reflexes are normal and there is no tremor. The anterior lobes of the lateral hemispheres, together with uvula and pyramid of the vermis form the palaeocerebellum. The palaeocerebellum connects to the spinocerebellar tracts and is involved with postural reflexes. Dysfunction leads to postural imbalance and increased reflexes. The posterior lobes of the lateral hemispheres form the neocerebellum, which connects to the cerebral hemispheres, basal nuclei and the pontine nuclei, via the middle cerebral peduncle. It is involved in the coordination of fine, voluntary movements. Dysfunction leads to nystagmus, intention tremor, dysdiadochokinesis, hypotonia and decreased or pendular reflexes. The vermis and surrounding nuclei of the cerebellum form the roof of the 4th ventricle. An expanding lesion may obstruct the cerebrospinal fluid (CSF) flow, with resultant hydrocephalus and truncal ataxia.

Table 8.5.1 Causes of acute ataxia in childhood

- Post-viral – acute cerebellar ataxia
- Poisoning/drug intoxication
- Tumours
  Posterior fossa, brainstem
  Paraneoplastic syndrome
- Trauma including non-accidental injury
  Haematoma
  Post-concussion
- Metabolic
  Hypoglycaemia
  Hyponatraemia
  Hyperammonaemia
  Inborn errors of metabolism
- Infections
  Meningitis – bacterial, viral
  Cerebral abscess
  Malaria
  Labyrinthitis
  Encephalitis
- Vascular
  Stroke
  Vasculitis
- Immune
  Multiple sclerosis
  Acute disseminated encephalomyelitis

Cerebellar peduncles and connections

The cerebellum receives inputs from the vestibular and peripheral nervous systems. Outputs, which coordinate muscle movements by modifying tone and contraction, travel in three sets of peduncles (superior, middle, and inferior) between each cerebellar hemisphere and the brainstem.

Differential diagnosis

The most common cause of acute ataxia in children is post-infectious, acute cerebellar ataxia. Drug intoxication and posterior fossa tumours are less common.

Acute cerebellar ataxia

Acute cerebellar ataxia is the most common diagnosis in acute ataxia in children, particularly between 2 and 7 years of age. It is a diagnosis of exclusion, after consideration of more sinister causes such as tumours. An autoimmune aetiology is likely, with autoantibodies demonstrated in acute cerebellar ataxia following infections with varicella,[1,2] Epstein–Barr virus (EBV),[3] mycoplasma and human parvovirus B19.[4] The clinical presentation is of a prodromal illness, frequently non-specific, with or without an exanthema, 5–10 days prior to the onset of acute ataxia, though the timing may show considerable variation. If a specific aetiology is present it is most commonly varicella,[5] though a number of other viruses have been implicated (Table 8.5.2).[6–22] Acute cerebellar ataxia usually presents with sudden onset of severe gait ataxia, though a small number of cases have an insidious onset. Most have dysarthric speech. Mild horizontal

Table 8.5.2 Causes of post-infectious acute cerebellar ataxia

- Varicella[6]
- Coxsackie A9[10]
- Epstein–Barr virus[8]
- Mycoplasma[9]
- Mumps[10]
- Poliomyelitis[11,12]
- Typhoid[13]
- Echovirus[14]
- Pertussis[15]
- Human parvovirus[16]
- Measles[15]
- Herpes simplex virus[17]
- Enterovirus 71[18]
- Malaria[19]
- Immunisation[20,21]
- Human herpesvirus-6[22]

nystagmus occurs in 50% of cases. Findings of intention tremor, dysdiadochokinesis, hypotonia and decreased or pendular reflexes are seen in two-thirds of cases, but are less pronounced than the gait disturbance. Truncal ataxia is uncommon. Unlike acute disseminated encephalomyelitis (ADEM) or multiple sclerosis, there are no focal neurological signs.

Investigations are aimed at excluding an alternative diagnosis, if the diagnosis is unclear. The computerised tomography (CT) scan is normal in acute cerebellar ataxia; however, magnetic resonance imaging (MRI) may be abnormal. In one series, inflammatory changes were seen in the cerebellum of one of nine children.[23,24] There is a slight elevation of CSF cell count by 4–50 cells per microlitre in 32%, though occasionally (in 8%) the elevation is higher. There may also be slightly elevated protein 410–900 mg L^{-1}.[25]

Acute cerebellar ataxia usually begins to improve within a few days, but full recovery may take from 10 days to 2 months. Patients who have a slower recovery are still likely to recover fully. In one series, 91% recovered fully from their ataxia, including all those with varicella, EBV or post-vaccination, but 8% had sustained learning problems. Varicella-associated ataxia recovered quicker than non-varicella.[24]

Poisoning

Ataxia is not uncommonly a presenting symptom of ingestion or excessive therapeutic drug levels, particularly anticonvulsants.

Accidental poisoning occurs most commonly in 1 to 4-year-old children. A wide variety of compounds are implicated, including alcohols, substances of abuse and essential oils, as well as medications (Table 8.5.3). In addition to ataxia, these children may have nystagmus, altered mental status and vomiting. This is different to acute cerebellar ataxia where consciousness is unimpaired.

Anticonvulsants

Phenytoin toxicity with serum levels of >20–30 mcg mL^{-1} may produce signs of ataxia, nystagmus on lateral gaze and drowsiness. Onset of symptoms following an acute ingestion is usually within 1–2 hours and may persist for 4–5 days. At >30 mcg mL^{-1}, the ataxia and drowsiness become more marked and the nystagmus vertical.[26–28]

Table 8.5.3 Drugs causing acute ataxia

- Anticonvulsants
  Phenytoin
  Carbamazepine
- Benzodiazepines
- Alcohols
  Ethanol
  Isopropanol
  Ethylene glycol
- Essential oils
  Eucalyptus oil
  Tea tree oil
  Pine oil
- Cough suppressants
  Codeine
  Dextromethorphan
- Drugs of abuse
  PCP
  Solvents, petrol, glue

Carbamazepine toxicity may also lead to ataxia. There are usually associated findings of drowsiness and nystagmus. There may be progression to seizures and coma, particularly if the level is >100 μmol L^{-1}.[29]

Benzodiazepines

Ataxia may be the sole presenting feature of benzodiazepine ingestion in children. In one series, it was an isolated finding in one-fifth of the cases who demonstrated ataxia. Other findings included lethargy (57%), GCS <15 (35%) and respiratory depression (9%).[30]

Alcohols

Ethanol intoxication produces ataxia, disinhibited behaviour and slurred speech. A serum ethanol level will aid clarification of the diagnosis.

Ethylene glycol is the main component of antifreeze. Early symptoms of ingestion are similar to those of ethanol intoxication. Delayed features include cardiopulmonary distress and nephrotoxicity. Ethylene glycol produces a raised anion gap metabolic acidosis with osmolal gap. Serum levels >20 mg dL^{-1} are toxic. The ethanol level will be zero. Isopropanol, a component of rubbing alcohol, is used widely as a solvent. Toxicity is evident between 0.5 and 2 hours post-ingestion and may include vomiting, ataxia, nystagmus, and altered mental state. Coma and apnoea may occur in severe poisoning.[31]

Essential oils

Eucalyptus oil is not an uncommon ingestion by children. In one series of 109 admitted children, 41% were asymptomatic. Those who were symptomatic demonstrated decreased conscious state (28%), vomiting (37%), ataxia (15%) and pulmonary disease (11%). There was a correlation between ingested dose and toxicity. An ingestion of >5 mL 100% oil was associated with a significantly decreased conscious state, whereas <2–3 mL was associated with minor depression of consciousness.[32] A second series of 41 presentations, however, only demonstrated effects in 20%, with no correlation with presumed dose. The clinical effects included ataxia (5%), decreased conscious state (10%) and gastrointestinal symptoms (7%).[33]

Other essential oils that may produce nystagmus include tea tree oil[34] and pine oil. In one small series of pine oil cleaner (35% pine oil, 10.9% isopropyl alcohol), symptoms developed within 90 minutes of ingestion. Lethargy was present in all symptomatic children and ataxia in four of five cases of children.[35]

Cough suppressants

Codeine is contained in a number of cough medicines as well as in analgesics. In one series of 430 children, ataxia was reported in 9% receiving codeine. Associated symptoms are somnolence 67%, rash 39%, miosis 30%, vomiting 27%, itching 10%, angio-oedema 9%.[36] Dextromethorphan is a common component of cough and cold medications, which acts through opiate receptors in the medulla. It may cause opisthotonus, ataxia and bidirectional nystagmus. Fatality is highly unlikely, even with one hundred-fold the therapeutic dose.[37,38]

Substances of abuse

Phencyclidine (PCP) and lysergic acid diethylamide (LSD) are rare causes of ataxia in children. 1,4-butanediol, which is metabolised to gamma-hydroxybutyrate (GHB) upon ingestion, was responsible for ataxia, vomiting and seizures in several children following the ingestion of Aqua Dots, from toy craft kits.[39]

More common, however, is the abuse of hydrocarbon solvents; toluene in glue, spray paints and petrol. Hydrocarbons may produce ataxia as a component of acute intoxication and also as a chronic central nervous system sequel.

Tumours

Cerebellar lesions may present with an acute, rather than insidious onset of ataxia as a result of either haemorrhage into a tumour or as a result of hydrocephalus. The ataxia may progress to chronic ataxia. Paraneoplastic syndromes including paraneoplastic cerebellar degeneration and opsoclonus-myoclonus-ataxia syndrome are uncommon causes of acute paediatric ataxia.

Clinical features suggestive of a brain tumour, and hence further investigation, include headache, vomiting, behavioural changes (particularly with frontal lobe lesions), papilloedema or cranial nerve dysfunction.

Posterior fossa tumours include medulloblastoma, astrocytoma and ependymoma. Medulloblastoma (20–25% of posterior fossa tumours) usually presents in a child of less than 6 years with symptoms of ataxia, which may be truncal, headache, irritability or vomiting. The tumour may be located in the 4th ventricle or vermis. Cerebellar astrocytoma (10–30% of paediatric brain tumours) is located in one of the cerebellar hemispheres. It is seen in primary-school-aged children who may display ipsilateral limb ataxia, headache and vomiting. The head may be held tilted to one side. Associated raised intracranial pressure may be life threatening. Ependymoma (8–10%), located in the 4th ventricle, causes obstruction of CSF flow and may present with headache, vomiting and ataxia, which may be truncal. Brainstem gliomas (10–15% of paediatric brain tumours) develop in the pons or medulla. They typically occur in early primary-aged children. Presenting symptoms include cranial nerve palsies, ataxia and vomiting.

Hydrocephalus may present with ataxia due to stretching of frontopontocerebellar fibres. Associated features are headache, vomiting and the late signs of raised intracranial pressure – altered conscious state, raised blood pressure and decreased pulse. Supratentorial tumours may also present with ataxia through involvement of the frontopontocerebellar fibres.

An occult neuroblastoma may present with a triad of acute ataxia, opsoclonus (jerky, random, chaotic eye movements) and myoclonus (severe myoclonic jerks of the head, trunk or limbs). The most common site for the tumour is in the abdomen.[40] The triad may also be seen with viral infections, including meningitis, particularly mumps, hence a lumbar puncture should be considered. Neuroblastoma may present with isolated ataxia and should be considered in cases of persistent or recurrent ataxia.[41]

Trauma

Head trauma is a frequent cause of ED presentations. While ataxia may be seen in post-concussion syndrome, intracranial injury requiring acute intervention, should be sought by CT scan. These include haemorrhage or cerebral oedema. A base-of-skull fracture may cause ataxia by direct damage to the vestibular apparatus. Non-accidental injury should be considered in all cases of paediatric trauma.

Infections

Meningitis and encephalitis may both have ataxia as a presenting feature.[42,43] Other features to suggest an infective cause, such as headache, vomiting, fever and neck stiffness in the older child, will usually be evident.

In labyrinthitis and vestibular neuronitis, vertigo and vomiting are prominent. Apart from nystagmus and hearing alterations, neurological examination is normal.

Vascular conditions

Vertebrobasilar stroke is a very uncommon cause of ataxia in children. Ataxia will not be an isolated finding. Other findings include ipsilateral cranial nerve palsies, contralateral weakness, vertigo and diplopia. Systemic lupus erythematosus vasculitis may rarely present with ataxia.[44]

Other neurological conditions

In ataxia there is preservation of muscle strength. A number of neurological conditions may present with an unsteady gait (pseudo-ataxia) because of weakness. These include Guillain–Barré syndrome in which areflexia and ophthalmoplegia (in Miller–Fisher variant) distinguish it from acute cerebellar ataxia. Tick paralysis should also be considered in cases where the patient has been in an appropriate area. Multiple sclerosis/transverse myelitis is usually not seen until adolescent years. It may present with ataxia, optic or retinal neuritis, regional paraesthesias or weakness.[45] ADEM, a post-infectious encephalomyelitis, where host myelin components become immunogenic, may have ataxia as one neurological sign. The diagnosis is made by abnormal CT and MRI findings.

Other neurological conditions that may present with ataxia include seizures and complex migraine phenomenon. Because of the episodic nature of these conditions, there will be a recurrent nature to the ataxia. Basilar artery migraine may demonstrate associated headache, blurred vision, visual field defects and vertigo. It tends to have a recurrent course. Epilepsy uncommonly presents with ataxia. Ataxia may be seen post-ictally or in minor motor status or partial complex seizures. Other clues to seizure disorders include altered consciousness or motor manifestations. Benign positional vertigo is uncommon in children. Ataxia accompanies severe, reproducible vertigo, nausea and vomiting. Cranial nerve examination is normal apart from nystagmus.

Metabolic disorders

A large number of metabolic disorders may have ataxia as a feature and should be kept in mind. Hypoglycaemia and hyponatraemia may present with ataxias but other signs will also be present. The inherited metabolic diseases will likely demonstrate episodes of ataxia, together with the other features of the conditions, which will point towards the diagnosis. There may be a progression to chronic ataxias. Other inborn errors are listed in Table 8.5.4.

Table 8.5.4 Causes of chronic ataxia

• Brain tumours
  Cerebellar astrocytoma
  Brainstem glioma
  Medulloblastoma
  Ependymoma
  Cerebellar haemangioblastoma
  (Von Hippel–Lindau)
• Hereditary ataxia
  Friedreich's ataxia
  Ataxia telangiectasia
  Dominant hereditary ataxia
  Olivopontocerebellar degeneration
  Roussy–Levy syndrome
• Hydrocephalus
• Congenital malformations
  Cerebellar aplasia/hypoplasia (autosomal recessive)
  Vermal aplasia, including Dandy–Walker malformations
  Arnold–Chiari malformations
• Inborn errors of metabolism
  Hartnup's disease
  Wilson's disease
  Refsum's disease
  Abetalipoproteinaemia
  Maple syrup urine disease
  Argininosuccinicaciduria
  Ornithine transcarbamoylase deficiency
  Multiple carboxylase deficiencies – biotinidase deficiency
  Pyruvate dehydrogenase deficiency
  Juvenile GM2 gangliosidosis
  Juvenile sulfatide lipidosis
  Leigh's syndrome
  Sphingolipidoses
  Neuronal ceroid-lipofuscinosis
  γ-Glutamyl cysteine synthetase deficiency
  Triosephosphatase isomerase deficiency
  Glucose transporter 1 deficiency syndrome
• Vitamin B_{12}, E or folate deficiency

Chronic ataxia

Chronic ataxia usually has an insidious onset but it may present as a progression of acute ataxia, or as recurrent episodes. Causes include fixed deficits as in ataxic cerebral palsy, which makes up 10% of cerebral palsy and progressive diseases such as the hereditary ataxia, inborn errors of metabolism and tumours. Some causes are amenable to treatment. Table 8.5.4 lists some of the causes.

Hereditary ataxias/ spinocerebellar degenerative

Friedreich's ataxia is an autosomal recessive condition, which manifests in a child less than 10 years of age with ataxia and nystagmus. There is usually rapid progression. On examination there is impaired position and vibration sense, positive Romberg's sign and absent tendon reflexes. The plantar response is up going. Dysarthria is present. Kyphoscoliosis, distal muscle wasting and contractures and cardiomyopathy may develop. Ataxia telangiectasia is also an autosomal recessive condition with neurocutaneous manifestations. Ataxia is predominantly truncal and becomes evident in early childhood. Ocular and cutaneous telangiectasia become evident between 2 and 6 years of age. Developmental delay, increased susceptibility to infection, due to thymic atrophy and IgA and IgE deficiency, and an increased incidence of neoplasia are seen.

Congenital malformations

Cerebellar aplasia/hypoplasia, Dandy–Walker malformations, Arnold–Chiari malformations or vermal aplasia may result in ataxic cerebral palsy which accounts for 10% of all cerebral palsy. Signs include, but are not limited to, ataxia, hypotonia and tremor.

Evaluation of the patient

The ED assessment includes history and a thorough examination to detect life-threatening conditions and to identify reversible factors. Investigation is dependent on the formulation of a differential diagnosis.

History Important aspects of the history include the timing of the ataxia. Is it acute, recurrent or chronic? What is mainly affected, is it the trunk or limbs? Are there other symptoms, such as headache, vomiting, blurred vision, altered mental status or nausea suggestive of a tumour or meningitis? The antecedent history is important; for example, a recent viral illness may suggest acute cerebellar ataxia, or there may be a history of trauma or possible drug ingestion. Other symptoms, for example paraesthesia, may suggest an alternative diagnosis such as ADEM.

Examination This should include a general examination to look for signs in need of urgent intervention, for example meningitis, shock, hypoglycaemia, raised ICP or head injury. A complete examination is required to detect signs that may aid in the diagnosis, such as abdominal masses, nystagmus, opsoclonus and myoclonus in neuroblastoma, or signs of infection or vasculitis.

A complete neurological examination should be performed and documented. Cerebellar signs should be carefully assessed. Dysmetria and intention tremor can be assessed in the younger child by asking him to point to the parts of a doll. Dysdiadochokinesis may, however, be difficult to perform. Gait should be assessed. If only the anterior lobe or the vermis are involved, gait may be affected but the upper limb spared. With truncal ataxia the child may have difficulty keeping balance whilst seated. This imbalance increases if sitting cross-legged, standing or walking. Heel–toe walking tests are useful in detecting cerebellar problems, but unsteadiness may also be due to weakness or sensory deficits. Sensory ataxia is differentiated from cerebellar ataxia by the presence of impaired position and vibration sense and a positive Romberg's test. Lesions of the ipsilateral cerebellar hemispheres cause ataxia prominent in one direction. The child will fall towards the side of the lesion. Dysmetria and hypotonia are seen on the side of the lesion. Cerebellar dysarthria (scanning speech) may be detected by repeating 'sizzling sausage'. The speech displays a slow onset and is a slurred, jerky sound with an explosive nature.

Reflexes are often decreased in cerebellar lesions and are absent in Guillain–Barré syndrome. Pendular knee jerks are seen in severe cases of cerebellar dysfunction and in those with associated pyramidal tract defects. Decreased tone is seen in cerebellar lesions with drift and static tremor on holding up the arms. Rebound may also be detected.

Nystagmus is horizontal in cerebellar lesions and maximal to the side of the lesion. It may be positional. In phenytoin intoxication, nystagmus is initially horizontal but becomes vertical at higher levels. Nystagmus in vestibular neuronitis is typically rotational. The cranial nerves should be carefully examined to look for brainstem involvement.

Investigations

Investigations are directed by the history and clinical features detected on examination. Acute cerebellar ataxia is primarily a diagnosis of exclusion and investigation may be required to detect alternative conditions where urgent intervention is required.

Appropriate drug assays may include ethanol, ethylene glycol, anticonvulsants or benzodiazepines. If the drug screen is positive in an appropriate clinical setting, no other tests may be required.

Imaging by CT and/or MRI is indicated urgently where there are signs of raised intracranial pressure. MRI is indicated in most cases of acute ataxia unless there is a clear alternative diagnosis.

A lumbar puncture should be considered when meningitis or encephalitis are possible. Differential of a space-occupying lesion or raised intracranial pressure may indicate that a CT scan be performed prior to the lumbar puncture. Treatment with antibiotics and antivirals, if indicated, should not be delayed whilst awaiting lumbar puncture results.

Electrolytes, glucose and ammonia are indicated to assess for metabolic causes. In recurrent ataxia, or where there are features of metabolic disease, further metabolic screening should be performed in consultation with a paediatric neurologist or metabolic physician. This may include arterial blood gas, urinalysis, liver function tests, thyroid function tests, lactate in blood and CSF, pyruvate, cholesterol and lipoproteins. Muscle biopsy may be required. If occult neuroblastoma is suspected, urinary homovanillic acid and vanillylmandelic acid levels are measured. Other investigations may include an electroencephalogram if seizures are suspected.

Management

Treatment is aimed initially at detecting and treating emergency conditions. For example, in hydrocephalus and tumours, raised intracranial pressure is treated in consultation with the neurosurgical unit. In meningitis, urgent antibiotics are given. Hypoglycaemia and other reversible metabolic causes are treated. Intoxications and poisonings are generally managed by supportive care.

Acute cerebellar ataxia usually resolves over weeks to months. Occasionally there is a persistent movement disorder or behavioural and speech disorders. There is insufficient evidence to recommend either immunoglobulin or steroid therapy and treatment is primarily supportive. Physiotherapy, occupational therapy and a wheelchair for mobility may be required.

Disposition

Most children with significant ataxia require admission for investigation and observation under a paediatrician. Some children who have mild ataxia, clearly due to postinfectious cerebellitis, are appropriate to be followed as an outpatient.

References

1. Adams C, Diadori P, Schoenroth L, Fritzler M. Autoantibodies in childhood post-varicella acute cerebellar ataxia. Can J Neurol Sci 2000;27:316–20.
2. Van der Mass AAT, Vermeer-de Bondt PE, de Melker H, Kemmeren JM. Acute cerebellar ataxia in the Netherlands: A study on the association with vaccinations and varicella zoster infection. Vaccine 2009;27(13):1970–3.
3. Uchibori A, Sakuta M, Kusunoki S, Chiba A. Autoantibodies in postinfectious cerebellar ataxia. Neurology 2005;65(7):1114–6.
4. Shimizu Y, Ueno T, Komatsu H, et al. Acute cerebellar ataxia with human parvovirus B19 infection. Arch Dis Child 1999;80(1):72–3.
5. Nussinovitch M, Prais D, Volovitz B, et al. Post-infectious cerebellar ataxia in children. Clin Pediatr 2003;42(7):581–4.
6. Dreyfus PM, Senter TP. Acute cerebellar ataxia of childhood. An unusual case of varicella. W J Med 1974;120(2):161–3.
7. Feldman W, Larke RP. Acute cerebellar ataxia associated with the isolation of Coxsackie virus type A9. Can Med Assoc J 1972;106(10):1104.
8. Erzurum S, Kalavsky SM, Watanakunakorn C. Acute cerebellar ataxia and hearing loss as initial symptoms of infectious mononucleosis. Arch Neurol 1983;40(12):760–2.
9. Steele JC, Gladstone RM, Thanasophon S, Fleming P. Acute cerebellar ataxia and concomitant infection with Mycoplasma pneumoniae. J Pediatr 1972;80(3):467–9.
10. Cohen HA, Ashkenazi A, Nussinovitch M, et al. Mumps-associated acute cerebellar ataxia. Am J Dis Child 1992;146(8):930–1.
11. Gupta PC, Gathwala G, Aneja S, Arora SK. Acute cerebellar ataxia: An unusual presentation of poliomyelitis. Indian Pediatr 1990;27(6):622–3.
12. Curnen EC, Chamberlin HR. Acute cerebellar ataxia associated with poliovirus infection. Yale J Biol Med 1962;34:219.
13. Thapa BR, Sahni A. Acute reversible cerebellar ataxia in typhoid fever. Indian Pediatr 1993;30(3):427.
14. Marzetti G, Midulla M. Acute cerebellar ataxia associated with echo type 6 infection in two children. Acta Paediatr Scand 1967;56:547.
15. Batton FE. Ataxia in childhood. Brain 1905;28:487–505.
16. Shimizu Y, Ueno T, Komatsu H, et al. Acute cerebellar ataxia with human parvovirus B19 infection. Arch Dis Child 1999;80(1):72–3.
17. Dano G. Acute cerebellar ataxia associated with herpes simplex virus infection. Acta Paediatr Scand 1968;57:151.
18. McMinn P, Stratov I, Nagarajan L, Davis S. Neurological manifestations of enterovirus 71 infection in children during an outbreak of hand, foot and mouth disease in Western Australia. Clin Infect Dis 2001;32(2):236–42.
19. Senanayake N, de Silva HJ. Delayed cerebellar ataxia complicating falciparum malaria: A clinical study of 74 patients. J Neurol 1999;241(7):456–9.
20. Sunaga Y, Hikima A, Ostuka T, Morikawa A. Acute cerebellar ataxia with abnormal MRI lesions after varicella vaccination. Pediatr Neurol 1995;13(4):340–2.
21. Deisenhammer F, Pohl P, Bosch S, Schmidauer C. Acute cerebellar ataxia after immunization with recombinant hepatitis B vaccine. Acta Neurol Scand 1994;89(6):462–3.
22. Hata A, Fujita M, Morishima T, et al. Acute cerebellar ataxia associated with primary human herpesvirus-6 infection: a report of two cases. J Paediatr Child Health 2008;44(10):607–9.
23. Maggi G, Varone A, Aliberti F. Acute cerebellar ataxia in children. Childs Nerv Syst 1997;13(10):542–5.
24. Connolly AM, Dodson WE, Prensky AL, Rust RS. Course and outcome of acute cerebellar ataxia. Ann Neurol 1994;35:673–9.
25. Siemes H, Siegert M, Jaroffke B, Hanefield F. The CSF protein pattern in acute cerebellar ataxia of childhood and intracranial midline tumours. Eur J Pediatr 1982;137(1):49–57.
26. Murphy JM, Motiwala R, Devinsky O. Phenytoin intoxication. S Med J 1991;84:1199–204.
27. Wilson JT, Huff JG, Kilroy AW. Prolonged toxicity following acute phenytoin overdose in a child. J Pediatr 1979;95135–8.
28. Booker HE, Darcey B. Serum concentrations of free diphenylhydantoin and their relationship to intoxication. Epilepsia 1973;14:177.
29. Tibballs J. Acute toxic reaction to carbamazepine: Clinical effects and serum concentrations. J Pediatr 1992;121(2):295–9.
30. Wiley CC, Wiley JF. Pediatric benzodiazepine ingestion resulting in hospitalization. J Toxicol 1998;36(3):227–31.
31. Stremski E, Hennes H. Accidental isopropanol ingestion in children. Pediatr Emerg Care 2000;16(4):238–40.
32. Tibballs J. Clinical effects and management of eucalyptus oil ingestion in infants and young children. Med J Aust 1995;163(4):177–80.
33. Webb NJA, Pitt WR. Eucalyptus oil poisoning in childhood: 41 cases in South-East Queensland. J Paediatr Child Health 1993;29:368–71.
34. Del Beccaro MA. Melaleuca oil poisoning in a 17-month-old. Vet Hum Toxicol 1995;37(6):557–8.
35. Brook MP, McCarron MM, Mueller JA. Pine oil ingestion. Ann Emerg Med 1989;18(4):391–5.
36. Von Muhlendahl KE, Kreinke EG, Scherrf-Rahne B, Baukloh G. Codeine intoxication in childhood. Lancet 1976;16:303–5.
37. Warden CR, Diekema DS, Robertson WO. Dystonic reaction associated with dextromethorphan ingestion in a toddler. Pediatr Emerg Care 1997;13(3):214–5.
38. Bem JL, Peck R. Dextromethorphan: An overview of safety issues. Drug Saf 1992;7(3):190–9.
39. Suchard J, Nizkorodov S, Wilkinson S. 1,4-Butanediol content of aqua dots children's craft toy beads. J Med Toxicol 2009;5(3):120–4.

40. Telander RL, Smithson A, Groover V. Clinical outcome in children with acute cerebellar encephalopathy and neuroblastoma. *J Pediatr Surg* 1989;**24**(1):11–4.
41. Blokker RS, Smit LME, van den Bos C, et al. *Ned Tijdschr Geneeskd* 2006;**150**(14):799–803.
42. Kaplan S, Goddard J, Van Kleeck M, et al. Ataxia and deafness in children due to bacterial meningitis. *Paediatrics* 1981;**68**:8–13.
43. Iff T, Donati F, Vassella F, et al. Acute encephalitis in Swiss children: Aetiology and outcome. *Eur J Paediatr Neurol* 1998;**2**:233–7.
44. Yaginuma M, Suenaga M, Shiono Y, Sakamoto M. Acute cerebellar ataxia of a patient with SLE. *Clin Neurol Neurosurg* 2000;**102**(1):37–9.
45. Rust RS. Multiple sclerosis, acute disseminated encephalomyelitis, and related conditions. *Semin Pediatr Neurol* 2000;**7**(2):66–90.

8.6 Headache

Alistair Murray • John Ryan

ESSENTIALS

1 The primary role of an emergency physician is to exclude a significant underlying cause for a headache, most urgently that of infection, raised intracranial pressure or an intracerebral bleed.

2 While the majority of headaches in children presenting to the emergency department (ED) are likely to be benign, appropriate investigation and follow up of patients will ensure that serious causes are unlikely to be missed.

3 A thorough history and examination is likely to provide a diagnosis in the majority of children presenting to an ED with a headache.

4 Chronic headaches need not necessarily be investigated on an emergent basis unless they are progressive.

5 *Red flags* prompting further investigation of headache include: occipital headache; meningism; focal neurological signs; seizures; progressive nature; papilloedema; persistent vomiting; ataxia; presence of a ventriculoperitoneal shunt; age younger than 3 years; or early morning headaches, especially those that wake the child from sleep.

Introduction

The aim of this chapter is to provide the reader with a basic understanding of the aetiology of headaches in a paediatric population presenting to an ED, while offering a functional and safe approach to the management of paediatric patients with headaches. Some key points should be remembered from the outset:

- Children may require different approaches, depending on factors such as age, ethnicity or socioeconomic status.
- Children under 3 years rarely complain of headache. This should prompt consideration of an organic cause.
- The classical history of migraine from a teenager may be more easily elicited than the history of symptoms from a shy 5-year-old.

Incidence

Approximately 1% of all presentations to emergency departments have headache as the presenting complaint.[1,2] Headaches in children are very common, with up to 75% of children having had a headache of some form by the age of 15.[3] Despite the frequency, very few paediatric patients with headaches ever consult their family physician or an ED. However, this does not take account of patients who present with a different complaint, such as a temperature, who might also have a headache as part of a concomitant illness.

Pathophysiology

The causes of headache are myriad, but the primary aim of the emergency physician should be to differentiate the patient with a headache which will run a relatively benign course, from that which may be a symptom of significant underlying pathology with immediate health implications.

The overwhelming majority of headaches will be diagnosed on history and examination alone, with little additional information arising from investigations.[3–5] Furthermore, the vast majority of children that present to the emergency department are likely to have headaches that are benign, but those that are not have the potential to be life threatening.

The classification of headaches is based on the underlying aetiology.[6] The International Headache Society has developed a classification of headache, the second edition of which was published in 2004 in *Cephalgia* and is also available on their website.[7] This classifies headache into three broad categories most notably, **primary or secondary headaches** and **cranial neuralgias central and primary facial pain and other headaches** (Table 8.6.1).

The causes of some headaches will be dealt with in other chapters, e.g. Chapter 8.7 on meningitis, while some of the primary headache disorders will be discussed in more detail later in this chapter. We recommend an approach whereby the emergency doctor considers each case by initially excluding the most sinister causes of the headache (Tables 8.6.2 and 8.6.3).

Clinical assessment

History

The first step in any medical assessment is the history and this is no less important in the case of headache. Depending on the age of the child, the history may be taken from the child, the parent or indeed both. Important features of the headache to explore in the history include:

Table 8.6.1   Summary of International Headache Society classification of headaches (ICHD-2)

Primary headaches

Migraine
Tension-type headache
Cluster headaches and other trigeminal-autonomic cephalgias
Other primary headaches

Secondary headaches

Headache attributed to head and/or neck trauma
Headache attributed to cranial and/or cervical vascular disorders
Headache attributed to non-vascular intracranial disorder
Headache attributed to a substance or its withdrawal
Headache attributed to infection
Headache attributed to disorder of homeostasis
Headache or facial pain attributed to disorder of cranium, neck, eyes, ears, nose, sinuses, teeth or other facial or cranial structures.
Headache attributed to psychiatric disorder

Cranial neuralgias, central and primary facial pain and other headaches

Cranial neuralgias and central causes of facial pain
Other headache, cranial neuralgia, central or primary facial pain

Table 8.6.2   Causes of headache in children

Infection

- Meningitis, encephalitis, abscess
- Influenza
- Systemic infection
- Sinusitis
- Dental infection

Vascular

- Migraine
- Intracranial haemorrhage
- Hypertensive encephalopathy

Post lumbar puncture

Raised intracranial pressure

- Brain tumour
- Hydrocephalus
- Benign intracranial hypertension
- Trauma – SDH, concussion

Toxic

- Carbon monoxide
- Lead

Functional

- Tension or cluster headache

Psychogenic

Table 8.6.3   Important causes of non-benign headache

- Brain tumours and hydrocephalus
- Benign intracranial hypertension
- Intracranial haemorrhage
- Meningitis encephalitis or abscess
- Hypertensive encephalopathy

Onset of the headache

Sudden onset headaches can be considered differently in children compared to adults. The classical history of sudden onset headache being suggestive of subarachnoid haemorrhage in an adult is less relevant in the case of the paediatric patient. In children, the most frequent underlying cause is an upper respiratory tract infection or primary headache.[2–4] There is a significantly higher proportion of underlying pathology in cases of acute headache, compared to chronic headaches. It should also be noted that the investigation of headache of acute onset is more properly the role of the emergency physician, while chronic headaches may be best investigated by the child's general practitioner or paediatrician.

Site

Classic migraine is typically unilateral. However, the case of childhood migraine is a little different, often being bilateral. The headache of meningeal irritation due to meningitis may involve neck pain. It should also be noted that occipital headaches are relatively uncommon in children and have been reported to be an independent predictor of underlying pathology, particularly of the posterior fossa.

Pyrexia

The presence of a fever will often be reported by a parent and should immediately raise the suspicion of an infectious origin. Other inflammatory disorders may also cause a pyrexia. Equally, the absence of pyrexia does not equal the absence of an infection. In the ED, a febrile child with a headache requires consideration of the possibility of meningitis or encephalitis.

Progression

The temporal progression is of relevance in children with headaches. For example, a classic migraine will last between 1 and 72 hours in a child, while a patient with a chronic headache that is becoming progressively more severe may well have an underlying organic cause. This should prompt the emergency physician who encounters a child with such a pattern, even if incidentally, to ensure that neuroimaging is performed and that urgent appropriate follow up is arranged.[5]

Nature

Headache of a throbbing nature is suggestive of migraine, while band-like headaches are often tension in type. It has also been suggested that the inability of a child to describe the nature of the headache may in itself be a predictor of underlying pathology.[3]

Behavioural change and avoidance behaviour

This is often noted in a collateral history. While entirely non-specific, it is particularly important in raising suspicion of other causes of a headache such as a school phobia, drug misuse in the adolescent or indeed may be a pointer towards sexual assault.[8]

Sleep disturbance

Benign causes of headache rarely wake patients from their sleep and if a child is being woken by a headache this should prompt the consideration of further investigation or referral.

Postural symptoms

A headache that is worse on lying flat or exacerbated by coughing may be related to raised intracranial pressure. Early morning headaches after recumbency of sleep may occur with raised intracranial pressure or space occupying lesions.

Neurological deficit

A history of neurological deficit, albeit temporary, should be considered highly significant and should always be sought. This is particularly important, as some children may have subtle objective neurological findings that could easily be overlooked in a hurried examination. Most mothers will have noticed an unusual posture or limp but may not immediately mention it unless prompted. The importance of this is reinforced by the evidence that it may take an average of 7 months for a brain tumour to be diagnosed, with as many as three different consultations with a physician. This is despite the fact that a significant proportion of children with tumours have abnormal neurological examinations.[9]

Family history (especially of migraine)

Approximately 70–90% of diagnosed cases of migraine have a positive family history. Therefore diagnosing a migraine in the absence of a family history should be done with caution.

Analgesic use

Abolition of a headache with simple analgesics or restoration of normal activities is more common in those with upper respiratory tract associated headaches. It should also be noted that chronic daily use of analgesics is in itself a cause of headaches.[10]

Examination

A number of specific points should be considered when examining the child with a headache. Headache may be a secondary symptom of a more generalised illness. A comprehensive physical examination is therefore mandatory. Observation of a child from a distance may be valuable. A child lying quietly, unresponsive to the environment, should prompt earlier assessment than an active child who interacts normally with healthcare staff. One must also consider other causes of headache that are not readily discernible. In some cases there may be few clinical signs, such as with carbon monoxide poisoning from houses with poorly ventilated gas boilers.[11] Heavy metal poisoning is another rare cause.

A focused examination should be directed on the basis of the history. Vital signs may provide valuable keys to the aetiology. A significant proportion of children who present with headache will have a diagnosis of respiratory tract infection, hence the importance of a thorough ear, nose and throat examination. Occasionally a child with tonsillitis will present with headache, without any complaint of a sore throat. Dental examination may reveal percussion tenderness of an infection that may cause a referred temporal headache. The presence of nasal discharge or respiratory symptoms should prompt the clinician to seek evidence of sinus tenderness. Likewise, it should be noted that, in most children, headaches due to uncomplicated upper respiratory tract infections can be expected to settle with simple analgesics. The persistence of headache should prompt the consideration of further investigation. The temperature should be recorded on more than one occasion. Likewise, it is important to measure the blood pressure as headache may be the presenting feature of coarctation of the aorta or underlying hypertension. The blood glucose is relevant if the history suggests hypoglycaemia. It is useful to measure head circumference and plot this on centile charts, even for the older child. A disproportionately large head should prompt further investigation[5] and the tension should be palpated in infants who have an open anterior fontanelle.

A careful examination may reveal subtle evidence of trauma, which may or may not have been sustained accidentally. A mild post-concussion headache may persist for a number of days after a head injury, but may require imaging to exclude a possible subdural haematoma, particularly where the headache is severe, responds poorly to analgesia, is associated with vomiting or is prolonged. Headache has been retrospectively described as being more common in victims of sexual abuse. The febrile, toxic-appearing child should be examined for evidence of nuchal rigidity and other signs of meningeal irritation, which may be present in meningitis. In the child who has a ventriculoperitoneal shunt, the reservoir should be assessed by palpation (see Chapter 8.1).[8]

Ophthalmological examination including fundoscopy is particularly important as it may influence immediate management. The presence or absence of papilloedema should be specifically sought as this may be the only objective finding in cases of benign intracranial hypertension (BIH). In this condition the computerised tomography (CT) scan may be normal and the diagnosis based on an elevated opening pressure >20 cmH$_2$O on lumbar puncture. This valuable test is frequently neglected in lumbar punctures performed in the ED, but should be done if one is considering benign intracranial hypertension. The cerebrospinal fluid (CSF) protein, glucose and cell counts are normal in BIH. These children may present with intermittent headache, vomiting, blurred vision or diplopia.

Retinal haemorrhages should be sought on ophthalmoscopy. Their presence is considered as evidence of significant trauma, in the absence of any other causes such as hypertension or diabetes mellitus. It is difficult, if not at times impossible, to achieve successful examination of the fundi and retina of the younger child. Occasionally one may require mydriatic eye drops to dilate the pupils or seek the opinion of a suitably qualified senior colleague. A deferred formal retinal assessment by an ophthalmologist may be required in cases where the possibility of non-accidental injury exists. Eye movements must be carefully examined as subtle nerve palsies may be apparent early in children presenting with a space-occupying lesion or hydrocephalus.

The main consideration in a cardiovascular examination should be directed at the exclusion of hypertension and the palpation of femoral pulses, checking for evidence of coarctation of the aorta.

Abdominal examination is usually normal but is nevertheless important, as nausea, vomiting and abdominal pain are frequently associated with headache in children. It is recognised by the International Headache Society that 'cyclical vomiting' and 'abdominal migraine' are distinct entities and not infrequently progress to the typical pattern of migraine in adulthood. Hypertension of renal origin may be suggested by the presence of polycystic kidneys.

A standard neurological examination should be performed. Specific features that should be sought include papilloedema, ataxia, hemiparesis, abnormal eye movements and abnormal tendon reflexes.[4]

The child should be fully undressed. In particular, a rash or abnormality of pigmentation should specifically be sought. The most urgent of these is the search for the petechial rash of meningococcal disease, but examination may also reveal neurofibromas and café-au-lait spots associated with neurofibromatosis or a pigmented patch associated with tuberous sclerosis.

Investigation

The issue of how to investigate a child with a headache in the ED is not clearly defined and remains contentious. It is clear that in the majority of cases the cause of children presenting to the emergency department with a headache is a respiratory tract infection or primary headache syndrome. The key role of the emergency physician is to diagnose those headaches that may have significant underlying pathology. Investigation should be driven by the history and by findings on examination, as the majority of diagnoses should be suggested by these and confirmed by appropriate diagnostic tests.

CT scanning

Numerous studies have assessed the value of investigating a child with headache, with most focusing on the relevance of neuroimaging.[3,12,13]

A CT scan cannot be considered a benign test as it carries with it a risk in relation to the sedation and transfer of a child and with regard to radiation exposure. A CT head scan carries a 1:1500 risk of developing a subsequent cancer directly related to that radiation exposure.[14]

In the setting of an acute atraumatic headache, the absence of focal neurology or other 'red flags' (as listed later in this chapter), a CT scan is unlikely to be of significant value (Table 8.6.4).

A guide to CT scanning in the context of trauma is considered separately.

In the context of a chronic, *non-progressive* headache with a normal neurological examination, CT is unlikely to be of value. This is different to a chronic *progressive* headache, which is a concerning feature and more likely to harbour underlying pathology. However, this artificially selects a cohort of patients that are unlikely to be seen in the emergency department. The investigation of chronic headaches is not the role of the emergency physician, and in the absence of an acute deterioration

Table 8.6.4 Red flags prompting further investigation of headache
Occipital headache
Meningism
Focal neurological signs
Chronic progressive headaches
Persistent vomiting
Seizures
Papilloedema
Focal neurological symptoms
Ataxia
Presence of a VP shunt
Age younger than 3 years
Abnormal eye movements
Early morning headaches especially those that wake the child from sleep.

VP, ventriculoperitoneal.

patients may be better served by redirection to their family physician or paediatrician.

Blood tests

Laboratory-based testing has a very low yield in children with headaches. Occasionally they can alert the clinician to more serious underlying pathology, but their value is diagnostically limited in the emergency setting. They should not delay the progression to more specific investigation and treatment. Indeed, with the increasing use of near patient testing much of the useful information in this regard can be obtained with the use of a venous blood gas, which provides information on pH, electrolytes, haemoglobin and even carboxyhaemoglobin levels.

Lumbar puncture

Lumbar puncture is mandatory in any case of suspected meningitis or encephalitis. It is a reassuring test when normal and often diagnostic when abnormal. It should be noted, however, that post lumbar puncture headache is also a recognised complication in children, as it is in adults.[15] Such an invasive procedure may often be emotionally traumatic for a child and should not be ordinarily recommended as a routine investigation in the diagnosis of headache. A lumbar puncture with measurement

of an elevated opening pressure is diagnostic in children with benign intracranial hypertension.

Other investigations

Magnetic resonance imaging (MRI) is an investigation that may show increasing utility in the future as its availability becomes more widespread. It has the advantage of no radiation dose and provides more detailed images of the brain.

Other investigations such as electroencephalogram, electromyogram, SPECT, positron emission tomography, autonomic testing and transcranial Doppler have not clearly demonstrated their utility in the acute setting.[13]

Management

Symptomatic treatment in the ED of most headaches in children can be achieved by use of oral analgesics such as paracetamol, codeine or ibuprofen. Headaches that require stronger analgesics to control pain are an indication for admission for further evaluation.

Disposition

The disposition of a patient from the ED should be considered on an individual basis, though some guidelines may be helpful in minimising the risk of missing a significant diagnosis. The increasing use of observation wards can prove helpful in selected cases. Such a facility is most useful in the case where an infective cause of the headache is suspected.

All patients who present to the ED with headache should have a follow-up appointment in the short term with either their family physician or a paediatrician, depending on each case. This will ensure that not only are high standards of care maintained, but unnecessary acute investigations can be avoided that would otherwise be ordered in order to exclude every possible cause of headache. Furthermore, there may be psychosocial aspects of relevance to childhood headaches that may be more appropriately dealt with by the family physician.

NEUROLOGY

8

MIGRAINE

ESSENTIALS

1 Family history of migraine is very common and a diagnosis of migraine in the absence of a family history should be carefully considered.

2 Unlike adult migraine, simple analgesics are often effective in the context of childhood migraine.

3 Childhood migraine is often bilateral.

4 Childhood migraine may be shorter-lived than in adults (1–72 hours).

5 Migraine is frontotemporal. Occipital headache suggests a sinister cause of headache.

Childhood migraine is a common condition presenting to the ED. The diagnosis is often based on an adequate history but the diagnosis can be a little more difficult to make in the younger age group. The emergency physician should not diagnose migraine in children less than 3 years old. Childhood migraine also has a wider spectrum of symptoms than adult migraine and should be considered in a patient who has recurrent abdominal pain, with normal investigations. It is important to remember that although the diagnosis of migraine is common, it is principally a diagnosis of exclusion.

Pathophysiology

The exact mechanism of migraine is complex and it has only recently become better understood. More recently, it is felt to be related to a hyperexcitable cerebral cortex, leading to cortical spreading depression (CSD), leading in turn to activation of the trigeminal nerve and its associated vessels. CSD can lead to areas of oligaemia of the cortex and may be responsible for the aura associated with migraine. Following this, the trigeminal nerve afferents appear to be sensitised and may account for the fact that ordinary activities can significantly exacerbate the migraine.[16]

It is also apparent that serotonin is integrally involved, hence the increasing popularity of the use of serotonin agonists such as sumatriptan in the acute treatment of adult migraine.

Clinical features

Migraine without aura is more common than migraine with aura in children.[17] A number of key features are listed below:

International Headache Society diagnostic criteria of migraine without aura:[7]

A. History of at least five attacks, fulfilling criteria B–D
B. Last 1–72 hours (untreated or unsuccessfully treated)
C. Headache with at least two of the following:
   ❶ Headaches pulsating in quality
   ❷ Headaches may be unilateral or bilateral (unlike adult migraine which is typically unilateral), *not* occipital
   ❸ Headaches exacerbated by routine activities (walking or climbing stairs)
   ❹ The headache is moderate or severe
D. At least one of the following
   ❶ Nausea and/or vomiting
   ❷ Photophobia or phonophobia (may be inferred from child's behaviour).

The presence of an occipital headache suggests a structural abnormality and not migraine.

In migraine with aura the headache is preceded by a period of altered perception that may take numerous forms. This period of altered perception can last up to 60 minutes. Examples are positive visual symptoms (flickering lights, spots, lines), negative visual symptoms (loss of vision, including partial), sensory symptoms (pins and needles) or fully reversible speech disturbances (dysphasia). This period of altered perception can last up to 60 minutes prior to the onset of the headache.[7]

Assessing the severity of headache in a child can prove challenging. Children almost universally point to the unhappiest face on a visual analogue scale when describing a headache. More reliable answers may be achieved by asking about quality of life issues such as ability to continue playing. Children who can continue playing during

a headache appear to have a more benign cause to their headache.

Up to 90% of patients with migraine have a positive family history, although it is noteworthy that only one migraine gene has been identified and this is associated with only 50% of the cases of familial hemiplegic migraine, a particularly rare condition.[5]

A number of other conditions are considered to be migraine disorders in childhood, most notably cyclical vomiting and abdominal migraine. In these conditions there may be recurrent episodes of severe abdominal pain with associated vomiting but the examination and investigation of the children is often normal. These conditions are a diagnosis of exclusion, but their consideration may lead to appropriate referral and follow up as they carry significant morbidity.

Migraine variant disorders may cause transient abnormal neurological findings, such as hemiplegia, ophthalmoplegia or confusional state. These conditions are rare and an abnormal examination should prompt the emergency physician to investigate further.

Investigation

Migraine as a distinct entity has no specific diagnostic test. Key to the diagnosis is the history, as described above, with a normal neurological examination. Investigations should be requested on the basis of excluding other pathology as the underlying cause of headache. It is notable that although a significant number of migraine sufferers have abnormal EEGs, these add little diagnostic value and on current evidence should remain a research tool.[13]

Treatment

Most cases of childhood migraine can be adequately managed with simple analgesics such as paracetamol (15 mg kg^{-1}) and ibuprofen (10 mg kg^{-1}), although ibuprofen appears superior.[18,19] As nausea can often be a significant feature, prochlorperazine appears to be of benefit.[20]

At present the triptan group of drugs remain unlicensed for paediatric use in many countries but there is now evidence for the use of nasal sumatriptan in adolescents and possibly even in those as young as 8.[18,21] The evidence behind the use of other triptans, or routes of administration, is currently limited in the paediatric population.

There are very limited data regarding prophylactic treatment of migraine in children and hence no clear recommendations can be given, other than ensuring appropriate follow up of these cases.

Disposition

All patients with a discharge diagnosis of migraine should be followed up to ensure that the headache resolves within the expected timeframe and also to ensure that it does not progress. Migraine can carry significant impairment to lifestyle, if unrecognised. Follow up should be arranged with the primary care physician, with review of medication and parental understanding of the condition. Children with frequent migraine warrant referral to a paediatrician.

Conclusions

Patients with headaches commonly present to paediatric EDs. Those children presenting with new onset symptoms, significant neurological symptoms/signs or evidence of abnormal physiology should be rapidly assessed, with early referral for diagnostic facilities and neuroimaging being a priority. Children with chronic symptoms or recurrence of chronic symptoms should have a thorough examination and treatment. Follow up should be arranged with the patient's paediatrician or general practitioner.

References

1. Conicella EMRU, Vanacore N, Vigevano F, et al. The child with headache in a pediatric emergency department. *Headache* 2008;**48**(7):1005–11.
2. Burton LJ, Quinn B, Pratt-Cheney JL, Pourani M. Headache etiology in a pediatric emergency department. *Pediatr Emerg Care* 1997;**13**(1):1–4.
3. Kan L, Nagelberg J, Maytal J. Headaches in a pediatric emergency department: etiology, imaging, and treatment. *Headache* 2000;**40**(1):25–9.
4. Lewis DW, Qureshi F. Acute headache in children and adolescents presenting to the emergency department. *Headache* 2000;**40**(3):200–3.
5. Lewis DW. Headaches in children and adolescents. *Am Fam Physician* 2002;**65**(4):625–32.
6. Society IH. International Headache Classification (ICHD-2). *Cephalalgia* 2004;**24**:1–160.
7. IHS. *International Classification of Headache Disorders 2 (ICHD-2)*. 2006. http://ihs-classificationorg/en/.
8. Golding JM. Sexual assault history and headache: five general population studies. *J Nerv Ment Dis* 1999;**187**(10):624–9.
9. Mehta V, Chapman A, McNeely PD, et al. Latency between symptom onset and diagnosis of pediatric brain tumors: an Eastern Canadian geographic study. *Neurosurgery* 2002;**51**(2):365–72; discussion 72–3.
10. Vasconcellos E, Pina-Garza JE, Millan EJ, Warner JS. Analgesic rebound headache in children and adolescents. *J Child Neurol* 1998;**13**(9):443–7.
11. Hampson NB, Hampson LA. Characteristics of headache associated with acute carbon monoxide poisoning. *Headache* 2002;**42**(3):220–3.
12. Lewis DW, Dorbad D. The utility of neuroimaging in the evaluation of children with migraine or chronic daily headache who have normal neurological examinations. *Headache* 2000;**40**(8):629–32.
13. Sandrinia GFL, Jänigc W, Jensend R, et al. Neurophysiological tests and neuroimaging procedures in non-acute headache: guidelines and recommendations. *Eur J Neurol* 2004;**11**:217–24.
14. Brenner D, Elliston C, Hall E, Berdon W. Estimated risks of radiation-induced fatal cancer from pediatric rCT. *Am J Radiol* 2001;**176**:289–96.
15. Janssens E, Aerssens P, Alliet P, et al. Post-dural puncture headaches in children. A literature review. *Eur J Pediatr* 2003;**162**(3):117–21.
16. Lewis D. Toward the definition of childhood migraine. *Curr Opin Pediatr* 2004;**16**:628–36.
17. Bulloch BTM. Emergency department management of pediatric migraine. *Pediatr Emerg Care* 2000;**16**(3):196–201.
18. Lewis D, Ashwal S, Hershey A, et al. Practice Parameter: Pharmacological treatment of migraine headache in children and adolescents. Report of the American Academy of Neurology Quality Standards Subcommittee and the Practice Committee of the Child Neurology Society. *Neurology* 2004;**63**:2215–24.
19. Lewis DW, Kellstein D, Dahl G, et al. Children's ibuprofen suspension for the acute treatment of pediatric migraine headache. *Headache* 2002;**42**:780–6.
20. Bailey B, Cummins McManus B. Treatment of children with migraine in the Emergency Department. A qualitative systematic review. *Pediatr Emerg Care* 2008;**24**(5):321–30.
21. Ahonen K, Hamalainen M, Rantala H, Hoppu K. Nasal sumatriptan is effective in the treatment of migraine attacks in children. *Neurology* 2004;**62**:883–887.

8.7 CNS infections: meningitis and encephalitis

Mike Starr

ESSENTIALS

1 Bacterial meningitis can be rapidly progressive, and result in substantial morbidity and mortality.

2 A high index of suspicion of the possibility of meningitis must be maintained in any sick infant or child.

3 Symptoms and signs are frequently non-specific, particularly with younger age.

4 Antibiotic treatment must not be delayed, although steroids can improve outcome if given before the first dose of antibiotic, and continued 6-hourly for 4 days.

5 Careful management of fluid and electrolyte balance is critical.

6 Careful evaluation for features suggesting raised intracranial pressure should be done at the initial assessment.

7 Conjugate haemophilus, meningococcal and pneumococcal vaccines have reduced the incidence of bacterial meningitis significantly.

8 HSV encephalitis must be considered in any child with features of meningitis with encephalopathy.

9 Empiric aciclovir must be given early when encephalitis is suspected.

Introduction

Meningitis and encephalitis are medical emergencies that require prompt assessment and treatment. Meningitis is inflammation of the meninges that surround the brain and spinal cord. Inflammatory cells invariably spill into the cerebrospinal fluid (CSF) from the meninges, producing an increased cell count. Encephalitis is inflammation involving the brain parenchyma, which may occur in conjunction with inflammation. There is considerable overlap between the features of meningitis and encephalitis, and the two may co-exist. Encephalitis should be considered if a child has encephalopathy, convulsions or neurological deficits.

Meningitis

Classification

Meningitis is usually broadly classified as bacterial or aseptic. Aseptic meningitis may be the result of a localised or systemic insult, but is most commonly caused by viruses. Fungal meningitis usually occurs in immunocompromised children.

Aetiology

Bacteria

The bacterial causes of meningitis vary with the age of the child. In infants less than 2–3 months old, organisms acquired from the maternal genital tract predominate: group B streptococci, *Escherichia coli* and *Listeria monocytogenes*. In older children and adults the most common causes are *Neisseria meningitidis* and *Streptococcus pneumoniae*. Other causes, including *Staphylococcus* species and Gram-negative bacilli, are occasionally seen in immunocompromised hosts or following trauma or neurosurgery. *Haemophilus influenzae* type b (Hib) is rarely seen as a cause now because of widespread immunisation. *Mycobacterium tuberculosis* is rare, other than in children who have spent prolonged periods in countries of high prevalence.

In Australia, meningococcal disease, particularly that caused by serogroup C, has declined since introduction of the meningococcal C conjugate vaccine (MenCCV) into the National Immunisation Program (NIP) schedule. The most common *N. meningitidis* serogroup causing invasive disease in those under 19 years is serogroup B (91%), followed by serogroup C (2–3%).[1] Until the introduction of 7-valent conjugate pneumococcal vaccine (7vPCV) into the NIP schedule, the most common pneumococcal serotypes causing invasive disease were those contained in 7vPCV (14, 6B, 18C, 19F, 4, 23F, 9V).[2] However, since then, it appears that serotype replacement is occurring; nasal carriage of 7PCV serotypes has been replaced by others, namely 19A and 16F,[3] and the rate of invasive pneumococcal disease caused by 7vPCV serotypes has decreased significantly.[4] However, the rate of invasive pneumococcal disease caused by serotype 19A increased in non-Indigenous people and in the population overall.[4] Antibiotic resistance is almost exclusively restricted to these serotypes (and remaining 7PCV serotypes).

Viruses

Enteroviruses, including coxsackie and echoviruses, cause 85–95% of cases of viral meningitis. Herpes simplex viruses 1 and 2 (HSV-1 and HSV-2) and other herpes viruses (human herpesviruses 6, 7 and 8, varicella-zoster virus, cytomegalovirus and Epstein–Barr virus) tend to cause meningoencephalitis. HSV-1 and HSV-2 are perhaps the most important causes to consider, as meningoencephalitis caused by these viruses is associated with high morbidity and mortality, which may be reduced with early treatment with antiviral medications.

Fungi

Cryptococcus neoformans is the most common fungal cause of meningitis, but occurs almost exclusively in immunocompromised hosts.

Clinical findings

The classical features of meningitis comprise fever, headache, vomiting, neck stiffness, photophobia and altered mentation. However, the clinical manifestations are often non-specific, particularly in infants and young children. They may include fever, irritability, lethargy, poor feeding or vomiting. Up to 58% of children with meningitis have received antibiotics before the emergency department (ED) presentation.[5] This may modify the clinical presentation of meningitis.[6] It is therefore important to consider the possibility of central nervous system (CNS) infection in any sick infant or child, particularly if they are already taking antibiotics.

If the fontanelle is still open, it may be bulging when examined with the infant in a sitting position. Photophobia is difficult to ascertain in young children, and other signs of meningeal irritation may be absent or difficult to elicit. Resistance to being picked up or distress on walking may be the only clues. Kernig's sign (inability to extend the knee when the leg is flexed at the hip), Brudzinski's sign (bending the head forward produces flexion movements of the legs) and nuchal rigidity may be present in older children, but have even been shown to have low positive and negative predictive value in adults with meningitis.[7]

Rashes may occur with any bacterial meningitis, although are less common with pneumococcal infection. Petechiae or purpura are suggestive of meningococcal sepsis, but may also occur in Hib and viral meningitis. Enteroviral meningitis may even be associated with florid purpura fulminans.

It is impossible to reliably differentiate between bacterial and viral meningitis on clinical grounds. However, children with enteroviral meningitis are more likely to present in summer or autumn with gradual onset of non-specific constitutional symptoms including diarrhoea, cough and myalgia, in addition to the more typical features.

Investigations

Definitive diagnosis of meningitis relies on examination of the CSF with biochemical analysis, microscopy and culture. Children with suspected meningitis should have a lumbar puncture (LP) performed, unless there is a clear contraindication. The only absolute contraindication is raised intracranial pressure (ICP). It may be difficult to determine whether ICP is raised, but the following signs may be indicative:

- coma (absent or non-purposeful response to painful stimulus);
- abnormal pupillary responses;
- abnormal posturing;
- focal neurological signs or seizures;
- recent (within 30 minutes), prolonged (over 30 minutes) or tonic seizures;
- papilloedema – although this is an unreliable and late sign of raised ICP.

A bulging fontanelle, in the absence of other signs of raised ICP, is not a contraindication to LP.

The threshold for performing an LP should be lower in young children with less specific signs or those who have been taking antibiotics prior to presentation.

Cerebral computerised tomography (CT) should not be used to decide whether it is safe to proceed with LP or not. In a prospective study of bacterial meningitis, CT findings obtained during the acute stages failed to reveal any clinically significant abnormalities that were not suspected on neurological examination.[8] Moreover, cerebral herniation can occur with a normal CT[9,10] and the true cause of coning and relationship to prior lumbar puncture is not clearly established.

Other relative contraindications to LP include:

- cardiovascular compromise or shock
- respiratory compromise
- coagulopathy or thrombocytopenia.

Examination of the CSF

A CSF specimen should always be sent for *urgent microscopy* to help guide empiric treatment. Normal CSF is clear and contains few cells (and no neutrophils). As few as 200×10^6 cells per litre will cause CSF to appear turbid. The CSF profile may help differentiate between bacterial and viral meningitis, but the findings vary. Table 8.7.1 indicates the typical profiles in normal children and those with meningitis. However, these should always be interpreted in the context of the clinical picture. In early bacterial meningitis, the CSF cell count may be normal. In enteroviral meningitis, there is typically a neutrophil predominance early,

and this may remain so for more than 24 hours.[11]

Organisms are seen on CSF Gram stain in 60–80% of cases of bacterial meningitis, provided that prior antibiotics have not been given. The sensitivity is highest in pneumococcal meningitis. Prior antibiotics may preclude culture of the causative organism, but the biochemistry and white cell count remain abnormal for several days whether or not antibiotics have been given.

A traumatic tap occurs in 15–20% of LP in children.[12,13] Several formulae have been devised for interpretation of CSF contaminated with blood, but the safest practice is to disregard the red cell count and treat if meningitis is suspected until culture and other studies are clearly negative.

Seizures do not result in increased CSF cell count in the absence of meningitis.

Bacterial or viral DNA can be detected in blood and/or CSF using polymerase chain reaction analysis (PCR). Sensitivity and specificity are high, particularly for *N. meningitidis*, HSV and enterovirus. PCR for *N. meningitidis* is particularly useful in patients with a clinical picture consistent with meningococcal meningitis, but who have received prior antibiotics.

Latex agglutination allows rapid detection of bacterial antigens in CSF and urine. However, it lacks sensitivity and specificity, other than for Hib, and is therefore not clinically useful.

Other investigations

- Culture of blood, throat swab, stool/rectal swab or of skin lesion may yield a causative organism.
- Gram stain on blood smear may be positive.
- Blood glucose should be measured at the same time as CSF glucose.
- A baseline sodium should be measured. Hyponatraemia occurs in about one third of children with meningitis, and may be due to increased antidiuretic hormone secretion, increased urine sodium losses, and excessive electrolyte-free water intake or administration.
- Full blood count and acute phase reactants (e.g. C-reactive protein) may provide supportive information, but are more useful when measured serially to monitor the response to therapy.

Table 8.7.1 CSF findings in meningitis

	White cell count		Biochemistry	
	Neutrophils ($\times 10^6 L^{-1}$)	Lymphocytes ($\times 10^6 L^{-1}$)	Protein ($g L^{-1}$)	Glucose (CSF:blood ratio)
Normal (>1 month of age)	0	≤5	<0.4	≥0.6 (or ≥2.5 mmol L^{-1})
Normal (<1 month of age)	0*	<20	<1.0	≥0.6 (or ≥2.1 mmol L^{-1})
Bacterial meningitis	↑ (but may be normal)	↑ (usually <100)	↑ (but may be normal)	↓ (but may be normal)
Viral meningitis	↑ (usually <100)	↑ (but may be normal)	0.4–1.0 (but may be normal)	Usually normal
Encephalitis	↑ (usually <100)	↑ (but may be normal)	0.4–1.0 (but may be normal)	↓ (but may be normal)

*Some studies have found up to 5% of white cells in neonates without meningitis comprise neutrophils.

Management

Antibiotics

Following initial fluid resuscitation, the emphasis is on prompt commencement of parenteral antibiotics. Delay in antibiotic therapy has been associated with adverse clinical outcome in adults with bacterial meningitis.[14]

Age <3 months:	Amoxicillin 50 mg kg^{-1} intravenously (IV) 12-hourly (week 1 of life), 8-hourly (week 2–4 of life), 4–6-hourly (> week 4 of life) *plus* Cefotaxime 50 mg kg^{-1} IV 12-hourly (week 1 of life), 6-hourly (>1 week of age).

Because of the morbidity associated with neonatal Gram-negative meningitis, and the high rates of recrudescence, some neonatologists add gentamicin to the above regimen.

Age >3 months:	Cefotaxime 50 mg kg^{-1} (max 2 g) IV 6-hourly

Rates of resistance to penicillin and cephalosporins amongst pneumococci have fallen in Australia since the introduction of the conjugate pneumococcal vaccine.[3,4,15] Vancomycin should be added if rates of resistance are high.

Steroids

Routine administration of steroids as adjunctive therapy has been controversial in the past. The evidence that they protect against neurological (particularly audiological) complications of childhood meningitis is strongest for Hib meningitis, when dexamethasone is given before the first dose of antibiotics, and when a third generation cephalosporin is used. A recent large European trial in adults with meningitis showed reduction in mortality and severe morbidity with pneumococcal meningitis.[16] A recent Cochrane meta-analysis including adult and paediatric trials concluded that adjuvant steroids are beneficial for children with bacterial meningitis.[17] Evidence from animal studies shows that dexamethasone reduces penetration of vancomycin into infected cerebrospinal fluid.[18] Thus, there is concern that use of dexamethasone with vancomycin could compromise the efficacy of vancomycin in third generation cephalosporin-resistant strains. Fortunately, the majority of cases of pneumococcal meningitis are still caused by strains that are susceptible to penicillin and third-generation cephalosporins.

Accordingly, children (>4 weeks old) who are being treated for possible meningitis (who have not yet received parenteral antibiotics, or who have received their first dose less than 1 hour previously) should be given dexamethasone 0.25 mg kg^{-1} IV (max 10 mg) (followed by 0.25 mg kg^{-1} 6-hourly). Steroids should preferably be given 15–30 minutes before antibiotics, although antibiotic administration should not be delayed for more than 30 minutes.

Fluids

Careful management of fluid and electrolyte balance is important in the treatment of meningitis. Over or under hydration are associated with adverse outcomes.[19–21] Many children have increased antidiuretic hormone secretion, and some will have dehydration due to vomiting, poor fluid intake or septic shock. Assessment of the clinical signs of hydration, including weight, measurement of the serum sodium, documentation of urine output, and clinical assessment of the neurological state should be monitored closely, and the total fluid intake adjusted accordingly.

Initial fluid resuscitation to treat shock should be with 20 mL kg^{-1} of isotonic (normal) saline. Thereafter, isotonic fluids should be given to maintain systemic blood pressure (and thereby cerebral blood flow). Previous guidelines have emphasised the importance of fluid restriction.[19] It may be necessary to restrict fluids if the serum sodium is <130 mmol L^{-1}, or if there are signs of fluid overload. However, fluid restriction does not generally improve outcome[20] and has even been associated with a worse neurological outcome.[21] Thus, most children should receive normal maintenance fluid volumes.

Prevention

Contacts of patients with meningococcal meningitis may require chemoprophylaxis to prevent secondary spread. Those who should receive chemoprophylaxis include:

- the index case if treated only with penicillin (does not eradicate carriage);
- all intimate, household or day-care contacts who have been exposed to the index case within 10 days of onset;
- any person who gave mouth-to-mouth resuscitation to the index case, or had direct contact with their airway secretions.

Although nosocomial transmission of meningococcal infection is rare, droplet precautions are recommended until the patient has received 24 hours of antibiotic therapy. As the aetiology is usually unknown during this period, all cases of suspected bacterial meningitis should be managed in this way. Preferred placement is in a single room. However, if a spatial separation of >1 metre can be achieved and curtains can be drawn between the infected patient and other patients and visitors, this may be sufficient.

Chemoprophylaxis
Rifampicin 10 mg kg^{-1} (5 mg kg^{-1} <1 month old) orally 12-hourly (max 600 mg) for 2 days *or*
Ceftriaxone 125 mg (≤12 years)/250 mg (>12 years) mg intramuscularly as a single dose *or*
Ciprofloxacin 500 mg orally as a single dose.

7vPCV and MenCCV vaccines are part of the routine NIP schedule for all children and should have a continuing impact on the number of cases of childhood meningitis.

Complications

Bacterial meningitis is associated with a 4.5% mortality rate, and intellectual, cognitive and auditory impairment in 10–20% of survivors.[22] The risk for sequelae is greatest in those who experience acute neurological complications at the time of their illness.[23]

Viral meningitis
Most cases are self-limiting, and treatment is symptomatic.

Brain abscess

Brain abscess classically presents with fever, headache and focal neurological deficit. Although rare, early recognition is vital, as early antibiotic treatment and drainage improve outcome. Diagnosis is by cerebral CT or magnetic resonance imaging (MRI). Aspiration for diagnosis and neurosurgical intervention are usually required. The most common causes are oral viridans streptococci, anaerobes, Gram-negatives and *S. aureus*.

Empiric treatment is:

Flucloxacillin 50 mg kg^{-1} (max 2 g) IV 4-hourly *plus*
Cefotaxime 50 mg kg^{-1} (max 2 g) IV 6-hourly *plus*
Metronidazole 15 mg kg^{-1} (max 1 g) IV stat, then 7.5 mg kg^{-1} (max 500 mg) IV 8-hourly.

Encephalitis

Aetiology

HSV is the most common cause of non-seasonal encephalitis in Australia. Other causes include enteroviruses, influenza virus, other herpes viruses and *Mycoplasma pneumoniae*. Several other viruses cause seasonal epidemics of encephalitis in specific geographic areas. Examples include Murray Valley encephalitis in the east Kimberley region, and Japanese B encephalitis in the Torres Strait Islands.

Clinical findings

There is considerable overlap between the features of meningitis and encephalitis, and the two frequently co-exist. Encephalitis should be suspected if there is encephalopathy, that is, a change of behaviour, altered conscious state or extreme drowsiness. Convulsions (particularly focal) and focal neurological deficits are also more common in encephalitis.

Investigations

CSF biochemistry and microscopy findings are non-specific (see Table 8.7.1). PCR testing for HSV and enterovirus is sensitive and specific. Cerebral CT or MRI of the brain and EEG may be suggestive of HSV encephalitis, particularly if they show temporal lobe involvement.

Management

It is vital to consider the diagnosis of HSV encephalitis early, because **early** treatment with aciclovir may improve the outcome. Treatment should be continued for 21 days unless HSV is excluded clinically or on subsequent investigations.

Aciclovir   20 mg kg^{-1} IV 8-hourly (age <3 months)
500 mg m^{-2} IV 8-hourly (age 3 months–12 years)
10 mg kg^{-1} IV 8-hourly (age >12 years)

Complications

Without treatment, mortality of HSV encephalitis is up to 80%, and 50% of survivors have long-term sequelae.[24] Outcome is worse if coma is present initially.

Conclusion

Meningitis and encephalitis are medical emergencies that must be assessed and treated urgently to reduce the likelihood of poor outcomes.

References

1. Annual report of the Australian Meningococcal Surveillance Programme, 2008. *Commun Dis Intell* 2009;**33**(3):259–67.
2. Liu M, Andrews R, Stylianopoulos J, et al. Invasive pneumococcal disease among children in Victoria. *Commun Dis Intell* 2003;**27**(3):362–6.
3. Leach A, Morris P, McCallum G, et al. Emerging pneumococcal carriage serotypes in a high-risk population receiving universal 7-valent pneumococcal conjugate vaccine and 23-valent polysaccharide vaccine since 2001. *BMC Infect Dis* 2009;**9**:121–9.
4. Giele C, Anthony K, Lehmann D, Van Buynder P. Invasive pneumococcal disease in Western Australia: emergence of serotype 19A. *Med J Aust* 2009;**190**:166.
5. Kallio MJ, Kilpi T, Anttila M, Peltola H. The effect of a recent previous visit to a physician on outcome after childhood bacterial meningitis. *JAMA* 1994;**272**(10):787–91.
6. Rothrock SG, Green SM, Wren J, et al. Pediatric bacterial meningitis: is prior antibiotic therapy associated with an altered clinical presentation? *Ann Emerg Med* 1992;**21**(2):146–52.
7. Thomas KE, Hasbun R, Jekel J, Quagliarello VJ. The diagnostic accuracy of Kernig's sign, Brudzinski's sign, and nuchal rigidity in adults with suspected meningitis. *Clin Infect Dis* 2002;**35**(1):46–52.
8. Cabral DA, Flodmark O, Farrell K, Speert DP. Prospective study of computed tomography in acute bacterial meningitis. *J Pediatr* 1987;**111**(2):201–5.
9. Rennick G, Shann F, de Campo J. Cerebral herniation during bacterial meningitis in children. *Br Med J* 1993;**306**(6883):953–5.
10. Shetty AK, Desselle BC, Craver RD, Steele RW. Fatal cerebral herniation after lumbar puncture in a patient with a normal computed tomography scan. *Pediatrics* 1999;**103**(6):1284–6.
11. Negrini B, Kelleher KJ, Wald ER. Cerebrospinal fluid findings in aseptic versus bacterial meningitis. *Pediatrics* 2000;**105**(2):316–9.
12. Mazor SS, McNulty JE, Roosevelt GE. Interpretation of traumatic lumbar punctures: who can go home? *Pediatrics* 2003;**111**(3):525–8.
13. Shah KH, Richard KM, Nicholas S, Edlow JA. Incidence of traumatic lumbar puncture. *Acad Emerg Med* 2003;**10**(2):151–4.
14. Aronin SI, Peduzzi P, Quagliarello VJ. Community-acquired bacterial meningitis: risk stratification for adverse clinical outcome and effect of antibiotic timing. *Ann Intern Med* 1998;**129**(11_Part_1):862–9.
15. McMaster P, McIntyre P, Gilmour R, et al. The emergence of resistant pneumococcal meningitis – implications for empiric therapy. *Arch Dis Child* 2002;**87**(3):207–10.
16. de Gans J, van de Beek D, the European Dexamethasone in Adulthood Bacterial Meningitis Study Investigators. Dexamethasone in adults with bacterial meningitis. *N Engl J Med* 2002;**347**(20):1549–56.
17. Brouwer M, McIntyre P, de Gans J, et al. Corticosteroids for acute bacterial meningitis. *Cochrane Database Syst Rev* 2010;(9):CD004405.
18. Martinez-Lacasa J, Cabellos C, Martos A, et al. Experimental study of the efficacy of vancomycin, rifampicin and dexamethasone in the therapy of pneumococcal meningitis. *J Antimicrob Chemother* 2002;**49**(3):507–13.
19. Shann F, Germer S. Hyponatraemia associated with pneumonia or bacterial meningitis. *Arch Dis Child* 1985;**60**(10):963–6.
20. Duke T, Mokela D, Frank D, et al. Management of meningitis in children with oral fluid restriction or intravenous fluid at maintenance volumes: a randomised trial. *Ann Trop Paediatr* 2002;**22**(2):145–57.
21. Singhi SC, Singhi PD, Srinivas B, et al. Fluid restriction does not improve the outcome of acute meningitis. *Pediatr Infect Dis J* 1995;**14**(6):495–503.
22. Baraff LJ, Lee SI, Schriger DL. Outcomes of bacterial meningitis in children: a meta-analysis. *Pediatr Infect Dis J* 1993;**12**(5):389–94.
23. Grimwood K, Anderson P, Anderson V, et al. Twelve year outcomes following bacterial meningitis: further evidence for persisting effects. *Arch Dis Child* 2000;**83**(2):111–6.
24. Whitley RJ, Lakeman F. Herpes simplex virus infections of the central nervous system: therapeutic and diagnostic considerations. *Clin Infect Dis* 1995;**20**(2):414–20.

INFECTIOUS DISEASES

Section editor *Gary Browne*

9.1 Infectious diseases

Mike Starr

ESSENTIALS

1 Fever is one of the most common reasons for children to present to the Emergency Department.

2 Serious bacterial infections need to be identified early and treated aggressively; these include meningitis, septicaemia, urinary tract infection, pneumonia, and bone and joint infections.

3 The majority of febrile children have a viral illness, requiring few if any investigations.

4 It is important to have a structured approach to the investigation and treatment of the febrile child without focus.

5 Most well-appearing febrile children over 3 months of age without a focus of infection do not require laboratory testing or treatment, apart from microscopy and culture of urine.

In this section, general infectious disease issues, including the appropriate collection of microbiological specimens, guidelines for empiric antibiotic therapy, post-exposure prophylaxis and immunisation are addressed.

Fever

Fever is one of the most common presenting complaints in children in both the primary care and emergency department settings. Of all children's visits to the emergency department (ED), 20–30% are with acute episodes of fever.[1] In children <1 year old presenting to EDs in Australia and New Zealand, fever without identifiable source is the diagnosis in over 3%.[2] In the first 2 years of life, children average four to six febrile episodes. Those in child care may have many more than this.

Defining and measuring temperature

There is controversy regarding the most appropriate thermometer and the best anatomical site for temperature measurement.[3] Parents often use touch to detect fever in their children. However, touch has only 50% specificity.[4] It tends to overestimate the incidence of fever, and is more useful to exclude fever. Rectal temperature has long been considered the gold standard for routine measurement of body temperature, but it does not in fact reflect true core temperature within the pulmonary artery.

Moreover, parents and patients generally prefer other temperature assessments. Nonetheless, rectal temperature remains the most widely used measure in infants under 3 months of age. Tympanic thermometers provide the most accurate assessment of core temperature, but the probe may be too large for an infant's auditory canal. Oral temperature requires patient cooperation, and is generally unsuitable for children under the age of 5 years. Axillary temperature measurement is inaccurate and insensitive.

The definition of fever is

- 38°C (rectal or tympanic);
- 37.5°C (oral); or
- 37.2°C (axilla).

Fever: to treat or not to treat?

The drugs most commonly used for treating fever are paracetamol, ibuprofen and aspirin. The routine use of these medications in the treatment of fever has been questioned.[5] In particular, there has been concern that the use of antipyretics may prolong viral shedding, impair antibody response to viral infection, and may increase morbidity and mortality.[5-7] Moreover, each of the commonly used antipyretics may have significant adverse effects such as hepatic dysfunction, metabolic acidosis, Reye syndrome and gastrointestinal bleeding. Treatment should therefore be focused on alleviation of discomfort or pain rather than on the height of the temperature. Either paracetamol or ibuprofen may be used.

It is important to note that the use of anti-pyretics has not been shown to prevent febrile convulsions.

Paracetamol may be given orally, rectally or intravenously at a dose of 10–15 mg kg^{-1} 4–6-hourly. In an unsupervised, community setting, the total daily dose should be limited to 60 mg kg^{-1}, although up to 90 mg kg^{-1} per 24 hrs can be used under medical supervision. Single doses of 30 mg kg^{-1} may be used for night-time dosing. Serious toxicity has been reported in children with chronic daily over-dosage, mostly occurring in children who have a febrile illness and associated anorexia, vomiting and/or dehydration.[8] A child should be reviewed after 48 hours if regular paracetamol has been 'required' for this period.

Ibuprofen can be used as an alternative to paracetamol at a dose of 5–10 mg kg^{-1} (maximum of 500 mg per dose), given 6- to 8-hourly (maximum daily dose of 40 mg kg^{-1} or 2 g). It is recommended that it be used alone, and not in combination with paracetamol, as this practice may lead to an increase in adverse effects, including gastrointestinal bleeding, renal dysfunction and anaphylaxis.[7] A theoretical risk of aggravating concurrent asthma has also been described, although these adverse effects are refuted in large prospective studies.[8] There is also a concern that ibuprofen may be associated with an increased risk of necrotising group A streptococcal infections.[9] There is no evidence that alternating paracetamol and ibuprofen is any better at reducing fever or spares the potential hepatotoxicity related to paracetamol administration.[9]

Practical approach to the febrile child

The majority of febrile children will have self-limiting viral infections. The challenge is to identify those children at risk of serious illness while avoiding unnecessary investigation and treatment of children with benign viral illnesses.

Fever in children may be classified into three groups:

- fever with localising signs;
- fever without focus;
- pyrexia of unknown origin.

Fever with localising signs

A careful history and examination will identify the source of infection in most patients. These children should be managed according to the individual condition and its severity.

Fever without focus

In a small number of children presenting with fever, no focus is found. While most will have a viral infection, a more serious illness such as a urinary tract infection (4–5%), occult bacteraemia (<1%) or meningitis (<0.2%) may be present.

Occult bacteraemia is the presence of bacteria in the bloodstream of a febrile child who has no apparent focus of infection and looks well. Diagnosis is by blood culture and exclusion of focal infection. The incidence of occult bacteraemia in febrile children has reduced dramatically to <1% since the introduction of conjugate pneumococcal vaccine.[10,11]

Most children who present with fever and no identifiable focus appear otherwise well. History should include details about immunisation status, infectious contacts, travel, diet and contact with animals or insects. A thorough physical examination should be performed, paying particular attention to general appearance (colour and level of activity) and vital signs (respiratory rate, pulse, peripheral perfusion and blood pressure).

It is difficult to assess whether a child is 'septic' or 'toxic'. A simple and effective approach that is useful in the ED is a combination of ABC, fluids-in and fluids-out.[12] An infant with one or more of these symptoms or signs has a higher risk of serious illness:

- A – poor arousal, reduced alertness and reduced activity.
- B – breathing difficulty.
- C – poor perfusion.
- Fluids in – the frequency of feeding over the 24 hours prior to presentation, <50% of normal over 24 hours prior to presentation, suggesting dehydration.
- Fluids out – significantly abnormal urine output of <50% of usual output.

Other features on examination that strongly suggest a seriously ill infant include pallor, purpuric rash, high-pitched scream and bulging fontanelle.

Patients with unexplained fever with a higher likelihood for serious infection include the following patient groups or conditions:

- neonates (<1 month of age);
- incompletely immunised children;
- immunocompromised (e.g. congenital immunodeficiency, human immunodeficiency virus (HIV), neutropenic and other oncology patients, cytotoxic drugs and steroids);
- asplenic children (congenital, post splenectomy or functional, e.g. sickle cell disease);
- patients who have received prior oral antibiotics; many of these patients have a viral infection, but meningitis or other serious bacterial infection must be considered;
- children with fever and prolonged convulsion;
- children with underlying medical conditions (e.g. cystic fibrosis, structural cardiac defects, etc.);
- children with central venous devices, shunts or other foreign material.

When considering management strategies for febrile infants, three age groups are generally assigned: <1 month of age, 1–3 months and >3 months (Table 9.1.1).

Table 9.1.1	Management of well-appearing febrile child without focus	
Age	Investigation	Management
<1 month	FBE; blood, urine and CSF cultures; CXR	Admit. Empiric IV antibiotics: amoxicillin and cefotaxime
1–3 months	Urine culture ± blood and CSF cultures ± CXR	Consider admission and observation. Discharge with arranged review
>3 months	Consider urine culture	Discharge with arranged review

CXR, chest X-ray; FBE, full blood examination; CSF, cerebrospinal fluid.

Infants less than 1 month of age, and those with any of the risk factors above require several investigations including full blood examination, culture of blood, urine and cerebrospinal fluid (CSF), and a chest X-ray if indicated. Empiric antimicrobial therapy should be based on the patient's clinical illness, risk factors, and the local epidemiology of potential pathogens and their antibiotic susceptibility.

Clinical scores, such as the Rochester and Boston criteria, have been devised to identify children at low risk of serious bacterial infection.[13] However, their utility has been questioned in the era of widespread Hib and conjugate pneumococcal vaccination.

Febrile infants between 1 and 3 months of age who appear well and do not have risk factors may not require blood tests or a lumbar puncture, although urine microscopy and culture is advisable. Those over 3 months of age do not routinely require laboratory testing or treatment, although urine microscopy and culture may still be appropriate.

There is no evidence that oral or parenteral antibiotics prevent the rare occurrence of focal infections from occult bacteraemia; instead, they result in delayed diagnosis, drug side effects, additional costs and the development of resistant organisms. What is required is a careful clinical assessment, parental education and review within 24 hours.

As urinary tract infection is the most common serious bacterial infection among febrile infants and children, urine microscopy and culture should be included in the investigation of most such children. In infants, a urine sample should ideally be obtained via suprapubic aspiration or catheter. A negative urinalysis does not exclude a urinary tract infection, which may occur in the absence of pyuria.[14,15]

Other rarer causes of fever should also be considered:

- Kawasaki disease;
- connective tissue disease (e.g. juvenile arthritis);
- inflammatory bowel disease;
- malignancy (e.g. leukaemia).

Pyrexia of unknown origin (PUO)

PUO is defined as prolonged fever (usually greater than 10 days) where history, examination and 'routine' investigations have not identified a cause. Occasionally, fever appears to occur in a repetitive or periodic pattern. In either case, a chronic or non-infectious condition should be considered, such as juvenile idiopathic arthritis and other connective tissue diseases, inflammatory bowel disease or malignancy. Infectious causes include systemic viral syndromes (such as infectious mononucleosis), upper or lower respiratory infections (e.g. sinusitis), urinary tract infection, central nervous system infection, bone infection, tuberculosis, abscess (e.g. parameningeal, intra-abdominal), endocarditis and enteric infections (e.g. typhoid fever).

More extensive investigations are often required, including specific investigations for mycobacterial, fungal or viral infections. Imaging may be required, looking for occult abdominal or central nervous system collection, for osteomyelitis or endocarditis.

Kawasaki disease is an important consideration in an infant or child presenting with prolonged fever, and diagnosis is often delayed. There is a degree of urgency in diagnosis, because treatment within 10 days of onset of fever with intravenous immunoglobulin and aspirin reduces the incidence of coronary artery lesions from around 20% to around 5%.[16]

Empiric antibiotic therapy

With the possible exception of bacterial meningitis, where Gram stain results may guide therapy, the most appropriate antibiotic therapy in children must be based on epidemiological grounds. The most important factors determining the likely pathogens, which should be targeted by empiric therapy, are:

- age;
- presumed focus of infection;
- presence of underlying disease or anatomical abnormality;
- whether the infection is hospital or community acquired.

In addition, the site of infection may have implications for the expected penetration of the antibiotic chosen (e.g. aminoglycosides do not penetrate into abscess cavities and are inactive in an anaerobic environment).

For presumed bacterial infection (including meningitis) in the first 3 months of life, empiric treatment must cover Group B streptococci, *Escherichia coli* and *Listeria monocytogenes* infections. Recommended antibiotics are: amoxicillin plus cefotaxime.

Amoxicillin 50 mg kg^{-1} per dose intravenous (IV) 12-hourly (week 1 of life), 8-hourly (week 2–4 of life), 4–6-hourly thereafter.

Cefotaxime: 50 mg kg^{-1} per dose IV 12-hourly (week 1 of life), 8-hourly (week 2–4 of life), 6-hourly thereafter.

For presumed bacterial infection (including meningitis) after 3 months of age, potential pathogens include *Neisseria meningitidis*, *Streptococcus pneumoniae*, Group A streptococci and *Staphylococcus aureus*. Recommended empiric therapy is: flucloxacillin plus cefotaxime.

Flucloxacillin 50 mg kg^{-1} per dose IV 6-hourly.

Cefotaxime 50 mg kg^{-1} per dose IV 6-hourly.

If meningitis has been excluded, recommended antibiotics are flucloxacillin plus gentamicin.

Gentamicin 7.5 mg kg^{-1} 24-hourly (<10 years), 6 mg kg^{-1} per dose 24-hourly (>10 years)

Antibiotic choice should also be modified once relevant culture results become available.

Antimicrobial resistance

Antimicrobial resistance is an increasing worldwide problem. Resistance of bacteria to antibiotics can conveniently be divided into two categories:

❶ Intrinsic – resistance due to inherent properties of the organism or antibiotic, and

❷ Acquired – resistance gained by the organism either before or during therapy.

Important examples of intrinsic resistance (which affects 100% of organisms) include enterococci to cephalosporins, enteric Gram negatives to penicillin and flucloxacillin and anaerobes to aminoglycosides and quinolones. A few important examples of increasing acquired resistance include:

- penicillin (and cephalosporin)-resistant *Strep. pneumoniae* (PRP) – of note, resistance rates have fallen since introduction of the conjugate vaccine;
- methicillin (multidrug)-resistant *Staph. aureus* (MRSA);
- *Staph. aureus* with intermediate sensitivity to vancomycin and teicoplanin (GISA);
- community acquired non-multiresistant MRSA (CA-MRSA);
- vancomycin-resistant *Enterococcus* (VRE);
- bacteria that produce extended-spectrum β-lactamases (ESBL), e.g. some *E. coli* and *Klebsiella* spp., which are associated with cephalosporin (and often gentamicin) resistance.

Common infectious exanthems

Most frequently, the cause of fever in children is a viral illness. This usually occurs in a seasonal pattern – in Australia particularly the months of April through to September when there is an increase of acute infections in the community. Most of these are due to respiratory and gastrointestinal pathogens, such as respiratory syncytial virus and rotavirus, respectively. However, there is an important group of viral infections that the emergency physician needs to be familiar with that commonly present with fever and rash.

A rash or other cutaneous manifestation accompanies a large number of presentations for childhood infectious disease. An exanthem is an acute infectious disease accompanied by a rash. The most common childhood exanthems are scarlet fever, measles, rubella, erythema infectiosum and roseola infantum. Rash and fever may be associated with many other viruses, bacteria, and even parasitic infections. In addition, a rash and fever may also be associated with a wide variety of non-infectious processes.

Scarlet fever

This infection is common amongst children 3–12 years of age. It is caused by Group A-β-haemolytic streptococci (GAS). The disease is transmitted by direct contact or respiratory droplets. It has a short incubation period of 2–5 days. The illness is characterised by an abrupt onset of fever, vomiting and a sore throat, with abdominal pain. The typical rash develops within 12–48 hours after onset, and is a generalised confluent erythematous papular rash giving the skin a sandpaper-like texture. The forehead and cheeks are red, smooth and flushed, with sparing of the area around the mouth (circumoral pallor). Petechiae may coalesce in linear form, particularly in skin folds such as axillae and antecubital fossae, forming pathognomonic Pastia lines. The tongue in scarlet fever is initially coated by a white fur, which after a few days is reddened by the projection of oedematous papillae through the coat. This white strawberry tongue loses its coating after 4 days, revealing a beefy red strawberry tongue. Resolution of the rash and other clinical manifestations usually occurs by the end of the first week, heralding a period of characteristic desquamation of skin. Desquamation progresses from face to trunk and finally to hands and feet after 3–4 weeks.

Complications of scarlet fever may be early local upper respiratory tract disease, including cervical adenitis and otitis media, and later immune-mediated disease including acute glomerulonephritis and rheumatic fever. A 10-day course of penicillin is effective in eradication of the bacteria; clindamycin may be added to inhibit toxin synthesis if there are associated features of shock.

Investigations are often unhelpful acutely. Isolation of GAS from a throat swab may reflect asymptomatic carriage and not necessarily invasive disease. Elevation of serial antistreptolysin O or anti-DNAse-B titres may aid diagnosis of recent streptococcal infection.

Measles

Measles is a highly infectious, acute viral illness, spread by respiratory droplets. It is characterised by fever, coryza, exudative conjunctivitis, cough and a pathognomonic buccal enanthem called Koplik's spots (white spots on a bright red buccal mucosa), followed 3–4 days later by a rash. The rash is erythematous and blotchy, starting at the hairline and moving down the body, before becoming confluent. It lasts up to a week, and may desquamate in the second week.

The average period from exposure to appearance of the rash is 14 days. The infectious period is from 1 to 2 days before the onset of symptoms to 4 days after the appearance of the rash.

Immunisation to measles using a live attenuated measles vaccine has been well established since the early 1960s, with an uptake rate increasing steadily to over 95% with the introduction of the measles, mumps and rubella (MMR) vaccine in 1988. Vaccination should be actively encouraged, given the potential complications due to measles infection of otitis media (2.5%), bronchopneumonia (4%), acute encephalitis (0.1% of cases, with a mortality rate of 10–15%) and late subacute sclerosing panencephalitis.

MMR may afford some protection if given within 72 hours of exposure to measles to those with doubtful immunity, as immunity from the attenuated vaccine virus is more rapid than that from natural measles. If MMR is contraindicated or if more than 72 hours have elapsed since exposure, normal human immunoglobulin may be given within 7 days of exposure, to prevent or modify disease.

Rubella (German measles)

Rubella is a mild acute infectious disease spread by droplets or direct contact. The incubation period is 14–21 days. Cases are infectious from 5 days before until 7 days after appearance of the rash.

Rubella is characterised by a 2–3-day prodrome of fever, malaise, upper respiratory tract symptoms, and lymphadenopathy, particularly postauricular and occipital. The rash consists of small fine pink maculopapules, starting on the face and spreading to the chest and upper abdomen and thighs, all within 24 hours. However, it is not diagnostic of rubella as a similar rash can be caused by other viruses, including parvovirus and enteroviruses.

The disease itself has rare complications such as encephalitis and thrombocytopenia, but the risk to the unborn fetus of exposure in the first trimester (especially 6–8 weeks' gestation) is significant, resulting in severe developmental and structural damage in 90% of affected cases (congenital rubella syndrome). The vaccine is contraindicated in pregnant women and post-exposure prophylaxis with immunoglobulin does not prevent infection in non-immune contacts, although it may modify the risk of abnormalities to in the fetus.

Erythema infectiosum

'Slapped cheek disease' or erythema infectiosum is caused by parvovirus B19. It is spread by droplets or direct contact, with an incubation period of 4–21 days. It is highly infectious until the rash appears, although 50–60% of adults are already immune. Fever occurs in up to 30% with a non-specific prodrome. The rash initially consists of red, flushed cheeks with circumoral pallor ('slapped cheeks'), followed after 7 days by a maculopapular rash on the limbs and trunk that clears centrally, leaving a lacy (reticular) pattern as it fades. The virus may precipitate a severe aplastic anaemic crisis in individuals with underlying haemolytic disease, such as hereditary spherocytosis, sickle cell anaemia and thalassaemia. It can cause fetal hydrops. Pregnant contacts should be offered serology and specialist review.

Roseola infantum (exanthem subitum, sixth disease)

Roseola infantum is caused by human herpesvirus 6 (HHV-6) or less commonly HHV-7. 95% of children are infected with HHV-6 by the age of 2, although only 30% present with roseola. Transmission is by direct contact or (asymptomatically shed) droplets. Initial presentation is with fever and few if any other symptoms (possibly a febrile convulsion). Fever resolves after 3–5 days, and a pink macular rash erupts over the trunk and arms, which then fades within 1–2 days.

Enterovirus infection

Enterovirus infections may present in a variety of ways, including malaise and fever, often accompanied by a non-specific rash, as occurs in Coxsackie and echovirus. In classical hand-foot-and-mouth disease, due to Coxsackie A16, vesicles occur in a typical distribution over the hands, feet and buttocks, with lesions in the anterior mouth often becoming painful ulcers. The lesions may be petechial, resembling those of meningococcal infection. Infections occur particularly through the summer and autumn and are usually self-limiting. The virus is shed in faeces and saliva for several weeks.

Varicella (chickenpox)

Chickenpox is caused by varicella zoster virus (VZV), which has an incubation period of 10–21 days. Patients are most contagious for 1–2 days before the rash and while new lesions erupt, which can be up to 5 days. It is more severe in adults and can be potentially fatal in immunocompromised patients, with a mortality rate of 7–10% in the latter. The clinical features include a 3–5-day prodrome of fever, irritability and lymphadenopathy. The itchy vesicular rash often begins on the scalp and spreads rapidly to involve the whole body. Cerebellitis, aseptic meningitis, transverse myelitis, thrombocytopenia and pneumonia may complicate the acute infection.

Most adults, including those with no history of chickenpox, are immune to varicella. Staff working in paediatric EDs who have no history of chickenpox should have VZV serology to determine their immune status. Those that spent their childhood in tropical countries are more likely to be non-immune as adults. Any non-immune staff should be vaccinated.

VZV vaccine can provide post-exposure prevention of chickenpox if given within 5 days of exposure. Zoster immune globulin can prevent or attenuate disease if given within 4 days of exposure. It is recommended for immunocompromised children, and for newborn infants exposed whose mothers had chickenpox in the 5 days before or 2 days after delivery.

Papulovesicular acrolocated syndrome (Gianotti–Crosti syndrome)

Papulovesicular acrolocated syndrome (PALS) is an exanthem in which papular (and often vesicular) lesions are located on the face, buttocks, and extensor surface of the extremities with truncal sparing. It is present for 2–4 weeks, though may take up to 4 months to resolve. It has been associated with a number of viral illnesses, including enterovirus, rotavirus, Epstein–Barr virus (EBV), some bacterial infections, and immunisation. More than 90% of patients are <4 years old.

What specimens and when should they be ordered?

Targeted and judicious use of laboratory investigations facilitates more rapid and accurate diagnosis of causes of infection in children presenting to the ED.

Collection of microbiological specimens

It is imperative that microbiological specimens be collected appropriately, taking care not to contaminate samples during collection. Samples should also be transported to the laboratory promptly, stored in appropriate laboratory environments and processed without undue delay.

Blood cultures
Collection

Proper hand washing technique and use of gloves will avoid contamination of the sample. Peripheral blood cultures are usually collected from veins, either direct puncture or immediately aspirated from a cannula after insertion. Arterial samples may also be used, but heel prick samples are inappropriate. It is imperative to disinfect the patient site for blood collection, usually with topical aqueous chlorhexidine or large alcohol swabs and to allow the disinfecting agent to dry, which is an important part of the disinfection process. Swab the rubber bung on the bottle with an alcohol swab and allow drying time before introducing blood into the bottle. Blood for cultures should be collected first, before placing blood into other, non-sterile bottles for additional investigations. Avoiding needle changes to inoculate the culture bottle minimises the risk of an accidental needlestick injury.

Volume of blood and collection media

It is important to remember that a minimum amount of blood must be collected, but also that more than a maximum amount of blood will decrease the sensitivity of the culture and thus the likelihood of identifying a microorganism. The optimum blood-to-culture broth dilution is 1:10 in most blood culture systems, and up to 5 mL of blood can be inoculated into older systems, but from 0.4 mL to 4 mL in newer collection media. Samples for anaerobic bacterial cultures are not routinely collected, with few exceptions:

- febrile neutropenic, immunocompromised patients;
- patients with suspected intra-abdominal or pelvic sepsis;
- neonates with a high risk of anaerobic sepsis, i.e. those with prolonged rupture of membranes, offensive liquor, or maternal fever in labour.

Blood culture bottles should be correctly labelled, and optimally stored in an appropriate incubator (never in a fridge).

Cerebrospinal fluid

See Chapter 8.7, p. 227–228, and also Section 23 (Common procedures).

Urine examination

A sterile urine sample enables a more accurate diagnosis of urinary tract infection (UTI) and as such the method of collection significantly influences the accuracy of the microscopic results obtained. If UTIs are overdiagnosed, other important diagnoses may be missed and the child may be subjected to unnecessary further investigations. A negative urinalysis does not exclude a UTI, and 16% of UTIs may be missed. The presence of white or red blood cells or protein does not either confirm or refute the diagnosis. All urine specimens should be sent for microscopy and culture if a UTI suspected, or if obtained via catheter/suprapubic aspirate in non-toilet-trained children. The laboratory should always be informed of the collection method as this influences the interpretation of results.

Bag urines

Urine collected is usually contaminated, and testing is neither sensitive nor specific.

Clean catch and midstream collection

Are both non-invasive and contamination is less likely, but care must be taken to reduce contamination. The 'best' clean catch possible is obtained from boys with the foreskin retracted, and girls with the labia spread after cleansing with soap and water and gentle drying. The patient or parent should avoid touching skin and the specimen should be collected in midstream.

Suprapubic aspiration

This is the most reliable means of collection of a sterile specimen, but the infant usually needs to have a reasonably full bladder. Bladder scanning/ultrasound improves the yield. The technique is safe.

Catheterisation

Quick 'in-out' urinary catheterisation is a reasonably reliable collection method and does not require the bladder to be filled. However, contamination of the specimen is common. It is very unlikely that infection can be introduced with an in-out procedure that is done with sterile technique. Only mild discomfort is usually experienced. Catheterisation should not be attempted in girls with significant labial adhesion, nor in boys with phimosis that prevents vision of the urethral meatus.

Interpretation

Reagent-impregnated dipstick A dipstick urinalysis can be used to detect the presence of nitrite-forming bacteria or estimate the presence of pyuria using a leucocyte esterase test strip, thereby allowing a quick presumptive diagnosis of a UTI and early treatment in an unwell child. Blood, protein and ketones can also be detected. The poor sensitivity for nitrites (40%) and pyuria (70%), however, means that a high false negative rate (of 50% and 20% respectively) for detection of true infection by this method exists.[14] Non-nitrite-forming bacteria such as *Enterococcus* spp. may also cause

UTIs, and pyuria is not always present in UTIs, which makes a negative urinalysis less likely to exclude a UTI.

Microscopy A urinary white cell count $>10 \times 10^6 \, \text{L}^{-1}$ together with a positive leucocyte esterase is a very sensitive screening test for UTIs, but still has a false negative rate of 15%. The presence of >10 leucocytes mm^{-3} on direct microscopy has been shown to have a low positive predictive value (56%) for UTI but, combined with the presence of bacteria, this constitutes the most accurate screening test in detecting positive urinary cultures.[15]

Culture UTI is ultimately diagnosed on demonstration of significant bacteriuria, which implies counts of $>10^8 \, \text{L}^{-1}$ of a single pathogen in a fresh, uncentrifuged clean catch or midstream urine sample. Any growth on a sample obtained by urinary catheter or suprapubic aspirate is also diagnostic.

Stool specimens

Viral gastroenteritis is the most common cause of paediatric hospital attendance during the spring and early summer months. The organism involved is usually rotavirus, which is usually self-limiting and is readily detected by enzyme-linked immunoassay or latex agglutination. Laboratory analysis is usually not warranted during seasonal endemic periods as most causes of diarrhoea are usually self-limiting and identification will not alter management in most cases. Indications for stool analysis are:

- persistent diarrhoea >7 days;
- blood in stool;
- recent overseas travel, particularly to typhoid endemic areas;
- immunocompromised children.

Collection

Diarrhoeal stool (5–10 g) should be collected in a sterile container with a secure fitting lid. Testing the stool pH using a reagent strip may be a useful indicator for rotavirus gastroenteritis as it causes an acidic stool (pH < 5). Similarly, testing stool for reducing substances may be positive in cases of secondary lactose intolerance.

Throat swab

Throat swabs may be performed both for bacterial and viral culture, although for the latter a nasopharyngeal aspirate or nasal swab is usually more helpful.

Nasopharyngeal aspirate (NPA)

NPA is the preferred method for recovering viruses from the upper respiratory tract. This may be helpful in children with the clinical syndrome of bronchiolitis, both for a specific diagnosis and to facilitate infection control procedures, although testing rarely affects patient management per se. Nasal lavage is an alternative to NPA, but swabs of the nose and throat are generally unsuitable for rapid immunofluorescence. Newer molecular techniques may be performed on nasal swabs.

Interpretation

Most respiratory viruses can be detected by direct immunofluorescence of exfoliated respiratory epithelium, as viral antigens are expressed on the cell surface. If available, this allows rapid diagnosis of infection. Viruses can also be cultured. The positive and negative predictive values of both NPA and nasal lavage in diagnosing respiratory syncytial virus infection are over 90%. *Bordetella pertussis* may be identified by PCR if a definitive diagnosis is required before culture results of NPA are available.

Nasal swab

A nasal swab is the classic method for collection of diagnostic specimens for diagnosis of pertussis. However, a nasopharyngeal aspirate is also satisfactory.

Collection

A small-tipped nasopharyngeal swab is passed into the posterior nasopharynx. Do not use a swab with a cotton tip as this may be inhibitory to the organism. The swab is left in place for at least 30 seconds, if possible.

Infection control in the ED

Adhering to strict universal precautions (i.e. treating all blood and body fluids as potentially infectious) is an integral part of containing the spread of infections in any healthcare setting. Nowhere more so than in paediatric EDs, where communicable viral respiratory and enteric infections are the most common causes of presentations. Cross-infection can be eliminated by strict hand-washing measures by both staff and parents, as well as avoiding toy sharing by patients in ward situations. Prophylaxis with normal or specific human immunoglobulin is sometimes indicated following significant exposure to communicable diseases such as hepatitis A and B, measles and varicella, and antibiotic prophylaxis may be indicated for significant exposure to meningococcal and Hib disease.

Needlestick injury (NSI)

The child presenting with a (community) needlestick injury

The risk of seroconversion to HIV, hepatitis B virus (HBV) or hepatitis C virus from a community acquired NSI is very low. Exposed individuals should be reassured. Immunity to hepatitis B should be confirmed, and if incomplete, hepatitis B vaccine should be given. Unless the injury is considered to be particularly high risk, no further management is required at the time. Follow up should be arranged for counselling and serology if required.

Hospital staff exposure to HBV

In general, NSIs occur more often in the hospital environment, where a lack of universal precautions in handling or discarding contaminated needles and sharps has occurred. It is advisable that all staff working in the hospital environment should be adequately immunised against hepatitis B and that serological confirmation of immunity is performed. If significant exposure (percutaneous, ocular, or mucous membrane) to blood or potentially blood-contaminated secretions has occurred in persons who are unimmunised, testing of the source should be done as well as of the recipient. A single dose of hepatitis B immunoglobulin (HBIG 400 IU for adults and 100 IU for children) is then offered to the recipient if HBsAb-negative, or if the source is HBsAg positive or cannot be identified. This should be given within 72 hours after exposure.

Immunisation

Immunisation of staff

It is in the best interests of all healthcare workers, and their patients, that staff in paediatric centres have a serologically proven immunisation record against communicable illnesses such as measles, mumps and rubella, varicella and HBV, and receive the relevant immunisation as appropriate. Pertussis-containing booster and annual influenza vaccine should also be given.

Opportunistic immunisation

The ED visit also presents an invaluable opportunity to monitor the immunisation status of children and offer 'catch-up' immunisation to those who have missed vaccinations, or commence the appropriate vaccination schedule. The current immunisation schedule is available in the Australian Immunisation Handbook.[20]

Acknowledgement

The contribution of Neil Smith as author in the first edition is hereby acknowledged.

References

1. Browne G, Currow K, Rainbow J. Practical approach to the febrile child in the emergency department. *Emerg Med* 2001;**13**:426–35.
2. Acworth J, Babl F, Borland M, et al. Patterns of presentation to the Australian and New Zealand Paediatric Emergency Research Network. *Emerg Med Austral* 2009;**21**:59–66.
3. El-Radhi A, Barry W. Thermometry in paediatric practice. *Arch Dis Child* 2006;**91**:351–6.
4. Ten C, Ng C, Nik-Sherina H, et al. The accuracy of Mother's touch to detect fever in children: A systematic review. *J Trop Pediatr* 2007;**54**:70–3.
5. Meremikwu M, Oyo-Ita A. Paracetamol for treating fever in children. *Cochrane Database Syst Rev* 2002;(2): CD003676 (2002).
6. Kramer M, Naimark L, Roberts-Brauer R, et al. Risks and benefits of paracetamol antipyresis in young children with fever of presumed viral origin. *Lancet* 1991;**337** (8741):591–4.
7. Russell F, Shann F, Curtis N, Mulholland K. Evidence on the use of paracetamol in febrile children. *Bull World Health Organ* 2003;**81**(5):367–72.
8. Riordan M, Rylance G, Berry K. Poisoning in children 2: painkillers. *Arch Dis Child* 2002;**87**(5):397–9.
9. Lesko S, O'Brien K, Schwartz B, et al. Invasive group A streptococcal infection and nonsteroidal antiinflammatory drug use among children with primary varicella. *Pediatrics* 2001;**107**(5): 1108–15.
10. Carstairs K, Tanen D, Johnson A, et al. Pneumococcal bacteremia in febrile infants presenting to the emergency department before and after the introduction of the heptavalent pneumococcal vaccine. *Ann Emerg Med* 2007;**49**:772–7.

11. Antonyrajah B, Mukundan D. Fever without apparent source on clinical examination. *Curr Opin Pediatr* 2008;**20**:96–102.
12. Hewson P, Humphries S, Roberton D, et al. Markers of serious illness in infants under 6 months old presenting to a children's hospital. *Arch Dis Child* 1990;**65**:750–6.
13. Baraff LJ. Management of infants and young children with fever without source. *Pediatr Ann* 2008;**37**:673–9.
14. Hoberman A, Wald E, Reynolds E, et al. Is urine culture necessary to rule out urinary tract infection in young febrile children? *Pediatr Infect Dis J* 1996;**15**:304–9.
15. Craig J, Irwig L, Knight J, et al. Symptomatic urinary tract infection in preschool Australian children. *J Paediatr Child Health* 1998;**34**:154–9.
16. Burns J, Glode M. Kawasaki syndrome. *Lancet* 2004;**364**:533–44.
17. Negrini B, Kelleher K, Wald E. Cerebrospinal fluid findings in aseptic versus bacterial meningitis. *Pediatrics* 2000;**105**:316–9.
18. Mazor S, McNulty J, Roosevelt G. Interpretation of traumatic lumbar punctures: who can go home? *Pediatrics* 2003;**111**:525–8.
19. Shah K, Richard K, Nicholas S, Edlow J. Incidence of traumatic lumbar puncture. *Acad Emerg Med* 2003;**10**:151–4.
20. *National Immunisation Program Schedule.* Available from: http://immunise.health.gov.au/internet/immunise/publishing.nsf/Content/nips2 [accessed 19.10.10].

10.1 Metabolic emergencies

Drago Bratkovic • Peter Francis

ESSENTIALS

1 Inborn errors of metabolism are individually rare but as a group are not uncommon.

2 The possibility of an inborn error of metabolism needs to be considered in any child with unexplained hypoglycaemia, acidosis, altered conscious state, neurological presentation or vomiting.

3 Prompt recognition is important to allow appropriate therapy and to avoid further decompensation.

4 Precise identification of the defect in the ED is not generally important as long as appropriate initial therapy is commenced and this usually consists of dextrose.

Introduction

Inborn errors of metabolism are a diverse group of disorders that result from a defect or absence of an enzyme or transport system. The presenting symptoms and signs are equally diverse; however, there are a number of common features that can alert the clinician to their presence. This chapter will concentrate on those metabolic conditions that present acutely to the emergency department (ED), but will also touch on those with more chronic presentations which could easily go unrecognised.

The majority of patients presenting with acute metabolic conditions to the emergency department will have already been diagnosed, particularly given the advent of extended newborn screening (see end of chapter). However, not all conditions can be screened for and some can be missed by screening, thus children and, indeed, adults can still present acutely with an undiagnosed metabolic condition.

Physiology and pathogenesis

The process by which living matter is built up (anabolism) or broken down (catabolism) is termed metabolism. Strictly speaking, an inborn error of metabolism (IEM) is an inherited defect in a metabolic pathway or enzyme. Generally, there is a defect in an enzyme that catalyses the conversion of one organic compound to another. However, not all defects in metabolic pathways give rise to pathology. Figure 10.1.1 shows that compound A is converted to B. If the enzyme that catalyses the reaction is not present or is functioning poorly, this can affect the body in any one of the following ways.

❶ There is accumulation of A, which is toxic – example: phenylketonuria.

❷ There is a deficiency of B, which results in cellular dysfunction – example: Smith–Lemli–Opitz syndrome, a disorder of cholesterol biosynthesis.

❸ Excess A is converted to C via an alternate pathway which is toxic – example: tyrosinaemia type 1.

❹ Excess A results in accumulation of metabolite E earlier in the pathway, which is toxic – example: maple syrup urine disease.

❺ Excess A is excreted by reacting/conjugating with D, which results in deficiency of D – example: carnitine deficiency in fatty acid oxidation defects.

The pathology seen in an IEM can result from any of the processes outlined in Figure 10.1.1, but in fact most IEM are the result of more than one mechanism. Genetic defects can also occur in the support processes of metabolic pathways such as transport proteins, enzyme chaperones and enzyme complex assembly proteins, which result in the block of a metabolic process and thus pathology.

Clinical features

The clinical features and presentations of IEM are many and varied due to the diverse nature of the enzymes and processes affected; however, Table 10.1.1 shows that there are a number of common features that should alert the clinician to the possibility of an IEM.

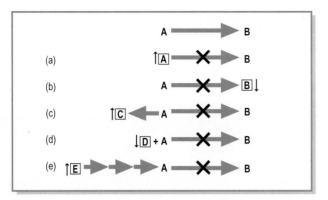

Fig. 10.1.1 Pathogenic mechanisms in IEM; refer to text for a full explanation.

Table 10.1.1 Groups of IEM that present to the ED and their common presenting features	
IEM group	**Common presenting features**
Glycogen storage disorders,e.g. GSD III, IV, VI, VII and IX	Hypoglycaemia, rhabdomyolysis, cardiomyopathy, hepatomegaly
Aminoacidopathies and organic acidaemia, e.g. maple syrup urine disease (MSUD)	Vomiting, acidosis, encephalopathy
Urea cycle defects, e.g. ornithine transcarbamylase deficiency (OTC)	Vomiting, encephalopathy, hyperammonaemia, respiratory alkalosis
Disorders of gluconeogenesis, e.g. glycogen storage disease type I	Lactic acidosis and hypoglycaemia
Fatty acid oxidation defects,e.g. medium chain acyl-CoA dehydrogenase deficiency (MCAD)	Hypoketotic hypoglycaemia, encephalopathy and rhabdomyolysis
Mitochondrial respiratory chain defects, e.g. Leigh disease, MELAS	Lactic acidosis, seizures, stroke-like events
Disorders of ketone production and utilisation, e.g. ketolytic defect	Severe ketoacidosis, hypoglycaemia

Table 10.1.2 can be used as a guide to identifying an IEM in the ED:

An IEM should be considered if there is both a clinical and a biochemical feature from each of the lists; however, considering an IEM should never take the place of the work up and treatment for more common causes of the above presentations, the most important being sepsis.

IEM are broken down into a number of groups of conditions, all of which affect a common metabolic pathway. The groups of IEM that are likely to present to the ED are outlined in Table 10.1.1, including the common presenting features of each.

Investigation

The metabolic markers of many IEM are present only at the time of presentation and may disappear with treatment. Thus, the timing of investigations is extremely important; if done incorrectly they could result in an incorrect or no diagnosis, with risky provocation testing, such as fasting or loading studies being the only option.

The following investigations are a good starting point when considering an IEM. They are all standard laboratory investigations

Table 10.1.2 Guide to identifying an IEM in the ED	
Clinical features	**Biochemical features**
Overwhelming illness in the neonatal period	Acute acidosis (with raised anion gap)
Recurrent vomiting	Hypoglycaemia
Coma or encephalopathy	Lactic acidosis (normal perfusion)
Apnoea and/or seizures	Ketoacidosis
Failure to thrive or malnutrition	Acute hepatic dysfunction
Presence of an unusual odour	Coagulopathy
Not responding to usual treatment	
Unusual odour	
FH of neonatal or infant death, SIDS or acute life threatening event (ALTE)	

with rapid turn-around times and are thus likely to be available to the physician in the emergency department.

Blood   acid–base, ammonia, urea, creatinine, electrolytes, liver function tests, laboratory glucose, lactate and calculated anion gap ($[Na + K] - [Cl + HCO_3]$).

Urine   ketone dipstick (will only detect acetoacetate).

In *all* cases of hypoglycaemia the following additional investigations are recommended and need to be collected *before* the hypoglycaemia is treated. Most tertiary paediatric emergency departments will have a hypoglycaemia investigation kit for use in this situation.

Blood   insulin, cortisol, growth hormone, adrenocorticotropic hormone (ACTH), free fatty acids (FFA), ketones (beta-hydroxy-butyrate and acetoacetate), acylcarnitine profile (collect a newborn screening card; NBS or Guthrie card).

Urine   organic and amino acids.

Once the results of the initial investigations are available, a possible diagnosis and further investigations may be suggested, depending on the profile (Table 10.1.3 and Figure 10.1.2). However, if this not helpful, all of the following second line investigations should be performed:

Blood   plasma amino acids, plasma ketones, acylcarnitine profile, creatine kinase, urate.

Urine   organic and amino acids.

Many of these investigations can take days for a result, and it is suggested that all suspected metabolic cases be discussed with a metabolic physician, so a treatment plan can be developed to keep the child stable while awaiting further results. The single most useful investigation in the suspected IEM work up is the urine organic and amino acids, which in some centres is referred to as the 'metabolic urine screen'. This can be performed even on a small non-sterile urine sample; however, for technical reasons most laboratories will not perform the test if there is faecal contamination.

Table 10.1.3 Biochemical profiles of the different IEM

Metabolic acidosis	Lactate	Ketones	NH₃	AST/AST	BSL	Defect/disorder	Further investigations
+ to +++	↑ to ↑↑↑	N to ↑↑	(↑)	N to ↑↑	N or ↓	Mitochondrial respiratory chain disorder	UO&AA, pre- and post-prandial lactate
+ to +++	N or ↑	↑↑	↑ to ↑↑	N or ↑	N or ↓	Organic aciduria	Plasma AA, UO&AA, ACP
++ to +++	N	↑↑↑	N	N	↓ or N	Ketolytic defect	Plasma ketones, UO&AA, ACP
+ to ++	↑ to ↑↑	N	N	N to ↑↑	↓↓↓	GSD I	Urate, triglycerides, cholesterol
+	N	↑ to ↑↑	N	N to ↑↑	↓↓↓	GSD III	CK, triglycerides, cholesterol
– to ++	N to ↑↑	N or ↑	(↑)	(↑↑)	↓↓↓	Fatty acid oxidation	UO&AA, ACP, CK
(+) OR alkalosis	N	N	↑↑↑	N or ↑	N	Urea cycle defect	Plasma AA
– to +	N	↑↑	N	N	N	MSUD	Plasma AA
(+)	N or ↑	N or ↑	N	↑↑↑	N or ↓	Galactosaemia, tyrosinaemia type 1	UO&AA, urine reducing substances

– = absent, + = present, ( ) = sometimes, N = normal, ↑ = elevated, ↓ = decreased
BSL = blood sugar level, GSD = glycogen storage disease, MSUD = maple syrup urine disease,
Plasma AA = plasma amino acids, UO&AA = urine organic and amino acids, ACP = acylcarnatine profile, CK = creatine kinase.

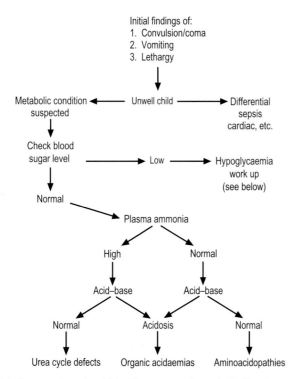

Fig. 10.1.2 Clinical approach to the child with a suspected metabolic disorder.

Management

The management of a child suspected of having an acute presentation of an IEM has three primary goals:

❶ Correction of altered homeostasis.
❷ Reduction of toxic compound production.
❸ Removal or enhancement of excretion of toxic compounds.

Correction of altered homeostasis

Hypoglycaemia and metabolic acidosis are the two most common biochemical abnormalities seen in IEM.

Hypoglycaemia should always be corrected immediately with an initial infusion of 5 mL kg^{-1} of 10% dextrose. This should be followed with an infusion of 10% dextrose at maintenance rates, equating to 5–6 mg kg^{-1} min^{-1} of glucose, and will be enough to meet basal endogenous glucose needs, however, to suppress catabolism higher rates of up to 10 mg kg^{-1} min^{-1} of glucose may be required. The requirement of infusion rates of dextrose higher than this suggests hyperinsulinism.

Persistent metabolic or lactic acidosis can be problematic; however, the management strategies outlined later in this section will help reduce acidosis as the patient recovers; occasionally sodium bicarbonate may be required; however, the effect of the associated sodium load needs to be considered and may make other clinical problems such a cerebral oedema worse.

Reduction of toxic compound production

This is generally achieved through dietary means and varies with the metabolic condition. A feature common to all dietary interventions in the acutely unwell patient with an IEM is the provision of increased calories. Many of the IEM are in catabolic pathways, and thus measures that help suppress catabolism, such as increased caloric intake, help reduce the production of toxic compounds.

The source of calories will vary depending on the condition (carbohydrate vs. fat vs. protein); however, in the acute emergency setting, extra calories from glucose are considered safe and preferable in the majority of IEM. However, protein-containing calories, which include all regular infant formulas, should be avoided in the undiagnosed IEM patient, given that most children presenting acutely with IEM are in pathways of amino acid degradation. Fat sources such as MCT oil or intralipid are a dense source of calories; however, they should only be used when a fatty acid oxidation disorder has been excluded.

Thus in the suspected IEM, dextrose at a high rate of between 5 and 10 mg kg^{-1} min^{-1} is the safest and best option while awaiting results and discussion with a metabolic clinician.

Removal/enhancement of excretion of toxic compounds

There are a number of pathways through which toxic metabolites are removed from the body in IEM. Renal excretion, usually conjugated to carnitine is a common pathway, but in some conditions there is no excretory pathway and the only treatment option is haemofiltration or dialysis. This is particularly the case in organic acidaemias such a maple syrup urine disease in order to remove the neurotoxic amino acid, leucine, and in the urea cycle disorders to help remove ammonia.

In the acute presentation of IEM, prompt institution of appropriate management is essential to achieve a good outcome for the patient; previously diagnosed patients should have a care plan for acute presentations, and in some centres pre-made supplements and formulas available for use. Thus, patients with a known IEM should always be seen promptly (ATS 2) and those with a suspected IEM should be discussed with a metabolic physician when the suspicion is first raised.

Chronic presentations

There are a number of IEM that do not present with acute symptoms, but in a progressive degenerative manner, frequently multisystemic. The early symptoms and signs in these conditions can be common presentations or incidental findings in the ED (Table 10.1.4). Appreciation of their significance can allow for early diagnosis and in a growing number of conditions an improved outcome for the patient, through innovative new therapies such as enzyme replacement therapy (ERT) and, in the future, gene and stem cell therapy.

Extended newborn screening

Many newborn screening programmes throughout the world now use a technique known as tandem mass spectrometry or MS/MS to screen for a large number of IEM from the one blood spot. The conditions screened vary between programs but generally cover most of the organic acidaemias, aminoacidopathies and fatty acid oxidation defects. The conditions a local program screens for affect the types of IEM that present both diagnosed and undiagnosed to the ED, remembering that these are population based screening tests and inevitably miss the occasional case.

Conclusion

The child with a metabolic condition may present in a variety of ways to an ED and the diagnosis should be considered in all children with an unexplained serious illness. There should be a low threshold for performing blood glucose in the young and initial investigations and management should be instituted expeditiously.

Table 10.1.4 Chronic presenting signs in IEM, the associated condition and appropriate investigation

Sign	Disorder(s)	Test
Recurrent abdominal hernia, especially umbilical	MPS, oligosaccharidoses	Urine MPS screen Oligosaccharides
Spinal deformity in infant or toddler	MPS, oligosaccharidoses	Urine MPS screen Oligosaccharides
Recurrent otitis media	MPS, oligosaccharidoses	Urine MPS screen Oligosaccharides
Persistent nasal discharge	MPS, oligosaccharidoses	Urine MPS screen Oligosaccharides
Recurrent pain attacks, particularly with fevers	Fabry disease	Lysosomal enzymes
Recurrent or bilateral avascular necrosis of the femoral head	Gaucher disease	Lysosomal enzymes
Hepatospelenomegaly	Any lysosomal storage disorder including MPS	Lysosomal enzymes Urine MPS screen
Interstitial lung disease	Niemann-Pick disease	Lysosomal enzymes

MPS = mucopolysaccharidoses.

10.2 Diabetic emergencies in children

Kam Sinn

> **ESSENTIALS**
>
> **1** Diabetes mellitus is one of the most common chronic diseases in childhood.
>
> **2** The incidence of childhood diabetes has been increasing over the last decade.
>
> **3** Diabetic ketoacidosis is defined as BGL >11 mmol L^{-1}, pH < 7.3 and bicarbonate <15 mmol L^{-1}.
>
> **4** As obesity becomes more prevalent in childhood, type II diabetes has started to present in younger and younger adolescents.
>
> **5** Type I diabetes remains the major ($>90\%$) cause of childhood diabetes.

Diagnosis

The classic symptoms of polyuria, polydipsia and weight loss may be present for a few weeks before parental concern is raised.

The diagnosis should be confirmed by a random blood glucose level (BGL >11 mmol L^{-1}) in addition to urine analysis for glucose and ketone.

Once the diagnosis is confirmed, initial management is dictated by the severity of dehydration, presence of shock, degree of acidosis, hyperglycaemia and osmolality.

In a child with no past history of diabetes the initial diagnosis may be misled by non-specific symptoms such as abdominal pain, weight loss, drowsiness, fever, secondary enuresis and dyspnoea. Beware of tachypnoea due to metabolic acidosis, intercurrent infection in a new diabetic, abdominal pain related to diabetic ketoacidosis (DKA) and drowsiness in a child. In such children, diabetes should be excluded as a possible cause with a random blood glucose.

Diabetic ketoacidosis

Diabetic ketoacidosis is the major cause of mortality in diabetic children. It often presents in newly diagnosed type I diabetic children. In established diabetics, it occasionally presents in the midst of intercurrent febrile illness or poor adherence to management.

Diabetic ketoacidosis is caused by insulin deficiency, leading to hyperglycaemia, osmotic diuresis, hyperosmolar dehydration, lipolysis, ketosis and acidosis. It may be defined by the combination of:

- hyperglycaemia;
- ketosis and ketonuria;
- acidosis (pH < 7.3, bicarbonate <15);
- dehydration and/or shock.

Management starts with rapid assessment, resuscitation and meticulous replacement of fluid, electrolyte and insulin infusion.

Like all medical emergencies, assessment of airway, breathing and circulation (ABC) is vital. Ketotic breath, degree of tachypnoea and respiratory distress should be noted. Degree of shock or dehydration should be assessed. Initial level of consciousness should be noted, and hourly neurological observation commenced. It is also important to look for a focus of infection and sepsis.

Initial investigations should include venous blood glucose, electrolytes, urea, creatinine, full blood count, venous or arterial blood gases. In addition, if sepsis is suspected, blood culture, urine culture and chest X-ray may be considered.

Resuscitation

Intravenous access should be established; ideally with two intravenous (IV) cannulae so that further venous sampling of BGL and electrolyte may be undertaken easily.

In children with shock, noted to be hypotensive and poorly perfused, resuscitation should start immediately with facial mask oxygen and intravenous fluid bolus. Normal saline (0.9% Na Cl) 10 mL kg^{-1} should be given as a bolus. The normal saline bolus (10 mL kg^{-1}) should be repeated if the child remains shocked upon reassessment in 10 minutes.

Careful and frequent monitoring should continue for the next 24–48 hours. Monitoring should include all vital signs, including neurological assessment, urine output and ECG monitoring.

Fluid

After the initial resuscitation, IV fluid consisting of maintenance fluid and deficit replacement should be calculated and replaced over 48 hours. The child's degree of dehydration should be assessed clinically, including an accurate weight.

The calculation of maintenance fluid is based on the child's weight or surface area.

Dehydration in the form of deficit in percentage of body weight would allow calculation of an estimated volume to be replaced over the next 48 hours. Maintenance and deficit replacement should be given as normal saline (0.9% Na Cl) until the BGL falls to 12–15 mmol L^{-1}. Once the BGL falls to 12–15 mmol L^{-1}, the IV fluid should be changed to half normal saline with glucose 5% (0.45% Na Cl with 5% glucose).

Beware of giving deficit replacement too rapidly, which decreases intravascular osmolality and may contribute towards cerebral oedema.

Insulin

Insulin infusion should only be started after shock has been resuscitated with normal saline intravenously as above. The BGL would fall rapidly during the resuscitation phase with fluid replacement alone.

Insulin infusion with short-acting insulin (soluble or regular) should be started with maintenance IV fluid. An initial bolus of insulin is not recommended, as it may reduce the BGL and osmolality too rapidly. The infusion is made up by diluting soluble or regular insulin in normal saline to a concentration of 1 U mL^{-1}, to be given in an electronic

IV syringe pump. The infusion is started at a rate of 0.05–0.1 U insulin kg^{-1} hr^{-1}. The insulin infusion rate can be titrated to achieve a fall in BGL of 4–5 mmol hr^{-1}.

Once the BGL falls to the normal range (5–10 mmol L^{-1}), the insulin infusion should continue until the child is ready to change over to subcutaneous insulin. As DKA is caused by Type I diabetes, the insulin infusion should not be stopped or decreased in rate of infusion below 0.05 U kg^{-1} hr^{-1} until subcutaneous insulin can be started, despite a normal BGL. Insulin is required to suppress lipolysis and clear ketosis. If there is a concern about hypoglycaemia, the glucose concentration in the maintenance IV fluid can be increased from 5% up to 10%.

The change over from IV insulin to subcutaneous insulin is often most conveniently performed at mealtime, when the child is no longer acidotic, is alert and able to tolerate an oral meal. At such time, rapid- or short-acting insulin can be given subcutaneously before a meal; the insulin infusion should continue during the meal and then cease 30 minutes after the meal.

Potassium

The initial serum potassium may be high, normal or low, despite a low total body potassium. Potassium replacement should be given intravenously once resuscitation is completed and there are no ECG changes of hyperkalaemia, anuria or severe renal impairment.

The measured serum potassium goes up by 0.6 mmol L^{-1} for every 0.1 drop in pH. As the acidosis gets corrected with fluid resuscitation and insulin, serum potassium will drop rapidly in exchange for H^{+} ions.

The potassium requirement may be as high as 4–5 mmol kg^{-1} day^{-1} in the first 24 hours. Initially, potassium chloride 40 mmol is usually added to each litre of normal saline for replacement. It is important that serum electrolyte is checked frequently every 2 to 4 hours in the first 12 to 24 hours of DKA management.

Sodium

Serum sodium is a major determinant of osmolality. Rapid change and fall in serum sodium should be avoided to minimise the risk of cerebral oedema. The measured sodium is initially affected by hyperglycaemia.

The corrected sodium can be calculated by:

$$corrected\ Na = measured\ Na + (BGL/3)$$

If there is hypernatraemia with a corrected serum sodium >150 mmol L^{-1}, rate of rehydration should be slowed down further to 72 hours, to minimise rapid changes in osmolality and fluid shift.

Bicarbonate

Bicarbonate is not indicated despite metabolic acidosis. Bicarbonate may increase central nervous system acidosis and worsen hypokalaemia and hypernatraemia. Blood gas should be repeated at frequent intervals if the initial pH is below 7.1.

Phosphate

Serum phosphate is often low initially. It is controversial whether replacement of phosphate makes any difference to outcome.

Complications

Approximately 0.5% children develop cerebral oedema as a complication of DKA. The warning signs are changes in level of consciousness, irritability, headache, cranial nerve palsies and seizures. Treatment includes slowing the rehydration infusion, IV mannitol, intubation and assisted ventilation.

Careful and close observation of vital signs, frequent review of clinical status and laboratory values of BGL, electrolytes, and acid–base status are vital in the first 24–48 hours of DKA to minimise complications.

Hypoglycaemia and hypokalaemia can be minimised by frequent monitoring of BGL and electrolytes, followed by the adjustment of rehydration fluid and insulin infusions.

Hypoglycaemia

Hypoglycaemia is a common complication in all diabetics. Education and ongoing support for the diabetic child and his/her family is the key to preventing and managing hypoglycaemia when it does occur.

Hypoglycaemia can be caused by insulin excess (e.g. 'honeymoon period'), overdose of oral hypoglycaemic (in type II diabetes), intercurrent illness (e.g. gastroenteritis), vigorous exercise and other metabolic/endocrine disorders (e.g. Addison's disease).

Hypoglycaemia is often defined as a BGL <2.5 mmol L^{-1}. However, symptoms of hypoglycaemia may appear with a BGL <4.0 mmol L^{-1} in a diabetic. Therefore, the level of BGL in a child with diabetes should be maintained above 4 mmol L^{-1}.

Hypoglycaemia may cause symptoms related to neuroglycopenia and autonomic activation.

In mild to moderate cases, where the patient remains conscious, treatments include ingestion of rapidly absorbed simple carbohydrate such as sugar or fruit juice, followed by more complex carbohydrate and medical review of the cause of the hypoglycaemia.

In severe hypoglycaemia, the patient may present with seizure or coma. Treatment includes stabilisation of airway, breathing and circulation.

- If IV access is available, 2–5 mL kg^{-1} of glucose 10% can be given as an IV bolus.
- If IV access is not available; intramuscular or deep subcutaneous infusion glucagon should be given.

The dose of glucagons is 0.5 U (0.5 mg) for children up to 8 years of age and 1 U (1 mg) for older children and adolescents.

In the recovery phase of severe hypoglycaemia, close monitoring of BGL, medical review of insulin dosage, diabetic control, IV infusion of glucose-containing crystalloid solution and/or additional oral complex carbohydrate would be required.

In all children with diabetes, education for the parents, patient, teachers and other carers on symptoms and management of hypoglycaemia, sick-day management, and the availability and use of glucagons are vital.

Some form of wearable identification (e.g. Medic-Alert bracelet) for the child would also help in the management of hypoglycaemic coma.

Long-term management

The key to good long-term management of children with diabetes is a team and holistic approach to education for the affected child and his/her parents.

Regular medical review of insulin dosage, diet, exercise, medium-term control and complications should be undertaken with a paediatrician, diabetic educator and dietician. It is beyond the scope of this chapter to deal with the details of long-term management of childhood diabetes.

Further reading

Australasian Paediatric Endocrine Group for the Department of Health and Ageing. *Clinical practice guidelines: Type 1 diabetes in children and adolescents.* Available from http://www.chw.edu.au/prof/services/endocrinology/apeg/apeg_handbook_final.pdf; 2005 [accessed 19.10.10].

National Collaborating Centre for Women's and Children's Health. *Type 1 diabetes diagnosis and management of type 1 diabetes in children and young people.* Available from http://www.nice.org.uk/nicemedia/live/10944/29394/29394.pdf; 2004 [accessed 19.10.10].

10.3 Thyroid emergencies

Malcolm Higgins

ESSENTIALS

1 Life-threatening paediatric thyroid emergencies are rare.

2 Children with undiagnosed thyrotoxicosis or hypothyroidism may present to the ED with a range of acute symptoms and signs.

3 The identification, appropriate management and referral of children with congenital hypothyroidism is important as this condition may cause severe neurological impairment if untreated.

4 The onset of clinical hypothyroidism in Hashimoto's thyroiditis may occur in adolescents.

Thyrotoxicosis

Hyperthyroidism is generally a disease of adult women but occasionally may present in adolescents. Although there are a number of causes the most common is Graves' disease, which is thought to have an autoimmune basis. In approximately 1–2% of cases the presentation of hyperthyroidism is acute and severe. This has been called the 'thyroid storm' and is potentially life threatening. Other causes of hyperthyroidism in children include thyroiditis, iodine-induced hyperthyroidism, thyroid-stimulating hormone (TSH) hypersecretion, excessive ingestion of thyroid hormone and thyroid neoplasms. Hyperthyroidism is one of several endocrinopathies associated with McCune–Albright syndrome.

Clinical features

Raised levels of circulating thyroid hormone have predictable clinical effects depending on the organ system and are similar to the symptoms and signs of catecholamine excess (see Table 10.3.1). The onset of symptoms in Graves' disease is usually insidious and variable in severity between patients. Severe ophthalmopathy or dermopathy is rare in children. Most patients with Graves' disease will have a goitre characterised by diffuse, non-tender and symmetrical enlargement of the thyroid gland.

The clinical presentation of thyroid storm is of abrupt onset of high fever and marked tachycardia and hypertension, with exaggerated features of hyperthyroidism (Table 10.3.1). Altered mental state is invariably present and may progress to seizures and coma.

Diagnosis

In most cases, low TSH with raised free T_4 and T_3 will be diagnostic of hyperthyroidism. Other investigations such as thyroid autoantibodies and radionuclear scans are not usually part of the emergency department (ED) assessment.

Thyroid storm is a clinical diagnosis and treatment should not be withheld while waiting for laboratory results.

Treatment

Further investigation and management of hyperthyroidism in children and adolescents will optimally occur following referral to a paediatric endocrinologist or general paediatrician. Therapy will depend on the cause but may include antithyroid drugs. β-Blockers are useful for initial control of symptoms, particularly in thyroid storm.

Thyroid storm is a medical emergency. Attention to airway, breathing and circulation are the initial priorities. Although antithyroid medications such as propylthiouracil (5–7 mg kg^{-1} day^{-1} in three divided doses given orally) or carbimazole (0.2 mg kg^{-1} $dose^{-1}$ in three divided doses, given orally) may be indicated, control of symptoms may be delayed. In patients with cardiac manifestations, propranolol (2–4 mg kg^{-1} day^{-1} in two divided doses given orally) should be considered.

Table 10.3.1 Signs and symptoms of thyrotoxicosis

Symptoms
- Nervousness/irritability
- Heat intolerance and increased sweating
- Weight loss
- Behaviour problems and poor school performance
- Fatigue
- Restless sleep/insomnia
- Palpitations
- Diarrhoea
- Menstrual irregularities

Signs
- Tachycardia, hypertension
- Thyroid enlargement with bruit or thrill
- Tremor
- Warm, moist skin
- Muscle weakness
- Eyelid lag and retraction
- Brisk tendon reflexes
- Growth acceleration

Neonatal thyrotoxicosis

This rare condition is usually due to the transplacental transfer of thyroid-stimulating antibodies from a mother with autoimmune hyperthyroidism. Importantly, antibody levels sufficient to cause neonatal thyrotoxicosis may not cause clinical hyperthyroidism in the mother.

The infant may develop clinical features of hyperthyroidism. Poor weight gain, cardiac dysfunction and hepatosplenomegaly may also be present. Cardiac failure and airway compression from the goitre may occur. Onset of symptoms may be delayed if the mother is on antithyroid medication. Although symptoms usually resolve spontaneously, this condition is associated with significant morbidity and mortality.

Hypothyroidism

Insufficient thyroid hormone leads to slowing of bodily functions and can impair the function of many organ systems. The most important causes in the paediatric patient are congenital hypothyroidism and autoimmune (Hashimoto's) thyroiditis.

Congenital hypothyroidism

Inadequate thyroid hormone production in newborn infants can occur from anatomic defects of the thyroid, an inborn error of thyroid metabolism, or from maternal iodine deficiency. Thyroid hormone is vitally important to brain growth and development. Profound mental retardation is the most serious effect of untreated congenital hypothyroidism.

Fortunately, the majority of infants with congenital hypothyroidism are diagnosed soon after birth via the newborn screening program. A small number of cases will be missed and present for medical attention because of symptoms of hypothyroidism. Suggestive symptoms and signs are listed in Table 10.3.2.

Table 10.3.2 Symptoms and signs of congenital hypothyroidism
• Poor feeding, growth and development • Constipation • Umbilical hernia, enlarged fontanelle • Enlarged, protruding tongue • Prolonged neonatal jaundice • Hypotonia • Hoarse cry • Bradycardia, cool extremities

Diagnosis of congenital hypothyroidism is confirmed by demonstrating decreased levels of serum thyroid hormone (total or free T_4) and elevated levels of TSH. Urgent referral for further investigation and initiation of therapy is important.

Hashimoto's thyroiditis

Autoimmune thyroiditis is generally a condition of adult women. Adolescents may be affected. The clinical features are of insidious onset (Table 10.3.3). Diagnosis is confirmed with a TSH assay supplemented by thyroid hormone levels, thyroid autoantibodies and a thyroid scan. Referral to an appropriate specialist is highly recommended.

Table 10.3.3 Symptoms and signs of Hashimoto's thyroiditis
• Weakness and lethargy • Weight gain • Cold intolerance • Constipation • Depression, emotional lability and personality changes • Forgetfulness and poor concentration • Hoarse/husky voice • Goitre • Menorrhagia and menstrual irregularity • Bradycardia • Hypothermia • Delayed relaxation of deep tendon reflexes

10.4 Adrenal crisis

Yuresh Naidoo

ESSENTIALS

1 The prompt recognition of the possibility of adrenal crisis or the risk of adrenal insufficiency is paramount to early and appropriate management.

2 Adrenal crisis should be considered as a possible contributor in any child with acute severe cardiovascular collapse.

3 In children, the majority of cases are due to primary adrenal failure, with congenital adrenal hyperplasia the most common cause.

4 A crisis can be precipitated in a child with known adrenal insufficiency who develops an intercurrent illness or other physiological stress.

5 Signs of glucocorticoid deficiency include hypoglycaemia, hypotension (absolute and postural) and refractory shock.

6 Signs of mineralocorticoid deficiency include dehydration (often out of proportion to estimated fluid losses), hyperkalaemia, hyponatraemia, acidosis, and pre-renal failure.

7 Patients are at risk of hypoglycaemia.

8 The management of adrenal crisis involves immediate fluid resuscitation, replacement of corticosteroid and treating hypoglycaemia.

9 The differential diagnosis of a collapsed neonate (particularly male) in the first 14 days includes adrenal insufficiency.

10 Prevention of adrenal crisis in susceptible children may be possible by following a predetermined action plan during intercurrent illnesses.

Introduction

Adrenal crisis is a life-threatening emergency caused by acute insufficiency of the adrenal hormones cortisol and aldosterone. This can occur in situations of stress where the adrenal gland would normally respond by an increase in glucocorticoid secretion. A crisis can be precipitated in a child with known adrenal insufficiency, who develops an inter-current illness or other physiological stress (e.g. burns, surgery, trauma, and sepsis). In this situation, the increased cortisol requirements of the stress or the altered oral intake of normal replacement therapy results in a relative insufficiency and rapid clinical deterioration. Alternatively, the emergency department (ED) visit may represent a new presentation of adrenal insufficiency in a child previously unrecognised to have the subtle, often non-specific

symptoms of lack of adrenal hormones or a child who is at risk due to suppression by prolonged steroid therapy. The prompt recognition of the possibility of adrenal crisis or the risk of adrenal insufficiency is paramount to early and appropriate management. These children are at risk of hypoglycaemia and this needs to be anticipated and managed accordingly.

Adrenal insufficiency can be primary, due to a failure of secretion of the adrenal cortex, or secondary to hypothalamic or pituitary dysfunction. In children, the majority of cases are due to primary adrenal failure, with congenital adrenal hyperplasia the most common cause. The incidence of neonatal congenital adrenal hyperplasia in Australia is estimated at 5.9 cases per 100 000 births.

❶ *Primary* causes include:
- congenital adrenal hyperplasia;
- Addison's disease (autoimmune);
- adrenal aplasia/hypoplasia;
- adrenal infarction secondary to haemorrhage/sepsis;
- other – trauma, tumour, post-surgical.

❷ *Secondary* causes include:
- central nervous system (CNS) tumour or trauma;
- idiopathic;
- exogenous steroid therapy – including inhaled corticosteroids.

Clinical presentation

Clinical features may be subtle; however, the diagnosis should be considered in all children with cardiovascular collapse. Features to look for in history, examination and investigation findings are listed below, with differential diagnosis.

History
- Prior steroid use, including inhaled steroids for asthma or other condition.
- Known congenital adrenal hyperplasia or other adrenal insufficiency on replacement therapy.
- Severe physiological stress (sepsis, trauma, burns, surgery).
- On anticoagulants, haemorrhagic diathesis.
- Neonate with collapse and/or hypoglycaemic event or ambiguous genitalia.
- Symptoms of glucocorticoid deficiency – weakness, fatigue, lethargy, anorexia, vomiting, diarrhoea, weight loss.

Examination
- Signs of glucocorticoid deficiency – hypoglycaemia, hypotension (absolute and postural), refractory shock.
- Signs of mineralocorticoid deficiency – dehydration (often out of proportion to estimated fluid losses), hyperkalaemia, hyponatraemia, acidosis, pre-renal failure.
- Signs of excess adrenocorticotropic hormone secretion – pigmentation of skin, lips, nipples, skin creases.

- Signs of glucocorticoid therapy – Cushing's syndrome.
- Signs of associated hypothalamic/ pituitary abnormality – growth abnormality, midline defects, hypogonadism, diabetes insipidus, hypothermia.

Investigations

- Bedside: finger-prick glucose (hypoglycaemia), electrocardiogram (ECG) (hyperkalaemia).
- Biochemical: glucose, urea and electrolytes, arterial blood gas, save clotted blood for cortisol level and 17-hydroxyprogesterone, if no underlying diagnosis is known.

Differential diagnosis

- Other causes of hyponatraemia – syndrome of inappropriate antidiuretic hormone hypersecretion, nephrogenic or cerebral salt wasting, gastrointestinal or urinary losses.
- Other causes of shock – septicaemia, profound dehydration, duct-dependent cardiac lesion.

Treatment

The management of adrenal crisis involves immediate fluid resuscitation, replacement of corticosteroid and treating hypoglycaemia. The underlying illness causing the stress needs to be treated on its merits. Potential complications, such as hyperkalaemia, may require intervention. In children not previously known to be adrenal deficient, blood (prior to administration of glucocorticoid) should be held for analysis to determine if an underlying condition exists.

Fluid management

Patients known to have adrenal deficiency who are not dehydrated or shocked can have a trial of enteral fluids in the ED. They should be considered to have vomited or potentially not absorbed normal replacement adrenal medication, and should be administered intramuscular (IM) hydrocortisone 2 mg kg^{-1} to ensure delivery.

Children who are dehydrated or shocked require intravenous resuscitation with crystalloid. Initial boluses of 20 mL kg^{-1} normal saline should be titrated to restore peripheral circulation in those children with shock.

Remaining estimated deficit plus maintenance volumes should then be replaced with 5% dextrose and normal saline over a 24-hour period. The maintenance fluid requirements are 1.5 times normal in this setting and clinical and biochemical (electrolytes and glucose) reassessment is required to tailor fluid therapy to the individual.

Replacement of corticosteroid

Hydrocortisone should be given intravenously, unless access is significantly delayed, where it should be administered IM as an interim alternative. The appropriate dose can be determined by age:

- neonate: 25 mg stat., then 10–25 mg 6-hourly;
- 1 month–1 year: 25 mg stat., then 25 mg 6-hourly;
- 1–3 years: 50 mg stat., then 50 mg 6-hourly;
- 4–10 years: 75 mg stat., then 75 mg 6-hourly;
- >10 years: 100 mg stat., then 100 mg 6-hourly.

Maintenance doses of glucocorticoid and mineralocorticoid are introduced after the child has been stabilised as an inpatient. Generally, glucocorticoid replacement dose is 10–15 mg m^{-2} day^{-1} orally and mineralocorticoid dose is 0.1–0.2 mg day^{-1} for salt-wasting children.

Hypoglycaemia

Hypoglycaemia is treated in the routine fashion using a lower concentration of intravenous dextrose in smaller children. Maintenance fluid will generally require 5–10% dextrose solution added to normal saline.

- neonate/infant: 5 mL kg^{-1} of 10% dextrose stat.;
- older child: 2 mL kg^{-1} of 25% dextrose stat.;
- maintenance fluid: 5–10% dextrose-containing solution.

Hyperkalaemia

Hyperkalaemia should be treated if K$^+$ >7 mmol L^{-1} with ECG changes.

- 0.5 mL kg^{-1} of 10% calcium gluconate over 3–5 minutes;
- 0.1 U kg^{-1} hr^{-1} of insulin + 2 mL kg^{-1} hr^{-1} of 50% dextrose infusion.

Disposition

All children with an established adrenal crisis require inpatient admission.

Discharge may be considered in milder cases, after a period of 6 hours observation, for those susceptible patients who respond well to treatment with oral fluids and increased dose of intramuscular hydrocortisone.

Prognosis

In the absence of bilateral adrenal haemorrhage, the survival rate of patients with adrenal crisis who are diagnosed and treated appropriately approaches that of patients without acute adrenal crisis with similar severity of illness. Because the true incidence of adrenal crisis and bilateral adrenal haemorrhage is unknown, the actual mortality rate is also unknown.

Prevention

At-risk children with an intercurrent illness may prevent an adrenal crisis with an action plan for parents:

- if moderately unwell and/or temperature is 38–39°C give 3× oral dose of oral hydrocortisone;
- if more unwell and/or temperature >39°C give 4× dose of oral hydrocortisone;
- if vomiting give IM 2 mg kg^{-1};
- If gastroenteritis or diarrhoea give 4× dose of oral hydrocortisone.

NB. Only the dose of hydrocortisone should be increased, not fludrocortisone. When the stress is over the previous dose should be resumed without tapering.

Controversies and future directions

❶ The role of screening for congenital adrenal hyperplasia (CAH) is controversial. In Australia there is currently no programme in place.

❷ Research indicates that early screening may reduce the morbidity or mortality associated with adrenal crisis.

❸ National newborn screening awaits the development of a more cost-efficient test.

❹ New research suggests that critically ill children with adrenal crisis may be best managed with a single intravenous bolus dose of hydrocortisone followed by a constant rate infusion. This in preference to the 6-hourly boluses used currently.

❺ A further recent research development is that CAH can be diagnosed and treated prenatally if a mother has previously had a child with CAH.

Further reading

Charmandari E, Lichtarowicz-Krynska EJ, Hindmarsh PC, et al. Congenital adrenal hyperplasia: Management during critical illness. *Arch Dis Child* 2001;**85**(1):26–8.

Fischer JE, Stalmach T, Fanconi S. Adrenal crisis presenting as hypoglycaemic coma. *Intens Care Med* 2000;**26**:105–8.

Gassner HL, Toppari J, Quinteiro Gonzalez S, Miller WL. Near-miss apparent SIDS from adrenal crisis. *J Pediatr* 2004; **145**(2):178–83.

Kirkland L. *Adrenal crisis.* eMedicine. www.emedicine.com; 2003.

Macdessi JS, Randell TR, Donaghue KC, et al. Adrenal crisis in children treated with high-dose inhaled corticosteroids for asthma. *Med J Aust* 2003;**178**(5):214–6.

Omori K, Nomura K, Shimizu S, et al. Risk factors for adrenal crisis in patients with adrenal insufficiency. *Endocr J* 2003;**50**(6):745–52.

Royal Children's Hospital. *Clinical Practice Guidelines.* Adrenal Crisis. Available from www.rch.org.au; 2005 [accessed 19.10.10].

The Children's Hospital at Westmead. *The New Children's Hospital Handbook. Acute adrenal insufficiency.* Available from www.chw.edu.au; 2005 [accessed 19.10.10].

Todd GRG, Acerini CL, Ross-Russell R, et al. Survey of adrenal crisis associated with inhaled corticosteroids in the United Kingdom. *Arch Dis Child* 2002;**87**:457–61.

Van der Kemp HJ, Noordham K, Elvers B, et al. Newborn screening for congenital adrenal hyperplasia in the Netherlands. *Paediatrics* 2001;**108**(6):1320–4.

10.5 Disorders of fluids, electrolytes and acid–base

Barry Wilkins • Wayne Hazell

ESSENTIALS

1 The most common causes of hypovolaemic shock in paediatric patients are sepsis, dehydration and trauma.

2 Vigorous restoration of the circulating volume reduces mortality in hypovolaemic shock.

3 Isotonic or near-isotonic fluids such as 0.9% saline, 4% albumin in 0.9% saline, blood products, Hartmann's or Ringer's solutions are appropriate for volume resuscitation. Hypotonic solutions including 5% glucose, 0.18%, 0.225% or 0.45% saline are inappropriate.

4 After resuscitation of circulating volume, residual dehydration should be corrected slowly with physiological solutions, such as Hartmann's solution or 0.9% saline, or 0.45% saline in the presence of hypernatraemia.

5 The degree of dehydration is easily overestimated.

6 The concept of maintenance fluids applies only after resuscitation of circulating volume and repair of dehydration or water overload. Even then fluids must be individualised to the patient's particular needs.

7 Hyponatraemia generally reflects water excess, and creates a risk for cerebral and pulmonary oedema. Hypotonic fluids are contraindicated until the plasma sodium is corrected. Cerebral oedema may develop rapidly in hyponatraemic children, especially after administration of hypotonic fluids.

8 Rapid correction of hyper- or hyponatraemia is contraindicated.

9 Hyperkalaemia with electrocardiogram (ECG) changes requires urgent potassium-lowering treatment.

10 Metabolic acidosis is common in sick children. The anion gap remains useful in determining the cause.

11 Treatment of acidosis is aimed at correcting the underlying cause. Alkali therapy is rarely indicated.

12 Metabolic alkalosis is caused by vomiting, especially pyloric stenosis, or as a compensation for chronic respiratory failure.

Introduction

Disorders of blood volume, body fluids, sodium, potassium and acid–base are common in acutely ill children. Always manage the airway and ventilation first, the 'ABC' principle of resuscitation, even in acute illness where shock and dehydration are dominant. In resuscitation of the circulation, vigorous replacement of blood volume deficit is urgent, but correction of residual dehydration is not. Maintenance fluids are the last consideration.

Physiology

There are many physiological differences between adults and infants, and a few specific features that must be taken into account in managing fluid therapy. Infants have greater total body water, up to 70% of body weight compared with 60% in adults, the extra fluid being mostly extracellular, 30% of body weight compared with 20%[1,2] (Fig. 10.5.1). The ionic composition of intracellular and extracellular fluid is shown in Table 10.5.1. Small children drink more to accommodate a higher metabolic rate and excrete a higher solute load, and thus urine volume is greater.

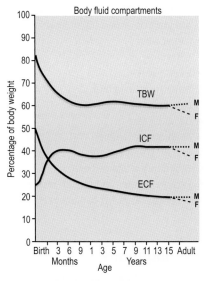

Fig. 10.5.1 Body fluid compartments in children. *Source:* Adapted from Henning, 1995.[1]

The following physiological differences apply to children:[1–3]

- Infants are more dependent on heart rate for cardiac output.
- Infants have less ability to increase myocardial contractility.
- The infant's ventricle is less compliant. Higher atrial pressures are required for the same degree of ventricular filling.
- The child is more dependent on the extracellular concentration of calcium.
- Storage and release of calcium from the sarcoplasmic reticulum in the infant's myocardium is less efficient.
- The infant tolerates more tachycardia and hypotension.
- Degenerative diseases are uncommon in children.

- The capacity of the infant's brain and heart for anaerobic metabolism is greater than the adult.
- The infant's kidney is less able to concentrate urine and to handle a sodium load in the first 2 years of life. Thus infants are less able to compensate for fluid loss.
- Renal blood flow and glomerular filtration rate are less per unit body surface area.
- Infants have less capability to acidify the urine and are thus less able to deal with a hyperchloraemic acidosis caused by too much chloride administration.
- Total body water and extracellular fluid are proportionally higher in the first 6 months of life. In later childhood extracellular fluid declines and intracellular fluid increases due to cell multiplication.
- Limited glycogen stores exist. Hypoglycaemia frequently occurs in periods of stress in infants and young children.

Clinical assessment

In assessing the degree of dehydration, sequential body weight measurement is the most accurate measure of water loss. However, previous normal body weight is seldom available in the emergency department (ED).

Capillary refill times were studied in 32 children, aged 1–26 weeks, admitted to hospital with dehydration.[4] The authors recommended a cut-off value of 2 seconds, below which minimal or no dehydration exists. A capillary refill time of 2–3 seconds suggests a 50–100 mL kg^{-1} water deficit; 3–4 seconds 100–120 mL kg^{-1}, and over 4 seconds >150 mL kg^{-1}. However, ambient temperature affects capillary return.[5]

In children less than 4 years old clinicians overestimate the degree of dehydration by 3.2%.[6] Other studies have suggested that the sensitivity of clinical examination for diagnosing dehydration is 74, 33 and 70% for mild, moderate and severe dehydration respectively.[7] See Tables 10.5.2 and 10.5.3 for clinical signs associated with dehydration and electrolyte imbalance.[8]

Plasma bicarbonate concentration may be the single most useful laboratory test; a level less than 17 mmol L^{-1} indicates moderate or severe dehydration. Addition of this to the clinical scale improves the sensitivity of diagnosing moderate and severe dehydration to 90 and 100% respectively. Plasma bicarbonate was a better predictor than plasma urea and creatinine.[7]

Shock is a disorder characterised by a decrease in end-organ oxygenation and/or perfusion. This does not solely depend on blood pressure and pulse rate. Blood pressure can be maintained in the infant with shock being present. Hypotension is a preterminal sign.

End-organ perfusion can best be assessed by the conscious state, capillary return, urine output and degree of metabolic acidosis.

Haemorrhagic shock

Clinical signs are of value in assessing degree of haemorrhage.[9] See Table 10.5.4. Hypotension is a preterminal sign.

Fluid deficit

In the case of dehydration, once the percentage loss of body weight (PLBW) is estimated from clinical and laboratory tests the fluid deficit can be estimated.

$$\text{Fluid deficit (litres)} = \text{PLBW \%} \times \text{estimated body weight (kg)}$$

Thus a 10 kg, 1- year-old who is 10% dehydrated has a fluid deficit of:

$$10\% \text{ of } 10 \text{ kg} = 1 \text{ kg} = 1000 \text{ g}$$
$$= 1 \text{ litre or } 1000 \text{ mL}$$

As this is an estimate, ongoing clinical parameters must be assessed including aiming for a urine output of >1.0 mL kg^{-1} hr^{-1}.

Table 10.5.1 Ionic distribution of body fluid compartments			
Cations and anions	*Intracellular fluid (mEq L^{-1})*	*Interstitial fluid (mEq L^{-1})*	*Plasma (mEq L^{-1})*
Sodium (Na$^+$)	10	145	140
Potassium (K$^+$)	150	4	4
Magnesium (Mg$^+$)	30	2	2
Calcium (Ca^{2+})	0	5	5
Chloride (Cl$^-$)	5	114	104
Bicarbonate (HCO$_3^-$)	10	24	24
Protein (Pr$^-$)	65	6	15
Phosphate (PO$_4^-$)	95 (organic)	4 (inorganic)	4 (inorganic)
Sulfate (SO$_4^-$)	20	1	1

Table 10.5.2 Degree of dehydration based on percentage of body weight lost*

Variable[a]	Mild (3–5%)	Moderate (6–9%)	Severe (10% or more)
Blood pressure	Normal	Normal	Normal to reduced
Quality of pulses	Normal	Normal or slightly decreased	Moderately decreased
Heart rate	Normal	Increased	Increased[b]
Skin turgor	Normal	Decreased	Decreased
Fontanelle	Normal	Sunken	Sunken
Mucous membranes	Slightly dry	Dry	Dry
Eyes	Normal	Sunken orbits	Deeply sunken orbits
Extremities	Warm, normal capillary refill	Delayed capillary refill	Cool, mottled
Mental status	Normal	Normal to listless	Normal to lethargic or comatose
Urine output	Slightly decreased	$<1\ mL\ kg^{-1}\ hr^{-1}$	$<<1\ mL\ kg^{-1}\ hr^{-1}$
Thirst	Slightly increased	Moderately increased	Very thirsty or too lethargic to indicate thirst

*For each dehydration category, the percentages of body weight lost varied among authors.
[a]See Table 10.5.3 for the physical signs of hypernatraemia and hypokalaemia in dehydration.
[b]Bradycardia may occur in children with severe dehydration.
Source: Based on Burkhart, 1999.[8]

Table 10.5.3 Signs of hypernatraemia and hypokalaemia in dehydration

Hypernatraemia

Cutaneous signs
Warm, 'doughy' texture
Possibly decreased skin-fold tenting in severe dehydration, thereby giving appearance of lower level of dehydration

Neurological signs

Hypertonia
Hyperreflexia
Lethargy common, but marked irritability when touched

Hypokalaemia

Weakness
Ileus with abdominal distension
Cardiac arrhythmias

Source: Based on Burkhart, 1999.[8]

Oedema

Oedema suggests that considerable water and salt retention has occurred. Mild sodium and water retention do not cause clinical oedema, nor does water retention without sodium retention, e.g. the syndrome of inappropriate antidiuretic hormone secretion rarely causes oedema. Oedema is most obvious in dependent and distensible subcutaneous tissue such as the genitalia, eyelids, lower legs and lower back. Firm pressure for at least 1 minute is needed to detect subtle cases. Causes include:

- Heart failure
  structural cardiac disease;
  myocarditis;

cardiomyopathy;
arrhythmias, especially supraventricular tachycardia;
effusion.
- Liver disease
  acute hepatic failure;
  chronic hepatic failure.
- Renal disease
  nephrotic syndrome.
- Protein-losing enteropathy
- Hereditary angio-oedema
- Excessive water and sodium intake
- Other causes of hypoalbuminaemia.

Investigations

Most children with gastroenteritis do not warrant an IV line or investigations. However, the following biochemical tests should be performed in children presenting with shock or significant problems of water and electrolyte imbalance that require intravenous treatment or where such disorders are expected, e.g. respiratory disease, renal disease, liver disease and encephalopathy:

- plasma sodium, potassium, urea, creatinine, osmolality, glucose, bicarbonate, lactate;
- plasma calcium, magnesium, phosphate, liver function tests, albumin;
- arterial and/or venous pH and gases if shocked.

Venous or intraosseous blood samples give a satisfactory measurement of electrolytes, and of respiratory and metabolic acid–base status.

- urine sodium, potassium, urea, creatinine, osmolality, glucose, and dipstick test for protein, red cells and casts (random spot sample).

A urine sample aspirated from a cotton wool ball placed at the perineum is satisfactory for all measurements except urine calcium.

Plasma osmolality can be calculated as well as measured in order to detect an osmolar gap.

$$Osmolality\ (mosmol\ kg^{-1}) = 1.86 \times (Na + K) + glucose + urea + 10\ (all\ in\ mmol\ L^{-1})$$

If measured osmolality is greater than this figure by 5 mosmol kg^{-1} or more, then an

Table 10.5.4 Classes of haemorrhagic shock[9]

Class of haemorrhage	Blood volume lost (%)	Signs
I	<15	Minimal, slight tachycardia
II	15–30	Tachycardia, tachypnoea, diminished pulse pressure, systolic BP unchanged, prolonged capillary refill, minimal decrease in urine output, anxiety
III	30–40	Tachycardia, tachypnoea, decreased BP, decreased urine output, mental status changes
IV	>40	Hypotension, anuria, loss of consciousness

Source: Based on Morgan and O'Neill, 1998.[9]

unmeasured solute is present such as an alcohol, e.g. ethanol or ethylene glycol. Ingestion of alcohols may cause a high anion gap ketoacidosis and hypoglycaemia.

Accurate timed urine collections are rarely possible in the ED. A useful indication of urine flow rate can be obtained from a spot urine sample, based on the relatively constant creatinine excretion between individuals. For example, a urine creatinine of 2000 μmol L^{-1} represents urine flow of 2–4 mL kg^{-1} hr^{-1}, and 8000 μmol L^{-1} represents 0.5–1 mL kg^{-1} hr^{-1}.

Fractional sodium excretion (FE$_{Na}$) is a useful diagnostic tool. It represents the proportion of filtered sodium that is not reabsorbed and is <1% in health. It is given by the formula:

$$FE_{Na} = \frac{Urine\ Na}{Urine\ creatinine} \times \frac{Plasma\ creatinine}{Plasma\ Na}$$

A high FE$_{Na}$ suggests any cause of natriuresis, including acute renal failure, a renal salt-wasting disorder or diuretics. Hyperosmolar urine with high urine creatinine and low FE$_{Na}$ suggests dehydration of non-renal cause. Diabetes insipidus causes hypo-osmolar urine (often <100 mosmol kg^{-1}), low urine creatinine (often <1000 μmol L^{-1}) and plasma hyperosmolality. Plasma urea is high in most cases of dehydration because of reduced urea clearance.

Treatment

Replacement of circulating volume

Also called volume resuscitation, this is an urgent priority in any cause of hypovolaemic shock, e.g. haemorrhage, sepsis, burns, anaphylaxis and dehydration. It requires isotonic fluids (Table 10.5.5). Hypotonic fluids are inappropriate. Crystalloids are inexpensive and readily available. Colloids have a theoretical advantage of increasing the colloid oncotic pressure of plasma, thus helping to maintain fluid in the vascular space. However, in a capillary leak syndrome such as septic shock, the colloid may pass into the interstitial space. In practice, albumin in saline solution has been tested against 0.9% saline in adult intensive care patients. There was no difference in mortality or intensive care unit (ICU) stay between the two therapies. More saline was administered than albumin (ratio 1.38:1), suggesting that albumin may be superior in patients where excessive water administration may be harmful, e.g. pulmonary oedema, pulmonary hypertension and encephalopathy. There was a suggestion that albumin may be superior in sepsis but inferior in traumatic brain injury.[10] A problem with saline is that it has no bicarbonate and relatively high chloride, so it can lead to hyperchloraemic acidosis. Hartmann's and

Ringer's solutions are more physiological, containing buffer and calcium.[10–12]

In dehydration, the loss of fluid and electrolytes is similar to the composition of extracellular fluid; this is predominantly where the loss comes from. Thus the deficit is best replaced with a solution that approximates extracellular fluid, i.e. 0.9% saline (normal saline).

However, as fluid replacement is not an exact science, and due to the fact that maintenance fluids also need to be given, a solution somewhere between 0.9% saline and 4% dextrose plus 0.18% saline is given. Saline (0.45%) with added glucose (2.5%) and sometimes potassium would be appropriate. Clinical parameters and serum biochemistry are sequentially measured and the fluid is adjusted accordingly.

Overall 24 – hour fluid requirement = fluid deficit + maintenance + ongoing losses

An initial bolus or boluses of 20 mL kg^{-1} to treat shock may be part of this initial fluid deficit.

Saline (but not Hartmann's, Ringer's and Plasmalyte) tends to cause a metabolic acidosis because of a dilution of bicarbonate by chloride, the principal extracellular buffer, and a relative hyperchloraemia.

Those containing lactate, gluconate or acetate are more physiological solutions,

Table 10.5.5 Common crystalloid and colloid IV fluids								
Content per litre	0.9% NaCl (normal saline)	0.45% NaCl (half-normal saline)	3% NaCl	5% glucose	Hartmann's solution	Plasmalyte	Albumin	Gelatine based products
Na$^+$ (mmol L^{-1})	154	77	500		130	140	140	145–154
K$^+$ (mmol L^{-1})					4–5	5	5	
Cl$^-$ (mmol L^{-1})	154	77	500		109	98	134	120–145
Ca^{2+} or Mg^{2+} (mmol L^{-1})					Ca^{2+} 2	Mg^{2+} 1.5		Ca^{2+} 0–6
Buffer (mmol L^{-1})					Lactate 28	Acetate 27 Gluconate 23	Octanoate 6	
Glucose (g L^{-1})				50				
Osmolarity (mosmol L^{-1})	285	145	900	278	274		280	280–293
Number average molecular weight (M$_n$)							69 000	23 000–24 500
Weight average molecular weight (M$_w$)							69 000	30 000–35 000
Duration of action							6 hours	3–4 hours
Survival in the body							21 days	7 days

Starches have not been included in this table because they are very infrequently used in children in Australia and the United Kingdom.

the buffer being rapidly metabolised to bicarbonate.

Glucose may be added to the sodium chloride preparations.

How much fluid?

Enough fluid should be given in shock to result in the improvement and disappearance of the signs of shock.

The blood volume of an infant is approximately 70–80 mL kg^{-1}. Decompensation in haemorrhagic shock starts to occur in class 3 haemorrhagic shock. At this stage it can be presumed that at least 30% or approximately 20 mL kg^{-1} of blood has been lost.

Thus a bolus dose of 20 mL kg^{-1} is a logical bolus dose of fluid with which to begin resuscitation.

However, in dehydration and sepsis much larger fluid losses and shifts have occurred and the total body water and extracellular fluid are likely to be depleted far more than 20 mL kg^{-1}. If crystalloid is given, not all of the fluid stays in the intravascular space. Capillary leakiness and third space losses in sepsis contribute to the ongoing loss of fluid from the vascular space.

Thus in dehydration repeated boluses may be necessary. Give a bolus, wait 10 minutes and reassess the patient again. Do not wait 10 minutes if it is clear that more than 20 mL kg^{-1} will be required.[13–15]

In severe sepsis such as meningococcaemia, 80–100 mL kg^{-1} may be required. Good evidence exists that early and vigorous resuscitation improves morbidity and mortality in paediatric sepsis and meningococcaemia.[16] The volume and the rapidity of resuscitation seems to be more important than the type of fluid used.[17–19]

In haemorrhagic shock, boluses of 10 mL kg^{-1} of whole blood or packed cells may be given. If fresh frozen plasma (FFP) is required this can also be given in 10 mL kg^{-1} aliquots.

How to administer fluid in shock

Intravenous access is often difficult in a shocked young infant, but it is essential that this is achieved as soon as possible. If intravenous access has not been achieved within 90 seconds and/or three failed attempts have occurred, intraosseous access should be gained.

Poiseuille's law states that the flow through a hollow tube is proportional to the radius to the power of four and inversely related to the

viscosity of the fluid and length of the tube. The small radius can be overcome by applying a larger pressure differential across the tubing. Fluid can be drawn up in a 20 or 50 mL syringe and injected rapidly. It is harder to push fluid through a small cannula with a 50 mL syringe.

A three-way tap can be connected to a normal giving set attached to the IV fluid of choice. The tap can be turned off to the patient allowing fluid to be drawn into the syringe. The tap can then be turned off to the giving set and fluid can rapidly be injected into the patient.

Ideally, blood should be given through the largest cannula that can be inserted. As well as the usual complications of blood transfusion, the paediatric patient is at risk of hyperkalaemia from cell lysis through the small cannula.

Infants have a higher surface area to body weight ratio and lose heat more quickly. Overhead radiant warmers or fluid warmers are recommended for large rapid volume replacement when hypothermia is a risk.

Investigation and management of fluids in different conditions
Gastroenteritis and dehydration

Dehydration is a common presenting feature in children. Causes are outlined in Table 10.5.6.

Oral rehydration either by mouth or nasogastric tube is the method of choice for rehydration unless shock exists. It is safe, cheap

---

Table 10.5.6   Causes of dehydration

Gastrointestinal loss
- Diarrhoea
- Non-obstructive vomiting
- Obstructive vomiting
- Third space loss into bowel wall and peritoneum

Renal loss
- Renal tubular disease
- Acquired tubulopathies
- Chronic renal failure including obstructive uropathy
- Adrenal failure
- Congenital adrenal hyperplasia (salt-losing)
- Diabetes insipidus (central and renal)
- Osmotic diuresis (e.g. DKA)
- Diuretics

Insensible loss
- Burns
- Sweating
- Hyperthyroidism
- Hyperventilation with reduced intake
- Ichthyosis, e.g. Netherton syndrome

Reduced intake (rarely causes dehydration)

---

and effective. It can be effective even in the case of vomiting.[21–26]

Recommendations for oral and intravenous hydration in gastroenteritis as given by the American Academy of Pediatrics are contained in Table 10.5.7. Oral

---

Table 10.5.7   American Academy of Pediatrics (AAP) recommendations for oral rehydration therapy (ORT) in children based on estimated degree of dehydration*

No dehydration
- Oral rehydration therapy: not generally needed unless the child is feeding poorly or is not taking other fluids well; then give 10 mL kg^{-1} of an oral rehydration solution for each diarrhoeal stool
- Feeding: continue age-appropriate diet[a]

Mild dehydration (3–5% body weight loss)
- Oral rehydration therapy: give 50 mL kg^{-1} of an oral rehydration solution plus replace ongoing fluid losses[b] over a 4-hour period; re-evaluate hydration and estimate ongoing fluid losses every 2 hours
- Feeding: resume age-appropriate diet[a] as soon as dehydration is corrected and emesis resolves

Moderate dehydration (6–9% body weight loss)
- Oral rehydration therapy: in a supervised setting, give 100 mL kg^{-1} of an oral rehydration solution plus replace ongoing fluid losses[b] over a 4-hour period; re-evaluate hydration and estimate ongoing fluid losses every hour
- Feeding: resume age-appropriate diet[a] when dehydration is fully corrected

Severe dehydration (10% or greater body weight loss; implies shock or near-shock)
- Intravenous therapy: give a rapid intravenous bolus of 20 mL kg^{-1} of normal saline solution or Ringer's lactate; repeat as needed until the child is haemodynamically stable and shock resolves; if the child does not respond to one or more boluses, consider causes of shock other than fluid loss from diarrhoea and emesis
- Oral rehydration therapy: when the child is stable and alert, begin administration of an oral rehydration solution; keep intravenous line in place until the child is drinking well
- Feeding: resume age-appropriate diet[a] when dehydration is corrected

*These recommendations cover children from 1 month to 5 years of age with no pre-existing comorbid conditions who live in developed countries. Specifically excluded are children who have diarrhoea lasting more than 10 days, diarrhoea associated with failure to thrive and/or vomiting in the absence of diarrhoea. If the physician is unsure of the dehydration category for a specific patient, the therapy for the more severe category should be used.
[a]The diet should emphasise complex carbohydrates, lean meats, yogurt, fruits and vegetables. Fatty foods, and foods and fluids that are high in simple sugars should be avoided.
[b]Replacement of ongoing fluid losses should include an amount for the estimated volume of emesis and 10 mL kg^{-1} for each diarrhoeal stool.
Source: Based on Burkhart, 1999.[8]

Table 10.5.8 Oral rehydration solutions

Product	Electrolyte content (mEq L^{-1})								
	Na$^+$	K$^+$	Cl$^-$	Citrate	Carbohydrate	Calories (per 30 mL)	Osmolality (mosmol kg^{-1})	How supplied
Commercial preparations	45–75	20–25	35–65	30–48	20–30 g L^{-1} of glucose (dextrose)* or rice syrup solids	3–4.2	250–310	60 mL freezer pops or 240–1000 mL ready-to-use, flavoured or unflavoured
WHO oral rehydration solution salts, mixed	90	20	80	30	20 g L^{-1} of glucose	2.5	310	Dry packets, mixed with 1 L water
Home mix (recipe developed by WHO)	90	20	80	30	20 g L^{-1} of glucose or 40 g L^{-1} of sucrose	2.5	310	Mix 3.5 g (one half teaspoon) of table salt, 1.5 g (one half teaspoon) of potassium chloride or potassium salt, 2.5 g (one half teaspoon) of baking soda and either 20 g (two tablespoons) of glucose or 40 g (four tablespoons) of sucrose in 1 L of water)

Na$^+$, sodium; K$^+$, potassium; Cl$^-$, chloride; WHO, World Health Organization.
*Some freezer pops also contain phenylalanine and aspartame.
Source: Based on Burkhart, 1999.[8]

rehydration should occur with one of the recommended oral rehydration solutions (Table 10.5.8). No evidence exists to show that one formula is more effective than another.[22] These fluids resemble 0.45% saline and 2.5% glucose with added potassium, a useful intravenous solution in this condition.[8]

Clear liquids or soft drinks are not to be encouraged. These may be high in carbohydrate and osmolality and lead to osmotic diarrhoea. Hyponatraemia may occur due to their low sodium content. Chicken broth is inappropriate as it may lead to hypernatraemia[8] (Table 10.5.9).

Some trials suggest frozen oral rehydration solution is better tolerated than the liquid form.[27] One study suggested that children with a serum bicarbonate greater than 13 mmol L^{-1}, and who were vomiting, could be treated with rapid intravenous rehydration (20–30 mL kg^{-1} of isotonic crystalloid over 1–2 hours) in the ED.[28] They could then tolerate oral rehydration and be discharged home. Shorter stays in the ED were also enabled compared to times reported with oral rehydration solution.

Hypernatraemia and hypernatraemic dehydration

Hypernatraemia is usually caused by water depletion, or water plus sodium depletion in dehydration states where there is relatively more water depletion. Most causes of dehydration (see Table 10.5.5) can cause hypernatraemia. Rarely, hyperaldosteronism or salt poisoning cause sodium excess.

The clinical features are usually those of dehydration. Coma and seizures may occur, especially if plasma sodium is >160 mmol L^{-1} at any time, and if there are rapid changes in circulating volume or plasma chemistry. Some neurological deficit may result from the encephalopathy of severe hypernatraemia.

Fractional sodium excretion is low because of a normal physiological response to dehydration, but may be high if the cause is an osmotic diuresis, excessive diuretic use or in salt poisoning. The urine is concentrated (osmolality >600 mosmol kg^{-1}) except in diabetes insipidus.

Shock is treated with isotonic fluids until haemodynamically stable, then 0.225–0.45% saline, with potassium as needed (40 mmol L^{-1} if not hyperkalaemic). The estimated dehydration should be corrected over 48 hours with slow correction of plasma sodium at no more than 0.6 mmol L^{-1} hr^{-1} (15 mmol L^{-1} day^{-1}).

If salt poisoning is suspected, obtain gastric fluid via nasogastric tube for sodium analysis. Features of dehydration are usually absent and FE$_{Na}$ is high, often >10%. If there is salt excess without dehydration, then give less than maintenance water with no sodium, aiming for a very slow correction of plasma sodium, <0.6 mmol L^{-1} hr^{-1}.

Table 10.5.9 Electrolyte and carbohydrate content of common 'clear liquids'

Liquid	Electrolyte content (mEq L^{-1})				
	Na$^+$	K$^+$	HCO$_3^-$	Carbohydrate (g L^{-1})	Osmolality (mosmol kg^{-1})
Cola	2	0.1	13	50 to 150, glucose and fructose	550
Ginger ale	3	1	4	50 to 150, glucose and fructose	540
Apple juice	3	20	0	100 to 150, glucose and fructose	700
Chicken broth	250	5	0	0	450
Tea	0	0	0	0	5
Sports drinks	20	3	3	45, glucose and other sugars	330

Na$^+$, sodium; K$^+$, potassium; HCO$_3^-$, bicarbonate.
Source: Based on Gremse, 1995.[23]

A diuretic may be considered and, in extreme cases, dialysis.[29–31]

Diabetes insipidus

Diabetes insipidus should be treated with glucose/water, replacing the previous hour's urine volume plus $10–20$ mL kg^{-1} day^{-1} for insensible losses. Hyperglycaemia may result. An intravenous vasopressin infusion may be needed, but only if the urine output is stable, which means usually after admission to a ward or ICU, and after consulting an endocrinologist.

Hyponatraemia and hyponatraemic dehydration

Hyponatraemia may be caused by water excess (e.g. water intoxication, inappropriate antidiuretic hormone (ADH)), water and salt retention where the water excess is greater than the sodium excess (e.g. nephrotic syndrome, heart failure, renal failure or liver failure), dehydration where sodium depletion is greater than the water depletion (e.g. renal loss, gastrointestinal loss, third-space loss, congenital adrenal hyperplasia, acute adrenal failure), or abnormal solute in extracellular fluid (e.g. glucose in uncontrolled diabetes) causing water shift from intra- to extracellular space.

Hyponatraemia may cause nausea, lethargy, depressed consciousness, raised intracranial pressure and seizures, especially if of rapid onset.

Urine osmolality and plasma urea are high in dehydration, but low in water intoxication. FE_{Na} is high in salt-losing states, inappropriate ADH and often in acute renal failure.

Treatment of shock is according to standard guidelines and can be instigated safely with normal saline. Severely symptomatic patients with plasma sodium less than 120 mmol L^{-1}, such as those with seizures or coma (which is likely to be associated with cerebral oedema), should have the sodium corrected rapidly to 125 mmol L^{-1} (but no higher), using 3% saline (0.5 mmol mL^{-1}).

The following formula may be useful:

$$\text{Sodium required (mmol)} =$$
$$(125 - \text{plasma sodium (mmoL/L)}) \times$$
$$0.6 \times \text{weight (kg)}$$

Excessive rapid correction of hyponatraemia can be associated with pontine or extrapontine myelinolysis, but it is not clear whether this relates to the severe hyponatraemia itself or the rapid correction. Convulsions and decreasing level of consciousness may occur at any time in treatment, especially if there are rapid changes in circulating volume or plasma chemistry. Some neurological deficit may result from the encephalopathy of severe hyponatraemia.

After treatment of shock, residual dehydration should be managed by replenishing extracellular space with 0.9% sodium chloride or one of the buffered isotonic solutions, slowly over 48 hours. Residual hyponatraemia should correct itself slowly.

Water intoxication needs water restriction to half maintenance and sodium supplementation if there is evidence of natriuresis.

Syndrome of inappropriate antidiuretic hormone secretion (SIADH)

This condition is over diagnosed. Plasma concentration of antidiuretic hormone, vasopressin, is elevated, despite physiological conditions which should suppress it, namely hypo-osmolality and water overload. Hyponatraemia and hypo-osmolality are accompanied by marked oliguria, but with high fractional sodium excretion and very high urine osmolality and sodium (often >200 mmol L^{-1}). The child is sodium depleted but water overloaded, so the management of choice is water restriction, the IV fluid being given as 0.9% saline. Furosemide causes a diuresis in SIADH and may contribute to management.

Pyloric stenosis

Shock is treated with 20 mL kg^{-1} boluses of 0.9% saline. Saline (0.9%) with 40 mmol L^{-1} of KCl is the appropriate rehydration solution. Glucose needs to be added. This remedies the loss of chloride and potassium, and slowly corrects the alkalosis.

Sepsis and meningococcal disease

There is no compelling argument for crystalloid or colloid.[18–21] A study of septic shock[14] found that fluid resuscitation in excess of 40 mL kg^{-1} in the first hour was associated with improved survival, decreased occurrence of persistent hypovolaemia and no increase in the risk of acute respiratory distress syndrome or pulmonary oedema. No restriction was placed on the type of resuscitation fluid used.

A study of severe meningococcaemia[17] looked at 336 patients retrospectively and found a decreased mortality, both in the general population and in high-risk groups, when FFP was not used.

Thus, early vigorous fluid management is the key.

Haemorrhagic shock

Initial resuscitation can take place with crystalloid or colloid. Whole blood at 10 mL kg^{-1} can be given and repeated as necessary until blood pressure is restored.

FFP should be thawed if a large transfusion is expected, and platelets requested. FFP only comes in adult-sized bags and doses of 10 mL kg^{-1} are appropriate with repeating of coagulation times.[9]

Head injury

Vigorous treatment of shock should be undertaken to maintain cerebral perfusion pressure.[32]

Interest has been generated in the use of 7.5% saline in head-injured patients. A prospective randomised study of 35 patients with head injury compared Ringer's lactate with 7.5% saline.[33] Children treated with hypertonic saline had a statistically significant decrease in complications, intracranial pressure and ICU stay. There was no difference, however, in survival or duration of hospital stay. Neurological outcome was not well documented. More evidence is required.[33–35]

Burns

The original Parkland formula of $3–4$ mL kg^{-1} per percentage burn is still applicable to burns patients. This is over the first 24 hours and starts at the time of the burn, not admission to ED.

Originally, 50% of this was to be given in the first 8 hours and the rest over the remaining 16 hours. However, recent evidence suggests that restoration of urinary output and vital signs occurs earlier if 50% is given in the first 4 hours. Many burns patients require more fluid than is provided by the Parkland formula. Aim for urine output greater than 1 mL kg^{-1} hr^{-1}.[35]

Some evidence also suggests that paediatric burns patients tolerate hypoalbuminaemia well and may not require albumin.[36]

Diabetic ketoacidosis

Treatment of shock should include boluses of 20 mL kg^{-1} of colloid or normal saline. Some solutions contain potassium and should ideally not be used in hyperkalaemic renal failure.

Rehydration over 48 hours is desirable so as to minimise the risk of cerebral oedema.

Cerebral oedema is almost exclusively a condition of the newly diagnosed young diabetic, with 95% of cases occurring under 20 years of age.

The fluid of choice is controversial. One article suggests that normal saline be used until restoration of glucose and then a change should be made to 0.45% saline. Potassium replacement should be started when the urinary output is adequate.[37]

Hyperkalaemia

Hyperkalaemia is often discovered incidentally on routine chemistry, but may be suggested by ECG changes. It may be associated with renal failure, hypoxia-ischaemia or acidosis. There may not be potassium excess but rather potassium shift from intra- to extracellular fluid), β-blockers, rhabdomyolysis, haemolysis, potassium sparing diuretics, acute adrenal failure and potassium poisoning.

Mild hyperkalaemia may be asymptomatic but potassium levels >6 mmol L^{-1}, especially when acute, may cause weakness, peaked T-waves and wide PR interval on ECG, and then loss of P wave, heart block and asystole.

Investigations should include a blood gas, creatine kinase (CK) and glucose.

Any plasma potassium >6 mmol L^{-1}, or <6 but rising fast, demands urgent treatment. If K$^+$ >7 mmol L^{-1} or there are ECG changes, consider giving calcium 0.1–0.15 mmol kg^{-1}, which does not change plasma potassium but protects cell membranes. Beware of subcutaneous infiltration of the infusion. Sodium bicarbonate may also be given, especially if the child is acidotic, 1–3 mmol kg^{-1} over 30–60 minutes, but its value is not certain. If plasma potassium is >6.5 mmol L^{-1}, consider arranging early dialysis. Discuss with the nephrology and intensive-care services.

Milder degrees of hyperkalaemia respond to 5–10 mcg kg^{-1} IV salbutamol over a few minutes (or 2.5–5 mg of inhaled nebulised salbutamol if there is no IV cannula), to promote potassium entry into cells. This is more effective and longer lasting than glucose/insulin (0.1 U kg^{-1} insulin plus 0.5 g kg^{-1} glucose over 30–60 minutes).

Resonium, 1 g kg^{-1} every 4–6 hours oral or rectal, may eliminate 1–2 mmol kg^{-1} of potassium.

All cases of hyperkalaemia should be admitted with ECG monitoring.

Hypokalaemia

Hypokalaemia is often an incidental finding on blood chemistry and usually represents potassium depletion. Causes of potassium depletion include vomiting, diuretics, secretory diarrhoea, ureterosigmoidostomy, renal tubular acidosis, hyperaldosteronism, anorexia nervosa and diabetic ketoacidosis. Causes of hypokalaemia without depletion include salbutamol use, alkalosis and familial periodic paralysis.

Mild hypokalaemia is often asymptomatic but tachyarrhythmias, ileus, weakness and rhabdomyolysis may occur. Hypokalaemia associated with alkalosis usually corrects itself as the pH corrects.

Treat potassium depletion by slow potassium supplementation at 2 mmol kg^{-1} day^{-1} or greater. Never give 0.5 mmol kg^{-1} in 1 hour without ECG monitoring and frequent repeat measurement. Concentration >40 mmol L^{-1} of infusion fluid should be given into a central venous catheter.

Maintenance fluids

The concept of maintenance fluids refers to healthy children, where the kidneys are able to conserve or excrete water and salt over a wide range, in each case according to intake and non-renal losses. 'Maintenance' is a volume of water intake which maintains urine output in the middle of the normal range with an osmolality about that of extracellular fluid. However, changes in total body water and sodium and other electrolytes are common in many diseases. Insensible skin loss of water may be high because of fever and the higher surface area:weight ratio in infants. Maintenance is only relevant after restoration of circulating volume and total body water, and is therefore relevant to ongoing rather than ED care. A maintenance amount should be a starting amount. It may be excessive for any sick child where there may be diminished ability to excrete water.

Maintenance rates of 0.18% sodium chloride with 20 mmol L^{-1} added potassium provide 40–100 mL kg^{-1} day^{-1} of water, 1.5–3 mmol kg^{-1} day^{-1} of sodium and 0.7–1.5 mmol kg^{-1} day^{-1} of potassium, which are normal quantities in healthy children.

A common formula for calculating 'maintenance' water requirements in a healthy child is as follows:

- for the first 10 kg of body weight: 100 mL kg^{-1} day^{-1} or 4 mL kg^{-1} hr^{-1};
- for the second 10 kg of body weight: 50 mL kg^{-1} day^{-1} or 2 mL kg^{-1} hr^{-1};
- for every subsequent kg of body weight: 25 mL kg^{-1} day^{-1} or 1 mL kg^{-1} hr^{-1}.

Reduce this by one-third initially, or even one-half if there is risk of cerebral oedema, e.g. in meningitis or brain injury, especially if hyponatraemia already exists. Less than 'maintenance' water should be given when water retention is likely, such as in sepsis and severe respiratory disease (0.7 × 'maintenance'), cardiac failure (0.5 × 'maintenance'), renal failure or other oliguric states without hypovolaemia (0.3 × 'maintenance' plus urine output) (Table 10.5.10). Greater than 'maintenance' is often advocated when water losses are expected, e.g. spontaneous hyperventilation or fever, but it is probably more appropriate to increase fluids only if urine output falls to 0.5 mL kg^{-1} hr^{-1}. The most appropriate maintenance IV fluid in the acutely ill child is 0.45% saline because at half-'maintenance' rates this provides 1–3 mmol kg^{-1} day^{-1} of sodium, but separate consideration should always be given to sodium and other electrolyte requirements. Do not include dehydration deficit in maintenance; consider this separately and use 0.9% saline or a buffered isotonic solution for replacement.

Acid–base disorders

Disorders of physiological control of acidity of body fluids are common in acutely ill children. The system of defining acid–base state by changes in pCO$_2$ (respiratory) and standardised base excess (metabolic) according to the Copenhagen school remains the most familiar way of analysing acid–base disorders. Base excess is mostly bicarbonate

Table 10.5.10 Guide to ongoing water therapy

Weight (kg)	0.7 × 'maintenance' – the commonest starting point		Full 'maintenance'	
	(mL hr^{-1})	(mL kg^{-1} day^{-1})	(mL h^{-1})	(mL kg^{-1} day^{-1})
4	11	70	16	100
6	17	70	24	100
8	22	70	32	100
10	28	70	40	100
12	31	62	44	88
14	34	57	48	82
16	36	55	52	78
18	39	53	56	75
20	42	50	60	72
30	49	39	70	56
40	56	34	80	48
50	63	30	90	43
60	70	28	100	40
70	77	27	110	38

deficit, but includes a small amount of buffering by albumin, and a larger amount by haemoglobin. Standardised base excess is provided by blood gas machines derived by microprocessor rather than the original nomograms. The philosophy of base excess has been challenged because it does not take into account the actual plasma albumin concentration and assumes a notional haemoglobin concentration of 50 g L^{-1} across blood and extracellular fluid in all patients. It can be argued that the bicarbonate concentration alone is a sufficient measure of the degree of metabolic acidosis or alkalosis.

The anion gap remains a useful tool in determining whether any bicarbonate deficit is caused by organic acid (high anion gap) or by chloride excess (normal anion gap). It is obtained from the formula:

$$\text{Anion gap} = Na^+ + K^+ - Cl^- - HCO_3^- \text{ (all in mEq L}^{-1})$$

The normal is 16 mEq L^{-1} and is essentially the negative charge on albumin and phosphate. Any excess is accounted for by abnormal unmeasured acid and/or lactate. Most modern laboratories, including blood gas machines, measure lactate. A more accurate way of determining the unmeasured component is from the formula:

$$\text{Unmeasured anion} =$$
$$Na^+ + K^+ + Mg^{2+} + Ca^{2+} - Cl^- -$$
$$HCO_3^- - \text{albumin} \times (0.123 \times pH -$$
$$0.631) - \text{phosphate} \times (0.309 \times pH -$$
$$0.469) - \text{lactate}^- \text{ (all in mEq L}^{-1})$$

Note that Mg^{2+} and Ca^{2+} are divalent and so are $2 \times$ mmol L^{-1}.

Albumin × (0.123 × pH – 0.631) is the negative charge on albumin, derived from its known buffer curve.

Phosphate × (0.309 × pH – 0.469) is the negative charge on phosphate, derived from its known buffer curve.

Plasma albumin at 40–45 g L^{-1} is 0.6 mmol L^{-1} but contributes 12 mEq L^{-1} to the anion at pH 7.4. Phosphate at 1.5 mmol L^{-1} contributes 2.7 mEq L^{-1}.

The normal value for unmeasured anion is 5–6 mEq L^{-1}, including 1 mEq L^{-1} of lactate. Any excess is abnormal. This may be lactate in hypoxia–ischaemia, acetoacetate or β-hydroxybutyrate in DKA, ketones in starvation, organic acids in inborn errors of metabolism or alcohol poisoning or toluene inhalation.

Most metabolic acid–base disturbances do not need treatment. Compensating mechanisms should generally not be treated, otherwise the primary disturbance is exacerbated. It is not necessary to restore pH to normal.

Metabolic acidosis

Normal physiology maintains extracellular pH close to 7.4 in health, but permits metabolic acidosis at times of anaerobic metabolism without danger. Metabolic acidosis may be advantageous because it is thought to protect cells against the effects of hypoxia, and assists oxygen unloading from haemoglobin by shifting the oxygen/haemoglobin dissociation curve to the right.

Acidosis is said to cause negative inotropy or failure of inotropes to work at pH < 7.2, but this has little experimental support. Acidosis causes pulmonary vasoconstriction and may predispose to arrhythmias caused by other electrolyte abnormalities.

In metabolic acidosis, bicarbonate deficit (mmol kg^{-1}) is given by:

$$\text{Weight (kg)} \times (24 - \text{plasma}$$
$$\text{bicarbonate [mmol L}^{-1}]) \times 0.5$$

Plasma lactate estimation should be performed if there is significant base deficit or high anion gap. Urine for drug screen may be indicated. For suspected inborn error of metabolism if the anion gap is greater than 20, send urine for metabolic screen.

First treat the underlying disease (Table 10.5.11), including general management of renal, hepatic failure, cardiac failure, hypoxia, shock and hypovolaemia. Alkali is not usually needed for mild acidosis (pH > 7.2) because the acidosis itself does not cause any compromise. Even extreme acidaemia (pH < 6.8) can be followed by full recovery, and bicarbonate therapy is only indicated if there is severe hyperkalaemia or tricyclic poisoning. Sudden changes in acid–base status should be avoided. Sodium bicarbonate has many adverse effects, especially when given rapidly, such as hypokalaemia, decreased plasma ionised calcium, sodium load, osmolar load, increased haemoglobin/oxygen affinity, exacerbation of effects of hypophosphataemia, and late metabolic alkalosis. There is no evidence for increased intracellular acidosis. Sodium bicarbonate is especially unhelpful in lactic

Table 10.5.11   Causes of acidosis

High anion gap	Normal anion gap
• Diarrhoea (starvation/ketosis) • Sepsis • Diabetic ketoacidosis • Renal failure • Hepatic failure • Drugs and poisons (e.g. salicylates, ethanol, methanol, ethylene glycol) • Inborn errors of metabolism (especially in babies) • Hypoxia • Circulatory failure	• Renal tubular acidosis • Other renal tubulopathies which include bicarbonate loss • Gastroenteritis • Intestinal fistulae or enterostomies • Excessive sodium chloride administration • Hypoaldosteronism

acidosis, resulting in sodium overload with a metabolic alkalosis as the lactic acid is metabolised to bicarbonate during recovery.

Slow sodium bicarbonate treatment may have a role in the management of normal anion gap acidosis where excessive chloride therapy would exacerbate hyperchloraemia. A suitable amount is 2 mmol kg^{-1} day^{-1}. In diabetic ketoacidosis bicarbonate is not recommended acutely, even in severe acidaemia with pH < 7.0. However, ketoacids are excreted by osmotic diuresis in preference to chloride, so it may be helpful to include about a fifth of the sodium replacement as bicarbonate given just as slowly as the rest of the fluid. This may avoid hyperchloraemia and tachypnoea after the metabolic disorder is corrected. There is, however, no intravenous fluid preparation available that contains bicarbonate.

Correct hypoglycaemia. If an inborn error of metabolism is suspected give glucose at >8 mg kg^{-1} min^{-1}, correct electrolyte imbalance, and partially correct acidosis with bicarbonate, giving this over at least 1 hour (see above).

Metabolic alkalosis

Metabolic alkalosis may be caused by chronic potassium and/or chloride depletion, e.g. vomiting, especially pyloric stenosis (accompanied by volume depletion) or renal (including diuretic use). It may be compensatory (chronic renal bicarbonate retention) in chronic respiratory failure, in which case it should not be treated. Acute alkalosis causing tetany by lowering plasma ionised calcium should be treated.

After correction of dehydration, chloride deficit is approximately 6 mmol kg^{-1} for every 10 mmol L^{-1} fall in plasma chloride. A suitable fluid for treating alkalaemic patients is 0.9% or 0.45% sodium chloride plus 40 mmol L^{-1} potassium chloride with added glucose. Hypotonic solutions, which may exacerbate hyponatraemia, should not be used. Intravenous hydrochloric acid (or arginine hydrochloride) is indicated in rare severe cases when alkalosis may be depressing respiratory drive, and when the chloride deficit is not accompanied by sodium deficit. Give hydrochloric acid (150 mmol L^{-1} solution) by central intravenous catheter. Give half-correction over at least 1 hour.

$$\text{Dose of HCl for full correction (mmol)} = \text{weight (kg)} \times (\text{plasma bicarbonate [mmol L}^{-1}] - 24) \times 0.5$$

Acidifying diuretics such as acetazolamide may be indicated in metabolic alkalosis where there is sodium and water retention.

Controversies and future directions

❶ There is debate about the use of albumin in sepsis and meningococcal disease.

❷ There is continuing controversy about whether crystalloid or colloid is preferable in paediatric resuscitation, and which colloid, if any.

❸ Hypertonic saline has been advocated in hypovolaemic shock but further research is required.

References

1. Henning R. Fluid resuscitation in children. *Emerg Med. Second Australian Symposium on Fluid Replacement* 1995;57–62.
2. Cullen P. Fluid resuscitation in infants and children. *Curr Anaesth Crit Care* 1996;7:197–205.
3. Tobias JD. Shock in children: The first 60 minutes. *Pediatr Ann* 1996;25:330–8.
4. Saavedra JM, Harris GD, Li S, Finberg L. Capillary refilling (skin turgor) in the assessment of dehydration. *Am J Dis Child* 1991;145:296–8.
5. Gorelick MH, Shaw KN, Baker N. Effect of ambient temperature on capillary refill in healthy children. *Pediatrics* 1993;92:699–702.
6. Mackenzie A, Barnes G, Shann F. Clinical signs of dehydration in children. *Lancet* 1989;ii:605–7.
7. Vega RM, Avner JR. A prospective study of the usefulness of clinical and laboratory parameters for predicting percentage of dehydration in children. *Pediatr Emerg Care* 1997;13:179–82.
8. Burkhart DM. Management of acute gastroenteritis in children. *Am Fam Phys* 1999;60:2555–63.
9. Morgan WM, O'Neill JA. Hemorrhagic and obstructive shock in pediatric patients. *New Horiz* 1998;6:150–4.
10. The SAFE Study Investigators. A comparison of albumin and saline for fluid resuscitation in the Intensive Care Unit. *N Engl J Med* 2004;350:2247–56.
11. Schierhout G, Roberts I. Fluid resuscitation with colloid or crystalloid solutions in critically ill patients: A systematic review of randomised trials. *Br Med J* 1998;316:961–4.
12. Emery EF, Greenhough A, Gamsu HR. Randomised controlled trial of colloid infusions in hypotensive preterm infants. *Arch Dis Child* 1992;67:1185–8.
13. Schexnayder SP. Pediatric septic shock. *Pediatr Rev* 1999;20:303–7.
14. Carcillo JA, Davis AL, Zaritsky A. Role of early fluid resuscitation in pediatric septic shock. *JAMA* 1991;266:1242–5.
15. Goh AYT, Chan PWK, Lum LCS. Sepsis, severe sepsis and septic shock in paediatric multiple organ dysfunction syndrome. *J Paediatr Child Health* 1999;35:488–92.
16. Pollard AJ, Britto J, Nadel S, et al. Emergency management of meningococcal disease. *Arch Dis Child* 1999;80:290–6.
17. Busund R, Straume B, Revhaug A. Fatal course in severe meningococcemia: Clinical predictors and effect of transfusion therapy. *Crit Care Med* 1993;21:1699–705.
18. McClelland B. Human albumin administration in critically ill patients. *Br Med J* 1998;317:882 [letter].
19. Cochrane Injuries Group Albumin Reviewers. Human albumin administration in critically ill patients: Systematic review of randomised controlled trials. *Br Med J* 1998;317:235–40.
20. Nadel S, De Munter C, Britto J, et al. Albumin: Saint or sinner? *Arch Dis Child* 1998;79:384–5.
21. Moyer VA, Elliott EJ. Evidence-based pediatrics: The future is now. *J Pediatr* 2000;136:282–4.
22. Mackenzie A, Barnes G. Randomised controlled trial comparing oral and intravenous rehydration therapy in children with diarrhoea. *Br Med J* 1991;303:393–6.
23. Gremse DA. Effectiveness of nasogastric rehydration in hospitalised children with acute diarrhea. *J Pediatr Gastroenterol Nutr* 1995;21:145–8.
24. Barnes GL. Oral rehydration solutions in gastroenteritis before and after admission to hospital. *J Paediatr Child Health* 1996;32:16–7.
25. Eliason BC, Lewan RB. Gastroenteritis in children: Principles of diagnosis and treatment. *Am Fam Physician* 1998;58:1769–76.
26. Wittenberg DF, Ramji S. Paediatric diarrhoea – rehydration therapy revisited. *S Afr Med J* 1995;85:655–8.
27. Santucci KA, Anderson AC, Lewander WJ, Linakis JG. Frozen oral hydration as an alternative to conventional enteral fluids. *Arch Pediatr Adolesc Med* 1998;152:142–6.
28. Reid SR, Bonadio WA. Outpatient rapid intravenous rehydration to correct dehydration and resolve vomiting in children with acute gastroenteritis. *Ann Emerg Med* 1996;28:318–23.
29. Ng PC, Chan HB, Fok TF, et al. Early onset of hypernatraemic dehydration and fever in exclusively breast fed infants. *J Paediatr Child Health* 1999;35:585–7.
30. Moritz ML, Ayus JC. The changing pattern of hypernatremia in hospitalised children. *Paediatrics* 1999;104:435–9.
31. Dunn K, Butt W. Extreme sodium derangement in a paediatric inpatient population. *J Paediatr Child Health* 1997;33:26–30.

32. Scalea TM, Maltz S, Yelon J, et al. Resuscitation of multiple trauma and head injury: Role of crystalloid fluids and inotropes. *Critl Care Med* 1994;**22**:1610–5.

33. Simma B, Burger R, Falk M, et al. A prospective, randomised, and controlled study of fluid management in children with severe head injury: Lactated Ringer's solution versus hypertonic saline. *Pediatr Crit Care* 1998;**26**:1265–70.

34. Sheikh AA, Matsuoka T, Wisner DH. Cerebral effects of resuscitation with hypertonic saline and a new low sodium hypertonic fluid in hemorrhagic shock and head injury. *Crit Care Med* 1996;**24**:1226–32.

35. Cocks AJ, O'Connell A, Martin H. Crystalloids, colloids and kids: A review of paediatric burns in intensive care. *Burns* 1998;**24**:717–24.

36. Sheridan RD, Prelack MS, Cunningham JJ. Physiological hypoalbuminemia is well tolerated by severely burned children. J Trauma: Injury. *Infect Crit Care* 1997;**43**:448–52.

37. Edge JA. Management of diabetic ketoacidosis in childhood. *Br J Hosp Med* 1996;**55**:508–12.

Further reading

Arieff AI. Postoperative hyponatraemic encephalopathy following elective surgery in children. *Paediatr Anaesth* 1998;**8**:1–4 [editorial].

Arieff AI, Ayus JC. Treatment of symptomatic hyponatremia: Neither haste nor waste. *Crit Care Med* 1991;**19**:748–51 [editorial].

Arieff AI, Ayus JC, Fraser CL. Hyponatremia and death or permanent brain damage in healthy children. *Br Med J* 1992;**304**:1218–22.

Bickell WH, Wall MJ, Pepe PE, et al. Immediate versus delayed fluid resuscitation for hypotensive patients with penetrating torso injuries. *N Engl J Med* 1994;**331**:1105–9.

Bohn D. Problems associated with intravenous fluid administration in children: Do we have the right solution? *Curr Opin Paediatr* 2000;**12**:217–21.

Brown WD, Caruso JM. Extrapontine myelinolysis with involvement of the hippocampus in three children with severe hypernatraemia. *J Child Neurol* 1999;**14**:428–33.

Chan JCM, Gill JR, editors. *Kidney electrolyte disorders*. New York: Churchill Livingstone; 1990.

Coulthard MG, Haycock GB. Distinguishing between salt poisoning and hypernatraemic dehydration in children. *Br Med J* 2003;**326**:157–60.

Doyle JA, Davis DP, Hoyt DB. The use of hypertonic saline in the treatment of traumatic brain injury. *J Trauma* 2001;**50**:367–83.

Duke T, Molyneux EM. Intravenous fluids for seriously ill children: Time to reconsider. *Lancet* 2003;**362**:1320–3.

Feld LG. Hyponatremia in infants and children: A practical approach. *J Nephrol* 1996;**9**:5–9.

Finberg L, Kravath RE, Hellerstein S, editors. *Water and electrolytes in pediatrics. Physiology, pathology and treatment*. 2nd ed. Philadelphia: WB Saunders; 1993.

Fraser CL, Arieff AI. Epidemiology, pathophysiology and management of hyponatremic encephalopathy. *Am J Med* 1997;**102**:67–77 [review].

Gerigk M, Gnehm HPE, Rascher W. Arginine vasopressin and renin in acutely ill children: Implication for fluid therapy. *Acta Paediatr* 1996;**85**:550–3.

Halberthal M, Halperin ML, Bohn D. Acute hyponatremia in children admitted to hospital: Retrospective analysis of factors contributing to its development and resolution. *Br Med J* 2001;**322**:780–2.

Holliday MA, Segar WE. Reducing errors in fluid therapy management. *Pediatrics* 2003;**111**:424–5 [Commentary].

Ichikawa I, Yoshioka T, editors. *Paediatric textbook of fluids and electrolytes*. Baltimore: Williams & Wilkins; 1990.

Kamel KS, Wei C. Controversial issues in the treatment of hyperkalemia. *Nephrol Dial Transpl* 2003;**18**:2215–8.

Kellum JA. Saline-induced hyperchloremic metabolic acidosis. *Crit Care Med* 2002;**30**:259–61.

Kelly A, Moshang T. Disorders of water, sodium and potassium homeostasis. In: Nichols DG, editor. *Rogers' textbook of pediatric intensive care*. Baltimore: Lippincott Williams & Wilkins; 2008, p. 1615–34.

Laureno R, Karp BI. Myelinolysis after correction of hyponatremia. *Ann Intern Med* 1997;**126**:57–62.

McClure RJ, Prasad VK, Brocklebank JT. Treatment of hyperkalemia using intravenous and nebulised salbutamol. *Arch Dis Child* 1994;**70**:126–8.

Meyers A. Fluid and electrolyte therapy for children. *Curr Opin Paediatr* 1994;**6**:303–9.

Myers CT. Minimal volume, hypotense resuscitation. *Emerg Med* 1995;**51**–6. Second Australian Symposium on Fluid Replacement.

Phin SJ, McCaskill ME, Browne GJ, Lam LT. Clinical pathway using rapid rehydration for children with gastroenteritis. *J Paediatr Child Health* 2003;**39**:343–8.

Rodriguez-Soriano J. Potassium homeostasis and its disturbances in children. *Paediatr Nephrol* 1995;**9**:364–74.

Ronco C, Bellomo R, Kellum J, editors. *Critical care nephrology*. Philadelphia: Saunders Elsevier; 2009.

Tuthill DP, Hewson M, Wilson R. Paediatric resuscitation – by phone. *J Paediatr Child Health* 1998;**34**:524–7.

Wilkins B. Fluid therapy in acute paediatrics: A physiological approach. *Curr Paediatr* 1999;**9**:51–6.

HAEMATOLOGY AND ONCOLOGY

11

Section editor *Jeremy Raftos*

11.1 The use of blood products in children

Joseph Ting

ESSENTIALS

1 Blood components are appropriately used when clinical benefits of administration outweigh potential hazards, provided the indication is appropriate. Although blood product administration is relatively safe, potential risks remain.

2 Use specific component(s) appropriate to a clinical problem whenever possible. Determine and document urgency for transfusion, the specific blood product to be administered, quantity and duration of transfusion and special instructions (e.g. premedication).

3 For safe use of blood products, hospitals must have a policy for blood product administration, including the staff responsible, credentialing, documentation, checking and administration procedures such as identity checks. The majority of adverse events result from administrative errors.

4 Blood loss with poor perfusion or/ and haemodynamic derangement requires rapid whole blood or packed red blood cell (PRBC) transfusion while a decision is made regarding the need for definitive haemostasis.

5 Anaemia that does not pose a hypoxic or metabolic risk to the asymptomatic child may not require transfusion; current guidelines use a Hb threshold $<70 \, \mathrm{g \, L^{-1}}$ in critically ill children, although well children without symptoms and/or where alternative therapy is available (e.g. erythropoietin) may tolerate lower levels.

Introduction

Successful and safe transfusion practice depends on administering a quality blood component of the right type, in the right amount, in the right way, at the right time to the right patient.[1]

Blood components should only be given when the expected benefits to the child outweigh the potential hazards. A range of clinical signs and symptoms viewed within the context of a clinical need is essential for the decision to transfuse. Transfusion triggers include both clinical (symptoms,

signs, comorbidities) and laboratory indications; benefit–risk of blood product use requires careful consideration. In the setting of massive haemorrhage whole blood could be used. Otherwise, there is no indication for the use of whole blood when specific component(s) appropriate to a clinical problem are available.

Emphasis on blood component safety, standardisation of appropriate guidelines for use of blood components and informed consent for blood component administration have led to a substantial reduction in the potential risks and complications of their use as well as increasing their appropriate usage. Informed consent with regards to the risks and benefits of blood component therapy needs to be obtained in the light of community concerns about transfusion safety, particularly the potential for infection transmission. The indication, risks, benefits, alternatives to transfusion, parental consent, response to treatment and any adverse event should be clearly documented. In non-urgent situations, parents and mature children can access publications such as 'Children receiving a blood transfusion: A parents' guide'[2] for more information.

Clinical guidelines for use of red blood cells (RBC) in children are consensus rather than evidence based,[3] with the latest National Health and Medical Research Council/ Australian Society of Blood Transfusion

Australian practice guidelines for blood product indication and administration available at www.nhmrc.gov.au, including haemoglobin (Hb) and platelet transfusion threshold triggers.[1] It is recommended that intravenous (IV) access be 22–24G or larger for children receiving blood products through a standard blood administration set primed with normal saline or the blood component. A blood warmer is indicated at flow rates >15 ml kg^{-1} hr^{-1} in children and for exchange transfusion in infants; very slow rates are recommended in small children if rapid volume expansion is not required. Blood products should not be warmed to above 41°C.[4]

The rate of administration should not be >5 mL min^{-1} in the first 15 minutes as severe reactions are most likely to occur then; all blood components should be infused within 4 hours unless fluid overload is a risk. The child and infusion need to be monitored during blood product administration, more closely if unconscious or anaesthetised. A severe reaction requires suspension of blood product administration pending further incompatibility or bacterial contamination checks, consideration of antihistamines/steroids, and be reported to the Australian Incident Monitoring System in Australia or the New Zealand Blood Service.

Whole blood

Whole blood is rarely used, being specifically used for massive blood loss requiring simultaneous restoration of oxygen-carrying capacity and blood volume, haemorrhage with uncontrolled coagulopathy and exchange transfusion. Eight ml kg^{-1} will increase a child's haemoglobin concentration by 10 g/dL^{-1}, and administration must be completed within 4 hours to avoid bacterial contamination.

Packed red blood cells (PRBC)

Indications

The child's Hb level, patient factors, signs and symptoms of hypoxia, ongoing blood loss, risk of anaemia and risk of transfusion should be considered. Each paediatric red cell unit is 25–100 mL (mean volume 50 mL) with a haemoglobin concentration of 100–150 g L^{-1}. PRBC is indicated if the oxygen-carrying capacity of blood is so reduced that the degree of anaemia poses a risk to the child or there is ongoing blood loss. Transfusion of PRBC in an asymptomatic child is not appropriate in most situations. PRBC transfusion is likely to be appropriate when haemoglobin is less than 70 g L^{-1} in critically ill children.[5] The haemoglobin threshold remains uncertain in stable children with anaemia. Use of PRBC with haemoglobin in the range 70–100 g L^{-1} is appropriate if the child is at risk of hypoxia (cardiac, respiratory disease) and should be supported by the need to relieve clinical symptoms and signs. Criteria for PRBC in patients aged less than 4 months are different from those for older children. Infants in the former group have smaller blood volumes, decreased erythropoietin production (especially if premature) and there may be physiological anaemia of infancy.

Additional indications for PRBC include:

- emergency surgery in a child with significant preoperative anaemia;
- anaemia related to chemotherapy or radiotherapy;
- sickle cell disease with ischaemic organ events to suppress endogenous Hb production;
- Chronic congenital or acquired anaemia such as B-thalassaemia.

Administration

If stored in optimal conditions, RBC have a shelf life of 35–42 days. In haemorrhagic shock, RBC infusion at an initial volume of 10–20 mL kg^{-1} should be considered when loss of blood volume approaches 30% (when hypotension first appears)[3] and shock is refractory to non-blood fluid resuscitation. A single Hb level is not reliable in acute haemorrhage.[3] If haemorrhage or haemolysis is accompanied by life-threatening hypoxia or rapid Hb decline then uncrossmatched group O rhesus negative packed cells may be required. In less urgent cases, type-specific or cross-matched RBC is preferred. Rh type specific blood takes 15 minutes to cross match. If the child has no immediate need for RBC replacement and there is no ongoing bleeding or haemodynamic instability, cross-matched RBC may be administered over 4 hours. The volume required for elective top-up transfusion in mL is:

$$\text{Weight (kg)} \times \text{haemoglobin rise required (gL}^{-1}) \times 3$$

Alternatives

Autologous blood (patient's own blood is collected before surgery) is suitable for elective surgery but has no role in urgent situations. Perioperative blood scavenging may be useful in reducing exposure to donor blood. Red cell substitutes such as cell-free haemoglobins and perfluorocarbon emulsions require 100% oxygen to be effective and are still being trialled.

Adverse reactions

Fatal acute haemolytic reactions occur in 1:250 000–1:1 000 000 transfusions, with half caused by ABO incompatibility as a result of mismatching the blood with the patient or other administrative errors. Another 1:260 000 patients have a haemolytic reaction due to minor red-cell antigen incompatibility and 1:1000 patients experience delayed haemolytic reactions.

Platelets

Indications

Platelets are appropriate in bleeding children in whom thrombocytopenia is a major contributory factor. In haemorrhagic shock, platelet infusion should be considered in massive transfusion associated with platelet count less than 50×10^9 L^{-1}. Platelet transfusion may be appropriate in children with failure of platelet production and platelet count less than 10×10^9 L^{-1}, as there is a risk of intracerebral bleeding. Platelets may be given prophylactically in children undergoing invasive procedures or surgery, to maintain platelet count $>50 \times 10^9$ L^{-1}. In children with platelet dysfunction (inherited or acquired), platelets are administered to treat active bleeding. Platelets are indicated in thrombocytopenic premature infants with active bleeding or prior to an invasive procedure.

Administration

Each paediatric unit is 40–70 mL and contains at least 5.5×10^{10} platelets.

Infusion of 5–10 mL kg^{-1} of platelets will lead to a rise in platelet count of 50–100 × 10^9 L^{-1}.

Adverse reactions and other problems

Platelets are stored at room temperature to maintain their ability to aggregate, and this promotes bacterial growth. Compared with other blood components, the risk of bacterial contamination of platelets is relatively high at 1:2000 units and sepsis is the most frequent severe complication of platelet use. Platelets older than 5 days lose their ability to aggregate and are therefore less effective. Alloimmunisation due to the development of platelet alloantibodies from repeated transfusions may lead to refractory thrombocytopenia.

Fresh frozen plasma (FFP)

FFP contains all coagulation factors, except VII, including approximately 150 units of factor VIII. FFP is used to treat bleeding related to coagulopathy associated with cardiac surgery or massive transfusion for haemorrhagic shock when 50% or more of circulating blood volume has been replaced. FFP may be considered for treatment of acute disseminated intravascular coagulation (DIC) and thrombotic thrombocytopenic purpura (TTP). Less urgent indications include children with coagulopathy undergoing invasive procedures/surgery, liver disease-related coagulopathy, replacement of single coagulation factor deficiency where a specific factor concentrate is not available, and reversal of life-threatening bleeding due to warfarin. FFP should not be used for volume expansion, plasma-exchange procedures or treatment of immunodeficiency states. Specific recombinant coagulation factors rather than FFP are used to treat specific inherited coagulation disorders.

Administration

In life-threatening exsanguination requiring massive transfusion, FFP may be required to minimise dilutional coagulopathy. One unit of FFP is required for every four units of packed cells but titrate FFP use against the coagulation profile if possible. FFP contains all coagulation factors including approximately one unit of factors VIII and V

for each mL of FFP. FFP is administered at an initial dose of 10–20 mL kg^{-1} from a 50 mL paediatric bag. This dose raises coagulation factor level by 20% immediately.[3] After thawing, FFP needs to be used immediately or stored at 2–6°C for up to 24 hours.

Cryoprecipitate

Cryoprecipitate is appropriate to use when clinical or potential bleeding (invasive procedure, trauma or DIC) is attributable to fibrinogen deficiency.[3] It contains factors VIII, XIII, fibrinogen, von Willebrand's factor and fibronectin. Approximately 200 units of each of these factors are contained in a 15 mL bag. This allows more rapid administration than FFP, whilst reducing the risk of fluid overload. In infants, a dose of 10–15 mL is sufficient to achieve haemostasis. Cryoprecipitate is not used to treat von Willebrand's disease, haemophilia and deficiencies of factor XIII or fibronectin.

Clotting factor concentrates

Bleeding or thrombosis in children with proven coagulation or antithrombotic factor deficiency may require specific factor replacement. These factors have become safer with the advent of synthesis using recombinant genetic technology. Recombinant factor VIII concentrate is used to treat haemophilia A whereas recombinant factor IX is the treatment of choice for haemophilia B. Antithrombin III, protein S and protein C concentrates are used to treat patients with these specific factor deficiencies.

Albumin

Indications

Albumin is derived from volunteer human plasma pools and is indicated for rapid volume expansion in children with evidence of shock or poor perfusion. In paediatric emergency practice, albumin may be used in the initial fluid resuscitation for hypovolaemic shock, although it is no better than crystalloids or other colloids in this setting in adults.[3] Other indications include the treatment of hypoproteinaemia, diuretic-resistant nephrotic syndrome, large

volume paracentesis, severe burns after the first 24 hours and plasma exchange. There is no evidence for albumin use as a nutritional supplement or for the treatment of ascites or oedema related to portal hypertension.

Administration

Albumin 4% (40 g L^{-1}) at 10–20 mL kg^{-1} is used for volume expansion. Albumin 20% (200 g L^{-1}) is used for plasma albumin repletion on a gram-for-gram basis.

Adverse effects and risks

There is evidence that albumin is associated with increased mortality and morbidity in critically-ill adults,[6] but no such evidence in young children. Complications of albumin use include circulatory and sodium overload, with the relative risk of viral disease transmission being less compared with cellular blood components.

Normal human immunoglobulin (NIGH)

Human immunoglobulin affords passive immunity against many infectious agents for several weeks. NIGH is derived by Cohn fractionation from pooled plasma and contains antibodies to viruses that are prevalent in the general population. Subclasses are present in the approximate proportions G1 60%, G2 30%, G3 6% and G4 4% but there is no such thing as generic IgG. The 'new' purified commercial products are all a little different, with different minor reaction rates. NIGH is administered IM for pre- or post-exposure prophylaxis against measles, varicella zoster and hepatitis A. IV NIGH (either Intragam or Sandoglobulin) is used to treat idiopathic thrombocytopenic purpura (ITP), Kawasaki's disease, perinatal acquired immune deficiency syndrome, Guillain–Barré syndrome, demyelinating disease, immunological disorders associated with antibody deficiency (such as primary hypogammaglobulinaemia) and sepsis with secondary immunodeficiency. Allergic reactions and, rarely, anaphylaxis may occur. NIGH is contraindicated in children with selective IgA deficiency and evidence for its role in the treatment and prevention of neonatal sepsis is conflicting. Immune response to live virus vaccines (with the exception of yellow fever vaccine) may be inhibited by NIGH given 3 weeks before or 3 months after immunisation.

Hyperimmune immunoglobulins (IG)

Maternal administration of Rhesus (Rh) Ig prevents the development of Rh antibodies in a Rh-negative mother who gives birth to a Rh-positive baby. This reduces the risk of maternal Rh sensitisation and maternal-neonatal Rh-incompatibility in subsequent pregnancies. Cytomegalovirus (CMV) Ig is used in the prevention and treatment of CMV in children at risk of adverse sequelae from CMV infection, such as with immuno-deficiency and following renal and bone-marrow transplantation. Zoster Ig (ZIG) is advisable within 72 hours after varicella exposure in children with cellular immune deficiency, immunosuppression, neonates whose mothers are susceptible to primary varicella infection and infants who are less than 28 weeks' gestation at birth. Infants born to HbsAg-positive mothers should receive hepatitis B Ig and commence pri-mary hepatitis B vaccination within 12 hours of birth. Respiratory syncytial virus (RSV) Ig is used prophylactically in infants at high risk of severe RSV infection, including those with bronchopulmonary dysplasia. Tetanus Ig passively protects non-tetanus immune children who sustain a tetanus-prone wound and a tetanus Ig infusion is used to treat clinical disease.

Risks of blood component use

These are categorised as acute or delayed, haemolytic or non-haemolytic, allergy-based or not. Mild non-haemolytic febrile reactions can occur with any blood component and need to be distinguished from major reactions. If a major reaction occurs, the transfusion is discontinued and threats to the airway, breathing and circulation are attended to. Specific treatment for anaphy-laxis, sepsis and blood group incompatibility may be required, in consultation with a haematologist. Recipient and donor blood samples are sent for immunological and microbiological testing. Critical adverse inci-dents should be notified to the blood bank

and followed up as a quality assurance activity with appropriate adjustments made to hospital transfusion protocols to reduce risk of recurrence.

Infections

Even though blood components are the safest they have ever been, infection trans-mission risk remains emotive and highly publicised, especially for human immunode-ficiency virus (HIV).[7] Infection acquired from a blood component is a rare occurrence when compared with non-infectious compli-cations. The estimated risks per actual blood unit transfused are 1:200 000–1:2 000 000 for HIV, 1:30 000–1:250 000 for hepatitis B and 1:30 000–1:150 000 for hepatitis C. Disease transmission occurs primarily during the window period when a blood donor is infectious and the infection is immunologi-cally silent and therefore undetectable on screening tests. Other infectious agents encountered include hepatitis A and G, human T lymphotropic virus 1 (HTLV I) and II, parvovirus B19, syphilis, malaria, babesiosis, *Salmonella* and *Trypanosoma cruzi*. There is no current evidence to sug-gest that variant Creutzfeldt–Jakob disease can be transmitted by blood transfusion. Donor selection and exclusion, donated blood screening, post-collection leucodeple-tion and viral inactivation help to minimise risk of infection transmission. Using pooled blood components allows contamination of the entire pool from one infectious donor and is therefore less safe than components derived from a single donor. Bacterial con-tamination of blood components, either from prolonged/faulty storage or acquired from the donor, is most frequently due to occult donor bacteraemia and donor skin organisms. *Yersinia enterocolitica* and other Gram negatives are most frequently implicated.

Transfusion-related acute lung injury (TRALI)

Acute respiratory distress syndrome with non-cardiogenic pulmonary oedema occurs within 4 hours in 1:5000 transfusions, with 90% of patients recovering. This reaction may be difficult to distinguish from fluid overload and is related to immune-mediated increased pulmonary capillary permeability.

Transfusion-mediated immunomodulation

Allosensitisation, disturbed immunomodu-lation (both due to contamination by donor leucocytes) as well as infection transmission may be reduced by leucocy-todepletion, psoralens and UV irradiation of blood components and using non-pooled blood components from a single donor. Immunomodulation is related to decreased cell-mediated immunity, with increased risk of reactivated viral infec-tion, solid tumour recurrence and post-operative sepsis.[8]

Transfusion-associated graft-versus-host disease (TA-GVHD)

This occurs as a result of transfused lym-phocytes engrafting and proliferating in the transfusion recipient. TA-GVHD is fatal in 90% of cases because of induc-tion of marrow hypoplasia. Irradiation of cellular blood components is effective prevention.

Other transfusion-related adverse reactions

These include donor-recipient incompati-bility, allergic reactions, anaphylaxis or anaphylactoid reactions, circulatory over-load, haemolysis (acute/chronic, intra-/extravascular, associated fever/no fever), complications associated with massive trans-fusion (hypothermia, dilutional coagulopathy and thrombocytopenia) and post-transfusion thrombocytopenia.[7]

Controversies and future directions

❶ The threshold for red cell transfusion at which benefits outweigh risk in stable children and non-critically ill adults remains unclear.

❷ The role and potential harm of albumin in adult resuscitation has not been investigated in paediatric resuscitation and the role of immunoglobulins in severe sepsis remains uncertain.

❸ Oxygen-carrying red cell substitutes such as modified haemoglobins and perfluorocarbon emulsions may offer the same benefits as red blood cells without the infection–transmission risk, but are not in clinical use at present.

❹ The role of non-blood alternatives such as autologous blood donation, perioperative blood salvage and directed parental transfusion is not clearly defined in children.

References

1. National Health and Medical Research Council/ Australian Society of Blood Transfusion. *Topics in Transfusion Medicine*. Available from: http://www.anzsbt.org.au/publications/TTM.cfm [accessed 19.10.10].
2. National Health and Medical Research Council/ Australian Society of Blood Transfusion. *Children receiving a blood transfusion: A parents' guide*. Available from:www.nhmrc.gov.au; and www.anzsbt.org.au [accessed 19.10.10].
3. Robitaille N, Hume HA. Blood products and fractionated plasma products: preparation, indications and administration. In: Arceci RJ, Hann IM, Smith OP, editors. *Pediatric Hematology*. 3rd ed. London: Blackwell Publishing Ltd; 2006. p. 693–723.
4. National Health and Medical Research Council/Australian Society of Blood Transfusion. *Guidelines for appropriate use of blood and blood components/Guidelines for the administration of blood components*. 2004. Available from: www.nhmrc.gov.au; and www.anzsbt.org.au [accessed 19.10.10].
5. Canadian Critical Care Trials Group; Pediatric Acute Lung Injury and Sepsis Investigators Network. Transfusion strategies for patients in pediatric intensive care units. *New Engl J Med* 2007;**356**:1609–19.
6. SAFE Study Investigators, Finfer S, Bellomo R, McEvoy S, et al. Effect of baseline serum albumin concentration on outcome of resuscitation with albumin or saline in patients in intensive care units: analysis of data from the saline versus albumin fluid evaluation (SAFE) study. *BMJ* 2006;**333**(7577):1044. Epub 2006 Oct 13.
7. Luban NLC, Wong ECC. Hazards of transfusion. In: Arceci RJ, Hann IM, Smith OP, editors. *Pediatric Hematology*. 3rd ed. London: Blackwell Publishing Ltd.; 2006. p. 724–44.
8. Goodnough LT, Shander A, Brecher RE. Transfusion medicine: Looking to the future. *Lancet* 2003;**361**: 161–9.

Further reading

American Association of Blood Banks. *Facts about blood and blood banking*. Availalble from http://www.aabb.org; 2003 [accessed 19.10.10].
Behrman RE, Kleigman RM. Intercontinental childhood ITP registry. In: *Nelson essentials of pediatrics*. 4th ed. Philadelphia: WB Saunders; 2002.
Christensen RD. *Hematologic problems of the neonate*. Philadelphia: WB Saunders Company; 2000.
Goodnough LT, Brecher ME, Kanter MH, AuBuchon JP. Transfusion medicine. Blood transfusion. *N Engl J Med* 1999;**340**:438–47.
Kruskall MS. The perils of platelet transfusions. *N Engl J Med* 1997;**337**:1914–5.
Miller DR, Bachner RL. *Blood diseases of infancy and childhood. In the tradition of Carl H Smith. Mosby-Year Book*. 7th ed. St Louis, MO: Mosby; 1995.
Regan F, Taylor C. Recent developments. Blood transfusion medicine. *Br Med J* 2002;**325**:143–7.
Sadowitz PD, Ammanullah S, Souid AK, et al. Hematologic emergencies in the pediatric ER. *Emerg Med Clin N Am* 2002;**20**:177–88, vii.
Smith H 1996 *Diagnosis in paediatric haematology*. New York: Churchill Livingstone.
Stainsby D, Jones H, Asher D, et al. Serious hazards of transfusion: a decade of hemovigilance in the UK. *Transfus Med Rev* 2006;**20**(4):273–82.

11.2 Anaemia

Jane Cocks

ESSENTIALS

1 The normal haemoglobin concentration and type is age and sex dependent.

2 Clinical effects of anaemia depend on the timing of its development, the magnitude of the anaemia and the underlying cause.

3 Iron-deficiency anaemia is the commonest cause of microcytic and hypochromic anaemia.

4 Autoimmune haemolytic anaemia (AIHA) is commonly caused by a variety of infective agents, although it can be triggered by a number of medications and systemic illnesses.

5 Non-immune haemolytic anaemia can be due to infective agents, medications and chemical exposures.

6 Haemolytic uraemic syndrome (HUS) is the commonest cause of acute renal failure in children, most frequently secondary to infection with *E. coli*.

7 Thrombotic thrombocytopenic purpura affects children over the age of 10 years. The clinical features are similar to HUS with the addition of neurological deficit.

8 G6PD deficiency is an X-linked enzymatic inborn error in which haemolysis is triggered by exposure to an oxidant.

9 Thalassaemia is a relatively common inherited defect in the synthesis of the globin chain.

10 Sickle cell disease is an autosomal recessive inherited condition with a globin chain that is unstable in the deoxygenated state, leading to haemolysis.

Introduction

Anaemia is defined as a reduction in the red blood cell (RBC) volume or haemo-globin concentration below normal values. The normal haemoglobin level is age and sex dependent, and racial differences exist. At birth, the haemoglobin level is 159–191 g L^{-1} and this falls to a trough level of 90–114 g L^{-1} between 8 and 12 weeks of age before rising again toward normal adult range.

Red blood cell production is regulated by erythropoietin, a hormone produced initially in the fetal liver and, after birth, in the renal peritubular cells. In normal erythropoiesis, erythropoietin stimulates differentiation of marrow stem cells into red blood cells. During this process there is a condensation of the cell's nuclear material with continual production of the hae-moglobin until it comprises 90% of the mass of the RBC. The nucleus is then extruded, leaving the RBC with no synthetic or replication ability, leading to a limited RBC lifespan of 120 days.

Haemoglobin is the major functional con-stituent of the RBC responsible for the task of carrying oxygen to the tissues, with the RBC acting as the carrier through the cardiovascular system. Haemoglobin is a complex protein consisting of iron-containing haem groups and polypeptide chains, known as globin. The haemoglobin molecule is made up of two pairs of polypeptide chains each coupled with a haem group. Chemical variations in the polypeptide chains lead to different types of haemoglobin being produced. At various stages of life, from the embryo to the adult, there are six different types of haemoglobin normally detectable. The normal adult haemoglobin, HbA, is comprised of two α-polypeptide chains and two β-chains, $(\alpha_2\beta_2)$. Haemoglobin F, or fetal Hb (HbF), is comprised of two α-chains and two γ-chains, $(\alpha_2\gamma_2)$ and constitutes 70% of the haemoglobin present at birth, reducing to trace levels by 6–12 months of age. Minor amounts of HbA2 $(\alpha_2\delta_2)$ are present at all ages. Pathological variations in the polypeptide chains can produce disease states, known as haemoglobinopathies (see below).

Anaemia is not a single disease, but may occur as a result of a variety of pathological processes. The anaemias of childhood can be usefully divided into two groups: (1) those caused by inadequate production of RBC or haemoglobin; and (2) those due to increased destruction or loss of RBC. Tables 11.2.1 and 11.2.2 outline the major causes of childhood and neonatal anaemias.

Overview

The principles of management of anaemia in the emergency department (ED) are:

❶ Resuscitate the patient with circulatory collapse.
❷ Remove or treat the precipitant if known.
❸ Treat the cause if treatment can be initiated in the ED.

Causes of *life-threatening anaemia* include uncontrolled haemorrhage, acute intravascular haemolysis in glucose-6-phosphatase deficiency (G6PD) or autoimmune haemolytic anaemia (AIHA), sequestration crisis in sickle cell disease (SCD) and acute decompensation in chronic anaemia.

Initial assessment is directed at respiration and circulation. The anaemic patient may be tachypnoeic with tissue hypoxia.

Table 11.2.1 Causes of childhood anaemia

Production defect

1. Primary bone marrow failure
   - Aplastic anaemia (congenital or acquired)
   - Diamond-Blackfan syndrome
   - Transient erythroblastopenia of childhood (TEC)
2. Erythropoietin production problem
   - Chronic renal disease
   - Hypothyroidism
3. Abnormal cytoplasmic maturation (microcytic anaemias)
   - Iron deficiency
   - Sideroblastic anaemia (congenital or acquired)
   - Lead toxicity
   - Thalassaemia syndrome
4. Megaloblastic anaemia
   - Vitamin B_{12} deficiency
   - Folate deficiency
   - Thiamine-responsive megaloblastic anaemia
   - Orotic aciduria (rare, associated with megaloblastic anaemia)
5. Others
   - Primary dyserythropoietic anaemias
   - Erythropoietic protoporphyria
   - Marrow infiltration, e.g. malignancy or myelofibrosis

Decreased RBC survival

1. Hereditary haemolytic anaemias
   a. Haemoglobin variants
      - Thalassaemias
      - Sickle cell disease
   b. Abnormal RBC membranes
      - Hereditary spherocytosis
      - Hereditary elliptocytosis
      - Hereditary stomatocytosis
   c. Abnormal enzymes
      - Glucose-6-phosphatase dehydrogenase deficiency (G6PD)
      - Pyruvate kinase deficiency
2. Acquired haemolytic anaemias
   a. Autoimmune haemolytic anaemia (AIHA)
   b. Non-immune haemolytic anaemia
   c. Fragmentation haemolysis
      - Haemolytic uraemic syndrome (HUS)
3. Haemorrhage
   - Traumatic
   - Non-traumatic – acute or chronic

Table 11.2.2 Causes of anaemia in the neonate

1. Physiological anaemia
2. Abnormal RBC production
   a. Nutritional deficiency
   b. Secondary to infection
3. Decreased RBC survival – blood loss
   a. Overt blood loss
      - Iatrogenic during delivery
      - Obstetric accidents
   b. Occult blood loss
      - Twin-to-twin transfusion
      - Fetoplacental haemorrhage
      - Fetomaternal haemorrhage
4. Decreased RBC survival – haemolysis
   a. Immune-related: isoimmunisation
   b. Infection-related
   c. Hereditary haemoglobin variants, enzyme abnormalities, membrane abnormalities

---

The adequacy of ventilation should be ascertained and supplemental oxygen provided. Circulatory compromise in acute haemorrhage and acute haemolysis requires cardiorespiratory monitoring and intravenous access for fluid resuscitation (see Chapter 2.5 on shock). Packed red blood cells are used if haemorrhage or haemolysis is life threatening. If tissue oxygenation is not critically affected, the circulatory volume should be sustained with colloid or crystalloid until group-specific or cross-matched RBCs are available. If the bleeding is controlled, with further bleeding unlikely, the signs mentioned above are stable and the haemoglobin concentration is greater than $70\,g\,L^{-1}$, a cross-match should be performed and the packed RBCs should be held in reserve for 24 hours. Early consultation with a haematologist is important in acute haemolytic anaemia especially if the underlying cause has not been diagnosed.

Anaemia is a clinical finding rather than a disease in its own right and symptoms depend on the timing of its development, the severity and the underlying cause. The presentation is frequently not specific to anaemia. Common presenting features consistent with insidious onset anaemia include:

- lethargy, irritability, sleep or settling difficulty;
- pallor or yellow skin hue;
- loss of appetite ± weight loss ± pica;
- bruising, bleeding or infection.

Patient factors to note are age, ethnicity and the presence of other significant disease. Iron-deficiency anaemia is uncommon in the first 6 months in term infants and sickle cell disease (SCD) is unlikely to present as anaemia under the age of 4 months. Haemolytic uraemic syndrome (HUS) mainly affects those under 4 years of age, whereas thrombotic thrombocytopenic purpura (TTP) affects children from 10 years of age. Iron deficiency is common in adolescent females, whereas G6PD deficiency occurs mainly in males. The association between ethnicity and various types of hereditary anaemia is shown in Table 11.2.3. Family history of anaemia may also suggest hereditary anaemia.

Dietary history can provide important clues. Iron-deficiency anaemia is likely in prolonged breast-feeding beyond 6 months of age in term infants and sooner in preterm infants if no iron supplementation is

Table 11.2.3 Ethnicity and anaemia

1. Thalassaemia syndromes
   - α-Thalassaemia – descendants from China, Malaysia, Indonesia and Africa
   - β-Thalassaemia – descendants from Africa, Middle East, Mediterranean, India, Pakistan, China
2. Sickle cell disease
   - Descendants from Africa, southern Arabia, Turkey, Greece, central India
3. Hereditary spherocytosis
   - Descendants from northern Europe
4. G6PD deficiency
   - Descendants from Africa, China, southeast Asia and the Mediterranean

provided, if there is excessive dependence on cows' milk as a food source or if food sources are restricted, e.g. food fads. Ingestion of clay and dirt may cause lead toxicity and iron deficiency. Ingestion of fresh uncooked broad beans is a potent precipitant of haemolysis in G6PD deficiency, along with medications.

Recent infections may precipitate AIHA, non-immune haemolytic anaemia, HUS and TTP. Hyperbilirubinaemia caused by haemolysis leads to jaundice, cholelithiasis, cholecystitis and dark urine. Mechanical destruction of RBCs is caused by vascular malformations, shunts, abnormal native or prosthetic cardiac valves. Septic shock, bleeding disorders, chronic renal disease, severe burns and hypothyroidism may all cause anaemia.

The salient physical findings in the context of anaemia relate to general appearance, cardiovascular status and abdominal examination. Frontal bone expansion and frontal bossing is due to expansion of the medullary spaces and may be seen in severe thalassaemias. Some hereditary anaemias may also have associated physical abnormalities (e.g. Diamond–Blackfan anaemia). Hepatosplenomegaly is a feature of some of the hereditary haemolytic anaemias. Purpuric or petechial rashes are due to coagulation disorders or vasculitis. Dark urine from bilirubinuria is consistent with haemolysis. Haematuria must be confirmed by microscopy to distinguish haemoglobinuria from haematuria.

Anaemia is confirmed by the lowered haemoglobin concentration and decreased RBC count. An age-related reference range must be used. Abnormalities in the other cell lines should be noted. The mean cell volume

(MCV) may suggest an underlying cause. The upper limit of normal in adults is 96 fL but MCV in children is less than in adults and average values may be estimated by adding 0.6 fL per year of age to 84 fl. The reticulocyte count is expressed as a percentage of the circulating RBC mass with a normal range of 0.5–1.5%. A low reticulocyte count is found in abnormalities of RBC production and a high reticulocyte count is found in increased destruction or from RBC loss, provided there is no concurrent bone-marrow pathology. Morphological features of RBC may be diagnostic of the underlying cause as shown in Table 11.2.4.

There are many additional investigations apart from full blood count to assist in identification of the underlying cause. Some that are undertaken in the ED include:

- bilirubin – elevated unconjugated bilirubin suggests haemolysis;
- urea and creatinine to detect renal failure in HUS and TTP;
- iron studies (serum iron, total iron binding capacity, transferrin saturation);
- Coombs' tests to identify immune-related haemolysis;
- haemoglobin electrophoresis.

Identification and treatment of the underlying precipitant, where appropriate and possible, is a crucial part of the management of anaemia in the ED. Packed RBCs are indicated in the treatment of severe anaemia with cardiovascular compromise. A dose of 4 mL kg^{-1} of packed RBCs raises haemoglobin concentration by 10 g L^{-1}. This dose can be given hourly or more slowly in the presence of cardiac failure. Furosemide 1 mg kg^{-1} may be given if there is evidence of volume overload. Involvement of a paediatric haematologist is recommended for all but the simple nutritional anaemias.

Table 11.2.4 Morphological features of RBCs to assist the diagnosis of anaemia

Schistocytes	Erythrocyte fragmentation syndromes
Sickle cells	Sickle cell disease
Spherocytes	Immune-meditated haemolytic anaemia Hereditary spherocytosis
Blister or bite cells with poikilocytosis	G6P deficiency

NEONATAL ANAEMIA

In the term neonate, the haemoglobin at birth is in the range of 159–191 g L^{-1} and rises in the first 24 hours. Subsequently it falls to a trough level of 90–114 g L^{-1} between 8 and 12 weeks of age. This decline is generally referred to as physiological anaemia of infancy, although it is an expected normal occurrence. The falling haemoglobin is due to a combination of rapid weight gain and blood volume expansion leading to relative haemodilution in the first 3 months of life, combined with a comparatively shorter life span of the fetal RBC and a sharp decline in erythropoiesis a few days after birth due to increased arterial oxygenation and a reduction in the production of erythropoietin. Following the nadir in Hb, erythropoiesis recommences and the Hb rises again.

Immune-related

Immune-related haemolysis is the commonest cause of anaemia in the neonate. Maternal antibodies pass through the placenta leading to fetal cell lysis. Haemolysis occurs when the target cells are the fetal RBCs. The commonest antigen responsible is the Rhesus antigen on the RBC surface, followed by ABO incompatibility. Sensitisation of the mother occurs when Rhesus incompatible fetal cells gain access to the maternal circulation. Fetal RBCs can be found from 8 weeks' gestation onwards. As little as 0.05–0.10 mL is enough to cause primary sensitisation but the volume and risk increases with obstetric procedures, miscarriages and toxaemia. Fetal harm occurs during subsequent pregnancies with a Rhesus positive fetus in a Rhesus negative mother. The resultant intravascular haemolysis in the fetus can be devastating. The clinical significance is due both to the severity of the anaemia and kernicterus from the hyperbilirubinaemia. ABO incompatibility produces less severe jaundice and anaemia during the second week of life.

Prevention relies on identification of the Rhesus status of all pregnant women. This is an essential task for any doctor involved in antenatal care. Prophylaxis therapy using anti-D immunoglobulin (Ig) is given to all Rhesus negative women with per vaginal bleeding or requiring any obstetric procedures that may lead to fetomaternal haemorrhage. The recommended dose is 250 IU if the sensitising event occurs in the first trimester and 625 IU beyond this gestation period. This passive immunisation is given intramuscularly. If required in the postpartum period the immunoglobulin is administered intravenously.

Neonatal infection

Infections cause anaemia by producing bone-marrow suppression of erythropoiesis or by haemolysis. The infections of relevance in the neonate are cytomegalovirus (CMV), rubella, toxoplasmosis and congenital syphilis. The human parvovirus may lead to spontaneous miscarriage in early pregnancy and, in late pregnancy, can selectively depress erythropoiesis, producing severe fetal anaemia. In the older child, parvovirus is the cause of Erythema Infectiosum (Fifth Disease), which can be complicated by aplastic crisis or chronic haemolysis. Vertical transmission of malaria to the fetus is a major cause of anaemia in the neonate in endemic regions. Human immunodeficiency virus (HIV) infection in the neonate is predominantly acquired via perinatal transmission from the mother. The transmission rate is in the range of 20–40%. The mechanism for subsequent anaemia is bone-marrow suppression and associated pancytopenia as well as chronic multisystem disease.

Haemoglobinopathies and enzymopathies

G6PD deficiency is an important global cause of neonatal jaundice. Haemolysis from other enzymopathies and haemoglobin variants, such as thalassaemias and SCD, is usually unmasked beyond the neonatal period when the proportion of fetal haemoglobin falls. It is important to consider congenital causes of anaemia in children with a family history of hereditary anaemia or persisting neonatal jaundice.

Blood loss

Blood loss may arise from twin-to-twin transfusion, or obstetric procedures, or as part of the delivery of the neonate in the perinatal period. Haemorrhage from an underlying haematological disorder must be considered. Vitamin K deficiency is normally present at birth but only a minority of neonates develop generalised bleeding. Breast milk has a small amount of vitamin K and, in the breast-fed baby, maternal medications such as warfarin, phenytoin, rifampicin and isoniazid, may compound the deficiency. Nutritional vitamin K deficiency has been associated with prolonged breast-feeding without supplementation, malabsorption, chronic diarrhoea, and prolonged use of oral antibiotics. Vitamin K prophylaxis is normally given at birth. Haemophilia can rarely lead to spontaneous haemorrhage in the newborn.

ANAEMIAS OF CHILDHOOD

Iron-deficiency

Iron deficiency is uncommon in the first 6 months in the term infant due to the efficient recycling of the iron from the haem component of haemoglobin when it is metabolised. In the preterm and low-birth-weight neonate, iron deficiency occurs earlier, often at the time of doubling of the birth weight. In the second 6 months of life, iron deficiency is found in 20% of Australian children, with associated anaemia in 3%. The respective figures in the second year are 35% and 9%. It is even more common in indigenous children and children from non-English-speaking backgrounds. In school-age children, iron deficiency is present in 1–2% but is found in up to 9% of adolescent girls.

Stages

The first stage of iron deficiency is a low serum ferritin level. Iron-dependent body functions, including erythropoiesis, are affected in stage two. Microcytes and an elevated erythrocyte protoporphyrin level are detectable and the serum iron falls. The third stage is the presence of a microcytic hypochromic anaemia.

Causes

The commonest cause globally is insufficient intake of dietary iron. In developing countries, the two most significant factors are the failure to obtain iron-rich nutrients and malabsorption from intestinal pathology. The aetiology is different in developed countries, such as Australia, where prolonged breast-feeding beyond 6 months of age without supplementation with iron-rich foods is a common finding. Breast milk has easily absorbable iron in modest amounts. The quantity is inadequate for the rapid growth in the second 6 months. Cows' milk has minimal iron content, which exists in a poorly absorbable form and is not recommended under the age of 12 months. Cows' milk can cause gastrointestinal bleeding in the immature gut and children who have an excess intake of cows' milk have a lower appetite for other foods. More than two servings of milk per day is not advisable. Iron-fortified cereals should be introduced from 5 months of age.

Adverse effects

Iron deficiency before 24 months can lead to impaired development of cognitive and psychomotor skills, which may be only partially reversible when the deficiency, and the associated anaemia, is corrected. Many parents report loss of appetite, irritability and inability to concentrate in affected children. Pica may be present. Iron deficiency affects neutrophil and lymphocyte function in vitro and is indicated as one of the investigations of recurrent infections.

Diagnosis

Iron deficiency is the commonest cause of microcytic hypochromic anaemia and is characterised by a low serum iron, a high total iron binding capacity and a low transferrin saturation. The reticulocyte count is less than 2% unless iron had been reintroduced into the diet. The diagnosis is not confirmed until iron supplementation is followed by a reticulocytosis within 1–2 weeks and a rise in the haemoglobin over 2–4 weeks. Other conditions producing microcytic anaemia must be considered if there is poor response to iron supplementation.

Treatment

Dietary advice and education are the basis of prevention and treatment in developed countries. If iron supplementation is required, the ferrous form is more effectively absorbed either as syrup or tablets at 2–3 mg kg^{-1} day^{-1}. The treatment dose for severe anaemia is up to 6 mg kg^{-1} day^{-1}, but side effects of nausea, vomiting, and constipation are dose-related. Transfusion is only ever required if there is cardiovascular compromise. Parents should be informed regarding the toxicity of iron in overdose so that they store the medication safely.

Haemolytic anaemias

RBC exist in the circulation for 100–120 days with up to 1% of the RBC population being removed by haemolysis and replaced per day. Pathological haemolysis is that which occurs outside of this normal process leading to reduced RBC survival. In response, bone marrow activity increases, leading to an increased reticulocyte count of >2%. In the older age group, the bone marrow's capacity to increase erythropoiesis can compensate for mild pathological haemolysis. In the infant and young child, the bone marrow is maximally active with minimal ability to increase erythropoiesis and anaemia accompanies pathological haemolysis.

The haemolytic anaemias of childhood may be classified as hereditary or acquired (Table 11.2.1). The hereditary haemolytic anaemias are caused by inherited traits that lead to abnormal haemoglobin chains (haemoglobinopathies), abnormal RBC membranes or abnormal RBC enzymes (enzymopathies). The acquired haemolytic anaemias may be immune or non-immune or as a result of fragmentation syndromes.

Acquired haemolytic anaemias

Autoimmune haemolytic anaemia (AIHA)

A variety of infectious agents (Epstein–Barr virus, CMV, mumps, mycoplasma and tuberculosis) can cause severe anaemia in the younger child. The antibody involved is mainly IgM, but may be IgG. Other diseases that trigger autoantibodies include systemic lupus erythematosus, rheumatoid arthritis, thyrotoxicosis, ulcerative colitis, malignancy and immunodeficiency syndromes. Idiopathic autoimmune anaemia can be rapidly progressive over days in the young infant and chronic and relapsing in the older child.

Haemolysis in these conditions occurs within the intravascular space. The Coombs' test in these conditions is positive. This test detects a coating of immunoglobulins or components of complement on the RBC surface. During haemolysis, free haemoglobin is liberated in plasma and combines with haptoglobin resulting in decreased serum haptoglobin. RBC fragmentation, spherocytes and sometimes tear-shaped cells are found on the peripheral blood film. Spherocytosis and other characteristic red-cell changes are due to membrane loss as splenic macrophages attack antibody-coated red blood cells. Lactose dehydrogenase, a RBC enzyme, is raised and free haemoglobin and haemalbumin may be found in the plasma.

In children the clinical pattern is most frequently an acute episode of severe anaemia with resolution within 3 months. Haemoglobin drops to less than $60 \, g \, L^{-1}$ in over 50%. A slower onset is more likely to follow a chronic and relapsing course with guarded prognosis.

A reticulocytosis may not be present initially due to rapid onset. Associated immune thrombocytopenia is present in a third. Direct Coombs' antiglobulin test is positive. Free antibodies may be detectable within serum. Antibodies that are maximally active at 37°C belong to the IgG class and are known as warm antibodies. Antibodies that are maximally active between 0 and 30°C belong to the IgM class and are known as cold antibodies. Serology may be useful in identifying the infective agent. Hyperbilirubinaemia is present.

IgG-induced AIHA responds to steroid therapy and variable regimes have been effective. This is not effective in cold agglutinin disease (IgM induced), which may require plasmapheresis. Both may respond to immunoglobulin, $1 \, g \, kg^{-1}$ IV, and require exchange transfusion if disease is severe. Splenectomy is a last resort in IgG-induced AIHA. A haematologist should be consulted regarding specific treatment.

Non-immune haemolytic anaemia

Non-immune haemolytic anaemia can also be caused by a variety of infectious agents (malaria, Gram-positive and Gram-negative organisms), medications (salicylates, sulfasalazine, nitrofurantoin) and chemicals (naphthalene). Clinical features are similar to AIHA but Coombs' test is negative. Treatment is supportive, focusing on the identification and treatment of the underlying cause.

Erythrocyte fragmentation syndromes

These are haemolytic anaemias due to direct physical or mechanical damage to the erythrocytes. They are characterised by red cell fragmentation with schistocytes and spherocytes in the peripheral blood film and features of intravascular haemolysis. There are two groups.

Macroangiopathic haemolytic anaemia

Macroangiopathic haemolytic anaemia results from RBC damage upon passage through large vessels and the heart and is associated with structural cardiac abnormality or large vessel disease (coarctation of the aorta). It can follow cardiac surgery but infection or failure of the prostheses must be considered if it occurs distinct from the surgical period. It is less likely with xenografts and also when prostheses are covered by endothelium. The damage is from a combination of shearing forces from turbulent flow and interaction between the cells and the abnormal surfaces. The anaemia is usually mild and severe haemolysis is uncommon. Treatment of the underlying cause is important.

Microangiopathic haemolytic anaemia

Microangiopathic haemolytic anaemia is due to RBC damage as they pass through diseased or partially occluded arterioles and capillaries and is often acute and severe, with associated thrombocytopenia. The commonest causes are HUS under 4 years of age and TTP in the child 10 years and older but connective tissue disease, haemangiomas and severe burns can all be causes.

Haemolytic uraemic syndrome

HUS is the commonest cause of acute renal failure in children. It is classically characterised by the triad of microangiopathic haemolytic anaemia, thrombocytopenia, and uraemia. In warmer climates it may be endemic but in cooler climates it occurs sporadically. More than 90% of affected children are under the age of 4 years, with peak incidence in children between the ages of 4 months and 2 years. Numerous infections can trigger HUS including *Shigella*, *Salmonella*, *Yersinia*, *Campylobacter*, *Streptococcus pneumoniae*, echovirus, Coxsackie virus A and B, and varicella. The commonest organism is *Escherichia coli* and verocytotoxin is the toxic agent. HUS may also develop in association with certain drugs, including oral contraceptives, mitomycin, or cyclosporin, and in diseases with significant endothelial cell injury such as systemic lupus erythematosus. A familial inherited version has been reported, although these occurrences are usually not associated with diarrhoea.

HUS is usually (80%) preceded by an infection with vomiting and bloody diarrhoea. Fever is present and oliguria occurs within days. Hypertension may be present. The thrombocytopenia is mild and severe bleeding is uncommon. Rarely, cardiomyopathy, cerebral infarcts or haemorrhage, bowel perforations and diabetes may complicate HUS.

The peripheral blood film shows the typical schistocytes. A leucocytosis with left shift often accompanies the anaemia and thrombocytopenia. Stool samples should be tested for verocytotoxin. Raised urea and creatinine indicate renal failure.

Treatment is directed at the acute renal failure with early dialysis indicated in some cases. Transfusion of packed RBCs may be required. Platelet transfusion is not indicated unless there is active bleeding. Careful monitoring is essential.

The long-term outcome for the acute renal failure is good, with 90% survival rate in the acute phase. Long-term monitoring is essential as chronic complications may not be apparent for several decades. Atypical HUS following an upper respiratory tract infection may manifest severe hypertension and renal failure. The prognosis for the latter is poor. The disease may recur.

Thrombotic thrombocytopenic purpura

This clinical syndrome is similar to that seen in HUS, with the addition of neurological deficit. The latter may take the form of an altered level of consciousness ranging from confusion, to seizure or coma. Cranial nerve palsies may also be present. The renal failure is not as severe compared to HUS but the thrombocytopenia is more severe. TTP usually affects children older than 10 years. Possible triggers include mycoplasma and viral infections, HIV and subacute bacterial endocarditis but none is evident in the majority of patients. Underlying immunological disease may be relevant, as is pregnancy, and genetic predisposition. Treatment is supportive, mainly via exchange transfusion using FFP. If there is no improvement in 24 hours then plasmapheresis is considered.

Transfusion of packed RBCs is rarely needed for severe anaemia. Involvement of a paediatric haematologist is mandatory.

Hereditary haemolytic anaemia

Glucose-6-phosphatase dehydrogenase (G6PD) deficiency

G6PD deficiency renders the RBC vulnerable to haemolysis when exposed to an oxidant. G6PD is the enzyme in the pathway leading to generation of reduced nicotinamide adenine dinucleotide phosphate, which maintains glutathione in its reduced form. Reduced glutathione is an essential factor in the degradation of cellular peroxides that may otherwise damage cellular proteins including haemoglobin. The enzyme activity is higher in the younger RBCs but deteriorates as the cell ages so older RBCs are more prone to haemolysis.

G6PD is an X-linked recessive condition with wide variability of expression depending on the biochemical type, the oxidant stress and the sex of the patient. Homozygous females are rare and the disease is predominantly found in males. The severity of the disease varies and levels of enzyme at or above 40% of normal will rarely result in clinically significant haemolysis. A number of different variants are found in patients of African, Chinese and Mediterranean descent.

Viral and bacterial infections can both cause acute haemolysis especially in children less than 2 to 3 years of age. Oxidant drugs and chemicals that commonly cause haemolysis include naphthalene, sulphonamides, antimalarials, nitrofurantoin, diazoxide and dapsone. Favism refers to the acute haemolysis resulting from the ingestion of broad bean (*Vicia faba*) or inhalation of the pollen in those with the Mediterranean variant but not those with the African variant. The haemolytic agent in the broad bean can be passed to the infant by breast milk. The anaemia is present within 3–36 hours and usually lasts for 2–6 days. Death can occur within 24 hours of the haemolysis. Definitive diagnosis of G6PD deficiency is via a quantitative assay of the enzyme. Treatment is non-specific. Prevention is crucial, with avoidance of oxidising medications and prompt treatment of infections.

Thalassaemias

Thalassaemia is one of the commonest inherited haemoglobin variants. Defective synthesis of globin chains leads to abnormal pairing of the globin chains in the haemoglobin molecule. Excess chains tend to aggregate, precipitate and cause damage to the RBCs. The nomenclature depicts the missing chain, e.g. β–thalassaemia refers to a deficiency of the β-chain. Haemoglobin electrophoresis defines the haemoglobin variants.

β-Thalassaemia major

Each carrier parent must donate one abnormal gene to the offspring and there is a 25% chance of a homozygote progeny with β-thalassaemia major. No β-chains are produced so presentation is in the first month of life when the fetal haemoglobin, HbF ($\alpha_2\gamma_2$), is falling, with an increasing reliance on adult haemoglobin, HbA ($\alpha_2\beta_2$). Excess unpaired α-chains aggregate to form an unstable tetramer, which is functionally useless. Haemolysis is increased and severe anaemia will occur. Extramedullary haemopoiesis leads to massive hepatosplenomegaly which may result in functional hypersplenism. Bone marrow expansion may result in skeletal changes (e.g. bossing of the frontal bone). The peripheral blood film shows a microcytic hypochromic anaemia with marked poikilocytosis, target cells and reticulocytosis. Basophilic stippling may be seen in the RBCs. Iron and folate deficiency may be demonstrated, although iron overload will eventually develop due to increased gastrointestinal tract absorption.

Treatment mainstay is regular (usually monthly) lifelong blood transfusions. Iron overload complicates this therapy and is managed with regular iron chelation therapy, but transfusion haemosiderosis is common, with its associated end-organ damage. HLA matched bone marrow transplantation has been curative.

β-Thalassaemia minor

Individuals with β-thalassaemia minor receive one abnormal gene only, thus demonstrating the heterozygote state. There is enough β-chain production and normal haemoglobin to avoid symptomatic anaemia. The life span of the RBCs is only slightly decreased. The anaemia is microcytic and hypochromic with target cells and elliptocytes. HbA$_2$ level in the range of 3.5–7.0% is almost diagnostic of the β-thalassaemia trait. The bone marrow is hyperplastic. Attention to potential iron and folate deficiency is important. The absence of an age-related rise in the MCV and major histocompatibility complex in a patient of the relevant ethnicity should prompt further investigations.

α-Thalassaemia

Two genes on chromosome 16 code for the α-chain, producing four possible phenotypes. Deletion of one α-gene is asymptomatic, with a minority having a microcytic hypochromic anaemia. Deletion of two α-genes produces mild anaemia. Deletion of three α-genes results in HbH disease due to aggregation of β-chains, which leads to an unstable haemoglobin. There is chronic haemolysis with anaemia in the range of 70–110 g L^{-1}, jaundice, cholelithiasis, hepatomegaly and leg ulcers. Deletion of four α-genes results in intrauterine death and stillbirths, usually after 25 weeks' gestation. Live births have severe anaemia, which may lead to congestive cardiac failure. The fetus is grossly oedematous. The haemoglobins present are HbH, Hb Barat (four γ-chains) and small amounts of Hb Portland (two ζ and two γ). None of these are functional.

Sickle cell disease

Sickle cell disease (SCD) is an autosomal recessive inherited condition in which glutamine in the sixth position of the globin chain is replaced by valine. In the homozygote with HbSS the haemoglobin is unstable in the deoxygenated state. It precipitates in the RBC and leads to a change in the biconcave shape to a configuration resembling a sickle. This change is initially reversible. The consequences are multiple. It is detrimental to the RBC and the end-organs. Sickle cells have a reduced life-span of 10–20 days and occlude the microvasculature, leading to end-organ ischaemia. The precipitants for the sickling are:

- tissue hypoxia;
- tissue acidosis;
- dehydration;
- vascular stasis;
- increased 2,3-diphosphoglycerate (2,3-DPG) levels in the RBC.

Diagnosis

Diagnosis is made on the family history and presentation. It is confirmed by haemoglobin electrophoresis and the 'sickle prep' test outside the neonatal age group. The 'sickle prep' uses sodium metabisulphite, which extracts oxygen from the RBC and causes sickling. Parents can be tested for further confirmation.

Clinical features

The baseline haemoglobin in SCD is in the range of 60–90 g L^{-1} with a reticulocytosis of 5–15%. Children with SCD have abnormal immune function. They have functional asplenism by age 5 years, although sometimes earlier, as well as abnormal complement components. Consequently, *fever* should be managed as a medical emergency with prompt medical evaluation and delivery of antibiotics because of the high risk of bacterial infection and mortality.

Dactylitis is frequently the first manifestation of pain in children with SCD, occurring in 50% of children by 2 years of age. Children present with symmetric painful swelling of the hands and/or feet and require careful management with pain medication. Differential diagnosis of osteomyelitis should be considered carefully if the presentation is unilateral.

Vaso-occlusive crises are acute episodes of severe pain from tissue infarction resulting from vessel occlusion by the sickled cells. The major organs involved are bones, lungs, liver, spleen, brain and the penis. Painful bone crisis is the commonest, with minimal signs on examination. Treatment is directed at effective pain relief. Intravenous fluids should be utilised only if clinical evidence of dehydration exists. Frequently recurrent episodes may be reduced by using hydroxyurea, but close monitoring is required.

In *aplastic crisis*, the reticulocytosis falls to less than 1%. The haematocrit may fall as rapidly as 10–15% per day. The precipitant is usually an infection. Spontaneous recovery is usual. Supportive therapy may involve transfusion of RBCs.

Acute splenic sequestration

Acute splenic sequestration (ASS) is a life-threatening complication of SCD occurring in 7–30% of patients under the age of 2 years with homozygous SCD. It has also been reported in heterozygous cases. ASS can occur suddenly with acute pallor, weakness, abdominal pain and distension with features of hypovolaemic shock. The precipitant is usually an intercurrent infection. The key finding is circulatory shock in a child with atraumatic abdominal pain and distension. A massive tender spleen is unmistakable.

The haematocrit is usually less than 50% of baseline. Reticulocytosis and moderately severe thrombocytopenia are present. Splenic sequestration of RBCs affects those SCD sufferers who are young enough to still have a spleen, as autosplenectomy from infarction commonly occurs. Hepatic sequestration may also occur but the volume of trapped RBCs is unlikely to lead to devastating hypovolaemia due to the tight hepatic capsule.

Treatment is resuscitation of the intravascular volume. Prevention of sickling of those RBCs remaining in the circulation is important as is the prompt treatment of the infective precipitant. ASS is recurrent in 50% of cases, with the interval between episodes being less each time. Splenectomy is the only method of preventing recurrent ASS.

Sickle cell trait

Sickle cell trait denotes the heterozygous or carrier state. The complete blood count is within the normal range. Haemoglobin analysis is diagnostic, revealing a ratio of HbS to HbA of 40:60. The RBCs have a normal lifespan. Serious complications in sickle cell trait are very rare, but may include sudden death during rigorous exercise, splenic infarcts at high altitude, haematuria, and bacteriuria. The life span of people with sickle cell trait is normal and children with sickle cell trait should not have any restrictions placed on activities.

Acknowledgement

The contribution of Marian Lee as author in the first edition is hereby acknowledged.

Further reading

Chang TT. Transfusion therapy in critically ill children. *Pediatr Neonatol* 2008;**49**(2):5–12.

Gera T, Sachdev HP, Nestel P, Sachdev SS. Effect of iron supplementation on haemoglobin response in children: systematic review of randomised controlled trials. *J Pediatr Gastroenterol Nutr* 2007;**44**(4):468–86.

Kleigman R, Behrman R, Jenson H, Stanton B. *Nelson's Textbook of Pediatrics*. 18th ed. Philadelphia: Saunders Elsevier; 2007.

Richardson M. Microcytic anemia. *Pediatr Rev* 2007;**28** (4):151.

HAEMATOLOGY AND ONCOLOGY

11.3 Disorders of coagulation

Evelyn Doyle

ESSENTIALS

1 Haemophilia and von Willebrand disease account for the majority of inherited coagulation disorders.

2 A positive family history of a bleeding disorder should be sought when a coagulation disorder is suspected.

3 Establishing disease severity (assayed factor levels), past history of bleeding, the nature of this bleed and presence of inhibitors will help guide replacement therapy in haemophilia.

4 Always consider 'hidden' potentially life-threatening bleeding: intracranial bleeding is a major cause of mortality in the haemophiliac patient.

Haemophilia

Introduction

Haemophilia A and B are coagulation disorders usually transmitted by X-linked recessive inheritance (70% of cases) but can occur as spontaneous gene mutations (30% of cases). Haemophilia A results from factor VIII deficiency and Haemophilia B (Christmas disease) is caused by factor IX deficiency. Acquired haemophilia is rare and occurs when autoantibodies develop against factor VIII.

Clinical presentation

Haemophilia A and B are clinically indistinguishable. Disease severity correlates well with assayed factor levels: severe disease occurs with factor levels <1% of normal, moderate and mild disease occur with levels between 1–5% and above 5%, respectively. In the absence of a positive family history, disease may go undetected for a variable period, depending on disease severity, with some cases of mild disease being diagnosed in adulthood.

Bleeding can occur in any tissue and may occur spontaneously or with minimal trauma. Most neonates, even those with severe disease, are born without significant bleeding, though intracranial haemorrhage may occur. As a child starts to ambulate bleeding episodes becomes more frequent. Unlike disorders of platelet function where mucosal bleeding typically occurs, bleeding into joints and soft tissues is characteristic, with large joints of the knee, ankle, hip, elbow, wrist and shoulder involved most frequently.

Other significant and potentially life-threatening bleeding can occur and should be considered in the haemophiliac patient: intracranial haemorrhage occurs with increased frequency after head trauma, retroperitoneal haematoma may occur spontaneously or following trauma and may mimic appendicitis, soft tissue haemorrhage in the head or neck is potentially life threatening due to the risk of airway obstruction. Gastrointestinal haemorrhage is a less common manifestation of haemophilia in children. Haematuria may be macroscopic or microscopic.

In the current paediatric haemophiliac population, transfusion-borne viruses including hepatitis B and C and human immunodeficiency virus are rare, as most cases of transmission occurred prior to 1985.

Investigations

Haemophilia A and B both cause a prolonged activated partial thromboplastin time (aPTT) with a normal prothrombin time and platelet count. Individual factor assays can then be performed to confirm the diagnosis. Haemophiliacs presenting with suspected intracranial or retroperitoneal bleeds need computerised tomography (CT) scanning. Plain radiographs will exclude fractures associated with traumatic haemarthroses.

Treatment

The primary treatment goal is control of bleeding by replacement of clotting factor. Factor concentrates are available as virus-inactivated plasma-derived product and recombinant factor concentrates. When available and expense allows, recombinant factor concentrates should be used. Factor replacement may be given following a confirmed bleed or as prophylaxis against potential bleeding; for example, prior to dental extraction. Prophylactic factor replacement, usually given two to three times a week at home, with increased doses given for any breakthrough bleeds, has led to a marked reduction in the number and severity of bleeding episodes.

The half-life of factor VIII is 8–12 hours and factor XI is up to 24 hours, so repeated doses may be needed. Many patients now initiate treatment for minor bleeds at home. Early and appropriate treatment reduces the risk of deterioration to disabling arthropathy and chronic pain. The amount of clotting factor required depends on the patient's weight, severity of disease, the location of the bleed and also previous bleeding in the same area and presence of inhibitors

Lacerations generally require factor replacement to prevent excessive bleeding. Head injury requires a high index of suspicion and a very low threshold for factor treatment. Continuous intravenous (IV) factor infusion may be required for major bleeding. A negative cranial CT scan does not preclude the need for factor replacement.

Analgesia should be provided as required but aspirin should be avoided. Other non-steroidal anti-inflammatory drugs may be used on the advice of the treating haematologist. Narcotic analgesia has limitations associated with use in treating a chronic condition.

Desmopressin (DDAVP), a synthetic analogue of vasopressin that elevates factor VIII levels for several hours after administration by stimulating release from endothelial stores, can be used to treat mild haemophilia A. In an emergency situation where no clotting factor is available, fresh frozen plasma (FFP) or cryoprecipitate can be administered.

Inhibitors are alloantibodies that develop against clotting factors and are present in 10–20% of those with haemophilia A and 3–5% of those with haemophilia B. Inhibitors may mean that large amounts of clotting factor are required, or that clotting factors will not work at all. Treatment options for patients with haemophilia are prothrombin complex concentrate (prothrombinex) or recombinant activated factor VIIa. Elimination of inhibitors is possible in a proportion of patients using immune tolerance therapy, where daily low-dose factor infusions will lead to the development of neutralising anti-inhibitor antibodies.

Von Willebrand disease

Introduction

Von Willebrand disease (vWD) is the commonest inherited disorder of coagulation and is present in 1% of the population in screening studies, though only a minority will present with clinically significant bleeding. In most cases inheritance is autosomal dominant with variable penetrance and expressivity, though autosomal recessive inheritance occurs (Type 2N and 3). Rarely, vWD may be acquired and has been described in conditions such as hypothyroidism, and SLE. Von Willebrand factor (vWF) is a large protein that has two roles in coagulation: it facilitates platelet adherence to the vascular endothelium enabling a platelet plug to be formed and also acts as a carrier protein for factor VIII. Quantitative or qualitative abnormalities of vWF occur. Three types of vWD and three subtypes have been described: Type 1, 2 (subtypes 2A, 2B, 2M, 2 N) and 3.

Clinical presentation

Mucosal and cutaneous bleeding, prolonged bleeding after surgical procedures and a positive family history of a bleeding disorder should prompt consideration of vWD. In children, bruising and bleeding out of proportion to the severity of the injury is typical. Haemarthroses, intracranial and intra-abdominal bleeds are much less common but can occur in more severe types 2N and 3 vWD. vWD is diagnosed in 10 to 20% of women and adolescents with menorrhagia and in 15% of children with recurrent epistaxis.

Type 1: The commonest form accounts for 60–80% of cases, and results from a partial quantitative deficiency of vWF. When bleeding occurs it ranges from mild to moderate, with only a minority having clinically significant bleeding episodes.

Type 2: (subtypes A, B, M and N) have qualitative defects of vWF. Bleeding tends to be moderate to severe. Type 2N may be misdiagnosed as haemophilia A until vWF testing becomes available.

Type 3: A total quantitative deficiency of vWF and decreased factor VIII activity occurs in this rare form of vWD. Clinically, bleeding is severe and indistinguishable from Haemophilia A, with mucosal, soft tissue and joint bleeding.

Investigations

A coagulation screen may be normal and does not rule out vWD. In most patients aPTT is normal, though a prolonged aPTT can occur in types 2N and 3, with reduced factor VIII levels. Bleeding time may be prolonged. Screening tests for vWD include: vWF assay, ristocetin co-factor assay and factor VIII activity. The diagnosis and typing of vWD is difficult and usually requires a specialist laboratory. Levels are affected by blood group and physiological factors such as stress and exercise. The patient's personal and family history of bleeding must also be taken into account in making this diagnosis.

Treatment

The main aim of treatment in vWD is replacement of deficient or defective vWF and factor VIII. Treatment is usually given in response to bleeding or prophylactically prior to surgical or dental procedures. Treatment options currently available are desmopressin and plasma concentrates

Desmopressin (DDAVP), a synthetic analogue of vasopressin releases factor VIII and vWF from endothelial storage sites, causing a transient rise in levels. DDAVP is effective in type 1 vWD and will increase plasma levels of vWF between three and five times from baseline within 30–60 minutes. It is usually ineffective in types 2A, M and N as vWF is functionally abnormal, and in type 3 vWD as an appreciable rise in levels may be clinically undetected. Desmopressin is contraindicated in type 2B vWD as it may cause thrombocytopenia and thus worsen bleeding. The dose is 0.3 mcg kg^{-1} given intravenously in 30–50 mL normal saline over 30 minutes. The most common adverse effects are facial flushing, headache and tachycardia, which usually respond to slowing the infusion. Repeat doses can be given at 12 to 24 hours if needed but tachyphylaxis occurs after approximately 48 hours. DDAVP should be used with caution in children under 3 years of age in whom there have been case reports of water intoxication and hyponatraemia. An intranasal DDAVP preparation is available but may be less reliable in children if part of the dose is swallowed. The dose is 2–4 mcg kg^{-1}.

Plasma-derived factor VIII concentrates contain both vWF and factor VIII. Recombinant factor VIII does not contain vWF and is ineffective. These plasma-derived products are the treatment of choice for type 2A, 2B (in which DDAVP is contraindicated) and type 3 vWD. They are virus inactivated and effective to control bleeding in most clinical situations. FFP contains both vWF and factor VIII but very large volumes would be required to raise vWF to satisfactory levels.

Adjunctive treatments include tranexamic acid for bleeding involving the oral or nasal mucosa, either alone or in conjunction with DDAVP. Synthetic oestrogens cause an unpredictable rise in vWF but may be useful in controlling menorrhagia.

Controversies and future directions

Haemophilia is particularly suited to gene therapy intervention because the disease is due to deficiency of a single gene product. Gene therapy is still at the stage of small human trials. Von Willebrand disease treatment options for the future include recombinant vWF, which has shown promising early results in animal trials, and interleukin-11 has also been shown to increase vWF, but human trials are needed.

Acknowledgement

The contribution of Fiona Reilly as author in the first edition is hereby acknowledged.

Further reading

Eikenboom J, Van Marion V, Putter H, et al. Linkage analysis in families diagnosed with type 1 von Willebrand disease in the European study, molecular and clinical markers for the diagnosis and management of type 1 VWD. J Thromb Haemost 2006;4:774–82.

Fischer K, van der Bom JG, Mauser-Bunschoten EP, et al. Changes in treatment strategies for severe haemophilia over the last 3 decades: Effects on clotting factor consumption and arthropathy. Hemophilia 2001;7:446–52.

Mannucci PM. Treatment of Von Willebrand's disease. N Engl J Med 12 2004;351(7):683–94.

National Hemophilia Foundation. www.hemophilia.org.

Rakel RE, Bope ET. Conn's Current Therapy 2009. 1st ed. Philadelphia: Saunders; 2009.

HAEMATOLOGY AND ONCOLOGY

11.4 Platelet disorders

Jane Cocks

ESSENTIALS

1 Abnormal bleeding can occur from disorders of total numbers of platelets or platelet function.

2 The normal platelet count is between 150 and $400 \times 10^9\,L^{-1}$.

3 Idiopathic thrombocytopenic purpura (ITP) is the commonest platelet disorder in childhood.

Introduction

The normal platelet count is between 150 and $400 \times 10^9\,L^{-1}$ and platelets usually exist within the circulation for 5–7 days. In normal haemostasis, blood loss is initially limited by the formation of a platelet plug and cross-linked fibrin at the site of injury. In platelet disorders this platelet plug is not formed or is ineffective, and abnormal bleeding occurs. Platelet abnormalities can be either quantitative or qualitative. Small petechial skin haemorrhages, less than 3 mm in diameter, are characteristic of platelet defects.

The commonest platelet disorder is thrombocytopenia (low platelet count). Significant thrombocytopenia has a characteristic bleeding profile of spontaneous bruising, petechiae, epistaxis and mucosal bleeding. Bleeding complications usually only occur at levels of less than $50 \times 10^9\,L^{-1}$, with spontaneous bleeding possible at levels below $10 \times 10^9\,L^{-1}$. As most platelet counts are performed by electronic particle counters, an inappropriately low platelet count can result from the spontaneous platelet clumping that can occur in EDTA collection tubes. This is confirmed by direct inspection of the peripheral blood smear for platelet clumping.

In qualitative disorders of platelet function the abnormal bleeding occurs despite a normal platelet count. Platelet dysfunction may occur in hepatic failure, chronic renal failure, myeloproliferative disorders, with some drugs (e.g. aspirin) and in rare inherited disorders of platelet function (Glanzmann, Portsmouth, Hermansky–Pudlak, May–Hegglin and Bernard–Soulier syndromes).

Thrombocytosis (elevated platelet count) is seen in inflammatory reactions including Kawasaki disease, patients with malignancy and polycythaemia rubra vera. Thrombocytosis of itself is rarely of clinical importance but platelet levels greater than $1000 \times 10^9\,L^{-1}$ can be associated with acute thrombosis or haemorrhage.

Idiopathic thrombocytopenic purpura

Introduction

Idiopathic thrombocytopenic purpura (ITP) is the commonest platelet disorder in children. It is an autoimmune disorder characterised by the development of platelet autoantibodies leading to decreased platelet survival. The incidence of ITP peaks in winter and spring due to the increased incidence of viral infections at those times. ITP in children is usually of the acute form, which lasts for less than 6 months, with a high rate of spontaneous resolution. ITP in children is most common between the ages of 2 and 6 years, but can occur in any age group. Up to 28% of children with ITP will develop a chronic form which lasts longer than 6 months.

Clinical presentation

ITP typically presents up to 3 weeks following a viral-type infection or vaccination. There is generally a short history of bruising, non-blanching rash (petechiae or purpura) or mucosal bleeding in an otherwise well child. The mucosal bleeding is usually from the gums or nose. Haematuria is also common. The petechial rash may appear in crops over several days. The physical examination is otherwise normal, with no signs of hepatosplenomegaly or lymphadenopathy.

Investigation

The blood count will demonstrate thrombocytopenia. Abnormally large and/or abnormally small platelets may be seen on the film. The blood count and film are otherwise usually normal. Anaemia may be present, dependent on the extent of previous haemorrhage. Eosinophilia may be noted, but is not consistent. Coagulation studies will be normal, bleeding time prolonged. There is no specific antiplatelet antibody test available for routine clinical use. Bone marrow aspiration is usually performed after 4 weeks if there is no evidence of remission, or earlier if the diagnosis is unclear.

Differential diagnosis

The diagnosis of ITP relies on the presence of laboratory-demonstrated thrombocytopenia, with a history, clinical examination and full blood count that do not suggest another cause. In the presence of a limp, hepatosplenomegaly or lymphadenopathy, consider the possibility of an underlying lymphoproliferative disorder. In infants with bruising, intentional injury must be excluded. In Wiskott–Aldrich syndrome eczema is present in the first year and the platelets are smaller than normal. The presence of other congenital abnormalities might be a clue to Fanconi's anaemia. In older children, particularly those with a chronic course, a systemic autoimmune disorder such as lupus or antiphospholipid syndrome should be considered. In infants, exclude cytomegalovirus and consider immunoglobulins and T/B lymphocyte subsets to exclude immune disorders.

Management

Most children recover spontaneously within 6 to 8 weeks and have only cutaneous or mild bleeding. They require no specialist treatment and can be managed as ambulatory patients. Parents should be supported with good written advice on the condition and given a telephone contact name and number. Written advice should include information about avoiding contact sports, bangs to the head, aspirin and other drugs that interfere with platelet function. They should watch for bleeding and report to hospital if new episodes occur. In the initial stages the platelet count can be reviewed weekly but this can be extended to every 2 to 4 weeks once it is improving. School can be recommenced when platelets are greater than $20 \times 10^9 \, L^{-1}$. By 6 months around 85% will have a normal platelet count. Patients with platelet counts greater than $150 \times 10^9 \, L^{-1}$ can be discharged but warned that occasional relapses are seen and to re-present if symptoms recur.

Consider admission of patients with initial platelet counts below $20 \times 10^9 \, L^{-1}$. Serious bleeding is rare in ITP, with intracranial haemorrhage occurring in ~1% of patients with platelet counts less than $20 \times 10^9 \, L^{-1}$. All children with counts less than $10 \times 10^9 \, L^{-1}$ during the course of the illness should be admitted. The decision to admit may be influenced by the social circumstances and parents' coping ability.

Consider treatment if bleeding is severe. There are a number of established options aimed at increasing the platelet count but there is no specific therapy to treat the underlying disorder.

Current treatments

Asymptomatic children with acute ITP and platelet count $<20 \times 10^9 \, L^{-1}$ should be carefully observed. In the presence of purpura, significant mucosal membrane bleeding or other haemorrhage, intravenous immunoglobulin (IVIG) infusion is recommended and high-dose oral glucocorticoids can be considered with the involvement of a paediatric haematologist.

IVIG infusion will lead to a rapid platelet count rise, usually within 48 hours, lasting for 2–4 weeks. As a pooled blood product IVIG carries the risk of viral transmission and is expensive. A range of side effects have been reported.

High-dose oral steroids may also be considered, although IVIG has been demonstrated to promote a faster response to get platelet numbers above $50 \times 10^9 \, L^{-1}$.

Anti-D is an effective alternative in Rh-positive children only, but the platelet increase is slower, taking 48–72 hours.

Splenectomy is reserved for life-threatening haemorrhage or children with significant bleeding who have failed to respond to medical treatment. Post-splenectomy patients have an increased risk of sepsis despite pneumococcal vaccination and antibiotic prophylaxis.

Medical emergencies

The risk of intracranial haemorrhage is less than 1% but persists as long as the platelet count is very low. Children with ITP and severe headache with neurological signs require urgent investigation with cranial computerised tomography scan and immediate treatment if indicated with IVIG and steroids. Life-threatening haemorrhage is the only instance where platelet transfusions should be used, as the antibodies in ITP target all platelets including donor transfusions. As a result the benefit of any transfusion is very short-lived. Emergency splenectomy may be used as a last resort.

Chronic ITP

Around 10–28% of children fail to remit within 6 months but spontaneous remission will occur in up to two-thirds of these patients in subsequent years. A chronic course is most often seen in older children, particularly adolescent girls. Some may have underlying conditions such as lupus. Most do not have significant bleeding problems or a need for regular treatment.

Controversies

The Intercontinental Childhood ITP Registry was established in 1997 to prospectively investigate the clinical course, management and outcome of children with ITP. Since then a Splenectomy Register and a prospective database on both paediatric and adult patients with chronic ITP have also been set up. Information from these databases should provide the evidence base for the optimum treatment strategy for individual children with ITP in the future.

Acknowledgement

The contribution of Kieran Cunningham as author in the first edition is hereby acknowledged.

Further reading

Pediatric Blood Cancer 2006;**47**(S5):649–745.
The Intercontinental Cooperative ITP Study Group (ICIS). website: http://www.itpbasel.ch/Home.90.0.html.
Greer JP, Foerster J, Rodgers GM, et al. *Wintrobe's Clinical Haematology*. 12th ed. Baltimore: Lippincott Williams & Wilkins; 2008.

11.5 Vasculitis

Evelyn Doyle

ESSENTIALS

1 The most common childhood vasculidites are Henoch–Schönlein purpura (HSP) and Kawasaki disease.

2 In HSP persistent renal disease occurs in a minority of children. Repeat urinalysis is recommended at intervals until resolution of symptoms, as nephritis may be delayed.

3 Kawasaki disease should be considered in all children with unexplained high fever for more than 5 days. All features may not be present simultaneously and a history of mucositis, cervical lymphadenopathy, conjunctivitis, rash and peripheral cutaneous manifestations should be specifically sought.

4 Vasculitis may occur secondary to a primary underlying disease, infections, drug reaction or malignancy and should be excluded.

5 Vasculitis should be considered in children with a non-specific febrile illness and exanthem without explanation that do not resolve as would be expected with a self-limited infectious illness.

Introduction

Childhood vasculitides are a group of disorders characterised by inflammation of blood vessels. Vasculitis is the common end point of several different disease processes and no one mechanism can explain the pathogenesis in this heterogeneous group of conditions. Distinguishing a primary vasculitis from a secondary underlying disease or from conditions that mimic vasculitis can be difficult. Most forms of vasculitis are rare in childhood. Henoch–Schönlein purpura (HSP) and Kawasaki disease (KD) are the two commonest childhood vasculitides.

Clinical presentation

The presentation varies widely according to the size of the affected blood vessel and the extent and nature of organ involvement. Constitutional symptoms are common to all vasculitides and include fever, weight loss, malaise, irritability and arthralgias. Skin manifestations are frequent and often give a clue to the size of the vessel involved; lesions are commonly purpuric but may be urticarial, ulcerative, vesicular or resemble erythema multiforme. In severe vasculitis, vessel destruction leads to tissue infarction, and can result in ischaemia and gangrene.

Classification

The primary vasculitic disorders can be divided according to the size of the vessel involved.

SMALL VESSEL VASCULITIS

HSP, Wegener's granulomatosis and Churg–Strauss syndrome predominantly involve small vessels; the latter two conditions are extremely rare in childhood.

Henoch–Schönlein purpura

HSP is the commonest vasculitis in childhood. It is immune mediated, associated with IgA complex deposition in tissues, and though several infective agents, drugs and immunisation have been implicated, the cause is unknown.

Clinical presentation

HSP is characterised by palpable purpura which is mandatory for diagnosis with one or more of the following: diffuse abdominal pain, arthritis or arthralgia, renal involvement, or a tissue biopsy showing predominantly IgA deposition.

Skin lesions begin as maculopapules that initially blanch and develop to palpable purpura, which may include macules, papules, vesicles, bullae, nodules and urticaria. Lesions are symmetrical and maximal on lower limbs and buttocks and may be painful. Local angio-oedema of face, hands, feet, back, scrotum and perineum is common in younger children.

Arthritis occurs in up to 80%, with one or more joints involved, and resolves leaving no residual joint deformity. Large joints of the lower extremity are usually affected but upper extremity joints may also be involved.

Gastrointestinal symptoms are common and include colicky abdominal pain, vomiting and bloody diarrhoea. Over half of patients have occult blood in stools. Intussusception (usually ileoileal) is the most common serious gastrointestinal complication and results from oedema and haemorrhage in the bowel wall acting as a lead point. Ultrasound is recommended when suspected, as contrast enema will not detect ileoileal pathology.

Some children present with isolated abdominal symptoms or arthritis and the diagnosis may only become apparent when the rash develops days to weeks later. Nephritis occurs in about half and may be delayed for up to 4 or more weeks. Other serious though uncommon conditions can occur including orchitis cerebral involvement, including seizures.

Investigations

There is no diagnostic test for HSP; the diagnosis is clinical but may be difficult in the absence of rash. Blood pressure measurement, urinalysis and renal function assessment at presentation are required in all patients. Renal biopsy is reserved for patients with nephritis complicated by nephrotic syndrome, hypertension or renal failure. Throat swab, C3/C4 and ASOT may be useful in distinguishing post-streptococcal arthralgia from HSP where the clinical picture is not full-blown.

Prognosis

It is generally a self-limited condition but can recur in one-third of patients. Resolution of symptoms occurs over a period of weeks. A small percentage of children develop persistent renal disease, with about 0.1% developing serious renal disease. Those with isolated haematuria and proteinuria without renal insufficiency completely recover.

Management

Most children are managed as outpatients with supportive care. Non-steroidal anti-inflammatory drugs are effective but use with caution in renal impairment. Steroids are not routinely used as the majority of patients' symptoms resolve spontaneously without sequelae, but may be considered in patients with severe renal or extrarenal symptoms. Steroids have not been found to prevent development of renal or gastrointestinal symptoms but may be effective in treating symptoms. Renal disease is the major concern long term and specialist consultation should be sought in severe disease. Follow up should involve blood pressure surveillance and urinalysis for 3 months as renal involvement can occur later even when initial urinalysis is normal.

MEDIUM VESSEL VASCULITIS

This group includes Kawasaki disease and polyarteritis nodosa (PAN).

Kawasaki disease

KD is an acute systemic vasculitis of unknown aetiology affecting predominantly medium muscular arteries, with a predilection for coronary arteries. It is the second most common vasculitic disease of childhood after HSP. The disease frequency varies globally, with highest rates in Japan and in Japanese children born overseas. It predominantly affects children under the age of 5 but can occur at any age. Coronary artery aneurysms develop in ~15–25% of untreated children and may lead to ischaemic heart disease or sudden death.

Clinical presentation

Diagnosis of KD is based on clinical criteria and the 'classic' form presents with unexplained high fever lasting at least 5 days and four of the following five clinical features, or fever with coronary artery involvement and three other clinical findings.

Some children may present with incomplete or 'atypical' Kawasaki disease: they have some but not enough features to meet classical criteria. In these children diagnosis can be difficult and consultation with an experienced physician should be sought.

❶ Cervical adenopathy.
❷ Bilateral non-suppurative conjunctival injection with perilimbal sparing.
❸ Polymorphous rash (maculopapular, multiforme or scarlatiniform).
❹ Peripheral cutaneous or perianal changes including erythema, swelling and induration. Desquamation may occur as a late sign, usually 2–3 weeks after the onset of illness, beginning in the periungal region.
❺ Mucous membrane changes to lips and/or oral cavity (fissuring of the lips, pharyngitis and strawberry tongue).

Fever is typically high, >39 with minimal response to antipyretics, and usually persists for 1 to 2 weeks if untreated. Extreme irritability in a toddler with persisting fever of unknown origin should always prompt consideration of KD. Other associated findings are carditis (pericarditis, myocarditis, valvular involvement), aseptic meningitis, arthritis, sterile pyuria, uveitis, hepatitis and hydrops of the gall bladder.

Investigations

There is no diagnostic test for KD. In the acute stage, laboratory findings may include leucocytosis with left shift, anaemia, and thrombocytosis (in the second to third week). Mild hepatitis with raised transaminases and elevated conjugated bilirubin, and cerebrospinal fluid analysis may show a mononuclear pleocytosis with normal glucose and protein and sterile culture. Mild proteinuria and pyuria may also be present.

If atypical KD is suspected laboratory tests, though non-specific, may be useful. The diagnosis is unlikely if platelet count, erythrocyte sedimentation rate (ESR) and C-reactive protein (CRP) are normal after day 7 of illness. A moderate to marked elevation in CRP or ESR is almost universal in children with KD. Leucopenia, lymphocyte predominance, and low platelet count in the absence of disseminated intravascular coagulation are also suggestive of an alternative diagnosis.

Echocardiography for coronary aneurysms should be performed in all children. Screening has shown that a substantial number of children with KD and coronary artery abnormalities are not identified by the classic case definition.

Management

Combined therapy with aspirin and high dose intravenous immunoglobulin (IVIG) has been shown to reduce the rate of coronary artery aneurysm from ~25% to ~5% when administered in the first 10 days of illness. High-dose IVIG 2 g kg^{-1}, is usually given as a single infusion. High-dose aspirin is given initially: doses varying from 30–100 mg kg^{-1} day^{-1} are used. Following defervescence, aspirin is given for its antiplatelet action in a dose of 2–5 mg kg^{-1} once daily.

Children who do not respond after the first dose of IVIG may respond to a second dose. A group of patients remain resistant to IVIG therapy and some novel therapies have been tried under specialist supervision. Follow up includes regular echocardiography, the duration of which will be determined by the degree of coronary artery involvement. Stress testing in adolescence is required if there has been cardiac involvement and angiography may be indicated. Long-term antiplatelet or anticoagulation therapy may be indicated.

Prognosis

In children without cardiac involvement recovery is usually complete though the long-term effects are largely unknown. Aneurysmal coronary artery dilatation occurs in ~25% of untreated KD, and half to two-thirds regress over time but stenosis in these vessels may progress independently of this. The worst prognosis occurs in large aneurysms (>8 mm), and risks include thrombosis, myocardial ischaemia and infarction; also late sequelae of KD may manifest in adulthood.

Polyarteritis nodosa

PAN is a necrotising vasculitis of unknown aetiology involving medium-sized muscular arteries. It is rare in childhood. PAN is a systemic illness with a wide spectrum of clinical presentations depending on the organs involved. Constitutional symptoms are common. Skin manifestations may resemble those of HSP or erythema multiforme or may be necrotic with peripheral gangrene. Other features include myalgia, ischaemic heart pain, nephritis and cerebral manifestations of stroke, visual loss and psychosis. Diagnosis relies on elevation of inflammatory markers (ESR and CRP) and biopsy showing characteristic histopathological changes or angiographic or magnetic resonance angiography evidence of aneurysm or occlusion in affected vessels. Antineutrophil cytoplasmic antibodies (ANCA) are present in some forms of PAN.

LARGE VESSEL VASCULITIS

Takayasu disease is a large vessel vasculitis of unknown aetiology involving the aorta and its main branches. It occurs 10 times more commonly in young women than men. Morbidity results from stenosis, ischaemia and aneurysmal dilatation of affected vessels. Presentation may be non-specific with constitutional symptoms or specific symptoms relating to inflammation of large vessels, including congestive heart failure, angina, myocardial infarction, stroke, limb claudication and renal artery hypertension may be found. In children, careful examination of pulses and blood pressures in all four extremities, with a search for asymmetry and bruits is essential. High-dose corticosteroids are first line therapy. In resistant or relapsing patients, cyclophosphamide and methotrexate have been used. Long-term immunosuppressive therapy is required in some patients.

SECONDARY VASCULITIS AND VASCULITIS MIMICS

Vasculitis is seen secondary to a primary underlying disease, infections, drug reaction or malignancy. Vasculitis occurs in connective tissue disorders such as systemic lupus erythematosus and dermatomyositis. There is an increased association with vasculitis in patients with familial Mediterranean fever, with several patients described with PAN and HSP features.

Many infectious diseases have been associated with vasculitis, predominantly with cutaneous manifestations. Papulovesicular acrolocated syndrome (PALS or Gianotti–Crosti syndrome) is a vasculitis associated with multiple viral and other triggers, including hepatitis B antigenaemia, Epstein–Barr virus, cytomegalovirus, human immunodeficiency virus, rickettsial diseases and streptococcal infections. Multiple skin-coloured or red, flat-topped papules occur in an acral distribution with sparing of the trunk.

Hypersensitivity angiitis is a serum-sickness-like reaction in infants that includes a rash, arthropathy and fever. It commonly follows the use of penicillin or cephalosporins (particularly Ceclor). Skin manifestations include oedema of the dorsum of the hands and feet and a nodular, purpuric, urticarial or erythema-multiforme-like rash. Arthralgia and arthritis are common and respond to non-steroidal anti-inflammatory drugs, with short-term oral steroids reserved for the more severe cases. The condition is self limiting but recurs on re-exposure to the same agent.

Any process that causes occlusion of a blood vessel can mimic vasculitis. In subacute bacterial endocarditis, the clinical appearance resembles a primary vasculitic process but is secondary to septic emboli.

Controversies and future directions

❶ Aspirin, though routinely used to treat Kawasaki disease, has not been shown to reduce the risk of coronary artery aneurysm in Kawasaki disease.

❷ Steroid use in HSP is not routine and remains controversial but recent studies appear to show benefit in terms of resolution of symptoms and may be considered in patients with severe disease.

❸ International collaboration to study rare disorders such as paediatric vasculitis may point toward new treatment approaches.

Acknowledgement

The contribution of Ruth Barker as author in the first edition is hereby acknowledged.

Further reading

Brogan PA, Bose A, Burgner D, et al. Kawasaki disease: an evidence based approach to diagnosis, treatment, and proposals for future research. *Arch Dis Child* 2002;**86**:286–90.

Dillon MJ, Ozen S. A new international classification of childhood vasculitis. *Pediatr Nephrol* 2006;**21**:1219–22.

Newburger JW, Takahashi M, Gerber MA, et al. Diagnosis, treatment, and long term management of Kawasaki disease: a statement for health professionals from the Committee on Rheumatic Fever, Endocarditis, and Kawasaki Disease, Council on Cardiovascular Disease in the Young, American Heart Association [Published correction appears in *Pediatrics* 2005;115:1118]. *Pediatrics* 2004;**114**:1708–33.

Weiss PF, Feinstein JA, Luan X, et al. Effects of corticosteroid on Henoch–Schönlein purpura: a systematic review. *Pediatrics* 2007;**120**:1079–87.

11.6 Acute leukaemia

Joseph Ting

ESSENTIALS

1 At its most severe, acute leukaemia leads to diffuse bone marrow infiltration and failure. Pancytopenia including neutropenia, anaemia and thrombocytopenia as well as extramedullary hematopoiesis give rise to classical symptoms of infection susceptibility, easy fatigability, bleeding diathesis and hepatosplenomegaly.

2 ED supportive treatment in conjunction with a paediatric haematologist includes broad spectrum antimicrobial administration or sepsis resuscitation, packed red blood cell transfusion for symptomatic or critical anaemia and platelet replacement if the child has high potential or actual risk of thrombocytopenia-related bleeding.

Introduction

The leukaemias are a group of diseases characterised by the clonal proliferation of malignant immature white blood cell precursors. They differ in the lineage and degree of differentiation of cells involved, being broadly divided into two groups: lymphoid and myeloid. These two categories are further subdivided into an acute form that progresses more rapidly than the chronic disease, which is relatively indolent. Preconceptional germ cell and postnatal environmental exposure to electromagnetic radiation and carcinogens may play a role,[1-3] with higher risk in children with congenital neutropenia, Down's syndrome and Fanconi anaemia.[4] Previous chemotherapy and radiotherapy are associated with increased risk of a secondary malignancy. Acute lymphoblastic leukaemia (ALL) comprises four-fifths of childhood leukaemia,[4] with acute myeloid leukaemia (AML) and chronic myeloid leukaemia (CML) accounting for 15% and 2%.[5] Together they account for one-third of all malignancies in children under 15 years old. Although children of all ages are affected, the peak incidence is between 2 and 6 years.

Classification

Leukaemogenesis represents clonal proliferation of white blood cells arrested at various stages of differentiation, lending itself to diagnostic and prognostic classification based on the cell line affected, degree of differentiation, immunophenotyping, cell receptor, cell antigen and chromosomal studies. Classification of leukaemia is complex, with the French–American–British (FAB) categories being useful for AML and immunotyping better suiting ALL.[4,5]

Clinical presentation

Signs and symptoms in ALL and AML are similar and depend on the degree of marrow infiltration and extent of extramedullary involvement. The first symptoms are non-specific including lethargy, bone pain and loss of appetite. Classic findings in acute leukaemia include fever/infection, pallor/lethargy/easy fatigability and bruising/mucosal bleeding due to febrile neutropenia, anaemia and thrombocytopenia, respectively. Marrow infiltration leads to bone pain and extramedullary spread leads to painless adenopathy (including mediastinal), hepatomegaly, splenomegaly, skin or periorbital infiltrates and rash. Difficulty with diagnosis arises in differentiating early acute from chronic disease, when symptoms (night sweats, arthralgia, bone pain, constitutional symptoms) and signs (enlarged liver and spleen, lymphadenopathy) are variable and non-specific. Central nervous system (CNS) involvement occurs in 4% of children (cranial nerve palsy, cord compression) and testicular leukaemia in 10% of boys (painless enlarged testes). Hyperviscosity results in tissue infarction (CNS, pulmonary) and rarely priapism results from leucocyte sludging and cavernosal obstruction.

Differential diagnosis

Pancytopenia may result from acute leukaemia, aplastic anaemia, marrow infiltration by non-haematological malignancy and collagen-vascular disease. However, hepatosplenomegaly and adenopathy is unusual with the alternative diagnoses. Viral infections may lead to lymphadenopathy and hepatosplenomegaly accompanied by atypical lymphocytes rather than blast cells. Leukaemoid reactions with leucocyte counts $>50 \times 10^9 \, L^{-1}$ may rarely occur with acute infections and inflammatory disease such as rheumatoid arthritis. Marked lymphocytosis without leukaemic cells occurs in pertussis. Isolated thrombocytopenia in childhood may follow a viral infection or be associated with idiopathic or thrombotic thrombocytopenic purpura rather than leukaemia.

Investigations

Full blood count reveals anaemia and thrombocytopenia in 80% of cases. The majority of children have leucocyte counts below $20 \times 10^9 \, L^{-1}$. Those with leucocyte counts up to $900 \times 10^9 \, L^{-1}$ usually have extramedullary involvement with hepatosplenomegaly and lymphadenopathy. The neutrophil count is often depressed to below $1.0 \times 10^9 \, L^{-1}$. Circulating blast cells are frequently present on blood film examination. Blood typing is necessary if red-cell transfusion is anticipated. A screen for atypical antibodies is warranted if there have previously been multiple occasions of blood product use. Cultures of blood and other potential infection sites are obtained prior to antimicrobial administration. Blood cultures may be positive in up to 25% of cases of newly diagnosed leukaemia. Tumour lysis syndrome due to massive cell death during treatment causes raised lactate dehydrogenase (LDH), liver enzymes, hyperkalaemia, hyperuricaemia, hyperphosphataemia, hypocalcaemia and acute renal failure. Anterior mediastinal masses are visible on chest X-ray in 5–10% of cases and pneumonia may require exclusion. Bone-marrow aspiration and trephine

(BMAT) is essential for specific diagnosis and prognostication, including complex tests such as immunophenotyping, cytogenetics, molecular studies and cell-cycle kinetics. AML is, rarely, complicated by a coagulopathy that progresses to disseminated intravascular coagulation, so that a coagulation profile and fibrinogen level may be helpful.

Prognosis

The cure rate for ALL is 80%,[4] compared with only 30–50% for AML,[5] depending on whether adverse prognostic factors are present. Poor-risk AML has a dismal outlook, with less than 20% achieving long-term remission. Adverse prognostic factors include age (ages <1, >10 years), certain chromosomal translocations (such as t(4;11) in infant ALL), a very high-presenting leucocyte count and poor response to first-course treatment. Although the cumulative risk of ALL relapse is 15–20%, the risk of developing second malignancies after successful treatment is low.[4,5]

Management

Management requires close collaboration with a paediatric haematologist. Emergency department supportive treatment focuses on the sequelae of acute leukaemia: febrile neutropenia and sepsis (broad-spectrum antimicrobial agents), actual or potential bleeding from thrombocytopenia (platelet transfusion) and correction of acute or symptomatic anaemia, which are described elsewhere. Chemotherapy may give rise to bone-marrow suppression, similar to the sequelae of acute leukaemia. Children who relapse or do not achieve remission are candidates for bone-marrow transplantation. Barrier nursing, isolation, antimicrobial and antiviral chemoprophylaxis, vaccination and post-exposure administration of immunoglobulin (e.g. varicella zoster virus) and careful monitoring for early infective complications help prevent complications related to immunosuppression. Psychosocial support of the child and family is important.

Controversies and future directions

❶ The future management of leukaemia will be influenced by new and improved risk stratified therapy to improve outcomes and minimise adverse effects. High-risk patients could be identified by molecular analysis, in vitro pharmacodynamic, pharmacogenetic, pharmacogenomic and drug resistance studies to receive more intensive and targeted therapy. [6–9]

❷ The increasing use of severely myelotoxic chemotherapy and unrelated bone-marrow transplantation has improved prognosis in acute leukaemia but has given rise to complications related to marrow suppression.

❸ Biological (e.g. monoclonal antibodies) rather than cytotoxic agents and agents with better specificity for leukaemic cells result in less 'collateral damage' [10] Gene therapy, although promising, remains experimental and clinically unproven.[11]

References

1. Schutz J, Ahlbom A. Exposure to electromagnetic fields and the risk of childhood leukaemia: a review. *Radiat Prot Dosimetry* 2008;**132**:202–11.
2. Infante-Rivard C. Chemical risk factors and childhood leukaemia: a review of recent studies. *Radiat Prot Dosimetry* 2008;**132**:220–7.
3. Greaves M. Infection, immune responses and the aetiology of childhood leukaemia. *Nat Rev Cancer* 2006;**6**:193–230.
4. Smith OP, Hann IM. Clinical features and therapy of lymphoblastic leukemia. In: Arceci RJ, Hann IM, Smith OP, editors. *Pediatric Hematology*. 3rd ed. London: Blackwell Publishing Ltd.; 2006. p. 450–81.
5. Kean LS, Arceci RJ, Woods WG. Acute myeloid leukemia. In: Arceci RJ, Hann IM, Smith OP, editors. *Pediatric Hematology*. 3rd ed. London: Blackwell Publishing Ltd.; 2006. p. 360–83.
6. Zwaan CM, Kaspers GJL. Possibilities for tailored and targeted therapy in paediatric acute myeloid leukaemia. *Br J Haematol* 2004;**127**:264–79.
7. Aplenc R, Lange B. Pharmacogenetic determinants of outcome in acute lymphoblastic leukemia. *Br J Haematol* 2004;**125**:421–34.
8. Harrison CJ. Cytogenetics of paediatric and adolescent acute lymphoblastic leukaemia. *Br J Haematol* 2009;**144**:147–56.
9. Pui CH, Robison LL, Look AT. Acute lymphoblastic leukemia. *Lancet* 2008;**371**:1030–43.
10. Blair A, Goulden NJ, Libri NA, et al. Immunotherapeutic strategies in acute lymphoblastic leukemia relapsing after stem cell transplantation. *Blood Rev* 2005;**19**:289–300.
11. Brown P, Smith FO. Molecularly targeted therapies for pediatric acute myeloid leukemia: progress to date. *Paediatr Drugs* 2008;**10**:85–92.

11.7 Febrile neutropenia

Joseph Ting

ESSENTIALS

1 Aggressive and early resuscitation of the child with overt or incipient septic shock is vital to avert hypoperfusion, even in the presence of normal mental state and blood pressure.

2 Careful physical examination and broad microbiological/radiological investigation to detect and eradicate the source of infection is essential.

3 Early institution of broad-spectrum antimicrobial therapy, followed by targeted culture-guided treatment contributes to improved outcome.

Introduction

Infection is a major cause of death in children with haematological malignancies following bone marrow or solid organ transplantation, iatrogenic immunosuppression, and chemotherapy. The major factor predisposing to infection in these patients is neutropenia, which is defined as decreased circulating neutrophils in the peripheral blood. The normal reference range for neutrophil counts varies with the age of the child, being highest in the neonatal period. In infants, the normal threshold is 1000 neutrophils per mL; the usual value is 1500 neutrophils per mL up to 10 years of age, with an adult threshold of 1800 neutrophils per mL applied thereafter.[1] Neutropenia is defined as ≤500 neutrophils per mL or an anticipated decline from 1000 to ≤500 neutrophils per mL. Infection risk increases when the neutrophil count is ≤500 neutrophils per mL and is highest when ≤100 neutrophils per mL. Febrile neutropenia requires an associated fever ≥38.3°C, or ≥38.0°C for at least 1 hour.[2] This chapter focuses on neutropenia associated with paediatric cancer or its treatment as this is the more frequent type encountered in the emergency department (ED).

Neutropenic children receiving chemotherapy for leukaemia or undergoing bone-marrow transplantation (BMT) are at significant risk from Gram-negative sepsis, including *Pseudomonas aeruginosa* and *Escherichia coli*. In BMT patients, half the infections are bacterial, evenly split between Gram-positives (such as *Staphylococcus aureus*) and Gram-negative organisms; 40% are due to viruses like cytomegalovirus; and 10% due to fungi, with up to a third of episodes due to systemic fungaemia being life threatening.[1] Vascular catheter-related infections are usually related to Gram-positive skin organisms. Although the overall mortality rate due to neutropenia-associated infection is 1%, children undergoing BMT with febrile neutropenia have a startling mortality up to 80%.[1]

Management priorities are:

- early recognition of the child with compensated septic shock before onset of hypoperfusion;
- aggressive and early resuscitation of the child with overt or incipient septic shock;
- careful physical examination and broad microbiological/radiological investigation to detect and eradicate the source of infection;
- Obtaining blood and other cultures prior to commencing antimicrobial therapy, followed by early institution of broad-spectrum antimicrobial therapy, followed by targeted culture-guided treatment;
- achieving optimal microcirculatory, metabolic and circulatory conditions using a combination of intravenous fluids, vasopressors/blood products and consideration of early mechanical ventilation; however, early goal-directed therapy has not been validated in septic children.

Presentation

Young children compensate for impending shock and remain normotensive in the early stages of systemic sepsis. The earliest reliable sign of vascular redistribution is delayed capillary return, because tachycardia and tachypnoea can be secondary to the fever. Neutropenic or immunosuppressed children may have attenuated or altered signs of infection. The absence of neutrophils to localise an infection makes it difficult to determine the source of infection by physical examination alone. Pay special attention to body regions vulnerable to bacterial infection, such as oropharynx, ears, skin, and perianal area. Evidence of respiratory, circulatory, renal, and metabolic derangement indicates severe sepsis.

Investigations

Microbiological samples from potential infection sources such as blood, urine, cerebrospinal fluid, throat, skin, and central access devices should ideally be obtained prior to, but not delay, treatment. Similarly, radiological investigation to localise infection source should not delay treatment commencement. Although no microbiological source is identified in one-half of febrile neutropenic children with cancer, a high proportion have culture-positive bacteraemia, respiratory tract infections and central access device infections.[1] Full blood count with white cell differential confirms neutropenia, and when followed serially tracks progress of neutrophil recovery. Thrombocytopenia and coagulopathy are early markers of disseminated intravenous coagulation. Chest X-ray may indicate lower respiratory involvement or cardiac decompensation.

Treatment

IV fluid resuscitation and vasopressor support may be required in septic shock. Urgent empiric intravenous therapy with combination broad-spectrum antimicrobials that have excellent Gram-negative cover is essential in febrile neutropenia. The pattern and severity of infection varies according to location, clinical context, and level of immune suppression. Regularly reviewed institution- and scenario-specific treatment protocols, developed in conjunction with infectious diseases physicians and microbiologists, that take into account local patterns of infection and their susceptibilities help to deliver and standardise optimal treatment.

The Victorian Drug Committee's Therapeutic Guidelines for Antibiotics[3] is an excellent resource for centres that do not have their own febrile neutropenia protocols but should ideally be adapted to local requirements. The recommended regimen in eTG 2010 includes: cefepime or ceftazidime 2 g (child: 50 mg kg^{-1} up to 2 g) IV, 8-hourly or piperacillin + tazobactam 4 + 0.5 g (child: 100 + 12.5 mg kg^{-1} up to 4 + 0.5 g) IV, 8-hourly in children with no immediate hypersensitivity to penicillin. Gram-positive bacteraemia from infected intravascular devices require addition of IV vancomycin (<12 years: 30 mg kg^{-1} up to 1.5 g IV, 12-hourly concentration monitoring) only if the child is shocked, known to be previously colonised with MRSA or has catheter-related infection in a treatment environment with high incidence of MRSA infection. Vancomycin is also indicated if a Gram-positive organism resistant to other drugs is isolated from blood cultures or the child worsens clinically despite broad spectrum antibacterials for 48 h.

If fevers persist in high-risk children after 96 hours of antibacterial therapy, consider empirically adding antifungal therapy after consultation with a paediatric infectious diseases physician. Antibiotics can be discontinued if there is clinical improvement, no proven infection, cultures remain negative, and neutrophil count improves to $\geq$500 mL^{-1}; this typically occurs at 3 to 7 days. Although inpatient management is associated with an excellent outcome, carefully selected children who are clinically well, with low-risk criteria, could be considered for early discharge or outpatient management with daily intravenous ceftriaxone or oral ciprofloxacin and daily reviews.[2,4-6]

Bone-marrow stimulation with colony-stimulating factors reduces the severity and duration of neutropenia and fever, and antibiotic requirements in children undergoing BMT, and may be effective in premature infants at high risk of infection as well as children with severe neutropenia and Gram-negative sepsis. Corticosteroids are effective in *Pneumocystis carinii* pneumonia and have been used in conjunction with immunoglobulin to treat immune-mediated neutropenia.[7]

Controversies and challenges

❶ Early goal-directed therapy, directed at optimising cardiac preload, afterload and contractility to balance oxygen delivery with oxygen demand as part of a sepsis bundle multimodal algorithm, was associated with reduced mortality in adults in a single-centre study which did not include children;[8] as such, it may not be relevant in septic children requiring further care in ICU.

❷ Granulocyte infusions are no longer used because of questionable efficacy but may have a role in refractory neonatal sepsis.

❸ Although colony-stimulating factor does not affect overall mortality in children with cancer-related febrile neutropenia, it is known to reduce length of hospital stay, infection rate and neutrophil recovery period.[9,10]

❹ The emergence of highly resistant and virulent organisms is increasingly recognised as a barrier to improved outcomes, especially in the context of immunosuppression.

References

1. Behrman RE, Kliegman RM, Jenson HB, editors. *Nelson textbook of pediatrics.* 17th ed. Philadelphia: Saunders; 2004.
2. Holdsworth M, Hanrahan J, Albanese B, Frost J. Outpatient management of febrile neutropenia in children with cancer. *Paediatr Drugs* 2003;**5**:443–55.
3. Victorian Drug Committee. *Therapeutic Guidelines for Antibiotics.* 14th ed. Victoria: Victorian Drug Committee; 2010 (etg32, November 2010).
4. Mullen CA. Ciprofloxacin in the treatment of fever and neutropenia pediatric cancer patients. *Pediatr Infect Dis J* 2003;**22**:1138–42.
5. Orudjev E, Lange BJ. Evolving concepts of management of febrile neutropenia in children with cancer. *Med Pediatr Oncol* 2002;**39**:77–85.
6. Paulus S, Dobson S. Febrile neutropenia in children with cancer. *Adv Exp Med Biol* 2009;**634**:185–204.
7. Hann IM. Management of infection in children with bone marrow failure. *Bailliere's Clinical Haematology* 2000;**13**:441–56.
8. Rivers E, Nguyen B, Havstad S, et al. Early goal-directed therapy in the treatment of severe sepsis and septic shock. *N Engl J Med* 2001;**345**:1368–77.
9. Sasse EC, Sasse AD, Brandalise S, et al. Colony stimulating factors for prevention of myelosuppressive therapy induced febrile neutropenia in children with acute lymphoblastic leukaemia. *Cochrane Database Syst Rev* 2005;(3): CD004139.
10. Clark OA, Lyman G, Castro AA, Djulbegovic B. Colony stimulating factors for chemotherapy induced febrile neutropenia. *Cochrane Database Syst Rev* 2003;(3): CD003039.

Further reading

Chakravorty S, Hann IM. Management of infection in children with bone marrow failure. In: *Pediatric Hematology.* 3rd ed. London: Blackwell Publishing; 2006.

12.1 Dermatology

Roderic Phillips • David Orchard • Mike Starr

ESSENTIALS

1 Look at the rash.

- Are there any blisters? Finding fluid-filled lesions greatly narrows the range of possible diagnoses.

- Is the rash red? Redness is from haemoglobin. Most red rashes blanch, i.e. the redness disappears with pressure. If not, the haemoglobin is outside the blood vessels giving purpura.

- Is the rash scaly? If so, the epidermis is involved in the disease process. The epidermis may be broken to give weeping, crusting or fissures ('eczematous rash'), or it may be intact ('red scaly rash').

2 Examine all the skin including the anogenital region.

3 Do not ignore a skin condition even if unrelated to the emergency visit. You may not deal with it yourself but you can organise appropriate follow up for it.

Introduction

Approximately 65 000 children a year attend the emergency department (ED) at the Royal Children's Hospital in Melbourne and about 15 000 of these have some skin findings relevant to their visit. For 4000 children (6%), skin findings are a primary reason for their visit. These figures are likely to be representative of other tertiary teaching hospital EDs in Australasia. Diagnosing and managing these children requires a careful history and astute observation, particularly focusing on the appearance, site and development of their rashes.

For children who present to the ED with the primary symptom in another organ, the physician has an opportunity to observe cutaneous signs of disease, which may be relevant or may be coincidental to the child's presentation, for example, a 5-year-old boy (Fig. 12.1.1) who presents with gastroenteritis. You notice the mild comedonal rash on his forehead and recognise that this is unusual at this age. Examination shows that he is tall for his age and has inappropriate penile (but not testicular) growth. His hyperadrenergic state can be investigated and treated years before it might otherwise have been recognised.

The discussion of diseases in this chapter is based on the features of the presenting rash and follows the algorithm given in Essentials. Diseases are grouped under their main morphology, e.g. vesicular, papular, eczematous, or purpuric. Mouth, anogenital, hair and nail problems are considered separately.

Erythroderma and skin failure

Erythroderma is one form of skin failure and refers to any condition that causes most of the skin surface to become red, often with some degree of scaling. Skin failure is rarely taught as a concept but is analogous to failure of any other organ system. Skin failure refers to the inability of the skin to adequately perform its functions, such as fluid and electrolyte balance, temperature control and protection from infection. Any child presenting with extensive areas of skin pathology or skin loss has some degree of skin failure. This may be well tolerated in otherwise healthy children but may be life threatening, especially in infants and those children with associated disorders.

Children presenting with erythroderma will usually be found to have one of the following: atopic eczema (with or without secondary staphylococcal infection); an allergic reaction; or sepsis with toxin-mediated skin involvement. Less common causes include: psoriasis; pityriasis rubra pilaris; several forms of inherited ichthyosis; some other genodermatoses; and internal lymphoid malignancies. In 10–20% of children with erythroderma, no cause can be found.

Management

- The aim is to restore and maintain the core functions of skin. Many sensible management decisions can be made before the diagnosis is clear.

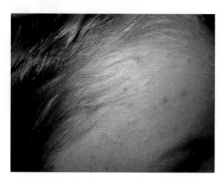

Fig. 12.1.1 Mild prepubertal acne on the forehead of a 5-year-old boy who presented with the unrelated problem of gastroenteritis. Examination and investigation confirmed that he had a variant of congenital adrenal hyperplasia requiring treatment.

- Have a low threshold for admission to hospital.
- Restore skin-barrier function by using an ointment emollient frequently.
- Monitor temperature, as the child may readily become hypothermic or, less commonly, hyperthermic.
- Monitor fluids and electrolytes.
- Monitor cardiac output, particularly if the child has known cardiac pathology.
- Skin and/or systemic sepsis may have caused the skin failure or may be secondary to it. Temperature control may be affected, so fever may not be present. Have a low threshold for giving systemic antibiotics, particularly to cover *Staphylococcus aureus* and streptococcal species.
- Local or systemic pain relief may be required.
- Cease all non-essential drugs.
- Identify and treat the underlying cause.
- Manage any associated conditions (e.g. diabetes, renal failure, congenital heart problems, metabolic disorders).

VESICULOBULLOUS RASHES

Vesicles are usually caused by infections (herpes simplex virus, varicella zoster virus, enterovirus, tinea, scabies or impetigo) or contact dermatitis. Also, consider drug reactions, erythema multiforme and photosensitivity. Dermatitis herpetiformis is a rare cause of itchy vesicles and papules. Larger blisters occur with staphylococcal infections, tinea, erythema multiforme, Stevens–Johnson syndrome, immune-mediated blistering disorders, arthropod bites, contact dermatitis, fixed and bullous drug reactions, mastocytosis, burns or trauma.

Many vesicles and blisters are fragile and rupture easily. A vesicular disease may present with a number of shallow monomorphic erosions but no vesicles. A bullous disease may present with several larger shallow erosions with surrounding loose epithelium but no bullae. Vesicles present for more than a couple of days become cloudy and vesiculopustular.

Varicella (chickenpox)

Varicella is caused by infection with varicella zoster virus. It usually occurs in children less than 15 years of age, and is highly contagious. The incubation period is 2–3 weeks. The contagious period begins 2 days before the rash and continues until the lesions are crusted. Clinical disease begins with a fever and malaise but these are usually mild. Lesions on the skin appear initially as erythematous macules, rapidly becoming small vesicles and then crusting. Over the next few days, anything from a few to hundreds of lesions may develop, initially on the face and trunk and gradually spreading onto the extremities. Superficial ulcers may be seen on all mucosal surfaces. Itch is not always present but may be marked. Vaccinated children may develop attenuated disease with fewer lesions and without constitutional symptoms. Diagnosis is clinical but can be confirmed by serology or immunofluorescence of vesicular scrapings for varicella-zoster virus antigen. Complete resolution occurs in most children but some scarring is common.

Children with varicella usually remain systemically well and afebrile after the first few days. If persistent fever and malaise is present, search for complications. In previously well children, the most common complications are:

- Bacterial skin infection with group A Streptococci or *Staphylococcus aureus*. Look for bullous, indurated, spreading or cellulitic lesions. Treat with oral antibiotics.
- Central nervous system (CNS) dysfunction. Encephalitis, meningitis, transverse myelitis, Guillain–Barré syndrome or Reye's syndrome (sudden onset of vomiting, coma and liver abnormalities) may occur. Cerebrospinal fluid (CSF) analysis, including polymerase chain reaction (PCR) assay for varicella-zoster virus DNA may be useful in suspected encephalitis.
- Pneumonia. Cough and respiratory distress begin a couple of days after onset of the rash.
- Cerebellar ataxia may appear as the rash is clearing and resolve within weeks.

In neonates, immunocompromised children and adolescents, varicella can be more severe and occasionally fatal.

Management

- Treatment of otherwise well children with varicella is supportive with bland emollients and oral antihistamine if necessary. If the child is unwell, look for secondary complications.
- Avoid aspirin or other salicylates because of the association with Reye's syndrome.
- Treat secondary skin infection with cefalexin 30 mg kg^{-1} (max 500 mg) three times daily.
- Immunocompromised children should be treated with intravenous aciclovir 20 mg kg^{-1} per dose (2–12 weeks), 500 mg m^{-2} per dose (12 weeks–12 years), 10 mg kg^{-1} per dose (adult) 8-hourly given over 1 hour.
- Premature neonates (less than 1 month old) with varicella should be treated with intravenous aciclovir.
- Term neonates should be admitted, and treated with aciclovir if they have severe disease.
- Give zoster immune globulin to at-risk contacts (immunocompromised children, those on prednisolone 2 mg kg^{-1} day^{-1} or more, newborns of mothers who have varicella any time from 5 days before until 2 days after delivery). Give within 4 days of exposure (6 mL for adults, 4 mL for children 6–12 years of age, 2 mL for children up to 5 years of age).
- Exclude from school until all lesions are crusted.
- Offer varicella-zoster vaccine to non-immune contacts – the vaccine has been shown to prevent or attenuate infection if given within 5 days of exposure.

Zoster

Zoster is uncommon in childhood but can occur at any age, even in the neonatal period. It occurs in children who have previously had primary varicella infection. Zoster in a young child is usually associated with primary varicella having occurred in infancy. The primary infection may have been mild and may even have gone unnoticed because of maternally-acquired IgG.

Radicular pain may be the first symptom of zoster but pain is less common than in adults and may not be present. Vesicles on an erythematous background appear in one or more groups aligned in a dermatomal distribution, frequently with a striking midline cut-off. The affected area can be an isolated group of a few vesicles suggestive of herpes simplex virus infection. Alternatively, there may be extensive involvement of one or more dermatomes. Lesions continue to appear for a few days and then resolve over 2 weeks, generally without sequelae. Postherpetic neuralgia is very uncommon after childhood zoster.

Complications include generalised dissemination during the first week of the rash, sometimes with pulmonary or brain involvement. This can be seen in both normal and immunocompromised children. Zoster on the head is occasionally accompanied by an aseptic meningitis, which resolves fully without treatment. Zoster lesions on the tip of the nose imply involvement of the nasociliary branch of the ophthalmic nerve and may accompany ocular involvement including keratitis and conjunctivitis. Facial nerve palsy and ear involvement can occur (Ramsay Hunt syndrome).

Immunocompromised children are much more likely to develop zoster. In such cases, zoster may be severe, extensive and prolonged. Significant dermatomal scarring can result.

Management

- If the diagnosis is unclear, collect epithelial cells from the base and roof of the vesicles for immunofluorescence and viral culture. This is not 'just a swab' and it requires some persistence to collect enough cells.
- In an otherwise well child, the occurrence of typical zoster does not require investigation for underlying immunodeficiency states. However, unusually severe or extensive zoster should raise this possibility.
- If a child has underlying chronic illness or immunodeficiency, give intravenous aciclovir or oral famciclovir or valaciclovir.

Oral antiviral agents can be considered in older adolescents but are not generally indicated in an otherwise well child as the risk of significant symptoms or postherpetic neuralgia is very small.

Hand, foot and mouth disease

Hand, foot and mouth disease is one presentation of enteroviral infection, usually Coxsackie A16 virus. There may be a mild prodrome of fever, malaise and sore throat. Discrete vesicles about 6 mm in diameter on an erythematous base appear first in the mouth, sparing the lips and usually sparing the gingiva. One to 2 days later, 3–7 mm vesiculopustules on an erythematous base appear on the palms, soles and around the fingers and toes. Lesions are also often found on the buttocks. They are often greyish and oval rather than circular in shape. In some cases, the mouth, hands or feet may not be involved. Resolution occurs within a week. The incubation period is about 5 days and epidemics are common. Virus is excreted in the faeces for weeks and exclusion is not recommended. Supportive care leads to complete recovery.

Herpes simplex infection (HSV)

Herpes simplex infection in childhood is common. Intrauterine, intrapartum and neonatal infection are considered elsewhere. Primary herpes infection after the neonatal period may be either primary herpetic gingivostomatitis or primary cutaneous herpes simplex. In children with impaired immune function, HSV infection can present as indolent, slowly growing, irregular ulcers. Most HSV infections in children are caused by HSV-1, but HSV-2 may also cause gingival and cutaneous infection.

Primary cutaneous herpes simplex can present at any age. There may be a history of a family member with a recently activated herpes simplex lesion on the lip ('cold sore'). However, the virus is ubiquitous and transmission more often occurs from an unknown source. At least 50% of the population have HSV-1 antibodies, and many of these have never had an obvious infection. Painful grouped vesicles on an erythematous base can appear at any site. Multiple lesions rupture, crust and coalesce into larger erosions with scalloped edges. There may be associated fever, malaise and lymphadenopathy.

Management

Management consists of the following;

- supportive care;
- bathing of crusts;
- analgesia;
- aciclovir is not routinely indicated unless risk factors for complications exist (e.g. underlying disease, immunosuppression).

Recurrent cutaneous herpes simplex can occur weeks or months after the primary episode. Recurrences usually get milder and less common with time but exacerbations can occur throughout childhood and later life (Fig. 12.1.2). Recurrences can lead to significant time off school. Antiviral prophylaxis may reduce the frequency and severity of recurrences, and should be used if recurrences are frequent or debilitating.

HSV infection can involve the fingers, especially the thumbs and index fingers (herpetic

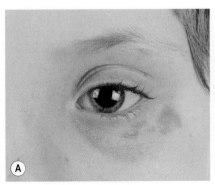
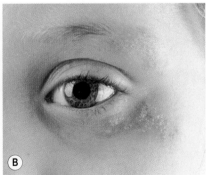

Fig. 12.1.2 (A) This erythematous, slightly vesicular rash around the eye of a 4-year-old boy had appeared over 12 hours. Because his other eye was blind, he was treated with oral aciclovir. Immunofluorescence confirmed herpes simplex virus. (B) One day later.

whitlow). At these sites, the thick skin does not readily rupture and children present with painful, coalesced pustular collections, often misinterpreted as bacterial abscesses. Any history of 'abscesses' occurring at the same site on a finger on more than one occasion is suggestive of herpes simplex. Management includes taking a swab for immunofluorescence and viral culture to confirm the diagnosis, analgesia and supportive care.

Eczema herpeticum

Herpes simplex infection in children with eczema is quite common. It occurs in children with any severity of eczema including children with mild eczema under excellent control. Many cases are misdiagnosed either as an exacerbation of the eczema or as bacterial infection (Fig. 12.1.3). Grouped vesicles may be prominent, but more often vesicles are rudimentary or absent and the infection may present as a group of shallow 2–4 mm monomorphic erosions on an inflamed base. In more severe cases, evolution is rapid and large crops of vesicles can arise daily. Ulcers may coalesce into larger erosions with scalloped edges. The infected area may not be painful or itchy.

In an atopic child, a high index of suspicion is needed about any patch of skin where small erosions or crusts are present and not responding to standard eczema therapy with moisturisers and topical cortisone derivatives. One reason for the under diagnosis of this condition is that even without treatment, resolution usually occurs in 1–4 weeks. However, dissemination may occur, leading to multifocal and extensive erosions, malaise and secondary bacterial infection. In the past, disseminated eczema herpeticum had a significant mortality but this has declined with the recognition and aggressive treatment of secondary bacterial infections.

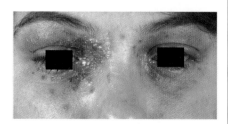

Fig. 12.1.3 Eczema herpeticum. Typical monomorphic vesicles can be seen away from the central weeping area.

After complete resolution, recurrences may occur at the same or different sites, sometimes as often as every few weeks. Recurrences can be widespread and severe but usually decrease in severity over 1 to 2 years.

Management

- Clinical differentiation between herpetic and bacterial infection may be difficult; investigation and empiric treatment for both may be necessary.
- Collect epithelial cells from the base and roof of the vesicles for HSV immunofluorescence and viral culture. This requires some persistence to collect enough cells.
- Local stable disease in an otherwise well child requires regular observation but does not need antiviral therapy.
- Milder cases demonstrating progression or facial involvement can be managed with oral aciclovir.
- Admission to hospital and treatment with intravenous aciclovir (20 mg kg^{-1} per dose (2–12 weeks), 500 mg m^{-2} per dose (12 weeks–12 years), 10 mg kg^{-1} per dose (adult) 8-hourly should be considered for children with any of fever, multiple sites of cutaneous herpes infection, widespread eczema, eye involvement, immunosuppression or age less than 6 months.
- Secondary bacterial infection is common. Swabs for microscopy and culture are usually unhelpful. If there is any suspicion of bacterial infection, add intravenous flucloxacillin 50 mg kg^{-1} (max 2 g) 6-hourly or oral cefalexin 30 mg kg^{-1} (max 500 mg) three times daily. Soak to remove excessive crusts.
- Monitor for eye involvement, particularly scleral redness. If present, this should be managed with topical or systemic aciclovir, or both, and urgent review by an ophthalmologist.
- The underlying eczema can be treated with moisturiser or wet dressings until the herpetic scabs have been removed and then it is important to restart topical cortisone treatment.
- Antiviral prophylaxis may reduce the frequency and severity of recurrences and is often warranted in older children with recurrent eczema herpeticum.

Impetigo (school sores)

This is caused by *Staphylococcus aureus* or group A *Streptococcus* or both.

Non-bullous impetigo presents initially as small erythematous vesicles that rapidly rupture to form yellow-crusted lesions, commonly on the face.

Bullous impetigo is due to *Staphylococcus aureus* and presents as flaccid blisters on normal skin. Lesions are rounded and well demarcated and may be single, grouped or widespread. Their onset and spread may be rapid or occur over days. New blisters appear and existing blisters rupture to give shallow moist erosions that can be many centimetres in size. There is often loose epithelium and/or brown crusting peripherally and some degree of central healing (Fig. 12.1.4). In more chronic cases, lesions may appear annular.

Impetigo is often secondary to itchy conditions such as scabies infection (especially hand impetigo), atopic eczema and head lice.

Post-streptococcal glomerulonephritis may occur in the ensuing 2 months. Contrary to long-held beliefs, it now seems likely that chronic streptococcal impetigo may also be a precursor of rheumatic heart disease in communities where medical conditions are poor and skin hygiene is suboptimal.[1]

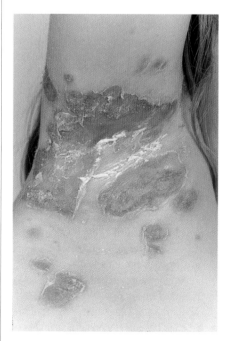

Fig. 12.1.4 Bullous impetigo in a 7-year-old girl.

Management

- Swab for microscopy and culture if the diagnosis is unclear or in widespread or complicated disease.
- Bathe off crusts.
- Apply topical mupirocin 2% ointment 8-hourly if very localised, or oral cefalexin 30 mg kg^{-1} (maximum 500 mg) three times daily if extensive.
- Isolate the child from other children or from sick adults unless all lesions are covered or antibiotic treatment has commenced.
- Treat any underlying condition such as scabies or eczema.
- Blisters or erosions often continue to occur for a couple of days after antibiotic therapy. If new blisters continue to form after this time, they may be caused by resistant *Staphylococcus aureus* infection, or the child may have an immune-mediated blistering disorder rather than impetigo.
- Children with chronic impetigo should be examined for any signs of heart disease. Families should be aware that rheumatic heart disease may be delayed by some years in this setting. Older siblings are likely to have had chronic impetigo in the past and therefore to also be at risk of heart disease and should be examined.
- In any child with chronic impetigo where ongoing care may be suboptimal, review with urinalysis to monitor for glomerulonephritis is warranted. In other cases, families should be aware of the possibility of renal involvement.

Staphylococcal scalded skin syndrome

This is usually seen in younger children or children with renal impairment. It is mediated by an epidermolytic toxin released from an often insignificant staphylococcal focus (e.g. eyes, nose or skin). Fever and tender erythematous skin are early features. Exudation and crusting develop, especially around the mouth. Wrinkling, flaccid bullae and exfoliation of the skin are seen and can be extensive. Nikolsky sign is present ('normal' skin separates if rubbed). Blisters are very superficial and heal without scarring.

Management

- Admit to hospital. Monitor temperature, fluids and electrolytes if large areas are

involved. Increase oral (or intravenous) fluids to increase toxin excretion. Give analgesia.
- Consider alternative diagnoses including Stevens–Johnson syndrome and toxic epidermal necrolysis. If the diagnosis is unclear, a skin biopsy will confirm the diagnosis by showing the split is in the granular layer in the upper epidermis.
- Flucloxacillin 50 mg kg^{-1} (maximum 2 g) IV 6-hourly if there is evidence of sepsis or systemic involvement.
- Look for a focus of infection. Drain any foci of pus if present.
- Handle skin carefully and use an emollient ointment.

Erythema multiforme

This is a specific hypersensitivity syndrome that occurs at any age, often preceded by facial herpes simplex virus infection. It is over-diagnosed in emergency departments. Most children diagnosed with erythema multiforme actually have urticaria, often with large lesions with annular or polycyclic borders. In erythema multiforme, the primary lesions are red papules, usually symmetrical and involving the forearms, palms, feet, face, neck and trunk. They can be found anywhere. There may be few or many lesions. At least some of the papules will form classical target lesions – these have an inner zone of epidermal injury (purpura, necrosis or vesicle), an outer zone of erythema and sometimes a middle zone of pale oedema (Fig. 12.1.5). These papules and target lesions are not migratory. The involvement of mucous membranes is common but unlike Stevens–Johnson syndrome, is limited to isolated patches. Most cases are caused by herpes simplex virus, including most of the cases that occur without prior symptoms. Drugs

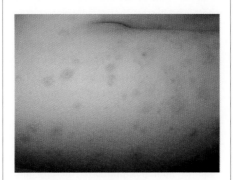

Fig. 12.1.5 Erythema multiforme target lesions.

are an uncommon cause. Erythema multiforme does not evolve into Stevens–Johnson syndrome. They are different conditions.

Management

- Fluid maintenance.
- Analgesia if required.
- Apply emollient ointment to the lips, if needed.
- If the condition is recurrent, it is highly likely to be related to herpes simplex virus. Prophylactic aciclovir prevents recurrences and should be considered if recurrences are frequent, severe and affecting the quality of life.
- Prednisolone alleviates symptoms but probably prolongs the duration of the condition and may cause recurrence of herpes simplex virus infection.

Stevens–Johnson syndrome/toxic epidermal necrolysis

Stevens–Johnson syndrome and toxic epidermal necrolysis are believed by many to be variants of the one condition. Most cases are thought to be triggered by medications, especially antibiotics (sulfonamides, penicillins), anticonvulsants (lamotrigine) and non-steroidal anti-inflammatory drugs. *Mycoplasma* and other infections may be the cause in some children. Fever, myalgia, arthralgia, headache and other organ involvement are usually present as a prodromal illness for several days. The rash evolves suddenly, characterised by widespread blisters on an erythematous or purpuric macular background, often with extensive mucous membrane haemorrhagic crusting. Lesions are usually on the face and trunk or generalised rather than acral, and typical target lesions are not seen. There may be tender erythematous areas with a positive Nikolsky sign ('normal' skin separates if rubbed). Mucous membrane involvement can be extensive, severe and painful. Conjunctivitis, corneal ulceration and blindness can occur. Anogenital lesions can lead to urinary retention.

Management

- See general advice under 'skin failure'.
- Admit to hospital. A multidisciplinary approach including dermatology, paediatrics, ophthalmology, surgery and paediatric intensive care is required. Good

nursing care is paramount. In severe cases, nurse in a specialised burns unit.

- Apply emollient ointment to the skin, lips and anogenital areas – this may be required many times a day.
- Regular eye examination with specialist review is required. Topical steroid eye drops may be needed.
- Give IV immunoglobulin 2 g kg^{-1}. Commence ciclosporin (5–6 mg kg^{-1} day^{-1} orally for a few days, then taper to 3–5 mg kg^{-1} day^{-1} for 2–3 weeks). Data about the efficacy of any treatment regimens are limited but are sufficent to justify treatment. Stevens–Johnson syndrome has a significant mortality and has a high rate of permanent visual scarring including blindness as well as other problems.
- Maintain good nutrition, with nasogastric feeding if needed.
- Intubation may be needed if the child is unable to protect the airway because of severe oropharyngeal involvement.

Note: Stevens–Johnson syndrome is *not* severe erythema multiforme. They are distinct conditions. Permanent sequelae are rarely seen in severe erythema multiforme and concurrent drug use is unlikely to be the cause. Skin lesion distribution and morphology are the best discriminating factors. Mucous membrane involvement can be seen in both conditions but is confluent in Stevens-Johnson syndrome.

Dermatitis herpetiformis

Dermatitis herpetiformis is an uncommon autoimmune blistering disease that may present at any age as itchy papules or vesicles. Rapid excoriation means that intact vesicles are rarely seen. Lesions occur on extensor surfaces of the limbs, buttocks, trunk and scalp. Most patients have gluten enteropathy (coeliac disease) and may have abdominal discomfort, diarrhoea or anaemia. Some degree of villous atrophy will be seen on small bowel biopsy in most cases, but coeliac disease is often asymptomatic at the time of presentation of dermatitis herpetiformis. Growth retardation has been reported with dermatitis herpetiformis, probably secondary to intestinal involvement.

Recurrence some years after successful treatment has been reported.

Management

- Perilesional skin should be biopsied for immunofluorescence to demonstrate the diagnostic granular IgA deposition.
- Investigate for coeliac disease with total IgA, anti-tissue transglutaminase IgA and anti-deamidated gliadin IgA. Anti-transglutaminase antibodies are the most specific for dermatitis herpetiformis. A small bowel biopsy is required but may be equivocal early in the disease course.
- Anaemia, usually megaloblastic secondary to malabsorption, may be found.

Skin lesions (but not intestinal symptoms) respond well to dapsone, but haemolysis and other side effects can limit its use. A gluten-free diet normalises gut function and, in most children, leads to eventual clearing of skin lesions.

Other immune-mediated blistering disorders

As with dermatitis herpetiformis, the many diseases in this group are characterised by circulating autoantibodies directed against one or other of the structural proteins that give the epidermis its integrity. All are uncommon in childhood, linear IgA dermatosis (chronic bullous disease of childhood) being the most common. An immune-mediated blistering disorder should be considered in an otherwise well child if vesicles, blisters, or crusted erosions continue to appear for more than a couple of weeks.

If there is a split below the basement membrane, lesions may be tense, long-lasting bullae, as seen in dermatitis herpetiformis, linear IgA dermatosis, systemic lupus erythematosus and pemphigoid. If the split is higher in the epidermis, lesions are flaccid, short-lived blisters that rapidly give crusted erosions with loose epithelium around the edges. These are seen in pemphigus variants. Lesions can mimic local or generalised impetigo. Mucous membranes may be involved. Despite the widespread and often dramatic appearance of the rash, the child is usually well. Accurate diagnosis always requires histology and immunofluorescence in addition to clinical findings. Management requires immunosuppressive therapy and long-term follow up.

Sunburn and photosensitivity

Excessive solar radiation to the skin causes erythema and tenderness commencing at least half an hour after the beginning of the exposure. Tenderness worsens for a day and resolves in 4 days. In more severe cases, oedema and blistering may be widespread. Healing is accompanied by desquamation and intense itch. Sunburn occurs more rapidly when the sun is overhead (summer, closer to the equator, 11 a.m. to 3 p.m.), and when the skin is less pigmented, but can occur with any skin type. Children with sensitive skin can burn significantly within 15 minutes of midday exposure in summer.

Any child presenting to the ED with sunburn or with a rash in sun-exposed areas may have an underlying photosensitivity disorder. These can be considered in four groups.

❶ Primary photosensitivity disorders.
❷ Inherited disorders including porphyrias.
❸ Diseases with a photosensitive component (systemic lupus erythematosus, dermatomyositis).
❹ Exogenous photosensitivity from drugs or plants.

A high index of suspicion is needed to diagnose photosensitivity. There have been examples of sunburn in children that were attributed to parental neglect but were actually due to a photosensitivity disorder. These diseases are common but diagnostic traps abound. For example, sun-induced rashes may develop in spring with the first sun exposure of untanned skin after winter, but not later in summer. The rash may develop on areas usually covered in winter such as the neck and arms and not on the face. Sun-induced rashes may require a few minutes or several days of sun exposure and may commence days after the exposure. In erythropoietic protoporphyria, sun exposure induces pain without skin changes initially. Viral exanthems may occur exclusively or mainly in areas of sun-exposed skin. Children with solar urticaria develop urticaria on sun-exposed areas.

Management

- Assess for associated causes (below) of increased sun sensitivity. Many children presenting to the ED with 'sunburn' have an associated photosensitive trigger. Any child who experiences symptoms within half an hour of sun exposure should be assumed to have an underlying condition.

- Assess the family situation, especially with younger children. Significant sunburn in a young child can occur in the setting of suboptimal child care, although usually it is due to an oversight by otherwise caring parents.
- Within the first few hours of exposure, before blistering has developed, application of topical potent steroid creams can considerably reduce the severity and duration of symptoms.
- Cool compresses and wet dressings will alleviate symptoms. Topical anaesthetics should not be used. Admission and oral analgesia may be required in severe cases. Maintain adequate fluid intake.
- Educate about prevention.

Prevention

Prevention of sunburn is important. Episodes of sunburn are linked to later development of naevi and melanoma.

Parents need to balance the psychological and physical benefits of activities associated with sun exposure (including increased fitness, increased independence, healthier bones and decreased obesity) with the increased risk of skin cancers of all types. In summer, children should minimise sun exposure during the middle 4 hours of the day, wear broad-brimmed hats and long-sleeved shirts in the sun, and use a sunscreen with SPF 30 or greater on exposed parts.

Sunburnt infants regularly present to the ED, partly because of widespread advice that sunscreens are not recommended below the age of 6 months. This recommendation is not based on any evidence of problems in infants. It is based on the premise that it is usually easy to protect young babies who can't crawl by keeping them out of the sun and appropriately dressed. However, if a young baby is going to be in the sun, sunscreen should be used.

Primary photosensitivity disorders

Polymorphous light eruption (PMLE)

Presents in spring or early summer as skin-coloured or erythematous itchy papules or vesicles on the face, ears, neck or arms. It is recurrent. Recurrences usually occur at the same sites in that child.

Juvenile spring eruption Is a specific variant of PMLE and is common in 4–12-year-old boys as a recurrent blistering of the ears each spring.

Hydroa vacciniforme Is rare and can begin at any age in childhood as a sun-induced vesicular eruption on the cheeks during spring and summer. The cheeks, ears, nose, dorsum of the hands and rarely the eyes can be involved. Recurrences occur for many years.

Diagnosis can be difficult and may require formal evaluation in a photobiology unit including assessment of the response to different wavelengths of light. Management requires sun avoidance and often both UVA and UVB sun protection.

Solar urticaria Presents as urticaria within minutes or hours of exposure and settles within 1 day. Sharp margins are seen at the edges of clothing. Skin chronically exposed to the sun, such as face and hands, is often spared.

Porphyrias and other inherited disorders with photosensitivity

The porphyrias are a group of inherited enzymatic defects in haem synthesis leading to increased levels of porphyrins, some of which cause photosensitivity.

Erythropoietic protoporphyria Is the most common childhood porphyria. Infants and young children present after brief sun exposure with acute discomfort, burning sensations, itching, erythema, oedema, urticaria and occasionally vesicles, particularly on the face and dorsum of the hands. Episodes are recurrent and with time affected skin appears prematurely aged. Erythrocyte protoporphyrin levels are elevated.

Congenital erythropoietic porphyria Is rare and presents in early childhood with extreme photosensitivity leading to painful blisters filled with red fluid on the face and dorsum of the hands. Progressive scarring can be severe.

Familial porphyria cutanea tarda Presents in childhood with chronic blistering on hands, arms and face leading to poorly healing ulcers, atrophic scarring and mottled hypo- and hyper-pigmentation.

If a porphyria is suspected, measure blood, urine and faecal levels of porphyrins. Management requires intensive avoidance of solar radiation including UVA and UVB. β-Carotene is useful in erythropoietic protoporphyria.

Many genodermatoses including xeroderma pigmentosum, Cockayne syndrome, Rothmund-Thomson syndrome and trichothiodystrophies are associated with photosensitivity and increased photo-damage to skin, but do not usually present with blistering.

Photosensitivity and bullous reactions to drugs

Blisters may be the presenting feature of a number of different types of drug reactions. A high index of suspicion is required to diagnose these conditions. Families must be asked about all ingested and topical products including herbal, recreational and prescription drugs and unusual food patterns (e.g. daily cups of celery juice). Families will occasionally not remember the causative drug and deny taking anything, only to recall the vital information days later.

Many medicines can cause increased sun sensitivity leading to erythema, oedema and blistering on sun-exposed areas. Doxycycline (particularly at doses higher than 100 mg day^{-1}), tetracyclines, griseofulvin, isotretinoin, non-steroidal anti-inflammatory drugs, sulfonamides, fluoroquinolones and diuretics are typical causes in children. In one series of children receiving naproxen, 12% developed photosensitivity reactions on the face. Other causes include tars, perfumes, cosmetics, sunscreens, artificial sweeteners and many dyes. As with other photosensitivity syndromes, the rash can occur rapidly or days after the sun exposure and is most prominent on sun-exposed areas. The photosensitivity can persist for up to 3 months after withdrawal of the medication. Prominent hyperpigmentation may persist for months after resolution.

Fixed drug eruptions in children are usually caused by paracetamol, non-steroidal anti-inflammatories or sulfonamides. They are quite common and present as single or multiple, usually circular red patches that may blister. With subsequent exposures, eruptions recur at the same site and sometimes at other sites. Post-inflammatory hyperpigmentation is prominent and may be the only sign of the drug reaction.

Many plants and herbal products contain chemicals that can induce drug reactions including fixed drug reactions, bullous drug reactions and photosensitivity reactions.

Management

- Recognise and stop the causative drug.
- Institute strict sun protection measures. Photosensitivity can persist for 3 months after cessation of the drug.
- If the patient is taking multiple drugs, the timing of the eruption and the frequency of reactions with each of the medications may suggest the causative drug.
- If continued drug ingestion is necessary, reducing the dosage may prevent the reaction.

Photosensitivity reactions to plants

Many plants contain furocoumarins, which are naturally occurring psoralens. UVA light induces covalent bonding of psoralen into DNA, leading to cell death. Typically, a child is playing outside in spring or summer and comes into close contact with a psoralen-containing species (e.g. species of celery, parsley, parsnip, fig, hogweed, limes and other citrus fruits). Several hours later, erythema, oedema and occasionally blistering develop. While contact dermatitis from plants can also present with streaky, often linear vesicular eruptions on areas of contact after exposure, photosensitivity reactions are more often painful, are usually sharply limited to sun exposed areas, and typically heal to leave striking patterns of hyperpigmentation that can persist for months or years.

Management

- Sun protection measures including a UVA sunscreen will prevent phytophotodermatitis.
- Offending plants can be removed.
- Treat as for sunburn.

Contact dermatitis – plants

In children, contact dermatitis reactions from agents other than plants usually do not blister and these conditions are discussed under eczematous rashes (p. 297).

Many plants, including *Rhus* and *Grevillea* species, can cause an allergic contact dermatitis. Some species only cause reactions at specific times of the year and contact with the plant at other times does not cause a rash. One to 3 days after exposure, erythema, oedema and vesiculation develop at sites of contact, often in linear distribution. Lesions may persist for 3 weeks. Periorbital erythema and vesiculation is often misdiagnosed in the ED as cellulitis needing antibiotics. Clues to the correct diagnosis are that pruritus is the main symptom, the degree of pain and tenderness is much less than would be expected for cellulitis, systemic features, such as fever, are absent, the outline of the rash often has irregular patterns corresponding to the contact areas and a careful examination will often reveal other lesions on sensitive parts of the body. In particular, genital skin may develop lesions from secondary spread of the allergen via the fingers. Patients with allergic contact dermatitis may be extremely uncomfortable. Treatment often requires a few days of oral prednisolone, topical potent steroid ointments, cool compresses and supportive care. Unlike plant-induced photosensitivity, contact dermatitis from plants does not induce long-term hyperpigmentation.

Irritant contact dermatitis to components of stinging nettles, chilli peppers, mustard, horseradish and other plant products can lead to irritation, stinging, and occasionally blisters. Burning, oedema and blistering in the oral cavity can occur in small children after chewing irritant plants.

Contact dermatitis – id reactions

Repeated exposure to an allergen can result in a papulovesicular eruption at sites distant from the area of contact. This is thought to be a result of systematised contact sensitisation. The id reaction may be local or generalised. Examples include non-infective blisters erupting on the hands of a child with chronic tinea infection of the feet,

and a severe generalised itchy vesicular rash on an adolescent using topical neomycin ointment.

Isolated blisters

For a child who presents with a single blister or a few blisters as an isolated finding, consider:

- Mastocytoma. Usually in an infant with a history of recurrent blistering or crusting at the site of a brownish macule, often misdiagnosed as recurrent localised impetigo. There may be one brownish lesion or as many as hundreds.
- Insect bite. There may be a few lesions in one area. Non-blistered papules may have a tiny central red bite punctum.
- Irritant contact dermatitis.
- Spider bite. These can grow over days to become a non-tender blister with a diameter of many centimetres. They are uncommon. Regular dressings may be required. Debridement is rarely necessary. White-tailed spiders and huntsman spiders do not cause chronic necrotic ulcers.
- Scalds or burns from cigarettes or other hot objects. Look for characteristic patterns in the burn, as well as other factors on the history or examination suggestive of non-accidental injury or suboptimal caring practices.
- Fixed drug eruptions, e.g. from tetracyclines, sulfonamides, non-steroidal anti-inflammatory drugs or paracetamol.
- Friction. If minor friction appears to cause more blistering than expected on hands and/or feet in children, consider the possibility of a mild inherited blistering disorder (e.g. mild epidermolysis bullosa simplex). There may be a positive family history of childhood blistering that settled in later life.
- Artefactual lesions caused by either the child or a carer.
- Bullous Sweet syndrome or pyoderma gangrenosum.

Chronic erosions or ulcers

Several primary skin conditions can cause chronic erosions or ulcers in children, including itchy conditions such as scabies and papular urticaria. Also consider:

- Immunodeficiencies. Recurrent boils can be seen in chronic granulomatous disease and hyper IgE syndrome. Poor wound healing is a feature of leucocyte adhesion defects.
- Skin fragility syndromes. In junctional and dystrophic forms of epidermolysis bullosa, chronic ulcers related to minimal skin trauma may be seen in association with failure to thrive, anaemia and gastrointestinal tract involvement.
- Porphyria. Several enzyme defects in haem metabolism are associated with chronic erosive lesions, photosensitivity and hyperpigmentation. Episodes of acute pain or neurological dysfunction are rarely seen in childhood porphyrias.
- Artefactual lesions caused by either the child or a carer.
- Pyoderma gangrenosum.
- *Mycobacterium ulcerans* infection.

Neonatal vesicles

A neonate with vesicles or blisters requires urgent assessment, as potential causes include infection with herpes simplex virus, varicella zoster virus and *Staphylococcus aureus*, including bullous impetigo. Neonates who acquire herpes simplex virus at birth usually present at a few days of age with grouped vesicles, often on the scalp. Lesions may rapidly spread and coalesce. Collect epithelial cells from the base and roof of a vesicle for immunofluorescence and viral culture. This is not 'just a swab' and it requires some persistence to collect enough cells. CSF must be examined for herpes simplex virus DNA, as 30% of neonates with apparently localised skin disease also have CNS involvement. Empiric intravenous aciclovir is essential until herpes infection has been excluded.

Non-infective causes of neonatal vesicles include:

- Epidermolysis bullosa. Over 40 inherited diseases are associated with skin fragility. Presentation ranges from a few isolated blisters in otherwise well children to extensive blistering at any site of handling, with associated systemic problems.
- Miliaria. Very superficial blistering in hot or occluded areas.

- Ichthyosis. Bullous subtypes present as blisters or erosions on red skin, which gradually becomes more scaly.
- Langerhans cell histiocytosis – vesicles and/or purpuric crusted lesions (see p. 294).
- Incontinentia pigmenti. This disease is X-linked and fatal in male fetuses. Girls present with lesions distributed in linear patterns. Lesions evolve through vesicular and warty phases to eventually leave permanent hyperpigmented streaks. Seizures and developmental, ocular and dental problems may occur.
- Mastocytosis. Urtication and blistering occur spontaneously or on top of oval brown macules.

PUSTULAR RASHES

Consider acne, folliculitis, drug reactions, pustular psoriasis, scabies, perioral dermatitis, tinea and localised bacterial infection. All vesicular rashes can become pustular if the vesicles persist for more than a couple of days. Vesicles on areas of thick skin can be white and look like pustules, e.g. on the toes in hand, foot and mouth disease. If in doubt, prick one lesion to reveal the clear fluid within.

Acne

Acne mainly affects the forehead and face but can involve other sebaceous gland areas (neck, shoulders and upper trunk). Early lesions include blackheads, whiteheads and papules. In more severe cases there may be pustules or inflammatory cysts that can lead to permanent scarring. Acne is common in adolescence. It is treatable and no person with acne should be told it is an inevitable part of adolescence. Several topical and oral acne therapies are available and should be used to treat the disease. Under-treated acne is a major medical cause of significant morbidity in adolescents and has a recognised mortality as a factor in teenage suicide. It can also lead to permanent scarring in 10% of untreated cases (Fig. 12.1.6). Significant acne in an adolescent attending the ED for another reason should not be ignored. The adolescent should be offered information, initial treatment and referral for ongoing management.

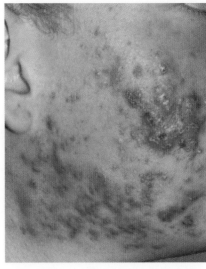

Fig. 12.1.6 Cystic acne. Acne should be treated with isotretinoin before reaching this stage.

Management

- Most cases are mild and either require no intervention or can be managed with topical treatments. A first-line topical treatment is benzoyl peroxide 2.5% applied once or twice a day. Warn the adolescent that improvement with topical therapy occurs steadily over 1–4 months (not in a few days). Other topical agents include topical antibiotics for inflammatory lesions (clindamycin, erythromycin or tetracycline), topical retinoids (isotretinoin, adapalene) or azelaic acid. These can be used singly or in combination and combination preparations are becoming more available. All of these topical agents have the potential to cause irritation.
- If there are prominent red papules or pustules, a course of oral antibiotics for 3–6 months in combination with a topical treatment is warranted (e.g. tetracycline 500 mg twice daily, erythromycin 500 mg twice daily, doxycycline 50–200 mg day^{-1}). Oral hormone therapy can help female patients.
- If the acne is severe, or if antibiotics and topical treatment have not resulted in considerable improvement in 3 months, oral isotretinoin (Roaccutane) is indicated. Prescription of isotretinoin is tightly controlled because it is expensive and because it is teratogenic, requiring

absolute avoidance of any pregnancy risk in girls. In boys, and in girls who do not become pregnant, it is safe and highly effective. Most adolescents with troublesome acne can be cured with oral isotretinoin.

- Some acne sufferers develop scarring. This can be quite subtle and can occur with otherwise fairly mild disease. Any scarring is an indication for oral antibiotics and early consideration of oral isotretinoin. Similarly, the presence of any cysts should alert you to the likelihood of scarring and the need for oral therapy.

Acne and depression

Both adolescence and acne can be associated with depression. Significant depression is an indication to consider oral isotretinoin therapy. For several years, the issue of whether isotretinoin can trigger depression and suicide has been investigated. Current medical evidence suggests that treatment of severe acne with oral isotretinoin may decrease the risk of suicide. Assessment and treatment of any depression is required.

Acne fulminans

Acne fulminans typically occurs in young males being treated for acne. There is sudden onset of fever, malaise, arthralgia, myalgia, lymphadenopathy and/or hepatosplenomegaly in association with a rapid worsening of acne over the trunk and shoulders. Many painful cystic lesions develop and become haemorrhagic and ulcerated. Many laboratory abnormalities have been noted, including elevations of white cell count, erythrocyte sedimentation rate, C-reactive protein and liver enzymes. The cause is unknown but may be an abnormal immunological response rather than a primary bacterial infection. The response to oral antibiotics is slow and indeed these adolescents are often taking oral antibiotics at the time of onset.

Management

- Oral prednisolone 0.5–1 mg kg^{-1} daily for 4–6 weeks (thereafter slowly reduced to zero).

- Oral isotretinoin being added to the regimen at the fourth week, initially at 0.5 mg kg^{-1} daily and gradually increased to achieve complete clearance.

Acne with Gram-negative folliculitis

This can develop in patients treated for acne with long-term antibiotics. It is more common in adolescents with an oily complexion. It presents as rapidly worsening acne with pustular lesions on the face. Several common Gram-negative pathogens may be involved. Treat with oral trimethoprim and oral isotretinoin.

Early onset acne

Acne normally appears after the onset of pubertal changes such as testicular enlargement, pubic hair and breast development. However, comedonal and occasionally papular lesions may be the first manifestations of puberty in a child. These changes can begin up to 2 years before other signs of puberty. Early onset of comedonal lesions, even if mild, is associated with more severe acne several years later.

If comedones or acneiform papules are noted before puberty (see Fig. 12.1.1), you should consider the possibility of pathological androgen secretion (see below). Look for increased growth, genital development and advanced radiological bone age.

Atypical acneiform rashes

Acne that is atypical in age of onset, distribution, morphology or severity may be associated with systemic disease. Consider:

- Glucocorticoid excess, either exogenous or endogenous. This can give a monomorphic acneiform rash on the face and trunk. Other cushingoid stigmata may be present. In children on corticosteroid treatment, the rash may appear as the dose of corticosteroid is being weaned. Glucocorticoid acne may be due to *Malassezia* folliculitis. If there is no response to tetracycline, treatment of *Malassezia* folliculitis with topical or oral

antifungals may be required (see Folliculitis below).

- Androgen excess. Other features depend on the age and sex of the child. In younger children accelerated growth, body odour, pubic hair, clitoromegaly (but not breast development) and penile (but not testicular) enlargement may be present. In teenage females, polycystic ovary syndrome is commonly the cause. Other causes include late-onset congenital adrenal hyperplasia, and virilising tumours. Investigations may include X-rays for bone age, pelvic ultrasound, plasma androgens, fasting glucose and insulin, and response to dexamethasone suppression.

- Precocious puberty.

- Several drugs can induce an acneiform rash with monomorphic papules and pustules in post-pubertal children. The distribution is different from acne vulgaris, often involving arms, legs or trunk, and comedones are not present. Affected individuals often have a history of troublesome acne vulgaris. Possible causative agents include anti-epileptic medications, especially phenytoin and phenobarbital, glucocorticoids, testosterone, isoniazid, lithium and iodides.

- Apert's syndrome and related craniofacial syndromes can present with more severe widespread acne.

Folliculitis

Infection of the hair follicles is usually due to *Staphylococcus aureus*. Predisposing factors include a moist environment, a heavy bacterial load (e.g. adjacent to wounds or anal region) and excessive occlusive ointment, particularly on the trunk. Treatment involves avoidance of the predisposing factors, use of topical cleansers such as chlorhexidine and, rarely, oral antibiotics. Folliculitis often occurs repeatedly over a period of months and may require continued topical measures for 3–6 months. In resistant cases, daily use of topical benzoyl peroxide lotion may be helpful.

Folliculitis can occur in a child with moderate or severe eczema. Oral antibiotics are usually beneficial in this setting.

In adolescents, *Malassezia* folliculitis is common and presents as a persistent itchy rash with many tiny monomorphic erythematous papules and pustules on the back, shoulders and upper trunk. It is often associated with occlusion or sweating. Daily application of ketoconazole 2% shampoo is effective in gaining control. For resistant cases, use oral ketoconazole 400 mg weekly for 6 weeks taken with a glass of grapefruit juice followed by indefinite weekly shampooing with selenium sulfide 2% shampoo.

Occasionally, pruritic papules and pustules can develop many hours after soaking in a hot spa. Lesions usually occur under the bathing costume and are caused by *Pseudomonas aeruginosa*. Oral antibiotics are not usually needed.

Acute generalised exanthematous pustulosis (AGEP)

AGEP appears as a rapidly developing facial or truncal erythema with hundreds of tiny sterile pustules. Oedema is often seen in the affected areas. Fever and malaise may be present. Healing is associated with extensive superficial peeling. In some cases, children presenting with acute generalised exanthematous pustulosis have an underlying psoriatic tendency.

Many common medications, including amoxicillin, erythromycin, azithromycin, sulfonamides, anticonvulsants (especially carbamazepine) and non-steroidal anti-inflammatory drugs can cause this. Acute generalised exanthematous pustulosis drug reactions often begin within hours of commencing the drug. Other causes include Group A streptococcal infection.

Treat by stopping any offending medication. Give oral antibiotics for underlying streptococcal infection if required.

Pustular psoriasis

Psoriasis can present with pustules on an erythematous background. The pustules are sterile. The affected area may be limited to fingers, palms and soles, or local areas of skin, often with an annular arrangement of pustules. Alternatively, there may be erythroderma, high fever, malaise and arthralgias with widespread pustules coalescing into sheets of pus. Local pustular psoriasis can be treated topically (see psoriasis, p. 295). Generalised pustular psoriasis requires admission to hospital, rest, skin emollients and/or wet dressings, monitoring of fluid balance, electrolytes, renal and cardiac function and oral therapy (see erythroderma p. 281 and psoriasis p. 295).

Neonatal pustules

In the neonatal period, pustules may be part of several transient benign conditions. Pustules or vesicles may also be a marker of serious underlying illness, even in the absence of fever and lethargy. Consider:

- Infection, either congenital or acquired, e.g. *Staphylococcus* species, Group B streptococci, *Haemophilus influenzae*, *Candida* species.
- Neutropenia from any cause. Superficial bacterial pustules may be the only sign of congenital neutropenia.
- Toxic erythema of the newborn. In this benign condition, well term babies develop many tiny papules or pustules on an erythematous macular background in the first few days of life. Lesions clear within several days.
- Transient neonatal pustular dermatosis. Loose pustules are present from birth, and disappear within two days. This condition is more common in dark-skinned babies.
- Acropustulosis of infancy. Itchy vesicles and pustules appear on the hands and feet, usually commencing in the first couple of months of life and continuing for some months. New crops appear each 2–4 weeks. Sleep disturbance is common. In some infants; it appears to follow previously treated scabies infection. Pustules contain neutrophils and are sterile. Multiple scrapings may be necessary to exclude active scabies infection. Potent topical steroids assist control of flares, and the condition remits over 1–2 years.
- Eosinophilic pustular folliculitis (scalp). Yellowish pustules appear on the scalp and face within the first days of life. Lesions crust over and new lesions develop for some weeks. Pustules contain eosinophils and are sterile but secondary infection can occur. Mid-potency topical corticosteroids are helpful to control itch.
- Milia (white papules on the face) and sebaceous hyperplasia (yellowish papules, particularly around the nose) can be misinterpreted as pustules. Both resolve within a few weeks of birth.
- Neonates with Down's syndrome can develop a leukemoid pustular reaction which is self-limiting.

Neonatal pityrosporum folliculitis

This extremely common eruption is referred to as 'milk spots', the '6-week eruption' or 'infantile acne'. It presents as a widespread papulopustular follicular eruption on the face and torso. This is not true acne and comedones are not present. It is due to an inflammatory reaction to *Pityrosporum* yeast as the newborn sebaceous glands, activated during pregnancy, are returning to their quiescent childhood state. It is self-limiting and often needs no treatment. In more severe cases, application of ketoconazole 0.2% solution (dilute the 2% shampoo) by cotton bud to affected areas twice daily leads to rapid clearing.

PAPULAR (RAISED) RASHES

If a child has itchy papules, consider scabies, urticaria, serum sickness, papular urticaria, molluscum, *Malassezia* folliculitis, dermatitis herpetiformis or Langerhans cell histiocytosis. If papules are not itchy, consider urticaria, molluscum, warts, acne, skin appendageal tumours, melanocytic naevi, Spitz naevi, pilomatricomas, keratosis pilaris, vasculitis and papular acrodermatitis. For raised red circles or rings, consider urticaria. For softer red, purple or blue swellings, consider haemangiomas or vascular malformations. For haemorrhagic papules, consider Henoch–Schönlein purpura and other causes of vasculitis. If papules are yellowish when blanched, consider juvenile xanthogranulomas or xanthomas.

Papules or nodules may also occur in a number of disorders including acute rheumatic fever, juvenile chronic arthritis, systemic lupus erythematosus and neurofibromatosis, but are rarely the presenting feature.

Scabies

Scabies infection occurs as a result of close, usually repeated, contact with an infected individual. Scabies mites eat into the upper skin forming burrows a few millimetres in length around the fingers, palms, wrists, elbows, axillae, nipples, penis, and soles. Early burrows may be vesicular. Usually only a few mites are present.

An intensely itchy secondary papular eruption develops 2–6 weeks after first exposure to the *Sarcoptes scabiei* mite or 1–4 days after subsequent reinfestation. This secondary eruption represents an immune response to the scabies antigen and does not mean that mites are spreading all over the body. Papules can occur anywhere, including the palms, soles, axillae and genitalia, but are most prominent on the abdomen, buttocks and thighs. The scalp and head may be involved in infants and young toddlers. Inflammatory nodules may also develop, especially on covered areas. Excoriations and secondary impetigo may be present. Scabies is pandemic and affects both adults and children.

Not all itchy parasitic rashes are scabies. Many species of parasite can cause small itchy papules on the skin, in some cases hundreds of lesions. Bird mites, fleas, body lice, mosquitoes, sand flies, horse flies, bed bugs, ticks, chiggers, midges and harvest mites can all masquerade as scabies. Parasites can be collected from the skin on transparent adhesive tape. The CSIRO Australian National Insect Collection provides an identification service on http://www.csiro.au/services/InsectID.html.

Management

- Treatment of scabies is expensive and upsetting. If there is any doubt about the diagnosis, confirm by scraping to find a scabies mite, or refer before treating.
- Permethrin 5% cream.
- An alternative, recommended for pregnant or neonatal cases, is sulfur 6% in yellow soft paraffin. This is unpleasant and has no proven safety advantages over permethrin in these groups. The following are *not* recommended: lindane 1% (contraindicated in infants or women who are pregnant or breast-feeding) or benzyl benzoate 25% (too irritant for children and ineffective if diluted).

- Apply to dry skin (not after a bath) from the neck down to all skin surfaces. For infants, apply to the scalp as well (not face). Use mittens if necessary to prevent finger-sucking.
- Leave the cream on for at least 8 hours.
- Wash the cream off. Wash clothing, pyjamas and bed linen at this time.
- Remove soft toys from the bed. The scabies mite cannot live for long periods away from the body, and insecticide sprays and cleaning of furniture and carpets are not warranted.
- Exclude from school until after treatment has commenced.
- Treat all family members and any other people who have regular close skin contact with the affected individuals.
- The itch takes a week or two to settle and can be treated with topical or oral corticosteroid. Nodules may take months to resolve despite successful treatment of the scabies infestation.
- Reinfestation is common. To minimise the risk of reinfestation, the family should notify all social contacts (e.g. crèche, school or close friends) to ensure that all those infected receive treatment.
- Treat secondary impetigo with oral cefalexin 30 mg kg^{-1} (max 500 mg) three times daily.

- Post-streptococcal glomerulonephritis may be seen after chronic impetigo secondary to scabies in the indigenous population. Oedema, hypertension and haematuria may occur over the next 2 months. In a child with long-standing infected scabies where ongoing care may be suboptimal, review and urinalysis to monitor for renal involvement is warranted. Examination of the child and siblings for signs of rheumatic heart disease is also warranted in this patient population.

Papular acrodermatitis of childhood

Papular acrodermatitis of childhood usually occurs in children aged 1–3 years but can occur outside this range. It is a reaction pattern to many infectious agents, including coxsackie viruses, echoviruses, *Mycoplasma* species, Epstein–Barr virus, adenovirus, respiratory syncytial virus, rotavirus, cytomegalovirus, hepatitis B virus and others. It has also been reported after all standard childhood vaccines. It is common and a regular source of confusion in EDs.

Papular acrodermatitis of childhood is characterised by the acute onset of monomorphic, red or skin-coloured papules mainly on the limbs, buttocks and face, with striking sparing of the trunk (Fig. 12.1.7). In any

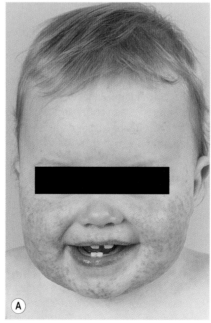
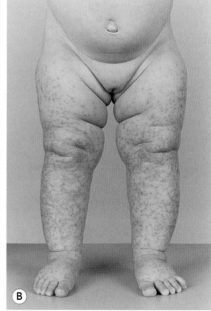

Fig. 12.1.7 Papular acrodermatitis of childhood showing almost complete sparing of the trunk.

given patient, the papules tend to all look the same, typically firm and dome shaped, measuring 2–4 mm in diameter. However, in different patients, the papules can vary from tiny, skin-coloured papules to larger urticarial plaques. Lesions may coalesce into patches on the extensor surfaces of the elbows and knees. Lesions may be papulovesicular (particularly on the limbs) or purpuric (particularly on the face). Hundreds of lesions may appear over several days. It is usually asymptomatic but may be itchy. Complete resolution occurs in 4–8 weeks.

Affected children may be otherwise well or may have features of the underlying infection, such as mild fever, malaise, coryza, sore throat, lymphadenopathy and splenomegaly. Lymphopenia or lymphocytosis may be present. In some cases, no history of a preceding or intercurrent illness can be found.

Papular acrodermatitis of childhood was formerly known as Gianotti–Crosti syndrome and was initially described as a manifestation of hepatitis B infection in Italy. This association has not been shown to be of general relevance, and papular acrodermatitis of childhood has been recognised as benign and much more common than previously thought.

Management

- Reassure and advise that clearing can take a few weeks.
- Children with papular acrodermatitis of childhood do not routinely require investigation to determine the underlying cause.
- Itch may require topical mid-potency corticosteroids and/or oral antihistamine.
- No exclusion from school or crèche is needed.

Papular urticaria

This is a clinical hypersensitivity to insect bites and may occur in just one child within a household, even though all family members may be bitten. New bites appear as crops of asymmetrical, small, red papules, usually in warmer weather. Older bites appear as 1–5 mm papules, sometimes with surface scale or crust, or with surrounding urticaria. Vesicles or pustules may form in the centre of lesions. Individual lesions

may resolve in a week or, if scratched, may last for months and may repeatedly flare up after fresh bites elsewhere. Itch is often intense and secondary ulceration or infection can occur. Full resolution usually occurs within 9 months. However, scratching can lead to secondary changes, with non-healing erosions, ulceration, scarring and nodule formation. These lesions remain itchy and a cycle of scratching and skin destruction can persist for years or decades if not treated. Improvements occur with new treatments but relapses are common without considerable medical support.

Management

- If the diagnosis is unclear, skin biopsy is useful as the typical histological findings are specific for insect-bite reactions.
- Prevent bites, e.g. by adequate clothing, modifying behaviour that leads to exposure, occasional use of repellent, and the treatment of pets and house for fleas and mites if necessary. The commonest source of bites is from mites in roof-dwelling animals such as birds, rats and possums. Surface spray of ceiling vents can be very useful.
- Treat the itch with an agent such as aluminium sulfate 20% (Stingose), liquor picis carbonis 2% in calamine lotion, potent steroid ointment or antihistamines.
- Protective dressings (e.g. Duoderm) can speed the healing of lesions. In older children, intralesional injection of corticosteroid is effective.
- Treat secondary infection with topical mupirocin ointment 2% or oral cefalexin 30 mg kg^{-1} (max 500 mg) three times daily.
- For more persistent and severe lesions, an intensive regimen may be necessary, including inpatient admission for moisturiser, potent topical steroid ointment and wet dressings, combined with continued intensive care of any relapse for weeks or months. Treatment needs to be modified according to response.

Molluscum

Molluscum is caused by a pox virus and is very common. Most children get at least a few molluscum at some stage between

the ages of 1 and 12 years. Uncomplicated molluscum lesions are easily recognised as firm, pearly, 1–4 mm dome-shaped papules with central umbilication. They are sometimes misdiagnosed as vesicles on initial examination. A child may develop a few or a great many lesions and individual lesions may last for months. Lesions can come and go for up to 3 years without causing any problems in most children. Complete resolution will not happen until an immune response develops, which may take from 3 months to 3 years.

Rarely, individual lesions can grow to over 1 cm in diameter. Individual lesions can become inflamed and, uncommonly, can develop secondary abscesses. More commonly, presentation to the ED is triggered by the development of widespread itchy and excoriated eczematous lesions in surrounding skin, usually on the lateral chest and axillary region or between the thighs. In such cases, recognition can be difficult, as the secondary changes can obliterate the primary lesions. A carefully taken history of the initial lesions is usually diagnostic.

Molluscum is common in the anogenital area and occurrence at this site does not suggest child sexual abuse. Molluscum is common on the face and occurrence at this site does not suggest underlying undiagnosed immunodeficiency.

Molluscum may occur on the eyelid margin or adjacent area. This can cause a persistent unilateral conjunctivitis. The molluscum may be isolated and subtle and go unnoticed for months during which the child may receive multiple courses of antibiotic treatment for conjunctivitis (Fig. 12.1.8).

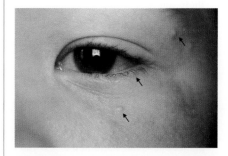

Fig. 12.1.8 This 6-year-old boy had presented to the ED four times in 6 months with recurrent unilateral conjunctivitis. Molluscum can be seen on the surrounding skin and a small papule towards the lateral end of his lower lid margin is also a molluscum. Treatment of the molluscum cured the conjunctivitis.

Management

- Most children with molluscum require no treatment.
- Children with molluscum should not share towels but should not be restricted in their activities. Swimming should not generally be restricted. It is possible that spread to other parts of the body and to other children may be reduced by advising the child not to soak in warm water (baths, spas, heated pools). This is a significant restriction for many children with long-term sequelae if they miss their school swimming lessons. If restrictions are imposed on the child, lesions must be actively treated to ensure rapid clearing.
- Any child having problems with molluscum should be treated.
- The treatment depends on the age of the child, the location of the lesions and any secondary changes. Uncomplicated lesions not causing problems and not spreading can be left alone.
- If the presenting problem is the itch from secondary eczema, treatment of the eczema with mild or mid-potency topical steroid ointment may be all that is required. Try not to overuse as it is possible that this may encourage spreading of molluscum lesions.
- It is not difficult to destroy molluscum lesions. Simply deroofing the central umbilication is almost painless and leads to the papule becoming inflamed and resolving. In older children, this can be achieved with superficial needle pricking or light cryotherapy. Benzoyl peroxide 5%, a variety of chemical irritants and tape stripping can all be used but these can tend to flare any surrounding eczema.
- Topical cantharidin (e.g. Cantharone) is the most rapid and effective way of dealing with molluscum in many situations. This is painless on application and causes small blisters at the site over the next several hours. Importation of cantharidin requires a personal TGA permit and is not warranted unless you see many children with troublesome molluscum.
- Imiquimod 5% cream nocte for several days is expensive but may be useful for small numbers of lesions at difficult-to-treat sites.

- Several treatment options exist for molluscum around the eye and causing conjunctivitis. One or two lesions in older non-anxious children can be treated physically as for elsewhere on the face. Imiquimod 5% cream can be tried. If there are many lesions elsewhere, treating all the other lesions away from the eyes often induces rapid resolution of the eye lesions as well. In anxious children with significant problems with conjunctivitis, sedation or a brief general anaesthetic may be warranted.
- Inflamed lesions rarely warrant antibiotic treatment or drainage.

Adnexal tumours – pilomatricoma

Many different benign tumours of the various cell types in hair follicles, sebaceous glands and sweat glands can present as papules during childhood. The most common by far are pilomatricomas. These present at any age in childhood as a slow-growing papule on the head, face or neck (or occasionally elsewhere) that can be 4–40 mm in size. They may be skin-coloured, white or bluish and are usually firm or hard, often due to calcification within the lesion. They may be lobulated. The main differential is an epidermal cyst. An ultrasound may confirm the diagnosis by demonstrating calcium shadows, which are not present in epidermal cysts. Pilomatricomas do not usually regress. Surgical removal is usually recommended because of the appearance but is not urgent.

Keratosis pilaris

This is a rough, somewhat spiky papular rash, mainly on the upper outer arms, thighs and/or cheeks with variable erythema. It affects 50–80% of all adolescents and approximately 40% of adults. About 30–50% of patients have a positive family history. Autosomal dominant inheritance with variable penetrance has been described. It appears in infancy and persists throughout life. However, it tends to improve towards adulthood. Rarely, the erythema and papules are florid and distressing and treatment is warranted.

Management

Reassure the patient that this is rarely a problem. Soap avoidance and moisturisers can improve the spiky feeling. Most children need no further treatment. Steroids do not help.

Granuloma annulare

Granuloma annulare is not common in children. It begins as a small skin-coloured or red papule that spreads outward over many weeks or months to give an annular, asymptomatic ring, usually on the hands or feet. Although often misdiagnosed as tinea, the epidermis is not scaly and discrete subcutaneous papules can be felt all around the ring. It is slow growing and takes months to reach a size of 2 cm. Resolution usually occurs within a year or two. No investigation is necessary. Most children should be reassured and don't need treatment.

Langerhans cell histiocytosis

Langerhans cell histiocytosis may present in several ways and should be considered as a possible diagnosis in any unusual, non-healing rash in infancy.

In neonates, Langerhans cell histiocytosis may present as a congenital self-healing form. One or a few papules are present at birth or shortly thereafter. They can be many millimetres in diameter and classically have a raised border and central necrosis. The papules usually show complete regression within months. Recurrence years later with visceral involvement or disseminated disease has been reported, and long-term monitoring is warranted.

In infants, Langerhans cell histiocytosis can present as recalcitrant 'cradle cap' with scaly, papular and petechial scalp lesions, often mistaken initially for severe seborrhoeic dermatitis. Flexural areas, especially the groin and anogenital area, can be involved, presenting as a chronic weeping 'nappy rash'. The presence of papules and/or petechiae, sometimes with ulceration, and the lack of response to treatment for napkin dermatitis should raise suspicion.

In infants and older children, there may be widespread, often itchy, small haemorrhagic papules mimicking a vasculitis. Erythematous and purpuric scaling and papules may be present on the hands and feet, and nails may become dystrophic. Mucosal involvement can lead to ulceration on the gums or palate.

Extracutaneous disease can involve the liver, lymph nodes, marrow, bone and CNS. Diabetes insipidus can occur.

Management

- Confirm the diagnosis with a skin biopsy.
- Investigate for other organ involvement with skull, chest and skeletal X-rays, dental examination, full blood examination and liver function tests.
- Skin lesions can be treated with topical corticosteroid application.
- While Langerhans cell histiocytosis can be self limited; it can also be rapidly progressive with progressive organ involvement and a poor prognosis, requiring intensive chemotherapy.

Juvenile xanthogranulomas

Juvenile xanthogranulomas are the commonest cause of yellow papules in children. Occurring in early childhood, lesions appear as low, dome-shaped papules 2–5 mm in diameter. They may be yellow or red-brown lesions that become yellow when blanched. They are often on the scalp but can occur elsewhere. There may be one or multiple papules appearing over weeks or months. Biopsy may be required to confirm the diagnosis. Resolution without treatment usually occurs within a few years. Juvenile xanthogranulomas are not associated with lipid disorders.

Children with neurofibromatosis have a considerably increased chance of having juvenile xanthogranulomas. The known increased risk of myelomonocytic leukaemia in a child with neurofibromatosis is probably not changed significantly if juvenile xanthogranulomas are also present, despite statements to the contrary in many texts.

Children less than 2 years old with multiple juvenile xanthogranulomas should have an ophthalmology assessment. Ocular juvenile xanthogranulomas leading to glaucoma have been reported in this subgroup of patients.

Xanthomas

True xanthomatous papules associated with elevated cholesterol levels are rare in childhood. They may present as multiple eruptive xanthomas, tuberous xanthomas (usually distributed over the elbows, knuckles, buttocks, knees and heels) and tendinous xanthomas (usually on tendons around the elbow, wrist, hand, or ankle). Investigation to exclude hyperlipidaemias is mandatory. Consider:

- Primary hyperlipoproteinaemias. Skin lesions may present between 5 and 15 years of age, sometimes as tendinitis or tenosynovitis. Look for signs of atherosclerotic disease, and a family history of high cholesterol, early myocardial infarcts or strokes.
- Secondary hypercholesterolaemia. This can occur in hypothyroidism, biliary cirrhosis, diabetes mellitus, glycogen storage disease and nephrotic syndrome.

Angiofibromas in tuberosclerosis

Facial angiofibromas may be the first sign of tuberosclerosis. They appear as small, red-brown papules (not pustules) on the cheeks from about 5–6 years of age and can be misinterpreted as flat warts or early-onset acne.

RED SCALY RASHES

Redness and scale indicate a combination of vasodilatation and epidermal involvement. Atopic eczema is the commonest cause of red scaly rashes in children (see p. 297). Other red scaly eruptions include seborrhoeic dermatitis (infants), psoriasis, tinea corporis, pityriasis rosea and pityriasis versicolor. If itch is present, consider any of the causes of eczematous rashes (p. 297).

Psoriasis

Psoriasis can occur at any age. Every year in a city of 2 million people, 400 children will present with psoriasis for the first time. Lesions typically begin as small, red papules that develop into circular, sometimes itchy, sharply demarcated, erythematous plaques with prominent silvery scale. However, psoriasis can present in many ways, including isolated thick scaly scalp lesions, scaly plaques on the hairline and behind the ears, annular lesions, pustular lesions, palmoplantar psoriasis, guttate psoriasis and flexural psoriasis. Therefore, psoriasis must be considered in the differential diagnosis of any red, scaly rash, particularly if well-demarcated and not particularly itchy.

Guttate psoriasis describes the eruption of hundreds of small, scaly papules on the trunk and limbs, often following a streptococcal throat infection.

Flexural psoriasis can involve any of the skin folds, particularly the anogenital area, and is more common in children than in adults. Psoriasis at flexural sites presents as moist, non-scaly erythema, often painless but sometimes with secondary fissuring or streptococcal infection.

Minor nail pitting is often seen in childhood psoriasis.

Management

- Presentation to the ED is often precipitated by the onset of guttate psoriasis or by secondary problems with long-standing anogenital psoriasis. The treatment depends on the site and extent of disease and the age of the child. Guttate psoriasis is often most easily managed with an extemporaneous tar cream, e.g. liquor picis carbonis (LPC) 3% and salicylic acid 2% in Sorbolene cream, 500 g. Adolescents are less tolerant of tar creams.
- Minimise skin trauma. Use regular moisturiser.
- Treat isolated skin plaques with either topical steroids (e.g. mometasone) or topical calcipotriol, or both, for 4 weeks, with clinical monitoring. Topical steroids are not used for large areas in childhood psoriasis because of the possible development of rebound pustular disease. Thick scalp plaques can be softened overnight with a tar cream and removed with a tar shampoo. Generally avoid tar cream on the face, flexures and genitalia as it can be irritating.
- Use hydrocortisone 1% or pimecrolimus 1% cream on the face, flexures and anogenital region.
- Palmoplantar psoriasis can be resistant to treatment. Initially treat with topical potent corticosteroid and calcipotriol ointment.

- Secondary infection including perianal streptococcal infection may require treatment with oral penicillin. Recurrent or persistent streptococcal infection or carriage should be considered but is uncommon.
- A mild normocytic (occasionally microcytic) anaemia of chronic disease can occur in more severe cases.
- Appropriate medical follow up is essential. Psoriasis will recur. Widespread or resistant psoriasis may need treatment with one or more of dithranol, ultraviolet therapy, acitretin, methotrexate or ciclosporin, all of which are effective.
- Widespread involvement may lead to erythroderma with metabolic and other complications (see erythroderma, p. 281).

Tinea corporis

Tinea corporis (often called ringworm) is a common skin disorder, especially among children, but it may occur in people of all ages. It is caused by mould-like fungi (dermatophytes). Tinea infections can be transmitted by direct contact with affected individuals or by contact with contaminated items such as combs, clothing, shower, or pool surfaces. They can also be transmitted by contact with pets that carry the fungus (cats are common carriers). The typical lesion is a slow-growing erythematous ring with a clear or scaly centre. Scale is usually most prominent on the outside of the annular ring. However, tinea corporis can present in a wide variety of ways. It can be pustular or vesicular, particularly on the soles (Fig. 12.1.9), or it can spread to many sites within days. Between the toes, it presents as an itchy, white, scaly and macerated rash. Previous treatment with steroid ointments often leads to partial improvement in symptoms but causes spreading of the rash, the development of papules and the masking of diagnostic features. Tinea should be considered in any red, scaly rash where the diagnosis is unclear, particularly if there is a gradually spreading eruption with inflammatory edges.

Management

- Confirm the diagnosis by scraping the scale for microscopy and culture.
- The family should identify and treat the source animal if any.

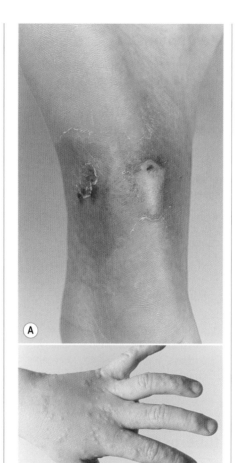

Fig. 12.1.9 Inflammatory bullous fungal infection. (A) The foot with (B) secondary id reaction involving the hands.

- Treat focal lesions with terbinafine cream (twice daily for 1 week) or an imidazole cream (e.g. clotrimazole, miconazole or econazole two to four times daily for 4 weeks).
- Rapidly spreading or widespread lesions, or involvement of hair-bearing areas usually requires oral griseofulvin (20 mg kg^{-1} day^{-1} in divided doses).
- Combined steroid and antifungal ointments (e.g. Kenacomb) are often ineffective for clearing tinea corporis.
- Exclude from school until 1 day after treatment has commenced.

Pityriasis rosea

Pityriasis rosea is common from 1–10 years. The cause is uncertain, but is thought to be viral. Human herpesvirus types 6 and 7 (HHV-6, HHV-7) have been implicated.

A similar eruption may occur in response to a number of drugs. A pink scaly patch 2–4 cm in diameter near the shoulders or hips (herald patch) is the first sign in about 50% of children and is often misdiagnosed as tinea corporis because of its central clearing. However, unlike tinea, the scale is usually most prominent on the inside edge of the inflammatory ring. A few days or weeks later (or as the first feature if no herald patch is present), many pink/red, scaly, oval macules appear, mainly on the trunk, arms and thighs. The face, palms, lower legs and soles are largely spared. There may be thin scale within the lesions and oval lesions may align with skin lines to give a 'Christmas tree' pattern on the back and trunk. Pityriasis rosea usually persists for 1–2 months. It may be mildly itchy but is often asymptomatic.

Pityriasis rosea may be atypical. Lesions may be papular, crusted, vesicular or purpuric. The distribution may involve neck and extremities.

Secondary syphilis can appear in a similar fashion, but mucosal and acral lesions are usually present. Secondary syphilis should be excluded in any adolescent at risk of sexually transmitted disease who presents with pityriasis rosea, particularly if palms and soles are involved.

Management

- Reassure the patient.
- Sunlight (or ultraviolet light in troublesome cases) will hasten clearing. Topical corticosteroids do not help. Emollients, or occasionally oral antihistamine, are useful for itch.
- In an adolescent at risk for sexually transmitted diseases, arrange VDRL test.

Secondary syphilis

Secondary syphilis presents 1–2 months after the primary chancre (which may be unreported). Erythematous, slightly scaly, macules or papules appear mainly on the trunk. There may be darker red macules on the palms and soles, as well as smooth or eroded papules on the tongue and oral mucosa, moist perineal papules (condylomata lata), annular lesions and pustules. Lymphadenopathy is usually present. Secondary syphilis can mimic pityriasis rosea and other red scaly disorders.

Seborrhoeic dermatitis

The term 'seborrhoeic dermatitis' has been used to describe a number of different clinical entities. It is most widely used for a particular dermatitis that occurs in areas of skin that have a high density of sebaceous glands, namely the scalp, the central 'T-zone' of the face, and the upper chest and back (not the anogenital area, see p. 316). It is due to a reaction to a *Pityrosporum* yeast, which is part of the normal flora at these sites.

As true seborrhoeic dermatitis can only occur in the setting of active sebaceous glands, the diagnosis should only be made in the first 3 months of life or after puberty has begun. The sites of predilection are the scalp, inner eyebrows and paranasal folds. The quality of the scale is more greasy than that of an eczema at other sites and the degree of pruritus and discomfort is usually minimal. The degree of erythema varies and mild cases present as neonatal cradle cap or adolescent dandruff.

Atopic eczema is common on the scalp of infants and is differentiated from seborrhoeic dermatitis by increased pruritus and discomfort, a harsher drier scale and occurrence after the age of two months. It is important not to diagnose scalp eczema as seborrhoeic dermatitis as eczema will be further irritated by shampoos and 'cradle cap' creams.

Management

- Gently debride any built-up crust with a non-irritating product such as olive oil, bath oil or a soap substitute. Only if very thick scale is present should salicylic acid creams be used.
- Settle erythema with 1% hydrocortisone cream.
- The use of an anti-yeast shampoo (e.g. 2% ketoconazole) may be helpful in more recalcitrant cases.
- Adolescents with seborrhoeic dermatitis may have to wash their hair more frequently.

Lichen striatus

Lichen striatus usually presents on a limb as a unilateral linear eczematous rash following the developmental lines of the skin. On close inspection, there are often collections of tiny flat-topped papules, coalescing into scaly lines that may stretch the full length of the limb. It may remain static for a period of months or a couple of years, before spontaneously resolving. It may be pruritic but usually not significantly so.

The cause of the eruption is an inflammatory reaction in a streak of skin that has a genetic abnormality (mosaicism). The genetic difference of the streak is so subtle that the skin is phenotypically and functionally normal until a trigger, mostly a viral infection, induces an inflammatory reaction against the abnormal skin. As the condition is self-limiting, no treatment is necessary if the condition is asymptomatic. Moderate-strength to potent topical steroid creams can help with any pruritus.

ECZEMATOUS RASHES

The term 'eczematous rashes' covers several common conditions that are characterised by erythema, itching and disruption to the epidermis with oozing, crusting, fissures or excoriations. The degree of epidermal disruption may be minimal so that the presentation of atopic eczema may be with just red dry patches. Alternatively, the degree of epidermal disruption may be severe, with oedema and widespread vesiculation (e.g. plant contact dermatitis, which is discussed under vesiculobullous rashes, p. 282).

Atopic eczema – general issues

The term 'atopic eczema' covers a range of presentations that depend on the age of the child and on the child's individual sensitivities. Several of these presentations are best seen as separate diseases. Clinical features and specific management suggestions are discussed under the individual headings below. However, some generalisations apply to most children with atopic eczema subtypes.

Atopic eczema usually begins in infancy. It commonly involves the face, and often the trunk and limbs as well. In older children, the rash may be widespread but is often localised to flexures. Erythema, weeping, excoriation and, rarely, vesicles may be seen in acute lesions. Chronic lesions may show scale and lichenification. In some children, the lesions are more clearly defined, thickened discoid areas that may intermittently be itchy. There is usually a cyclical pattern of improvement and exacerbation.

Families who present to the ED with atopic eczema often have children with chronic and severe disease requiring frequent, time-consuming applications of topical medicines and wet dressings. These children may have recurrent infections, particularly with *Staphylococcus aureus* or herpes simplex. Failure to thrive may be present. A mild, normocytic (occasionally microcytic) anaemia of chronic disease can occur. Severe psychosocial and behavioural problems are common in these children although often hidden from medical staff. Parents may be under enormous stress with financial, marital and other problems secondary to the child's eczema. These problems need to be identified and addressed.

Atopic eczema – general management principles

- *Education*. Parents need to know that treatments are effective in controlling the disease. They should be aware of the principles of avoiding relevant triggers and settling the inflammation.
- *Avoid irritants*. The following may worsen atopic eczema: soaps, bubble baths, prickly clothing, including clothing worn by adults carrying babies, seams and labels on clothing, car seat covers, sand, carpets, overheating or contact with pets. Smooth cotton clothing is preferred.
- *Avoid heat*. Overheating increases itch. Most parents overdress young children. Outer clothing should be removed when entering warm environments. Bedding and baths should be kept comfortably cool.
- *Keep the skin moist*. Use a moisturiser such as sorbolene with 10% glycerine, aqueous cream or paraffin ointment (50:50 white soft paraffin/liquid paraffin) as often as a few times a day if necessary.
- *Treat inflammation*. In mild or moderate cases, steroid creams can be used intermittently with good effect. Hydrocortisone 1% is usually adequate. If not, moderate potency (e.g. betamethasone valerate 0.02%) or

potent (e.g. mometasone 0.1% or methylprednisolone 0.1%) ointment can be used for exacerbations. Widespread long-term use of moderate potency steroids to the skin can cause atrophy or striae, especially on the face, the nappy area of infants, and sites of rapid growth such as the thighs of pubertal girls. Although expensive, pimecrolimus 1% is a useful alternative in some situations. Oral steroids are rarely indicated in atopic eczema. For chronic atopic eczema on the limbs, zinc and tar combinations are alternatives to steroids. Topical calcineurin inhibitors (tacrolimus and pimecrolimus) are increasingly used as an adjunct to topical steroid therapy but are expensive.

- *Control itch.* Advise parents to avoid saying 'stop itching' all the time and to distract the child instead. Wet bandaging is very helpful if warranted. Antihistamines are often unhelpful but if the itch is not controlled by other measures, they may be tried.
- *Wet dressings.* Wet dressings are bandages applied over topical moisturiser or corticosteroid ointments two to four times a day. They cool the skin and are effective in controlling flares of eczema, settling troublesome focal patches of eczema and reducing the need for corticosteroid. They are well tolerated by children although cumbersome to apply. However, if the initial application is done by a parent at home, acceptance of the treatment may be prejudiced by pre-existing conflict between the child and parent over treatment regimens. If possible, wet dressings should ideally be commenced by trained staff in hospital.
- *Treat infection.* Weeping and yellow crusted areas that do not respond to therapy may indicate secondary bacterial or herpetic (see p. 328) infection. Take cultures and treat with simple wet dressings and oral cephalexin 30 mg kg^{-1} (max 500 mg) three times daily. For recurrent bacterial infection, use bleach baths, e.g. White King Bleach (4.2%) 3 tablespoons (= 45 mL) in a quarter full bath (approx 60 L).
- *Severe cases.* Do not accept that nothing more can be done. Children with chronic severe eczema need to be referred for psychosocial support and for assessment

as to whether they warrant admission to hospital, oral prednisolone, narrow-band ultraviolet B therapy or other systemic immunosuppressive therapy.[2]

Atopic eczema – dietary principles

A normal diet is indicated in most children with eczema. If a child has immediate urticarial reactions to a particular food, that food should be avoided. No alteration should otherwise be made to an infant's or child's diet unless appropriate conventional therapy, as above, has not worked. In difficult cases, particularly in infants, consider a formal allergy assessment. Restrictive diets without professional supervision should be avoided.

Babies with a first-degree relative with eczema have a 50% chance of developing eczema. For these babies, no modifications to the mother's diet are recommended during pregnancy and breast-feeding. Exclusive breast-feeding for the baby is recommended for a minimum of 4 months for a number of reasons. If exclusive breast-feeding is not possible, supplementation with partially hydrolysed formula may reduce the risk of eczema. The use of soy formula has no role in the prevention of allergy but is to be considered if there is clinical suspicion of dairy allergy. Peanuts and other nuts should be avoided until 1 year of age.

Atopic eczema – admission to hospital

Children with eczema who attend EDs often do so because the parents have become increasingly desperate to get their child's skin under control. Admission to hospital can be very helpful. You should consider admitting the child if any of the following circumstances apply.

- A child is missing school because of atopic eczema. If so, they should generally be admitted to hospital for intensive treatment.
- A child has severe impetiginisation or you have concerns about sepsis.
- A child has widespread eczema herpeticum.
- The family has social, financial or mental health issues that make home treatment difficult.

- Education of the parents in an emergency setting is difficult because they speak a language other than English.
- The parents exhibit significant stress or impending breakdown.
- Outpatient management has not given a satisfactory response.
- An adolescent has widespread chronic eczema that affects their lifestyle (wears long clothing in summer, won't swim, etc.).

Atopic eczema – use of topical steroid preparations

The use of topical steroids remains a pivotal component of eczema management. It is important to settle the eczema and restore the natural integrity of the skin. If eczema is left untreated, the natural barrier of the skin remains disrupted and the skin is more prone to react to other eczema triggers. Any scratching will further flare the skin and a worsening cycle is created. Topical cortisone preparations are used to break this cycle and heal the skin. They should not be used as prophylaxis on normal skin. The preparations are best prescribed in ointment formulation as these are more moisturising. Creams may be used if ointments are poorly tolerated. As a general rule, topical corticosteroids are extremely safe. Side effects are very uncommon if used appropriately.

Always ask parents if they are treating their children with herbal creams. Any herbal cream that gives dramatic clearing should be assumed to contain corticosteroid products until proven otherwise. A British study in 2003 looked at a number of herbal creams given to children for eczema.[3] Over 80% of those tested had illegal potent or very potent corticosteroid additives. Similar results have been found in previous studies.

Systemic effects of topical steroid use Suppression of the pituitary-adrenal axis can occur if potent topical corticosteroids are used over most of the skin surface continuously for many weeks, but this is an uncommon clinical scenario. If a child is using large amounts of topical corticosteroids in combination with inhaled corticosteroids and/or occasional oral cortisone therapy, you should consider adrenal suppression. Steroid therapy should not be abruptly stopped in this situation.

Local effects of topical steroid use

Irritation or allergy to one of the constituents of the topical steroid occurs in a few children. Apart from this, local side effects rarely occur. Inappropriate use can lead to atrophy, striae, telangiectasia, purpura, cataracts and juvenile rosacea. Care is required when treating the face, anogenital areas, flexures and any areas of rapid growth where the skin is already under tension (e.g. breasts in adolescent females). In these situations, permanent striae can occur within weeks. Precipitants of eczema should continue to be sought if the need for topical corticosteroids is ongoing. It should be explained to patients that once the eczema has cleared, the topical corticosteroids should be ceased. This is more important in darker-skinned individuals, where post-inflammatory hyperpigmentation may be mistaken by the patient for active disease.

The topical calcineurin inhibitors, tacrolimus and pimecrolimus, are now available as steroid-sparing agents. However, their expense currently limits their use for widespread disease.

Atopic eczema – generalised infantile

Some infants present in the first 6 months of life with red, scaly and excoriated lesions covering much of the trunk and often the limbs, scalp and face as well. These infants are typically irritable and often sleeping and feeding poorly. The parents are often highly stressed by the difficulties with managing the child. Appropriate treatment usually leads to a dramatic change in the baby's behaviour and the family dynamics.

A detailed history should be taken to identify any exacerbating factors in the child's environment. Examination will often reveal considerable dermographism and urticarial change. Allergy to foods is common in this setting and allergy testing is useful. Foods in the maternal diet can trigger allergy in a breast-fed baby. Consider whether admission for wet dressings is required. Consider whether secondary bacterial or herpes infection is present. Treat with a bland emollient such as paraffin ointment once or twice daily. Use hydrocortisone 1% ointment on the face and methyl-prednisolone 0.1% to the body daily to gain rapid control of the skin. Arrange follow up within a week or two if using significant amounts of potent topical steroid preparations. Skin prick testing and appropriate allergen avoidance may be useful in the longer term.

Atopic eczema – facial

Some infants will present with facial lesions. There may or may not be eczema elsewhere. Facial eczema may be secondarily infected with *Staphylococcus aureus*, resulting in weeping and crusting (Fig. 12.1.10). Saliva is often a significant exacerbating factor. Herpes simplex virus infection needs to be considered (look for the typical monomorphic erosions, see p. 284). Treat with ointment moisturiser several times daily and, if indicated, oral cefalexin 30 mg kg^{-1} (max 500 mg) three times daily for 1 week. If appropriate follow up can be assured, use methyl-prednisolone 0.1% ointment for a few days to gain rapid control of the skin. Arrange follow up within a week to avoid problems from prolonged steroid use. Avoidance of irritating factors such as using napkin wipes on the face and general management measures are required to prevent relapse.

Atopic eczema – perioral eczema vs. juvenile rosacea

Perioral eczema Refers to eczema round the mouth. This is common in infancy and early childhood. Irritation from saliva is the main cause. Occasionally, intolerance or allergy to foods can play a role in the older child. Confluent patches of erythema with weeping and superficial erosion occur in

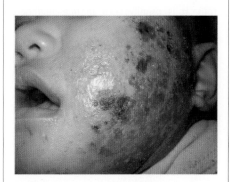

Fig. 12.1.10 Facial eczema with secondary impetiginisation in a 10-month-old boy.

acute eczema. Management involves settling the active patches with a brief period of topical corticosteroid ointment and then trying to minimise irritation from saliva. This is difficult in the dribbling infant. Thicker moisturisers such as 50% white soft/liquid paraffin (Dermeze) may be used both as a moisturiser and as a barrier on the skin. In persistent cases, use pimecrolimus 1% cream or tacrolimus 0.03% ointment.

Juvenile rosacea Is often called 'perioral dermatitis' and confused with perioral eczema but it is not a true dermatitis. It is better thought of as a subset of rosacea. The most common clinical setting is following the use of topical steroids in a young child who is genetically predisposed to develop this condition. The morphology is quite different from perioral eczema. Erythematous papules occur around the mouth but spare the skin immediately adjacent to the lips. Other facial areas may be involved. The papules are essentially distinct from each other but may coalesce at times. Topical steroids tend to temporarily settle the inflammation and then cause a rebound flare, and patients are often under the false impression that the topical steroids are the only effective therapy. Treatment involves the cessation of all topical steroids on the skin in this area and the introduction of an appropriate antibiotic. Use erythromycin in children or tetracyclines in adolescents. Pimecrolimus 1% cream may give added benefit. Resolution usually takes 3–4 weeks of therapy. It is important to warn patients who have been actively using topical steroids that there will be a rebound flare before they begin to see improvement.

Atopic eczema – periorbital

Periorbital eczema is usually associated with sensitivity to airborne allergens, especially house dust mites, cat dander and pollens. Consideration of the occasions when the itch is worst will often indicate the causative agent. Formal skin prick testing, allergen avoidance measures, moisturiser, pimecrolimus 1% cream and follow up are required. In atypical cases, consider allergic contact dermatitis, irritant contact dermatitis and molluscum.

Atopic eczema – sudden worsening or urticarial flare

Children with eczema occasionally present to the ED with an acute worsening of previously stable eczema. This should prompt a search for an underlying cause. Look for any evidence of scabies, which can easily be overlooked amongst the background eczema – other family members may be itchy. Look for secondary bacterial infection. Consider if herpes simplex virus infection (p. 283) may be present. Small papules in widespread patches of eczema may be from subtle molluscum lesions. The child may have developed an irritant or allergic contact sensitivity to their topical treatments or other agents. Search for and treat any exacerbating factors. Arrange early follow up for management of the underlying eczema.

Often a sudden worsening with a dramatic increase in itch in a child with previously mild eczema is caused by viruses or allergy to drugs, food or environmental agents. They are often dermographic (i.e. they urticate in response to pressure on the skin) and it is likely that the cause of the flare is a subtle urticaria. When they itch, the scratching causes more urticaria, thereby causing more itch and escalating problems. These flares will often abate over a few days or weeks and the addition of a regular antihistamine will considerably help to control the symptoms. Uncommonly, metabolic triggers such as iron deficiency or thyroid disease may present with increased itch and worsening of eczema.

Atopic eczema – molluscum

Molluscum infection can trigger a marked local or generalised reaction in children. Presentation to the ED follows the development of widespread itchy and excoriated eczematous lesions in surrounding skin, usually on the lateral chest and axillary region or between the thighs. If the child has a previous history of atopic eczema, the molluscum lesions may be overlooked or hidden in the eczema. A careful history may reveal that clear, firm papules were present at some stage. A careful examination may reveal some typical molluscum or some residual papules in the centre of eczematous patches. Treat as previously described (under molluscum, p. 293).

Atopic eczema – flexural

While flexural eczema is the most common form of atopic eczema in children, it is rarely a cause for attendance at the ED unless sudden worsening has been triggered by secondary bacterial infection, secondary herpetic infection, acute irritant or allergic contact sensitivity or molluscum infection. Search for and treat any exacerbating factors. General principles of moisturisation, reducing overheating and avoiding irritants are usually adequate to regain control.

Atopic eczema – discoid

Discoid eczema is characterised by chronic focal circular crusted lesions 1–5 cm in diameter. These children may have an associated psoriatic tendency. The discoid lesions are thickened, oozing and itchy. They are relatively resistant to therapy. Secondary staphylococcal infection is present in most cases. Intensive and prolonged therapy is needed to break the cycle of itch, lichenification and infection. Oral cephalexin 30 mg kg^{-1} (max 500 mg) three times daily, ointment moisturiser, potent topical steroid ointment and regular wet dressings for 2 weeks may be adequate, but therapy may need to be prolonged. Follow up is mandatory. Hospital admission, intralesional steroid injections, ultraviolet light therapy or oral ciclosporin may all be considered.

Atopic eczema – juvenile plantar dermatosis

Juvenile plantar dermatosis is characterised by erythema, dryness and cracking of the anterior sole and the under surface of the toes. It is usually seen in mid-childhood and tends to occur in children with a tendency for increased sweating. The child may or may not have atopic eczema elsewhere. Both feet are usually symmetrically involved in the weight-bearing skin on the soles. Juvenile plantar dermatosis may persist for years and exacerbations may be associated with painful fissures. The differential includes tinea (which should be excluded by culture), psoriasis and contact dermatitis, which can all present with red scaly lesions on the soles. Cotton socks, leather shoes

and regular ointment moisturiser three-times daily should be used. Cotton socks can be worn over the moisturiser. Minimise exposure of cracked skin to carpets and other irritants. Topical potent corticosteroid ointments may be necessary. Follow up is needed.

Atopic eczema with systemic associations

Eczematous skin lesions can also be associated with:

- Immunodeficiency syndromes. Thrombocytopenia, immunodeficiency and eczema are seen in Wiskott–Aldrich syndrome. Petechiae, failure to thrive, recurrent infections, diarrhoea or haematological abnormalities may suggest this or other immunodeficiencies that are variably associated with eczema. Netherton's syndrome should be considered if neonatal-onset eczema is associated with failure to thrive and sparse hair.
- Multiple food allergies with consequent dietary restrictions and secondary nutritional and psychosocial problems.
- Metabolic or nutritional disorders. Phenylketonuria often presents with eczema. Less typical eczematous lesions, more prominent in periorificial areas, are seen in biotin, essential fatty acid and zinc deficiency syndromes. Malnutrition and organoacidaemias, e.g. methylmalonicacidaemia, can result in similar lesions.

Irritant contact dermatitis

The most common forms of irritant contact dermatitis in children are irritant napkin dermatitis (p. 317), juvenile plantar dermatosis (see above) and lip licking. Lip licking refers to a dermatitis caused by chronic exposure to saliva. Usually the application of saliva by the child is presumed by the carers to be secondary to the dermatitis rather than causative, and may not be mentioned. Lip licking often presents with a clearly defined ring of dermatitis around the mouth but the pattern of involvement may vary considerably depending on the behaviour of the child. Any habit that spreads saliva in a particular direction will affect the pattern of the dermatitis. Acidic foods, artificial colours, preservatives and toothpaste may contribute to the irritation. Treatment requires education, frequent topical ointment barrier applications (initially many times daily) and immediate treatment of any relapse. A short period of topical pimecrolimus 1% cream may be needed. Secondary bacterial or candidal infection is rarely present.

Allergic contact dermatitis

Acute allergic contact reactions (e.g. to plants) often cause vesiculation and are considered under vesiculobullous rashes (p. 282). Chronic exposure to a contact allergen presents with erythema, itch and lichenification. The site of reaction usually suggests the cause: axillary rashes from deodorants, ears from earrings, lips and eyes from make-up, lower abdomen from nickel buttons on pants, wrist from watch, perioral from toothpaste and so on. However, the trigger may be overlooked. For example, an itchy eczematous patch on the scalp may be due to a metal stud in a cap that is not being worn at the time of presentation to the ED. Consider allergic contact dermatitis if a child has persistent eczema in an unusual distribution.

Allergic contact dermatitis – 'black henna' reactions

In recent years, several children have presented to EDs with an allergic reaction to 'black henna'. Henna is widely used in Asian countries as a traditional skin colouring agent. It is dark brown. Many street vendors use cheap black hair dye instead, calling it 'black henna', often mixing this with other agents such as petrol to enhance absorption. These tattoos last for some weeks. These tattoos contain paraphenylenediamine, a strong contact sensitiser that should not be applied to the skin.

Three to 10 days after the application of the tattoo, the child may notice discomfort, itch, erythema and swelling. This may progress over the next 2 weeks to blistering and scabbing of the tattoo site, sometimes with ulceration. Generalised itch and urticaria may be present and it may take months

for complete resolution to occur. These children may develop a long-lasting cross-sensitivity to sun screens, hair dyes, black clothing and cosmetics.

Treat with ointment moisturiser and potent topical corticosteroid or oral prednisolone if warranted.

Generalised dry skin – ichthyosis

Ichthyosis refers to generalised scaly skin. There are several forms. Some ichthyoses only affect the skin but several have associated abnormalities in other organs.

Ichthyosis vulgaris is the commonest of the ichthyoses. It has autosomal dominant inheritance, and occurs as an isolated finding in 1 in 200 children.

X-linked ichthyosis is less common and may be undiagnosed for years or decades. About one-third of affected boys are diagnosed for the first time by an observant clinician during an emergency attendance for an unrelated problem. A fine scaling at birth is later replaced by larger brown scales. Diagnosis is confirmed by enzyme analysis for the affected steroid sulfatase gene. Boys with X-linked ichthyosis are usually otherwise normal but need to be monitored for hypogonadism, cryptorchidism, anosmia, short stature and mental retardation. Female carriers may have obstetric difficulties leading to prolonged labour.

In Sjögren–Larsson syndrome, a yellow-brown lichenified appearance is present in infancy. This evolves into a more florid scaling with a symmetric spastic paralysis and mental retardation. In some trichothiodystrophies, ichthyosis is associated with brittle hair and mental and growth retardation. Several ichthyoses are linked with deafness, cataracts or other eye problems. Mild, generalised scaling may be the first feature in later-onset Refsum disease, before development of multiple visual problems, deafness and neuropathy.

Eczema does not usually present as generalised dryness in babies. Unless there is a clear history of familial ichthyosis vulgaris, an infant with significant dryness should be referred for assessment by a skin specialist.

Ectodermal dysplasias are a heterogeneous group of conditions characterised by congenital, non-progressive abnormalities of

hair, teeth, nails and sweat glands. The skin is dry and may be hyperpigmented. Deficient sweating may cause overheating in infants at any time and in older children in summer. Children may present with undiagnosed recurrent fevers or with heat prostration, collapse or death. Teeth are often poorly developed or absent. Cleft lip and palate, limb abnormalities and mucous retention in the upper airway and ear may be present. Accurate diagnosis, genetic counselling, dental and audiological review, appropriate moisturiser and topical cortisone use if needed, education about avoiding overheating and regular follow up are all required.

RED BLANCHING RASHES (ERYTHEMATOUS)

Erythematous rashes are common in children. They are most commonly caused by viral infections (e.g. Coxsackie virus, echovirus, Epstein–Barr virus, adenovirus, parainfluenza, influenza, parvovirus B19, HHV-6, rubella and measles) or by a drug reaction. Consider also septicaemia, scarlet fever, Kawasaki disease and *Mycoplasma* infection.

Fever and exanthem

Fever and rash is a common presentation to the ED. The most common cause is a viral illness. Some infections have specific clinical features that aid diagnosis, e.g. measles and erythema infectiosum. However, in most instances, a specific viral diagnosis cannot be made with certainty. To manage such a child, consider:

- Is the child sick? Is the child lethargic, or peripherally cold? Are they young? Consider meningococcal disease, other bacterial sepsis, Kawasaki disease. These children require resuscitation if needed, urgent investigation and appropriate treatment guided by the findings.
- Is the child taking medications? Consider ceasing any medication.
- Are there other people at risk? If relatives are immunosuppressed or pregnant, consider serology, stool viral culture, and advising the at-risk person to consult their doctor.

- Is the rash papular? Consider papular acrodermatitis (p. 292).
- Is the rash itchy? If so, it may be primarily urticaria or a dermatitis.
- If the answer to all the above is 'no', reassurance and review is probably appropriate.

Scarlet fever

Group A streptococci cause a variety of diseases including scarlet fever, pharyngotonsillitis, impetigo, cellulitis, otitis media, streptococcal toxic shock syndrome, necrotising fasciitis, glomerulonephritis and rheumatic fever. Group A streptococcal infection usually occurs in school-age children.

Scarlet fever begins with a prodrome consisting of sudden onset of high fever, vomiting, malaise, headache, and abdominal pain. This is followed within a few hours by rash. The typical rash is a diffuse, pink-red generalised 'flush' with pinhead spots, that feels like sandpaper. The rash blanches. It is first noted on the upper chest, before spreading to the trunk, skin folds, neck, and extremities. The face is often flushed with circumoral sparing. It does not usually involve the palms or soles. Other features include strawberry tongue (initially white, then red day 4–5), pharyngotonsillitis and tender cervical and submaxillary nodes.

Confirm diagnosis by throat swab and serology. Notification is not required. Transmission occurs by direct contact. Isolate the child from school or crèche for 3 days after the start of treatment. Treat with phenoxymethylpenicillin (penicillin V) 250 mg orally (under 10 years), 500 mg orally (over 10 years) twice daily for 10 days. For penicillin-sensitive patients, use roxithromycin.

Toxic shock syndrome

Toxic shock syndrome is an acute, febrile illness with a characteristic rash and multiple system involvement. It has potential complications that include shock, renal and myocardial failure, coagulopathy and respiratory distress syndrome. Toxic shock syndrome has been associated with *Staphylococcus aureus* and group A streptococcal infection.

Presentation is initially similar to that of scarlet fever, but other features include myalgia, profuse diarrhoea, conjunctival injection and hypotension. Desquamation of digits, palms, soles and perianal region occurs 7–21 days later.

Initial management should focus on resuscitation. Antibiotic treatment should include intravenous flucloxacillin 50 mg kg^{-1} (max 2 g) 4–6-hourly. Clindamycin 5–10 mg kg^{-1} 6–8-hourly oral or IV should be added as it has been shown to inhibit the release of toxin in vitro.

Kawasaki disease

Kawasaki disease (see Chapter 5.8) is mainly seen in children between the ages of 6 months and 5 years. It is an acute, self-limiting vasculitic illness and a major cause of acquired coronary artery disease in Australian children. An understanding of the timing of clinical features aids diagnosis. The cardinal feature is a high fever persisting for 1–4 weeks with unusually severe irritability unresponsive to antipyretics. Dilatation of conjunctival vessels is seen within a few days of the onset of fever in 90% of children but may be subtle and evanescent and there is no conjunctivitis or purulent discharge. In 60% of children, cervical lymph nodes are enlarged as a firm mass at the onset of fever. In older children, there may be striking, unilateral tender lymphadenopathy thought to be cervical adenitis but unresponsive to antibiotics.

Within a few days of onset of fever, 90% of children develop a widespread erythematous rash. This may include urticarial and maculopapular lesions that increase to several centimetres in diameter. There is usually involvement of the anogenital area. There are no vesicles or crusting but there may be a few pustules on elbows or knees. The rash lasts for 1–7 days.

Within a day or two of the rash, 90% of children develop changes of the lips and mouth. The lips become red, dry, fissured and occasionally crusted and bleeding. The oral mucosa is red without ulceration. These changes can persist for 2–3 weeks.

Within a day or two of the development of a rash, about 95% of children develop erythema of the palms and soles, often with associated oedema to give a shiny swollen appearance to the hands. The swelling can persist until the fever resolves. About 2 weeks after the onset of fever, desquamation begins at the finger tips and spreads to involve the palms, followed a few days later by desquamation of the toes then soles. Fingertip desquamation will usually be seen even if no palm or sole involvement was noted earlier. This is an important feature as palm and sole involvement in a widespread eruption is otherwise uncommon.

Less common features include arthritis, diarrhoea, vomiting, coryza, cough, and hydrops of the gall bladder.

In babies under 6 months of age, and sometimes in older children, Kawasaki disease may present as prolonged fever with only one or two of the above features. Untreated, about 25% of children with Kawasaki disease develop coronary artery changes. These can occur up to 6–8 weeks after the onset of fever and may ultimately be fatal. Any child with persistent fever of unknown cause should be carefully screened for any manifestations of Kawasaki disease. Investigations should include full blood count, erythrocyte sedimentation rate, liver function tests and Group A streptococcal and other serology to exclude possible differential diagnoses. If Kawasaki disease is suspected, echocardiography should be performed at least twice: at presentation and again at 6–8 weeks. Treatment with intravenous immunoglobulin (2 g kg^{-1}, repeated if fever persists) and aspirin (10 mg kg^{-1} 8-hourly while febrile, then 3–5 mg kg^{-1} orally daily for at least 6–8 weeks) may be life-saving. Regardless of the initial echocardiogram result, treatment should be given as early in the course of the illness as possible, to minimise the risk and severity of cardiac problems.

Erythema infectiosum

Erythema infectiosum, also known as slapped cheek disease or fifth disease, is caused by parvovirus B19. It begins with a non-specific prodrome of fever (15–30% of cases), malaise, myalgia and headache. The distinctive rash has three stages:

❶ Slapped cheek appearance (1–3 days).
❷ Maculopapular blanching rash on the proximal extensor surfaces, flexor surfaces and trunk. This fades over several days with central clearing and then forms a reticular pattern (after 7 days).
❸ Reticular rash reappears with heat, cold and friction (weeks/months).

Arthralgia and arthritis occur infrequently in infected children, but are common in adults. Other potential complications include aplastic crises in children with haemoglobin abnormalities and chronic anaemia in children with human immunodeficiency virus (HIV) infection.

Treatment is supportive. Children with erythema infectiosum are highly infective before the onset of illness and are probably not infective once the rash appears. They do not need to be excluded from school or childcare. Seek specialist advice if the child is known to have a blood disorder or to be immunosuppressed.

Pregnant women who contract parvovirus B19 have a small risk of fetal anaemia and death but do not have an increased risk of fetal abnormalities. It is not practicable to prevent exposure at home, and exclusion of pregnant women from work is not recommended.[4] Pregnant women in contact with a child with parvovirus B19 infection should be advised to consult the doctor supervising their pregnancy.

Roseola infantum

This common viral exanthem is caused by HHV-6, and in some cases by HHV-7. Ninety-five percent of children have been exposed to HHV-6 by the age of 2 years. Up to 30% of all infants will present with the clinical features of roseola. Typically, an infant has a high fever for 2–4 days and is often prescribed oral antibiotics. Despite the high fever, the child remains well and active. Occipital and cervical lymphadenopathy is frequently present. The fever then disappears, but at the same time a widespread erythematous rash appears on the face and trunk. This commonly leads to presentation to the ED. Recognition of this condition is important so that both doctor and family realise that the rash is not a reaction to the antibiotics. After the appearance of the rash, the child remains well and no isolation is necessary.

Enteroviruses

Coxsackie A, B and echoviruses are all enteroviruses that cause a range of childhood illnesses, particularly in the summer months. They can cause several types of exanthem, including maculopapular, erythematous, vesicular and petechial rashes. Hand, foot and mouth disease represents one particular syndrome, usually caused by coxsackie A16 virus, and less commonly by other group A and group B coxsackie viruses and enterovirus 71 (EV71) (see p. 283). Pharyngitis is a frequent feature of enteroviral infection. Encephalitis is a less-common accompanying presentation.

Infectious mononucleosis

This syndrome is most commonly caused by Epstein–Barr virus, but may also be associated with cytomegalovirus and other viruses. Clinical features include fever, generalised lymphadenopathy, exudative tonsillopharyngitis, palatal petechiae, and hepatosplenomegaly. Children usually have milder disease than adults.

Rash occurs in up to 20% of children in the first few days of the illness. The rash may be erythematous, maculopapular or morbilliform. There is an increased incidence of rash in children with infectious mononucleosis if treated with amoxicillin or other penicillins. This rash is typically maculopapular and pruritic, and occurs mainly over the trunk.

Epstein–Barr virus has a number of other less-common dermatological manifestations, including papular acrodermatitis, oral hairy leukoplakia and cutaneous lymphoproliferative disorders.

Diagnosis can be confirmed by full blood examination, liver function tests and serology. Isolation is not required. Children with significant throat symptoms may need admission for supportive care. Oral prednisolone for 5 days may assist resolution of symptoms. Children with splenomegaly should be advised to avoid contact sports until improved.

Measles

As a result of widespread measles immunisation, this disease is now seen infrequently. However, outbreaks continue to occur in most parts of the world. The hallmarks of measles are cough, conjunctivitis and rash. The rash appears 3–4 days after the prodrome of fever, conjunctivitis, coryza, cough and Koplik spots (white spots on a bright red buccal mucosa). The rash is initially red, blanching and maculopapular. It begins around the ears and hairline; and spreads to the trunk and the proximal arms and legs. It becomes confluent by the third day. High fever often persists after onset of the rash. Uncommonly, a child will develop otitis media, pneumonia or encephalitis. Subacute sclerosing panencephalitis is a rare, fatal, late complication.

Measles vaccination gives a transient mild exanthem in about 5% of cases. If a child has been previously immunised with killed measles vaccine and later contracts measles, the presentation may be unusual. This 'atypical measles' often has high fever and malaise, no cough, no eye signs, no Koplik spots, and a rash that is more distal and often purpuric.

Measles is highly contagious and spread by airborne droplets or direct contact with infected nasal or throat secretions. Suspected cases presenting to the ED should be managed in a separate area to other patients in the department, preferably in a negative pressure room. Diagnosis should be confirmed by immunofluorescence (rapid) and culture of a nasopharyngeal aspirate or throat swab and serology. Laboratory confirmation and notification to the health department is essential to prevent epidemics. The child should be excluded from school or crèche for 5 days.

If an unimmunised child over 9 months of age has contact with measles, measles infection can be prevented by MMR vaccination within 72 hours. This is because the incubation period of the vaccine strain is shorter (4–6 days) than the incubation period of wild measles virus (10–14 days). Older contacts who do not have documentation of immunisation with measles vaccine, should be tested for measles IgG if this can be performed within 72 hours. If seronegative, or if serology cannot be performed, contacts should be immunised within 72 hours. Infants under 9 months old who have contact with measles should be given normal human immunoglobulin within 7 days.

Rubella

Rubella infection is asymptomatic in 25–50% of children. Affected children are usually only mildly unwell. The prodrome lasts up to 5 days and consists of low-grade fever, malaise, headache, coryza, and post-auricular, occipital and posterior triangle lymphadenopathy. The rash is characterised by small, fine, discrete, pink maculopapules. It starts on the face and spreads to the chest and upper arms, abdomen and thighs, all within 24 hours.

If a child is over 1 year of age and known to have received rubella vaccination, a subsequent exanthem is highly unlikely to be rubella and investigation is not required. If rubella is suspected in younger children or you cannot confirm that the child has been previously vaccinated, immunofluorescence (rapid) and culture of a nasal or throat swab should be performed. If diagnosis is confirmed, notification to state health departments is required in most states. The child should be excluded from school or crèche for 5 days. Pregnant women in contact with a child with rubella infection must consult the doctor supervising their pregnancy without delay.

Unilateral laterothoracic exanthem

Unilateral laterothoracic exanthem has only been well recognised in the past decade but is another common presentation to the ED. It usually occurs between 1 and 4 years. There is often a mild fever with gastrointestinal or upper respiratory symptoms 1 to 3 weeks before the onset of rash. The rash begins in one axilla or on one side of the chest as erythematous, urticarial, eczematous or papular lesions. Uncommonly, the rash may start in the inguinal region or on the thigh. Over a period of a week, the rash spreads to give a strikingly unilateral involvement of the lateral chest, axilla and arm. Over the next 2 weeks, there may be some spread to the other side and other areas. Itch may be present but is not marked. Coryza, pharyngitis, and regional lymphadenopathy may occur. Complete resolution occurs without sequelae within a total of 4 to 6 weeks.

Although the epidemiology of unilateral laterothoracic exanthem suggests an infective cause, no causative agent has been identified despite exhaustive searching. No isolation or restriction of activities is needed. Moderate potency topical corticosteroids may give some relief but often no treatment is needed.

Urticaria

Urticaria is common. It is characterised by the rapid appearance and disappearance of multiple raised red wheals on any part of the body. Circular erythematous macules or swellings, sometimes with central pallor, appear, migrate and disappear over minutes or hours. Individual lesions are often itchy and resolve within 1 day. There may be central clearing to give ring lesions. (These are not the target lesions of erythema multiforme, which always persist for several days.)

In some children the urticarial wheals do not fully blanch with pressure. As the lesions migrate or grow circumferentially, they leave a purplish non-blanching tinge on the skin, indicating some degree of leakage of red cells from capillaries. Frank purpura is not usually present. Typically, these children are otherwise well and are reacting to the same group of possible triggers as children with normal urticaria. Occasionally, this may be a presentation of serum sickness or cutaneous or systemic vasculitis. Features that raise suspicion about an underlying vasculitis include weals lasting more than 24 hours, bruising within weals, painful lesions or associated fever, arthralgia, abdominal pain or haematuria.

Urticaria usually occurs in otherwise well children as an isolated finding. The most common trigger for acute urticaria is a viral infection, but it may be triggered by any environmental or food allergen, or by prescription and non-prescription drugs. In most cases of short duration the urticaria resolves rapidly and the cause cannot be determined. Occasionally, the parents will strongly suspect some food or environmental agent that the child contacted before the onset of the urticaria.

Urticarial drug reactions in children are often associated with penicillin group antibiotics, cefaclor, other antibiotics, aspirin, other non-steroidal anti-inflammatory drugs and latex. Latex allergy is most common in children with recurrent exposure to latex such as repeated catheterisations or surgery, and may present as local urticaria, oedema or anaphylaxis. Banana, avocado and kiwifruit can cross-react with latex and after ingestion, children may present with itch, oedema, urticaria and wheezing.

Urticaria can be precipitated by sunlight, pressure, water, cold, heat and other physical factors.

Urticarial episodes usually resolve over days or weeks and rarely last longer than 3 months. Chronic urticaria refers to lesions being present virtually every day for more than 3 months. Rarely, this can last for many years. Urticaria may be recurrent with individual episodes resolving quickly but occurring many times over weeks, months or years. Recurrent or chronic urticaria is usually of unknown aetiology but rarely may be related to underlying inflammatory conditions such as systemic lupus erythematosus, juvenile chronic arthritis, other vasculitic diseases, and parasitic infection. Painful urticaria may be a presenting feature of erythropoietic protoporphyria.

In a child who is very unwell with urticaria, consider anaphylaxis or Kawasaki disease. If individual lesions last longer than 2 days or are tender or purpuric, consider investigation for cutaneous vasculitis including Henoch–Schönlein purpura and urticarial vasculitis.

Management

- Urticaria may be the first sign of anaphylaxis. If there is associated angio-oedema (prominent subcutaneous swelling) or wheeze, continued observation and appropriate treatment is required (see Chapter 22.5 on anaphylaxis).
- Investigation is usually not required.
- Identify the cause if possible. Ask about illnesses, medications, recent unusual foods and environmental contacts. Document these clearly.
- Treat the itch with oral antihistamine. Oral prednisolone, 1 mg kg^{-1} per day (maximum 50 mg), for a few days may be warranted by the severity of the itch but is usually not needed.
- If any purpura is present or the child is significantly lethargic or less responsive than usual, assess and investigate to exclude meningococcal sepsis and other causes of purpura. Check urine for blood.
- For recurrent or chronic urticaria, look for trigger factors. Consider mast-cell-degranulating drugs (including opiates, aspirin, and other non-steroidal anti-inflammatory drugs), foods, alcohol, animals, parasitic infections, heat, cold, sunlight and physical pressure. Consider investigating with a throat swab (for Group A streptococcal carriage), full blood examination (for eosinophilia and

anaemia), IgE, antinuclear antibodies, urine culture for bacteraemia, nocturnal check for threadworms and a possible challenge with any suspected agent. Assessment of erythrocyte protoporphyrin is warranted in young infants with sun-induced, painful urticaria.

- For recurrent or chronic urticaria that is unresponsive to conventional H1 antihistamine antagonists, adding cimetidine 10–15 mg kg^{-1} (maximum 200 mg) orally 6-hourly, to the antihistamine may help in a few cases.
- For recurrent urticaria, or for chronic urticaria where there is a clear history of regular exacerbations in the severity of the lesions, a diary recording all happenings in the 24 hours before each relapse may be rewarding in identifying the cause.

Serum sickness

Serum sickness (sometimes called 'serum-sickness-like-reactions') consists of the triad of fever, urticaria and arthralgias. It can occur at any age. Historically, about 50% of serum sickness reactions in Australian children are idiopathic and 50% have been associated with a recent course of cefaclor. Other medications may also be implicated.

Symptoms begin 5–21 days after commencement of the cefaclor and persist for 5 to 10 days. Previous courses of cefaclor may have been taken uneventfully, but more rapid onset can be seen in those children previously exposed. The child presents with an urticarial rash, which can be dramatic in appearance and cause considerable alarm to parents. The lesions may be more fixed than typical urticaria and may bruise or be tender. Arthralgia and joint swelling, possibly with effusion, is observed. Polyarthralgia occurs in up to 80%. Fever, lymphadenopathy, malaise, nausea, vomiting and abdominal pain are less common. Symptoms resolve fully in a few days. Laboratory investigations are unrewarding and infectious studies negative.

Management (see also urticaria)

- If associated with cefaclor, or another medication, cease the medication and give written information about this to the family and treating doctor.
- Joint symptoms may require analgesia and bed rest.

- Oral antihistamines may provide symptomatic relief. A few days of oral prednisolone, 1 mg kg^{-1} day^{-1} (maximum 50 mg), may be warranted by the severity of the symptoms.
- Hospitalisation and supportive care may occasionally be needed.
- Rechallenge with cefaclor may result in a recurrence of serum sickness although the risk of recurrence is unknown. A serum sickness reaction to cefaclor is not a contraindication to having another cephalosporin.

Lupus erythematosus

Systemic lupus erythematosus may present as erythematous, well-demarcated facial lesions, occasionally urticarial or slightly scaly. These lesions occur most commonly in a characteristic butterfly distribution over both cheeks and the base of the nose. In children, the facial rash may be the only manifestation (cutaneous lupus) or there may be systemic involvement. There is usually an epidermal and a dermal component. Therefore the lesion is usually more indurated than a dermatitis and more scaly than an urticaria.

In more widespread disease, patchy lesions may be present over the ears, neck and less commonly the limbs. Erythematous macules, petechiae and small infarcts can also be seen around the nail beds and on the tips of the fingers and toes. Erythematous macules may appear on the palms of the hands and soles of the feet. Florid urticaria, blistering and erythema nodosum are uncommonly seen.

Fever, arthralgias and arthritis affecting many joints imply systemic involvement. Lymphadenopathy, anorexia, weight loss, muscle weakness, pulmonary disease (especially pleuritis), cardiac disease (myocarditis and coronary artery disease), nephritis and a wide range of neuropsychiatric symptoms can be seen in childhood systemic lupus erythematosus.

If lupus is suspected, a detailed history and examination should look for systemic organ involvement, and investigations should include antinuclear and anti-double-stranded DNA antibodies, erythrocyte sedimentation rate, full blood count, renal assessment and/or brain imaging as indicated. Localised

cutaneous lesions generally respond well to moisturiser, sun protection and potent topical corticosteroid preparations. Systemic disease requires oral corticosteroid therapy initially. Regular follow up and monitoring for renal and other organ involvement is essential in all cases.

Neonatal lupus erythematosus

Neonatal lupus erythematosus occurs in infants whose mothers are positive for anti-Ro(SSA) and/or anti-La(SSB) antibodies. Most of these mothers are asymptomatic and unaware of their antibody status. About 5% of infants of antibody-positive mothers develop neonatal lupus.

Skin lesions in neonatal lupus can first appear from a few days to a few months after birth. Widespread, erythematous, often annular and growing lesions develop on the face, scalp, trunk, extremities and neck. These can be misdiagnosed as tinea or eczema. They persist for months before clearing as the maternal antibodies clear. Moderate potency topical steroid assists clearing. Sunlight and ultraviolet light can precipitate or worsen the rash.

The other major manifestation of neonatal lupus is complete heart block (from the third trimester). This is permanent and often fatal and requires a pacemaker. Interestingly, about half of all babies with neonatal lupus have complete heart block and about half have the characteristic skin lesions but only a small proportion have both.

All infants with neonatal lupus presenting with skin lesions require ongoing follow up as they appear to have an increased risk of developing autoimmune thyroid or rheumatological disorders during childhood. Subsequent siblings may be normal but 25% develop neonatal lupus in either the skin or cardiac form. Subsequent pregnancies should therefore have serial echocardiogram monitoring. Most mothers eventually develop rheumatological disease and they also require referral for follow up.

Dermatomyositis

Childhood dermatomyositis affects skin and muscle. Children may present with skin changes years before any muscle involvement or may present with acute or subacute development of fever, rash, pain and weakness. The earliest features in many children are an erythematous, sometimes violaceous, rash on the eyelids, periorbital oedema, a malar erythematous rash, and erythematous papules over the extensor surfaces of the joints of the hands. In more severe cases, there may be widespread desquamation and ulceration around the eyes, fingers and skin folds.

Muscle weakness may not have been noticed at presentation but may be present on testing. Investigations should include erythrocyte sedimentation rate, full blood count, and creatine kinase. Magnetic resonance imaging has replaced muscle biopsy as a means of assessing muscle inflammation. Therapy involves high-dose oral corticosteroid therapy initially, maintenance immunosuppression for a couple of years, and regular follow up.

Juvenile chronic arthritis

An erythematous maculopapular rash is often seen in the systemic form of juvenile chronic arthritis. This rash usually has a salmon pink colour, and tends to come and go, being particularly evident at the time when the fever is at its height. It may be urticarial.

Erythema nodosum

Erythema nodosum can occur at any age and presents with the fairly abrupt onset of painful and tender subcutaneous erythematous lesions up to 5 cm in diameter, mainly on the anterior lower legs. The arms, soles and trunk may be affected. Malaise, fever, and arthralgia may be present. Histologically there is a septal panniculitis.

In about 50% of children, erythema nodosum occurs in association with another condition, either as the presenting feature or as part of the evolution of an already diagnosed disease. Causes include chronic streptococcal disease, tuberculosis at any site, inflammatory bowel disease, chronic gastrointestinal infections, sarcoidosis, *Mycoplasma* infection, lymphoma, secondary syphilis, deep fungal infections and the oral contraceptive pill.

Lesions pass through colour changes similar to aging bruises. Resolution occurs in 3 to 6 weeks in most cases. Chronic or recurrent erythema nodosum can persist for months or years, particularly if an underlying cause has not been removed.

Management

- Search for any underlying cause.
- Investigations may include throat swab, full blood examination, erythrocyte sedimentation rate, serology for Group A *Streptococcus*, *Mycoplasma* and Epstein–Barr virus, stool culture, Mantoux testing and chest X-ray.
- Depending on the severity of symptoms, bed rest or limitation of activities for a few days may be required.
- Non-steroidal anti-inflammatory treatment will help settle inflammation and pain. The use of oral prednisolone is controversial.
- In troublesome, prolonged or recurrent cases, potassium iodide (10% solution, 2.5 mL = 250 mg three-times daily for older children, taken with milk or juice for 2 weeks) is effective.[5]

Necrobiosis lipoidica

This presents as large, irregularly shaped, red-yellow patches on the lower legs, usually in adolescents. With time, the central area may become atrophic or sclerosed. Necrobiosis lipoidica may be the first sign of diabetes in childhood and a fasting serum glucose should be arranged with follow up.

Palmoplantar hidradenitis

Palmoplantar hidradenitis, (previously known as childhood neutrophilic eccrine hidradenitis or plantar erythema nodosum), occurs in otherwise well children, typically aged 2–14 years, during spring or autumn. There may be a history of considerable physical exertion in the days before the lesions appear, often with exposure to cold or water. Erythematous, dusky tender lesions appear on the soles (Fig. 12.1.11), and sometimes on the hands. *Pseudomonas* infection within the sweat glands may be the cause in some or most cases. Antibiotics are not needed and spontaneous resolution occurs within 3 weeks. If you are confident of the diagnosis, no investigation is necessary.

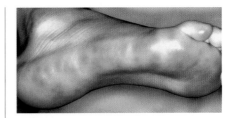

Fig. 12.1.11 **Palmoplantar hidradenitis.** (Photo courtesy of Dr Cremer.)

Pernio (chilblains)

Pernio usually presents after exposure to cold, such as playing outdoor sport in winter. Tender red/purple swellings occur on the fingers and or toes. Initially there is no epidermal change but lesions can persist for weeks and dusky scaling can develop. Symptoms are usually mild. Most children presenting with pernio are otherwise well and do not routinely need investigation. In persistent and troublesome cases, baseline investigations may include anti-Ro, antinuclear and anti-phospholipid antibodies, rheumatoid factor and cryofibrinogens. Recurrences are common. Manage by avoiding cold exposure to hands and using adequate clothing to stay systemically warm.

Spider telangiectasia

A spider naevus presents as a tiny red macule or papule with a surrounding network of fine telangiectasias, best appreciated by compressing the lesion to make it disappear then watching it reappear in the characteristic centripetal pattern, filling from the centre. These appear during mid-childhood in about 50% of children, typically on the face, hands or arms. Most resolve within a few years. Investigation is not needed. If the cosmetic concern is severe, removal by electrodessication or laser can be arranged.

Multiple spider naevi are of no medical significance in healthy children. Multiple telangiectatic vessels of non-spider type may raise suspicion of hereditary haemorrhagic telangiectasia or a photosensitivity syndrome.

Other erythematous rashes

Many conditions that present with red, scaly or purpuric rashes may appear erythematous initially, including guttate psoriasis, pityriasis rosea and Henoch–Schönlein purpura. Sometimes, most of the lesions may be erythematous but a few may reveal the more typical features of the underlying condition, such as scale or purpura.

Many haemangiomas (vascular tumours) will initially present as erythematous macules. This possibility should be borne in mind in any infant presenting with an erythematous macule on the face. Early review may show some progression of the lesion. If so, urgent referral for treatment may minimise potentially severe long-term problems from florid facial haemangiomas (p. 309).

PURPURIC RASHES

Purpuric rashes in childhood may be due to vascular dysfunction, coagulation disorder or a low platelet count. Fever may or may not be present. Purpuric rashes are associated with several life-threatening diseases and require urgent assessment.

Fever and petechiae

Petechiae are pinpoint, non-blanching spots, less than 2 mm diameter. There are many causes of fever and petechiae. These include:

- Viral infections including enteroviruses and influenza.
- *Neisseria meningitidis* (meningococcal) disease.
- Other causes of bacteraemia including *Streptococcus pneumoniae* and *Haemophilus influenzae.*
- Other diseases including Henoch–Schönlein purpura, idiopathic thrombocytopenic purpura and leukaemia.
- Illness associated with vomiting or coughing causing petechiae around the head and neck.

The majority of children with fever and petechiae do not have a cause identified – they are presumably due to viral infections. Few children with fever and petechiae (<5%) will have meningococcal disease. Recognition and early treatment of these children with meningococcal disease is paramount. Clinical signs and laboratory investigations will help determine those who should be treated for suspected meningococcal disease. All children with fever and petechiae should be reviewed by a senior doctor.

Fever and petechiae in an unwell child (including meningococcal sepsis)

If a child with fever and petechiae meets any of the following criteria, they should be presumed to have meningococcal sepsis until proven otherwise and treated accordingly (see meningococcal and other septicaemia below, this page).

- impaired conscious state (lack of alertness, lethargy, irritability);
- abnormal signs (tachycardia, tachypnoea, desaturation in air, widened pulse pressure);
- poor perfusion (cold extremities);
- any purpuric lesions greater than 2 mm (unless the clinical picture is suggestive of Henoch–Schönlein purpura, see below);
- abnormal blood indices (including WCC $>15 \times 10^9 \, L^{-1}$ and $<5 \times 10^9 \, L^{-1}$ or raised CRP >8).

Fever and petechiae in a well child

If a child with fever and petechiae is well and does not meet any of the criteria for meningococcal sepsis in the preceding paragraph, the petechiae may be due to an obvious mechanical cause. These children do not require investigation and may be discharged with review planned within 12–24 hours. Mechanical causes of petechiae include:

- coughing or vomiting leading to petechiae around the head and neck;
- local physical pressure such as a tight tourniquet or being held tightly for procedures;
- the practice seen in some ethnic groups of treating a febrile child by rubbing or suctioning the skin with a variety of implements, producing bizarre circular and linear patterns of petechiae.

If no mechanical cause is identified in a well child with fever and petechiae, the child is likely to have a viral infection, and should be managed as follows:

- investigate with a full blood count, C-reactive protein and blood cultures;

- observe for 4 hours;
- if the initial test results are normal and there is no clinical deterioration or progression of the rash over the 4 hours, discharge with review the next day.

Children who have received antibiotics prior to presentation can be managed the same way, but the possibility of partially treated meningitis or sepsis may lead to a lower threshold for admission or early review.

Meningococcal and other septicaemia

Septicaemia with purpura is usually due to meningococcal disease. There may be an upper respiratory prodrome followed within hours by high fever, malaise and headache. Skin lesions may begin as tender erythematous macules or as petechiae on the skin and mucous membranes. Lesions develop purpuric centres and large haemorrhagic areas may form. Purpura may also be due to sepsis with *Haemophilus influenzae*, group A streptococci, *Staphylococcus aureus* and some Gram-negative organisms. Infective endocarditis, typhus, typhoid fever and certain viral haemorrhagic fevers may cause purpuric lesions.

Early management (a detailed protocol for meningococcal management can be accessed online[6]):

- Give oxygen.
- Gain intravenous or intraosseous access.
- Immediate investigations (if blood can be obtained without delay) including blood culture, blood smear, blood PCR, full blood count/differential, glucose, urea and electrolytes, clotting, if appropriate.
- Administer cefotaxime ($50 \, mg \, kg^{-1}$ per dose – maximum 3 g, 6-hourly).
- Meningococcaemia is often associated with hypovolaemia: give $20 \, mL \, kg^{-1}$ of normal saline. More fluid will often be needed to improve blood pressure and peripheral perfusion ($40 \, mL \, kg^{-1}$ in the first hour is common).
- Isolate cases (if possible) until they have had >12 hours antibiotic treatment.
- Subsequent investigations include throat swab, lumbar puncture (unless contraindicated). Urinary or CSF 'rapid antigen' testing is not recommended because of poor sensitivity and specificity.

Vasculitis and Henoch–Schönlein purpura

Vasculitis is a reaction pattern that presents as non-itchy, painless macules, papules or urticarial lesions with purpuric centres. There are many causes of vasculitis including infections (streptococcal, hepatitis viruses and others), autoimmune diseases (systemic lupus erythematosus, Behçet disease), allergy (drugs) or idiopathic.

Henoch-Schönlein purpura is an IgA-mediated condition and is the commonest cause of vasculitis in children. It can occur at any age but is most common between the ages of 2 and 10 years. There is sometimes a preceding streptococcal or non-specific viral illness. Over a couple of days, lesions occur in a symmetrical distribution, mainly on the buttocks and lower legs, and occasionally on the genitalia, arms and elsewhere (Fig. 12.1.12). In many children, most lesions are purpuric, ranging from pinpoint petechiae to 2 cm in diameter. In other children, only a few purpuric areas may be noted amongst many erythematous or urticarial lesions. There may be associated abdominal pain, arthralgia, arthritis or haematuria. Renal involvement leading to chronic renal failure is rare, but can occur irrespective of the severity of the rash and other symptoms, and may be delayed until weeks or months after the onset of the illness.

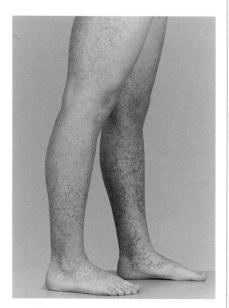

Fig. 12.1.12 Vasculitis. Henoch–Schönlein purpura.

A child with Henoch–Schönlein purpura may warrant a full blood examination to exclude thrombocytopenia. Check blood pressure and urine for blood or protein. Bed rest and analgesia may be needed if discomfort is considerable. Oral prednisolone may reduce the duration of abdominal pain and may reduce the likelihood of renal problems. Severe renal involvement may require immunosuppression, plasmapheresis or hypertensive therapy but this is rare. In children with no renal involvement at presentation, blood pressure and urinalysis should be done weekly for 1 month, then each 2 months for 6 months. Children who have not developed urinary abnormalities within 6 months do not require further regular follow up.

Thrombocytopenic purpura

Idiopathic thrombocytopenic purpura (ITP) is the most common cause. This is an acquired thrombocytopenia due to immune-mediated shortened circulating platelet survival in the absence of other disturbances of haemostasis or coagulation. Most children present with bruising and petechiae alone. Oral bleeding, epistaxis, rectal bleeding or haematuria are less common. There is often a history of a recent viral infection. The child is otherwise well. More serious causes, such as leukaemia or aplastic anaemia should be excluded. Full blood examination will be normal apart from a low platelet count.

Thrombocytopenia may be drug-induced (e.g. secondary to chloramphenicol, antithyroid medications).

Leukaemia

Leukaemia should be suspected in a child with generalised petechiae or purpura in the absence of trauma. Features may include tiredness, pallor, limb pain, malaise and gum hypertrophy. Thrombocytopenia is usually present. An urgent full blood examination should be obtained (see Chapter 11.6 on acute leukaemia).

Two subtypes of acute myeloid leukaemia typically present with skin lesions. Acute monocytic leukaemia may present with skin infiltrates and gum hypertrophy. Acute pro-myelocytic leukaemia often presents with a purpuric rash anywhere on the body in association with disseminated intravascular coagulation.

Coagulation disorders

Extensive purpuric lesions in a well child without a history of significant trauma may be due to an underlying coagulation disorder. This may be inherited or acquired. There may be a history of joint pain or swelling, or bleeding from other sites.

Child abuse

Twisting, compression, pinching and hitting can all cause petechial or purpuric lesions. Look for bruises of bizarre shapes and different ages or evidence of fractures or other injuries. Assess the child's affect and relationship with carers. A complete examination is mandatory. If child abuse is suspected, admission or immediate referral to a paediatrician may be needed for complete assessment and further investigations (see Chapter 18.2 on child abuse).

Artefactual purpura

Older children sometimes present with self-induced purpuric lesions. These are often in bizarre, non-physiological shapes, sometimes with obvious marks of finger trauma. They occur in exposed areas. Lesions may have recurred for months or longer in an otherwise well and generally unconcerned child or adolescent. The history typically has inappropriate or contradictory details and a lack of concern about the lesions. The diagnosis and management of artefactual disease in children may be difficult and requires confidence in interpretation of the skin findings and ongoing paediatric and psychological follow up of the child and family. Occasionally, admission to hospital may be required.

Papular-purpuric gloves and socks syndrome

Papular-purpuric gloves and socks syndrome is caused by parvovirus B19 and probably by several other common viruses. Adolescents develop vague symptoms of fever, fatigue and pains. Redness and swelling of the palms and soles progresses rapidly to petechial and purpuric lesions that do not extend onto other body parts. There may be oral vesicles or erosions. The adolescent remains generally well and the eruption clears in 2 weeks. Interestingly, unlike erythema infectiosum, adolescents with papular-purpuric gloves and socks syndrome are thought to be infective during the period of rash.

Dusky purple nodules on hands and feet

For tender red/purple areas (not usually purpuric) on hands and feet in otherwise well children, consider pernio (p. 306) and palmoplantar hidradenitis (p. 306).

Chronic pigmented purpura

Chronic petechiae in childhood are usually due to chronic pigmented purpura. This typically presents as several 2–3 cm patches of petechiae. In each patch, both new and old petechiae can be seen giving red, purple and brown dots (like cayenne pepper). Patches may be subtle, the child is otherwise well, the condition is benign, but lesions recur for months or years.

Other causes of childhood purpura

Unusual patterns or presentations of purpura in childhood may be associated with vasculitic diseases, glucocorticoid excess, any cause of abnormal skin elasticity and scurvy. In children with scurvy, irritability, bone pain, gum sponginess and bleeding may be present. Wrist X-rays are diagnostic.

Langerhans cell histiocytosis may present with persistent anogenital or scalp petechiae in infants, or with widespread, itchy, haemorrhagic papules, including on the hands and feet (see p. 294).

Neonatal purpura

Purpuric rashes in the neonatal period may be an early presentation of any cause of childhood purpura (see above). In addition, consider:

- congenital infection including rubella, cytomegalovirus, toxoplasmosis, and herpes simplex.
- haemolytic disease of the newborn.
- malignancy, including neuroblastoma, Langerhans cell histiocytosis and leukaemia.
- iatrogenic injury, including birth trauma, extravasation of drugs and arterial injury during catheterisation.
- protein C or S deficiency.

VASCULAR TUMOURS – HAEMANGIOMAS AND HAEMANGIOMA VARIANTS

Haemangiomas of infancy

Haemangiomas are tumours of vascular endothelial cells. While haemangiomas may be present at birth, most appear in the first days or weeks of life. The appearance depends on whether the haemangioma involves the skin. If the skin is involved, the first sign is often a patch of pallor, followed by the development of an erythematous macule. Over a few weeks, this may grow and thicken into a soft, partly compressible, well defined, crimson or purple nodule (the so-called 'strawberry haemangioma'). There may be a substantial subcutaneous mass. Haemangiomas that do not involve the skin are often first noticed as firm, blue or skin-coloured swellings. Haemangiomas can occur anywhere on the body and may involve internal organs such as the liver or trachea.

Haemangiomas may remain as tiny 1-millimetre lesions or involve extensive areas of the body. Growth may be slow but can be rapid and frightening, even with intensive treatment.

Haemangiomas usually grow for 3–9 months and then slowly involute over the next 2–10 years. Involution is first noticed as a decrease in the intensity of the surface crimson colour with development of small islands of greyish skin. The haemangioma becomes softer and gradually shrinks in size. Half resolve by age 5, and 90% by age 9. Resolution may not be complete. Particularly with larger lesions, there may be residual telangiectatic vessels, fibro-fatty tissue or

redundant skin. Some haemangiomas show little resolution.

Most haemangiomas never cause problems and are best left alone and allowed to involute spontaneously. However, haemangiomas can rapidly lead to problems such as extreme disfigurement, ulceration, blindness, destruction of cartilage, respiratory obstruction, coagulation failure or death. Urgent assessment by a clinician experienced in this field is needed in the following circumstances:

Association with stridor Stridor, especially increasing stridor of recent onset in a child of a few months of age, may be due to a laryngeal or tracheal haemangioma. This risk is greatest in children with a superficial haemangioma involving the beard area. About half of all children with an airway haemangioma will have a visible superficial haemangioma.

Eye involvement Even quite small haemangiomas on the eyelid or adjacent to the globe of the eye can cause impaired vision on that side, either by directly obstructing the visual axis or more commonly by pressing on the globe to cause astigmatism. In both cases, amblyopia may result and may lead to permanent blindness if not treated.

Involvement of facial structures Haemangiomas may deform structures such as the lip, ear cartilage, nasal cartilage, dentition or jaw growth. This deformity will remain after resolution of the haemangioma. Deforming lesions require aggressive treatment.

Ulceration Ulceration is more common in haemangiomas at sites exposed to trauma, including areas of friction, anogenital lesions and lesions involving the lips. Ulcers may be very painful and can spread within days to give necrotic lesions several centimetres in size. There may be full tissue loss of lips, nose and eyelids with permanent disfigurement and loss of function. Early treatment with topical metronidazole and paraffin ointment several times daily usually leads to healing. Laser to the ulcer base or surgical excision may be warranted.

Macular facial lesions A macular (flat) capillary lesion on the face of a neonate is likely to be a capillary malformation, not a haemangioma, and does not require urgent treatment. However, it may be the first sign of an extensive facial haemangioma. This can commence as a large macular capillary lesion that is indistinguishable from a capillary malformation until thickening and rapid growth occurs (Fig. 12.1.13). These haemangiomas cause extreme disfigurement and after thickening has commenced, treatment is difficult. Treatment with vascular laser can dramatically help if given during the brief macular phase, but is of little value after thickening has commenced. If you are suspicious about a large macular capillary lesion in a neonate (e.g. onset after birth, changing colour, any sign of thickening), monitoring and/or referral should be done with an awareness of the possible urgency of treatment.

Sudden onset of swelling and bruising in a large haemangioma This may presage the development of a consumptive coagulopathy – see Kaposiform haemangioendothelioma/tufted angioma (p. 310).

Multiple haemangiomas (diffuse neonatal haemangiomatosis) Infants with five or more cutaneous haemangiomas have a considerably higher risk of haemangiomas at other sites, including liver, gut and lungs. Investigations should include a hepatic ultrasound, full blood examination, platelet count, fibrinogen level, clotting profile, urinalysis, liver function tests, and stool analysis for blood. An electrocardiogram and chest X-ray may be needed. Liver haemangiomas in particular are associated with high flow cardiac failure and a significant mortality. If small hepatic lesions are found on imaging, follow up is required to ensure that undetected rapid growth does not occur.

Management

- Most parents just need education and reassurance about the inherently benign nature of these lesions.
- If complications, as described above, are considered likely, the initial treatment option was oral prednisolone for 6 weeks, 3–5 mg kg⁻¹ day⁻¹ for some weeks before slow weaning. Since 2008, the initial treatment of choice has been oral propranolol (e.g. 1 mg kg⁻¹ bd). For some

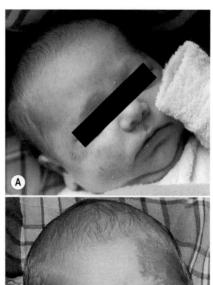
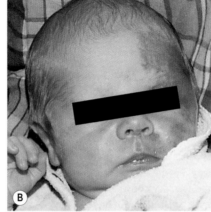
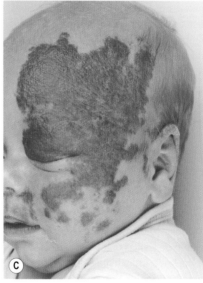

Fig. 12.1.13 Untreated segmental facial haemangioma. (A) At 1 week; (B) at 2 weeks (easily misinterpreted as a capillary malformation); and (C) at 6 weeks, by which time thickening has occurred. Urgent assessment for possible laser and oral propranolol treatment can minimise morbidity.

types of lesions, such as large facial tumours, propranolol has led to remarkable shrinking and fading. Not all haemangiomas respond as well. Other beta blockers may also be effective. As more experience is gained with propranolol treatment, optimal protocols for pre-treatment investigations and for monitoring while on treatment will be better understood. Intralesional corticosteroids, intravenous vincristine, subcutaneous α-interferon, vascular laser, surgery and embolisation may all be warranted in individual patients, either at presentation or if the response to initial treatment is insufficient. Early treatment will prevent or minimise complications in most cases.

- Any infant with a midline lumbosacral or anogenital haemangioma or other vascular malformation should be checked for genitourinary abnormalities and have imaging to exclude a tethered cord. To image the spine prior to 3 months of age, an ultrasound examination is generally satisfactory. In older children, a magnetic resonance imaging (MRI) examination is warranted.

Rapidly involuting congenital haemangioma

Rapidly involuting congenital haemangiomas have recently been recognised as a distinct type of haemangioma. They are present at birth as raised violaceous vascular tumours, often many centimetres across. They can be associated with high-flow cardiac failure, and can be mistaken both on clinical and radiological assessment for arteriovenous malformations or vascular sarcomas. The distinction is important because they resolve within 12–18 months without treatment.

Kaposiform haemangioendothelioma/ tufted angioma

These tumours may be present at birth. Growth can be rapid and extend over much of a leg and buttock. The texture is often firmer than felt with typical infantile haemangiomas. Kaposiform haemangioendothelioma and tufted angioma are associated with platelet trapping and a consumptive coagulopathy (Kasabach–Merritt syndrome). This has a significant mortality if untreated. Crises usually manifest clinically as rapid swelling of the lesion with the lesion appearing bruised and becoming hard and tender. Assess platelet count, clotting profile and fibrinogen level. High-dose oral corticosteroids may not be effective and vincristine for many months is commonly required to achieve and maintain control and reduction in tumour size. Alpha-interferon may be needed, sometimes for years.

Pyogenic granuloma

Pyogenic granulomas are benign acquired vascular tumours that often present to EDs with a history of bleeding. They usually occur after infancy, on the face and neck, hands, or elsewhere on the body. There may be a history of preceding trivial trauma to that site. Over several days, a dark red/bluish papule appears and grows to 10 mm in height. The surface may be moist, scaly or warty. Bleeding is common and may be recurrent.

Management

Bleeding will stop with the application of pressure. Pedunculated lesions can be ligated at the base without anaesthetic. Alternatively, or if recurrence occurs, surgical curettage is curative. Usually, local anaesthesia is adequate. Any solitary feeding arteriole beneath the papule may need cautery. A protective dressing will minimise the risk of rebleeding before surgery.

Vascular malformations

Vascular malformations are developmental lesions composed of dilated blood vessels and/or lymphatic channels. They are present at birth but may not become evident until infancy or occasionally later in childhood. Malformations include common capillary malformations on the face (port-wine stain), more extensive capillary lesions, localised venous malformations, venous malformations involving large areas with associated overgrowth and other changes, arteriovenous malformations, lymphatic malformations (e.g. cystic hygroma) or any combination of these.

They are not tumours and do not have a growth phase or resolution phase as haemangiomas do. They are generally static lesions. However, changes can occur over time, leading to increasing problems. Particularly at puberty, there may be growth of the malformation leading to its appearance for the first time, or leading to problems such as pain in a previously asymptomatic lesion.

The appearance depends on the nature and site of the malformation. Purely capillary malformations appear as red macules on the skin. They blanch partially or fully. Venous involvement manifests as dilated veins or soft compressible bluish lumps that empty when elevated. Phleboliths are common and may be palpable. Significant arterial involvement may allow a thrill to be felt on examination. Lymphatic lesions give diffuse swelling of a limb or soft subcutaneous masses. Lymphatic involvement on the skin surface results in a mass of firm warty 2 mm papules that may be clear but often are dark blue or black because of haemorrhage into the lesions.

Vascular malformations can be associated with many chronic and acute problems that can precipitate attendance at an ED. Chronic problems include concerns about the appearance, psychological problems, social isolation, pain, deformity, dental problems, overgrowth, leg length discrepancy, arthritis and bone erosion. Acute problems may be related to any of these and also include pain, haemorrhage, infection, thrombosis and pulmonary emboli.

Neonatal vascular malformations

A neonate with a substantial vascular malformation should be examined thoroughly for associated malformations, for high-flow cardiac compromise and for other abnormalities in any system. Investigation includes ultrasound and radiological imaging.

Facial capillary malformations ('port wine stain')

Facial capillary malformations are usually present at birth and persist throughout childhood, becoming darker and thicker during adolescence. Treatment with vascular laser in early childhood leads to clearing of most of the lesion in most children.

Children with vascular malformations around the eye should be screened for glaucoma and other eye abnormalities. Children with capillary malformations involving the forehead and upper eyelid have a 10% risk of intracranial involvement and a smaller risk of developing epilepsy, strokes, hemiplegia or mental retardation (Sturge–Weber syndrome).

Beware of any facial 'capillary malformation' that appears after birth or becomes darker or thicker in the first weeks of life. This may actually be a haemangioma requiring urgent treatment (see 'macular facial lesions', p. 310).

Pain, swelling

Chronic discomfort and pain is common with large venous malformations, particularly those involving the legs. Pain is worse after standing for prolonged periods. Sudden onset or worsening of pain is also common. In venous malformations, it may arise from localised microthrombi and microinfarction. In venous and lymphatic malformations, it may be due to secondary infection. Sudden pain may be accompanied by a sudden increase in swelling and may lead to a rapid compromise of a body function, depending on the site. Sudden, severe pain in an adolescent, with or without fever, may be the presenting feature of Fabry disease (see below). Complex regional pain syndrome should also be considered.

High flow lesions

Arteriovenous malformations are dangerous. Any vascular lesion with a thrill should be presumed to be an arteriovenous malformation. They can present in many ways to the ED – as a new swelling, an area of skin necrosis, skin ulceration, bleeding, or with the sequelae of internal bleeding, including intracranial bleeding. They can expand and erode surrounding structures. If a high-flow lesion is suspected, Doppler ultrasound should be arranged to confirm this. Expert follow up is essential.

Bleeding, coagulopathy

Large venous malformations are associated with chronic consumption of clotting factors, low fibrinogen, somewhat reduced platelet count and bleeding. (This is not Kasabach–Merritt syndrome, which is associated with vascular tumours.)

Intestinal bleeding

Multiple cutaneous and visceral vascular malformations occur in blue rubber bleb syndrome and may cause intestinal bleeding. In hereditary haemorrhagic telangiectasia, telangiectasias usually appear on the face, mouth and nose. Nose bleeds become frequent in late childhood and gastrointestinal bleeding occurs in adult life.

Bladder or bowel dysfunction in older children

Congenital lesions over the lumbosacral area may be associated with occult spinal abnormalities such as a tethered cord. These spinal anomalies may not cause problems until later in childhood when they can present insidiously with irreversible bladder, bowel or limb dysfunction. These problems can be prevented by early screening with MRI and surgical correction. Congenital lesions that have been associated with underlying spinal problems include haemangiomas, capillary malformations, lipomas, dimples, sinuses and hairy patches.

Leg length discrepancy

Children with a significant vascular malformation involving a leg need to be monitored for unequal leg growth. This can present as a limp or as a secondary problem including scoliosis, back pain, joint pain and headache.

Multiple telangiectatic vessels

Multiple telangiectatic vessels of non-spider type may raise suspicion of hereditary haemorrhagic telangiectasia or some photosensitivity syndromes. Multiple spider naevi do not require investigation.

Fabry disease

Fabry disease is X-linked and primarily affects males. Females can be variably affected. Angiokeratomas (flat or raised, slightly warty, red/purple lesions) appear in mid-childhood on the lower trunk, pelvis and thighs. Tiny vascular lesions may be seen on the lips or in the mouth. Corneal opacities are invariably present. Children or adolescents may present to the ED with paraesthesia of the hands and feet, or with sudden severe pain involving the limbs. Renal, cardiac and central nervous system problems occur later.

Management of vascular malformations

- Management of vascular malformations can be demanding and complex. For example, interventional embolisation of a large venous malformation of a limb may achieve an excellent result but only after perhaps 20 or more general anaesthetics each of a few hours duration.
- Management requires a multidisciplinary approach using expertise from surgical, paediatric, dermatological, radiological and psychological fields.
- Children with lumbosacral vascular malformations should have magnetic resonance imaging to exclude a tethered spinal cord.
- Compression stockings may reduce chronic pain in venous malformations. Low-dose aspirin may reduce episodes of pain in venous malformations. Heparin will minimise the coagulopathy from large venous malformations (but does not help the coagulopathy associated with Kasabach–Merritt syndrome seen with some vascular tumours).
- Partial or complete surgical resection may be needed for venous, lymphatic or arteriovenous malformations.
- Orthotic or surgical correction may assist with a leg length discrepancy.

HYPERPIGMENTATION

Diffuse hyperpigmentation

Diffuse hyperpigmentation is rare in children and investigation to identify the cause is required. Generalised darkening of the skin is often most obvious on the palmar creases, linea alba and areola, on the buccal mucosa and on the sun-exposed areas of the face, neck and extremities. Consider:

- Endocrine disease. Addison disease (also thickening of the skin and signs of increased androgen production), Cushing syndrome of pituitary origin (also acne, hirsutism, striae, purpura), exogenous adrenocorticotropic hormone administration, acromegaly (thickened, greasy, more hairy and often with many skin tags) and hyperthyroidism can all cause hyperpigmentation.
- Renal failure may cause greying of the skin.
- Haemochromatosis. In children, this is usually secondary to transfusions.
- Lipoidoses. A yellow-brown darkening of skin, most prominent in sun-exposed areas, can occur in the Niemann–Pick diseases. Look for waxy indurated skin, purpura, hepatosplenomegaly and neurological deterioration. Although a similar colour can be seen in adult-onset Gaucher's disease, it is not a feature of the earlier onset forms.

Localised macular hyperpigmentation – including café-au-lait macules

Many normal children have one or two well-defined pigmented macules, generally not present at birth but appearing in the early years. In a child with pigmented macular lesions of normal texture, consider:

Neurofibromatosis Six or more café-au-lait spots greater than 0.5 cm in diameter are strong evidence for neurofibromatosis. Examine for other features including axillary 'freckling' (usually not seen until mid-childhood), pigmented or thickened skin over plexiform neurofibromas (present in early childhood), iris pigmentation, optic tumours, skeletal abnormalities, short stature, skin neurofibromas, hypertension, macrocephaly and learning difficulties. The diagnosis may be uncertain early in life but full penetrance of neurofibromatosis is usually seen by 8 years of age. Regular follow up is needed, including assessment of intellectual progress and audiological and ophthalmological review. In children under 5 years old, magnetic resonance imaging of optic tracts to exclude optic glioma is warranted. Other investigations are not required unless suggested by clinical findings. The risk of myelomonocytic leukaemia in a child with neurofibromatosis is several hundred times higher than in other children. It is still sufficiently low (0.05%) that routine testing is not warranted but any unexplained hepatomegaly, splenomegaly, lymphadenopathy, pallor or infiltrative skin lesions requires investigation. Most children with neurofibromatosis never develop any of the significant medical associated features.

McCune–Albright syndrome A child with one or more large unilateral brown macules may have McCune–Albright syndrome. Endocrine or bony abnormalities should be looked for on examination. A bone scan should be performed at 3 years of age, and the child should be monitored for any signs of increased hormonal secretion. Routine endocrine investigations are not warranted in the absence of abnormal clinical signs.

Incontinentia pigmenti If the earlier phases have occurred in utero, hyperpigmented linear streaks may be present at birth.

Peutz–Jeghers syndrome Small, pigmented macules present on the lips and mucosa from birth are associated with intestinal polyposis. Care must be taken when assessing any episodes of abdominal pain as these children are at higher risk of intussusception and collapse. Intestinal bleeding may be the presenting feature.

Segmental pigmentary disorder (including linear and whorled hyperpigmentation and hypopigmentation of Ito) Streaks, lines and whorls of hyperpigmentation and/or hypopigmentation may be present from birth. These patterns reflect mosaicism. Usually these children are otherwise normal but a wide range of associated malformations in other systems have been reported, particularly eye, teeth, brain and skeletal malformations. Apart from audiological and ophthalmological examination, investigations are not required unless suggested by clinical findings, but these children should be reviewed until settled in school.

Post-inflammatory hyperpigmentation This occurs particularly in dark-skinned people. Many inflammatory skin disorders may heal leaving diffuse, hypo- or hyperpigmented macules that can persist for months or years.

Pellagra Hyperpigmentation and erythema on sun-exposed areas, cheilitis, perineal inflammation and diarrhoea may be seen in niacin deficiency.

Naevus of Ota This presents at birth or during childhood as a bluish brown patch around the eye, sometimes involving the sclera. Glaucoma has been reported with naevus of Ota.

Localised raised hyperpigmentation

If local areas of hyperpigmentation are roughened, raised or warty, consider:

- Congenital and acquired pigmented naevi (see below).
- Genodermatoses such as dyskeratosis congenita. Congenital nail dystrophy, pancytopenia, skeletal and eye anomalies may be present.
- Acanthosis nigricans. Rough 'dirty' skin on the neck or axillary folds is associated with obesity, polycystic ovary syndrome, other insulin resistance syndromes and hypothyroidism. Early acanthosis nigricans can be seen in many overweight children. If weight continues to increase, the acanthosis nigricans will progress to become cosmetically obvious and widespread. Early intervention and follow up is required.

Congenital pigmented naevi

Congenital melanocytic naevi are thickened, sharply defined, tan, dark brown or black birthmarks. They range in size from common small lesions less than 2 cm in diameter to rare giant lesions that may cover entire parts of the body, such as the trunk. Larger lesions may have irregular colour, texture and hairiness with areas of thick redundant skin. Large congenital melanocytic naevi often are associated with many smaller lesions elsewhere on the body, some of which appear in the first 2 years of life.

Management

- The risk of malignancy in isolated small congenital melanocytic naevi is very small and does not require surgical excision. Decisions about removal are based on the site and potential effects of the child's psychosocial development. Excision, if desired, can be done early in life, or later if undecided.
- Giant congenital melanocytic naevi are associated with major psychosocial problems. Early dermabrasion can markedly decrease the colour of the naevus and is usually warranted. Results may be better if surgery is performed within the first 3 months of life. Urgent contact with a plastic surgeon experienced in this area is necessary. Pigment lasers have also recently been used and may be useful for some lesions.
- A second concern is malignancy. The lifetime risk of melanoma in a giant congenital melanocytic naevus is small (less than 5%). Parental instruction about reporting changes in the naevus will allow early biopsy of changing areas.
- Giant congenital melanocytic naevi of the scalp or spine can be associated with neurocutaneous melanosis and other CNS abnormalities. Most of these abnormalities remain asymptomatic, and screening with MRI is controversial. A reasonable approach is to screen if there is any suggestion of obstructive hydrocephalus, if there are large lesions involving the axial spine and posterior scalp or multiple cannonball-shaped lesions (look for Dandy–Walker malformations), or if there are lesions over the lower spine (look for tethered cord). Early imaging in the first weeks of life allows the use of ultrasound where possible and the use of MRI without the need for a general anaesthetic.
- Regular follow up is needed throughout childhood to monitor the naevi and psychosocial development.

Acquired pigmented naevi

During childhood, most children develop multiple acquired melanocytic naevi. Sun exposure in white children is associated with the development of an increased number of naevi. Acquired melanocytic naevi begin as small, flat, well-demarcated pigmented lesions (junctional melanocytic naevi). A small percentage of junctional melanocytic naevi become raised and dome shaped (compound melanocytic naevi) often with a darker centre. Enlargement and darkening of naevi just before and during puberty is common.

Melanoma is very rare in childhood and uncommon in adolescence. Children and adolescents continue to acquire new melanocytic naevi until age 20. Therefore, the presence of a new naevus is not in itself suspicious. You do need to be concerned if atypical features are present, particularly in adolescents. Any rapid change over a few weeks leading to an increase in asymmetry, an irregular border, multiple colours especially with non-brown areas within brown areas, and growth beyond 10 mm may suggest malignancy.

Immune-suppressed children and those who have had chemotherapy are at greater risk of skin malignancy and should have regular skin review.

Children with a great many lentigines (small, dark brown 1–2 mm macules) may have associated findings (e.g. LEOPARD syndrome) and require screening for hearing and cardiac problems and regular follow up.

Dysplastic naevi

These are a subtype of acquired pigmented naevi. Dysplastic naevi are usually macular, greater than 5 mm in diameter, with a less-regular border, some erythema, and some variability in colour. They may develop during childhood or after puberty. The presence of multiple dysplastic naevi is associated with a significant increased risk of melanoma. However, the great majority of melanomas that occur in this population are found in unaffected skin or normal moles rather than in pre-existing dysplastic naevi. Removal of a dysplastic naevus is only indicated if there is concern that a naevus may represent a melanoma. Regular photography and follow up are indicated to aid in the detection of melanoma at an early stage.

Children with a family history of malignant melanoma and/or multiple dysplastic naevi are at a higher risk of developing melanoma and require regular skin review.

Halo naevi

Halo naevi appear as a sharply defined area of depigmentation 5–15 mm in diameter, centred on a regressing mole. They are common in childhood and benign.

Spitz naevi

Spitz naevi are fairly common, benign melanocytic lesions. They usually present prior to puberty as single, red or red/brown papules that can grow to 1 cm in diameter. They are vascular and blanch to reveal the underlying pigmentation.

Management is controversial. Spitz naevi are benign but usually do not resolve. Removal may be indicated because of uncertainty about the clinical diagnosis or for cosmetic reasons. Lesions on the central face that are only a few millimetres in diameter at presentation are likely to grow considerably and early surgical excision may be desirable. Histological interpretation is sometimes difficult with findings that overlap with malignant melanoma. Assessment by an experienced dermatopathologist is required.

Naevus of Ota

Naevus of Ota is present at birth in 50% of cases and appears at puberty in most others. It can occur in any racial group and is one manifestation of dermal melanocytosis. It presents as a unilateral, well-demarcated, blue-black patch of skin on the cheek, forehead and periorbital area. The sclera of the associated eye may also be pigmented. Cover-up cosmetics or laser depigmentation have been used to treat the discolouration.

Mongolian spots

Mongolian spots are another manifestation of dermal melanocytosis. They are extremely common and can be found on most Asian and dark-skinned babies as poorly-circumscribed, blue-black patches. The most common site is on the lower back, but they can occur elsewhere, and may be multiple and widespread. They are benign and usually fade over many years. No treatment is required. When at unusual sites, they can be mistaken for bruises.

HYPOPIGMENTATION

Localised patches of depigmentation (total loss of pigment of skin or hair) can be seen in vitiligo, halo naevi, naevus depigmentosis and piebaldism. Localised patches of hypopigmented skin may be due to pityriasis versicolor (usually in adolescence), pityriasis alba (representing post-inflammatory change following mild eczema, usually in mid-childhood) and post-inflammatory loss of pigment. Focal pale patches may be the only marker of leprosy in an individual from an endemic area.

Pityriasis versicolor

This is common in adolescents, and caused by an increased activity of commensal yeasts. Multiple oval macules, 3–10 mm in diameter and usually covered with fine scale, appear on the trunk or upper arms. The lesions coalesce and may appear paler or darker than the surrounding skin. It is distinguished from vitiligo by the presence of scale and residual pigment. Scrapings can be sent for microscopy to confirm the diagnosis. Treat with topical imidazole creams or with anti-yeast shampoos. For example, apply selenium sulfide 2% shampoo or ketoconazole 2% shampoo. Leave on for 30 minutes, if tolerated, rinse, and treat daily for 1 week and then monthly. If there are cosmetic concerns, a short course of oral ketoconazole followed by the above measures may be warranted. The yeast is readily treated, but the post-inflammatory hypopigmentation takes months to resolve. Relapses are common unless ongoing monthly treatments are used for a year or so.

Pityriasis versicolor is extremely uncommon in young children but, when it occurs, lesions may be on the face or neck. If found in a young child, examine the child for other markers of an underlying congenital adrenal hyperplasia.

Pityriasis alba

This condition is common in prepubertal children and simply represents post-inflammatory hypopigmentation secondary to mild eczema. Single or multiple, poorly demarcated hypopigmented (but never completely depigmented) 1–2 cm macules are seen on the face or upper body. Lesions are not itchy but often have a fine scale. Usually no treatment is needed. If desired, treat with emollients. Treat any erythema with hydrocortisone 1%. Resolution takes weeks and requires sun exposure for full repigmentation.

Vitiligo

This condition is characterised by sharply demarcated, often symmetrical areas of complete pigment loss. Eventual repigmentation in childhood vitiligo is common and is helped by topical steroids or pimecrolimus cream. In troublesome cases, corrective cosmetics or ultraviolet therapy may be required. The association in children between vitiligo and other organ-specific autoimmune conditions (e.g. diabetes, thyroid disease) is very small. Investigations for these are not necessary unless there is a clinical suspicion of an associated disorder.

Post-inflammatory hypopigmentation

This condition occurs particularly in dark-skinned people. Many inflammatory skin disorders may heal leaving diffuse, hypo- or hyperpigmented macules that can persist for months or years. Repigmentation eventually occurs.

Linear and whorled hypopigmention ('hypomelanosis of ito')

See linear and whorled hyperpigmentation and hypopigmentation, p. 313.

Tuberous sclerosis

Hypopigmented patches may be the first sign of tuberous sclerosis. These patches can be regular or irregular in shape. A couple of isolated hypopigmented patches in a young child are far more likely to be simple achromic naevi than to be the first sign of tuberous sclerosis. Tuberous sclerosis becomes much more likely if the child has

a history of epilepsy. Look also for forehead plaques (pink, initially flat but later slightly raised) and shagreen patches (rough, slightly thickened skin usually over the back). Other skin findings such as periungual fibromas and facial angiofibromas usually appear in older children. The diagnosis of tuberous sclerosis may require imaging of eyes, brain, heart and kidneys and investigation of relatives. Regular paediatric follow up is required.

Generalised hypopigmentation

Generalised hypopigmentation, blonde hair and grey-blue eyes are seen in several geno-dermatoses involving chromosomes 11 or 15. The clinical presentations vary from mild to complete loss of pigmentation and individuals may go undiagnosed unless compared to their siblings and parents. Early diagnosis and investigation is important to ensure early ophthalmological intervention and rigorous sun protection. Look for:

- Poor vision, photophobia and nystagmus. Type 1 oculocutaneous albinism usually results in more severe disease than type 2.
- Bleeding diathesis, due to a platelet defect in Hermansky–Pudlak syndrome.
- Recurrent infections in Chédiak–Higashi syndrome.
- Mental retardation and obesity. Both Angelmans' and Prader–Willi syndromes can present with albinism.

SKIN TEXTURE

Lax skin

Lax, hyperextensible skin is seen in the several Ehlers–Danlos syndromes. There may be bruising, scarring at sites of minor trauma, joint hyperextensibility and arthritis, and recurrent urinary infections.

Firm or thickened skin

Scleredema (do not confuse with scleroderma) is a rare condition in childhood, which presents over some weeks with gradual thickening of the skin of the head, neck and upper trunk. It may be related to preceding streptococcal infection. Diagnosis can be

confirmed by skin biopsy showing mucopolysaccharide intradermal staining. Resolution usually occurs over months.

Unusually firm skin is an early feature of systemic sclerosis. In children, there is usually widespread skin involvement. Raynaud phenomenon may be present and involvement of lungs, heart, kidneys and gastrointestinal tract usually occurs within a few years.

Waxy indurated skin may accompany neurological degeneration and hepatosplenomegaly in type A Niemann–Pick disease. Thickened skin may be seen in acromegaly and Addison's disease.

MOUTH DISORDERS

Most of the conditions covered in the section on vesicular disease can involve the oral mucosa. Oral vesicles break rapidly so that usually only erosions or small ulcers are seen. Oral involvement is often the first feature of hand, foot and mouth disease, manifesting as a few lesions involving the tongue and palate, followed a day or two later by vesicles on the extremities. Oral erosions may be seen occasionally in varicella and rarely in zoster.

Primary herpetic gingivostomatitis

Primary herpetic gingivostomatitis (see p. 283) presents in infants and young children with malaise, high fever, soft-tissue swelling, lymphadenopathy and vesicles and erosions on the buccal mucosa, gingivae, lips and adjacent face. Drinking and eating is painful. Management includes supportive care, bathing of crusts and analgesia. Aciclovir is not routinely indicated unless risk factors for complications exist (e.g. underlying disease, immunosuppression).

Herpangina

Several echoviruses and Coxsackie viruses can cause the sudden onset of malaise, high fever, sore throat and vomiting, sometimes with abdominal pain. Examination of the pharynx and posterior mouth reveals a large number of small, 2-mm vesicles or erosions coalescing on an erythematous background to form painful ulcerations. Diagnosis can be confirmed by throat or faecal swab. Complete resolution occurs with supportive care over 5 days.

Transient lingual papillitis

Transient lingual papillitis is probably the same condition as eruptive familial lingual papillitis. It was first described in 1996 and is not mentioned in major paediatric or dermatology texts but is much more common than generally realised. Most reported cases have been in the families of hospital staff. In one survey of 200 hospital staff, 50% of families appeared to have experienced this condition.[7] In most cases, an infant appears to be the index case and many other family members are then affected. Older children present with a burning sensation on the tip or sides of the tongue. Younger children present with irritability and poor feeding of unknown cause. The tongue is normal apart from small papules or 'scalloping' along the anterior and lateral tongue margins without ulceration. Affected individuals are otherwise well without any fever, lethargy, respiratory or gastrointestinal problems. Symptoms and signs last from 2–20 days. Recurrent episodes may occur for many weeks and again years later. Manage with symptomatic treatment and education.

Angular cheilitis

Angular cheilitis can occur during childhood and is common in older children. It presents as persistent erythema, scaling and fissuring at the corners of the mouth and surrounding skin, sparing the buccal mucosa. Discomfort and pain may be worsened by stretching, during yawning for example, and by salty or tart foods. Most cases are primarily attributable to atopic eczema but are multifactorial. Contributing factors include saliva, licking, drooling at night, significant dental malocclusions, irritant and allergic dermatitis (e.g. cosmetics, medicated lip balms, sunscreen lip creams, toothpaste, fluoride and sucked or chewed lollies). *Staphylococcus aureus*, *Candida albicans* or streptococcal species may all be cultured from affected skin.

Rarely, angular cheilitis may be the presenting feature of nutritional deficiencies including riboflavin, iron, zinc, pyridoxine, biotin and protein metabolic disorders. Malabsorption, malnutrition, oral corticosteroids and oral antibiotics may contribute.

- Management requires avoidance as much as possible of any factors that may be contributing.
- Minimise acidic foods such as tomatoes and citrus fruit.
- A trial of non-fluoride toothpaste and supervised rinsing after teeth cleaning helps in some children.
- Topical unmedicated ointment or paste up to several times a day will assist recovery. Topical 1% hydrocortisone ointment is useful. If microscopy reveals evidence of *Candida* or bacterial pathogens, topical miconazole or mupirocin, respectively, can be added.
- Allergy to a component of the treatment schedule should be suspected if the condition persists despite treatment, and patch testing may be warranted.
- In difficult cases, consider an uncommon underlying cause as above, and a trial of iron, vitamin and mineral supplementation.

Geographic tongue

Geographic tongue is typically seen under 4 years of age but can occur in older children. Most children are asymptomatic but some complain of tenderness or pain with salty foods. Irregular smooth patches are seen on the tongue in a pattern that changes from day to day. The cause is unknown. Geographic tongue is more common in psoriasis but most children (>90%) who have geographic tongue never develop psoriasis. No treatment is needed unless some foods cause discomfort, in which case avoidance of those foods for a while is usually sufficient. If needed, topical corticosteroid can alleviate symptoms.

Recurrent mouth ulcers

These are most often due to aphthous stomatitis. Aphthous ulceration usually presents as a few, painful, 4–8 mm ulcers on an erythematous base on the non-keratinised mucosa (the 'softer' areas) rather than the gums or hard palate. They resolve in a few days. Less commonly, ulcers can be larger and persist for weeks. Any atypical features should lead to a consideration of less-common causes of recurrent mouth ulcers including:

- Iron, folate or vitamin B_{12} deficiency.
- Recurrent erythema multiforme.
- Pemphigus, pemphigoid and other immune-mediated blistering conditions.
- Gastrointestinal disorders. Coeliac disease, Crohn's disease and ulcerative colitis are all associated with mouth ulceration. Recurrent abdominal pain, intermittent diarrhoea and failure to thrive may be present.
- Connective tissue disorders. Patients with Behçet's disease usually present in late childhood with ulcers at one site (mouth or genitals) and it may be many years before a second site is involved. Systemic lupus erythematosus and juvenile rheumatoid arthritis may cause recurrent mouth ulcers.
- Immunodeficiency states, HIV infection, cyclic neutropenia and periodic fevers.
- Malignancy and chemotherapy. Lymphoma and Langerhans cell histiocytosis can present with non-healing mouth ulcers.
- PFAPA syndrome of periodic fever, aphthous stomatitis, pharyngitis, cervical adenitis.

Troublesome episodes of aphthous ulceration can be managed by:

- investigating for an underlying cause as above;
- topical anaesthetic gels;
- topical steroid paste (e.g. triamcinolone acetonide);
- oral colchicine.

ANOGENITAL RASHES

Anogenital rashes are common in infancy. Most anogenital rashes seen in infants that wear nappies are primarily caused by reaction to urine or faeces (irritant napkin dermatitis). Soaps, detergents and secondary yeast infection may contribute. In atypical or persistent anogenital rashes in infancy, consider psoriasis, Langerhans cell histiocytosis, zinc deficiency and malabsorption syndromes. In older children, consider perianal streptococcal infection (if painful), psoriasis, lichen sclerosis, and atopic eczema. Kawasaki disease may be associated with a tender anogenital rash in an unwell child.

Treatment of rashes in the anogenital area requires caution. The moistness and occlusion of these areas increases the penetration and effectiveness of topical agents. For example, the absorption of topical hydrocortisone per square centimetre of anogenital skin can be several times greater than trunk skin. Adrenal suppression may occur after use of excessive topical hydrocortisone under the nappy area in small infants. Anogenital skin is also more likely to develop local steroid side effects, such as atrophy and striae. Any child using cortisone products in this area should have written instructions and appropriate medical follow up.

Irritant napkin dermatitis

Irritant napkin dermatitis is the most common cause of napkin dermatitis in infants and typically presents as confluent erythema that spares the groin folds. Variant presentations include multiple erosions in the natal cleft secondary to diarrhoea, scaly or glazed erythema, and satellite lesions at the periphery. Satellite pustules are suggestive of secondary *Candida* infection. *Candida* infection is much less common with breathable disposable nappies.

Gluteal granulomas are purple/brown papules or nodules, often oval shaped, which can develop around the skin folds in infants with troublesome napkin dermatitis. Most cases are associated with the inappropriate use of potent topical steroid in this area. These lesions slowly resolve over several months provided the underlying irritant napkin dermatitis is treated.

Irritant or traumatic anogenital rashes may be seen in circumstances of suboptimal care, emotional abuse or physical abuse.

Management
- Keep the area clean and dry. Leave the nappy off whenever possible.
- Clean the anogenital area by hand under warm water or with diluted bath oil on cotton wipes. Avoid commercial 'wipes', which can be irritating.
- Gel-based disposable nappies or a non-wettable under-napkin can be helpful. Cloth nappies should be thoroughly washed and rinsed.
- Use topical zinc cream or paste for mild eruptions. This functions as a barrier and should be applied thickly so that some is still present at the next nappy change. The cream or paste does not need to be completely removed at each change.
- Add hydrocortisone 1% cream if inflamed. Do not use stronger steroids.
- Consider mupirocin 2% cream if not settling. Antifungal therapy is usually not needed even if *Candida* is present.

Candida napkin dermatitis

This occurs secondary to irritant napkin dermatitis and antibiotic use, leading to erythema and white material in the folds and satellite pustules. Treat the underlying cause as above and add topical imidazole cream if necessary.

Anogenital seborrhoeic dermatitis

The term 'seborrhoeic dermatitis' has been used to describe an anogenital eruption in infants, with or without scalp or flexural involvement. Traditionally, it is differentiated from irritant napkin dermatitis by accentuation in the skin folds. However, this distinction is far from clear. The napkin area is not a seborrhoeic site. Many presentations with anogenital 'seborrhoeic dermatitis' represent either atopic eczema with irritant napkin dermatitis or psoriasis with anogenital involvement, or a combination of the two. Treat as for irritant napkin dermatitis, or anogenital psoriasis if suspected.

Anogenital psoriasis

Anogenital psoriasis can present at any age from infancy to adolescence. Sharply demarcated, non-scaly, brightly erythematous plaques can be seen and may involve any or all of the perianal and intragluteal region, inguinal folds and the genital area in both

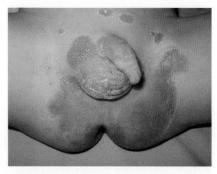

Fig. 12.1.14 Anogenital psoriasis in a 1-year-old boy.

boys and girls (Fig. 12.1.14). Symptoms are often surprisingly minimal. If pain and/or fissuring are present, swab for secondary streptococcal infection. This leads to a marked increase in discomfort and pain and is often the cause for presentation in an older child who may have had months or years of asymptomatic redness. Anogenital psoriasis may be an isolated finding or there may be similar lesions in other intertriginous areas, such as the axillae, or more typical signs of psoriasis elsewhere. Occasionally, in infants, anogenital psoriasis will lead to a few lesions on the lower trunk and then a rapid eruption of lesions elsewhere including scalp, face and trunk. This settles within weeks.

Manage by treating streptococcal infection, if present, and then treat as for irritant napkin dermatitis (this page). Medical follow up is essential to ensure clearing, as children and adolescents are often unaware of quite significant asymptomatic anogenital psoriasis or fail to report it because of embarrassment.

Perianal streptococcal dermatitis

A painful, red, perianal rash in a child between the ages of 1 and 10 is likely to be due to perianal streptococcal dermatitis. The usual presentation is a child who has had a sore anal region for weeks or months. Defecation is painful and constipation is present, but treatments aimed at relieving the constipation have not helped. Bright red blood may be present on the stool or toilet paper. On examination, a localised, well-demarcated erythema that covers a circular area of 1–2 cm radius around the anus can be seen. Fissures or macerated skin may be seen.

Perianal group A streptococcal dermatitis may be secondary to any cause of perianal itching. Concurrent pinworm infestation should be considered. Constipation usually follows painful defecation, rather than being the cause of it. It takes a long while for the child to recover confidence in defecation after successful treatment.

Management

- Take perianal and throat cultures to confirm the presence of group A *Streptococcus*.
- Apply paraffin ointment three-times daily to the perianal area for symptomatic relief. Topical mupirocin three-times daily has a role. Treat with phenoxymethylpenicillin (penicillin V) orally BD 250 mg (under 10 years), 500 mg (over 10 years) for a minimum of 2 weeks. Several weeks of therapy may be required. Intramuscular benzathine benzylpenicillin can be used if there are concerns about compliance.
- Consider treatment for pinworm with mebendazole or pyrantel.
- Keep stools soft with oral liquid paraffin.
- Perianal emollient ointment and stool softeners should be continued for a further 2 months after resolution of symptoms to prevent relapse, which is otherwise common.

Staphylococcal-mediated anogenital rashes

Bullous impetigo may present in the anogenital area as small vesicles or pustules that coalesce to give areas of peeling skin with peripheral margins of loose epidermis. These may be asymptomatic and the infant is otherwise well. Provided the baby is well, the disease is localised and the parents will follow instructions regarding follow up, an alternative is to treat with topical mupirocin 2% and general measures for napkin care. Oral cefalexin 30 mg kg^{-1} (max 500 mg) three times daily may be required for more widespread disease.

Herpes simplex virus

Primary herpes simplex virus infection and eczema herpeticum can both occur in the anogenital area. Initially, small vesicles on an erythematous base may be seen but these rapidly become small monomorphic erosions, crusting and coalescing, sometimes into an extensive, painful, erosive rash. Herpes simplex virus infection in the anogenital area of young children is usually innocent, contracted from a cold sore on a carer but the possibility of child sexual abuse should be considered. The possibility of child sexual abuse is higher in older children. For management see p. 283.

Varicella

Varicella lesions may initially be localised to the anogenital area in young children. Immunofluorescence and culture may be required to avoid an incorrect diagnosis of herpes simplex.

Threadworms

In older children, threadworms (*Enterobius vermicularis*) are a common cause of an itchy anogenital rash. Look for the worms at night and treat with oral mebendazole 50 mg (<10 kg), 100 mg (>10 kg) (not in pregnancy or less than 6 months) or oral pyrantel 10 mg kg^{-1} (maximum 500 mg) as a single dose. A repeat dose 2 weeks later helps reduce the high rate of reinfestation. Emphasise the importance of wearing clean underwear at night, preventing perianal scratching at night, hand washing immediately on awakening, avoidance of thumb sucking and good toileting hygiene.

Lichen sclerosis

Lichen sclerosis presents with chronic itch, discomfort or pain in the vulval area of girls aged 3 years or older. On examination, there may be an area of atrophy with white shiny skin, purpura or telangiectasia in the perivulval region. Cases have been misdiagnosed as sexual abuse. Management is with moisturisers and brief courses of moderately potent or potent steroid ointment. About 50% of cases resolve spontaneously. Relapses after successful treatment are common and children with this condition may have ongoing troublesome symptoms and vulval abnormalities into adulthood. Long-term follow up is required.

Vulval itch/vulvitis in prepubertal girls

Prepubertal girls with vulval itch usually have an identifiable dermatological condition. (Do not call this 'vulvovaginitis' as the vagina is not involved.) Girls between the age of 2 and 10 present with months or years of vulval itch, occasionally with stinging or pain on micturition. On examination, the labia majora may appear normal or may show erythema, scale, lichenification and excoriation. The introitus is normal. The great majority of these girls have atopic eczema. There may be signs of this elsewhere or signs may be limited to the vulval area. Management is as for atopic eczema at other sensitive sites and involves avoidance of chemicals, soaps, bubble baths and other irritants, and use of cotton underwear and ointment moisturiser. Use of corticosteroid or pimecrolimus creams is appropriate to settle the erythema and itch. Measures to 'oestrogenise the vagina' are either irrelevant or counterproductive and oestrogen creams should not be used.

Less common causes of vulval itch include psoriasis, lichen sclerosis, staphylococcal folliculitis or infection with group A streptococci. In all these cases, clinical signs suggestive of the associated condition are likely to be present.

ZINC AND OTHER NUTRITIONAL DEFICIENCIES

Zinc deficiency may be due to an inherited defect in zinc handling or may be an acquired deficiency as a result of prematurity, malabsorption syndromes or abnormally low maternal breast-milk zinc levels. Breast milk normally provides some protection from the inherited form, so presentation of inherited zinc deficiency is usually after breastfeeding has ceased. By contrast, acquired zinc deficiency can present earlier, in the neonatal period.

Zinc deficiency causes acrodermatitis enteropathica. A sharply defined, red, often extensive, anogenital rash is an early and prominent manifestation. Look for perioral, perinasal and acral (hand and foot) dermatitis, alopecia, diarrhoea, and failure to thrive.

Serum zinc levels do not correlate well with body zinc status. Oral zinc leads to a rapid improvement of the rash within days. Long-term follow up to monitor the child's zinc and copper status is essential.

Biotin deficiency and various other metabolic deficiency syndromes can give a similar picture, although usually in the setting of an unwell acidotic baby.

Malabsorption

Malabsorption from any cause (e.g. cystic fibrosis) can present with diarrhoea, erosive dermatitis and failure to thrive. There may be a progressive intractable napkin rash contributed to both by the diarrhoea and by secondary nutritional deficiencies. If malabsorption continues, the rash may become glazed and generalised in association with oedema and malaise. Identify and treat the cause of the malabsorption. Manage the anogenital area as for irritant napkin dermatitis. Topical pastes are thicker than ointments and may be required.

Langerhans cell histiocytosis

Langerhans cell histiocytosis may present in infancy as a chronic inguinal or anogenital rash, with brownish/red scale and petechiae, which is often erosive and unresponsive to treatment. A scaly, papular, eruption on the scalp or trunk may appear. Purpura, fever, diarrhoea or hepatosplenomegaly may be present, see p. 294.

Constipation

Constipation by itself does not cause perianal erythema and pain. Look for another cause, e.g. eczema, psoriasis or streptococcal infection.

ANOGENITAL PAPULES AND LUMPS

Anogenital warts Are soft fleshy warts that occur at the mucocutaneous junctions, especially around the anus. They may be isolated, flesh-coloured nodules or may coalesce into large cauliflower-like masses.

Management options include awaiting resolution, topical podophyllotoxin, imiquimod, curettage and diathermy and carbon dioxide laser.

The presence of genital warts in a young child is not an indication for mandatory reporting to government protective services. Genital warts in young children should prompt consideration of the possibility of sexual abuse, but transmission is usually by normal intimate parent-child contact, including at birth. Unless there are other risk factors for sexual abuse on history or examination, referral for sexual abuse investigation is inappropriate. If in doubt, seek paediatric advice. In children older than 5 years, the association between anogenital warts and sexual abuse increases and assessment by a paediatrician is warranted.

Molluscum In the anogenital area are often misdiagnosed as warts. Close examination of all lesions usually reveals a few to have the classical umbilicated pearly appearance. Molluscum in the anogenital region are common and are not a marker of child sexual abuse.

Congenital syphilis Erosions and moist warty lesions in the perianal area may be seen in infants with congenital syphilis. There may be erythema on the palms and soles, fever, failure to thrive and hepatosplenomegaly.

IMMUNODEFICIENCY STATES

Immunodeficiency from any cause may present in infancy as diarrhoea with a chronic erosive napkin dermatitis, widespread seborrhoeic dermatitis or neonatal erythroderma. Secondary infection with bacteria and/or viruses can complicate the clinical appearance. Look for other features of immunodeficiency including failure to thrive, erythroderma, lymphadenopathy, unusual infections and petechiae with eczema.

HAIR PROBLEMS

For an itchy scalp, consider tinea capitis, atopic eczema and head lice. For patches of hair loss, consider alopecia areata, traumatic alopecia, tinea capitis and kerion. For diffuse hair loss, consider telogen effluvium and nutritional causes. Longstanding sparse hair can be associated with ectodermal dysplasias and with many primary genetic abnormalities of hair and hair anchoring.

Head lice

Head lice infestation is common. Epidemics of head lice regularly sweep through primary schools in all areas. Nits (eggs) can be seen as small white specks firmly attached (unlike dandruff flecks) to hairs. Adult lice may occasionally be seen as small brown insects, about 4 mm long, walking across the scalp. Itching and excoriation are common. Presentation to an ED usually follows secondary eczematisation and infection causing extending weeping and crusted scalp lesions and neck lesions.

Suitable treatments include pyrethrin 0.165% (e.g. Pyrifoam), maldison 0.5% and permethrin 1% (e.g. Nix and Lyclear cream rinse). Wash the hair with soap and water. Thoroughly moisten the hair with the treatment and leave for 10 minutes. Rinse well and comb out with a fine-toothed lice comb. Reapply 1 week later to kill any eggs that have subsequently hatched. Reinfestation is common. A regular physical inspection, use of conditioner and combing of the hair are as important as chemical treatment. Resistance to chemical preparations is increasingly common and a combination of chemical and physical therapies is generally required. A shorter hair cut can make this more manageable.

Tinea capitis

In Australia, tinea capitis is usually caused by *Microsporum canis* contracted from cats or dogs or by *Trichophytum* species contracted from other infected children or animals. The incidence of tinea capitis is much higher in children with racially determined tightly curled black hair. Any child of African background with an itchy scalp should be assumed to have tinea until proven otherwise. Apart from itch, tinea capitis is characterised by patches of hair loss with some short, lustreless, broken hairs a few millimetres in length. Redness and scaling are present in the patch. Occasionally, inflammatory pustular swellings may be present (see kerion below). Hair loss without any epidermal changes is not likely to be fungal.

Confirm the diagnosis by greenish fluorescence of the hair shafts (not present with some fungi) with Wood's light and with microscopy and culture of hair and scale. Treatment usually comprises griseofulvin orally 20 mg kg^{-1} in divided doses (maximum 1 g, after meals with milk) daily for 8–12 weeks or until non-fluorescent. Terbinafine and itraconazole are also effective. Ketoconazole 2% shampoo twice-weekly can be used by all family members for 6 weeks to reduce cross-infection. Exclude from school until 2 days after treatment has commenced.[2]

Kerion (inflammatory ringworm)

This represents an inflammatory scarring immune response to tinea capitis. It is an erythematous, tender, boggy swelling, often several centimetres in diameter, which discharges pus from multiple points. The swellings appear fluctuant and are often misinterpreted in EDs as pyogenic abscesses. Skin incision and drainage should be avoided as it leads to delayed healing and increased scarring. Scrapings and/or some extracted hairs should be sent for microscopy and culture. Treatment is as for tinea capitis combined with a brief course of oral steroids to suppress the immune response. Antibiotics for secondary infection may occasionally be useful. Other inflammatory granulomas can mimic kerions. Exclude from school until 2 days after treatment has commenced.

Alopecia areata

Typically one or more oval patches of hair loss develop over a few days or weeks. These patches are usually completely bald but some hairs may remain within the patches. Rarely, the hair loss is diffuse. The scalp appears normal and does not show scaling, erythema or scarring. Most cases in childhood resolve spontaneously but progression

to total scalp or body-hair loss or recurrent alopecia can occur. Regrowth can occur decades later.

Management

- For isolated small patches present for weeks without further progression, no treatment is needed.
- In older children who are bothered cosmetically, intralesional corticosteroid injections are the treatment of choice.
- For recent or progressive hair loss, treatment with potent topical steroids may be trialled but is rarely useful as penetration into the deeper dermis to the hair follicle bulb is small. In difficult cases, other therapies, including contact sensitisation, irritant agents and pulsed corticosteroids, need to be considered.

Traumatic alopecia

This condition is usually caused by rubbing (as on the occiput of many babies), cosmetic practices (e.g. tight braiding) or hair pulling as a habit (trichotillomania). Trichotillomania may be largely nocturnal and parents are often unaware of it. The affected areas are usually angular and on the anterior or lateral scalp. The areas contain hairs of different lengths and are never completely bald, unlike alopecia areata. Presentation to EDs may be triggered by the hair loss or by the sequelae of eating the hair, including acute intestinal obstruction (trichobezoar) in severe cases.

Management

- Recognition of the problem and a careful explanation to the family is often sufficient. Alert the family to the risk of trichobezoar.
- Trichotillomania in younger children does not usually indicate that significant psychological problems are present. It is a habit similar to thumb-sucking or nail-biting and a low-key approach similar to that used in those conditions is appropriate. In older children, it may be part of an obsessive trait or other psychological problems that require professional and pharmacological support.

Diffuse hair loss

Diffuse hair loss in children is usually from telogen effluvium. This is characterised by an increased number of hairs going synchronously into the resting (telogen) phase and subsequently being shed several weeks later. Shed hairs have a small club-like appearance at the proximal end. Telogen effluvium presents as diffuse, often quite dramatic hair loss 4–16 weeks after the causative event. In children, this is commonly a high fever for a few days. Other causes include car accidents, operations and acutely stressful events. Complete regrowth always occurs.

Dramatic widespread diffuse hair loss may be from alopecia areata.

Diffuse hair loss occurs after cancer chemotherapy. More chronic, diffuse hair loss without an obvious cause may require investigation to exclude treatable causes, such as zinc or iron deficiency, malnutrition, excess vitamin A, oral retinoids for acne, hypothyroidism or antithyroid medications, hypopituitarism, hypoparathyroidism, diabetes, and thallium poisoning.

Long-standing sparse or irregular hair is a feature of many genetic diseases. In some, such as monolethrix, the child is otherwise normal. In others, such as ectodermal dysplasias, many associated features may be present. These include decreased or absent sweating, pointy or missing teeth, dysplastic nails and dry skin. Clinical findings may be subtle. In any young child with unusual nails, skin or teeth who presents with fever and collapse, ectodermal dysplasia with inability to sweat and dysfunctional temperature control should be considered. Treatment includes cooling to restore normal body temperature, ongoing parental education and support to avoid similar overheating crises.

Hypertrichosis

Generalised hypertrichosis (increased hair in all areas) may be an isolated finding or may be related to inherited syndromes (including Hurler's and De Lange's syndromes), medications (especially minoxidil, phenytoin and ciclosporin), gastrointestinal disease (including coeliac disease), anorexia nervosa, hypothyroidism, and porphyria (look for photosensitivity and blisters).

Local patches of hypertrichosis can be seen as an isolated finding, or in association with lichenified eczema (temporary), pigmented lesions (congenital pigmented naevi, acquired naevi, Becker's naevi), plexiform neurofibromas, other naevoid lesions, chronic rubbing or over the sacral area in association with underlying spinal anomalies ('Faun's tail'). A small degree of increased hair growth over the sacral area is common in many racial groups and this is not a marker of spinal anomalies.

Hirsutism

Hirsutism refers to an increase in male pattern terminal hair. Increased pubic or axillary hair in young children may be due to adrenal, gonadal or CNS disease and requires investigation. Hirsutism in adolescent females may be an isolated finding or may be seen with obesity and amenorrhea in polycystic ovary syndrome. Cushing syndrome, mild congenital adrenal hyperplasia, virilising adrenal and ovarian tumours, exogenous androgens and thyroid dysfunction may cause hirsutism.

NAIL PROBLEMS

Infants' nails are often thin and exhibit a degree of koilonychia (spoon shape) that requires no investigation. Congenitally abnormal nails are usually atrophic and can be the presenting feature of rare inherited conditions, such as ectodermal dysplasias (these children may present with fever and heat prostration), dyskeratosis congenita, pachyonychia congenita (thickened nails), congenital malalignment of the great toenails and the nail-patella syndrome. Nails may have appeared normal at birth and become dystrophic over the first year of life.

Acquired nail disease is usually a result of paronychia, fungal infection, psoriasis, ingrown toenails or 20-nail dystrophy. It may also be seen in association with diseases, such as alopecia areata and lichen planus. Nail-biting and picking can lead to marked deformity of involved nails.

Paronychia

Acute paronychia (inflammation of the nail fold) Is usually caused by *Staphylococcus aureus* or group A *Streptococcus*. It can be seen during therapy with oral isotretinoin for acne. One or more nail folds become red painful and swollen. Pus may be present at the nail margin. Any cause of prolonged wetness or minor trauma (e.g. finger sucking, nail picking, finger eczema, preceding chronic paronychia) predisposes to acute infection by breaching the cuticle between nail and skin. Treatment requires identification and avoidance of the trigger factors, warm compresses, drainage if needed, oral cephalexin 30 mg kg^{-1} (max 500 mg) three times daily, topical paraffin ointment and ongoing nail care. If due to oral isotretinoin, dose reduction and treatment as above usually resolves the problem.

Chronic paronychia Is traditionally associated with *Candida albicans*, which can be found in specimens from most cases. However, *Candida* is now seen by many authorities as a secondary feature that may not be particularly relevant to the onset and maintenance of the condition. The primary event is disruption of the nail cuticle resulting in inflammation of the proximal nail fold. Chronic paronychia may be a primarily eczematous condition caused by many factors including finger sucking, nail picking, finger eczema and any increased exposure to moisture. Affected nail folds are often dusky red or purple with loss of the cuticle and without significant pain. The nail often has several horizontal ridges corresponding to episodes of inflammation of the proximal nail fold. The nails may become increasingly dystrophic with time but do not tend to thicken. Chronic paronychia may be present for months or years with occasionally acute exacerbations that respond to oral antibiotics without clearing the underlying problem.

Management
- Management requires topical potent corticosteroid application daily for several weeks.
- Avoid all factors that predispose to continuing irritation or allergen exposure. Nails should be kept dry. Repeated applications of Vaseline or even a hydrocolloid dressing over the cuticle can assist in this. Cotton gloves under rubber gloves should be used for wet work.
- In difficult or unresponsive cases, consider an unusual infection or rare underlying cause such as mucocutaneous candidiasis (especially if oral *Candida* infection is present), hypoparathyroidism and malignancy.

Nail psoriasis

Psoriasis can present as isolated nail disease and can mimic acute or chronic paronychia and onychomycosis. Features of nail psoriasis include pitting, thickening and brownish subungual discolouration. There may be repeated episodes of pain associated with the collection of pus under the nail. Drainage leads to relief but antibiotics don't help. Cultures are sterile. Detailed history and examination of the rest of the child may reveal other features of psoriasis. Initially treat with potent topical steroid ointments.

Ingrown toenail

The nail of the large toes can grow into the lateral nail fold and cause pain, redness, swelling and occasionally pus secondary to *Staphylococcus aureus*. The chronic inflammatory process leads to progressive granulation tissue formation. Management involves avoidance of shoes where possible, avoidance of tight-fitting shoes, careful cutting of the nails and use of pledgets between the nail and lateral nail fold. Oral antibiotics are not usually required. Surgical removal of granulation material is helpful. Trimming of the lateral nail alone usually results in recurrence of the problem. In troublesome cases, surgical ablation of the lateral nail plate may be warranted.

Tinea unguium (onychomycosis)

Dermatophyte infection may affect one or more nails. White or yellow patches develop at the distal and lateral nail edges. The rest of the nail may become discoloured, friable and deformed with accumulation of subungual debris. Multiple nails may become involved over years. Tinea may also present on the adjacent skin, particularly in the interdigital folds. It can be difficult to clinically distinguish between psoriasis and fungal infection in nails. Always confirm the diagnosis by microscopy and culture of nail clippings before commencing treatment. If cultures are negative, repeat the cultures but do not start oral treatment. In very mild cases only, treatment with physical debridement and antifungal nail lacquer (e.g. amiolfarone) may be effective. Most cases require oral therapy with terbinafine or griseofulvin for months. School exclusion, although specified in some states, is not medically warranted or appropriate.

ITCH WITHOUT RASH

Some children present with an itch without an obvious rash. Other children may have multiple excoriations without obvious cause, or they may have much more severe pruritus than would be expected for the eruption present. All such children need to be evaluated for:

- atopy;
- scabies;
- symptomatic dermographism;
- dermatitis herpetiformis;
- iron deficiency;
- food allergy;
- drug use. Most pharmaceutical, recreational and herbal drugs can cause itch;

- systemic disease, including hepatitis C infection, diabetes, uraemia, conjugated hyperbilirubinaemia, paraproteinaemia, polycythaemia and thyroid disease.

Collection of specimens

Bacterial swabs (Gram stain and culture)

- Swab lesion with a plain dry swab and roll over a glass slide. Discard swab and air dry slide.
- Swab lesion with second swab. Wet swab with sterile saline if lesion is dry. Place swab in charcoal medium (maintains organism viability).

Swabs for HSV or VZV

- Roll dry swab over base of suspicious lesion (to collect cells for immunofluorescence). Roll over appropriate slide (3 wells). Swab can then be cut off and placed in viral transport medium for culture.
- Fluid from vesicles is not suitable for immunofluorescence, but may be collected into viral transport medium for culture.

Swabs for PCR (for pertussis, VZV, HSV, *Mycobacterium ulcerans*, etc.)

- Dry (flocked) swab

Swabs for *Chlamydia trachomatis*

- Dry swab for PCR.
- For culture, swab lesion with two dacron or rayon-tipped swabs. Smear one onto 'microtrak' well and break tip of other into *Chlamydia* transport medium.

Skin scrapings for fungal/dermatophyte culture

- Use scalpel blade to scrape the surface of the lesion. Collect flakes of skin in specimen jar.

References

1. McDonald M, Currie BJ, Carapetis JR. Acute rheumatic fever: a chink in the chain that links the heart to the throat? *Lancet Infect Dis* 2004;**4**:240–5.
2. Borchard KL, Orchard D. Systemic therapy of paediatric atopic dermatitis: an update. *Australas J Dermatol* 2008;**49**:123–34.
3. Ramsay HM, Goddard W, Gill S, Moss C. Herbal creams used for atopic eczema in Birmingham, UK, illegally contain potent corticosteroids. *Arch Dis Child* 2003;**88** (12):1056–7.
4. Gilbert G, Starr M. Parvovirus. In: Palasanthiran P, Starr M, Jones C, editors. *Management of perinatal infections.* Australas Soc Infect Dis Sydney; 2002. p. 30–2.
5. Sterling JB, Heymann WR. Potassium iodide in dermatology: A 19th century drug for the 21st century uses, pharmacology, adverse effects, and contraindications. *J Am Acad Dermatol* 2000;**43** (4):691–7.
6. Royal Children's Hospital Melbourne. *Clinical Practice Guidelines.* Available from http://www.rch.org.au/clinicalguide [accessed 20.10.10].
7. Whitaker SB, Krupa JJ, Singh BB. Transient lingual papillitis. *Oral Surg Oral Med Oral Pathol Oral Radiol Endod* 1996;**82**:441–5.

EYES

Section editor *Jeremy Raftos*

13.1 Ophthalmological emergencies

Toby Fogg

ESSENTIALS

1 A history of contact lens use should always be sought.

2 Visual acuity should always be assessed.

3 Neonatal conjunctivitis may have severe sequelae if inadequately treated.

4 The suspicion of keratitis should prompt urgent ophthalmic review.

5 The distinction between orbital and preseptal cellulitis should always be made.

6 Local anaesthetic drops should never be given to a patient to take home.

Introduction

Few ophthalmological emergencies relate exclusively to children. Although the pathology may be the same, the general approach, examination and compliance with treatment is very different depending on the age and development of the child. Also, the long-term sequelae of serious eye injury or disease are much greater.

History

As with other paediatric encounters, it is important to gain the child's confidence in you whilst obtaining the history from the parents or carers. A detailed history should be obtained from an adult witness. If this is unavailable, injury will be the likely cause of a painful red eye. Other conditions presenting with a red eye are listed in Table 13.1.1. Always enquire about the use of contact lenses or glasses.

Examination

The approach to the examination of a paediatric eye may differ from that of an adult in that an opportunistic strategy should be taken. Leave touching the child until last, particularly if it will result in fear, pain or discomfort.

Some form of assessment of acuity must be made. In pre-verbal children, assess their ability to fix and follow interesting objects and then reach for them. In older children, monocular testing should be carried out using picture cards, single letter matching or a standard Snellen chart. Use of the slit lamp is not essential for a detailed examination, but even small children may co-operate if they remain seated on their parent's knees.

If the child is compliant, a logical sequence of examination would be from outside to inside thus:

- visual acuity – using Snellen chart with letters or pictures;
- extraocular movements – follow a finger, a small toy or a face;
- visual fields;
- lids, lashes and lacrimal apparatus;
- conjunctiva and sclera;
- cornea;
- anterior chamber;
- pupil and iris;
- lens;
- red reflex, posterior chamber and retina.

All drops will sting, except for fluorescein. However, once the pain has subsided, the effects of local anaesthetic may allow for a much more meaningful examination than would otherwise have been possible. If, however, this remains impossible, consideration should be given to examination under anaesthetic.

Eyelid disorders

Blepharitis

Blepharitis is an inflammatory process of the eyelids that is characterised by crusting at the base of the eyelashes. There may be oedema of the lids themselves and occasionally the conjunctiva is also injected. Staphylococci are the usual organisms. Treatment should involve the removal of the crusts using a warm flannel, cleansing with dilute baby shampoo and application of antibiotic ointment to the lid margin.

Hordeolum (stye)

A hordeolum is an acute infection, usually staphylococcal, of an eyelash follicle. It causes

Table 13.1.1 Differential diagnosis of the red eye

Normal visual acuity	
Conjunctivitis (bacterial, viral, allergic, chemical)	Gritty, itchy, injected conjunctiva, discharge
Foreign body	Pain, grittiness, epiphoria, photophobia
Episcleritis	Mild pain, localised conjunctival injection
Scleritis	Severe pain, diffuse conjunctival injection
Subconjunctival haemorrhage	Consider trauma or pertussis
Reduced visual acuity	
Corneal abrasion	Pain, grittiness, epiphoria, photophobia. Corneal defect seen with fluorescein staining
Keratitis	Photophobia, epiphoria, ciliary injection, flare in anterior chamber, corneal infiltrate
Corneal ulcer	Photophobia, epiphoria, corneal injection, flare in anterior chamber, defect on fluorescein staining. History of contact lens use?
Anterior uveitis	Photophobia, epiphoria, ciliary injection flare in anterior chamber, miosis, posterior synechia

a small, tender swelling, often with a head of pus, which is seen at the lid margin. Treatment is with warm compresses and chloramphenicol ointment until resolution occurs.

Chalazion (meibomian cyst)

This is caused by inflammation of the lipid-secreting meibomian glands of the lid, probably due to ductal obstruction. It presents as a slowly progressing, mildly painful red lump in the eyelid. Most settle with conservative treatment, namely warm compresses for 10 minutes four times a day with light massage and chloramphenicol ointment for up to 4 weeks. If this treatment fails, or the cyst is excessively large causing visual disturbance, it can be incised. It may become complicated by preseptal cellulitis that may require systemic antibiotics.

Disorders of the lacrimal apparatus

Nasolacrimal duct obstruction

This condition occurs in 6% of infants and almost invariably resolves within the first year. It may cause epiphoria (watering), a mucoid discharge or some erythema of the lids. There may be a minor mucopurulent discharge and rarely a bluish palpable mass will be seen overlying the drainage system, which represents a dacryocele. Treatment of simple obstruction consists of gentle massage four times a day and cleansing. Should

spontaneous resolution not occur, the child should be referred for probing of the duct after 6 to 12 months of age. If there is a mucopurulent discharge, topical antibiotics should be added for 2 weeks.

Dacryocystitis

This is defined as infection of the nasal lacrimal duct and presents with pain, redness, swelling and tenderness of the overlying skin and the adjacent nasoperiorbital area. There may also be tearing, discharge and fever. Pressure over the lacrimal sac may express pus from the punctum. This should be sent for culture. *Staphylococcus aureus* and *Staphylococcus epidermidis* are the commonest organisms. Treatment should be with cefalexin orally or cefazolin intravenously (IV) if unwell. Gentle massage in the more minor cases may well aid in clearing the infection and unblocking the duct, as dacryocystitis is invariably associated with ductal obstruction that may be congenital or acquired. Probing or irrigation of the lacrimal system should be avoided in the acute setting and in infants less than 6 months old. Complications include preseptal cellulitis; orbital cellulitis and cavernous sinus thrombosis occur very rarely.

Dacryoadenitis

Infection of the lacrimal gland, found in the superotemporal orbit, is called dacryoadenitis. Acute disease is characterised by abrupt onset of pain, swelling and erythema in the superotemporal region. There may also

be chemosis, conjunctivitis and a mucopurulent discharge. Rarely there is proptosis, fever, malaise and a reduction in ocular motility, making clinical differentiation from orbital cellulitis difficult, and thus requiring a computerised tomography (CT) scan or magnetic resonance imaging (MRI).

The disease is usually viral in origin but a mucopurulent discharge makes a bacterial infection more likely so swabs should be taken before starting cephalexin.

Conjunctival and scleral disease

Neonatal conjunctivitis (ophthalmia neonatorum)

This condition is defined as conjunctivitis occurring within the first 30 days of life. The causative organisms are usually passed from mother to fetus during passage through the birth canal and are commonly *Neisseria gonorrhoeae*, *Chlamydia trachomatis*, staphylococci, streptococci or herpes simplex.

Gonococcal infection presents within 24 to 48 hours of birth with acute eyelid oedema, bulbar conjunctivitis, chemosis and a profound purulent discharge. Both eyes are usually affected. As the presentation may overlap with other infectious agents, a swab should be taken before treatment is commenced. An urgent Gram stain may show Gram-negative intracellular diplococci. Urgent ophthalmology consultation should be sought and treatment should not be delayed due to the risk of rapidly progressive corneal ulceration and perforation. Ceftriaxone 50 mg kg^{-1} IV for 7 days is used, with the addition of erythromycin orally to cover for infection with *C. trachomatis* until cultures are negative.

Chlamydial infection is classically associated with a watery then mucopurulent discharge 5 to 14 days after delivery. There is also palpebral conjunctival injection, but less lid oedema is seen than with gonoccocal infection. Swabs are sent for culture and polymerase chain reaction and then treatment is commenced with oral erythromycin 10 mg kg^{-1} qid for 21 days. This disease is complicated by pneumonitis in 10–20% of cases.

For both of these conditions, the mother will also need treatment and her partner will need screening.

The same organisms that affect older children can also cause neonatal conjunctivitis. These organisms typically present from day 5 to 7. Clinical findings do not distinguish the pathogen so cultures should be taken and treatment commenced with broad-spectrum antibiotic ointment. Herpes simplex virus (HSV) conjunctivitis is the exception and should be suspected if there is a maternal history of infection, vesicular blepharitis or dendritic ulceration. In this instance, treatment should be with topical and systemic aciclovir after urgent ophthalmological consultation.

Conjunctivitis in older children

Conjunctivitis represents the commonest paediatric ophthalmic emergency presentation. Unlike the adult population, bacterial infections predominate.

Bacterial conjunctivitis

This is characterised by epiphoria and a foreign body sensation that progresses to diffuse conjunctival injection and a purulent discharge that may glue the lids together. The onset is usually abrupt and spreads to the other eye within 48 hours. Staphylococci, *Streptococcus pneumoniae* and *Haemophilus influenzae* are the commonest organisms. After swabbing, therapy is with chloramphenicol 0.5% 1 to 2 drops every 2 hours initially, tapering to 6-hourly as symptoms improve.

In sexually active teenagers and isolated communities in central and northern Australia, *N. gonorrhoeae* or *N. meningitidis* may be the causative organism and will require systemic treatment with ceftriaxone 1 g intramuscularly for 3 to 5 days.

Viral conjunctivitis

This is usually adenoviral in origin and findings include itching or grittiness, tearing, oedematous lids and a characteristic palpable pre-auricular lymph node. It usually spreads to the other eye after a few days. There may be corneal involvement as well, when it is known as epidemic keratoconjunctivitis. Adenovirus can also cause pharyngoconjunctival fever that, intuitively, comprises pharyngitis, conjunctivitis and fever. It is a self-limiting disease but may very rarely disseminate and cause multiorgan failure.

Other viral infections known to cause conjunctivitis include rhinovirus, enterovirus, influenza and respiratory syncytial viruses.

The diagnosis of adenoviral conjunctivitis is clinical but swabs should be taken in most cases to exclude a bacterial cause. It is a highly contagious disease so household or other social contact spread is likely. Treatment should be with cold compresses several times a day, artificial tears and good hygiene. If there is difficulty ruling out bacterial conjunctivitis clinically, antibiotic ointment should be used. Parents should be advised that the child will be contagious for 12 days from onset.

Allergic conjunctivitis, e.g. hay fever

Presentation is similar to viral conjunctivitis although a preauricular lymph node is not present and there is usually a good history of atopy. Treatment should consist of artificial tears, oral antihistamines and removal of the trigger.

Atopic conjunctivitis

This is commonest in male adolescents with a history of atopy. It occurs in spring and summer and causes itching and a thick, ropy discharge. Large subtarsal papillae may also be seen. Treatment should be as for allergic conjunctivitis, with the addition of sodium cromoglycate drops.

Herpes simplex conjunctivitis

Patients complain of a foreign body sensation, pain or burning and may give a history of past ocular or perioral herpetic lesions. Examination will reveal a unilateral conjunctivitis with vesicles on the eyelid or periorbital skin and a palpable preauricular lymph node. Treatment is with topical antiviral medication and close ophthalmic follow up.

Trachoma

Trachoma results from recurrent infections of *Chlamydia trachomatis*. In Australia, it affects remote indigenous communities, whilst internationally it is a leading cause of blindness in the third world.

Infection manifests as a mild mucopurulent conjunctivitis that is self-limiting. However, recurrent episodes result in a chronic inflammatory state affecting the palpebral conjunctiva and cornea. Eyelid deformities due to scarring include entropion and ectropion whilst corneal complications include scarring (known as cicatrization), vascularisation, ulceration and perforation.

Treatment for children under 6 is by erythromycin 10 mg kg^{-1} orally qid for 21 days. For older children and adults use azithromycin 1 g (20 mg kg^{-1} up to 1 g for children) as a single dose. In prevalent areas, consideration should be given to treating all household contacts.

Episcleritis

This condition presents with acute redness to a section of the sclera. There is usually minimal discomfort or tenderness and it is only the more superficial episcleral vessels that are engorged. Although it is associated with connective tissue disorders, HSV, varicella zoster virus (VZV) and inflammatory bowel disease, most presentations are idiopathic in nature.

Treatment is symptomatic with artificial tears and oral non-steroidal anti-inflammatoriy drugs (NSAIDs) but if severe, topical steroids can be used. Ophthalmic follow up should be arranged to ensure resolution.

Scleritis

In contrast to episcleritis, scleritis usually presents with pain that gradually becomes severe and a diffuse redness due to injection of the scleral, episcleral and conjunctival vessels. When viewed in daylight, the affected sclera may have a bluish hue and vision may be reduced. There is a strong association with connective tissue disorders. Treatment consists of oral NSAIDs and steroids and should be initiated by an ophthalmologist.

Corneal disease

Keratitis

Keratitis is defined as inflammation of one or more layers of the cornea. It appears as a focal white corneal opacity without an overlying defect. If ulceration is also present it will stain with the use of fluorescein. Symptoms include pain, redness, photophobia and poor vision. The lids may be erythematous or oedematous whilst chemosis, tearing, conjunctival injection, hypopyon or flare in the anterior chamber may all be seen on examination.

Causes of keratitis

Bacterial infection is the commonest cause of keratitis and this is considered to be one of the leading causes of blindness in the developing world. Organisms include Gram positives, such as staphylococci, streptococci and bacilli, as well as Gram negatives. Of these, *Pseudomonas aeruginosa* is of significance as it is the commonest cause of keratitis in the contact lens wearer. Other organisms include:

- Fungi, particularly after trauma from vegetable matter. The course is usually more gradual in comparison to bacterial keratitis.
- Acanthamoebic keratitis is a parasitic infection seen in contact lens wearers, especially if they have poor lens hygiene. It is also a complication of a corneal injury contaminated by soil. Patients often present with pain out of proportion to early clinical findings which progress over several weeks.
- HSV may cause a punctate keratitis before the classical dendritic ulcer manifests. It may affect both eyes and corneal scarring may be permanent.
- VZV is associated with a dermatomal skin rash.

Management

All patients with suspected infectious keratitis should be urgently referred to an ophthalmologist for culture by corneal scraping before starting antibiotic treatment.

Recurrent corneal erosion

This manifests with recurrent attacks of pain, photophobia, grittiness and tearing, which occur on waking or rubbing the affected eye. There is often a prior history of corneal abrasion. Examination may often reveal a corneal defect but minor epithelial changes may have resolved by the time the patient is reviewed. Treatment consists of antibiotic ointment and then artificial tears once the corneal defect is healed. Ophthalmic follow up is recommended.

Uveitis

Inflammation of the uveal tract is subdivided according to location of disease (anterior, intermediate or posterior) or structure involved (iris, choroid, retina).

The most frequently encountered of these conditions is that of traumatic iritis. This presents with photophobia, epiphoria, blepharospasm, perilimbal injection and blurring of vision 1 to 3 days after a blunt globe injury. The pupil may be miotic or irregular and cellular flare may be seen in the anterior chamber upon slit lamp examination with an oblique beam. Relief of pain with topical local anaesthetic is a relatively sensitive way of excluding the disease. Other causes include juvenile rheumatoid arthritis,

inflammatory bowel disease, and psoriasis. Referral to an ophthalmologist should be made to rule out any involvement of posterior structures. Treatment is with a cycloplegic agent and steroid drops.

Intermediate and posterior uveitis may present with flashes, floaters and decreased vision.

Glaucoma

Glaucoma is very rare in children. An enlarged, clouded cornea is seen associated with tearing (epiphora) and photophobia. It may be associated with a hyphaema, lens subluxation, retinoblastoma or systemic disease (neurofibromatosis or Sturge–Weber syndrome) or high dose steroid use. Ophthalmological referral should be made immediately as prompt diagnosis is essential to prevent visual loss.

Orbital and preseptal (periorbital) cellulitis

The fibrous orbital septum is a continuation of the periosteum of the orbital rim. It connects to the tarsal plates and separates the eyelids and other preseptal structures from the orbital space, acting as a barrier to the spread of infection. It is important to distinguish clinically or radiologically between the two conditions, as missing the diagnosis of orbital cellulitis may have grave sequelae.

Preseptal cellulitis

Of these two conditions, preseptal cellulitis is far more common, accounting for 95% of infections around the eye. It presents with lid oedema and erythema, mild pain and a low-grade fever. The child is unlikely to appear ill. There is usually a portal of entry for the organism such as a nearby wound or insect bite, lid lesion or a pre-existing dacryocystitis. Rarely, haematogenous spread can occur. *Staph. aureus*, *Strep. pneumoniae* or *H. influenzae* in the unvaccinated are the commonest organisms in the under 5s. Cultures should be taken as appropriate and if the child is well and the symptoms minor, treatment can be as an outpatient with augmentin or cefalexin for 7 days as long as appropriate follow up will occur to ensure that symptoms are improving. This is, however, contentious and some advocate

admission for IV antibiotics, as for orbital cellulitis, for all cases of presumed preseptal cellulitis, particularly in the under 5s.

Orbital cellulitis

The orbit is surrounded on three sides by paranasal sinuses. The migration of organisms from an infected sinus into the orbital cavity causes orbital cellulitis in the majority of cases. Haematogenous or dental spread can also occur and there may be an associated subperiosteal abscess. Infection is usually poly-microbial and causative organisms are as for preseptal disease, with the addition of Gram negatives and anaerobes. Orbital infection presents with swollen, erythematous lids but, unlike preseptal cellulitis, the swelling should be limited to the orbital rim due to the septum preventing anterior spread. The fever is likely to be higher than that seen with preseptal cellulitis and the child usually appears toxic. There may be chemosis and proptosis and eye movements are likely to be restricted and painful. A raised white count is expected but will not aid differentiation from preseptal infection. Blood culture should be taken and then a CT scan or MRI will confirm the diagnosis and guide drainage of the offending sinus or subperiosteal abscess. Therapy should be with IV flucloxacillin and ceftriaxone and urgent referral should be made to ophthalmology as well as ear, nose and throat for consideration for a sinus drainage procedure. Complications include optic nerve compression, reduced visual acuity, cavernous sinus thrombosis, osteomyelitis, meningitis and cerebral abscess.

Acknowledgement

The contribution of Adrienne Adams as author in the first edition is hereby acknowledged.

Further reading

Bravermann RS. Eye. In: Hay WW, Levin MJ, Sondheimer JM, Deterding RR, editors. *Current pediatric diagnosis & treatment.* 19th ed. New York: McGraw Hill; 2008.

Christiansen K, Currie B, Ferguson J, et al., editors. *Antibiotic Guidelines 2006.* Version 13. Therapeutic Guidelines Limited.

Ehlers JP, Shah CP. *The Wills Eye Manual.* 5th ed. Baltimore: Lippincott Williams & Wilkins; 2008.

Greenberg MF, Pollard ZF. The red eye in childhood. *Paediatr Clin N Am* 2003;**50**:105–24.

Prentiss KA, Dorfman DH. Pediatric ophthalmology in the Emergency Department. *Emerg Med Clin N Am* 2008;**26**:181–98.

Rubenstein JB, Virasch V. Conjunctival disease. In: *Yanoff & Duker: Ophthalmology.* 3rd ed. New York: Mosby; 2008.

13.2 Congenital, developmental and neoplastic conditions

Greg Stevens

ESSENTIALS

1 These conditions are most likely to present with a concern from a parent or caregiver who has noted that there has been a change in the appearance of their child's eyes, or that they are not responding to visual cues in an expected way.

A detailed examination will help to further define the abnormalities or deficits noted. These conditions require specialised investigations and management, and as such consultation with a paediatric ophthalmologist is advised.

Deficits in visual acuity

This may reflect a deficit anywhere from the visual cortex to the cornea and a careful examination including pinhole testing in children old enough to co-operate will help localise this and guide appropriate referral.

Strabismus

Abnormalities of the binocular alignment of the eyes, strabismus, may present with a concern from a parent that their child has a squint, and this may be confirmed by careful examination of the corneal reflex and use of the cover-uncover test.

Strabismus may be convergent (esotropia), divergent (exotropia), upwards (hypertropia) or downwards (hypotropia).

Strabismus may be a dynamic process, occurring in relation to alterations in the accommodative reflex with refractive errors.

The importance of strabismus lies in the development of amblyopia, which is the decrease in visual acuity occurring in visually immature children due to the lack of a clear image provided to the retina. It is usually unilateral. Strabismus may also be an early sign of significant visual pathology, e.g. retinoblastoma, retinitis of prematurity and Coats' disease.

Paediatric cataracts

These can be detected as an abnormality of the red reflex. There is an association with several chromosomal, metabolic and intrauterine infective causes.

Congenital nasolacrimal duct obstruction

This is a common disorder, occurring in up to 6% of children. It presents with excessive overflow of tears. It has a good outcome, with 96% resolving by the age of 1 year.

Infantile glaucoma

Glaucoma in children is rare, but if undetected may cause blindness.

Because of the elasticity of the paediatric eye, significant enlargement of the cornea may occur, with subsequent clouding of the cornea. Excessive lacrimation and photophobia may be present. It is a cause of irritability in the infant.

The treatment is usually surgical.

Ocular tumours

Tumours may present with an evident deformity, with proptosis, or with an alteration in the visual axis. Any of the tissues in the orbit and eyelids may give rise to tumours. Children treated in infancy with radiotherapy for an intraorbital tumour are at increased risk of developing malignancies in the radiated area in later life.

Retinoblastoma

This is the most common primary intraocular tumour in childhood.

Hereditary and non-hereditary forms exist. The heredity forms are usually bilateral and multifocal. There is a defect of a tumour suppressor gene located on chromosome 13.

When the tumour is confined to the eye there is a good survival rate (>90%).

Rhabdomyosarcoma

This is the most common primary intraorbital tumour in childhood and usually occurs in the first decade.

Presentation may be rapid with associated eyelid oedema, and can lead to confusion with an infective process.

Neuroblastoma

The orbit is a common site of metastasis of neuroblastomas. The primary is usually abdominal and usually known at the time of orbital metastasis. Most occur in the first 5 years of age.

13.3 Ocular trauma

Jennie Martin

ESSENTIALS

1 Anxiety is pronounced in the carer, be calm in your approach.

2 Consider hidden injury.

3 Never apply pressure to an eye that may be ruptured or penetrated.

4 Commence immediate treatment with chemical injury.

Introduction

Injury is the leading cause of visual disability and blindness in children and has the following features

- severe eye injury is not uncommon;
- all age groups may be affected, peak 11–15 years;
- male predominance after infancy;
- usually unintentional, age-related patterns;
- causes include sports activities (balls or clashes); projectiles; plant thorns; pet bites/scratches; elastic/bungee cords; fireworks;
- education is important as up to 90% of injuries are preventable;
- visual impairment results in an emotional, social and economic cost;
- there are unique challenges to obtaining a history and examination in the child.

Trauma to the eye engenders a marked anxiety reaction in the carer who is always concerned about long term visual impairment. Use a careful and calm approach to enable co-operation so a thorough examination may be performed. Ensure the parent/carer is with the child at all times.

Always consider what may lie beneath an injury that appears to be superficial. Even in an unco-operative child, extensive information can be obtained by observation alone. Uncommonly, mild sedation may be required; however, when there are genuine concerns, referral for general anaesthesia to enable adequate examination is preferred. If gentle restraint has not facilitated examination or a particular procedure, repeated and forcible restraint should not be performed.

Begin by taking a careful history. In addition to aspects of history common to all presentations, ask specifically about existing eye disorders, the mechanism of injury and subsequent events.

Often the injury is unwitnessed or the child may be frightened and so the history may be vague or concealed. Have a high index of suspicion for hidden injury. Specifically ask for visual symptoms of reduction or change in vision. Children are prone to the oculocardiac reflex and a history of bradycardia, nausea, somnolence or syncope strongly suggests a significant injury.

Perform the non-invasive aspects of the examination first. Reassure the patient and carer that you will not hurt them. Dim the room lights if possible, keep the ophthalmoscope light to a minimum. Be systematic and touch last. Importantly, know when to stop and refer.

Document the visual acuity in each eye. Visual acuity testing should be adjusted to the age and ability of the child. Fix and follow testing, ability to reach for a small toy with one or the other eye covered, an Allen chart using pictures (allow the child to identify the pictures closely first), a Tumbling E chart (described as table legs pointing in different directions) or a formal Snellen chart. A difference of two or more lines is significant. Remember the child has a low attention span, so do not insist on them reading every line. If acuity is markedly reduced, use finger counting or light perception at close range.

Follow with a visual inspection. If appropriate, relieve pain with topical anaesthesia early to assist examination.

Examine and document:

- the pupillary shape, size and reaction to light;
- ocular movements in all directions of gaze (nystagmus, diplopia, pain or limitation of movement);
- inspect the lids;
- palpate orbital rims for steps or tenderness;
- test for infraorbital nerve sensation;
- the position of the globes (exophthalmos, enophthalmos);
- the conjunctival surface of eye lids (the deep superior fornix requires lid eversion for viewing);
- conjunctiva and sclera for laceration or foreign body;
- red reflex;
- corneal surface (use fluorescein staining where possible);
- examine the anterior chamber depth and clarity.

Trauma

Lid lacerations

A laceration to the eyelid may be partial or full thickness and may involve the lid margins, canthal tendons, levator complex or canalicular system.

Perform a thorough and complete eye examination to exclude an injury to the globe (see 'ruptured globe' below). Pressure exerted by attempts at cleaning and repair may apply pressure to a potentially ruptured globe. Children who are unable to co-operate enough to allow accurate assessment of wound depth should be referred for examination under anaesthesia. If a globe injury is suspected, apply a rigid shield, fast the patient and refer immediately.

The mechanism of injury should be determined to assess the risk of a foreign body (e.g. windscreen shattering), whether a bite (human or animal) and whether significant contamination may have occurred.

Indications for emergency ophthalmologic consultation include:

- bites and those with significant contamination requiring debridement;

- lacerations involving the eyelid margin to prevent notching;
- lacerations on the nasal side of the eyelid punctum – due to the risk of injury to the canalicular system;
- lacerations with involvement of the levator aponeurosis of the upper eyelid (which produces ptosis) or the superior rectus muscle.
- exposure of orbital fat – this suggests the orbital septum has been lacerated as there is no subcutaneous fat in the lids themselves;
- lacerations with significant tissue loss.

Wounds requiring referral should be cleaned with normal saline and have foreign material removed as much as possible. Following cleansing, the wound should be covered with a saline soaked dressing, prophylactic antibiotics commenced for bites or significantly contaminated wounds and tetanus status considered.

If the laceration is suitable for repair in the emergency department, the eyebrow should not be shaved as long-term cosmetic alterations may result and the hair direction assists in correct alignment of the wound. Tissue should not be removed, as the good blood supply of the eyelid generally ensures viability. Partial thickness lacerations should be repaired with 6/0 synthetic suture and full thickness lacerations should be repaired in layers. In general, non-absorbable sutures should be removed in 4–7 days. Tissue glue is not advised due to proximity to the lashes and cornea.

Ecchymosis

A black eye is a common injury and may be limited to a minor ecchymosis of the lid or extend to a periorbital haematoma with significant oedema. Always consider a blow-out fracture of the orbit, globe injury and/or base of skull fracture or anterior fossa fracture (suggested by a subconjunctival haemorrhage without posterior limit). Always document the ocular motility. Care must be exercised when opening the lids so that pressure is not exerted on the globe until a ruptured globe is excluded. If the eyelids are markedly swollen, examination of the eye is difficult. Placing one's thumb on the infraorbital and supra orbital rims, the swollen eyelids can be separated without placing pressure on the globe. The eyelids should not be forcibly opened. If a strong index of suspicion exists, place a rigid shield and refer. When swelling limits direct visualisation of the eye, ocular ultrasound is used in some centres to allow non-invasive assessment.

After other injury is excluded, the eyelid haematoma requires no specific management. Cold compresses may provide analgesia for the first 24 hours. The eye should be re-examined in 24 hours to ensure an injury has not been missed. Swelling and bruising may appear to extend down the cheek or to the other eye.

Orbital fracture

Suspect fracture when there is tenderness of the orbital rim or crepitus of the lid indicating a sinus fracture. There is often a haematoma of the eyelid. 'Blow-out' fractures (fracture of the orbital floor ± the medial wall) from blunt trauma are typically seen in adolescents.

Look for

- restricted ocular movements which may produce diplopia, usually on upward gaze;
- enophthalmos; and
- infraorbital nerve anaesthesia.

Nausea and vomiting may occur. Facial computerised tomography (CT) with axial and coronal views, ophthalmological and faciomaxillary referral is required. Ensure a globe or central nervous system (CNS) injury is not present, as this will have greater priority. Eye injury may occur in over 50% of these fractures, with globe rupture in 5–10%. If prominent symptoms of the oculocardiac reflex are present, immediate repair is indicated. If not, surgery may be arranged nonurgently. Instruct the patient not to blow the nose, as orbital emphysema may occur.

Conjunctival haemorrhage, lacerations

Subconjunctival haemorrhage presents as a red eye with a painless collection of bright, smooth blood confined to a sector of the bulbar conjunctiva which is sharply demarcated at the limbus and does not pass beyond the limbus. The visual acuity is normal.

Causes include:

- trauma;
- idiopathic;
- hypertension;
- bleeding diathesis;
- Valsalva (cough, heaving lifting, straining).

Pain with extraocular movement, reduced vision, hyphaema, pupil abnormality and/or bloody chemosis raise suspicion of a globe injury. A 360 degree subconjunctival haemorrhage should be referred urgently for ophthalmological review as the globe may be ruptured posteriorly. No specific treatment is required for an isolated subconjunctival haemorrhage. The haemorrhage will clear spontaneously within 1–2 weeks.

Conjunctival lacerations present as a red eye with a foreign body sensation and usually a history of trauma. Conjunctival and subconjunctival haemorrhages are often associated. The conjunctival edges can be separated gently with a moist cotton tipped applicator following topical anaesthesia to assess the depth of injury. If the diagnosis is uncertain, refer to ensure a scleral perforation or subconjunctival foreign body is excluded. If the conjunctival laceration is isolated, treatment with antibiotic ointment or drops is required for 4–7 days. They rarely require repair.

Corneal lacerations may be partial (not into the anterior chamber) or full thickness (ruptured globe). Complete examination is required to exclude a penetrating injury of the cornea or sclera. Ensure the anterior chamber is of normal depth and there is no hyphaema. Superficial partial thickness lacerations will heal spontaneously with antibiotic cover; however, daily review is necessary to exclude the development of infection until healing is complete. Deep partial thickness lacerations should be referred for consideration of repair. Seidel's test can be used (see ruptured globe). For management of full thickness lacerations refer to ruptured globe.

Corneal abrasions: 75% of ED visits are related to corneal abrasions, conjunctival or corneal foreign bodies and conjunctivitis. Corneal abrasions are very painful. Fingernails, sticks or foreign body may be the cause.

They may present with:

- tearing;
- a foreign body sensation;
- photophobia;
- visual acuity may be reduced, dependent on the size of the abrasion and the position over the visual axis;
- conjunctival injection, iritis and eyelid swelling may be associated.

The application of a topical local anaesthetic provides temporary pain relief and will assist in allowing the eye to be opened for examination. In a non-compliant child, place a drop at the medial canthus and when the eye is opened, the drops flow in. The non-verbal child may present simply with undifferentiated distress with or without refusal to open the eye and topical anaesthetic may be diagnostic.

Topical anaesthesia should never be provided to the patient for continued installation and home use as this may impair healing, inhibit protective reflexes and permit further injury.

Abrasions may be associated with a foreign body on the lid conjunctiva, which must be everted to be examined fully. An upper lid foreign body is suggested by a linear vertical abrasion. The inner surface of the upper lid is examined by asking the patient to look down, applying a cotton bud to the lid crease and applying light pressure. Use the eyelashes to pull the everted lid over the bud, away and up from the globe. Hold the lashes against the orbital rim to keep the lid everted. To return the lid, release the pressure and ask the patient to look up. The lower fornix is easily inspected by applying downward pressure to the lower lid while the patient looks up.

Diagnose the abrasion by demonstrating a staining defect with fluorescein using either an ophthalmoscope (+12 magnification) or a slit lamp. Use only a small amount of fluorescein as excessive dye can mask the defect. The abrasion will appear bright green when viewed under a blue light.

Conjunctival foreign bodies (palpebral or bulbar) should be removed after topical anaesthesia, with gentle irrigation or a moist cotton tipped swab.

Corneal foreign bodies: Assess for and refer those with an intraocular foreign body immediately (see penetrating injury). Always document the visual acuity. Topical anaesthesia is usually required to relieve pain and blepharospasm, enabling examination.

Removal requires adequate magnification and illumination. Foreign bodies may be removed by irrigation; a cotton tipped applicator or needle removal. Needle removal of a superficial foreign body must occur at the slit lamp and this will require a co-operative child. Approaching from the temporal side, use a 25-gauge needle attached to a 1–3-mL syringe, bevel angled away from the eye, to gently scrape the foreign body from the cornea. Referral should be made if the foreign body is central or deep or if the child is not co-operative. Post removal, complete examination of the eye using fluorescein.

If a rust ring or residual foreign body remains, next day referral should be arranged. Refer patients with central or large abrasions for daily review. Topical antibiotic treatment should be commenced. A topical non-steroidal anti-inflammatory drug (NSAID) provides effective analgesia and if there is severe pain, a cycloplegic (tropicamide 0.5–1%, cyclopentolate 0.5–2%) may be prescribed to relieve ciliary spasm (avoid in infants). Ensure tetanus prophylaxis. Eye patching does not reduce pain or aid healing, may cause difficulty walking in children and thus should be avoided.

Contact lens wearers should be referred for follow up and require pseudomonal coverage (tobramycin or ciprofloxacin). The lens should not be worn until the defect has been healed for a week.

Chemical burns are unusual in childhood, but are potentially very serious. For all chemical burns, irrigation should begin immediately. Anaesthetise the eye (procedural sedation may be required in young children) and then copiously rinse the eye with at least 1–2 litres of Hartmann's or normal saline (warm if possible) for at least 30 minutes. Use IV tubing connected to the bag of solution and direct the flow from medial to lateral onto the conjunctiva, not cornea. Ensure the fornices are irrigated by everting the lid. A Morgan lens (a moulded lens applied to the eye) allows continuous irrigation if available. Five minutes after irrigation has been completed, check the pH with litmus paper and continue irrigation until a pH > 7 is achieved A urine dipstick can be used (trim with scissors to retain the pH section). Check the pH again 20 minutes after irrigation to ensure there is no rebound fall. Once irrigation is completed, examine for retained foreign bodies. Particulate matter requires removal (moist cotton bud or toothed forceps) and this may require general anaesthesia. Alkali burns (dishwasher liquid, oven cleaner) produce liquefactive necrosis and are often more severe than acid burns.

Once irrigation has been completed, assess injury severity and document acuity. Assess with a slit lamp and fluorescein stain. Moderate or severe burns are suggested by significant epithelial loss, chemosis, corneal oedema or haziness, blanching of the conjunctival vessels or opacification. Refer immediately. All patients require treatment with antibiotic drops/ointment and analgesia ± cycloplegics.

Thermal burns are managed similarly to abrasions. UV keratitis may result from welding, sun lamp exposure or excessive sunlight. The symptoms develop several hours after exposure with pain, tearing and red eye. There are usually bilateral superficial corneal defects seen on fluorescein staining. Treatment is with topical antibiotics ± a cycloplegic.

Traumatic iritis presents with the onset of a dull, aching pain, photophobia, and tearing within 3 days of trauma. Possible signs: small pupil; perilimbal injection of the conjunctiva and pain in the affected eye when a light is shone into either the affected or non-affected eye; reduction in visual acuity; hyphaema. White blood cells and a flare are seen within the anterior chamber when examined under the slit lamp. This is best seen by placing the slit lamp beam at 45 degrees with full intensity and a short narrow slit. The appearance is like dust in a room illuminated with a torch. Refer immediately.

Hyphaema is blood in the anterior chamber and may result from blunt or penetrating trauma. Presents with pain, photophobia, mydriasis/miosis, reduced visual acuity or blurred vision. The red reflex will be intact. If the pupil is dilated, it is important to differentiate between traumatic mydriasis (present only in the affected eye) and an afferent pupillary defect (swinging light test – paradoxical initial dilatation of the affected pupil occurs when light is shone quickly from the unaffected to the affected eye); this may suggest an optic nerve or severe retinal injury. The size may vary from microscopic hyphaema to blood involving the whole anterior chamber. Urgent ophthalmological referral is required for all children. Treatment includes restricted activity, eye shield, anti-emetic, cycloplegic and topical steroid in some children. NSAIDs and aspirin should be avoided. Always consider non-accidental injury. Rebleeding occurs in up to one-third of patients, usually after a few days.

Ruptured globe and penetrating eye injury: A ruptured globe occurs when the integrity of the sclera or cornea is disrupted by blunt trauma or direct perforation. There may be surprisingly few signs. Suspect if there is a peaked pupil (apex of the teardrop points to the perforation), which may be the only clue to occult rupture. Chemosis overlying the laceration, subconjunctival haemorrhage, corneal or scleral laceration, distortion of the anterior chamber (deep or shallow), bubbles in the anterior chamber, extrusion of the intraocular contents, hyphaema, or loss of ocular motility may be indicative. A Seidel's test can be used if the diagnosis is unclear. Apply a moistened fluorescein strip over the potential site of perforation. Use the blue light of the slit lamp and the leak from a perforation will manifest as a green dilute aqueous stream within the darker, concentrated orange dye.

Once perforation or penetration of the eye is suspected, further emergency department examination is unnecessary.

- DO NOT apply pressure to the globe if penetration or rupture is suspected.
- NEVER attempt to remove a protruding foreign body from the globe.
- NEVER force the lids open.
- Do not use further eye drops and never use eye ointment on an open globe.

Rest the child in bed, head up. Protect the eye with a rigid eye shield. If a formal eye shield is unavailable, one can be created from the base of a polystyrene cup. Keep nil by mouth. Commence an anti-emetic and analgesia, ensure tetanus prophylaxis and systemic antibiotic prophylaxis. Contact the ophthalmologist urgently. If an intraocular foreign body or globe rupture is suspected CT will usually be required.

Non-accidental injury may result in any eye injury. A high index of suspicion is required if the injury is inconsistent with the given history or the history is inadequate. Retinal haemorrhage due to inflicted injury is typically seen in the child <1 year and often there are associated injuries.

Further reading

American Academy of Pediatrics. Policy Statement. Eye Examination in Infants, Children, and Young Adults by Pediatricians. *Pediatrics* 2003;111(4):902–7.

Babineau MR, Sanchez LD. Ophthalmologic procedures in the emergency department. *Emerg Med Clin N Am* 2008;26:17–34.

Curryn KM, Kaufman LM. The eye examination in the pediatrician's office. *Pediatr Clin North Am* 2003;50 (1):25–40.

Ehlers JP, Shah CP, editors. *Wills Eye Manual: Office and Emergency Room Diagnosis and Treatment of Eye Disease.* 5th ed. Baltimore: Lippincott Williams & Wilkins; 2008. p. 12–48.

Danis RP, Neely D, Plager DA. Unique aspects of trauma in children. In: Kuhn F, Pieramici DJ, editors. *Ocular Trauma: Principles and Practice.* Chap 30. Stuttgart: Thieme; 2002. p. 307–17.

Levine LM. Pediatric ocular trauma and shaken infant syndrome. *Pediatr Clin N Am* 2003;137–48.

NSW Health. *Eye Emergency Manual, An Illustrated Guide.* NSW Health; 2007.

14.1 The ear

Stuart Lewena • Gervase Chaney

ESSENTIALS

1 Otitis externa usually results from excessive exposure to heat and moisture and is usually very painful. Treatment involves cleaning, keeping dry and topical antibiotics.

2 Acute otitis media is a very common emergency presentation, but not all red ear drums are due to otitis media. Management with adequate analgesia is essential. However, antibiotic use should be restricted to specific circumstances.

3 Discharging otitis media due to chronic suppurative otitis media usually presents with painless and offensive discharge. Treatment is with ear toilet and topical antibiotics. Oral antibiotics have little or no role.

4 Otitis media with effusion is very common in children, but treatment is unnecessary in the majority, with resolution over 3 months.

5 Mastoiditis continues to be a problem in the antibiotic era and in many cases is the first presentation of ear disease. Admission, myringotomy and IV antibiotics constitute the mainstays of medical management.

6 Ear trauma is uncommon. Accidental ear injuries are usually unilateral and isolated. Ear trauma is rare in the first year of life and may indicate non-accidental injury. Haematomas should be removed by aspiration or excision.

Otitis externa

Introduction

Otitis externa includes various conditions from the most common acute diffuse otitis externa (swimmer's or tropical ear) to otomycosis, localised (furunculosis) or chronic otitis externa. It occurs commonly in hot, humid climates or in the summer of temperate climates. Risk factors also include swimming and other water exposure, local trauma, loss of the protective coating of the ear canal, including cerumen and obstruction of the ear canal. Allergy may also play a role.

History

It may initially present with aural fullness or itch, but usually progresses to pain with or without discharge. The pain is often severe and is worse with chewing.

Otomycosis or fungal otitis externa makes up 10% of cases and has a more insidious onset.

Examination

Oedema and erythema of the canal with serous or purulent discharge is usual. The tragus is tender to manipulation. With increased severity, the canal becomes occluded with periauricular oedema and may progress to otitis externa with cellulitis when the child becomes febrile with a toxic appearance.

Differentiation from acute otitis media with perforation or chronic suppurative otitis media is important. Usually in these conditions, the tragus and canal are not tender and there is no erythema and oedema of the canal.

Acute localised otitis externa (furunculosis) occurs in the posterosuperior aspect on the ear canal. Otomycosis has only mild canal wall inflammation and thick otorrhoea.

Investigations

Investigations are largely unnecessary and rarely alter empiric treatment. The organisms found in diffuse otitis externa are most commonly *Pseudomonas aeruginosa* and *Staphylococcus aureus*. Furunculosis is usually *S. aureus* and otomycosis – *Aspergillus* or *Candida* species. Consideration of cultures – aerobic, anaerobic and fungal – is worthwhile in cases resistant to routine therapy or if there is more extensive disease – such as associated cellulitis.

Treatment

Acute diffuse otitis externa is managed with frequent gentle cleaning of the canal, along with avoidance of water (swimming prohibited). Ototopical medications are the mainstay of treatment, usually topical antibiotics such as framycetin/gramicidin/dexamethasone combinations. Ciprofloxacin is also effective. Insertion of a wick or ribbon gauze is also helpful. Close follow up for repeated cleaning with or without wick reinsertion may be required.

Furunculosis treatment is by local heat application and oral antibiotics (flucloxacillin or cephalexin) or incision and drainage. Otomycosis will require canal cleaning and antifungal drops or gentian violet.

Prevention

Keeping the ear canal dry and avoidance of trauma to the canal are the mainstays of prevention.

Complications

Progression to cellulitis of the nearby skin/soft tissue and/or lymphadenitis may occur. Oral antibiotics are usually then indicated, with cephalexin a reasonable first choice, but antipseudomonal antibiotics may be necessary. Progressive cellulitis and a toxic-appearing child will require admission for intravenous antibiotics, including pseudomonas cover. Less commonly, involvement of the parotid gland, temporomandibular joint or base of skull may occur.

Chronic otitis externa may occur, and may be a sign of an underlying dermatological disease such as seborrhoeic or atopic dermatitis.

Acute otitis media

Introduction

Acute otitis media (AOM) is one of the most common primary care paediatric presentations. It occurs as a result of infection of the middle ear cavity by both viral and bacterial organisms. It is frequently over diagnosed and remains a common cause for excessive antibiotic use. Adequate analgesia and a selective approach to antibiotic use are the mainstays of management.

History

Classic symptoms include fever, malaise and ear pain. The pain can be severe and during the night may wake the child. Other systemic features such as nausea and vomiting can occur. In younger children, presentation is often non-specific, with crying and irritability. Eardrum perforation and otorrhoea

may occur (see complications). These symptoms may present as a primary complaint or frequently occur in the course of an upper respiratory infection.

Examination

A red, bulging, non-mobile tympanic membrane is the most reliable constellation of signs. Redness of the eardrum is a non-specific finding and may be seen with a high fever or following crying. Alone, therefore, it is not diagnostic of otitis media and is an inadequate finding to make the diagnosis.

Investigations

The diagnosis of otitis media is made solely on clinical grounds and investigations are rarely performed. In cases where tympanostomy has been performed, two-thirds are bacterial-culture positive, with a predominance of *Streptococcus pneumoniae*, *Moraxella catarrhalis* and *Haemophilus influenzae*.

Treatment

The administration of adequate analgesia is paramount to the management of acute otitis media. Paracetamol alone may not be adequate and the combination with codeine may be required. Topical instillation of lidocaine 2% has been shown to be a useful adjunct for rapid pain control but should be combined with longer-acting oral analgesia. Decongestants and antihistamines have not been shown to be effective and are not recommended.

The majority of cases of otitis media will resolve spontaneously. However, antibiotics continue to be widely used. In an otherwise healthy child over 2 years, most authorities now recommend deferring antibiotic use for 2 to 3 days, and to commence treatment only if the child remains symptomatic at review. Approximately 80% of children will avoid antibiotic use with this approach. Provision of a prescription upfront, with advice to commence antibiotics in 2 to 3 days if the child remains unwell, has been shown to result in approximately 50% of children avoiding antibiotics. Both strategies are reasonable, with the latter chosen in cases where access to timely medical review is uncertain. Early antibiotic therapy continues to be advocated in the very young or those with comorbidity.

Amoxicillin is a reasonable first-line antibiotic choice. The usual recommended dose

is 45 to 90 mg kg^{-1} per day. Amoxicillin + clavulanate is the next choice for poor responders. Cefaclor has a significant rate of serum sickness reactions in children and should not be used.

Topical otic antibiotic preparations may be used instead of oral antibiotics in cases with tympanic membrane perforation or those with intact tympanostomy tubes when purulent otorrhoea is the prominent finding.

Complications

The most common complication is perforation of the drum and otorrhoea. Other complications are very unusual but potentially severe. Most are due to bacterial spread and include extracranial complications such as mastoiditis, cholesteatoma and facial nerve paralysis and intracranial complications such as epidural abscess, meningitis and lateral sinus thrombosis.

Persistent middle ear effusions are almost universal after an episode of acute otitis media and should not be viewed as a complication. Complete resolution over several months occurs in 90% of cases.

Prevention

Prophylactic antibiotics confer a small decrease in recurrence at best, and are likely to contribute to increasing antibiotic resistance and generally are not recommended. More appropriate means of reducing recurrence include avoidance of passive smoke exposure, reducing day-care attendance and immunisation (pneumococcal and influenza).

Discharging otitis media – chronic suppurative otitis media

Introduction

Persistently discharging otitis media is most common in developing countries and certain high-risk populations in developed nations, such as Aboriginal Australians. It generally occurs following perforation of the eardrum from acute otitis media. It may also occur as a complication of tympanostomy tube (grommet) placement.

History

There is usually an absence of pain and a variable history (often weeks) of discharge that is purulent and offensive. It is often recurrent.

Examination

The canal is usually non-tender and there is usually no inflammation or some chronic inflammation. If the tympanic membrane can be visualised, usually only after ear toilet, there will be a perforation or tympanostomy tube in situ.

Investigations

Investigations are largely unnecessary. If performed, the organisms found on ear swabs are most commonly *Pseudomonas aeruginosa* and *Staphylococcus aureus*.

Treatment

Ear toilet (using a dry tissue spear) and topical antibiotics, particularly quinolones (such as ciprofloxacin with hydrocortisone) or framycetin/gramicidin/dexamethasone combinations, have been demonstrated to be effective in acute resolution of otorrhoea. Long-term outcomes are still to be determined. Systemic antibiotics alone are not as effective and addition to topical treatment does not improve outcome.

Complications

Chronic perforation and discharge are the main issues, although hearing impairment may be a problem. Cholesteatoma occurs in a small proportion of affected children.

Otitis media with effusion

Introduction

Otitis media with effusion (OME) is the presence of a middle-ear effusion in the absence of acute inflammation. It is unlikely to be a presenting complaint in an emergency department (ED) setting. It is more likely to be an incidental finding. It is extremely common, particularly in pre-school children. Its significance is in relation to its effect on conductive hearing.

History

Older children may present with aural fullness or reduced hearing. OME is usually asymptomatic in young children.

Examination

The eardrum may appear dull and non-erythematous and the effusion is most easily recognised by the presence of bubbles or a fluid level. If these are not present, pneumatic otoscopy will demonstrate impaired mobility.

Investigations

No acute investigations are indicated. In persistent cases, referral for audiology is recommended to determine any significant hearing loss.

Treatment

As the majority of OME cases will resolve spontaneously (90% by 3 months) a period of observation is recommended. Persistent OME is more likely to follow acute otitis media in the first year of life.

Trials of many different treatments including antibiotics, nasal decongestants, nasal insufflation, and corticosteroids have failed to show benefit. Persistent OME with concerns of significant hearing loss is an indication for audiology and referral to an ear, nose and throat (ENT) surgeon for consideration of tympanostomy tubes (grommets).

Complications

The principal concern for persistent OME is conductive hearing loss and potential impact on language and cognitive development. There are potential long-term changes to the tympanic membrane and middle ear that may cause hearing loss (e.g. tympanosclerosis).

Mastoiditis

Introduction

Mastoiditis is the infection of the mastoid air cells. It is an infrequent illness with a rate of between 1.2 and 4.2 per 100 000 person years in developed nations. Presentation can occur at any age, with a median of 12–48 months. There is some evidence that decreased use of antibiotics for AOM has resulted in a small increase in cases of mastoiditis. However, it is estimated that approximately 5000 children with otitis media would need to be treated with antibiotics to prevent 1 case of mastoiditis.

History

Symptoms at presentation with mastoiditis are very similar to AOM, with pain, irritability and fever. Mean time from onset of illness to signs of acute mastoiditis has been reported as just over 4 days.

Examination

Examination findings differentiating mastoiditis from AOM include protrusion/displacement of the auricle, post-auricular inflammation and tenderness, and narrowing of the external auditory canal. The tympanic membrane is usually abnormal and may be perforated.

Investigations

Increased routine use of computerised tomography scanning is due to the difficulty in diagnosis of subperiosteal abscess by clinical examination alone. Magnetic resonance imaging may also be valuable. Bacteriological diagnosis can be made at the time of operative treatment. Cultures show *Streptococcus pneumoniae*, *Strep. pyogenes* and *Staph. aureus* to predominate but many organisms are possible. *P. aeruginosa* can be seen in chronic or recurrent cases.

Treatment

Management has historically been cortical mastoidectomy. However, a number of series report successful treatment in the majority of cases with myringotomy and intravenous antibiotics. Broad-spectrum antibiotics such as third-generation cephalosporins are generally recommended, although antipseudomonal antibiotics may be required.

Complications

Complication rates are significant (13–35%) and include subperiosteal abscess, facial nerve paralysis, sigmoid sinus thrombosis, epidural abscess and meningitis.

Trauma

Introduction

Paediatric ear trauma is an uncommon presentation to an ED. Accidental ear trauma is almost always unilateral. There is the usual male predominance, with a majority between 1 and 7 years of age. Accidental ear trauma is rare in the first year of life and such presentations should be assessed for possible non-accidental (inflicted) injury. Other suggestive findings are bilateral ear injuries and associated injuries, particularly retinal haemorrhages and subdural haematoma.

History and examination

The most common mechanism is falls, followed by blows from an object and self-inflicted penetrating injuries which may result in perforation of the tympanic membrane. The most common objects inserted are cotton buds. Dog bites of the ear also occur. Lacerations are the most common injury, followed by bruising, abrasions and haematomas. Blood in the canal is a common finding in the penetrating injuries, making assessment of the eardrum difficult at the time of initial presentation. Burns are rare and are likely to be associated with more extensive burns. Barotrauma from explosions and loud noises are uncommon compared to industrial injuries in adults.

Assessment should include assessment of the facial nerve and hearing.

Investigation

Acute investigations are rarely required. However, audiology and ENT referral is indicated in penetrating and barotrauma injuries.

Treatment

Minor lacerations may be managed with steristrips, glue or suturing under local anaesthesia. Complex or larger lacerations will often require a general anaesthetic and surgical repair. Haematomas can lead to cartilage necrosis, infection and chondritis or fibrous organisation. All of these have potential to cause significant deformity. Therefore removal of the haematoma is indicated. Smaller haematomas can be aspirated and larger or recurrent collections should be evacuated. Appropriate contoured pressure dressings are then required to avoid reaccumulation. Penetrating injuries will often require ENT referral. Unless minor, burns will require evaluation by a burns specialist.

Complications

The main concerns are cosmetic deformity from haematomas, lacerations and burns, and hearing loss from penetrating injuries.

Controversies and future directions

❶ Acute otitis media:

- Antibiotic usage for acute otitis media in Australia, the UK and USA remains high. Due to concerns over the emergence of antibiotic resistance, the Netherlands has limited antibiotic use (31%), with good results leading to a review of use in high-prescribing countries. The concern about lower rates of antibiotic use is the potential for

increased complications (see mastoiditis).

❷ Discharging otitis media – chronic suppurative otitis media:

- Concern has arisen with the use of potentially ototoxic antibiotic ear drops in the presence of a tympanic-membrane perforation, despite routine use by ENT specialists with few reported cases of ototoxicity.
- A series of nine cases of iatrogenic topical vestibulotoxicity, all secondary to gentamicin-containing eardrops, has been reported. As a result, agents such as ciprofloxacin are being increasingly used.

❸ Otitis media with effusion

- Ventilation-tube (grommet) insertion remains one of the most common surgical procedures performed in children.
- It is effective at improving hearing in the short term. There has been conflicting evidence for its long-term benefit on language and cognitive development.

Further reading

Acuin J. Extracts from 'concise Clinical evidence': Chronic suppurative otitis media. Br Med J 2002;325(7373):16.

Acuin J, Smith A, Mackenzie I. Interventions for chronic suppurative otitis media. Cochrane Database Syst Rev 2000;2. John Wiley & Sons, Chichester.

Ah-Tye C, Paradise JL, Colborn DK. Otorrhea in young children after tympanostomy-tube placement for persistent middle-ear effusion: Prevalence, incidence, duration. Paediatrics 2001;107(6):1251–8 [comment].

Bitar CN, Kluka EA, Steele RW. Mastoiditis in children. Clin Paediatr 1996;35(8):391–5.

Bolt P, Barnett P, Babl FE, Sharwood LN, et al. Topical lignocaine for pain relief in acute otitis media: results of a double-blind placebo-controlled randomized trial. Arch Dis Child 2008;93(1):40–4.

Brook I. Treatment of otitis externa in children. Paediatr Drugs 1999;1(4):283–9.

Butler CC, Van Der Voort JH. Oral or topical nasal steroids for hearing loss associated with otitis media with effusion in children. Cochrane Database Syst Rev 2002 2000;4 [update of Cochrane Database of Syst Rev 4:CD001935, PMID: 11034736].

Byington CL. The diagnosis and management of otitis media with effusion. Paediatr Ann 1998;27(2):96–100.

Cantor RM. Otitis externa and otitis media. A new look at old problems. Emerg Med Clin N Am 1995;13(2):445–55.

Cohen-Kerem R, Uri N, Rennert H, et al. Acute mastoiditis in children: Is surgical treatment necessary? J Laryngol Otol 1999;113(12):1081–5.

Combs JT. Diagnostic accuracy of otitis media. Paediatrics 2003;112(1):205–6.

Dagan R, McCracken Jr GH. Flaws in design and conduct of clinical trials in acute otitis media. Paediatr Infecti Dis J 2002;21(10):894–902 [comment].

Del Mar CB, Glasziou PP. Should we now hold back from initially prescribing antibiotics for acute otitis media? J Paediatr Child Health 1999;35(1):9–10.

Dowell SF, Marcy SM, Phillips WR, et al. Principles of judicious use of antimicrobial agents for pediatric upper respiratory tract infections. Paediatrics 1998;101(1):163–5.

Dowell SF, Marcy SM, Phillips WR, et al. Otitis media – Principles of judicious use of antimicrobial agents. Paediatrics 1998;101(1):165–71.

Flynn CA, Griffin G, Tudiver F. Decongestants and antihistamines for acute otitis media in children. Cochrane Database of Syst Rev 2002 2001;1 [update of Cochrane Database Syst Rev 2:CD001727, PMID: 11406002].

Froom J, Culpepper L, Green LA, et al. Antimicrobials for acute otitis media? A review from the international primary care network. Br Med J 1997;315(7100):98–102.

Garbutt J, Jeffe DB, Shackelford P. Diagnosis and treatment of acute otitis media: An assessment. Paediatrics 2003;112(1):143–9.

Glasziou PP, Hayem M, Del Mar CB, et al. Antibiotics for acute otitis media in children. Cochrane Database Syste Rev 2000 2000;4 [update of Cochrane Database Syst Rev 2: CD000219, PMID: 10796513].

Holmes RE. Management of traumatic auricular injuries in children. Paediatr Ann 1999;28(6):391–5.

Hughes E, Lee JH. Otitis externa. Paediatr Rev 2001;6:191–7.

Kozyrskyj AL, Hildes-Ripstein GE, Longstaffe SE, et al. Short course antibiotics for acute otitis media. Cochrane Database Syst Rev 2000;2.

Little P, Gould C, Williamson I, et al. Pragmatic randomised controlled trial of two prescribing strategies for childhood acute otitis media. Br Med J 2001;322(7282):336–42.

Little P, McCormick DP, Chonmaitree T, et al. Predictors of poor outcome and benefits from antibiotics in children with acute otitis media: Pragmatic randomised trial. Br Med J 2002;325(7354):22 [commentary: research directions for treatment for acute otitis media].

Pond F, McCarty D, O'Leary S. Randomized trial on the treatment of oedematous acute otitis externa using ear wicks or ribbon gauze: Clinical outcome and cost. J Laryngol Otol 2002;116(6):415–9.

Rovers MM, Straatman H, Ingels K, et al. The effect of ventilation tubes on language development in infants with otitis media with effusion: A randomized trial. Paediatrics 2000;106(3):e42.

Rovers MM, Straatman H, Ingels K, et al. Randomised controlled trial of the effect of ventilation tubes (grommets) on quality of life at age 1–2 years. Arch Dis Child 2001;84(1):45–9 [comment].

Ruohola A, Heikkinen T, Meurman O, et al. Antibiotic treatment of acute otorrhea through tympanostomy tube: Randomized double-blind placebo-controlled study with daily follow-up. Paediatrics 2003;111(5–1):1061–7.

Segal S, Eviatar E, Lapinsky J, et al. Inner ear damage in children due to noise exposure from toy cap pistols and firecrackers: A retrospective review of 53 cases. Noise & Health 2003;5(18):13–8.

Spratley J, et al. Acute mastoiditis in children: Review of the current status. Int J Pediatr Otorhinolaryngol 2000;56(1):33–40.

Steele BD, Brennan PO. A prospective survey of patients with presumed accidental ear injury presenting to a paediatric accident and emergency department. Emerg Med J 2002;19(3):226–8.

Straetemans M, Sanders EA, Veenhoven RH, et al. Pneumococcal vaccines for preventing otitis media. Cochrane Database Syst Rev 2002;2.

Thompson PL, Gilbert RE, Long PF, et al. Effect of antibiotics for otitis media on mastoiditis in children: a retrospective cohort study using the Unitied Kingdom general practice research database. Pediatrics 2009;123(2):424–30.

Van Zuijlen DA, Schilder AG, Van Balen FA, Hoes AW, et al. National differences in incidence of acute mastoiditis: Relationship to prescribing patterns of antibiotics for acute otitis media? Paediatr Infect Dis J 2001;20(2):140–4 [comment].

Vassbotn FS, Klausen OG, Lind O, Moller P, et al. Acute mastoiditis in a Norwegian population: A 20 year retrospective study. Int J Paediatr Otorhinolaryngol 2002;62(3):237–42.

14.2 The nose

Stuart Lewena • Gervase Chaney

ESSENTIALS

Rhinitis and sinusitis

1 Acute rhinitis is common and largely due to viral infections.

2 Mucopurulent discharge does not mean bacterial infection.

3 Antibiotics might be indicated in prolonged cases of nasal discharge ($>$ 10–14 days duration), indicating possible sinusitis.

4 Constant nasal discharge may be due to perennial allergic rhinitis.

Epistaxis

1 Epistaxis is common and largely responds to simple first aid – compression of the nose.

2 Severe cases are uncommon, but are a medical emergency, requiring nasal packing and urgent ENT referral.

3 Underlying bleeding tendency should be excluded in cases with a family history of bleeding tendency or those with severe recurrent epistaxis.

Nasal trauma

1 Nasal trauma is common.

2 Most injuries will require little or no intervention. However, a careful examination to exclude septal haematoma is essential.

3 Septal haematoma requires urgent ENT referral.

4 Acute assessment can be difficult and a review, once the swelling has settled, is required to manage any deformity.

Rhinitis and sinusitis

Introduction

Viral upper respiratory tract infections causing rhinitis and inflammation of the upper respiratory tract are a frequent cause of febrile illness presentations amongst children to emergency departments. Children will commonly experience three to eight of these infections per year, even more if attending day care. After exclusion of more significant illness, education and symptomatic treatment is all that is required. Despite recommendations against such practice, many children will have been prescribed antibiotics. Bacterial sinusitis has been estimated as complicating only 0.5–5% of upper respiratory tract infections. Most of these will resolve without antibiotic treatment.

History

The common cold usually commences with a throat irritation and clear, thin nasal discharge and progresses to a thick, mucopurulent discharge after a few days. This does not indicate bacterial infection. Sneezing, nasal obstruction, systemic features such as malaise and low-grade fever, and cough are common. Generally the duration is about 7 days.

Persistence of mucopurulent nasal discharge without improvement for longer than 10–14 days, or more severe acute symptoms, such as high fever, headache, facial pain and/or swelling are more indicative of bacterial sinusitis.

Persistent clear nasal discharge is more likely due to perennial allergic rhinitis. This may be associated with sneeze, and itchy eyes and/or nose. Unilateral nasal discharge, particularly offensive, is suggestive of a nasal foreign body.

Examination

In rhinosinusitis, nasal discharge is the usual finding. This may be clear or mucopurulent and, as already discussed, is not indicative of cause. A red throat is a common association. In allergic rhinitis, the nasal mucosa will be pale and swollen. Facial swelling, such as orbital/periorbital and/or facial tenderness may occur in sinusitis.

Investigations

Investigations are not indicated for the common cold. Sinusitis is also a clinical diagnosis. Radiological investigations for acute sinusitis are difficult to interpret, as similar findings may be found in the common cold or even asymptomatic children. Also, the sinuses of young children are poorly developed, with frontal and sphenoid sinuses not appearing till 5–6 years of age. Radiological investigations should be reserved for those cases with suspected complications of orbital/intracranial extension, or possibly in recurrent cases.

If aspirated under general anaesthesia, sinusitis fluid most commonly cultures *Pneumococcus*, followed by *Haemophilus influenzae*, *Moraxella catarrhalis* and then viruses. Nasopharyngeal cultures are not predictive and therefore not useful.

Treatment

Antibiotics are not indicated for the common cold and have been shown neither to alter the course of the illness nor prevent the development of complications. Perennial allergic rhinitis responds best to intranasal corticosteroids, but these are often not tolerated well by children.

Even in bacterial sinusitis, the majority of cases will resolve spontaneously. Nasal decongestants may provide some short-term relief. If antibiotics are used, amoxicillin is recommended as first-line treatment for 10–14 days duration. Amoxicillin + clavulanate can be kept for those cases failing to respond in 48–72 hours.

Complications

Bacterial complications of the common cold do occur, such as otitis media, but cannot be prevented by antibiotic use. Asthma is frequently precipitated by upper respiratory tract infections.

Ethmoid sinusitis can spread to cause orbital cellulitis or intracranially, causing an abscess or cavernous sinus thrombosis.

Prevention

Breast-feeding has a protective effect on the number of upper respiratory tract infections experienced by young children. Day care attendance and environmental tobacco exposure increase the number of episodes.

Epistaxis

Introduction

Although epistaxis is common in childhood (affecting about 6–9%), it is usually mild and usually does not require any medical intervention, let alone presentation to an emergency department (ED).

History

The frequency and severity of episodes should be determined together with first aid measures undertaken. A history of abnormal bleeding/bruising, infections or trauma should be sought.

Examination

In the majority of cases, positive examination findings are limited to the nose. Bleeding can be unilateral or bilateral. Crusting and vessels in Little's area are commonly seen. The remainder of the examination should exclude hypertension, abnormal bruising or petechiae and findings of lymphadenopathy or hepatosplenomegaly.

Investigations

Investigation for bleeding disorders is frequently performed. However, the vast majority of these will be normal unless there are other indications of bleeding tendency or family history. A more severe history of epistaxis, with frequent bleeds of greater volume and duration, is more suggestive of a bleeding disorder such as von Willebrand disease and warrants appropriate testing.

Treatment

First aid treatment of epistaxis is firm compression of the alar nasae, applying pressure over Little's area. This will result in cessation of bleeding in the majority of cases. The use of anaesthetic/vasoconstrictor spray or soaked pledgets may assist in haemostasis. If these measures fail, nasal cautery can be used for a well-identified bleeding site or an anterior nasal pack inserted. Purpose-made self-expanding nasal packs have made this procedure much easier. These packs should be lubricated with antibiotic ointment before insertion. Children with epistaxis that has required packing should be considered for investigation of underlying bleeding problems and have an ear, nose and throat (ENT) referral. Posterior nasal packing or other more invasive procedures are rarely required in children, but may be needed in severe epistaxis in the context of resuscitation and urgent ENT consultation.

Complications

Rarely, recurrent epistaxis is sufficient to cause anaemia. Care should be taken when applying nasal cautery to avoid damage to the underlying septal cartilage. Bilateral cautery should be avoided for this reason.

Nasal trauma

Introduction

Nasal trauma is common in children. It can occur at any age, but is most frequent in early primary-age groups. Like most injuries, there is a male predominance.

History and examination

The most common mechanism of injury is falls, usually at home, followed by sports injuries. Child abuse (inflicted injury) should be considered, particularly in the younger (non-mobile) child. A careful history is therefore required.

The types of injury are varied, from abrasions and lacerations of the soft tissues to fractures, dislocations and cartilage damage. More than minor epistaxis is unusual. Due to swelling it is often difficult to make a thorough assessment of the extent of injury in the acute setting – particularly for deformity. Examination must include an examination of the nasal cavities. Deviation, swelling and/or discolouration of the nasal septum may indicate a septal haematoma and urgent ENT consultation for evacuation is indicated.

Investigations

Nasal X-rays offer no benefit. A young child's nose is predominantly cartilage, and even when a fracture of the nasal bones is identified, this information does not influence management. Facial X-ray or computerised tomography (CT) should be limited to those suspected of more serious facial bony injury.

Treatment

Most nasal injuries require no acute intervention beyond analgesia. However, follow up may be required to determine the extent of deformity. The timing of this is recommended to be about 1 week post-injury, as the swelling has usually resolved by then, and, if required, further treatment can be instituted.

Complications

Septal haematoma, ± abscess formation, is the main complication that causes long-term damage and therefore concern. It may present later down the track and may have been missed on earlier assessment. Haematomas can be very painful and frequently cause nasal obstruction. On its own, a septal haematoma can cause nasal cartilage damage, including aseptic necrosis. However, the development of an abscess is almost always associated with cartilage damage and potentially severe nasal deformity. *Staphylococcus aureus*, *Streptococcus pneumoniae* and *Strep. pyogenes* have all been cultured. Meningitis or cavernous sinus thrombosis may also complicate a septal abscess.

Controversies

Epistaxis

The choice of which children to test and extent of investigation for bleeding disorders is still uncertain. For the severe and recurrent cases, thorough coagulation testing, including for von Willebrand disease, is appropriate.

Nasal trauma

Open rhinoplasty for nasal deformities may affect nasal growth in itself and should be used as conservatively as possible.

Further reading

Canty PA, Berkowitz RG. Hematoma and abscess of the nasal septum in children. *Arch Otolaryngol Head Neck Surg* 1996;**122**(12): 1373–1376.

Crockett DM, Mungo RP, Thompson RE. Maxillofacial trauma. *Paediatr Clin N Am* 1989;**36**(6): 1471–1494.

East CA, O'Donaghue G. Acute nasal trauma in children. *J Paediatr Surg* 1987;**22**(4): 308–310.

Ghosh A, Jackson R. Towards evidence based emergency medicine: Best BETs from the Manchester Royal Infirmary. Cautery or cream for epistaxis in children. *Emerg Med J* 2001;**18**(3): 210.

Ginsburg CM. Nasal septal hematoma. *Paediatr Rev* 1998; **19**(4): 142–143.

Katsanis E, Luke KH, Hsu E, et al. Prevalence and significance of mild bleeding disorders in children with recurrent epistaxis. *J Paediatr* 1988;**113**(11): 73–76.

Makura ZG, Porter GC, McCormick MS. Paediatric epistaxis: Alder Hey experience. *J Laryngol Otol* 2002;**116**(11): 903–906.

Nyquist A-C, Gonzales R, Steiner JF, et al. Antibiotic prescribing for children with colds, upper respiratory tract infections, and bronchitis. *JAMA* 1998;**279**(11): 875–877.

O'Brien KL, Dowell SF, Schwartz B, et al. Acute sinusitis—Principles of judicious use of antimicrobial agents. *Paediatrics* 1998;**101**(1): 174–177.

Rosenstein N, Phillips WR, Gerber MA, et al. The common cold—Principles of judicious use of antimicrobial agents. *Paediatrics* 1998;**101**(1): 181–184.

Ruddy J, Proops DW, Pearman K, et al. Management of epistaxis in children. *Int J Paediatr Otorhinolaryngol* 1991;**21**(2): 139–142.

14.3 The mouth and throat

Stuart Lewena • Gervase Chaney • Richard P. Widmer

ESSENTIALS

Stomatitis

1 Acute herpetic gingivostomatitis is the most common cause of stomatitis in young children.

2 Early treatment with aciclovir is effective if commenced in the first 72 hours.

3 Aphthous stomatitis or ulcers are more common in young adults, but do occur in children.

Pharyngitis/tonsillitis

1 Most sore throats in children are due to viral infections.

2 Bacterial tonsillitis is more likely in older children with isolated sore throat, high fever and tender cervical lymphadenopathy.

3 Ten days of penicillin is the recommended course of treatment for bacterial infection.

Peritonsillar abscess

1 Peritonsillar abscess is the most common abscess of the head and neck.

2 Diagnosis is not always straightforward.

3 Management is analgesia, antibiotics, fluids and draining the abscess.

Post-tonsillectomy haemorrhage

1 Tonsillectomy remains a relatively common procedure.

2 Post-tonsillectomy bleeding occurs in about 1.5% and although most may be managed conservatively, for some, transfusion and/or surgery are necessary.

Oral/dental trauma

1 Oral/dental trauma is common in children.

2 A careful examination of the orofacial structures is required.

3 Dental consultation is indicated for all but the minor cases.

Oral/dental infection

1 Dental infections are the most common cause of facial cellulitis.

2 There are usually underlying dental caries and tooth extraction is often required.

Stomatitis

Introduction

Acute herpetic gingivostomatitis is the most common cause of stomatitis in young children (1–3 years). It is also the most common clinical presentation of primary herpes simplex infection in young children. It can also occur in older children and adults. Untreated, the course of the illness is 10–14 days. Aphthous ulcers usually occur as single ulcers and are often recurrent.

History

Acute herpetic gingivostomatitis may present suddenly or insidiously – initially with fever and irritability. Mouth pain, often severe, plus drooling and refusal to eat will usually follow. Dehydration can occur if the child refuses to drink. Gingival bleeding can occur

Aphthous ulcers present as recurrent painful lesions of the oral mucosa, usually single and less than 1 cm diameter.

Examination

Early herpetic lesions are vesicles, but usually not seen, due to early rupture. Multiple ulcers up to 1 cm then occur on any part of the oral mucosa and initially are covered with a yellow-grey membrane. Associated gingivitis is usual.

Investigations

Viral swabs and immunofluorescence or viral culture for herpes simplex can confirm the diagnosis if required. However, if this is not readily available, clinical diagnosis is reasonably accurate.

For recurrent aphthous ulcers, checking a neutrophil count to exclude cyclical neutropenia is appropriate.

Differential diagnosis

Initially presentation is non-specific and can be confused with a general viral infection. If the tonsils are involved early, acute tonsillitis or herpangina may be suspected. Some cases are misdiagnosed as oral candidiasis.

Aphthous ulcers are easily distinguished, as these are usually single. Recurrent aphthous ulcers can be seen in cyclical or congenital neutropenia and PFAPA syndrome (fever, malaise, aphthous stomatitis, tonsillitis, pharyngitis and cervical adenopathy).

Treatment

Traditional treatment has been symptomatic, in the form of analgesia and hydration. Analgesia usually requires a combination of topical anaesthetic agents and oral analgesics, such as paracetamol or ibuprofen. Topical lidocaine gel can be very effective. Rehydration may require the use of nasogastric or intravenous fluids.

Recent studies, including a placebo-controlled study, have demonstrated the efficacy of oral aciclovir, if commenced in the first 72 hours of the illness. They have shown a significant reduction in duration of fever, feeding and drinking difficulties and viral shedding. A dose of 15 mg kg^{-1} per dose (up to 200 mg) five times a day for 5–7 days is recommended.

Aphthous ulcers with an adherent/dental base can be treated with topical corticosteroids (e.g. triamcinolone).

Complications

Acute dehydration has been mentioned. Secondary bacterial infection is uncommon. Primary herpetic infection may progress to generalised vesicular eruption. Also, auto-inoculation can occur, particularly to the eye.

Recurrent labial herpes is common and more of an inconvenience. It occurs following exposure to sunlight, stress, trauma or cold. Topical aciclovir may be of use, when applied with the first evidence of symptoms.

Pharyngitis/tonsillitis

Introduction

Sore throat is an extremely common presentation and is predominantly viral in cause. Group A streptococcal infection accounts for 10–20% of cases, and is even less frequent in young children (infants < 1 year < 5%). The concern over potential complications from streptococcal infection, such as rheumatic fever and glomerulonephritis, has led to many children being prescribed unnecessary antibiotics. Most people do not seek medical care for sore throats and the problem resolves spontaneously.

History

Older children will present with a complaint of sore throat, while younger children may be non-specifically unwell. A reluctance to take food or drinks may indicate a sore throat. Associated symptoms include fever, headache, vomiting and abdominal pain, but are not predictive whether bacterial or viral.

Examination

Ulcerative pharyngitis (herpangina) is a helpful finding indicating viral infection, such as coxsackie. Otherwise, it is difficult to differentiate between bacterial and viral causes. Features that suggest bacterial infection are tender cervical lymphadenopathy and absence of other symptoms such as coryza, cough, conjunctivitis and diarrhoea. Tonsillar exudate or pus is not an accurate predictor of bacterial infection and is frequently seen in viral causes such as infectious mononucleosis, Epstein–Barr virus (EBV) and adenovirus. EBV infection may be suggested by the presence of more widespread lymphadenopathy, particularly if there is associated splenomegaly.

Scarlet fever is suggested by a widespread, fine, maculopapular rash with a sandpaper-like feel, with associated pharyngitis and possibly a 'strawberry-tongue'. Although the scarlatiniform rash is highly specific for streptococcal infection, it only occurs in a minority of cases.

Investigations

Throat swab and culture may be used to assist differentiation between viral and bacterial aetiology. Opinion varies with regard to the value of throat swabs and they should probably only be performed in cases with a high clinical index of bacterial aetiology. (Child older than 4 years, significant fever, pharyngitis in the absence of other upper respiratory tract infection signs, tender tonsillar lymph nodes.)

Blood tests are usually done for investigation of infectious mononucleosis, although in children, the monospot/monotest has a high false-negative rate and serology is more reliable.

Treatment

For the majority of sore throats due to viral pharyngitis/tonsillitis, no antibiotics are necessary. Analgesia in the form of paracetamol or ibuprofen will provide symptomatic relief. For streptococcal pharyngitis, phenoxymethylpenicillin (250 mg or 500 mg) twice daily for 10 days is the recommended treatment, with a cure rate of approximately 90%.

Antibiotics should be routine in groups at high risk of rheumatic fever, those with existing rheumatic heart disease and those with scarlet fever.

Complications

Complications from sore throats are uncommon. Suppurative complications of streptococcal infection include peritonsillar abscess, sinusitis and otitis media. The principal concerns, however, are with the non-suppurative complications: rheumatic fever and glomerulonephritis. Acute tonsillitis can cause airway obstruction, particularly with pre-existing tonsillar hypertrophy and may even warrant admission for monitoring.

Peritonsillar abcess

Introduction

Peritonsillar abscess is the most common deep space head and neck infection in children. It is likely to be an extension of acute tonsillitis. However, it has been suggested that some cases may arise from obstruction and infection of Weber's glands (mucous glands located in the superior tonsillar pole). It can occur at any age.

History and examination

Presentation is usually with sore throat or neck pain, which is often severe. Odynophagia, dysphagia, and fever are also common. A muffled (or hot potato) voice and trismus occurs in about one-third of cases. Only a minority will have a prior history of tonsillitis (20–30%).

Examination findings include cervical lymphadenopathy, unilateral tonsillar erythema, bulging of the superior aspect of the tonsil and uvular deviation. The differential is peritonsillar cellulitis, where there is no abscess. Clinical differentiation between the two is difficult.

Investigations

The definitive investigation is needle aspiration, but not all children will be co-operative. Computerised tomography scan or ultrasound may assist diagnosis. Microbiological identification of abscess contents probably does not alter management. If performed, the predominant organism found is *Streptococcus pyogenes*.

Treatment

Initial treatment is rehydration, analgesia and antibiotics (penicillin). Acute drainage is generally recommended, with either intraoral drainage, abscess tonsillectomy or needle aspiration. Needle aspiration alone would appear to be effective in a majority of cases (>90%). Sedation or general anaesthesia may be required.

Abscess tonsillectomy should be reserved for recurrent tonsillitis abscess, but many of these can still be managed with aspiration and delayed tonsillectomy.

Complications

Dehydration is common and will require medical intervention. Uncommon, but dangerous, complications include infection spread, such as to the parapharyngeal space, airway obstruction and aspiration of pus causing pneumonia.

Post-tonsillectomy haemorrhage

Introduction

Tonsillectomy remains a very commonly performed procedure. The most common complication of tonsillectomy is bleeding. Secondary (delayed) haemorrhage, which occurs after the first 24 hours following surgery, complicates about 1.5% of tonsillectomies. The mean time of presentation is about 7 days, with a range up to 15 days. Rarely, haemorrhage is catastrophic and life threatening.

History

Bleeding is usually obvious, although occasionally will be swallowed and not immediately apparent. A history of bleeding or bruising tendency should be sought, although ideally will have been identified prior to surgery.

Examination

Initial assessment should focus on signs of shock or haemodynamic compromise. Examination of the tonsillar fauces for evidence of active bleeding is then important.

Investigations

Full blood examination to monitor for a drop in haemoglobin and taking blood for cross match is recommended in any significant post tonsillectomy bleed. Coagulation profile testing rarely demonstrates abnormality, but is warranted in major haemorrhage.

Treatment

Immediate, preferably large-bore, intravenous access is indicated with cross-matching of blood and commencement of fluid resuscitation as required. Early involvement of an ear, nose and throat surgeon for children with active bleeding is indicated. Transfusions have been reported as being required in 10–12% of secondary haemorrhage. However, a more conservative approach is probably possible with the use of other intravenous fluids and close monitoring. Surgical intervention under general anaesthesia is less frequently required according to a retrospective Australian study (4.3%).

Complications

Post-tonsillectomy bleeding is potentially life threatening, largely from hypovolaemic shock. Massive bleeding may also cause airway obstruction.

Oral/dental trauma

Introduction

The most common reasons for infants and children to present to the emergency department (ED) with oral/dental trauma are falls and sporting injuries. Most of these are relatively minor. Occasionally, higher impact trauma including motor vehicle accidents will produce severe injury requiring maxillofacial reconstructive surgery and early problems of haemostasis and airway compromise.

History

Make specific enquiry with regard to the time and mechanism of trauma and the nature of the dentition prior to injury. This includes the number of deciduous teeth that were present and the presence of any secondary dentition. Determine whether any teeth have been avulsed and their current location and method of storage. Consider the possibility of aspiration if a tooth is missing.

Examination

The physical examination should review all orofacial structures with careful scrutiny, digital palpation and observation of normal function. Externally and internally the orofacial region should exhibit consistent symmetry and any departure from this, be it an area of altered facial soft tissue architecture associated with a swelling or altered bony architecture associated with a fracture, will be important. For example chinpoint trauma is a common injury associated with mandibular condylar fracture. Assessment of mandibular opening and malocclusion is vital. In cases where the child has fallen with an object in their mouth, careful assessment for palatal or pharyngeal penetrating trauma is required.

The key points in recognition of a facial fracture are pain, facial swelling, stepping (of the bony border), limited jaw opening, palatal or sublingual haematoma, malocclusion and paraesthesia. The need for tetanus prophylaxis and antibiotics should be considered. Usually, antibiotics (penicillin and metronidazole) should be given for a compound fracture in the mouth.

A common error when assessing a child's occlusion is to fail to recognise that an anterior open bite (associated with a prior digit or object sucking habits) is a normal anterior relationship for that child and not necessarily evidence of a fracture in the maxilla/mandible. Check the posterior teeth for appropriate occlusion in this situation. The older child will usually be able to tell you if the teeth 'feel right' when they bite.

Investigations

The most relevant extraoral radiograph is an orthopantomogram (OPG). This radiograph will give an excellent view not only of the body of the mandible, the dentoalveolar area, but also of the temporomandibular joints (TMJ). However, the child's co-operation is required. If a TMJ view is specifically required it will be important to notify the radiographer.

Treatment

Management will obviously depend upon the exact diagnosis, which may include the following five factors:

Luxation

This is defined as a slight movement of the teeth as a result of trauma, with or without associated gingival bleeding. These injuries can occur in either the primary or permanent teeth and can be in any direction, i.e. internal, external or lateral. Active intervention may or may not be needed, depending on the extent of movement and interference with the occlusion or risk to the development of the underlying secondary dentition.

The appropriate treatment in luxation may be conservative in minor cases or involve extraction of the damaged primary tooth/teeth or repositioning of displaced teeth and placement of a dental splint with associated suturing of damaged soft tissues.

Avulsion

This is defined as the complete loss of a tooth, primary or permanent. In all situations, if there is any doubt about the nature of the tooth (that is, whether it is primary or not) and given that permanent teeth are always re-implanted, it is prudent, as first-line advice, to suggest that all avulsed teeth are placed in milk or an appropriate tissue-culture medium, if available. The appropriate tissue-culture medium is Hanks' balanced salt solution. This can be kept frozen in the ED in a small vial. It will provide up to 12 hours' working time before replanting the avulsed tooth is necessary. It is important not to store the tooth in water. If milk or tissue-culture medium is not available, it is crucial to keep the tooth moist by wrapping it in clingfilm or a gauze that is kept moist with saline or the patient's saliva. As a general rule, the primary teeth are not

re-implanted. Reasons include the potential damage to the developing permanent teeth, difficulties in securing the tooth/teeth in place and the level of co-operation that is required.

Ideally, avulsed permanent teeth should be repositioned/reimplanted in the tooth socket as soon as possible. It is crucial not to handle the root of the tooth. Manipulate using the crown only. This avoids damage to the periodontal ligament cells, which line the root surface and are critical in re-establishing the tooth back in the mouth as a functioning unit. Once re-implanted, avulsed teeth need to be splinted in place. Temporary splints can include moulded aluminium foil around the teeth or a fishing line and super glue. It will be crucial to stress dental follow up to try and avoid the sequelae that lead to tooth loss.

Root factures

The root of the tooth, which is buried in the alveolar bone, can also be fractured, often with minimal damage to the crown of the teeth. This may present at review, if not initially obvious. A particularly mobile or loose tooth/teeth, that is/are slightly extruded are classic signs of associated root fractures.

Hard tissue injuries

This involves a chip off the tooth, whether it is just enamel or involves the deeper layers – such as the dentine. It may involve all three layers of the tooth and 'expose' the dental pulp. If a tooth is exposed, then it is important that the exposure is treated immediately so as to preserve the vitality of the dental pulp and thus enable the root to grow to its full length and thickness. This is very important for the tooth's long-term maintenance as a useful member of the dentition.

Soft-tissue injuries

The soft tissues of the mouth involve the gingival tissues, mucosa and muscle. The soft tissue lacerations, especially of the gingival tissues, need to be carefully assessed for degloving and may need to be repositioned and sutured. Where teeth are significantly displaced there will be associated displacement and laceration of soft tissue and it is very important for the long-term periodontal health of the traumatised teeth

that displaced soft tissues are adequately repositioned and sutured. Alveolar bone should not be left exposed to granulate over.

Prevention

Advice on prevention is never misplaced and recommendation of well-made and fitted mouth guards is encouraged.

Oral/dental infection

Introduction

Dental infections are the most frequent cause of acute facial cellulitis, accounting for about 50% of all cases. Therefore, for children presenting with a facial swelling associated with fever and general malaise, a dental cause must be high on the list of differentials.

History

Facial cellulitis will present as above, with facial redness and tenderness. The upper face is affected more frequently, particularly in younger children. The lower face is affected relatively more often in older children, probably related to caries patterns.

Examination

A thorough examination, particularly intra-orally is required and early dental involvement is very helpful in determining a dental source.

Investigations

Appropriate radiographs are frequently indicated to determine a dental aetiology. These may be extraoral, e.g. an OPG, and/or intraoral.

Treatment

The usual treatment involves the use of antibiotics (usually penicillin will be adequate) and repair or removal of the offending tooth/teeth. Metronidazole may be added in cases of significant infection requiring hospitalisation.

Prevention

Lifting the upper lip in all children seen is a useful way of detecting early dental decay, which presents with whitening of the teeth at the gum margins and later staining. A significant cause of tooth decay in infants and young children is inappropriate feeding habits based on the use of a night-time feeding bottle containing sweetened liquids, which end up causing extensive dental damage. Advice should be given to parents to go from breast to cup with their babies or to wean from the bottle by 12 months. Also, infants should not be put to bed with a bottle.

Other dental issues

Spontaneous oral haemorrhage

Oral bleeding is still a very important sign for the diagnosis of underlying generalised bleeding disorders. It is important to determine the actual site of the bleeding and consequently a through oral examination will be required. Try to rinse the child's mouth with water or saline and use gauze to remove any blood clots and identify the source of the oral bleeding. In many instances this may be a tooth socket associated with a recent extraction. However, life-threatening disorders such as haemangiomas and arteriovenous malformations may present in the same fashion.

If a tooth-extraction socket is identified as the cause of bleeding, local measures to control the bleeding will usually be sufficient. This involves applying digital pressure to the bleeding socket or having the child bite down on a gauze pad for 15 minutes. Bleeding disorders such as von Willebrand's disease and haemophilia should be considered in cases that continue to bleed.

Controversies

Pharyngitis/tonsillitis

Although antibiotics have a protective effect in the prevention of rheumatic fever, the evidence does not support a similar effect on prevention of glomerulonephritis.

Tonsillectomy

Antibiotics post-tonsillectomy do lessen morbidity, in particular pain, analgesic use and delay in resumption of oral diet. Amoxicillin and amoxicillin + clavulanate have been shown to be effective. The studies have not had the numbers to demonstrate whether this is also true for post-tonsillectomy haemorrhage.

Oral/dental trauma

❶ The management of avulsed permanent teeth centres on the prescription of routine antibiotics post-re-implantation in an effort to limit the unwanted side effects associated with re-implantation, such as an ankylosis of the teeth and inflammatory root resumption. This prescription of antibiotics is not universally accepted.

❷ The immediate disimpaction of the traumatically intruded permanent tooth/teeth using orthodontic appliances is proposed as the most appropriate care, especially when trying to limit the unwanted sequelae of poor alveolar bone height and gingival attachment. However, there is a school of thought that proposes to partially disimpact surgically, and then complete the job of realignment orthodontically.

Oral/dental infection

Antibiotic choice is not universally agreed in either delivery (oral vs. intravenous) or type (penicillin vs. cephalosporins).

Further reading

Amir J, Harel L, Smetana Z, et al. Treatment of herpes simplex gingivostomatitis with aciclovir in children: A randomised double blind placebo controlled study. *Br Med J* 1997;**314** (7097):1800–3 [comment].

Cmejrek RC, Coticchia JM, Arnold JE. Presentation, diagnosis, and management of deep-neck abscesses in infants. *Arch Otolaryngol Head Neck Surg* 2002;**128**(12):1361–4.

Dawes LC, Bova R, Carter P. Retropharyngeal abscess in children. *Aust N Z J Surg* 2002;**72**(6):417–20.

Del Mar CB, Glasziou PP, Spinks AB. Antibiotics for sore throat. *Cochrane Database Syst Rev* 2000;**4** [update of *Cochrane Database Syst Rev* 2000;**2**:CD000023; PMID 10796471].

Delaney JE, Keels MA. Paediatric oral pathology Soft tissue and periodontal conditions. *Paediatr Clin N Am* 2000; **47**(5):1125–47.

Edmond KM, Grimwood K, Carlin JB, et al. Streptococcal pharyngitis in a paediatric emergency department. *Med J Aust* 1996;**165**(8):420–3.

Febres C, Echeverri EA, Keene HJ. Parental awareness, habits, and social factors and their relationship to baby bottle tooth decay. *Paediatr Dentistry* 1997;**19**(1):22–7.

Gianoli GJ, Espinola TE, Guarisco JL, Miller RH. Retropharyngeal space infection: Changing trends. *Otolaryngol Head Neck Surg* 1991;**105**(1):92–100.

Goldenberg D, Golz A, Joachims HZ. Retropharyngeal abscess: A clinical review. *J Laryngol Otol* 1997;**111** (6):546–50.

Graham DB, Webb MD, Seale NS. Paediatric emergency room visits for nontraumatic dental disease. *Paediatr Dentistry* 2000;**22**(2):134–40.

Herzon FS, Nicklaus P. Paediatric peritonsillar abscess: Management guidelines. *Curr Probl Paediatr* 1996;**26** (8):270–8.

Irani DB, Berkowitz RG. Management of secondary hemorrhage following paediatric adenotonsillectomy. *Int J Paediatr Otorhinolaryngol* 1997;**40**(2–3):115–24.

Myssiorek D, Alvi A. Post-tonsillectomy hemorrhage: An assessment of risk factors. *Int J Paediatr Otorhinolaryngol* 1996;**37**(1):35–43.

Nussinovitch M, Finkelstein Y, Amir J, Varsano I. Group A beta-hemolytic streptococcal pharyngitis in preschool children aged 3 months to 5 years. *Clin Paediatr* 1999;**38** (6):357–60.

Ripa LW. Nursing caries: A comprehensive review. *Paediatr Dentistry* 1988;**10**(4):268–82.

Schraff S, McGinn JD, Derkay CS. Peritonsillar abscess in children: A 10-year review of diagnosis and management. *Int J Paediatr Otorhinolaryngol* 2001;**57**(3):213–8.

Schwartz B, Marcy SM, Phillips WR, et al. Pharyngitis: Principles of judicious use of antimicrobial agents. *Paediatrics* 1998;**101**(1):171–4.

Schwartz SS, Rosivack RG, Michelotti P. A child's sleeping habit as a cause of nursing caries. *J Dentistry Child* 1993;**60** (1):22–5.

Sharma HS, Kurl DN, Hamzah M. Retropharyngeal abscess: Recent trends. *Auris, Nasus, Larynx* 1998;**25**(4):403–6.

Spruance SL, Stewart JC, Rowe NH, et al. Acyclovir cream for treatment of herpes simplex labialis: Results of two randomized, double-blind, vehicle-controlled, multicenter clinical trials. *Antimicrob Agents Chemother* 2002;**46**(7): 2238–43.

Tsevat J, Kotagal UR. Management of sore throats in children: A cost-effectiveness analysis. *Arch Paediatr Adolesc Med* 1999;**153**(7):681–8 [comment].

Unkel JH, Mckibben DH, Fenton SJ, et al. Comparison of odontogenic and nonodontogenic facial cellulitis in a paediatric hospital population. *Paediatr Dentistry* 1997;**19** (8):476–9.

van Everdingen T, Eijkman MA, Hoogstraten J. Parents and nursing-bottle caries. *J Dentistry Child* 1996;**63**(4): 271–4.

Wilson S, Smith GA, Preisch J, Casamassimo PS. Nontraumatic dental emergencies in a paediatric emergency department. *Clin Paediatr* 1997;**36**(6):333–7.

Windfuhr JP, Chen YS. Hemorrhage following paediatric tonsillectomy before puberty. *Int J Paediatr Otorhinolaryngol* 2001;**58**(3):197–204.

14.4 Retropharyngeal abscess

James Tilleard

ESSENTIALS

1 The potential for airway compromise and other complications mandates early diagnosis and treatment.

2 Retropharyngeal abscess should be suspected in children with sore throat, neck pain, fever, dysphagia, dysphonia, neck swelling or torticollis.

3 The differential diagnosis includes meningitis and epiglottitis.

4 Antibiotics must be initiated early.

5 Patients should be managed in an institution with appropriate paediatric medical, surgical, anaesthetic and intensive-care facilities.

Introduction

Retropharyngeal abscess is an uncommon condition with the potential for significant complications including airway compromise. Retropharyngeal abscess formation occurs in the space between the fascia covering the posterior pharyngeal wall and the prevertebral fascia. The related parapharyngeal abscess occurs in the deep neck space lateral to the pharynx containing the carotid sheath and cranial nerves.

Retropharyngeal abscess in the paediatric population is usually secondary to upper respiratory tract infection and suppuration in retropharyngeal lymph nodes. Other causes include infection following trauma, foreign body ingestion or dental problems. While abscess formation may occur at any age, the peak incidence is in children aged less than 6 years.

The most common causative organisms are group A β-haemolytic streptococci and *Staphylococcus aureus*. Anaerobes, especially *Bacteroides*, Gram-negative and mixed infections also occur.

History

Children with retropharyngeal abscess may present with a history of recent upper respiratory tract infection, fever, neck pain, sore throat, dysphagia, poor oral intake, trauma or other infective focus of the head and neck.

Examination

Examination may reveal fever, a neck mass, lymphadenopathy, limitation of neck extension, torticollis, dysphonia or bulging of the pharyngeal wall. There may be evidence of complications, including respiratory compromise, dehydration or spread of infection.

Investigations

Computerised tomography (CT) scanning is the investigation of choice. It is essential to ensure the patient is stable and safe for this procedure, with special attention to the airway. The CT result will assist with diagnosis and the differentiation of cellulitis from abscess formation which is essential in determining the need for surgery.

Lateral soft tissue neck X-ray may reveal prevertebral swelling, gas, foreign body, air fluid level or bony erosion but is not sensitive or specific. Both magnetic resonance imaging and ultrasound have also been used. A chest X-ray may reveal evidence of aspiration or mediastinitis.

Laboratory studies typically reveal an elevation of white blood cell count and inflammatory markers. Microbiology specimens, including blood cultures and culture of pus obtained at the time of surgery, are important in guiding subsequent antibiotic therapy.

Treatment

The initial priority in treatment is to ensure an adequate and stable airway. The potential for upper airway obstruction and a difficult intubation should be planned for. Consideration should be given to performing intubation in the operating theatre with both anaesthetic and surgical assistance available.

Once resuscitation is complete, antibiotics must be commenced as soon as possible. Empiric treatment must cover the most likely causative organisms and account for possible resistance. Antibiotic combinations include a third-generation cephalosporin, flucloxacillin and metronidazole. Clindamycin, penicillin, vancomycin and ticarcillin + clavulanate are also considered in some references. Attention must also given to analgesic needs, fluid and metabolic resuscitation. Complications should be excluded and these include airway compromise, septic shock, aspiration, mediastinitis, septic emboli, osteomyelitis and involvement of vessels or cranial nerves.

Controversies and future directions

Current debate centres on the need for surgery or initial medical treatment with antibiotics and close observation.

Further reading

Brook I. Microbiology and management of peritonsillar, retropharyngeal and parapharyngeal abscess. *J Oral Maxillofacial Surg* 2004;**62**(12):1545–50.

Cmejrek RC, Coticchia JM, Arnold JE. Presentation, diagnosis and management of deep-neck abscesses in infants. *Arch Otolaryngol-Head Neck Surg* 2002;**128**(12):1361–4.

Craig FW, Schunk JE. Retropharyngeal abscess in children: Clinical presentation, utility of imaging and current management. *Paediatrics* 2003;**111**(6):1394–8.

Dawes LC, Bova R, Carter P. Retropharyngeal abscess in children. *ANZ J Surg* 2002;**72**(6):417.

Shefelbine SE, Mancuso AA, Gajewski BJ, et al. Paediatric retropharyngeal lymphadenitis: differentiation from retropharyngeal abscess and treatment implications. *Otolaryngol Head Neck Surg* 2007;**136**(2):182–8.

ESSENTIALS

Nasal foreign bodies

1 Foreign body removal from the nasal passage requires good preparation and lighting.

2 The appropriate method of removal depends upon the type of object and its location.

Aural foreign bodies

1 Foreign bodies in the medial two-thirds of the ear canal are difficult to remove and frequently require sedation or general anaesthesia.

Caustic ingestion

1 Caustic ingestion is usually accidental in children.

2 The children are often asymptomatic and are at minimal risk of complications such as stricture.

3 Airway management is the priority in resuscitation.

4 There is no proven treatment to prevent stricture formation.

Nasal foreign bodies

Introduction

Nasal foreign bodies are a relatively common presentation to a paediatric emergency department (ED), although there is little published literature on the subject. They are not life threatening, but can cause significant morbidity.

History

Nasal foreign bodies predominantly present in children from 2 to 5 years of age. Children with nasal foreign bodies are usually brought in within 24 hours of insertion/impaction. Delayed presentation is mostly with unilateral purulent nasal discharge, which is usually offensive. Other possible symptoms include foul breath, nasal pain, sneezing, snoring and mouth breathing.

Examination

The type of foreign body is extremely variable, although it is most commonly a plastic toy or bead. The foreign body is usually readily visible.

Investigations

Investigations are not usually required. Imaging is usually indicated for other possible causes such as tumour.

Treatment

Except for button batteries (see also Chapter 7.6), removal of the foreign body is not urgent. Most foreign bodies can be successfully removed in the ED with adequate preparation and planning. Prior to the attempted removal, use of a topical anaesthetic nasal spray, such as lidocaine + phenylephrine, is recommended. Sedation and/or appropriate restraint of the child may be required. A good light source and an assistant to hold the child's head still are essential.

The appropriate procedure for removal will depend upon the foreign body size, shape, consistency and location in the nares. These include:

- Right-angle hooked probes can be passed alongside and past larger objects, rotated and then drawn back gradually, removing the object.
- Forceps (alligator or bayonet) are useful for smaller objects near the anterior nares.
- Positive pressure ventilation using bag–valve–mask is effective, particularly for larger objects that occlude the nasal cavity. An alternative to a bag–valve–mask is for the parent to blow into the child's mouth with their own. Air is 'bagged' or blown rapidly through the mouth while the unaffected nostril is occluded with a finger. The high pressure generated in the upper airway expels the foreign body from the nose. There is an unreported theoretical risk of barotrauma.
- Suction catheters can be used. Generally a soft, pliable end is required, and this can be made up using soft tubing, although commercially available kits are now available.
- A balloon catheter can be used if passed beyond the foreign body, inflated and drawn back.
- Application of cyanoacrylate glue via a wooden swab stick or similar is described, but requires patience and a very steady hand. It may adhere to the mucosa.

General anaesthesia and removal by ear, nose and throat (ENT) staff is required for the failed removal and the unco-operative child.

Complications

Possible complications include epistaxis, local and more widespread infection. Uncommonly, septal perforation has occurred secondary to a button battery. Mucosal injury may occur within hours.

Aural foreign bodies

Introduction

Aural foreign bodies in children are also a relatively common presentation to EDs. Again morbidity can be significant.

History

A greater proportion of children present beyond 24 hours from insertion compared with nasal foreign bodies and in many cases the time frame may not be determined. It may be a result of the event being witnessed, reported by the child due to irritation or pain, or as an incidental finding. The object may have been placed due to existing ear canal irritation due to wax impaction or otitis. Live insects are a common finding, and may result in marked discomfort.

Examination

Visualisation of the foreign body is usually by otoscopy. The type and location of the object has a significant role in the difficulty of removal.

Investigation

Investigations are not indicated.

Treatment

Removal of foreign bodies from the lateral one-third of the external auditory canal is much easier and more successful than from the medial two-thirds. The latter is the osseous portion and is narrower, more vascular and very tender. Therefore removal is more likely to require sedation or general anaesthesia and ENT expertise.

- Appropriate, restraint of the child and a good light source are always necessary;
- Sedation may have a role in some children;
- Choice of method of removal will depend upon the object and its location;
- Irrigation is the simplest method, but is contraindicated if there is a tympanic perforation, or for soft objects or vegetable matter that may swell;
- Suction via a small catheter;
- Forceps – alligator, Hartmann;
- A right-angled hook passed beyond the object and pulled out.

Button batteries are again a risk (see also Chapter 7.6), causing necrosis of the ear canal or tympanic membrane and should be removed as soon as possible. A live insect should be killed or immobilised with microscopic immersion oil, mineral oil or local anaesthetic solutions (2% lidocaine). It can then be removed using irrigation or forceps. Putty is often very difficult to remove and may require otomicroscopic removal. Sharp objects also usually require ENT removal.

Failure to remove in the ED will require ENT referral. Inspection following removal is advised to ensure there is no persisting foreign body and to assess for trauma or inflammation. Aural antibiotic drops with steroid are often recommended, particularly if there is evidence of trauma or inflammation.

Complications

Trauma to the ear canal is common as a result of the foreign body and/or its removal. More seriously, trauma to the tympanic membrane or ossicles can occur. Otitis externa can occur as a result of trauma.

Caustic ingestion

Introduction

Caustic ingestion in children is an uncommon presentation and significant injury with stricture formation is rare because the volume ingested is usually small. The ingested agents are variable and include alkalis (more common) and acids in liquid, granule or solid form. The likelihood of significant injury is dependent upon how alkali or acidic the agent is (i.e. its pH). Strong liquid alkali is particularly dangerous.

History

In children, in contrast to adults, ingestion is largely accidental and, as a result, significant injury far less common. Most cases occur in children less than 3 years of age and, like accidents in general, occur in boys more frequently than girls. Most ingestions occur at the home of the child. The most common alkali agent ingested is dishwasher detergent and commonest acidic agent is acetic acid. Button batteries have a significant corrosive and burn risk if lodged or impacted in the oesophagus (see Chapter 7.6).

Many children are asymptomatic. If they do occur, symptoms include vomiting, drooling, pain on swallowing and dysphagia, chest pain and refusal to drink. Less commonly, stridor may occur secondary to upper airway burns and obstruction.

In one series, the most predictive symptoms of significant injury and scar formation were prolonged drooling and dysphagia (100% sensitivity and 91% specificity). In another, haematemesis and respiratory distress were always associated with severe injury.

Examination

Many children will have normal examination findings, but oral burns may be demonstrated by inflammation, oedema or white areas. In at least half of these, that will be the limit of injury. Occasionally, significant burns occur beyond an unaffected oral cavity.

Investigations

Chest X-ray has demonstrated pulmonary irritation in up to 13% in some series. However, there is evidence that radiological investigations have little impact upon management and therefore cannot be recommended routinely, except to localise a button battery.

Oesophagoscopy may be performed according to symptoms, particularly ongoing drooling and dysphagia, vomiting/haematemesis and stridor. The type of caustic substance, its form and pH should be considered.

Treatment

Resuscitation, involving airway and breathing management, is the priority in severely affected cases. Upper airway obstruction may warrant intubation. However, there is a case report of successful use of nebulised adrenaline (epinephrine) for acute marked stridor following hypochlorite ingestion.

Dilution using water or milk may be useful for solid or granule ingestions. Children who remain asymptomatic may be discharged. Button batteries should be removed endoscopically, followed by a period of observation.

There is no proven effective treatment for oesophageal burns, especially in the prevention of stricture development. Antibiotics and corticosteroids have been commonly used, but have not been shown to be of any value.

Complications

Stricture formation is rare and, in a combination of nine series giving a total of 1961 children who had caustic ingestions, occurred in only 3.2%. This was despite a mean incidence of oesophageal burns of 21.4% and of deep burns of 4.7%. Upper airway obstruction has been mentioned and is potentially life threatening.

Prevention

Labelling, formulation, and child-proof containers and caps, have proved effective in prevention, when legislated. Storage of strong caustics should be in locked cupboards or similar, and handling should occur out of the reach of children. More hazardous caustics are available in developing countries and severe injury occurs more frequently.

Controversies

In caustic ingestion, acute oesophagoscopy has been advocated as critical to the early diagnosis and management of burns. This may help assess severity of injury and likelihood of stricture formation. However, as there is no clearly effective treatment and stricture formation is uncommon, it is difficult to recommend this routinely.

Further reading

Anderson KD, Rouse TM, Randolph JG. A controlled trial of corticosteroids in children with corrosive injury of the esophagus. *N Engl J Med* 1990;**323**(10):637–40 [comment].

Ansley JF, Cunningham MJ. Treatment of aural foreign bodies in children. *Pediatrics* 1998;**101**(4):638–41.

Christesen HB. Epidemiology and prevention of caustic ingestion in children. *Acta Paediatr* 1994;**83**(2):212–5.

Cox RJ. Foreign bodies, nose. eMedicine 2001.

de Jong AL, MacDonald R, Ein S, et al. Corrosive esophagitis in children: A 30-year review. *Int J Pediatr Otorhinolaryngol* 2001;**57**(3):203–11.

Karnak I, Tanyei FC, Buyukpamukou N, et al. Pulmonary effects of household bleach ingestion in children. *Clin Pediatr* 1996;**35**(9):471–2.

Kiristioglu I, Gurpinar A, Kilic N, et al. Is it necessary to perform an endoscopy after the ingestion of liquid household bleach in children? *Acta Paediatr* 1999;**88**(2):233–4.

Lamireau T, Rebouissoux L, Denis D, et al. Accidental caustic ingestion in children: Is endoscopy always mandatory? *J Pediatr Gastroenterol Nutr* 2001;**33**(1):81–4.

Lovejoy FH Jr, Woolf AD. Corrosive ingestions. *Pediatr Rev* 1995;**16**(12):473–4.

Mantooth R. Foreign bodies, ear. eMedicine 2001.

Nuutinen M, Uhari M, Karvali T, Kouvalainen K. Consequences of caustic ingestions in children. *Acta Paediatr* 2001;**83**(11):1200–5.

Samad L, Ali M, Ramzi H. Button battery ingestion: Hazards of esophageal impaction. *J Pediatr Surg* 1999;**34**(10):1527–31.

Tong MC, Ying SY, van Hasselt CA. Nasal foreign bodies in children. *Int J Pediatr Otorhinolaryngol* 1996;**35**(3):207–11.

Ziegler DS, Bent GP. Upper airway obstruction induced by a caustic substance found responsive to nebulised adrenaline. *J Paediatr Child Health* 2001;**37**(5):524–5.

OBSTETRICS AND GYNAECOLOGY

Section editor **Jeremy Raftos**

15.1 Paediatric gynaecology

Pamela Rosengarten • Sonia Grover

ESSENTIALS

Prepubescent girls

1 Vaginal examination is inappropriate in paediatric patients and usually provides little information. Ultrasound may provide further information or, if necessary, an examination under anaesthesia (EUA) is more appropriate.

2 Vulvovaginitis is the most common gynaecological problem in prepubertal girls and in most cases a specific infectious cause cannot be identified.

3 Vaginal bleeding in the prepubertal female is abnormal after 3–4 weeks of age.

Adolescents

1 Laboratory confirmation is required to make an accurate diagnosis of a vaginal discharge.

2 Pregnancy-related conditions need to be considered for all adolescents with pelvic pain or abnormal vaginal bleeding.

3 Abnormal vaginal bleeding may be secondary to an underlying haematological condition.

PREPUBESCENT GYNAECOLOGY

Vaginal discharge

Introduction

Vaginal discharge in neonates and prepubertal girls can be physiological. In neonates, a white mucoid vaginal discharge is present in most baby girls and is due to the effects of maternal oestrogens; it disappears by about 3 months of age. The second period where physiological discharge may occur is at the time ovarian activity commences with the onset of puberty.

Other conditions that cause vaginal discharge in the prepubertal girl include vulvovaginitis, lichen sclerosis, foreign body, eczema and pinworms.

Vulvovaginitis

This is the most common gynaecological problem in childhood, usually occurring in girls aged between 2 years and prior to the onset of puberty.[1,2] Most vulvovaginitis in this age group is non-infectious in origin and results from irritation of the vaginal and vulval skin, particularly where there is contact between the labial surfaces.[2,3] Factors that contribute to genital inflammation include the vaginal and vulval skin of children being thin and atrophic due to low oestrogens and therefore easily irritated. In addition, lack of protective labial hair and fat pads as well as moisture from wet swimming costumes, obesity and poor hygiene may play a role.[2–4] Additionally, the presence of bowel flora, which is the normal flora in the atrophic vagina, may contribute to skin irritation and the other related common symptom of offensive smell.

Infectious vulvovaginitis is less common and is due to an overgrowth of one organism, for example Group A *Streptococcus*, *Staphylococcus*, enterococci and *Escherichia coli*. In this instance, profuse discharge is usually present with marked skin inflammation, often beyond the contact surfaces of the labia.[3] Isolation of an organism that has strong sexual transmission, such as *Neisseria gonorrhoeae* or *Chlamydia trachomatis*, generally indicates sexual abuse or sexual activity and therefore warrants further investigation.[3,4]

Lichen sclerosis is an uncommon condition of unknown aetiology. It may present in childhood with vulval irritation, pruritus, dysuria or bleeding.[1,2] Examination reveals pale atrophic patches on the labia and perineum. The patches can be extensive and coalesce, and with scratching lead to chronic inflammation and purpuric haemorrhage into the skin. The condition usually persists with intermittent exacerbations. Most resolve before puberty although some may continue to have problems into adult life.[5]

Eczema may contribute to the symptoms of vulvovaginitis with the addition of itch. In these cases eczema is usually present elsewhere on the body and can be superimposed on the irritation due to the discharge.

Foreign bodies are a potential cause for a persistent, unresolving, often bloodstained offensive discharge.

Candida is very uncommon in the prepubertal girl unless there has been significant antibiotic use or they are still in nappies.[2,4] (Thrush thrives in an oestrogenised environment, not in the atrophic setting.) In this age group, recurrent or unexplained candida requires exclusion of diabetes mellitus or other causes of diminished immune function.

History

The child or parent/caregiver usually describe:

- an offensive vaginal discharge;
- erythema (redness)/irritation of the labia and perineal skin;
- itch, dysuria and urinary frequency may also be present.

These symptoms often fluctuate in severity.

A general medical history is required, with specific history of the symptoms and their duration including nature of discharge as well as any previous treatments. Also important is past history of urinary tract infection, encopresis, constipation, enuresis, the presence of skin disorders, and any other illness, including antibiotic use in the previous 4 weeks. Although a history of perineal hygiene (e.g. wipe front to back, frequency of bathing, type of underwear/clothes, specific irritants, such as bubble baths or use of feminine hygiene sprays in the adolescent population, etc.) should also be established, there is limited evidence to support the role of this in the pathogenesis of vulvovaginitis.[3] Where itch is the dominant symptom, pinworms should be considered and questions asked about family symptoms.

Although uncommon, the possibility of sexual abuse should always be considered in a child that presents with genital symptoms, and check for other signs that may be present including alterations in behaviour such as phobias, eating or sleeping disorders.

Examination

A general examination including sexual development is required. Perineal, vulval and introital examination may be required for the above conditions. Attempts must be made to ensure it is not a traumatic event for the child. The perineum is best examined either with the girl supine with heels together and knees flexed and hips abducted or in the lateral position with knees drawn up to the chest.[6] Vaginal examination is inappropriate in paediatric patients and usually provides little further information. Specific external examination of the perineum usually reveals mucoid discharge and reddened introitus, particularly on the contact surfaces between the labia.

The presence of a profuse discharge or marked skin inflammation, especially if it extends beyond the contact surfaces of the labia, suggests an infectious cause. An offensive discharge can occur with vulvovaginitis or foreign body. A bloody discharge can occur with vulvovaginitis (particularly with *Shigella* or Group A streptococci).[6] The presence of perianal excoriation suggests pinworm.

Investigations

Swabs are generally not required. If taken in mild cases, they usually reveal a growth of mixed coliforms.[3] If discharge is visible or profuse or marked erythema is present, introital swabs should be taken for culture. Vaginal swabs are painful and distressing and are not required.

If urinary symptoms are present, the urine (midstream urine; MSU) should be checked to exclude urinary tract infection. A pinworm test should be taken if itch is a prominent symptom. This requires briefly placing clear sticky tape on the perianal skin in the morning and viewing under a microscope for eggs. Otherwise worms may be seen in the perianal region at night.

Ultrasound may provide further information, especially if there is a possibility of foreign body, or if necessary an EUA may be more appropriate.

Management

Vulvovaginitis

Management consists of:

❶ Explanation and reassurance.
❷ Toileting/hygiene advice:

- avoidance of potential irritants such as soaps and bubble baths and other causal factors, such as tight/synthetic clothing and wet bathers;
- vinegar (add one cup white vinegar in a shallow bath and soak) or the use of a simple barrier cream to the labial area (e.g. zinc-castor oil or nappy rash cream) or both.

Rarely, if the problem persists, further action may be required. The natural history of vulvovaginitis is for recurrences to occur up until the age when oestrogenisation begins. If a primary bacterial cause is suspected, cultures should be taken and treatment commenced with the appropriate antibiotics, e.g. initial amoxicillin, and adjusted when culture results are available.

Where itch is a dominant symptom consider:

- Pinworms, especially if perianal excoriation is present, and treat the child and their family with pyrantel 10 mg kg^{-1} (maximum 500 mg) orally or mebendazole 50 mg ($<$10 kg), 100 mg ($>$ 10 kg) orally (contraindicated in pregnancy and $<$6 months of age) as a stat. dose and repeat 2 weeks later.[7]
- Lichen sclerosis in the asymptomatic patient does not require treatment other than
- reassurance. In symptomatic patients, avoidance of irritants, improved hygiene, reduced trauma and barrier ointments, e.g. nappy rash creams. In more severe cases, a brief course of topical steroid (1% hydrocortisone) and referral to a dermatologist or paediatric gynaecologist is required.
- Eczema, especially if skin disease is present elsewhere. Combined treatment of the vulvovaginitis (as above) and hydrocortisone or Diprosone may be indicated.

Foreign body

If foreign body is suspected then an examination under anaesthesia with vaginoscopy is usually required. If the presence of a foreign body is questionable then an ultrasound may be beneficial to visualise the object. The most common foreign bodies are tiny pieces of tissue paper. The possibility of sexual abuse should be borne in mind.

Vaginal bleeding

Introduction

Vaginal bleeding in the prepubertal child is abnormal after 3–4 weeks of age.[6]

Causes of vaginal bleeding in the prepubertal girl can be classed as hormonal and non-hormonal.

Hormonal causes

Neonates A withdrawal bleed from maternal oestrogens is common and does not require investigation or treatment. This will cease after approximately 4 weeks of age.

Onset of menstruation Consider as premature (precocious puberty) if this occurs at less than 8 years of age.[7]

Non-hormonal causes

Vulvovaginitis In prepubescent girls, vaginal bleeding in this age group is most commonly due to more severe vulvovaginitis (the most common pathogens are *Shigella* or Group A β-haemolytic streptococci).[6] The discharge is brown and often offensive (see above under vaginal discharge, vulvovaginitis).

Trauma Accidental injury usually results from straddle injuries where the girl falls on a narrow object (e.g. bicycle cross bar, jungle gym). Non-accidental injury/sexual abuse should be considered in trauma, especially where there is a hymenal tear without a history of accidental penetrating injury.

Foreign body Vaginal foreign body may also result in bloodstained discharge and should be considered if no infectious cause is identified or there is failure to respond to appropriate treatment. In bleeding secondary to excoriation from pinworms, lichen sclerosis or eczema, examination should demonstrate eczema and lichen sclerosis. The presence of anal and perineal excoriation suggests pinworms and treatment as previously described under vulvovaginitis.

Tumours Although rare, the possibility of a genital tumour should be considered when there is chronic genital ulceration, non-traumatic swelling, tissue protruding from the vagina or foul smelling, bloody, vaginal discharge. Vaginal bleeding associated with genital enlargement, premature sexual maturation or virilisation may be associated with hormonally active ovarian or adrenal tumour.

Non-vaginal causes of bleeding

Haematuria may stain the underwear or nappy and be reported as vaginal bleeding. This will become evident upon urinalysis. Urethral prolapse often presents with bleeding thought to be vaginal in origin. The peak age is 5–8 years. Bleeding disorders are an uncommon cause of vaginal bleeding but should be considered when there are other systemic signs of a bleeding tendency, e.g. bruising and petechiae.

History

A general medical history including family and past history should be taken.

The history of vaginal bleeding should focus on the amount and circumstances of bleeding, the times of recurrences and the presence of associated pain. A history regarding any perineal trauma should be elicited as well as the possibility of a foreign body. Other medical disorders and symptoms of blood dyscrasias, such as epistaxis and bruising should also be noted.

Examination

Vital signs and haemodynamic stability should be established. General examination, including sexual development, should be performed. On examination, excessive bruising or petechiae and generalised skin disorders, such as eczema, should be noted.

Specific examination requires abdominal and vulval/perineal examination. Abdominal examination should note abdominal tenderness and the presence of a mass. Perineal examination should note the presence of vulvovaginitis, other skin disorders, such as eczema, or traumatic injury.

The common perineal injuries in trauma are bruising/haematoma of vulva and periclitoral folds and superficial lacerations of the labia minora and periurethral tissue. If a hymenal tear is present, a history of penetrating injury, e.g. broom handle or bed post should be sought. If there is no history of penetrating trauma then sexual abuse needs to be considered.

A foreign body in the vagina may be evident on examination of the perineum.

A urethral prolapse will be evident on examination of the perineum as a friable, red-blue (doughnut-shaped) annular mass.

Investigations

Full blood examination should be performed if the child appears clinically anaemic or bleeding has been prolonged. Coagulation studies may be indicated. Perineal swabs should be taken for microscopy and culture where there is evidence of severe vulvovaginitis.

In trauma, where there is a history of penetrating injury or where it is not possible to perform adequate perineal examination, an examination under anaesthesia is required. Midstream urine for micro and culture should also be performed where haematuria is present.

In the child less than 8 years of age who has signs of puberty evident, referral to a paediatric endocrinologist or gynaecologist is required.

Management

Trauma

A warm bath several times a day to help voiding as well as assist in keeping the perineum clean is all that is required. The girl may find voiding in a bath more comfortable. Antibiotics are rarely required. Examination under anaesthesia is only required if there is persistent bleeding, uncertain origin of bleeding, massive bruising or history of a fall on a potentially penetrating object. Suspected sexual abuse must be referred.

Urethral prolapse

The management is conservative as long as voiding is normal. Warm baths may be of assistance. Topical oestrogen cream assists in the resolution.

Labial adhesions

Labial adhesions are seen in infancy, and usually resolve by about 8 years, although they may occasionally persist through to puberty when they will resolve around the time of menarche. The adhesion is not congenital, but it is acquired from a secondary adherence of the atrophic surfaces of the labia minora, presumably as a result of irritation.[1,2]

Labial adhesions are usually asymptomatic in children and do not need to be divided as long as the child is able to void. When symptoms occur they usually relate to difficulty with urination or pooling of urine behind fused labia, which results in irritation.[1,2,5] Urinary tract infections are seldom a complication.[5] Parents should be reassured that separation of the labia will occur when oestrogenisation commences as the child grows. Although it is possible to divide the adhesions with lateral traction this is frequently distressing for the child and the parents, and unnecessary. There is a considerable recurrence rate after this approach.[5]

The use of topical oestrogen cream is likewise unnecessary, and is associated with significant failure and recurrence rates, but may occasionally be indicated when catheterisation is required for a micturating cystoureterogram.

Associated nappy rash or vulvovaginitis is managed as described above.

Distressing vaginal or perineal pain

Severe perineal or vaginal pain, often described as a vaginal shooting pain that is very distressing, is reported in the prepubertal girl. It predominantly occurs in the evening – waking from sleep. The likely cause for this is pinworms (Enterobius vermicularis). The worms, usually found in the perianal region, can become 'lost' within the vagina. When they crawl onto the thin atrophic hymen in the prepubescent girl they cause the distressing pain. Treatment with mebendazole, with repeated treatments (usually ×3 at weekly intervals), is required to ensure clearance.

ADOLESCENT GYNAECOLOGY

Vaginal discharge

Introduction

Vaginal discharge in an adolescent female may be physiological, a symptom of vaginal or cervical infection or secondary to a vaginal foreign body. Under the influence of oestrogen there is an increase in the glycogen production by the vaginal epithelial cells, which supports the growth of lactobacilli in the vagina, which leads to lowering of the vaginal pH to 3.8–4.5. The acidic environment helps to inhibit the growth of bacteria seen in the prepubertal female. Oestrogen also influences the cervix, resulting in increased mucous production, which is largely responsible for the physiological vaginal discharge.[8]

Vaginal infections include candidiasis, bacterial vaginosis and trichomoniasis, with only the latter being sexually transmitted. Chlamydia and gonorrhoea are sexually transmitted infections of the cervix and/or the upper genital tract, which may also result in a vaginal discharge.

History

Diagnosis can often be suspected from the history and the appearance of the discharge.

- *Candida* infections typically present as a cheesy white discharge and are associated with vulval and vaginal itching, dysuria or superficial dyspareunia in sexually active girls. They are commonly associated with antibiotic use, stress and diabetes mellitus.
- Bacterial vaginosis generally presents as a homogenous white discharge associated with a fishy odour. Symptoms of vaginal irritation are uncommon.
- Trichomoniasis is a sexually transmitted infection (STI) and typically presents with a frothy, green vaginal discharge.
- *Chlamydia* and gonorrhoea infections may present as vaginal discharge, intermenstrual or post-coital bleeding, urethritis or pelvic inflammatory disease (PID). *Chlamydia* and gonorrhoea may also be identified incidentally due to the high incidence of asymptomatic infections. The presence of lower abdominal pain and/or dyspareunia in the history increases the likelihood of PID, with a positive and negative predictive value of 17% and 100% respectively.[9] STIs may be contracted by oral or digital contact and do not necessarily require penetrative intercourse for transmission.
- The most common vaginal foreign body in adolescent girls is a retained tampon. The presenting symptom is often a malodorous discharge.

Examination

Inspection of the external genitalia should be performed, specifically looking for evidence of warts, herpetic lesions, the nature of the discharge and evidence of excoriation.

Adolescent girls who have never been sexually active and/or who have not used tampons should not be examined internally. If there is a suspicion of a vaginal foreign body, vaginal trauma or PID in a girl who is sexually active or uses tampons, a gentle vaginal examination may be considered. However, even sexually experienced girls may be unable to proceed with the examination and alternative forms of assessment may need to be considered.

Investigations

Microscopy, culture and wet-preparation analysis of a vaginal discharge will help to confirm the diagnosis of candidiasis, bacterial vaginosis and trichomoniasis.

The gold standard for diagnosis of both *Chlamydia* and gonorrhoea is culture from a cervical sample. However, both infections can readily be detected with a high degree of sensitivity using a molecular replication technique (either PCR or LCR) performed on samples collected from either the cervix or a first-catch urine.

Management

- *Candida albicans* is the most common cause of vaginal thrush. One treatment option is clotrimazole 10% cream inserted vaginally as a single dose at night. An alternative, if the patient, is intolerant of topical therapy and not pregnant, is fluconazole 150 mg orally as a single dose.[10]
- Bacterial vaginosis should be treated in symptomatic patients and in those at high risk of acquiring other STIs. Oral metronidazole 400 mg bd for 5 days is recommended in non-pregnant patients.[10]
- Trichomoniasis can be treated with oral metronidazole 2 g orally as a single dose.[10]
- *Chlamydia* treatment is with either a 7-day course of doxycycline (100 mg bd) or a single oral dose of 1 g azithromycin.[10]
- Gonorrhoea has developed resistance to a number of antibiotics and therefore treatment should be based on local sensitivities. In urban Australia a single dose of 250 mg ceftriaxone intramuscularly in combination with

cover for *Chlamydia* is currently recommended.[10]

- A retained tampon can generally be removed in the ED. However, occasionally the swollen tampon cannot be extracted due to a hymenal ring and removal under general anaesthesia is required. If the tampon is removed in the ED it should be immediately placed into a container of water to limit exposure to the often offensive odour.

Disposition

Adolescents with a sexually transmitted infection should have a follow-up communicable disease consultation to discuss prevention of further STIs. Ongoing contraception and contact tracing should also be addressed.

Gonorrhoea and *Chlamydia* are notifiable diseases in some Australian states.

Abnormal vaginal bleeding

Introduction

Abnormal vaginal bleeding may be caused by a complication of pregnancy, trauma, infection or it may be secondary to contraceptive use. The most common causes of heavy vaginal bleeding are anovulatory bleeding or an underlying haematological condition.[11]

Menstrual cycles in adolescents are often anovulatory due to the gradual maturation of the hypothalamic–pituitary–ovarian axis, which can take up to 5 years after the menarche.[11–14] Anovulatory or dysfunctional uterine bleeding generally presents as irregular, often heavy, blood loss. Anovulatory bleeding may result from a relative deficiency of either oestrogen or progesterone. Relative oestrogen deficiency is more common in thin young women who have just commenced their menstrual cycles. The relative oestrogen deficiency results in a thin, atrophic endometrium, which can bleed profusely.

In girls with higher endogenous oestrogen levels, anovulatory menstrual cycles are more likely to result in a relative progesterone deficiency due to failure of the luteal phase. In this case the unopposed oestrogen results in thickening of the endometrial lining, which can bleed erratically.

Menorrhagia, whether associated with ovulatory or anovulatory cycles, may be a marker of systemic illness. Up to 20% of patients admitted with menorrhagia have been found to have an underlying haematological disease, the most common of which is a coagulopathy, half of which are von Willebrand's disease and the other half due to platelet problems or dysfunction – other factor deficiencies are very rare.[11,14]

Chronic untreated menorrhagia may also present with signs and symptoms of anaemia.

Examination

The haemodynamic status of the patient and the severity of the bleeding should be assessed. A general examination should be performed, particularly noting evidence of a haematological disorder or anaemia.

Investigations

A full blood count, iron studies and coagulation screen will assist in identifying anaemia, an underlying coagulopathy or haematological cause for the bleeding(although caution needs to be taken in interpreting these results as stress may result in apparent 'normalising' of the test results, particularly in von Willebrand's disease[11]). A pregnancy test should also be performed.

Ultrasound may be helpful when ovarian pathology is suspected and can sometimes be used to assess the thickness of the endometrium, although transabdominal views may be limited. An STI screen should be obtained if clinically indicated, as *Chlamydia* in particular can cause intermenstrual or heavy bleeding.

Dilation and curettage is very rarely indicated for a diagnosis and is not a recognised treatment for dysfunctional uterine bleeding.[15]

Management

Heavy bleeding, either acute or chronic, should be treated with fluid and blood products as clinically indicated.

Oestrogens and progestins are generally used in the management of anovulatory bleeding. Suggested regimens vary with respect to the route of administration, the dose and the type of hormone used. Currently there is no convincing evidence in favour of any particular regimen.[16]

For both the acute and non acute bleed tranexamic acid should be used. This can be used in combination with hormonal approaches. If using progestogens first line, regimens include oral norethisterone 5–10 mg every 2 hours for four doses, followed by 5 mg two to three times a day for 14 days.[8] Commencing the oral contraceptive pill once the bleeding has ceased may be sensible, as cessation of the progestogens will almost invariably result in bleeding recommencing.

Alternatively, treatment may include oral conjugated oestrogens 0.625–1.25 mg every 4–6 hours or oral oestradiol 1–2 mg every 4–6 hours until the bleeding stops, which is usually about 24 hours. The dose is then reduced to once or twice daily. Intravenous conjugated oestrogens are no longer available in Australia and have been associated with thromboembolic complications, consequently oral regimens are generally preferred.[17] This approach is worth taking when progestogens have already been used and failed, but can be used first line. Again, the oral contraceptive pill should be commenced for ongoing control, particularly if there is a need to allow some time before further menses in the context of a low haemoglobin. Supplement with iron therapy.

Menorrhagia, in the absence of a coagulation disorder or other underlying pathology, can be treated with non-steroidal anti-inflammatory agents or tranexamic acid, which reduce the menstrual loss by 33% and 50% respectively,[11,18] or, alternatively, low-dose oral contraceptive therapy.[12]

Disposition

The identification of a coagulation disorder will necessitate review by a haematologist. Pregnancy-related bleeding should be reviewed by an obstetrician/gynaecologist. Anovulatory bleeding and simple menorrhagia can be managed by either a primary care physician or a gynaecologist.

Pelvic pain

Introduction

The differential diagnosis of acute pelvic pain in an adolescent includes both gynaecological and non-gynaecological causes. Common gynaecological causes include pregnancy-related pain, dysmenorrhoea, ovulation pain (Mittelschmertz), ovarian cysts and their complications, torsion of the ovary, pelvic inflammatory disease

(PID), endometriosis and congenital uterine abnormalities, such as imperforate hymen.

History

A general gynaecological history should be taken, with particular note made of the relationship of the pain to the menstrual cycle. History should also include the nature of onset of the pain and a history of similar episodes. The pain of dysmenorrhoea, Mittelschmertz, endometriosis and imperforate hymen may be cyclical. However, they may also present during the first episode or as an unusually severe exacerbation. An ectopic pregnancy is not excluded by the history of a recent menstrual period.

- Primary dysmenorrhoea is common in the adolescent population; it refers to pain associated with menstruation in the absence of underlying pathology. The pain is generally described as crampy, occurring in the lower abdomen, often with radiation to the back or to the inner thighs. Associated features may include nausea, vomiting, diarrhoea, headache and syncope. The symptoms have been attributed, in part, to an increased release of, or increased sensitivity to, prostaglandins. The diagnosis is generally made on the basis of history and limited physical examination findings.
- Mittelschmertz is pelvic pain related to ovulation. The pain is generally dull in nature and located in either of the iliac fossae. The pain may last from a few hours to 2–3 days. The pathological basis of the pain is unclear but may be due either to distension of the capsule of the ovary prior to ovulation or to spillage of a small amount of follicular fluid at the time of ovulation.[8,19]
- Simple ovarian cysts are a normal physiological consequence of ovulation. They can be up to 6 cm in diameter. The pain may be from irritation of surrounding structures or stretching of the wall of the cyst. Corpus luteal cysts can reach up to 10 cm in size and may present as acute pain secondary to haemorrhage into the cyst. Both simple and corpus-luteal cysts can present as acute pain they rupture. Although uncommon, a ruptured corpus-luteal cyst may continue to bleed and be associated with significant

haemoperitoneum.[8] Bleeding disorders need to be considered if recurrent haemorrhagic cysts occur or a significant haemoperitoneum.

- Complex ovarian cysts include dermoid cysts, which are often asymptomatic but may cause local pressure symptoms.
- Ovarian torsion is an uncommon condition and is almost exclusively seen in association with ovarian pathology. The history is typically an acute onset of colicky iliac fossa pain, with the right being affected more than the left. There may be associated nausea, vomiting and a leucocytosis. Ultrasound has a high degree of sensitivity and specificity in making the diagnosis of an enlarged ovary – however, doppler studies are not necessarily conclusive and presence of flow does not exclude torsion.[20,21]
- Pelvic inflammatory disease can have a range of clinical presentations, depending on the location and the severity of the infection. The pain can range from mild to severe; systemic features of infection are not always present. Due to the significant complications associated with untreated PID, the isolated findings of adnexal, uterine or cervical motion tenderness in the young woman who is sexually active, for which no other cause can be found, have been suggested as a basis for the diagnosis and treatment of PID.[22]
- Endometriosis is reputed to cause a range of menstrual disorders and pain syndromes. However, the symptoms do not appear to correlate well with the degree of disease identified at laparoscopy. The diagnosis should be made with caution due to the risk of labelling a patient with what may be seen as a sentence for chronic pain and infertility.
- Congenital obstructive abnormalities include an imperforate hymen or obstruction of one side of a double uterine, cervical or vaginal system. An imperforate hymen may present as cyclical or irregular lower abdominal pain in a girl with well-developed secondary sexual characteristics and the absence of menstruation. Unilateral obstruction in a double system more typically presents with dysmenorrhoea that commences

several days after the onset of menses and persists beyond the end of the menstrual period.

Examination

Examination should include vital signs and abdominal examination. Pelvic examination can give additional information regarding the location of the pain and its relationship to pelvic organs. Uterine, adnexal or cervical motion tenderness should be sought if pelvic examination is performed. The identification of an adnexal mass is clinically imprecise. However, it should prompt consideration of such conditions as ovarian torsion, tubo-ovarian abscess or ectopic pregnancy.

Investigations

A pregnancy test and a pelvic ultrasound are the most valuable tests for excluding pregnancy-related conditions. Ultrasound is the investigation of choice for the definition of masses and in the identification of ovarian cysts.[23] If a congenital anomaly is suspected, information regarding the kidneys at the time of the ultrasound can be helpful.

Laparoscopy is reserved for pain that cannot be adequately explained or has failed to respond to appropriate treatments. Laparoscopy may be required to exclude torsion where a cyst is present combined with a suspicious history.[21] It may also have a role in the investigation of chronic pelvic pain.

Management

- Dysmenorrhoea will generally respond to antiprostaglandin agents, such as mefenamic acid 500 mg orally 8-hourly or ibuprofen 400 mg orally 8-hourly. The response is improved by commencing treatment prior to the onset of symptoms.[24] Lifestyle issues, such as increasing physical exercise and decreasing stress, may also improve symptoms.[25] For patients who fail to respond to treatment, combined oral contraceptive therapy is considered second-line therapy and further investigation, such as ultrasound and laparoscopy, may be considered to identify other pathology, for example significant endometriosis.[24]
- Mittelschmertz and simple ovarian cysts can often be treated by reassurance. However, if this is not adequate, simple analgesia and non-steroidal anti-

inflammatory drugs may be required. If the pain is recurrent then consideration should be given to the use of the combined oral contraceptive pill in an attempt to suppress ovulation. Failure of resolution of a cyst after 2 months or a simple cyst greater than 8 cm diameter may require surgical exploration.[8]

- Complex ovarian cysts, including dermoids and endometriomas, are generally treated surgically.
- Ovarian torsion requires urgent operative intervention with the aim to preserve ovarian tissue. [21]
- PID can be treated with either oral or parenteral antibiotics. However, there should be a low threshold for admission in adolescents.[26]

Disposition

Most forms of pelvic pain will require further management or investigation and should be referred accordingly.

Controversies

❶ The management of anovulatory vaginal bleeding.

❷ The diagnosis and management of ovarian torsion.

❸ The diagnostic criteria and optimal management of PID.

Acknowledgement

The contribution of Sheila Bryan as author in the first edition is hereby acknowledged.

References

1. Mroueh J, Muram D. Common problems in paediatric gynaecology: New developments. *Curr Opin Obstet Gynecol* 1999;**11**(5):463–6.
2. Fiorillo L. Therapy of paediatric genital diseases. *Dermatol Ther* 2004;**17**:117–28.
3. Jaquiery A, Styianopoulos A, Hogg G, Grover S. Vulvovaginitis: Clinical features, aetiology, and microbiology of the genital tract. *Arch Dis Child* 1999;**81**:64–7.
4. Farrington P. Paediatric vulvo-vaginitis. *Clin Obstet Gynaecol* 1997;**40**(1):135–40.
5. Fischer G. Vulval disease in pre-pubertal girls. *Australas J Dermatol* 2001;**42**:225–36.
6. Quint E. Vaginal bleeding and discharge in the paediatric and adolescent age groups. In: Pearlman M, Tintinalli J, editors. *Emergency care of the woman*. New York: McGraw-Hill; 1998. p. 395–407.
7. Grover S. Gynaecological conditions. In: Smart , editor. *Paediatric handbook*. 6th ed. Melbourne: Blackwell Science Asia; 2000. p. 342–50.
8. Mackay E, Beischer N, Pepperell R, Wood C. *Illustrated textbook of gynaecology*. 2nd ed. London: WB Saunders; 2000.
9. Blake DR, Fletcher K, Joshi N, Emans SJ. Identification of symptoms that indicate a pelvic examination is necessary to exclude PID in adolescent women. *J Paediatr Adolesc Gynaecol* 2003;**16**(1):25–30.
10. *Therapeutic Guidelines. Antibiotic Version 13.* Therapeutics Guidelines Ltd; 2006.
11. Grover S. Bleeding disorders and heavy menses in adolescents. *Curr Opin Obstet Gynecol* 2007;**19**: 415–9.
12. Sandofilippo JS, Lara-Torre E. Adolescent gynaecology. *Obstet Gynaecol* 2009;**113**:935–47.
13. Apter D, Viinikka L, Vihko R. Hormonal pattern of adolescent menstrual cycles. *J Clin Endocrinol Metab* 1978;**47**(5):944–54.
14. Claessens EA, Cowell CA. Acute adolescent menorrhagia. *Am J Obstet Gynecol* 1981;**139**(3): 277–80.
15. Duflos-Cohade C, Amandruz M, Thibaud E. Pubertal metrorrhagia. *J Paediatr Adolesc Gynaecol* 1996;**9** (1):16–20.
16. Hickey M, Higham J, Fraser IS. Progestogens versus oestrogens and progestogens for irregular uterine bleeding associated with anovulation. In: *Cochrane Review. The Cochrane Library.* Issue 3. Oxford: Update software; 2003.
17. Richlin SS, Rock JA. Abnormal uterine bleeding. In: Carpenter SEK, Rock JA, editors. *Paediatric and adolescent gynaecology.* 2nd ed. Philadelphia: Lippincott Williams & Wilkins; 2000. p. 207–24.
18. Prentice A. Fortnightly review: Medical management of menorrhagia. *Br Med J* 1999;**319**:1343–5.
19. Hann LE, Hall DA, Black EB, Ferrucci JT. Mittelschmerz. Sonographic demonstration. *JAMA* 1979;**241** (25):2731–2.
20. Ben-Ami M, Perlitz Y, Haddad S. The effectiveness of spectral and color Doppler in predicting ovarian torsion. A prospective stud. *Eur J Obstet Gynecol Reprod Biol* 2002;**104**(1):64–6.
21. Grover S. Pelvic pain in the female adolescent patient. *Aust Fam Phys* 2006;**35**(11):850–3.
22. Centers for Disease Control and Prevention. Sexually transmitted diseases treatment guidelines. *MMWR* 2002;**51**(NoRR-6):32–6, 69–71.
23. Arbel-Derowe Y, Tepper R, Rosen DJ, et al. The contribution of pelvic ultrasound to the diagnostic process in paediatric and adolescent gynaecology. *J Paediatr Adolesc Gynaecol* 1997;**10**: 3–12.
24. Sanfilippo J, Erb T. Evaluation and management of dysmenorrhoea in adolescents. *Clin Obstet Gynecol* 2008;**51**(2):257–67.
25. Bolton P, Del Mar C, O'Connor V. Exercise for primary dysmenorrhoea (Protocol for a Cochrane Review). In: *The Cochrane Library.* Issue 3, Oxford: Update Software; 2003.
26. Hemsel DL, Ledger WJ, Martens M, et al. Concerns regarding the Centers for Disease Control's published guidelines for pelvic inflammatory disease. *Clin Infect Dis* 2001;**32**:103–7.

15.2 Emergency contraception

Alastair D.McR. Meyer • Jacqueline E.L. Parkinson

ESSENTIALS

1 Emergency contraception (EC) should be made available to an adolescent who has had unprotected sexual intercourse within 72 hours prior to presentation, regardless of the stage of her menstrual cycle.

2 Pregnancy must be excluded by urinary β-HCG testing.

3 Commonly prescribed treatment is with levonorgestrel (LNE) EC, two 0.75 mg tablets, 12 hours apart.

4 Follow up is essential.

Introduction

Emergency contraception (EC) or post-coital contraception can be defined as preventing pregnancy after sexual intercourse. Every year over 3.5 million unintended pregnancies occur in the United States alone, mostly to teenage mothers. It is believed that half of these unintended pregnancies could be avoided by the judicious use of EC. Indications for the provision of EC are shown in Table 15.2.1.[1]

Many of these unintended pregnancies are later surgically terminated. Estimates of as many as 170 000 such terminations are performed in England and Wales annually.[2] These surgical terminations are not without clinical risk and cost, as well as being a major social, religious and political issue.

Clinical assessment

EC should be made available to an adolescent who has had unprotected sexual intercourse within 72 hours prior to presentation, regardless of the stage of her menstrual cycle. Pregnancy must be excluded by urinary β-human gonadotrophin hormone (β-HCG) testing.

Depending on the age of the young person, issues of child protection and consent to treatment may need to be explored.

Available medications

Historically, the Yuzpe method of EC was commonly practised in Australasia. This involved a high-dose oestrogen/progestogen preparation. Two doses of 100 mcg of ethinylestradiol combined with 500 mcg of levonorgestrel given 12 hours apart resulted in withdrawal bleeding within 21 days for 98% of women.[3]

Simple anti-emetics such as metoclopramide were routinely prescribed for nausea associated with the high oestrogen dose. This method of EC disrupted the natural hormone patterns necessary to sustain pregnancy. The high oestrogen and progestogen levels were believed to alter the endometrium, thereby preventing implantation. The fertilised ovum had implantation prevented by blocking oestrogen and progestogen receptors, which made the endometrium hostile to implantation. Endometrial biochemistry and glandular and stromal development were affected such that the environment was hostile to the fertilised ovum. The therapy therefore prevents implantation and can consequently be described as a contraceptive rather than an abortifacient.

In June 2002, levonorgestrel (LNE) became the first drug licensed for use in Australia specifically as an EC agent. The first dose of 0.75 mg LNE is taken as soon as possible after unprotected sexual intercourse. This dose is repeated 12 hours later.

While the precise mechanism by which LNE prevents pregnancy is not clear, it is believed to work by preventing ovulation and by altering the tubal transport of sperm and ova. Fertilisation is thus prevented. When used within 72 hours of unprotected sexual intercourse, LNE EC prevents 85% of expected pregnancies. Efficacy falls with time (Table 15.2.2).

LNE EC is contraindicated in unexplained vaginal bleeding, current breast cancer and pregnancy. Care should be taken with patients taking anticoagulants. Adverse reactions include fatigue, abdominal pain, gastrointestinal discomfort, dizziness, headache, breast tenderness and vaginal bleeding. LNE is primarily metabolised in the liver.

Conditions regarded as relative contraindications include: severe hypertension; diabetes with nephropathy; retinopathy; neuropathy; ischaemic heart disease; and past history of breast cancer.

LNE contraception has fewer side effects than the traditional Yuzpe method. Only 20% of patients experience nausea, which usually responds to standard anti-emetics. LNE EC results in 60% of women commencing their next menstruation within 3 days of their expected date. Fifteen percent of women can be up to 7 days late with their period. It is essential that women have pregnancy testing if their period is more than 7 days late.[6]

If unprotected sexual intercourse has occurred more than 72 hours but less than 5 days before presentation, insertion of a

---

Table 15.2.1 Indication for providing EC

- Unprotected intercourse
- Barrier contraception failure
- Intrauterine contraceptive device (IUCD) expulsion
- Missed contraceptive pills
- Sexual assault

Table 15.2.2 Efficacy of LNE EC[4,5]

Hours post-coital	Pregnancies prevented (%)
<24	95
24–48	85
49–72	58

copper-based intrauterine contraceptive device (IUCD) should occur. These devices prevent implantation. IUCDs should be inserted in consultation with the gynaecology service.

If inserted up to 5 days after predicted ovulation, IUCDs can prevent 99% of expected pregnancies.[5] Relative contraindications are nulliparity and patients who are at high risk of sexually transmitted infection.

All women presenting to EDs following unprotected sexual intercourse should be counselled regarding sexually transmitted infections, ongoing contraception and the need for follow up.

Controversies

❶ Is the ED an appropriate site for dispensing EC, as these patients are essentially well?

❷ There may be a place for non-medical providers of the EC, given its safety.

❸ The place of follow-up termination, should EC fail, is important to consider.

All patients receiving EC from EDs must have clear follow-up arrangements made. The patient's usual doctor or the hospital female health clinic are the most appropriate facilities.

References

1. Trussel J, Stewart F, Guest F, et al. Emergency contraceptive pills. Simple proposal to reduce unintended pregnancies. *Family Planning and Prevention* 1992;**24**:269–73.
2. Anonymous. Hormonal emergency contraception. *Drug Ther Bull* 1993;**31**(7):27–8.
3. Yuzpe AA, Percivalsmith R, Rademaker AW. A multicentre clinical investigation employing ethinylestradiol combined with dinorgestrel as a post-coital agent. *Fertil Steril* 1982;**37**:508–13.
4. Rodrigues I, Grou F, Joly J. Effectiveness of emergency contraceptive pills between 72 and 120 hours after unprotected sexual intercourse. *Am J Obstet Gynecol* 2001;**84**:531–7.
5. Bryan S. Female sexual health. *Emerg Med* 2003;**15**: 223–6.
6. Task force on postovulatory methods of fertility regulation. Randomised controlled trial of levonorgestrel versus the Yuzpe regimen of combined oral contraceptives for emergency contraception. *Lancet* 1998;**352**:428–33.

OBSTETRICS AND GYNAECOLOGY

16.1 Acute kidney injury

Barry Wilkins

ESSENTIALS

1 Acute kidney injury (AKI, or acute renal failure) is acute reduction in glomerular filtration rate.

2 A high or rising plasma creatinine is the hallmark, but this does not necessarily distinguish it from chronic renal failure.

3 A normal plasma creatinine does not exclude AKI.

4 The commonest causes of AKI presenting to the ED are haemolytic uraemic syndrome and post-streptococcal glomerulonephritis.

5 Not all AKI is oliguric or anuric.

6 Most cases of oliguria are not AKI.

7 Most cases of elevated plasma urea are not AKI.

8 The most important treatment areas are circulating volume, potassium, and blood pressure.

9 Hyperkalaemia in acute kidney injury is not necessarily caused by potassium retention, especially when of short duration, but by potassium redistribution from cells.

10 Posterior urethral valves should be suspected in male infants with unexplained acute kidney injury.

11 Do not continue diuretics if two IV doses of furosemide of 1 mg kg^{-1}, then 5 mg kg^{-1} (over 1 hour) produce no urine.

Introduction

Acute kidney injury (AKI), or acute renal failure (ARF), means any acute reduction in glomerular filtration rate (GFR), i.e. in the excretory function of the kidneys, with oliguria (<0.5 mL kg^{-1} hr^{-1} in children or <1 mL kg^{-1} hr^{-1} in infants) or anuria, and a rise in plasma creatinine. Occasionally it is non-oliguric. It may evolve over hours (e.g. hypoxic–ischaemic cause) or days (e.g. glomerulonephritis). AKI caused by acquired renal disease presenting to the emergency department (ED) is rare. However, it is common in hospitalised critically ill children, where it is associated with significant mortality. AKI caused by shock states may be preventable by attending to circulating volume.

Classically, AKI has been divided into three broad categories, but pathophysiological processes overlap, and the first and second groups can lead to the third when severe or prolonged.

❶ **Prerenal.** Hypovolaemia, hypotension and low cardiac output reduce renal blood flow and cause elevation of plasma urea and a mild reduction in GFR and elevation in creatinine. This is not true renal failure, but a normal physiological adaptation to reduced renal blood flow, which responds to rehydration or other treatment of the cause.

❷ **Postrenal.** Obstruction in the renal tract anywhere from the pelvicalyceal system to the urethra may lead to AKI or chronic renal failure (CRF). Crystalopathy (obstructing the tubules) is usually regarded as a 'renal' cause.

❸ **Renal.** Primary disease in the glomerulus, which may be intrinsic (e.g. glomerulonephritis (GN)) or imposed (e.g. hypoxia, ischaemia, toxins).

Table 16.1.1   Causes of AKI

1. Reduced renal blood flow
   - Severe shock from hypovolaemia or myocardial failure
   - Rarely, the following may cause acute tubular necrosis (ATN) or cortical necrosis, and are more common in children with pre-existing cardiac, renal or liver failure:
     - Severe gastroenteritis
     - Nephrotic syndrome[a]
     - Burns
     - Diuretic use
     - Haemorrhage
     - Salt-wasting tubulopathies
     - Hypoaldosteronism
   - Cardiogenic shock
   - Pericardial tamponade
   - Coarctation of the aorta or renal artery stenosis
   - Septic shock
   - Anaphylactic shock
   - Systemic inflammatory response syndromes (e.g. severe trauma, pancreatitis)
   - Hepatorenal syndrome (rare)
   - Malignant hypertension
   - Arterial or venous thrombosis
   - Disseminated intravascular coagulation (DIC)
   - Drugs (e.g. angiotensin-converting enzyme (ACE) inhibitors, non-steroidal anti-inflammatory drugs (NSAIDs), tacrolimus, ciclosporin)

2. Intrinsic renal disease
   - Haemolytic uraemic syndrome (HUS)[b]
   - Thrombotic thrombocytopenic purpura (TTP)
   - Acute proliferative glomerulonephritis (GN), including post-streptococcal and other post-infectious[c] glomerulonephritis
   - Acute tubular necrosis (ATN) caused by hypoxia plus ischaemia
   - Systemic lupus erythematosus (SLE) or vasculitis
   - IgA nephropathy
   - Wegener's granulomatosis
   - Anti-glomerular basement membrane (anti-GBM) disease
   - Pyelonephritis
   - Toxins (e.g. petrol, carbon tetrachloride, heavy metals)
   - Drugs (e.g. aminoglycosides, vancomycin, cisplatin, tacrolimus, ciclosporin, ACE inhibitors, non-steroidal anti-inflammatory drugs (NSAIDs), amphotericin B)
   - Acute tubulointerstitial nephritis (TIN); drugs (e.g. furosemide, NSAIDs, penicillin, rifampicin, thiazides, allopurinol), immune-mediated diseases (e.g. IgA nephropathy, SLE) and infections (bacterial including *Yersinia*, viral, fungal, rickettsial) are causes
   - HIV nephropathy
   - Snake or arachnid envenomation
   - Renal trauma
   - Myoglobinuria from crush injury or rhabdomyolysis
   - Haemoglobinuria (acute intravascular haemolysis, e.g. in G6PD deficiency)
   - Sickle cell disease
   - Leukaemic infiltration
   - Shunt nephritis (ventriculoperitoneal shunt infection)
   - Radiographic contrast agents (rare in children)
   - Renal dysplasia, hypoplasia, and agenesis in neonates (chronic but acute presentation)

3. Urinary tract obstruction
   - Posterior urethral valves (chronic but acute presentation)
   - Urethral stricture
   - Ureterocele
   - Pelvic or retroperitoneal tumours
   - Neurogenic bladder
   - Retroperitoneal fibrosis (rare)
   - Stones, sludge (metabolic disease), pus, fungal ball, sloughed renal papilla, clots, proteinaceous material or crystals (uric acid, calcium oxalate, aciclovir, methotrexate, purines, sulphonamides) in the ureters or renal tubules

4. Acute presentation of end-stage renal failure

[a]Sometimes nephrotic syndrome caused by mesangiocapillary GN may present with features similar to acute post-streptococcal GN.
[b]In developed countries HUS and post-streptococcal GN are the commonest causes presenting to the ED, whereas in tropical countries 'prerenal' causes predominate outside the hospital environment.
[c]Various infectious agents can produce nephritis similar to that of post-streptococcal GN (e.g. *Mycoplasma*, *Leptospira*, atypical *Mycobacterium*, *Varicella*, cytomegalovirus, Epstein–Barr virus, *Toxoplasma*, *Rickettsia*, hepatitis B and C).

Table 16.1.2   Causes of oliguria

- AKI
- Hypovolaemia
- Dehydration
- Low cardiac output
- Intrarenal vasoconstricting drugs when renal impairment is mild
- Syndrome of inappropriate antidiuretic hormone secretion (SIADH)

Table 16.1.3   Causes of polyuria

- AKI
- CRF
- Diuretics
- Osmotic diuresis, e.g. diabetic ketoacidosis
- Obstruction of the urinary tract
- Nephrogenic diabetes insipidus (DI)
- Nephrocalcinosis
- Interstitial nephritis
- Renal tubular disorders, e.g. Bartter's syndrome
- Hypoaldosteronism, e.g. Addison's disease, congenital adrenal hyperplasia
- Cerebral salt wasting
- Sickle cell disease
- Psychogenic polydipsia

Table 16.1.4   Causes of water retention and oedema

- AKI
- CRF
- Nephrotic syndrome (also has hypovolaemia and oliguria)
- Chronic liver disease
- Other causes of hypoproteinaemia (e.g. protein-losing enteropathy)
- Inappropriate ADH secretion or administration (oedema rare)
- Congestive heart failure (congenital or acquired structural heart disease, tachyarrythmias, pericardial effusion)
- Excess sodium and water intake

Table 16.1.5   Causes of uraemia

- AKI
- Increased dietary protein load
- Catabolic states with fever, e.g. sepsis, rhabdomyolysis
- Gastrointestinal or internal haemorrhage
- Hypovolaemia, dehydration, low cardiac output (increased reabsorption by the renal tubules)

Causes

See Table 16.1.1.

There are many causes of oliguria other than AKI. Beware of urine retention or a blocked bladder catheter before assuming true oliguria (Table 16.1.2).

There are many causes of polyuria other than AKI (Table 16.1.3).

There are many causes of oedema other than AKI (Table 16.1.4).

There are many causes of elevated plasma urea (P_{Urea}) other than AKI (Table 16.1.5).

Pathophysiology

Physiology

The kidney has three principal areas of function:

❶ Excretion of waste products of metabolism (e.g. urea and non-volatile acid) and excess ingested elements (e.g. potassium). This is effected by glomerular filtration, measured by the GFR.

❷ Regulation of the volume and mineral composition of body fluids. This is effected by tubular function, by absorption of >90% of filtered water, >99% of filtered sodium and 100% of glucose.

❸ Endocrine functions, e.g. erythropoietin, renin.

Normal GFR is around $1\,mL\,kg^{-1}\,min^{-1}$ in newborn infants, rising to $2\,mL\,kg^{-1}\,min^{-1}$ in adults, but there is wide variation between and within individuals, reflected in wide variations in plasma creatinine (P_{Cr}) in normal children. Measurement of GFR is unhelpful in the acute situation. Creatinine clearance approximates to GFR. Plasma creatinine reflects GFR because creatinine production is remarkably constant, both within and between individuals, and is related to muscle mass. It is around $100\,\mu mol\,kg^{-1}\,day^{-1}$ in infants, rising to around $200\,\mu mol\,kg^{-1}\,day^{-1}$ in adults. There is a little absorption from, or secretion into, the tubule and this is abolished by Histamine-2 (H2) receptor antagonists. In AKI with complete cessation of glomerular function, plasma creatinine (P_{Cr}) increases by up to $150\,\mu mol\,L^{-1}\,day^{-1}$ in infants and $300\,\mu mol\,L^{-1}\,day^{-1}$ in adults. In less severe AKI, P_{Cr} rises by $>50\,\mu mol\,L^{-1}\,day^{-1}$. In stable renal function, GFR can be estimated by the formula: $70/P_{Cr}\,mL\,kg^{-1}\,min^{-1}$ in infants or $140/P_{Cr}\,mL\,kg^{-1}\,min^{-1}$ in adults, but this is an approximation. The formula does not hold true if GFR is changing.

Although there are published tables of P_{Cr} and GFR according to age, gender and size, the variability and different P_{Cr} assays in use preclude their being of much use in interpreting isolated creatinine results. A normal plasma creatinine does not exclude AKI. Generally any creatinine $>100\,\mu mol\,L^{-1}$ is abnormal, but in infants > 50 should raise a suspicion of impaired GFR, in a 5-year-old >70, in a 10-year-old >80, and in a 15-year-old >100. More important is the rate of increase of plasma creatinine in AKI, which takes 12–24 hours to become evident.

Renal blood flow (RBF) is normally very high (one quarter of cardiac output) in order to effect glomerular filtration. It is auto regulated over a wide perfusion pressure range. Normally 20% of the renal plasma flow is filtered. Up to 50% of urea is reabsorbed, more in oliguric states; hence plasma urea may reflect dehydration more than GFR. The high metabolic rate (for tubular reabsorption) and high endothelial mass (greater than any other organ by weight) make the kidney vulnerable to hypoxia and ischaemia.

Pathogenesis of AKI

Most AKI presenting to EDs has a single identifiable cause, in contrast to hospital acquired AKI, which may be multifactorial.

In acute tubular necrosis (ATN), there is a generalised hypoxic or ischaemic insult affecting the glomerulus and tubules. Tubular injury leads to failure of electrolyte absorption and a tendency to loss of extracellular fluid, which would be rapidly fatal if not limited by a reduction in GFR. ATN is a term that is not strictly correct. Rarely is there histological necrosis, though individual tubular cell apoptosis does occur. Acute tubular dysfunction (at a subcellular level) is a better term. This process was once termed 'acute renal success' because of the saving of the patient's life by the kidney 'taking itself out'. Pre-existing haemodynamic compromise, CRF, age, hypovolaemia, diuretics, diabetes, or proteinuria favour the induction of ATN with any insult.

Vasoconstricting local mediators, including adenosine, angiotensin II, endothelin, thromboxane, leukotrienes, urotensin, platelet activating factor, heat shock proteins, oxygen free radicals and superoxides, together with deficiency of vasodilating mediators, including prostacyclin, atrial natriuretic peptide (ANP) and nitric oxide, are causes of the intense glomerular vasoconstriction in ATN. In future, endothelin A receptor antagonists may play a role in moderating renal injury.

Inflammatory infiltrate, interstitial oedema, up-regulation of adhesion molecules, tubule cell swelling, loss of epithelial surface area, loss of epithelial cell polarity, compression of peritubular capillaries, impaction of debris in tubules, increased intratubular pressure, back-leak of urea, aggregation of erythrocytes, leucocytes and fibrin in peritubular capillaries, all contribute to the established state of reduced GFR.

The following pathological processes may contribute to other causes of AKI.

- In snake and arachnid envenomation, haemolysis, disseminated intravascular coagulation (DIC) and the venom itself may contribute to renal injury.
- Sickle cell haemoglobinopathy causes papillary necrosis by red cell sickling in medullary blood vessels. This may cause gross haematuria. Sepsis and volume depletion may contribute to renal injury. Recurrent episodes often lead to a nephropathy with an irreversible urine concentration defect in teenagers. Approximately 10% of sickle cell crises have AKI.
- In hypovolaemia, hypotension and low cardiac output states the combination of decreased renal perfusion pressure and afferent arteriolar constriction reduces GFR.
- In ATN, increased tubular hydrostatic pressure due to obstruction caused by casts and injured tubular cell debris, and back-leak of filtrate through injured tubular epithelium reduces effective GFR further. Influx of calcium into renal tubular cells may activate enzyme systems, leading to membrane and organelle dysfunction.
- Birth asphyxia may precipitate renal vein thrombosis in neonates, commencing within the kidney, spreading into larger veins, but thrombogenic states (e.g. protein S or protein C deficiency) are rare causes. There are firm palpable kidneys with haematuria.
- Renal function may deteriorate suddenly in some patients without an oliguric phase. Obstruction, sepsis, hypercalcaemia and some drugs and other nephrotoxins may be causes. Functioning nephrons have reduced reabsorption capacity, thereby maintaining urine output. It has a better prognosis than oliguric renal failure.
- Although minimal change nephrotic syndrome rarely causes AKI, hypovolaemia, peritonitis, septicaemia, renal vein thrombosis and drug toxicity may precipitate AKI that is histologically ATN and may be reversible.
- Human immunodeficiency disease (HIV) disease may first present as AKI, nephrosis or CRF. Minimal change, mesangial proliferation and focal segmental glomerulosclerosis (FSGS) may be seen.
- After initiation of AKI by glomerular or tubular injury there is a maintenance

phase where GFR remains relatively low for several days or weeks, then a recovery phase characterised by gradual and progressive restoration of GFR and tubular function.

Presentation

See Table 16.1.6.

A careful history and examination may give clues to the cause of AKI. Ask about diuretic and other drug use, recent hospitalisation or radiographic investigations, diarrhoea or vomiting (may be the presenting symptom of UTI or HUS), weight change, musculoskeletal symptoms, abdominal or flank pain, urinary dribbling, arthralgia and myalgia, recent upper respiratory tract infrction. Enquire for family history of renal disease or hypertension. Examine for signs of heart failure. Look for fever and rash that might be signs of GN or tubulointerstitial nephritis (TIN), vasculitic signs, palpable bladder. Important features of hypovolaemia or low cardiac output include tachycardia (for normal pulse rates, see Chapter 1.1), prolonged capillary refill time >2 s (but beware of cold ambient temperature), postural hypotension (remember that supine blood pressure can be preserved until late in hypovolaemia and dehydration – for normal blood pressures, see Chapter 16.3) and possibly a gallop rhythm. Oedema, when present, can be hard to find – press firmly

Table 16.1.6 Possible presenting features of AKI

- Oliguria
- Anuria
- Polyuria
- Haematuria
- Brown urine
- Hypertension
- Pulmonary oedema
- Water retention (but oedema less common)
- Recent weight gain or weight loss
- Acidosis
- Electrolyte abnormalities, especially hyperkalaemia, hyperphosphataemia
- Arrhythmias
- Pericarditis
- Gastrointestinal symptoms (e.g. anorexia, nausea, vomiting, haemorrhage)
- Neuro-psychiatric manifestations (confusion, agitation, seizures, headache, visual disturbances)[a]
- Itching (uraemia)
- Generalised systemic illness with malaise, anorexia and fatigue
- Acute respiratory distress syndrome (ARDS)

[a]Neurological manifestations are usually late and may represent hypertensive encephalopathy.

on the shin for at least 1 minute. Haematuria may suggest renal parenchymal disease. Poor urinary stream and palpable bladder points to obstruction but in the very young this can be only excluded by thorough investigation. Monitor cardiac electrical rhythm and oximetry.

Investigations

Tests in AKI include the following.

- Full blood count.
- Plasma Na, K, Cl, Ca, PO_4, Mg, osmolality.
- Plasma glucose.
- Plasma uric acid.
- Plasma urea and creatinine.
- Plasma albumin.
- Plasma pH, bicarbonate and lactate.
- Liver function tests.
- Coagulation screen.
- Blood cultures.
- Plasma creatine kinase (CK) and troponin.
- Urinalysis for protein and blood by dipstick.
- Urine microscopy, Gram stain and culture.
- Urine chemistry (Na, K, urea, osmolality, creatinine). Only 1 mL is needed and can be aspirated from a cotton-wool ball placed in the nappy (calcium and phosphate may be falsely elevated).
- Urine protein (quantitative – protein: creatinine ratio >20 mg mmol^{-1} is abnormal).
- Urine urate.

Examination of urine sediment by microscopy is often neglected. Normal urine indicates a pre- or post-renal cause of AKI. Cells, casts or protein suggest intrinsic renal pathology. In ATN there are granular and epithelial cell casts. White cell casts or eosinophils occur in acute TIN. Red blood cell casts and heavy proteinuria occur in GN or vasculitis. A dipstick positive for blood in the absence of red cells in urine is suggestive of haemoglobin or myoglobin. Nitrite in urine may suggest UTI. Obstruction and UTI may cause pyuria.

Calculate the plasma anion gap, corrected for hypoalbuminaemia:

$$\text{Anion gap (corr·)} = Na + K - Cl - \text{Bicarbonate} + \frac{(45 - \text{Albumin})}{4}$$

NB. Albumin is in g L^{-1}, the electrolytes in mmol L^{-1}.

Normal is 16 mEq L^{-1}.

Calculate the plasma osmolal gap:

$$\text{Osmolal gap} = (Na + K) \times 1.86 + \text{Urea} + \text{Glucose} + 10 - \text{Osmolality}$$

NB. Electrolytes, urea and glucose are in mmol L^{-1}, osmolality in mosmol kg^{-1}.

If osmolal gap is >5 mosmol kg^{-1} then unmeasured solute such as ethanol or ethylene glycol may be present.

Chest X-ray will detect pulmonary oedema, pleural effusions or cardiomegaly.

Abdominal X-ray may detect nephrocalcinosis and spinal abnormalities.

All children with AKI should have a urinary tract ultrasound examination to check for two kidneys. This may diagnose polycystic kidneys, renal vein thrombosis, nephrocalcinosis, hydronephrosis or other causes of obstruction. The kidneys are likely to be normal in size or enlarged in AKI, but small in CRF. A non-dilated system does not necessarily exclude an obstructive uropathy in anuria; hence retrograde pyelography may be needed.

Further tests if there is any suspicion of GN or vasculitis include:

- Antistreptolysin O titre.
- Complement C3, C4, CH50.
- Serology for hepatitis.
- Autoantibodies, especially anti-nuclear antibodies (ANA), anti-double-stranded DNA (anti-ds-DNA) antibodies, anti-neutrophil cytoplasmic antibodies (ANCA), anti-glomerular basement membrane (anti-GBM) antibody.
- Consider HIV serology.
- Consider isotope renal scans and angiography. Dimercaptosuccinic acid (DMSA) scan assesses functioning renal tubular mass and shows scars, while diethylene-triamine-penta-acetic acid (DTPA) and mercaptoacetyl glycylglycylglycine (MAG3) scans assess glomerular filtration and renal blood flow. They may be useful in distinguishing ATN from other causes of AKI.
- Echocardiography assists in assessing myocardial function or in excluding bacterial endocarditis.
- If the cause of renal failure still remains obscure, the paediatric nephrologist will consider a percutaneous renal biopsy, generally after admission. This may show

various types of acute GN, vasculitis or TIN that may need immunosuppression and/or plasmaphaeresis.

Urine chemistry is often neglected. Protein: creatinine ratio >20 mg mmol^{-1} diagnoses significant proteinuria, but may be falsely elevated by fever, trauma, recent surgery, upright posture and exertion; early morning sample is best. Haematuria plus proteinuria strongly suggests a renal parenchymal lesion. Urate:creatinine ratio >1 mmol mmol^{-1} suggests catabolic state, or tumour lysis, and uric acid nephropathy.

Urine electrolytes and osmolality are helpful in differentiating causes of uraemia. Always measure the urine creatinine. Calculate fractional excretion of sodium (FE$_{Na}$). This is the fraction of filtered sodium that ends up in the urine, and is calculated by:

$$FE_{Na} = \frac{\dfrac{Urine\ Na}{Urine\ creatinine}} \times \frac{Plasma\ creatinine}{Plasma\ Na}$$

N.B. this formula does work even if the GFR is increasing or decreasing rapidly (Table 16.1.7).

In health, FE$_{Na}$ is <1% except in high-salt diet. In dehydrated patients, hypovolaemia or low cardiac output it is <0.1% (representing normal renal physiology). In general, FE$_{Na}$ >2% is seen in most cases of intrinsic renal failure. However, not all low FE$_{Na}$ represents normal physiology; it may also be low in some causes of oliguric AKI (e.g. ciclosporin toxicity). Not all high FE$_{Na}$ with oliguria represents AKI with tubular injury. In prerenal uraemia, FE$_{Na}$ may be higher in the presence of glycosuria,

bicarbonaturia or use of diuretics. Also, in syndrome of inappropriate antidiuretic hormone there is oliguria with a high FE$_{Na}$. High FE$_{Na}$ and polyuria suggest natriuresis, possible causes being a renal salt-wasting disorder, polyuric AKI, diuretics (including osmotic diuretics) and volume overload (mediated via natriuretic hormones). FE$_{Na}$ is also unreliable in preterm newborns and in obstructive uropathy. Fractional urea excretion (FE$_{Urea}$) may be more useful in distinguishing low renal perfusion forms of oliguria from ATN, especially after diuretics. FE$_{Urea}$ is <35% in 'prerenal' syndromes even after diuretic use, and >50% in ATN. FE$_{Urate}$ is >15% in ATN and many tubulopathies, and <7% in 'prerenal' states.

The urine calcium:creatinine ratio will help identify hypercalciuria as a cause of calculi or nephrocalcinosis (normal <0.7 mmol mmol^{-1}).

Treatment

The principles of treatment of AKI involve:

Treat established causes and complications First, pay attention to the airway, breathing and circulation. Treat life-threatening conditions (e.g. hypoxia, hypovolaemia, hyperkalaemia and seizures). Ventilation may be needed for pulmonary oedema not responsive to diuretic. Monitor continuous electrocardiogram.

Minimise further renal injury Avoid excessive fluids and electrolytes (especially Na and K). Attempt to establish a diuresis to wash out intra-tubular debris. Use diuretics

in small doses initially, because acute hypovolaemia can occur. Furosemide 1 mg kg^{-1} IV is appropriate, and then 5 mg kg^{-1} over 60 minutes if there is poor response. Give no more if there is no response. Remember that furosemide is itself nephro- and ototoxic. Mannitol is not recommended as it may worsen the situation by acute intravascular expansion, especially if there is no diuresis.

Remove the cause Treat sepsis. Remove nephrotoxic agents (e.g. drugs and poisons). Treat low cardiac output with inotropes, e.g. dopamine or dobutamine at 5–10 mcg kg^{-1} min^{-1} IV, but note that there is no evidence that low-dose dopamine either improves prognosis or reduces the incidence of AKI in patients at risk. Avoid potentially nephrotoxic drugs, e.g. aminoglycosides, peptidoglycans, ACE inhibitors. Pure obstructive AKI is commonly reversible and always treatable. It is usual to treat urethral obstruction (posterior urethral valves) by urethral catheterisation (by urologist), or suprapubic catheterisation, initially. In proven vascular thrombosis, tissue plasminogen activator (TPA) may be of benefit, but renal vein clot removal is unlikely to speed recovery.

Compensate for the reduced GFR and impaired tubular function Avoid or reduce the dose of renally excreted drugs. Pay strict attention to water and electrolyte balance.

Remove accumulated water and minerals Water and sodium input should be reduced. Begin an accurate water balance chart. Replace each previous hour's urine

Table 16.1.7	Using plasma and urine biochemistry to distinguish causes of oliguria						
Cause	Plasma urea	Plasma creatinine	Plasma Na	Urine Na (FE$_{Na}$)	FE$_{Urea}$	Urine creatinine	Urine osmolality
Low cardiac output Hypovolaemia Dehydration Renal vasoconstriction (e.g. ciclosporin toxicity)	Moderate–marked increase	Mild–moderate increase	Normal, low or high	<10 mmol L^{-1} (<0.5%)	<35%	>4 mmol L^{-1}	> 400 mosmol kg^{-1}
ATN	High	Mild increase on 1st day, then progressive increase to high	Normal or low	>20 mmol L^{-1} (>3%)	>50%	<1 mmol L^{-1}	Similar to plasma osmolality
SIADH	Normal or low	Normal or low	Low	Often 100–200 mmol L^{-1} (>1%)	–	Very high, often >10 mmol L^{-1}	Inappropriately high for plasma osmolality, > 300, often > 800 mosmol kg^{-1}

output plus insensible losses (10–20 mL kg^{-1} day^{-1}). Refer early to the nephrology service for renal substitution therapy if diuretic is ineffective, for control of water, urea (plasma urea >30 mmol L^{-1}), phosphate, metabolic acid and potassium retention, and to remove any toxic drugs or poisons. Oral calcium carbonate, calcium acetate (600–1800 mg elemental calcium per meal) or phosphate binding resin helps to control hyperphosphataemia. Aluminium is now avoided.

Optimise nutrition Supply adequate energy.

Disposition

All children with AKI should be admitted to a paediatric intensive-care or high-dependency facility under joint care of intensivist, nephrologist and any other relevant specialties. This may involve discussions with those specialties in a children's hospital and with an emergency retrieval service.

Acute presentation of CRF

Occasionally a child with CRF (also called chronic kidney insufficiency), that may have been previously undiagnosed, may present acutely with any of the symptoms of AKI. Anaemia, poor growth, clinical or radiological evidence of osteodystrophy, or small kidneys on ultrasound may suggest CRF (though polycystic kidneys are large). Elevated P$_{Cr}$, rising by <40 μmol L^{-1} day^{-1} is also suggestive that the renal failure is chronic. AKI can occur in a child with CRF, which may be a flare of the original disease or genuine AKI. Most CRF patients will already be under the care of a nephrologist, who should be contacted early. Symptoms such as anorexia, nausea, vomiting, malaise and sleep disturbances are common, but be alert for acute deterioration in any of these.

History should be sought regarding medications (diuretics, antihypertensive agents, steroids, erythropoietin, salt supplements, alkali, vitamin D, calcium carbonate phosphate binder), type and frequency of renal support (if appropriate), other illnesses and usual follow up. When CRF is previously undiagnosed, a family history of Alport disease, haemophilia, polycystic kidney disease, sickling or stones should be sought. Ask for family history of 'kidney failure', 'dialysis machine', deafness, and blood or protein in urine.

The same investigations as in AKI are mandatory.

Acute problems in chronic renal failure include the following.

- Hypertensive crisis, possibly hypertensive encephalopathy with convulsions and coma.
- Salt depletion, especially with superimposed gastroenteritis.
- Dehydration can lead to irreversible deterioration in GFR caused by hypovolaemia. Urine output cannot be used to judge circulating volume. Hypertension may be normal for the child.
- Volume overload and heart failure.
- Hyperkalaemia. See hyperkalaemia protocol in Chapter 10.5.
- Arrhythmias.
- Acidosis. Chronic acidosis may be managed by oral alkali administration (2–3 mmol kg^{-1} day^{-1}).
- Hyper- or hypocalcaemia.
- Urinary tract infection.
- Urinary tract obstruction.
- Haemodialysis catheter or shunt, or peritoneal dialysis catheter malfunction.
- Haemodialysis catheter or shunt infection.
- Peritonitis in a child on continuous cycling or ambulatory peritoneal dialysis.
- Acute gastrointestinal haemorrhage caused by platelet dysfunction. Desmopressin (DDAVP) is a therapeutic agent that may be useful, together with platelets, fresh frozen plasma or cryoprecipitate.
- Anaemia is often tolerated very well, even down to haemoglobin levels of 30–50 g L^{-1}. Do not transfuse without consulting the nephrologist, except in emergency. Transfusion, especially of platelets, may actually worsen prognosis in HUS (see Chapter 16.5).
- Fractures secondary to renal osteodystrophy.

AKI in the renal transplant recipient

The cause of a rising creatinine or sudden oliguria must be diagnosed without delay as a transplant carries high stakes. AKI in the transplanted kidney is often reversible with prompt management. Contact the transplant/nephrology service urgently for all transplants presenting to the ED for any cause. Prerenal uraemia must be excluded in any intercurrent illness.

Possible causes include:

- volume depletion – the transplanted kidney compensates less well to dehydration;
- delayed, antibody mediated rejection;
- ciclosporin or tacrolimus toxicity (a glomerulopathy with hyaline arteriolar thickening);
- urine leak at the ureteric-vesical anastomosis;
- ureteric obstruction;
- ATN (rare in the child presenting to ED);
- vascular thrombosis, including microangiopathic thrombosis diagnosed only on renal biopsy;
- infection;
- aciclovir.

Controversies and future directions

❶ Acetylcysteine has been shown to ameliorate the acute progression of some causes of AKI, but its role is not yet defined.

❷ Low-dose vasopressin is being evaluated for a role in improving renal blood flow and GFR.

❸ Dopamine A1 receptor agonists, e.g. fenoldopam, are being evaluated for a role in improving renal blood flow and GFR.

❹ Adenosine A1 receptor agonists are being evaluated for a role in improving renal blood flow and GFR, especially in association with furosemide.

❺ Anaritide (atrial natriuretic peptide) may improve renal perfusion, particularly in oliguric renal failure.

❻ Melanocyte stimulating factor, insulin-like growth factor, epidermal growth factor and hepatocyte growth factor, anti-adhesion molecule compounds, free radical scavengers and antioxidants are also being evaluated.

❼ Endothelin A receptor antagonists may in future play a role in moderating renal injury.

❽ Stem cells to produce new renal tissue.

❾ More accurate markers of GFR may become available, e.g. cystatin C.

❿ Plasma and urinary biomarkers of AKI, e.g. NGAL, NAG, KIM 1.

Further reading

Andreoli SP. Acute renal failure. *Curr Opin Pediatr* 2002;**14**:183–8.

Andreoli SP. Clinical evaluation and management. In: Avner ED, Harmon WE, Niaudet P, editors. *Pediatric nephrology*. 5th ed. Baltimore: Lippincott, Williams & Wilkins; 2003. p. 1233–52.

Benfield MR, Bunchman TE. Management of acute renal failure. In: Avner ED, Harmon WE, Niaudet P, editors. *Pediatric nephrology*. 5th ed. Baltimore: Lippincott, Williams & Wilkins; 2003. p. 1253–66.

Better OS, Stein JH. Early management of shock and prophylaxis of acute renal failure in traumatic rhabdomyolysis. *N Engl J Med* 1990;**322**:825–9 [review].

Bidani AK, Griffin KA. Calcium channel blockers and renal protection: Is there an optimal dose? *J Lab Clin Med* 1995;**125**:553–5 [review].

Chan JCM, Gill JR, editors. *Kidney electrolyte disorders*. New York: Churchill Livingstone; 1990.

Cronan K, Kost SI. Renal and electrolyte emergencies. In: Fleisher GR, Ludwig S, Henretig FM, editors. *Textbook of pediatric emergency medicine*. 5th ed. Philadelphia: Lippincott, Williams & Wilkins; 2006. p. 873–920.

Finney H, Newman DJ, Thakkar H, et al. Reference ranges for plasma cystatin C and creatinine measurements in premature infants, neonates and older children. *Arch Dis Child* 2000;**82**:71–5.

Griffin KA, Bidani A. Guidelines for determining the cause of acute renal failure. *J Crit Illness* 1989;**4**:32.

Mathew A, Berl T. Fractional excretion of sodium: Use early to assess renal failure. *J Crit Illness* 1989;**4**:45.

Miller PD, Krebs RA, Neal BJ, McIntyre DO. Polyuric prerenal failure. *Arch Intern Med* 1980;**140**:907–9.

Ronco C, Bellomo R, Kellum J, editors. *Critical care nephrology*. Philadelphia: Saunders Elsevier; 2009.

Schrier RW. Acute renal failure. In: Schrier RW, editor. *Section VII Diseases of the kidney and urinary tract*. 8th ed. Lippincott, Williams and Wilkins; 2007. p. 930–1209.

Siegel NJ, Van Why SK, Devarajan P. Pathogenesis. of acute renal failure. In: Avner ED, Harmon WE, Niaudet P, editors. *Pediatric nephrology*. 5th ed. Baltimore: Lippincott, Williams & Wilkins; 2003. p. 1223–32.

Siegler RL. The hemolytic uremic syndrome. *Pediatr Clin N Am* 1995;**42**:1505–29 [review].

Soni SS, Ronco C, Katz N, Cruz DN. Early diagnosis of acute kidney injury: the promise of novel biomarkers. *Blood Purif* 2009;**28**(3):165–74.

Stein JH. Acute renal failure. Lessons from pathophysiology. *W J Med* 1992;**156**:176–82 [review].

Taylor CM, Chapman S. Handbook of renal investigations in children. London: Wright; 1989.

Thadani R, Pascual M, Bonaventre J. Acute renal failure. *N Engl J Med* 1996;**334**:1448–60.

Thurau K, Boylan JW. Acute renal success. The unexpected logic of oliguria in acute renal failure. *Am J Med* 1976;**61**:308–15.

Venuto RC. Pigment-associated acute renal failure: Is the water clearer 50 years later? *J Lab Clin Med* 1992;**119**:452–4.

Wilkins BH, Goonasekera CDA, Dillon MJ. Chapters 2.10 and 3.5. In: Macnab AJ, Macrae DJ, Henning R, editors. *Care of the critically ill child*. London: Churchill Livingstone; 1999.

16.2 Haematuria

Frank Willis

ESSENTIALS

1 In children haematuria usually originates from the kidneys.

2 Haematuria can be caused by urinary infection, glomerular disease, tumours, congenital abnormalities and coagulopathies.

3 All paediatric haematuria should be investigated.

4 All patients with haematuria require follow up.

Introduction

Blood in the urine (haematuria) may be visible to the naked eye (macroscopic) or be detected only on dipstick testing and/or urine microscopy (microscopic). It may be found in isolation or associated with other urine abnormalities such as proteinuria, crystals and casts. It is essential to consider urinary tract infection (UTI) as a possible cause and, if confirmed, to manage accordingly (see Chapter 16.4).

Microscopic haematuria may be defined as >10 red blood cells (RBCs) per high-power field, or >50 RBCs mL^{-1} of urine (confirmed on three separate occasions).

Note that small numbers of red cells are normally excreted in urine.

Macroscopic haematuria exists when visible to the naked eye and confirmed on testing as being blood.

Haematuria can originate at any site in the urinary tract but, in contrast to adults, lower tract haematuria is relatively uncommon in children (and therefore cystoscopy is rarely indicated).

Remember:

❶ Microscopic haematuria in the setting of an acute febrile illness can be normal. UTI should be excluded by urine culture and the urine tested again after the acute illness has passed.

❷ Asymptomatic micro-haematuria in children without other signs of renal disease (hypertension, oedema, proteinuria, urinary casts, poor growth or renal impairment) is also relatively common.

❸ Consider idiopathic thrombocytopenic purpura (ITP), Henoch–Schönlein purpura (HSP) and coagulation disorders.

Causes of glomerular haematuria include:

- glomerulonephritis (GN) (including nephritis in multisystem disorders, e.g. systemic lupus erythematosus (SLE));
- familial nephritis (Alport's disease);
- thin basement membrane disease ('benign' familial haematuria);
- IgA nephropathy;
- polycystic kidney disease.

Causes for non-glomerular haematuria include:

- UTI;
- idiopathic hypercalciuria;
- stones;
- anatomical abnormalities;
- tumours;
- trauma;
- sickle cell disease (in relevant ethnic groups).

History

As in all cases attending the emergency department (ED), a relevant and thorough general and specific history should be taken.

It is important to obtain a family history of renal tract disease in patients with isolated micro-haematuria. Considerations include the possibility of familial haematuria. Check for a family history of renal tract stones (suggesting hypercalciuria) or sensorineural deafness and nephritis (with Alport's disease).

Ask about previous episodes of haematuria and/or features of HSP or SLE.

Historical features of upper tract haematuria include:

- brown urine;
- frothy urine, which may indicate proteinuria.

Features of lower tract haematuria include:

- pink or bright red colour;
- blood in the initial part of the urine stream suggests a urethral origin;
- blood towards the end of the urine stream suggests bladder origin.

Examination

Physical examination should seek to elicit signs of renal disease. A thorough general examination is essential, concentrating on the following in particular:

- *cardiovascular status* (pallor, BP, hypovolemia and/or fluid overload including gallop rhythm, pulmonary oedema, ascites, peripheral, scrotal/perineal oedema);
- *abdominal examination* (loin tenderness, ascites, petechiae or purpura);
- *neurological status* (anaemia, hypertensive encephalopathy, uraemia).

Investigations

In children presenting to the ED with haematuria, investigations should focus on identifying the anatomical source of the haematuria as well as its clinical significance.

Urine dipstick testing, microscopy and culture should always be performed as part of the initial evaluation of a child with haematuria.

Features suggestive of upper tract haematuria include the following:

- protein is often present;
- RBCs are often small and misshapen (dysmorphic);
- RBC casts and tubular casts may be seen.

Features suggestive of lower tract haematuria include:

- RBCs of normal shape (non-dysmorphic);
- no proteinuria.

NB. Urinary RBC morphology alone is an inaccurate method to determine the site of origin of haematuria and should not be relied upon in isolation.

The extent and type of other investigations done while in the ED will be determined by the clinical scenario. The following tests may be considered:

- urine calcium:creatinine ratio >0.7 mmol nmol^{-1} (hypercalciuria);
- urine protein:creatinine ratio > 20 mg nmol^{-1} (glomerulonephritides, chronic renal failure);
- plasma urea, creatinine + electrolytes (abnormal renal function);
- plasma calcium, PO$_4$, albumin (chronic renal failure);
- FBC, platelets, film (thrombocytopenia, anaemia);
- coagulation screen (coagulopathy);
- streptococcal serology (post-streptococcal GN);
- pharyngeal swab culture (post-streptococcal GN);
- complement C3, C4 (post-streptococcal GN, mesangiocapillary GN (MCGN), SLE);
- anti-nuclear antibody (ANA), (screening for SLE);
- abdominal X-ray (renal calculi, nephrocalcinosis);
- renal ultrasound (structural abnormalities, stones, etc.);
- sickle screen (sickle cell disease);
- schistosomiasis serology (schistosomiasis infection).

Differential diagnosis

It is important to remember that blood in urine may come from somewhere other than the urinary tract, e.g. vaginal haemorrhage, rectal fissure or contamination by the child or another person (such as in Münchausen syndrome by proxy).

Not everything staining the urine pink, brown or red is haematuria.

Urine dipstick tests for haematuria are very sensitive and will also be positive in the presence of haemaglobinuria and myoglobinuria. Dyes and foodstuffs (e.g. beetroot, blackberries) can colour the urine pink/red. Urates in the urine of neonates may also stain the nappy pink. Drugs (e.g. rifampicin, phenothiazines, phenolphthalein) and porphyria may also discolour the urine.

Treatment/disposition

- Treatment of patients presenting to ED with haematuria will obviously depend on clinical factors such as the presence or absence of hypertension, anaemia, problems of fluid balance and fluid distribution and pain or discomfort. Biochemical, haematological and imaging results may also be important.
- Whatever the ED management, all cases of haematuria should be followed up by the family doctor, a paediatrician or paediatric nephrologist (as appropriate).

Further reading

Andreoli SP. Management of acute renal failure. In: Barratt TM, Avner ED, Harmon WE, editors. *Pediatric nephrology*. 4th ed. Baltimore: Lippincott, Williams & Wilkins; 1999. p. 1119–34.

Renal Unit – Royal Hospital for Sick Children. *Guidelines on the management and investigation of haematuria*. Glasgow, UK: Yorkhill. Available at http://www.clinicalguidelines.scot.nhs.uk/Renal%20Unit%20Guidelines/Haematuria.pdf; [accessed 21.10.10].

Leticia UT, Fildes RD. Hematuria and proteinuria. In: Barakat AY, editor. *Renal disease in children – clinical evaluation & diagnosis*. New York: Springer-Verlag; 1990. p. 133–56.

Royal Children's Hospital – Melbourne Clinical Practice Guidelines – Haematuria. Available at http://www.rch.org.au/clinicalguide/cpg.cfm?doc_id=5208; [accessed 21.10.10].

Willis FR, Geelhoed GC. Haematuria. In: *Management guidelines – Emergency Department*. Perth, Western Australia: Princess Margaret Hospital for Children; 2002.

16.3 Hypertension

Frank Willis

ESSENTIALS

1 Hypertension is blood pressure that is consistently above the 95th percentile.

2 Severe hypertension is blood pressure that is consistently above the 99th percentile (i.e. 1% of children).

3 All hypertension should be investigated.

4 The most common secondary cause is renal disease.

5 Accelerated hypertension with encephalopathy is an emergency.

6 In malignant hypertension blood pressure should be lowered slowly.

7 Borderline hypertension is of uncertain significance, but needs follow up.

Introduction

In children, blood pressure (BP) is a continuous variable that is influenced by age, sex, body size, and genetic, circadian and environmental factors.

Hypertension is defined as BP that is consistently above the 95th percentile for age, gender and height (nomograms are available with these data and should be present in both the emergency department (ED) and paediatric wards) (Table 16.3.1).

Severe hypertension is BP consistently above the 99th centile with signs of end-organ damage such as retinopathy, nephropathy or left ventricular hypertrophy.

Accelerated hypertension occurs with severe hypertension plus neurological signs and symptoms (hypertensive encephalopathy) and severe hypertensive retinopathy.

Prevalence of hypertension is around 1–3% of children (note that this is to some extent a statistical issue related to use of BP centiles in defining hypertension). The most common secondary cause of hypertension in children is renal disease, though with increasing age (and the pandemic of childhood obesity) essential hypertension assumes more significance.

Ideally, all children presenting to ED should have a BP measurement.

History and examination

History

Ask about signs or symptoms of underlying disease, urinary tract infection (UTI), drugs, family history of renal disease or hypertension (essential or otherwise).

Non-specific signs and symptoms of hypertension in infants may include vomiting, irritability, respiratory distress, failure to thrive and congestive heart failure.

In older children, also consider polyuria, polydipsia, fatigability, headache, epistaxis, chest pain, abdominal pain and neurological abnormalities such as Bell's palsy or impaired vision. Enquire regarding any noted deterioration in school performance and/or change in personality, as these can be seen in chronic hypertension.

Examination

Measurement of BP is 'classically' performed using a mercury sphygmomanometer (though these are no longer universally available, e.g. in the United Kingdom), with the largest possible cuff (do not be misled by labels on cuffs). The inflatable part should encircle the arm and the width should cover 75% of the length of the upper arm.

Increasingly, oscillometric BP machines (e.g. Dinamap) are routinely used in EDs and elsewhere. Automated devices need regular service and calibration. Elevated measurements should (if possible) be confirmed with a mercury sphygmomanometer.

BP should be checked in both arms and at least one leg to exclude the possibility of aortic coarctation. BP should be repeated after an interval in an attempt to exclude 'white coat' hypertension.

Ambulatory blood pressure monitoring is available for children and is a useful method of further evaluating BP as well as for monitoring treatment effects.

Feel all pulses. As well as a thorough general examination, physical assessment following identification of elevated blood pressure should consider specifically: presence or absence of encephalopathy, growth, hydration, signs of chronic disease and presence of abdominal masses or bruits (cardiac, cranial and abdominal). The optic fundi must be visualised, specifically looking for papilloedema and vascular changes.

Investigations

Investigations to be considered in ED include:

- full blood count, electrolytes, urea and creatinine, liver function tests (LFTs), calcium, phosphate, magnesium, alkaline phosphatase;
- urinalysis by dipstick for protein and blood;
- urine microscopy and culture;
- urine catecholamines;
- chest X-ray, electrocardiogram and echocardiography;
- abdominal and renal ultrasound scan, including grey-scale sonography to identify parenchymal and collecting system disease and tumours, colour and duplex Doppler sonography to identify vessel disease;
- plasma renin and aldosterone (refer to lab regarding collection);
- complement C3, C4, anti-nuclear antibody (ANA);

Table 16.3.1 Upper limit of systolic blood pressure by age

Age	Upper limit for normal systolic BP (95th percentile)	
	Males	Females
1 month	104	102
2 months	109	106
3 months	111	108
4 months	110	109
6 months	110	110
1 year	110	110
2 years	110	110
3 years	111	110
4 years	112	111
5 years	113	112
6 years	115	114
7 years	117	116
8 years	118	117
9 years	120	119
10 years	122	121
11 years	124	123
12 years	127	125
13 years	129	128
14 years	130	129
15 years	133	130
16 years	136	131

Data obtained with permission from the National Heart, Lung and Blood Institute of the United States National Institutes of Health.

- drug screen, (e.g. amphetamines);
- cranial computerised tomography (CT) scan.

Subsequent investigations will depend on results of preliminary investigations and on the underlying diagnosis.

Causes

There are many possible causes of hypertension:

Renal
- Reflux nephropathy.
- Obstructive uropathy.
- Glomerulonephritis.
- Haemolytic uraemic syndrome.
- Nephrotic syndrome.
- Renal artery stenosis.
- Renal vein thrombosis.
- Acute and chronic renal failure.
- Polycystic disease.
- Renal tumours.
- Renal dysplasia.

Endocrine
- Catecholamine excess (neuroblastoma, phaeochromocytoma).
- Corticosteroid excess (congenital adrenal hyperplasia).
- Hyperthyroidism.

Vascular
- Aortic coarctation.
- Arteriovenous fistula.
- Takayasu arteritis.
- SLE.

Metabolic
- Diabetes.
- Porphyria.
- Hypercalcaemia.

Neurological
- Guillain–Barré syndrome.
- Raised intracranial pressure.

Drugs
- Steroids.
- Oral contraceptives.
- Stimulant medications (methylphenidate and dexamphetamine).
- Recreational drugs.
- Liquorice.

Toxins
- Heavy metals.

Miscellaneous
- Anxiety and pain.
- Burns.
- Essential hypertension.

Treatment

Hypertensive encephalopathy

Treatment for encephalopathy/accelerated hypertension is urgent. The blood pressure should be treated before proceeding with investigation of the underlying cause. Such patients should be discussed with a paediatric intensivist and nephrologist and will generally be admitted to the paediatric intensive care unit.

Aim initially for 25% reduction towards target BP (upper limit of normal systolic – see Table 16.3.1) in the first 12–24 hours, then the reduction should be slow, over 24–48 hours. Neglecting to lower the blood pressure can lead to permanent disability or death. Acutely lowering the blood pressure to normal is also contraindicated, because a rapid drop in blood pressure to normal can produce tissue ischaemia. This may manifest as shock (despite normal to slightly elevated blood pressure values), encephalopathy leading to cerebral injury, retinopathy or optic nerve infarction leading to blindness, hypoventilation and apnoea.

Peripheral vasodilators
- Intravenous (IV) nitroprusside infusion. Starting dose $1 \, mcg \, kg^{-1} \, min^{-1}$, increment by $1 \, mcg \, kg^{-1} \, min^{-1}$ every 5–10 minutes to maximum $5 \, mcg \, kg^{-1} \, min^{-1}$. Beware of cyanide toxicity above this dose, or with lower doses in renal failure. Check a plasma thiocyanate level every 12 hours. Half-life is very short.
- IV nitroglycerine infusion. Starting dose $1 \, mcg \, kg^{-1} \, min^{-1}$, increment by $1 \, mcg \, kg^{-1} \, min^{-1}$ every 5–10 minutes to maximum $5 \, mcg \, kg^{-1} \, min^{-1}$. Half-life is very short.
- IV hydralazine. $100–200 \, mcg \, kg^{-1}$ IV bolus followed by $4–6 \, mcg \, kg^{-1} \, min^{-1}$ infusion.
- IV clonidine. $3–6 \, \mu g \, kg^{-1}$ as slow injection followed by $0.5–2 \, \mu g \, kg^{-1} \, hr^{-1}$ infusion. Clonidine is a centrally acting vasodilator acting on spinal cord α_2-receptors.

Avoid diazoxide because it has a too-rapid, large and sustained effect.

Beta-blockers
- IV labetalol infusion. Starting dose $1 \, mg \, kg^{-1} \, hr^{-1}$, increment by $0.25–0.5 \, mg \, kg^{-1} \, hr^{-1}$ (to maximum $3 \, mg \, kg^{-1} \, hr^{-1}$) every 30 minutes until desired rate of reduction in BP is achieved. Monitor BP every 15 minutes

initially. Half-life is approx 4 hours and not altered in chronic renal insufficiency. Be aware of negative inotropic and chronotropic effect in patients with cardiac failure or bradycardia, and risk of asthma exacerbation. Lower acceptable limit of heart rate is 120 in neonate, 100 in children up to 3 years, 80 in children 3–10 years, 60 in children >10 years old.

- IV esmolol infusion. Starting dose 200 mcg kg^{-1} min^{-1}, increment by 50 mcg kg^{-1} min^{-1} every 5–10 minutes to maximum 1000 mcg kg^{-1} min^{-1}. Half-life is very short – only a few minutes, because of plasma esterase metabolism.

Beta-blockers and vasodilators may be used in combination. Beta-blockers and calcium channel blockers together are absolutely contraindicated. The combination is severely negatively inotropic.

Diuretics

In situations of clinical fluid overload, diuretics can be helpful. Furosemide 0.5–1 mg kg^{-1} IV bolus, which may be repeated after 4 hours, is first choice. If no response in patients with renal failure, try 2 mg kg^{-1}, then 5 mg kg^{-1} infusion over 1 hour once only. Avoid inducing hypovolaemia.

Less severe hypertension and oral management after control of malignant hypertension

When target blood pressure is reached, nitroprusside can be slowly withdrawn and other intravenous agents replaced by oral drugs as follows. Oral antihypertensive agents should be used to treat less severe hypertension because of their slower and more sustained effect. Drugs that may be used include:

Vasodilators

- Calcium channel blockers.
  oral or sublingual nifedipine, initial dose 0.25 mg kg^{-1}, then 0.5–1.5 mg kg^{-1} day^{-1} in 3–4 doses per day, or

isradipine 0.1 mg kg^{-1} 8-hourly, amlodipine 0.05–0.3 mg kg^{-1} once daily.
- Angiotensin converting enzyme (ACE) inhibitors. Captopril, initial test dose 0.1 mg kg^{-1}, then 0.3–4 mg kg^{-1} day^{-1}. Be aware that ACE inhibitors may decrease intrarenal blood flow and induce or worsen renal failure.
- Angiotensin II receptor (AT$_1$) blockers, e.g. losartan 0.5–2 mg kg^{-1} as a once-daily dose.
- Clonidine, 1–6 mcg kg^{-1} 8-hourly.

Beta-blockers

- Metoprolol, initial dose 1 mg kg^{-1} 12-hourly, incrementing to 2.5 mg kg^{-1}.
- Atenolol, initial dose 1 mg kg^{-1} 12–24-hourly, incrementing to 2 mg kg^{-1} 12-hourly.

NB. Where available, local guidelines should be referred to when using antihypertensive agents, especially when given by the intravenous route. Early consultation (as appropriate) with a paediatric intensivist or nephrologist is wise.

Treatment is less urgent in severe hypertension (without encephalopathy), but such patients should be admitted for investigation and treatment. Early liaison with the admitting consultant is prudent.

What to do about borderline hypertension is less clear, though such children should be referred for follow up by a paediatrician or paediatric nephrologist.

Controversies and future directions

❶ Significance of borderline hypertension.

❷ Routine or selective BP measurement in paediatric EDs.

❸ Obesity and blood pressure in paediatric populations.

❹ Pharmacology and pharmacokinetics of antihypertensive drugs in children.

❺ Speed of reduction in hypertensive encephalopathy/accelerated hypertension.

❻ The role of ambulatory BP measurements.

❼ CT and MR angiography to identify small intrarenal vessel disease.

❽ Angiotensin converting enzyme inhibitor renography to identify small vessel disease.

❾ Assessment of the impact of rigorous treatment of hypertension in childhood on the later development of vascular disease, stroke, renal disease and congestive heart failure.

❿ Evaluation of the role of dietary salt intake in childhood on the development of hypertension.

⓫ Further evaluation of genetic factors and the link with obesity and insulin resistance.

⓬ The role of newer angiotensin II inhibitor and angiotensin converting enzyme inhibitor drugs.

Further reading

Flynn JT. What's new in pediatric hypertension. *Curr Hypertens Rep* 2001;**3**:503–10.

Julius S. Clinical and physiological significance of borderline hypertension in youth. *Paediatr Clin N Am* 1978;**25**: 35–45.

Mouin GS, Arant BS. Hypertension. In: Barakat AY, editor. *Renal disease in children – clinical evaluation and diagnosis*. New York: Springer-Verlag; 1990. p. 307–28.

Report of the second task force on blood pressure control in children. *Paediatrics* 1987;**79**:1–25.

Report of the task force on blood pressure control in children. *Paediatrics* 1977;**59**:797–820.

Rocchini AP. Pediatric hypertension 2001. *Curr Opin Cardiol* 2002;**17**:385–9 [review].

Sorof JM, Portman RJ. White coat hypertension in children with elevated casual blood pressure. *J Paediatr* 2000;**137**: 493–7.

Vogt BA. Hypertension in children and adolescents. *Curr Thera Res Clin Exp* 2001;**62**:283–97.

Wells TG. Trials of antihypertensive therapies in children. *Blood Pressure Monitor* 1999;**4**:189–92.

Appendix

Age-specific percentiles of BP measurements

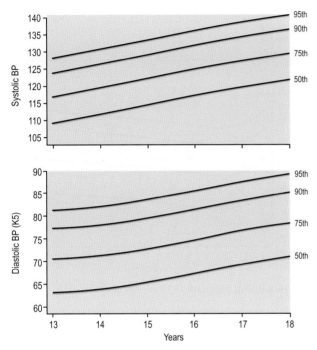

Fig. 16.3.1 Boys 13–18 years of age.

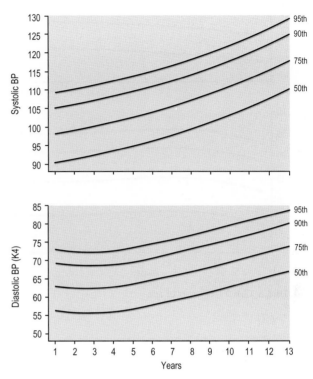

Fig. 16.3.2 Boys 1–13 years of age.

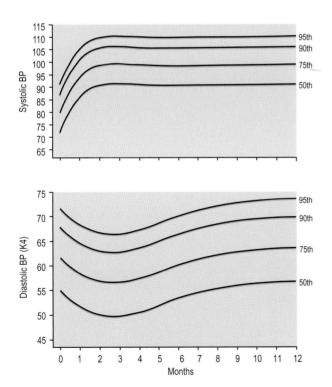

Fig. 16.3.3 Boys from birth to 12 months of age.

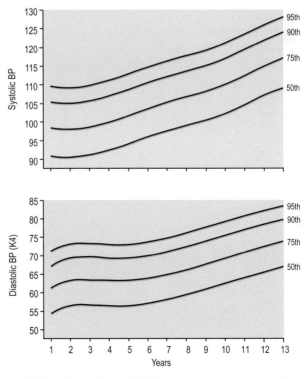

Fig. 16.3.4 Girls 1-13 years of age.

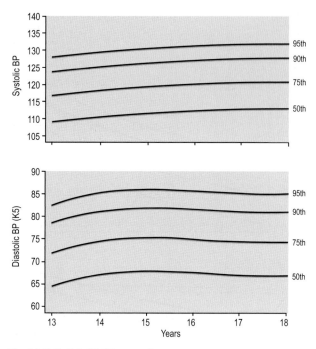

Fig. 16.3.5 Girls 13-18 years of age.

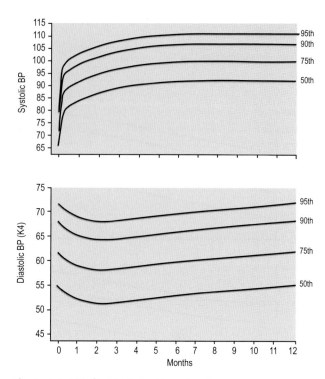

Fig. 16.3.6 Girls from birth to 12 months of age.

16.4 Urinary tract infection in pre-school children

Frank Willis

ESSENTIALS

1 Urinary tract infection is common and potentially serious.

2 Septicaemia may occur in babies.

3 Renal scarring is a serious and potentially preventable complication.

4 Urinary tract infection should be considered in all febrile infants and young children, as well as babies who are non-specifically unwell.

5 In young children, urinary tract infection cannot be diagnosed reliably or excluded on clinical grounds.

6 Dipstick urinalysis is an unreliable method of ruling out urinary tract infection in infants.

Introduction

Bacterial infection of the urinary tract (UTI) is common in the paediatric age group. Its significance is greatest in young children, particularly in the first year or two of life, where the high incidence of upper tract infection (pyelonephritis) and the presence of immature kidneys lead to significant potential for renal scarring (reflux nephropathy). It is unlikely that new scarring occurs after age 5 years.

Data from Sweden suggest that in the first 2 years of life, up to 3% of infants may suffer UTI. Between 1 and 10 years of age 3–8% of girls and < 1% of boys will have at least one urine infection. It is important to remember that recurrences are common. UTI is more frequent in boys than girls in the first months of life, partly because of a higher incidence of obstruction including pelviureteric junction obstruction, thereafter occurring significantly more often in girls (Fig. 16.4.1).

UTI is caused by organisms normally resident in the gut. It is thus an ascending infection that may affect the bladder (cystitis) or upper renal tract (pyelonephritis), which may in turn result in scarring. Neonates are unusual as they may also develop UTI following haematogenous dissemination of organisms.

Renal involvement is associated with:

- young age (especially <1 year);
- symptoms > 5 days;
- systemic upset, fever, leucocytosis;

- presence of vesicoureteric reflux (VUR) or other anatomical abnormality.

Long-term complications of renal scarring include: pregnancy-associated problems; hypertension; and, rarely, chronic renal insufficiency (see prognosis section below).

History and examination

In infants and young children with UTI, the clinical history is frequently non-specific and may include irritability, jaundice (neonates), poor feeding or fever without apparent source. Symptoms and signs become more specific with increasing age (Table 16.4.1).

Don't forget to obtain a family history of renal tract disease, in particular regarding UTIs, VUR (probably an autosomal dominant condition) and renal impairment.

Physical examination of young children with UTI is often unremarkable or non-specifically abnormal. Septicaemia, however, does occur with UTI in infancy and must be considered in babies up to around 6 months of age. Fever is the best clinical marker of pyelonephritis in infants with UTI, but is non-specific.

Diagnosis

A reliable urine sample is required to establish the diagnosis of UTI. In older children this is usually accomplished by obtaining a midstream sample. Difficulties arise in children too young to have been toilet trained, who are also the group at highest risk for pyelonephritis and renal scarring.

In infants and toddlers, urine bag samples are unreliable (very high false-positive rate) and should not be used. Clean catch samples are more reliable and are the preferred method for non-invasive urine collection. If samples are required urgently, bladder catheterisation is the most reliable method, though those familiar with the technique can consider suprapubic aspiration (SPA). The yield from SPA is markedly improved by using ultrasound to confirm a full bladder.

Samples should be sent to the laboratory for urinalysis, microscopy and culture. Findings supportive of the diagnosis of UTI include presence of leucocytes and organisms on microscopy and leucocyte esterase and nitrites on dipstick urinalysis. Organisms may be seen on Gram stain. In centres without 24-hour laboratory services, after-hours samples should be sent using a urine dipslide.

Dipstick urinalysis may be helpful in making a provisional diagnosis of UTI. However, a negative result does not rule out UTI in infancy. One study showed that urinalysis was normal in 50% of infants <8 weeks with confirmed UTI. Another study suggested that dipstick urinalysis was a reliable method of ruling out UTI only after age 2 years.

The traditional definition of pyuria is >5 white blood cells (WBC) per high-power field (centrifuged urine). Another definition is >10 WBC mm^{-3} (uncentrifuged urine).

The definition of significant bacteriuria is guided by the method by which the urine specimen was collected (Table 16.4.2), though on occasion genuine UTI may be present with lower colony counts than would usually be considered significant, especially in babies – interpret results in light of history and clinical findings.

Treatment

ED treatment recommendations for UTI vary. However, one approach is as follows.

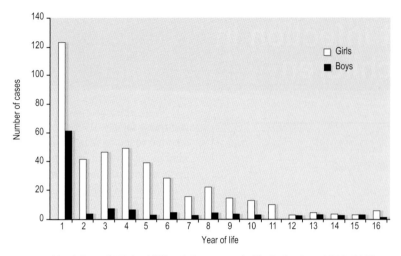

Fig. 16.4.1 Epidemiology of UTI in childhood. Cases recorded in Gothenburg 1960–1966.
Source: Winberg J, Andersen HJ, Bergström T, et al. Acta Paediatrica Scandinavia Supplement 1974;63 (Suppl. 252):1–20.

Table 16.4.1 UTI symptoms by age

Age	0–2 years	2–5 years	5–12 years
Failure to thrive	✓		
Feeding problems	✓		
Screaming	✓		
Irritability	✓		
Diarrhoea	✓	✓	
Vomiting	✓	✓	
Fever	✓	✓	✓
Convulsions	✓		
Haematuria		✓	✓
Urinary frequency		✓	✓
Dysuria		✓	✓
Enuresis		✓	✓
Abdominal pain		✓	✓
Loin pain			✓

Table 16.4.2 Definition of significant bacteriuria

Method of collection	Colony forming unit count (CFU mL^{-1})
Clean catch	> 10^5
Catheter	>5 × 10^4
Suprapubic	>0

Age <6 months
- Admit all for intravenous (IV)/ intramuscular (IM) antibiotics (septicaemia occurs in this age group).

- Admit to medical ward (observation ward only if systemically well).
- If discharged from observation ward, arrange general practitioner (GP) or ED follow up at 24–48 hours.
- Ensure urine culture and sensitivity results are checked at 48–72 hours.

Age 6–12 months
- If systemically unwell, admit to observation ward or medical ward for IV/IM antibiotics.
- If not systemically unwell, consider single IM/IV dose of ceftriaxone or gentamicin, followed by oral antibiotics.

- Arrange GP or ED follow up at 24–48 hours.
- Ensure urine culture and sensitivity results are checked at 48–72 hours.

Age >12 months
- Treat on clinical merits, i.e. admit or allow home, parenteral or oral antibiotics.
- Overnight admission to observation ward for IV/IM antibiotics may be worth considering if unwell.
- Ensure urine culture and sensitivity results are checked at 48–72 hours.

Which antibiotic?
Empirical antibiotic choice, dose and duration should be guided by local sensitivity patterns and antibiotic guidelines. However, consideration may involve the following:

Parenteral treatment (IV/IM)
- Ceftriaxone 25 mg kg^{-1} twice daily IV (may not cover enterococci in young infants), or
- Amoxicillin 10–25 mg kg^{-1} 8-hourly IV + gentamicin 7.5 mg kg^{-1} once daily IV/IM (reduce gentamicin to 2.5 mg kg^{-1} as a single dose in patients with known or suspected renal impairment and check a level before repeat dosing).

Oral treatment
- Amoxicillin 20 mg kg^{-1} with clavulanic acid 8-hourly, or cefalexin 15 mg kg^{-1} twice daily.
- Cotrimoxazole (1.5–3 mg kg^{-1} trimethoprim) twice daily is generally less good.
- Amoxicillin is not recommended.

Duration of treatment?
- Infants up to 12 months: treat for 10 days at full dose.
- Older children: generally treat for 5–10 days at full dose.
- Courses as short as 3 days may be used in older children with uncomplicated lower tract UTI.

Management after discharge from ED or observation wards
Most centres will have a referral, management and investigation protocol which should be followed. Many of these are based on the National Institute for Clinical Excellence Guidelines from the United Kingdom,[1] though significant variation

exists from place to place. In the absence of local guidelines, the following approach is reasonable.

Arrange a 'proof of cure' urine culture after stopping antibiotic.

In pre-school children (both sexes), following the first documented UTI (or if previous UTI not investigated), start low-dose nocturnal prophylactic antibiotics. Co-trimoxazole (because of its long shelf life) and nitrofurantoin are reasonable choices. The dose is $1-2$ mg kg^{-1} at night for both drugs (expressed as the trimethoprim component in the case of co-trimoxazole). Trimethoprim suspension is unavailable commercially in Australia, but is a better choice than co-trimoxazole in countries where it is readily obtainable.

A practical note – after the full course of treatment, if any antibiotic is left over, continue this as a *nocte* dose until finished, and then change to a nocte dose of the chosen prophylactic antibiotic.

Arrange a renal tract ultrasound (although some would restrict this to children <3 years), and refer to medical outpatients, hospital UTI clinic or paediatric nephrology clinic (depending on local organisation) all those discharged home from ED/observation wards who have not previously been investigated.

It is generally not necessary to book other imaging studies as consultants will differ in the investigations that they prefer, e.g. micturating cystourethrogram (MCUG) and/or dimercaptosuccinic acid (DMSA) isotope scan, though this can be expedited by speaking to the consultant or unit to whom the child has been referred.

Prognosis

UTI in preschool years may be associated with renal damage. Risk factors are listed in the introduction to this section. While most children with UTI will not suffer any long-term sequelae, a number will do so. Examples include:

- 10–20% of children with VUR and scars develop hypertension during childhood;[2]
- 34% of adults with reflux nephropathy are hypertensive;[3]
- 30–50% of children with VUR have scarring at initial evaluation;[4]

- 5–15% of end-stage renal disease (ESRD) in adults <50 years is due to reflux nephropathy.[4]

At least some of these consequences may be preventable by early and effective diagnosis and treatment of UTI in very young children (though even this has been questioned by some authors[5]).

Prevention

The 'basics' of good fluid intake, regular and complete voiding, avoidance of constipation and proper (front to back) bottom wiping (in toilet-trained females) should be encouraged in order to reduce the likelihood of repeat infections. There is also some evidence of benefit from the regular use of cranberry juice (which acidifies urine and reduces bladder wall adhesiveness). Prophylactic antibiotics should be considered in cases of VUR in pre-school children, recurrent pyelonephritis, recurrent symptomatic UTI in older children and in pre-school children awaiting renal tract imaging.

Controversies and future directions

❶ 'There is no subject in which there is so little uniformity of opinion and so much confusion.' This statement made in 1916 is seemingly just as pertinent in the early 21st century, with many questions about paediatric UTI management still the subject of debate and controversy. On the specific subject of VUR, one author, considering 'the effect of scientific evidence on clinical decision making in children with VUR during the past 40 years' (since its description), suggests that 'reported data have been overlooked in favour of unfounded speculation or clinical tradition.'[5]

❷ Current controversies and areas for potential investigation in paediatric UTI include:

- Parenteral or oral antibiotic treatment.
- Duration of antibiotic treatment.
- Outpatient or inpatient management.

- Post-UTI imaging protocols.
- The role of antibiotic prophylaxis.
- Diagnosis and management of vesicoureteric reflux.
- 'Complementary' therapies such as lactobacillus and bifidus consumption.
- Cranberry juice as prophylaxis.
- Recognition of dysfunctional voiding.
- Recognition of sphincter and detrusor dyssynergia.

References

1. NICE Guidelines. *Urinary tract infection: diagnosis, treatment and long-term management of urinary tract infection in children.* Available at http://www.nice.org.uk/CG054 [accessed 21.10.10].
2. Smellie J, Edwards D, Hunter N, et al. Vesico-ureteric reflux and renal scarring. *Kid IntSuppl* 1975;4:65–72.
3. Malek RS, Svensson J, Neves RJ, Torres VE. Vesicoureteral reflux in the adult. III. Surgical correction: benefits. *J Urol* 1983;130:882–6.
4. Noe HN. The current status of screening for vesicoureteral reflux. *Paediatr Nephrol* 1995;9:638–41.
5. Hewitt IK, Zucchetta P, Rigon L, et al. Early treatment of acute pyelonephritis in children fails to reduce renal scarring: data from the Italian renal infection study trials. *Pediatrics* 2008;122(3):486–90.

Further reading

Bachur R, Caputo GL. Bacteraemia and meningitis among infants with urinary tract infection. *Paediatr Emerg Care* 1995;11:280–4.

Crabtree EG, Cabot H. Colon bacillus pyelonephritis: Its nature and possible prevention. In: *Transactions of the Section of Genitourinary Diseases of the American Medical Association*, vol 57.1916. p. 209–17.

Crain EF, Gershel JC. Urinary tract infections in febrile infants younger than 8 weeks. *Paediatrics* 1990;86:363–7.

Doley A, Neligan M. Is a negative dipstick urinalysis good enough to exclude urinary tract infection in paediatric ED patients? *Emerg Med* 2003;15:77–80.

Hodson EM, Wheeler DM, Vimalchandra D, et al. Interventions for primary vesicoureteric reflux. *Cochrane Database Syst Rev* 2007;(3):CD001532.

Jakobsson B, Esbjorner E, Hansson S. Minimum incidence and diagnostic rate of first urinary tract infection. *Paediatrics* 2000;106:620–1.

Kinney AB, Blount M. Effect of cranberry juice on urinary pH. *Nurs Res* 1979;28:287–90.

Montini G, Zucchetta P, Tomasi L, et al. Value of imaging studies after a first febrile urinary tract infection in young children: data from Italian renal infection study 1. *Pediatrics* 2009;123(2):e239–46. Epub 2009 Jan 12.

Pollack CV, Pollack ES, Andrew ME. Suprapubic bladder aspiration versus urethral catheterisation in infants: Success, efficiency and complication rates. *Ann Emerg Med* 1994;23:225–30.

Shihab ZM. Urinary tract infection. In: Barakat AY, editor. *Renal disease in children – clinical evaluation & diagnosis.* New York: Springer-Verlag; 1990. p. 157–70.

Sobota AE. Inhibition of bacterial adherence by cranberry juice: Potential for treatment of urinary tract infections. *J Urol* 1984;131:1013–6.

Willis FR, Geelhoed GC. Urinary tract infection. In: *Management guidelines – Emergency Department.* Perth, Western Australia: Princess Margaret Hospital for Children; 2002.

16.5 Haemolytic uraemic syndrome

Karen McCarthy

ESSENTIALS

1 Diagnosis is based on the presence of microangiopathic haemolytic anaemia, thrombocytopenia and renal impairment.

2 Diarrhoea-associated haemolytic uraemic syndrome accounts for 90% of cases.

3 The cornerstone of treatment is careful attention to fluid and electrolyte balance.

4 Most patients with haemolytic uraemic syndrome have some degree of encephalopathy.

5 Hypertension is present in up to 50%.

6 Long-term follow up is necessary.

7 Use of antibiotics, antimotility agents and non-steroidal anti-inflammatory drugs should be avoided in children acutely infected with Shigatoxin *Escherichia coli*.

Introduction

Definition

Haemolytic uraemic syndrome (HUS) is the commonest cause of acute renal failure in infants and young children <5 years of age in developed countries. There is multisystem involvement in this syndrome, which is characterised by sudden onset of non-immune microangiopathic haemolytic anaemia, thrombocytopenia and acute renal failure. Various degrees of severity occur. One-third of patients are anuric at presentation.

An inherited form, which is transmitted in an autosomal dominant manner, may present in the newborn period.

Epidemiology

The commonest form of HUS in children is the one that occurs following a prodromal illness of acute gastroenteritis with bloody diarrhoea. This diarrhoea-associated haemolytic uraemic syndrome (D+HUS) accounts for 90% of cases. D+HUS is most often caused by Shiga toxin (verotoxin) producing *Escherichia coli* (STEC, also called VTEC). Other cytotoxin-producing bacteria such as *Shigella dysenteriae* type 1, *Salmonella typhi* and *Campylobacter* are less common causes of HUS. *Streptococcus pneumoniae* also causes HUS but does so via a completely different mechanism, which involves neuraminidase rather than cytotoxin production.

D+HUS occurs in epidemics as well as sporadically. Outbreaks can be traced to contaminated food, especially undercooked hamburger and contaminated water.

There are over 100 different serotypes of STEC with different phage typing and subtyping. STEC O157:H7 is the commonest subtype producing disease in North America, the British Isles and Japan. It is rare as a causative agent of HUS in Australia, where other types, including O111:H, are pathogenic. *E. coli* can be spread by person to person contact. The incubation period to onset of diarrhoea is 1–8 days.

Non-diarrhoeal-associated HUS (D–HUS) cases account for 10% of cases. These are secondary to:

- non-enteric infections, e.g. streptococcal pneumonia;
- immunosuppression: malignancy-associated, following bone-marrow transplant, and drug-related, e.g. mitomycin, ciclosporin and FK-506 (tacrolimus);
- immunodeficiency and pregnancy may also be associated with HUS.

Pathophysiology

The primary process in the pathogenesis of HUS is vascular endothelial cell injury. *E. coli* is ingested and colonises the gut. These bacteria attach to the epithelium of the distal ileum and large intestine by complex mechanisms. Cytotoxins are produced and they damage the microvasculature of the intestinal wall, causing haemorrhagic and ulcerative intestinal lesions. Once the intestinal–blood barrier has been compromised, the toxins gain entry to the circulation. It is presumed that the toxin then initiates microvascular damage in the glomerular endothelium of the kidneys. Intravascular and intraglomerular fibrin clot is formed and at the same time there is activation of the coagulation system, which leads to occlusion of the vessels and glomerular loss. Erythrocytes passing through these vessels become damaged. Microvascular endothelial cell injury is central to the renal thrombotic microangiopathy that is characteristic of HUS. Thrombocytopenia results from intrarenal platelet adhesion and platelet survival is shortened. Renal dysfunction results from this process.

History

A child who has previously been healthy presents with a history of gastroenteritis within the previous 2 weeks. There is subsequent development of vomiting, bloody diarrhoea and crampy abdominal pain. The child is usually afebrile at presentation. The presentation may resemble an acute surgical abdomen. The child then becomes pale and develops haematuria and oliguria and is noted to become lethargic. Not uncommonly, the patient appears to be improving from his/her gastroenteritis but then deteriorates suddenly, becoming quite ill.

Examination

The child appears pale, lethargic and dehydrated. Petechiae may be noted on the skin, which may also appear jaundiced.

Most patients have some degree of encephalopathy. Central nervous system involvement can range from irritability and restlessness to seizures or coma. Seizures can be present in up to 40%. Hemiparesis and cranial nerve dysfunction may be seen.

Hypertension is present in up to 50% and is likely secondary to increased renin levels. Evidence of cardiac involvement may present as myocarditis, cardiomyopathy or high-output failure. Oliguria occurs often. Hepatomegaly and oedema develop (reflecting fluid overload) if the oliguria is not recognised and fluid intake is not restricted. Splenomegaly is not as common as hepatomegaly.

Investigations

Diagnosis of HUS is based on the presence of microangiopathic haemolytic anaemia, thrombocytopenia and renal failure.

- Anaemia is usually severe and is normochromic normocytic in type with a haemoglobin level of 50–90 g L^{-1}.
- White cell count is non-specific and often raised with increased number of immature forms.
- Platelet count is low in 95% and can be as low as 20×10^9 L^{-1}. Subsequent increase in platelet count may be the first indication of resolution of the microangiopathic process.
- Reticulocyte count is mildly elevated.
- Evidence of schistocytes, burr cells and helmet cells on blood film.
- Coombs test is negative – indicating anaemia is not immunologically mediated.
- Coagulation tests are usually normal but may show mild disseminated intravascular coagulation.
- Serum haptoglobin is low, lactic dehydrogenase (LDH) is elevated along with indirect bilirubin level – all indicators of intravascular haemolysis.
- Elevated serum blood urea, creatinine and phosphate reflect renal involvement, occurring at the same time as the urine output is declining and the haemolysis developing.
- High triglycerides.
- High lipase/amylase reflecting pancreatic involvement.
- Low albumin even without nephrosis.
- Electrolyte derangement may result from the renal abnormalities, including hyponatraemia, hyperkalaemia, hypocalcaemia and metabolic acidosis (which can be severe).
- Urinalysis shows haematuria that can be gross and the red blood cells are dysmorphic. There can be evidence of proteinuria (mild to severe) and leucocytes. Granular and hyaline casts may be present.

Renal biopsy is rarely indicated in children who have the characteristic features of HUS.

Differential diagnosis

- Intussusception.
- Disseminated intravascular coagulation (DIC) in patients with sepsis and multi-organ failure.
- Idiopathic thrombocytopenic purpura (ITP).
- Systemic lupus erythematosus (SLE) with nephropathy.
- Leukaemia.
- Toxic syndromes and encephalitis may have similar presentation.
- Post-infectious glomerulonephritis.

Findings on blood film, coagulation profile, urinalysis, stool and blood cultures assist in differentiating all these conditions from HUS. There is no evidence of haemolysis in intussusception. The complete blood count in leukaemia would reveal low haemoglobin, thrombocytopenia and a white cell count that was depressed or markedly elevated with the presence of blasts.

Patients with DIC have sepsis and prolongation of the prothrombin time and partial thromboplastin time. ITP has isolated thrombocytopenia with a normal coagulation profile.

Treatment

There is no specific therapy for Shiga toxin-producing *E. coli* and prevention of the disease is therefore of utmost importance.

Supportive therapy may include dialysis, antihypertensive therapy, blood transfusions and management of neurological complications. With supportive therapy, 85% of children recover renal function.

The cornerstone of treatment is careful attention to electrolyte and fluid balance. Once intravascular volume has been restored, the amount and type of fluid administered should be limited to ongoing losses, i.e. insensible loss, urine output and gastrointestinal losses.

No added potassium is required unless serum levels are below normal values. Hyperkalaemia must be anticipated and treated in a timely fashion (refer to management of hyperkalaemia in Chapter 10.5 on electrolytes).

Anaemia should be treated with packed red blood cell transfusion (10 mL kg^{-1}) when anaemia is severe, the patient is symptomatic or the haematocrit is falling rapidly. In general, an attempt is made to maintain Hb > 70 g L^{-1} when possible.

Platelet transfusion is avoided because of precipitous worsening of the patient's clinical status. This results from the aggregation of platelets, which are a major constituent of microthrombi and thus induce further damage. Newly formed platelets in HUS function very well and platelet transfusion is not required, even prior to the surgical insertion of a central venous catheter or peritoneal dialysis catheter.

Hypertension responds well to treatment with short-acting calcium channel blockers, e.g. nifedipine. Intravenous nitroglycerine can be used if oral medication is not tolerated. Nitroprusside is not favoured because of the danger of cyanide poisoning in renal failure. Labetalol by intravenous bolus or continuous infusion can also be used to manage hypertension (see Chapter 16.3). Treatment of hypertension can prevent development of encephalopathy and congestive heart failure.

Seizures should be treated with short-acting benzodiazepines initially, followed by intravenous infusion of phenytoin or phenobarbital.

There is some evidence that early dialysis may improve outcome in HUS. Dialysis should be commenced in the following situations:

- severe hyperkalaemia uncontrollable by medical means;
- fluid overload and pulmonary oedema;
- significant uraemic symptoms;
- blood urea >36 mmol L^{-1} even if electrolyte and water balances are satisfactory;
- anuria.

Peritoneal dialysis is generally used in infants and preschool-age children unless there is evidence of severe colitis or abdominal tenderness is present. This management strategy is dependent on the resources and preferences of the managing team/unit.

There are no controlled clinical trials demonstrating efficacy of antibiotic therapy on the prevention and amelioration of HUS. In fact, the use of antibiotics should be avoided in children infected with Shiga toxin *E. coli*.

There are no controlled randomised studies on plasmapheresis as treatment for D+HUS. Plasmapheresis may be beneficial in patients with drug-induced HUS. Vincristine and ciclosporin A are known to cause drug-induced HUS.

Nutritional requirements must be addressed aggressively, as these patients are catabolic and hypoalbuminaemic. Enteral feeds can be commenced once the diarrhoea has settled. Total parenteral nutrition is required in some cases.

No evidence exists for the use of aspirin, heparin, warfarin, streptokinase, urokinase, vitamin E or immunoglobulin G in the treatment of HUS.

Prognosis

Overall prognosis for D+HUS is better than that for D–HUS. However, long-term prognosis for those D+HUS who recover, but have persistent proteinuria 1 year following recovery, is guarded. There is an early mortality rate of about 5%. Another 5% require lifelong dialysis because of the development of chronic renal failure and anuria.

The improved prognosis has resulted from careful correction of electrolyte abnormalities, judicious fluid management and earlier institution of dialysis.

The risk of renal sequelae in children is higher in males, and those with hypertension, prolonged anuria and haemoglobin <100 g L^{-1} at onset of disease.

Other poor prognostic indicators include:

- elevated white cell count ($>20 \times 10^9$ L^{-1}) at presentation;
- elevated white cell count at presentation, which remains elevated;
- age < 1 year or > 5 years;
- central nervous system involvement (seizures, coma, etc.);
- the degree and duration of renal dysfunction.

Complications

Children with D+HUS should be followed for many years following full recovery as some long-term studies have shown late complications developing in patients who had fully recovered initially. These complications include hypertension, proteinuria, reduced glomerular filtration rate and late development of end-stage renal disease (ESRD). ESRD was shown to develop in 10–15% as late as 15–25 years following recovery.

The frequency of complications is higher in D–HUS patients.

HUS can recur in transplanted kidneys regardless of the aetiological agent. Recurrence of disease following renal transplant is infrequent in D+HUS in comparison with D–HUS.

Occasionally, children can be left with chronic sequelae due to HUS, which are not renal related. Almost any organ system can be involved. Stroke is the most serious sequela and occurs in 3–5% of patients. Colitis can result in bowel infarction, leading to colostomy/colectomy or stricture formation.

Pancreatitis can develop, sometimes with diabetes, and hepatic involvement can occur.

Prevention

D+HUS is an infectious disease and the most effective prevention strategy would be to prevent ingestion of the *E. coli*. Avoidance of undercooked meat can assist in this area. There are, however, other vectors for the transmission of the *E. coli* and these include contaminated water and beverages. Food handlers, vendors and consumers must be made aware of proper food-handling techniques.

Controversies and future directions

❶ In one study, a strategy was developed in which a recombinant *E. coli* was generated that had on its surface a lipopolysaccharide (LPS), which mimicked the Shiga toxin receptor. These recombinant *E. coli* bind to the Shiga toxin thus preventing the binding of Shiga toxin to target cells.

❷ Strategies for immunisation have been explored. The first steps in evaluation of development of a vaccine against Shiga-toxin-producing strains of *E. coli* have been undertaken in a preclinical study.

❸ An oligovalent water-soluble carbohydrate pentamer with five pairs of trisaccharide ligands linked to a central dendrimer, and called 'Starfish', neutralises all five B subunits of Shiga toxin and protects human cells from Shiga toxin in culture.

❹ Administration of intravenous γ-globulin IgG and gabexate mesilate, a synthetic serine protease inhibitor used as an anticoagulant resulted in amelioration of disease in five children with D+HUS. The IgG itself has no proven benefit on the course of D+HUS.

❺ The use of angiotensin-converting enzyme inhibitors in conjunction with controlled intake of protein (to recommended daily allowance) may help preserve renal function in children with persistent proteinuria during the chronic stages of Shiga toxin HUS.

❻ New DNA probes to detect Shiga toxin in stool have been developed but are not yet clinically available.

Further reading

Corrigan Jr JJ, Boineau F. Hemolytic uremic syndrome. *Pediatr Rev* 2001;**22**:365–8.

Cronan K, Norman M. Renal and electrolyte emergencies. In: Fleisher GR, Ludwig S, editors. *Textbook of pediatric emergency medicine*. 4th ed. Philadelphia: Lippincott, Williams & Wilkins; 2000. p. 847–8. Chapter 86.

Elliott EJ, Robins-Browne RM, O'Loughlin EV, et al. Nationwide study of haemolytic uraemic syndrome: Clinical, microbiological, and epidemiological features. *Arch Dis Child* 2001;**85**:125–31.

Garg AX, Suri RS, Barrowman N, et al. Long-term renal prognosis of diarrhoea-associated hemolytic uremic syndrome: a systematic review, meta-analysis and meta-regression. *JAMA* 2003;**290**(10):1360–70.

Kaplan B, Meyers K. The pathogenesis of hemolytic uremic syndrome. *J Am Soc Nephrol* 1998;**9**:1126–33.

Ray P, Liu X. Pathogenesis of Shiga toxin-induced hemolytic uremic syndrome. *Pediatr Nephrol* 2001;**16**:823–39.

Ring GH, Lakkis FG, Badr KF. Microvascular diseases of the kidney. In: Brenner B, editor. *The kidney*. 6th ed. vol. 2. Philadelphia: WB Saunders; 2000. p. 1597–603. Chapter 35.

Siegler RL. The hemolytic uremic syndrome. *Pediatr Clin N Am* 1995;**42**(6):1505–22.

Stewart CL, Tina LU. Hemolytic uremic syndrome. *Pediatr Rev* 1993;**14**(6):218–24.

Tarr PI, Gordon CA, Chandler WL. Shiga-toxin-producing *Escherichia coli* and haemolytic uraemic syndrome. *Lancet* 2005;**365**(9464):1073–86.

Trachtman H, Christen E. Pathogenesis, treatment and therapeutic trials in hemolytic uremic syndrome. *Curr Opin Pediatr* 1999;**11**:162–8.

16.6 Nephrotic syndrome

Karen McCarthy

ESSENTIALS

1 Nephrotic syndrome refers to the clinical findings of hypoalbuminaemia, heavy proteinuria, oedema and hyperlipidaemia. Every child has albuminaemia but not all features are necessary for diagnosis.

2 Despite the presence of oedema, shock still needs to be treated with 20 mL kg^{-1} 0.9% saline or albumin boluses.

3 Renal function is usually normal though serum creatinine may be slightly elevated at presentation.

4 There is 1–2% mortality despite good long-term prognosis.

5 The physical findings of peritonitis in nephrotic syndrome may be very subtle, thus the emergency physician must have a very high index of suspicion for peritonitis.

6 Death from peritonitis and thrombosis can occur despite very good care.

7 All children with nephritic syndrome should receive pneumococcal vaccine.

8 All non-immune children on steroid therapy who are exposed to varicella require prompt administration of zoster immune globulin. Should they develop lesions, they require treatment with intravenous aciclovir.

Introduction

Definition

Nephrotic syndrome (NS) refers to the findings of heavy proteinuria, hypoalbuminaemia, oedema and hyperlipidaemia, which result from a massive loss of protein in the urine secondary to glomerular disease. All components of the disease do not need to be present for diagnosis. The protein lost in the urine includes plasma proteins of molecular weight up to and including albumin. Generalised glomerular leak to macromolecules does not occur in most cases, but can occur in severe disease. In severe disease, as there is progressive loss of glomerular permselectivity, renal clearance of IgG approaches that of albumin. Protein selectivity is seen mainly in minimal change nephrotic syndrome. The determination of protein selectivity has little clinical value but does increase the likelihood of response to steroid therapy.

The hallmarks of nephrotic syndrome are hypoalbuminaemia (serum albumin <30 g L^{-1}), heavy proteinuria (>50 mg kg^{-1} body weight per 24 hours, or >1000 mg m^{-2} per 24 hours), generalised oedema and hyperlipidaemia (triglycerides and cholesterol).

Primary nephrotic syndrome (idiopathic) represents disease limited to the kidney. Disease is classified by responsiveness to steroid therapy (steroid sensitive, steroid dependent or steroid resistant) and histology on renal biopsy (minimal change, mesangial proliferative glomerulonephritis (GN) and focal segmental glomerulosclerosis, FSGS).

Secondary nephrotic syndrome represents multisystem disease that has kidney involvement, e.g. lupus nephritis, hereditary nephritis and Henoch–Schönlein purpura.

Certain drugs and chemicals can cause nephrotic syndrome, e.g. phenytoin, non-steroidal anti-inflammatory drugs, and captopril.

Epidemiology

Minimal change nephrotic syndrome (MCNS) is more common in males. Mean age of onset is <6 years for primary nephrotic syndrome, and >6 years for secondary. It is usually sporadic. A congenital form, inherited in an autosomal recessive manner, presents in the newborn period.

Aetiology

The cause of primary nephrotic syndrome is unknown and hence is referred to as idiopathic. The commonest form is minimal change disease (85%). Renal biopsy findings in this form show no abnormality of the glomeruli on light microscopy. Electron microscopy shows effacement of the epithelial foot processes. Biopsy findings of FSGS (10%) reveal normal appearing glomeruli but may show some mesangial proliferation. Some biopsy specimens may demonstrate segmental scarring. Mesangial proliferative disease (5%) shows diffuse increase in mesangial cells and matrix on biopsy.

Pathophysiology

An immune basis for MCNS was proposed in 1974 but no primary immune abnormality has been identified. Studies have shown increased levels of circulating soluble interleukin-2 receptor in patients with active MCNS and FSGS. This soluble interleukin-2 receptor is shed by activated lymphocytes and may therefore indicate generalised activation of the immune system. However, this circulating soluble interleukin-2 receptor could serve as a neutraliser of circulating interleukin-2. It is unknown whether circulating levels represent evidence of activation or an attempt to down-regulate the immune responses.

There is hypercoagulability resulting from serum protein abnormalities introduced by renal protein wasting. All children with acute NS have increased platelet aggregation. Blood viscosity is increased and blood flow is reduced. Fibrinogen concentration is increased and antithrombin III is lost in the urine. All these factors contribute to this problem in NS.

The cause of cholesterolaemia and hypertriglyceridaemia remains uncertain. One theory is that reduced plasma oncotic pressure may stimulate lipoprotein synthesis and perhaps lipolytic factors may be lost in the urine.

Oedema reflects retention of salt and water. Reduced serum albumin causes a reduction in plasma oncotic pressure. When plasma oncotic pressure falls, intravascular volume is reduced, which stimulates proximal tubular reabsorption of sodium. The renin–angiotensin system is also stimulated, raising the serum aldosterone, which further increases distal tubular reabsorption of sodium. There is an increase in filtration capacity in patients with nephrotic syndrome along with an increase in glomerular permeability, resulting in proteinuria.

There is also evidence in some patients for primary salt and water retention by the kidney.

History

The presence of the following may be noted on history:

- recent flu-like illness;
- anorexia;
- abdominal pain;
- diarrhoea;
- recent ant bites or bee stings.

Examination

Periorbital oedema is noted initially, but in time oedema becomes generalised. Oedema of the lower extremities is usually 'pitting' in type and accumulates in dependent sites. The rate and degree of oedema formation is directly related to salt intake and to the degree of hypoalbuminaemia and therefore can vary from child to child. Ascites may be present. Pleural effusions or pulmonary oedema may develop. Scrotal or perineal oedema may be very distressing to the patient. Blood pressure may be decreased when hypovolaemia exists or may be elevated if there is significant renal disease by activation of the renin–angiotensin system or primary salt retention.

Investigations

- Hypoalbuminaemia (serum albumin <30 g L^{-1}) occurs in every child with nephrotic syndrome.
- Reliably timed 24-hour urine collections are difficult to obtain in children (protein excretion exceeds 50 mg kg^{-1} per 24 hours or 1000 mg m^{-2} per 24 hours in nephrotic syndrome), so the proteinuria is generally quantified by the ratio of urine protein to urine creatinine. Spot urine protein:creatinine ratio is >300 mg $nmol^{-1}$ in nephrotic syndrome.. Normal is <0.2 mg protein per mg creatinine (or protein per mmol creatinine).
- Microscopic haematuria is seen in $< 15\%$ but macroscopic haematuria is rare.
- Urinalysis by dipstick reveals $+ 3$ or $+ 4$ proteinuria.
- Urine specific gravity is usually high at >1.020, but may be lower.
- Haematocrit is often elevated due to intravascular depletion and can be followed to assess fluid status.
- Hyperlipidaemia is present with elevated serum cholesterol and triglyceride levels.
- Serum sodium can be low due to decreased free water excretion but is rarely symptomatic and does not require treatment. Total body sodium is high.
- Hypocalcaemia is a common finding and reflects the low serum albumin. The ionised calcium is usually normal, however, and the hypocalcaemia is asymptomatic.
- Plasma urea and creatinine are elevated in approximately 25% of patients.
- Serum complement levels are normal in MCNS, FSGS and mesangial proliferative glomerulonephritis.

Steroids can be used as a diagnostic tool in the management of NS. The patient is said to be steroid responsive when the urine becomes free of protein. If the child continues to have proteinuria ($>2 +$) after 4–8 weeks of compliance with continuous daily prednisone, the nephrosis is termed steroid resistant and renal biopsy is indicated to determine the precise cause, e.g. FSGS.

Renal biopsy is not indicated during the initial episode of acute nephrotic syndrome. The need for, and timing of a renal biopsy is determined by the subsequent disease course, e.g. poor or no response of initial episode to steroid therapy after 4–8 weeks of treatment or if other signs or symptoms are present that indicate a systemic disease.

Differential diagnosis

Other causes of oedema need to be excluded: congestive heart failure; starvation; protein-losing enteropathy; cystic fibrosis; hypothyroidism; vasculitis; and steroid therapy.

Treatment

- It can be difficult to assess volume status in patients with NS. The patient may be in shock despite the presence of oedema. Attention to detail on clinical examination can assist with the assessment. Clues to hypovolaemia are: tachycardia; peripheral vasoconstriction with poor capillary refill time; and orthostatic hypotension, i.e. positive tilt test. Other clues to volume status include a history of oliguria and evidence of renal insufficiency on laboratory investigations.
- Albumin infusions transiently increase plasma volume and are most useful in patients with profound volume depletion. Plasma volume is increased using 4% albumin rather than 0.9% saline. It is important to note that this is only a temporising measure. The infused albumin is rapidly lost in the urine, especially when the original albumin level is very low because of high renal albumin clearance (rate of loss is proportional to albumin clearance and serum albumin level). The patient can develop acute pulmonary oedema requiring admission to an intensive-care unit.
- In a patient symptomatic from massive oedema, a trial of diuretics may be given, provided the patient is not hypovolaemic, and only after discussion with a nephrologist. Diuretics may induce hypotension, severe volume depletion, ARF and hyperkalaemia if there is already incipient hypovolaemia. An infusion of 20% salt-deficient albumin 0.5–1 g kg^{-1}, followed 30 minutes later by furosemide 0.5–1 mg kg^{-1} intravenously can be effective. In occasional circumstances, ultrafiltration or haemofiltration may be used to manage fluid overload.
- The natriuretic effect of furosemide is thought to be diminished in NS. Increasing the dose or using furosemide in combination with a diuretic acting at another site, such as a thiazide diuretic (hydrochlorothiazide 1 mg kg^{-1} day^{-1} in two divided doses) is recommended to overcome the hyporesponsiveness. Metolazone (diuretic activity on the distal tubule) is a powerful diuretic and is occasionally employed but must be used

with caution. If serum albumin is <15 g L^{-1}, diuretic therapy is ineffective.

- Oral fluids, when offered, should be given in small aliquots, especially in hyponatraemic patients, in whom any free water will tend to lower the plasma sodium further.

- Therapeutic paracentesis may be indicated for acute respiratory distress but is rarely necessary. Respiratory distress is due to reduced lung capacity secondary to the increased abdominal pressure. Paracentesis should only be used when there is no other way to support respiration, because of the association of complications with the procedure, e.g. infection and the re-accumulation of the fluid.

- Prednisolone is started at 2 mg kg^{-1} day^{-1} (60 mg m^{-2} day^{-1}) in two divided doses. A divided daily dose is used in preference to a single dose as some children who fail to respond to a single daily dose respond to divided doses. Disappearance of proteinuria is seen in 90% within 4–6 weeks.

- If the child is unwell or peritonitis is suspected, antibiotics are commenced after appropriate cultures are taken. Prophylactic antibiotics are generally recommended for all patients whilst nephrotic and on high-dose steroids.

- Some units advocate routine use of low-dose aspirin, though this is not commonly done.

- Angiotensin-converting enzyme (ACE) inhibitors are good antihypertensive drugs in those patients who have hypertension from their primary disease or as a result of steroid therapy. ACE inhibitors are useful as most of the hypertension is due to activation of the renin–angiotensin system. If the hypertension is a result of steroid therapy, the patient may respond better to a β-blocker.

- Some children with MCNS who are steroid-responsive either relapse frequently or require a high daily dose of steroids to maintain remission. These children are at risk of development of serious side effects from the steroids, including growth failure, hypertension, osteoporotic bone disease and posterior sublenticular cataracts. The alkylating

agents cyclophosphamide or chlorambucil can produce prolonged and sometimes permanent remission and are considered to be 'steroid-sparing'. These alkylating agents are not commonly needed in patients with MCNS but when needed they are very effective. Some patients with MCNS may not respond to the alkylating agents and will respond to ciclosporin (<5.5 mg kg^{-1} per 24 hours or <200 mg m^{-2} per 24 hours) if there is steroid responsiveness. Dependence on ciclosporin is common, the effect lasting only as long as treatment continues. Some nephrologists consider the limited risk of ciclosporin nephrotoxicity in this population to be preferable to the side effects of chronic steroid toxicity or the risk of sterility from a second alkylating agent when one course of an alkylating agent is insufficient therapy.

- In FSGS ciclosporin is more effective in steroid-dependent rather than in steroid-resistant disease and may even be more nephrotoxic in this latter group.

- Whilst on steroid therapy, non-immune children exposed to chickenpox require prompt administration of zoster immune globulin.

- Immunisations: Live-virus vaccines should not be administered to children on high-dose corticosteroid therapy. Children receiving <2 mg kg^{-1} per 24 hours of prednisolone or its equivalent, can be immunised. Those children receiving >2 mg kg^{-1} per 24 hours daily or alternate daily prednisolone or its equivalent for more than 14 days, should have live-virus vaccine administration deferred for at least 1 month after discontinuation of the steroids. Resonse to treatment – see Table 16.6.1.

Disposition

Outpatient management is appropriate for children with the first presentation of NS, if the oedema is not massive and there is no suspicion of infection or life-threatening complications and the physician can be assured of close follow up. The rest are best managed as inpatients to permit further work up and treatment and to provide education and support for the patient and family.

Admission is warranted in a child with known history of nephrotic syndrome if there are signs of severe dehydration, unexplained fever, renal insufficiency (i.e. elevation in serum creatinine), refractory oedema (e.g. respiratory distress) or suspected peritonitis. Discuss admission of frequent relapsers, or > 1st relapse, with the nephrologist.

Prognosis

Long-term prognosis is good for children with steroid-responsive primary nephrotic syndrome, though 1–2% mortality is associated. Most deaths are due to peritonitis or sepsis (pneumonia), and thrombus, which may occur despite good care. Relapses may recur for many years, often until puberty, with a small number continuing to relapse through to adulthood. These relapses are not usually severe and can be treated with short courses of oral steroids. Though these children with steroid-responsive disease may require steroid therapy intermittently throughout childhood, serious sequelae of steroid toxicity are uncommon.

When in remission, the child should have unrestricted diet and activity.

Recovery is considered permanent if the child remains asymptomatic and has no requirement for medications for more than 2 years.

Table 16.6.1	Definitions of response to treatment
Remission	Urine protein excretion <4 mg hr^{-1} m^{-2} or urine protein negative/trace for 3 consecutive days
Relapse	Urine protein on Dipstix 2+ for 3 consecutive days having previously been in remission. This occurs in up to 75% of patients
Frequent relapse	2 more relapses within 6 months or >4 relapses in 12 months
Steroid dependence	2 consecutive relapses occurring during steroid treatment or within 14 days of its cessation
Steroid resistance	Failure to achieve response after 28 days of steroid at 60 mg m^{-2} day^{-1}

Complications

As MCNS is a self-limited disease in most children, a distinction must be made between the complications of the disease itself and those that are related to the treatment. Major complications of the disease itself are infection, dislipidaemia and thrombosis. Treatment with steroids may increase body mass index and impair growth.

Acute complications occur in two groups of patients:

❶ Those who present de novo or in relapse but not taking steroids.

❷ Those who present in relapse or remission while still receiving pharmacological doses of steroids.

The tendency to develop infections is a true complication of the disease.

Hypogammaglobulinaemia Is a factor in the reduced defences against bacterial infections. IgG is the immunoglobulin most severely depleted. This may be a consequence of it being the smallest of the immunoglobulins and the one with the greatest renal excretion.

Bacterial infections occur in both groups but are more common in the steroid-treated group

Spontaneous bacterial peritonitis is a major source of morbidity in children with NS. Main causative organisms are *Streptococcus pneumoniae* and *Escherichia coli*. Diagnosis of peritonitis should always be considered in a child with nephrotic syndrome who complains of abdominal pain. The physical findings of peritonitis in NS may be very subtle. The patient does not necessarily have a rigid abdomen. The physician must have a high index of suspicion when assessing these patients. Steroid therapy, especially high dose (2 mg kg^{-1} day^{-1} of prednisolone) can mask the typical signs and symptoms of infection. Children with NS can develop other infections such as pneumonia, cellulitis and sepsis.

Thromboembolism from hypercoagulability is the second major contributor to morbidity and mortality. The thrombus is usually venous and is located in the deep vessels of the extremities, renal vein, pulmonary venous system and cerebral cortical system. For this reason, it is recommended that femoral or deep venepuncture is avoided if possible in children with nephrotic syndrome. The risk of thromboembolus is real and exists even in the first acute presentation with NS. This is due to increased platelet aggregation, and in part also due to the urinary loss of several proteins that inhibit blood coagulation, especially antithrombin-III, protein C and protein S. Increased blood viscosity and reduced blood flow also play a role. Renal vein thrombosis should be suspected if flank pain, haematuria and decreased renal function occur. Occlusion of the arterial system is uncommon.

Hyperlipidaemia associated with NS rarely gives rise to clinical complications as it usually reverses with steroid therapy. It may become problematic in patients with chronic NS.

Symptomatic hypovolaemia Despite the presence of oedema, symptomatic hypovolaemia leading to shock can develop if fluids are restricted injudiciously with or without diuretic therapy

Respiratory compromise can rarely be caused by massive ascites, warranting emergency paracentesis in some cases

Hypertensive encephalopathy Acute increase in blood pressure may occur in steroid-treated children at any stage of their illness. The diagnosis of hypertensive encephalopathy is based on the degree of change in the blood pressure and rate of increase rather than on a specific level of systolic and/or diastolic blood pressure.

Benign intracranial hypertension can be precipitated by abrupt reduction in steroid doses

Growth can be impaired in nephrotic syndrome. Insulin-like growth factor (IGF-1)-binding protein is lost in the urine, which may account for the reduced serum levels of IGF-1 and IGF-2. Growth impairment is also a consequence of steroid therapy.

Prevention

As the primary causes of idiopathic nephrotic syndrome are unknown, there is no means of prevention.

There is some evidence supporting a role of the immune system in paediatric minimal change disease. Relapses can be triggered by minor infections.

Vaccination against varicella, influenza and pneumococcus would seem prudent, given the relapsing nature of nephrotic syndrome. Some susceptibility to infection may result from loss of opsonising factors in the urine so even if the child has been immunised, vigilance is warranted against the possibility of any bacterial infection.

Controversies and future directions

Cyclo-oxygenase inhibitors are a class of drugs that may be of assistance in reducing proteinuria in patients with NS, although, unlike ACE inhibitors, they generally cause a reduction in GFR.

Further reading

Bergstein J. Conditions particularly associated with proteinuria. In: Behrman R, Kliegman R, Jenson H, editors. *Nelson's textbook of pediatrics*. 16th ed. Philadelphia: WB Saunders; 2000. p. 1592–6.

Cronan K, Norman M. Renal and electrolyte emergencies. In: Fleisher G, Ludwig S, editors. *Textbook of pediatric emergency medicine*. 4th ed. Philadelphia: Lippincott Williams & Wilkins; 2000. p. 832–5.

Falk RJ, Charles Jennette J, Nachman PH. Nephrotic syndrome. In: Brenner B, editor. *The kidney*. 6th ed. vol. 2. Philadelphia: WB Saunders; 2000. p. 1266–83.

Gipson DS, Massengill SF, Yaol L, et al. Management of childhood onset nephrotic syndrome. *Pediatrics* 2009;**124**:747–57.

Grimbert P, Audard V, Remy P, et al. Recent approaches to the pathogenesis of minimal-change nephrotic syndrome. *Nephrol Dial Transpl* 2003;**18**:245–8.

Kaysen GA. Proteinuria and the nephrotic syndrome. In: Schrier RW, editor. *Renal and electrolyte disorders*. 6th ed. Philadelphia: Lippincott, Williams & Wilkins; 2003. p. 580–614.

Roth KS, Amaker BH, Chan JCM. Nephrotic syndrome: Pathogenesis and management. *Pediatr Rev* 2002;**23**: 237–47.

16.7 Henoch–Schönlein purpura

Karen McCarthy

ESSENTIALS

1 There is no diagnostic laboratory test for the diagnosis of Henoch-Schönlein purpura.

2 The diagnosis is clinical and consists of the tetrad: palpable purpura in patients with neither thrombocytopenia or coagulopathy, arthritis/arthralgia, abdominal pain and renal disease.

3 Urinalysis, and blood pressure should be measured at presentation.

4 Clinical hallmark of Henoch–Schönlein nephritis is haematuria.

5 Onset of nephritis may be delayed for weeks or months after onset of other symptoms.

6 All patients with Henoch–Schönlein nephritis need follow up for 6 months even if urinalysis is normal at presentation.

7 There is no need for follow up beyond the first 6 months if urinalysis remains normal.

8 Recurrence of Henoch–Schönlein purpura is common and is normally observed within 4 months of resolution of original symptoms.

Introduction

Henoch–Schönlein purpura (HSP) is the most common acute vasculitis affecting children. It has a prominent cutaneous component. It is a leukocytoclastic vasculitis that affects small vessels (arterioles and venules). The aetiology is unknown. The disease is more common in males, with mean age of occurrence 4–7 years. Infants tend to have milder disease and those less than 2 years of age are less likely to have nephritis and abdominal pain in comparison with older children. With the exception of nephritis, it is generally an acute self-limited illness lasting from several days to several weeks.

The characteristic histological finding on skin biopsy is neutrophil infiltration in and around dermal vessels. Histological changes in the kidney range from minimal change to focal or diffuse mesangial proliferation that may be accompanied by glomerular crescent formation. The characteristic finding on immunofluorescence is diffuse mesangial deposition of immunoglobulin A (IgA) and complement 3 (C3). IgA plays a central role in the pathogenesis of HSP.

The reported incidence of nephritis is 20-50% but may in fact be higher. Renal involvement may manifest with haematuria ± proteinuria and occasionally with nephritic or nephrotic syndrome or with renal failure associated with rapidly progressive glomerulonephritis. Risk factors for renal progression are nephrosis, hypertension, renal impairment at presentation, and haematuria.

History

There is usually a history of antecedent upper respiratory tract infection. The characteristic rash is the most frequent presentation. Arthritis is the second most frequent manifestation, occurring in approximately 80% and though it may be incapacitating, it is self-limiting and non-deforming. Gastrointestinal involvement occurs in 50–75% of patients and is potentially the most serious complication of HSP due to the possible development of gastrointestinal bleeding and intussusception.

The clinical hallmark of HSP nephritis is haematuria. In contrast to arthritis and abdominal pain, it is extremely uncommon for nephritis to precede the appearance of the rash. The onset of nephritis may in fact be delayed for weeks or months after the onset of other symptoms. Approximately 80% of patients manifest nephritis within 4 weeks and 95% within 3 months of the onset of other symptoms.

Examination

The clinical features of HSP may be atypical in the extremes of age. The clinical manifestations can develop over days or weeks. The characteristic rash consists of crops of palpable purpura and is symmetric in distribution and located on the extensor surfaces of the arms, legs and buttocks. It is worth noting that the rash is not restricted to these areas. The rash may begin with urticaria that progresses over 24 hours to palpable purpura. The arthritis involves the knees, ankles or feet and may result in refusal to weight bear. Periarticular swelling and tenderness are often noted.

Gastrointestinal symptoms of nausea, vomiting and abdominal pain occur in approximately 50%. These symptoms are caused by submucosal haemorrhage and oedema. Asymptomatic microscopic haematuria occurs in most but up to 40% have gross haematuria. Proteinuria occurs in conjunction with haematuria in two-thirds of patients but the occurrence of proteinuria alone is rare.

Investigations

- Diagnosis of HSP is straightforward when the typical rash is present.
- Diagnosis of HSP requires a normal platelet count by definition.
- There is no diagnostic laboratory test for HSP – routine laboratory tests are neither specific nor diagnostic.
- Urinalysis should be performed to establish the presence of microscopic haematuria, with or without proteinuria.

- Serum creatinine should be checked when HSP nephritis is present.
- Blood pressure should be measured and recorded at presentation for baseline evaluation.

Differential diagnosis

The differential diagnosis of a purpuric rash is broad. Purpura may be the initial manifestation of an infectious process.

Meningococcaemia Palpable purpura (as opposed to the usual non-palpable purpura) can occur if there are pre-existing coagulation abnormalities (such as protein S or protein C deficiency). This diagnosis must be considered in any child with purpura.

Kawasaki disease Considered in the patient with an unremitting fever with a maculopapular rash that is prominent on the lower extremities. This rash, however, does not appear in crops and is not associated with arthritis. The eye findings in Kawasaki disease are usually absent in HSP.

Bacterial endocarditis, infectious mononucleosis, rubeola and streptococcal infection may present with a purpuric rash. HSP can occur with other forms of vasculitis or autoimmune disease, such as inflammatory bowel disease or familial Mediterranean fever.

Rocky Mountain spotted fever should be considered in endemic areas when there is a history of tick exposure.

Treatment

Treatment is mainly supportive with hydration, rest and analgesics.

There is suggestive evidence that corticosteroids enhance the rate of resolution of the arthritis and abdominal pain but do not appear to prevent recurrence of disease. Available data, though considered somewhat controversial, suggest that patients with severe nephritis (haematuria, nephrotic syndrome, decreased glomerular filtration rate (GFR) and crescent formation involving >50% of the glomeruli) should receive a combination of high-dose intravenous methylprednisolone (30 mg kg^{-1} day^{-1}) for 3 days followed by oral steroids plus an immunosuppressive agent, either azathioprine or cyclophosphamide.

Plasmapheresis has been reported to be of benefit in a few patients with rapidly progressive HSP glomerulonephritis i.e. severe disease.

Hypertension – angiotensin blockade by use of angiotensin-converting enzyme (ACE) inhibitors like enalapril may decrease proteinuria and result in slower deterioration in renal function as well as providing effective control of blood pressure.

Disposition

Outpatient management is appropriate for most patients with HSP.

Inpatient management may be required for management of abdominal pain and the arthritis/arthralgia, especially if the child is unable to ambulate. Urinalysis should be performed weekly whilst the disease is active. Provided there is no evidence of nephritis during this period, patients should have a urinalysis on a monthly basis for 6 months after all other manifestations have resolved.

Patients who develop nephritis at any time should have blood pressure and serum creatinine monitored periodically until the nephritis has resolved.

Children with overt renal disease, e.g. complicated by nephrotic syndrome, hypertension or renal insufficiency at presentation should be referred to the renal physicians for management, as a renal biopsy may be required to predict prognosis more precisely. These patients usually require prolonged follow up.

Recurrence

A recurrence rate of 40% has been reported for symptoms of HSP. The recurrences tend to resemble the original episode but are usually milder and of shorter duration.

Recurrences appear to be more common in those patients with nephritis.

With each recurrence of disease, patients should have urinalysis and blood pressure checked.

HSP nephritis may recur in transplanted kidneys. Recurrence of the nephritis and extra-renal manifestations are more likely in recipients of living related-donor kidneys than of cadaveric kidneys. It is recommended that transplantation is delayed for 12–24 months following disappearance of the purpuric lesions.

Complications

- Acute renal insufficiency with elevation of serum creatinine can develop in patients with HSP nephritis.
- Patients can also develop nephrotic syndrome. In this situation the urine protein excretion is >50 mg kg^{-1} per 24 hours, with oedema and hypoalbuminaemia.
- End-stage renal disease (ESRD) is a possible complication of HSP nephritis.
- Orchitis is a well-described complication of HSP and it may mimic testicular torsion.
- Testicular torsion can be an infrequent complication of scrotal oedema.
- Gastrointestinal bleeding and intussusception can complicate HSP.

Prognosis

Though the overall prognosis is excellent for HSP, nephritis is the one manifestation that can become chronic. Renal disease develops in 5%. Prognosis depends on the severity and extent of renal involvement. In general, patients with isolated haematuria, with or without trivial proteinuria, have a uniformly good prognosis. However, up to 50% of children with nephritis associated with nephrotic syndrome may progress to renal insufficiency. Approximately 20–50% will have persistent urinary abnormalities on long-term follow up but only 1% of patients progress to ESRD.

Clinical presentation is helpful but is not a precise determinant of prognosis. Severity of renal disease and the ultimate outcome correlate more closely with histopathological changes on renal biopsy and the degree of proteinuria at presentation. Poor prognosis is associated with crescent formation involving more than 50% of the glomeruli.

Regardless of clinical presentation or histological changes, all patients with nephritis need prolonged follow up since deterioration in renal function may occur in some patients many years later.

Prevention

There appears to be no single pathogen or environmental agent that has emerged as an important precipitating cause of HSP, thus there is no means of preventing HSP.

Controversies and future directions

❶ A number of studies have addressed the question of whether early corticosteroid treatment prevents the delayed appearance of nephritis but the results are conflicting.

❷ Further work is needed to explore the role of cytokines in determining the exclusive involvement of IgA1 in the immunopathogenesis of HSP. IgA has two subclasses, IgA1 and IgA2, but HSP is associated with abnormalities involving IgA1 rather than with IgA2.

❸ The fundamental abnormality responsible for HSP and IgA nephropathy needs to be elucidated.

❹ Role of other immunosuppressives?

Further reading

Chang W-L, Yang YH, Wang LC, et al. Renal manifestations in henoch Schonlein purpura: a 10 year clinical study. *Ped Nephrol* 2005;**20**:1269–72.

Cronan K, Norman M. Renal and electrolyte emergencies. In: Fleisher G, Ludwig S, editors. *Textbook of pediatric emergency medicine*. 4th ed. Philadelphia: Lippincott Williams & Wilkins; 2000. p. 851.

Meulders Q, Pirson Y, Cosyns JP. Course of Henoch–Schönlein nephritis after renal transplantation. *Transplantation* 1994;**58**:1179–86.

Narchi H. Risk of longterm renal impairment and duration of follow up recommended for Henoch Schonlein Purpura with normal or minimal urinary findings: a systematic review. *Arch Dis Child* 2005;**90**:916–20.

Oner A, Tinaztepe K, Erdogan O. The effect of triple therapy on rapidly progressive type of Henoch–Schönlein nephritis. *Paediatr Nephrol* 1995;**9**:6–10.

Saulsbury FT. Henoch–Schönlein purpura in children – Report of 100 patients and review of the literature. *Medicine* 1999;**78**(6):395–406.

17.1 Paediatric psychiatric emergencies

Raymond Chin • Michael Fairley

ESSENTIALS

1 Children with psychological problems often present with somatic complaints and at times of family crisis. The treating emergency physician should be aware of this.

2 Early identification of psychological illness can reduce prolonged investigations and expedite specific psychiatric treatment.

Introduction

Paediatric patients and, at times, their parents can provide complex diagnostic and logistic challenges to staff in a busy emergency department (ED). They often present in a time of life crisis. However, the complaint may be primarily emotional. The majority of cases have no clear diagnosis and may be complicated by multiple visits to previous medical practitioners.

Assessment requires time and patience and unique clinical skills. Intent listening with directed questioning is required. It is important to avoid drawing premature conclusions, and emotional factors should be considered, even when the problem appears predominantly organic.

General approach

Assessment

In the case of children, parents generally initiate medical contact, so it is important to seek the child's opinion early. If possible, a history from both the parent and the child should be obtained. Reassurance needs to be provided that the visit is not a punishment. Playing and drawing may put the child at ease.

In adolescents, self-referral for psychological problems is more likely, but is usually associated with reluctance to identify and discuss the problem. Physical complaint may point to a psychological issue, e.g. headache and panic attack. As the patient is usually unco-operative, reassurance should be provided about confidentiality.

History

A thorough medical history is imperative. In addition, the six Ps of collateral history should be explored.

Collateral history

❶ Pre-existing psychological disorders, life experiences, medical conditions, family vulnerability.
❷ Precipitants – trigger for presentation.
❸ Presentation – why now, who is most troubled by the symptom.
❹ Perpetuation – factors that operate to prevent recovery.
❺ Positives – strengths and resources, coping with previous problems.

❻ Preconceptions – belief system, expectations from medical consultation. What the child and parent really want.

Synthesis of assessment

It should be possible for the emergency physician to determine why the child is attending, who wants something done, and where the main pathology rests; in the patient, the parent or their relationship.

Examination

Examination includes obtaining vital signs, and a physical and mental state exam.

Investigations

Special tests should be confined to the differential diagnosis of assessment.

COMMON PAEDIATRIC PSYCHIATRIC PRESENTATIONS

The acutely disturbed child

See separate chapter dealing with this presentation.

Suicidal patients

It is important to establish:

❶ Risk of suicide or repeat attempt.
❷ Nature of current crisis and meaning of the event.
❸ Presence of psychiatric disorder.

❹ Background history, personality style, coping mechanisms.
❺ Social supports.
❻ Source of appropriate help.

Introduction

The presentation of a child or adolescent with self-directed harm or injury constitutes a medical and psychiatric emergency, even if the need for medical urgency appears low. The presentation of a child or adolescent with suicidal ideation but no apparent physical injury similarly constitutes a psychiatric emergency. More people die in Australia by suicide than by motor-vehicle accidents. The ratio of male to female suicides is currently approximately 4:1 and the figures representing ratios of male to female attempted suicides vary generally from being equal to up to 15:1 in favour of females.[1]

The rate of suicide in older teenagers has increased, especially over the past 30 years. Although rare in prepubertal children, it is always indicative of a severe disorder.

In young persons who commit suicide, up to 46% have made a prior threat or attempt, and of those who attempt suicide, some 10% eventually kill themselves, often within 2 years.

The most important contribution that can be made to the prevention of suicide is the recognition of the early signs of mental illness, in particular, depression and schizophrenia. Depression can present as school failure after normal achievement, hypochondriasis, social withdrawal and aggressive behaviour, more often than verbal complaints of depression and anxiety.

Energetic, persistent and effective treatment is required once a suicide attempt has been made.

Risk factors

Theories abound to explain these high suicide rates although many of the assumptions about causality are not proven but based only on occasions. Nevertheless, a thorough review of the literature[2] leads to the conclusion that the risk of suicidal behaviour is increased among young people who:

- have previously attempted suicide;
- have a mood disorder or are involved in harmful use of drugs (including alcohol);
- have problems involving violence;

- are from a socially disadvantaged background characterised by low socioeconomic status, limited educational achievements, low income, poverty and associated factors;
- experience parental loss through separation and divorce;
- have experienced physical or sexual abuse;
- have experienced impaired parent–child relationships;
- have parents with a mental illness such as mood disorders, harmful drug use (including alcohol) or problems involving violence;
- experienced loss through suicide in their family or peer group;
- experience a greater number of life stresses than normal.

Evaluation of the suicidal crisis
Suicidal act
- Intent (wish to die).
- Lethality (danger to life).
- Mitigating circumstances (factors interfering with the person's ability to assess the consequences of the act).

Specific enquiry into:

- Degree of isolation, probability of intervention, precautions against discovery.
- Actions to gain help during, or after, an attempt.
- Degree of planning, level of impulsivity.
- Communication of intent, suicide note.
- Expectations of method's lethality.
- Conception of reversibility with medical attention.
- Use of alcohol or other drugs.

Circumstance of the act
- Precipitants – bereavement, separation, custody, disciplinary crisis.
- Immediate past history.
- Interpersonal relationships.
- Social support systems.
- Impact on others – e.g. rescue or rejection.
- Family diseases.

Mental state examination
Look for:

- suicidal ideation;
- ongoing depression;
- psychotic features (delusions, hallucinations);

- pervasive hopelessness;
- quality of interaction with the interviewer.

Document:

- appearance;
- behaviour during interview;
- communication (content, themes, structure);
- affect (mood);
- perception;
- cognition (orientation level, formal thought disorder);
- insight into present situation;
- judgement;
- rapport.

Hazards during assessment
- Use of denial by parents, doctors and nurses.
- Refusal to be interviewed.
- Lack of insight.
- Negative influence of relatives.
- Pressure and hostility from other staff.

Management following an attempt
❶ Comprehensive medical assessment for extent of injury as soon as possible. This should occur prior to psychiatric examination.
❷ Admission to a medical unit if outcome of assessment indicated that physical safety has been adversely affected.
❸ If medical status is stable, referral to psychiatry for assessment is required in all cases.

Anxiety disorders

Anxiety is a complex feeling of apprehension, fear, and worry often accompanied by pulmonary, cardiac, and other physical sensations. It is a ubiquitous condition that varies from the physiological to the pathological in its presentation. Panic disorder has a lifetime prevalence of 1.5–3.5%.

In school refusal, the child often presents with a somatic complaint such as abdominal pain. Cases of syncopal collapse may manifest as a panic attack. Early identification can reduce the number of medical investigations and commence early psychiatric referral.

Acute anxiety can effectively be treated with a comprehensive approach utilising psychotherapy, counselling, and a wide spectrum of anxiolytics (e.g. benzodiazepines, buspirone, and antidepressants).

Autism

A syndrome of early childhood characterised by: abnormal social relationships; language disorder with impaired understanding, echolalia; rituals and compulsive phenomena; and uneven intellectual development with mental retardation in most cases.

Autism is two to four times more common in boys than girls.

Autism usually is manifest in the first year of life; its onset is not later than age 3 years.

Treatment

For the most severely impaired children, systematic application of behaviour therapy, a technique that can be taught to parents, helps manage the child in the home and at school. Butyrophenones provide limited benefit, mainly in controlling the most severe forms of aggressive and self-destructive behaviour – they do not resolve the psychosis. Fenfluramine, a serotonergic antagonist, is no longer available.

Speech therapy should begin early. For mute children, the value of learning sign language is not yet established. Children in the near-normal or higher IQ range often benefit from psychotherapy and special education.

Childhood schizophrenia

Psychotic states usually have onset after age 7 years and with behavioural similarities to adult schizophrenia. Evidence suggests that environmental stress precipitates manifest illness in children with a genetic predisposition.

The prevalence of this disorder increases with age. Whereas autism and pervasive developmental disorder are distinctly different from the adult schizophrenias, childhood schizophrenia forms a continuum with the adolescent and adult forms.

It is characterised by withdrawal, apathy, flat affect, thought disorder (blocking and perseveration), ideas of reference, hallucinations and delusions, and complaints of thought control. Diagnosis is based on descriptive clinical phenomena.

Treatment

Combined psychotropic and psychotherapeutic treatment is required. Phenothiazines (e.g. thiothixene 0.10–0.40 mg kg^{-1} day^{-1}) and butyrophenones (e.g. haloperidol 0.05–0.15 mg kg^{-1} day^{-1}) may be effective in controlling acute psychotic symptoms, but relapse is common. Hospitalisation is useful in managing acute exacerbations; some children require continuing inpatient psychiatric care.

Eating disorders

Anorexia nervosa occurs in approximately one out of 100 adolescent females and is most frequently found in middle-to-upper socioeconomic groups. Most recent studies have suggested no increased incidence of anorexia nervosa over the last four decades. A familial component appears to be present.

Mortality/morbidity The mortality rate for anorexia nervosa ranges from 5–10% and is greater (5–40%) among bulimic patients.

Race Anorexia nervosa is significantly more frequent in white populations than in people of other races. The co-existent effect of socioeconomic class, however, is difficult to isolate.

Sex Female to male ratio is 10–50:1 in developed countries.

Age Anorexia nervosa is primarily a phenomenon of puberty and early adulthood, although premorbid determinants and long-term outcomes are still being defined.

Anorexia nervosa is an eating disorder characterised by severe weight loss to the point of significant physiological consequences. Patients with anorexia nervosa generally fall into two categories: (1) those who practise extreme food restriction behaviours; and (2) those who display food binge/purge behaviour.

Complications

Complications of anorexia nervosa may result in ED presentation.

Cardiovascular effects include supraventricular and ventricular dysrhythmias, long QT syndrome, bradycardia, orthostatic hypotension, and shock due to congestive heart failure.

Renal disturbances include decreased glomerular filtration rate, elevated creatinine, oedema, acidosis with dehydration, hypokalaemia, hypochloraemic alkalosis with vomiting, and hyperaldosteronism.

Gastrointestinal findings include constipation, delayed gastric emptying, gastric dilation and rupture, dental enamel erosion, palatal trauma, enlarged parotids, oesophagitis, Mallory–Weiss lesions, diminished gag reflex, and elevated transaminases.

Finally, bone marrow suppression may occur, leading to platelet, erythrocyte, and leucocyte abnormalities.

History

- Patients may present to the ED with extreme weight loss, food refusal, dehydration, weakness, or shock.
- Affect may be flat or nearly catatonic.
- Patients may be depressed and should be questioned to gauge risk of suicide.
- Obtain a mental history because there is a strong association with depression and substance abuse.
- Often, the family will bring in the patient because many patients may refuse to seek help or may have no insight into their problem.
- Recurrent patients may recognise their problem and present spontaneously for therapy.

Physical

- Physical examination may reveal hypothermia, peripheral oedema, thinning hair, and obvious emaciation.
- Behaviourally these patients often have a flat affect and display psychomotor retardation.

Care

ED care may include rehydration, correction of electrolyte abnormalities (e.g. hypokalaemia), and institution of appropriate disposition for continuing medical and psychiatric treatment.

Consultations

As appropriate, consult with psychiatry and adolescent medicine specialists in order to optimise inpatient care and facilitate outpatient follow-up care.

Problem parents

Parents with a mental illness
Depression
Mothers with postnatal depression may present frequently in a 'cry for help'.

Münchausen's syndrome by proxy
In 1977, Englishman Roy Meadow published[3] the first report of a new form of child abuse. He coined the term Münchausen's syndrome by proxy (MSBP) after the syndrome that first had been reported by Asher in 1951. This term is applied when an adult, usually the mother, presents a false history to the physician regarding a child who is not suffering from any of the fabricated symptoms. This history causes the physician to perform unnecessary diagnostic procedures that do not result in any specific diagnosis. (MSBP has also been called Polle syndrome, after Baron von Münchausen's only child, who died when aged 1 year.)

In 1994, the DSM-IV[4,5] included a definition for factitious disorder by proxy, which is now the accepted psychiatric category for MSBP. The definition includes the following:

❶ Intentional production or feigning of physical or psychological signs or symptoms in another person who is under the individual's care.
❷ The motivation for the perpetrator's behaviour is to assume the sick role by proxy.
❸ External incentives for the behaviour, such as economic gain, avoiding legal responsibility, or improving physical well-being, are absent.

Children at risk for MSBP abuse are aged 15 months to 6 years. The emergency physician often is confronted with baffling symptoms. Frequently, the child has been taken to many care providers before the diagnosis is finally established. Warning signs that are suggestive of MSBP include the following:

- illness is multisystemic, prolonged, unusual, or rare;
- symptoms are inappropriate or incongruent;
- patient has multiple allergies;
- symptoms disappear when parent or caretaker is absent;

- in children, one parent, usually the father, is absent during hospitalisation;
- history of sudden infant death syndrome in siblings is noted;
- parent is overly attached to patient;
- patient has poor tolerance of treatment (e.g. frequent vomiting, rash, and problems with intravenous lines);
- general health of patient clashes with results of laboratory tests;
- parent shows inordinate concern for feelings of the medical staff;
- seizure activity is unresponsive to anticonvulsants and is witnessed only by parent or caretaker.

Tests that emergency physicians may consider include the following:

- urine toxicology screening;
- chemistry panels;
- electrocardiogram;
- drug levels for suspected poisoning agents (e.g. aspirin, paracetamol (acetaminophen), anticonvulsants);
- cultures;
- coagulation tests;
- head CT scan.

Parents with substance abuse
Parents with significant substance abuse, i.e. alcohol and other drugs have significant impact on the child's presentation. The parental behaviour can be inappropriate, threatening and aggressive towards the practitioner. This makes the assessment of the child much more difficult and unreliable.

Miscellaneous

Night terrors
Sleep disruption is a parent's most frequent concern during the first 2 years of a child's life. Half of all infants develop a disrupted sleep pattern serious enough to warrant physician assistance. Night terror disorder is characterised by recurrent episodes of intense crying and fear, and by difficulty arousing the child. Children also can experience signs of autonomic arousal (e.g. tachycardia, tachypnoea, sweating) during episodes. Children do not recall a dream after a night terror and typically do not remember the episode the next morning. Night terrors are frightening episodes that disrupt family life and cause the child significant distress and impaired everyday function. Usually onset is in children aged 3–12 years; the disorder generally resolves during adolescence.

An estimated 1–6% of children experience night terror episodes. Recurrent night terror episodes accompanied by significant distress and impairment are less frequent.

Peak frequency in children younger than 3.5 years is at least one episode per week; among older children, peak frequency is 1–2 episodes per month.

History
The most important step toward diagnosing this disorder is to obtain a detailed history.

- Approximately 90 minutes after falling asleep, the child sits up in bed and screams. Prominent autonomic activity (e.g. tachycardia, tachypnoea, diaphoresis, flushing) occurs. The child appears awake but confused, disoriented, and unresponsive to stimuli.
- Most episodes last 1–2 minutes, but the child may remain inconsolable for 5–30 minutes before relaxing and returning to quiet sleep.
- If the child awakens during the night terror, only fragmented pieces of the episode may be recalled.
- In the morning, the child typically has no memory of the experience.

Management
This consists of educating the family about the disorder and reassuring them that episodes are not harmful.

References

1. Aghababian RV, Allison EJ, Braen GR, et al., editors. *Emergency medicine: The core curriculum*. Philadelphia, PA: Lippincott, Raven; 1998.
2. Baeutrias A. Risk factors for suicide and attempted suicide among young people. *Setting the evidence-based research agenda for Australia: A literature review*. Canberra: National Health and Medical Research Centre, Commonwealth Department of Health and Aged Care; 1999.
3. Meadow R. Munchausen syndrome by proxy. The hinterland of child abuse. *Lancet* 1977;**2**(8033):343–5.
4. DSM-IV. *Diagnostic and statistical manual of mental disorders*. 4th ed. Washington, DC: American Psychiatric Association; 1994.
5. ICD-10-AM. *The international statistical classification of diseases and related health problems, 10th revision, Australian modification*. 2nd ed Lidcombe, NSW: National Centre for Classification in Health; 2000.

17.2 The treatment of the behaviourally disturbed adolescent

Kenneth Nunn

ESSENTIALS

1 Emergency psychiatry is treating the underlying neurobehavioural processes NOT the cognitive content or psychiatric diagnosis.

2 When thinking about management it is worthwhile to move back through the ABCC from the most disrupted young people, through to the early levels of distress and dysfunction.

C – If cognitive processes are very disrupted, hospital admission will be necessary irrespective of the eventual diagnosis.

C – If containment is threatened - offer co-operative sedation early and put security on notice. If it is actually being breached, all other treatment must wait until containment is addressed voluntarily or involuntarily.

B – If behaviour is extreme, actively offer relief with calm reassurance, nursing presence and medication while consciously preparing for escalation to a containment breach.

A – If arousal is high, establish whether this can be readily managed by calmness and co-operative use of medication. If calm is not forthcoming, be prepared for behavioural escalation.

Introduction

Emergencies fragment clinician thought, unless they are transformed into routine. No area of medicine is more difficult to conform to routine without practice than psychiatry and no area of psychiatry is more 'inconvenient' in this regard than adolescent psychiatry.

Just as in paediatrics, the first question is not 'which illness?' but 'how sick are they?' There is currently too much emphasis on whether or not there are signs of a particular mental illness, not whether there are the crucial elements of neurobehavioural disorder and the disruption of basic neurobehavioural systems. Despite this, once the essentials are understood and applied, the emergency physician can provide consistent, high quality care in triage, initial stabilisation and management of immediate risks before preparing for transfer for definitive management and ongoing treatment where needed.

This chapter is written with the underlying premise that psychiatrists will be in short supply, sometimes not trained in Emergency Psychiatry, or unaccustomed to adolescent psychiatry. For the present, emergency adolescent psychiatry largely falls to emergency physicians.

The principles of psychiatric triage

Purpose of triage

Triage aims to enable the earliest possible identification and treatment of factors that may threaten the immediate safety and well-being of the patient, others and staff in triage and the emergency department (ED). The aim is to put safety first, management of distress and behaviour second, and diagnosis third. It is critical that the task of definitive diagnosis does not delay acute management. Whether or not a young person has a *particular* psychiatric disorder is of secondary importance. Accurately identifying the components of threat, the complexity of the threat (that is the number of

domains of risk), the level of the threat, the emotional and behavioural identifiers of risk and the performance indicators for risk management, all within a rapid time frame, requires training, skill and experience.

Time is risk

The time taken before treatment begins in psychiatric triage is related to increasing risk, as impulsivity, agitation and lack of relief of distress converge with the sensory over-stimulation of most ED waiting areas. Time passing constitutes an escalating risk of a loss-of-control, or loss-of-containment, event. Where agitation is present, motor activity increased and cognitive processes clearly altered, the risk rises dramatically after even short periods of waiting. The commonly encountered slide down the spectrum of distress to disruption – anxiety, agitation, anger, together with demanding, impatient, impulsive and explosive behaviour – leaves few options once in full progress. On the other hand, the rapid initiation of triage and the commencement of an altogether less disruptive process – seen, relieved, treated, monitored, transitioned – are each associated with a reduced risk of loss-of-control.

Pre-triage
Early warning signs – subjective

- Identifying a safety threat to staff and others.
- Questions such as 'Do I feel unsafe?' 'Am I anxious for their welfare?' 'Is there a sense of threat?' may all provide useful clues, if considered (Table 17.2.1). It is worthwhile acting on this as a given until reassured otherwise.

Early warning signs – observed

Some behaviour stands out as 'out of control', unusual, potentially dangerous, conflicting, or distressing, before the patient and those attending them sit down and you begin to listen. Sitting down is a helpful first step to reducing arousal and activation. A louder than usual voice, an argument between parent and child, a surly withdrawn

Table 17.2.1	A triad of subjective early warning signs	
Threats to safety	Syndromes of distress	Organic flags
If you feel unsafe or moved to protect others	If you feel distressed at watching	If you can't make sense and the child looks unwell

father, a seemingly drunken teenager, may all catch our attention.

An immediate threat to others, an immediate threat of patients to themselves or an immediate threat to medical safety, all require immediate action analogous to a cardiac arrest. Practising commonly encountered scenarios with acceptance of 'error and inefficiency' is essential.

The hierarchy of needs

All triage involves addressing a hierarchy of needs (Table 17.2.2).

Safety, symptom relief and initial investigation (SSRI) and working or provisional diagnosis (PD) form the underpinnings of emergency psychological care. The establishment of mental state monitoring and the active exclusion of medical contributors commence immediately upon completing the initial stabilisation.

Signs of threat to safety

❶ Behaviour potentially injurious to others requiring – PROTECTION & RESTRAINT.
❷ Disruptive behaviour with a threat to safety requiring – CONTAINMENT.
❸ 'Out of control' behaviour that requires CONTAINMENT.

Signs of intense distress

By way of analogy with the provision of acute life support, it is helpful to employ the ABCC mnemonic.

The ABCC of rapid psychiatric assessment

Arousal – autonomic and cortical arousal
Behaviour – behavioural activation
Containment – behavioural control within a social setting

Cognitive processes – the coherent communication of reality-based thinking and feeling.

Identifying the triad of early changes, rate of change and the extremity of change to each component of assessment will be used throughout.

Arousal The triad of early signs of change in arousal, volatility of arousal and extremes of arousal are our focus. Thus, early autonomic signs of either sympathetic or parasympathetic shift include pallor, flushing, tachycardia, bradycardia, tremulousness, mydriasis and tachypnoea. Marked hypervigilance and clouding of consciousness or rapid excursions between the two are very helpful in identifying the need to intervene rapidly. Anxieties may be more difficult to assuage with lack of fine social and emotional tuning with either unresponsiveness, or exquisite responsiveness, to the environment, or a rapidly changing mixture of both. If the arousal is sufficiently disruptive, the child or young person may have a functional overflow of their arousal into their behaviour.

Behaviour Again, early signs of change in behaviour, volatility of behaviour and extremes of behaviour are our focus. Sitting with one leg constantly shaking, wringing of hands or stroking of hair as part of anguish or anger all portend an imminent deterioration in behaviour. Constant pacing or refusal to move, a loud voice or speaking very quietly, swearing excessively and particularly offensively, or refusing to talk as part of a broader picture of social disinhibition or extreme inhibition, reflect extremes of response and lack of fine social and emotional tuning. If these

are sustained, they may overflow and have an impact on the other patients, staff and the functioning of the ED. If this impact is sufficiently disruptive, they may constitute a containment threat or demand for containment.

Containment Behavioural control within a social setting so as to reduce major threat and disruption, that is in an acute medical setting, is termed containment. While containment is usually a physical process, which reduces the capacity of a patient to disrupt the ED, it is primarily aimed at reducing risk to others, risk to self and risk to the environment in the ED. The acute and open nature of the ED means that any disruptive threat may constitute a broader threat to the provision of urgent medical treatment to the young person in question or to others.

It follows that, since changes in arousal normally precede changes in behaviour, which precede changes in the likelihood of containment, the early warning signs of a loss of containment event have already been covered under the headings of arousal and behaviour. However, frequently these early features will have happened prior to being seen in the ED and the demand for containment is the presenting request.

Running away, disrupting the ED, damaging property and creating an atmosphere of threat and menace would all constitute a containment threat or a containment failure event. In extreme cases this may involve weapons, the police and the clearing of the ED, with cessation of medical activities while a local Disaster Response is put into place. In most cases, some form of containment was in place before being brought to the ED and it is important that this containment is not lost in the transition process into the ED or in transfer from the ED. If containment failure is the external manifestation of maximal disruption to the individual, the fragmentation of thought processes or pathological coalescence of thinking into paranoid or self-destructive ideation is the inner manifestation shown in arousal, behaviour, including speech, and containment.

Cognitive processes The early manifestations of thought disruption are changes in arousal, behaviour, especially speech, and containment that belie a loss of coherence in the *process* of thought and other cognitive processes. Other cognitive processes such as

Table 17.2.2	The hierarchy of patient needs	
Threat	*Need*	*Sign for observation*
Danger	Safety	Signs of threats to safety
Distress	Relief	Signs of intense distress
Disease	Treatment	Signs of organic cerebral, and long-term psychiatric dysfunction

attention, executive function (planning, judgment, problem solving and insight) and perception, underpin thinking and consequent action. This is not to say that thought or speech *content* is irrelevant. The young person may be worried, fearful, self-loathing, bizarre, threatening and angry. However, the processes of *perceived threat* (in the extreme, paranoia) and the pursuit of relief (in the extreme, self-harm and suicide) are the underpinning cognitive processes foremost in any emergency assessment.

Extremes of incoherence or coherence apply here as well. Jumbled, accelerated, guarded, slowed down, rigidly preoccupied, fixedly convinced or non-communicative speech and thought are all more worrying process variables, irrespective of what or who is upsetting the patient.

Managing the ABCC, including restraint and acute sedation

It is inappropriate to attempt to obtain a detailed developmental history, systems review or full exploratory psychiatric history from an acutely distressed and very ill young person. When thinking about management it is worthwhile to move back through the ABCC from the most disrupted young people, through to the early levels of distress and dysfunction.

C – If cognitive processes are very disrupted, hospital admission will be necessary, irrespective of the eventual diagnosis.

C – If containment is threatened, offer co-operative sedation early and put security on notice. If it is actually being breached, all other treatment must wait until containment is addressed voluntarily or involuntarily.

B – If behaviour is extreme, actively offer relief with calm reassurance, nursing presence and medication while consciously preparing for escalation to a containment breach.

A – If arousal is high, establish whether this can be readily managed by calmness and co-operative use of medication. If calm is not forthcoming, be prepared for behavioural escalation.

There are only six essential things which must be attempted:-

❶ Rapport and respect – even where they cannot be achieved.

❷ Identify the immediate issue of concern to the young person and to others while establishing a formulation in medical terms.

❸ Identify risks – to self and others, including, maltreatment, *medical* and reputation risks.

❹ Symptomatic relief – provide immediate treatment with whatever biological, psychological and social supports and resources are available. The provision of relief is the single biggest factor in reducing risk.

❺ Identify psychosocial supports and stressors (immediate), i.e. who is the consenting authority for the young person and where do they normally live. None of these may be available in the acute situation. However, they will save a great deal of time in determining the disposition of the patient.

❻ A plan of action for the next 24 hours.

Sedating the adolescent brain

When attempting to provide reduction in arousal and behavioural agitation, or to manage a breach of containment, it is helpful to consider which parts of the brain – or neurobehavioural systems – are being targeted. The neurobehavioural systems are referred to here as subbrains as a useful shorthand.

The thinking brain (the cortex) – easiest to sedate, especially in children – inhibits the other two brains. When the cortical brake is sedated, the two lower brains (disinhibition) are released. Benzodiazepines are often enough to sedate this brain.

Target arousal and preoccupation – for example, the inability to stop thinking about distressing events despite sustained talking through and reassurance.

The feeling brain (the limbic system) – takes longer and more medication to sedate, especially when distress is established. Benzodiazepines may be enough, but often antipsychotics are needed.

Target arousal and distress – for example, the inability to find emotional relief despite sustained and skilled reassurance.

The moving brain (the basal nuclei) – takes longest to sedate and is first to awaken from sedation. Antipsychotics are almost always needed.

Target behaviour and agitation – for example, the inability to be able to move in an emotional paralysis or to sit still due to agitation, despite sustained reassurance.

Tracking the seven stages of sedation

❶ Fixation – immobilising the body to enable vascular access and a safe medical procedure.

❷ Induction – commencing sedation with the steady reduction of consciousness.

❸ Disinhibition – loss of emotional and behavioural control associated with loss of cortical inhibition before limbic and basal nuclei are similarly inhibited.

❹ Stabilisation of arousal depth – titrating to a level of sedation that maintains gag reflexes, pharyngeal patency and adequate breathing and oxygenation.

❺ Maintenance – high-level observation with clear parameter thresholds and specification of appropriate responses when thresholds are breached.

❻ Emergence – the period of decremental lowering of medication to allow a transition to the fully conscious state with an awareness that disinhibition may occur during this process as during the establishment of sedation.

❼ After care – the psychological explanation and support required specifically in relation to the sedation process.

Five tips on sedating adolescents

❶ Start high (without bolus) and titrate down in an emergency.

❷ If there is definite motor agitation, do not use a benzodiazepine alone, which may disinhibit the patient. Add haloperidol and monitor for extrapyramidal side effects such as dystonia.

❸ If re-sedation is likely, move to regular doses rather than p.r.n., 'ebb and flow prescribing'. Less medication is needed if non-p.r.n.

❹ Initiate sedation away from the main ED (more private and less disruptive) and maintain and monitor close to the main ED.

❺ Plan for emergence risks – ensure security presence during emergence from sedation or be prepared to re-sedate.

Signs of organic dysfunction syndromes

- Elevated temperature in a psychotic patient.
- *Appearance* – Looking lost or 'out of it' with lowered eyelids, glazed eyes and 'in a world of their own'.
- *Behaviour* – Recent personality change with loss of social fine tuning and reversal of sleep rhythms.
- *Speech* – Muddled speech and thinking, often with paranoid but fragmented themes.
- *Perception* – Visual illusions, i.e. misidentifying actual stimuli, e.g. shadows mistaken for people or frank visual and tactile hallucinations (especially with antihistamine or anticholinergic overdose).
- *Ideation* – Often paranoid in thinking.
- *Cognition* – Clouded and fluctuating levels of consciousness with disorientation.
- *Judgement and insight* – Impaired markedly.

Differential diagnosis

❶ Specific toxidromes and syndromes of adverse drug reaction
  - substance abuse
  - accidental ingestion.
❷ Delirium – generalised acute brain syndrome.
❸ Frontal lobe syndromes (including TBI and intellectual disability).
❹ Seizure-related disorders.
❺ Starvation-related syndromes.
❻ Cerebellar dysfunction
  - slurred speech;
  - ataxic gait;
  - incoordination;
  - substance abuse, e.g. benzodiazepine;
  - toxicity from prescribed medications, e.g. anticonvulsants;
  - ingestion of poisons, e.g. alcohol, phenytoin.
❼ Dementia – generalised chronic brain syndrome.

The management of acute risk including medical risk

Managing threat to staff and others

- Do not ask medical or nursing staff to carry out unsafe practice.
- Offer co-operative oral sedation early, such as olanzapine or quetiapine.

- Work closely with security staff.
- Ask early and provide sedation back-up.

Behaviours that usually de-escalate aggression

Nothing works all the time and nothing works in every case, but some of these are likely to be helpful.

Ten DOs

❶ Do be respectful, friendly and open (single most important strategy, especially respect).
❷ Be quicker to listen than to speak.
❸ Do speak clearly, quietly, gently and calmly with an expectation that they will respond.
❹ Use humour that shows we accept we have things about us that are not ideal, perfect or completely 'respectable', especially when we are derided or spoken to rudely.
❺ Do declare desire to be helpful even if it is not always known how to help or what it is they want.
❻ Do relax posture, voice and face, even if preparing internally for fight and/or flight.
❼ Move slowly, predictably and with due respect for distance.
❽ Distract to details that they might be interested in as well, especially things about them and what they like.
❾ Acknowledge any faults in our behaviour (not someone else's) that might be contributing to them being upset.
❿ Acknowledge tiredness, a hearing problem (if they are withdrawn, hostile, talking quietly), irritability or crabbiness after a busy shift, which emphasise our humanity.

Ten DON'Ts

❶ Try to shame them into good behaviour by telling them they are childish, silly or stupid.
❷ Try to get above them (so-called 'towering') physically, by position, verbally, intellectually or socially.
❸ Talk without listening or 'nag'. Don't all talk at once – one person only.

❹ Issue ultimatums – 'do this or else' – almost always leads to 'or else' in this population.
❺ Back into corner either physically or psychologically (unless everything else has failed and safety demands we must).
❻ Adopt a 'thou shalt' tone of voice instead of a reasonable request.
❼ Raise voices in a counter 'arc-up' to the patient.
❽ Mock, criticise or accuse the patient at any time.
❾ Rush the process or create time pressure.
❿ Hark back to previous behaviour or try to sort out longstanding issues unless this is a previously agreed treatment goal.

The four main themes are to

❶ Communicate respect.
  Many of them have not been treated with respect.
❷ Communicate our desire to keep everyone safe.
  We want them, and us, to be safe. Many of our patients have not lived in safe environments.
❸ Be willing to acknowledge we may have contributed to their distress by what we have done or not done.
  Many of the young people who will present have lived with people who have never accepted blame, use denial a great deal and blame others.
❹ Appreciate their distress even though it may not be fully understood why they feel like this or how bad they feel.
  Many of the patients have been told they don't or do feel a certain way (even if they did not) and had the legitimacy of their distress invalidated. They may never have been in a situation where high distress is tolerated, validated and appreciated so long as safety is high as well.

Identify patients' threat to themselves?

- If the patient or those with them feel unsafe, they probably are unsafe.
- If your ABCC evaluation says they are unsafe, they are unsafe.
- If a colleague outside the hospital says they have been behaving unsafely, be very wary of not honouring their assessment.

Managing a threat to themselves

- Remain calm, firm, enlist security, maintain constant observation and, if actually attempting to hurt themselves during the assessment, intervene immediately.
- Identify treatable disorders and social predicaments while waiting for suicidality to settle (attenuates over several days usually).

Identify medical risks

- The broader medical needs of the patient need to be recognised.
- Psychiatric disorder does not protect against medical disorder.
- It is possible to do a great deal with a non-co-operative patient to clarify medical status.

Manage specific medical risks

- Obtundation - due to panic sedation in response to previous failed sedation in adolescents who became disinhibited.
- Extrapyramidal side effects – nuchal spasm with headache is common in the young as a form of dystonia.
- Respiratory – laryngeal dystonia – especially in younger patients but still rare, especially if benzodiazepines are not used with butyrophenones.
- Cardiac – prolonged QTc, especially in poor 2D6 metabolisers (5% of normal population).
- Neurological – delirium (common, especially substance abuse), serotonergic syndrome, neuroleptic malignant syndrome (rare) (NMS).
- Concurrent medical disorder – asthma, diabetes, traumatic brain injury, epilepsy, atopy and anorexia.
- Dermatological – lamotrigine-induced Stevens–Johnson syndrome.
- Metabolic – lithium toxicity – especially chronic.

Sentinel nursing observations post intramuscular or intravenous sedation

Respiratory rate, O_2 saturation, pulse, blood pressure and level of consciousness should be checked continuously *during* the maintenance of sedation – *each 15 minutes for 2 hours, then each 30 minutes for 2 hours.*

An electrocardiogram should be performed as soon as possible after any sedation with zuclopenthixol acetate or droperidol and the medical officer contacted if QTc is above 440 ms in males and 460 ms in females. These are conservative figures and represent nursing thresholds for alerting doctors, not thresholds for medical algorithms, which may be considerably higher.

Three tips for monitoring adolescents

❶ Expect the medication to be metabolised quicker.

❷ They become disinhibited more easily going into sedation and coming out of sedation.

❸ Maintaining a sedation intravenously (IV) should be done with a slow injection over several minutes – avoid boluses to avoid respiratory depression (benzodiazepines) or cardiac (butyrophenones).

Specific medications

Intramuscular injection (IMI) will often be the route of choice and the agent should be relatively quick, effective and safe:

- Haloperidol IMI – 0.05–0.20 mg kg^{-1} per dose with doses up to 6-hourly.
- Midazolam IMI – 0.05–0.20 mg kg^{-1} per dose with doses up to 6-hourly.
- Diazepam IVI

  - 0.05–0.20 mg kg^{-1} per dose;
  - give slowly. Dilution enables greater control of injection, monitoring respiration for bradypnoea, pause between inspiration and expiration and paradoxical respiration;
  - can be given in divided doses (2.5 mg quanta) alternating with haloperidol and flush;
  - several minutes between doses initially;
  - 4-6 hours between doses once initial sedation has been established.

Transfer is a potential escalation of risk

The leaving – are they stable?

The transfer – are they monitored with an adequate response to thresholds strategy?

The arriving – are the recipients prepared?

Conclusion

Emergency psychiatry is treating the underlying neurobehavioural processes *not* the cognitive content or psychiatric diagnosis. Process psychiatry requires a different mind-set. Emergency physicians are ideally trained to adopt that mind-set.

Further reading

Glick RL, Berlin JS, Fishkind AB, Zeller SL. *Emergency Psychiatry – Principles and Practice.* Philadelphia: Lippincott Williams & Wilkins; 2008.

Hillard R, Zitek B. *Emergency Psychiatry.* New York: McGraw Hill Professional; 2004.

Nunn KP, Dey C, editors. *The Clinician's Guide to Psychotropic Prescribing in Children and Adolescents – Second Edition.* Child and Adolescent Mental Health Statewide Network, (CAMHSNET) Publications; 2004.

Petit JR. *Handbook of Emergency Psychiatry.* Philadelphia: Lippincott Williams & Wilkins; 2004.

Slaby AE, Lieb J, Tancredi LR. *Handbook of Psychiatric Emergencies.* New York: Medical Examination Publishing Co; 1975.

CRISIS INTERVENTION

Section editor **Gary Browne**

18.1 Sexual assault

Matt Ryan

ESSENTIALS

1 Sexual assault occurs when a child is engaged in sexual activity that the child cannot comprehend, for which the child is developmentally unprepared and cannot give consent, and/or that violates the law or social taboos of society.

2 Sexual assault includes a spectrum of activities ranging from rape to physically less intrusive sexual activity.[1,2]

3 Assessment and management of children following alleged or suspected sexual assault is a highly specialised area and requires a multidisciplinary, multiagency team approach.

Introduction

Assessment of child sexual assault (CSA) requires a dedicated, well-trained and experienced doctor who is able to spend a significant amount of time making an unhurried and thorough assessment and detailed documentation of history and examination findings. The doctor must have an accurate knowledge of genital anatomy, and experience in performing gynaecological examinations. Skills and experience in this field are developed through postgraduate studies, significant case numbers, a knowledge of current literature and involvement in peer-review practices.[3]

Inexpert assessment of such cases may have a profound negative influence on the child and family. It may potentially lead to inappropriate removal of the child from the family or wrongful imprisonment.[4]

The roles of the emergency physician in this process are:

- recognition of the *possibility* of sexual assault;
- treatment of acute physical injury;
- provision of emergency contraception and/or antibiotic and antiviral prophylaxis;
- protection of the child and referral to local child protection agencies;
- referral to a paediatrician;
- ensuring appropriate psychological support is provided to the child and family.

In the majority of cases, determination of whether or not sexual assault has occurred is not possible within the emergency department (ED). In the majority of cases, physical examination will neither confirm nor refute an allegation of sexual assault. The most important indicator of possible CSA is disclosure by the child.

Definitions

CSA is the use of a child for sexual gratification by an adult or significantly older child/adolescent.[5] It may involve a range of activities that vary from exposing the child to sexually explicit materials to anal or vaginal penetration of the child. Central to the definition is the limitation of the child to provide truly informed consent for sexual activity with adults.

Sexual play between children of similar age does not fit into this description.

The term 'assault' is preferred over 'abuse' as it highlights the criminal nature of the activity and avoids minimisation of such abusive acts.

Attitudes/myths surrounding CSA

The subject of CSA is an emotive one. Emergency physicians will often have strongly held opinions and attitudes on this subject. These attitudes may be shaped by past experience and/or social taboos. In order to approach CSA in a calm, non-judgemental and objective manner it is important that emergency physicians are cognisant of their own opinions and emotional responses. In dealing with victims of CSA, expressions of anger, sadness or surprise are not helpful and potentially stigmatising and harmful to the child. With emergency physicians infrequently encountering CSA, it is useful to reflect on the following, sometimes poorly understood, statements.

- A broad range of sexual behaviours has been observed in 'normal' children.
- Most children are not abused by strangers.[6]

- As historians, children are no less reliable than adults.
- CSA is not normally an isolated incident.
- CSA uncommonly produces severe genito-anal injury.[3,7–10]
- CSA often occurs in the context of other family problems, including physical abuse, emotional maltreatment and substance abuse.[11]

Epidemiology of CSA

There has been a significant increase in the recognition of CSA,[3,11,12] which has been reflected by a substantial increase in the number of reports made to child protection services across Australia and overseas, particularly in the last 5 years.

Sexual assault has been documented as occurring on children of all ages and both sexes, and is committed predominantly by men, who are commonly members of the child's family, family friends or other trusted adults in positions of authority.[11]

Sexual abuse by family members or acquaintances usually involves multiple episodes over periods ranging from a week to years.

Victims of unknown assailants tend to be older than children who are sexually abused by someone they know and are usually only subjected to a single episode of abuse.

The estimated proportion of children exposed to some form of sexual assault varies depending on the definition of sexual abuse and methodology used. In the United States, literature surveys provide estimates of 9–52% for females and 3–10% for males.[6] There is no comprehensive comparative Australian literature.

CSA and emergency medicine

Children who are victims of sexual assault may present to EDs in a variety of circumstances:

❶ They may be seen for an unrelated matter when routine history and physical examination produce information where sexual assault forms part of the differential diagnosis.
❷ They are brought by a parent or carer to the ED for evaluation of suspected abuse.

❸ They are brought to the ED by social services or the police for a medical evaluation for possible sexual abuse as part of an investigation.
❹ They are brought to an ED after a suspected acute sexual assault for evaluation, evidence collection, and crisis management.

Recognition of CSA

Recognition of the possibility of CSA is dependent on history and examination findings, both of which are normally non-specific.

History from the child remains the single most important diagnostic feature in coming to the conclusion that a child has been sexually abused.[13]

Signs and symptoms

Non-specific
Children who have been sexually assaulted may develop a variety of emotional and physical complaints, often unrelated to the genital area. These include:

- developmentally regressive behaviour;
- deterioration in school performance;
- sleep disturbances;
- abdominal pain;
- enuresis, encopresis;
- phobias;
- sexualised behaviour.

Specific
- Disclosure by child.
- Genitoanal injury.
- Sexually transmissible disease.
- Pregnancy.

Genitoanal injury

Only 4% of all children referred for medical evaluation of sexual abuse have abnormal examinations at the time of evaluation. Even with a history of severe abuse, such as vaginal or anal penetration, the rate of abnormal medical findings is only 5.5%.[13]

The physical examination of sexually abused children should not result in additional emotional trauma.

When the alleged sexual abuse has occurred within 72 hours, or there is

bleeding or acute injury, the examination should be performed immediately. In this situation, protocols for CSA victims should be followed to secure biological trace evidence such as epithelial cells, semen, and blood, as well as to maintain a 'chain of evidence'. When more than 72 hours has passed and no acute injuries are present, an emergency examination usually is not necessary. An evaluation, therefore, should be scheduled at the earliest convenient time for the child, physician, and investigative team.[17]

In the child presenting with genitoanal injury or abnormality, CSA is only one of a number of diagnoses that should be considered. The differential diagnosis of genitoanal injury includes:

- accidental injury;
- falls astride;
- sexual assault;
- medical/dermatological condition, e.g. lichen sclerosis/drug reaction.

Genital findings in children are difficult to interpret. Such interpretation is generally beyond the expertise of most emergency physicians.[14] Whilst acute trauma may be easily recognised, interpretation of such findings may be problematic for the occasional examiner.[14]

Genitoanal anatomy

Knowledge of what constitutes normal and abnormal anatomy has evolved over recent years. This has been driven partly by several highly publicised cases where misinterpretation of normal findings led to inappropriate separation of children from parents and wrongful conviction.

Hymen
There is considerable variation in the shape of the hymen. In the prepubertal girl it is thin and relatively inelastic. In this age group, blunt penetrating trauma to the vagina may result in tearing of the hymen. Such tears when healed may manifest as a notch or defect in the hymenal tissue.

As an oestrogen-dependent/responsive tissue, at puberty the hymen becomes thick, irregular and elastic and distensible. It is less likely to sustain injury during penetration than in the prepubertal state.

Table 18.1.1 Guidelines for decision making

Data available				Response
History	Physical examination	Laboratory findings	Level of concern about sexual abuse	Report decision
None	Normal	None	None	No report
Behavioural changes	Normal	None	Variable depending upon behaviour	Possible report; follow-up closely (possible mental health referral)
None	Non-specific findings	None	Low (worry)	Possible report; follow-up closely
Non-specific history by child or history by parent only	Non-specific findings	None	Intermediate	Possible report; follow-up closely
None	Specific findings	None	High	Report
Clear statement	Normal	None	High	Report
Clear statement	Specific findings	None	High	Report
None	Normal, non-specific or specific findings	Positive culture for sexually transmissible disease, presence of semen, sperm acid phosphatase	Very high	Report
Behaviour changes	Non-specific findings	Other sexually transmitted diseases	High	Report

Sexually transmitted diseases

The diagnosis of a sexually transmitted disease in a child may be highly suggestive but is not diagnostic of sexual contact. Rectal and genital *Chlamydia* infections in young children may be due to a persistent perinatally-acquired infection, which may last for up to 3 years.[15,16]

Diagnostic considerations

The diagnosis of CSA can often be made based on a child's history. Physical examination is infrequently diagnostic in the absence of a history and/or specific laboratory findings. Physical findings are often absent even when the perpetrator admits to penetration of the child's genitalia. Many types of abuse leave no physical evidence, and mucosal injuries often heal rapidly.

On examination, findings which are suggestive, but not diagnostic, of CSA include:

- abrasions or bruising of the inner thighs and genitalia;
- scarring or tears of the labia minora;
- enlargement of the hymenal opening.

Findings that are of greater concern include:

- scarring, tears, or distortion of the hymen;
- a decreased amount, or absence, of hymenal tissue;
- injury to, or scarring of, the posterior fourchette;
- anal lacerations.[17]

Many cases of alleged sexual abuse involve parents who are in the process of separation or divorce and who allege that their child is being sexually abused by the other parent during custodial visits. Although these cases are generally more time consuming, they should not be dismissed because a custody dispute exists. Allegations of abuse that occur in the context of divorce proceedings should either be reported to the child protective services agency or followed-up closely.

Role of the emergency physician

The emergency physician (EP) has many roles in CSA. The EP should ensure that any physical injuries are detected, accurately documented and correctly treated.

Medical issues, such as sexually transmitted diseases and emergency contraception, should be discussed and managed.

The EP should collect, or provide opportunity for collection of, forensic specimens, ensure appropriate psychological support is provided to the child and family, and report the case to protective agencies within the legislation of the local jurisdiction.

Documentation

Because the likelihood of civil or criminal court action is high, detailed records, and/or drawings should be kept.

Mandatory reporting legislation

Some form of mandatory reporting legislation exists in all Australian jurisdictions. Although this legislation varies from state to state, the basic principles are similar. Doctors are mandated to report cases where there is reasonable suspicion that CSA will occur, or is occurring, and the guardian is unlikely to prevent such acts (Table 18.1.1). The reporting practitioner has statutory protection from prosecution if a report is made in good faith.

References

1. American Academy of Pediatrics. Committee on Adolescence. Sexual assault and the adolescent. *Paediatrics* 1994;**94**:761–5.
2. American Academy of Child and Adolescent Psychiatry. Practice parameters for the forensic evaluation of children and adolescents who may have been physically or sexually abused. *J Am Acad Child Adolesc Psychiatry* 1997;**36**:423–42.
3. Donald T, Wells D. *Graduate Diploma in Forensic Medicine, Subject guide.* Melbourne: Monash University Centre for Learning and Teaching Support; 2000. p. 253.
4. Butler-Sloss E. *Report of the Enquiry into Child Abuse in Cleveland 1987.* London: HMSO; 1988.
5. Kempe CH. Sexual abuse, another hidden paediatric problem: The 1977 C. Anderson Aldrich lecture. *Paediatrics* 1978;**62**:382–9.
6. Tomison A. *Update on child sexual abuse.* National Child Protection Clearinghouse; 1995. Issues in child abuse prevention number 5. Available from *http://www.aifs. gov.au/nch/pubs/issues/issues5/issues5.html* [accessed 26.10.10].

7. Adams JA, Harper K, Knudson S, Revilla J. Examination findings in legally confirmed child sexual abuse: It's normal to be normal. *Paediatrics* 1994;**94**:310–7.
8. Finkel MA. Anogenital trauma in sexually abused children. *Paediatrics* 1989;**84**:317–22.
9. McCann J, Voris J, Simon M. Genital injuries resulting from sexual abuse: A longitudinal study. *Paediatrics* 1992;**89**:307–17.
10. McCann J, Voris J. Perianal injuries resulting from sexual abuse: A longitudinal study. *Paediatrics* 1993;**91**:390–7.
11. Finkelhor D. The international epidemiology of child sexual abuse. *Child Abuse Negl* 1994;**18**(5):409–17.

12. Leventhal JM. Epidemiology of child sexual abuse. In: Oates RK, editor. *Understanding and managing child sexual abuse.* Sydney: Harcourt Brace Jovanovich; 1990.
13. Heger A, Ticson L, Velasquez O, Bernier R. Children referred for possible sexual abuse: Medical findings in 2384 children. *Child Abuse Negl* 2002;**26**(6–7):645–59.
14. Makoroff KL, Brauley JL, Brandner AM, et al. Genital examinations for alleged sexual abuse of prepubertal girls: Findings by pediatric emergency medicine physicians compared with child abuse trained physicians. *Child Abuse Negl* 2002;**26**(12):1235–42.

15. Hammerschlag MR. Sexually transmitted diseases in sexually abused children. *Adv Pediatr Infect Dis* 1988;**3**:1–18.
16. Hammerschlag MR, Doraiswamy B, Alexander ER, et al. Are rectogenital chlamydial infections a marker of sexual abuse in children? *Pediatr Infect Dis J* 1984;**3**:100–104.
17. American Professional Society on the Abuse of Children. *Guidelines for psychosocial evaluation of suspected sexual abuse in young children.* Chicago, IL: American Professional Society on the Abuse of Children; 1990.

18.2 Child at risk

Simon Young • Raymond Chin • Gervase Chaney

ESSENTIALS

1 Non-accidental injury occurs when an adult responsible for the care of the child either harms the child or fails to protect the child from harm.

2 A child may be at risk from physical abuse, sexual abuse, emotional abuse or neglect.

3 Medical and nursing practitioners are often mandated by law to report suspicions of non-accidental injury.

Introduction

Non-accidental injury is increasingly recognised as a major public health and social welfare problem with important short-term and long-lasting effects for children and adolescents. As Australian and New Zealand Emergency Departments (ED) provide care for many hundreds of thousands of children and adolescents each year, departments and their staff play an important role in the detection of abuse and initiation of a medical and community response. This response is aimed primarily at treating the child, minimising psychological effects and ensuring their safety.

Children and adolescents are, by virtue of their developing intellectual, emotional and physical state, a vulnerable group. The environment within which they develop is influenced by many factors outside their control: the economic and social status of their family, the personality and values of family members and friends, and the extent of physical and intellectual stimulation that they receive may all have profound influence upon their development. The potential variability in these factors and the recognition that negative experiences often have serious short- and long-term implications for the child has led to a general acknowledgment that children and adolescents need protection.

The United Nations Convention on the Rights of the Child recognises that:

> . . . for the full and harmonious development of his or her personality, [a child] should grow up in a family environment, in an atmosphere of happiness, love and understanding . . .

The Convention continues, stating in Article 19 that governments shall:

> . . . take all appropriate legislative, administrative, social and educational measures to protect the child from all forms of physical or mental violence, injury or abuse, neglect or negligent treatment, maltreatment or exploitation, including sexual abuse, while in the care of parent(s), legal guardian(s) or any other person who has the care of the child . . .

It is this philosophy that has driven the creation of the social and legal framework of child protection. Doctors, nurses and other healthcare workers who deal with children are an integral part of this system that acts to protect children and adolescents. Every health professional that has contact with children needs to be aware of the possibility of non-accidental injury, must be able to detect when it is occurring and know how to act in the best interests of the child once it is suspected.

Definition

The child at risk is not a medical diagnosis but rather a description of certain forms of behaviour displayed by adults responsible for the care of a child. The child is at risk when an adult responsible for the care of the child harms, threatens to harm or fails to protect the child from harm. Harm may be either physical (e.g. inflicting an injury, causing pain or poisoning), psychological (e.g. causing feelings of being unloved or worthless) or both.

A child may be at risk from:

- physical injury;
- sexual abuse;
- emotional abuse;
- neglect.

These are not exclusive and a child may be subjected to more than one type of abuse.

Physical injury

This is the commonest type of abuse that is reported to child protection agencies. Many thousands of children present to EDs around Australia each year with a wide range of physical injuries, the vast majority of which are caused accidentally. It is a difficult but essential task to identify children within this group who have been injured as a consequence of abuse. While medical and nursing staff must be alert for the possibility of any non-accidental injury, there are specific circumstances that may raise suspicion. These include:

- situations where there are direct allegations of violence directed against the child made by the child or any other person;
- the type and pattern of injury observed at the examination;
- an explanation being offered for an injury that does not fit the type or pattern of injury;
- delayed presentation for medical care with an injury that a reasonable person would have recognised as needing care sooner;
- multiple presentations, often to different healthcare providers, seeking medical attention.

Once the possibility of non-accidental injury has been raised the priorities of the treating doctor are:

❶ To diagnose, treat and document the child's injuries.
❷ To interpret the pattern of injury or behaviour as to the possible causes.
❸ To notify and involve the agency responsible for ensuring safety of the child.
❹ To provide a written or verbal report and advice to that agency or the police.

Presentation

Physical abuse may present to the ED in many different ways. Most commonly it will present as a child with an obvious injury and a suggestive history but in some situations it will be more subtle, such as a younger child who presents not using a limb.

Children who present with a decreased conscious state with no obvious cause may have a head injury from a blow or a fall or may have been poisoned. If the child is very young, the decreased conscious state may be a result of being shaken.

History

It is necessary to collect as much information as possible on the events that led to the child sustaining the injuries. Specifically, enquire as to when, where and how the injury happened, who was present at the time and what happened after the injury. The child's medical, developmental and social history, with specific information on past injuries, is important.

This history must be sought in an open and non-judgemental fashion, which encourages the participants to reveal all the important information. Unfortunately, the ED is often not the ideal place to conduct a lengthy and in-depth forensic interview with the parents or carers and it may be prudent to limit the information gathering to items that will enable specific issues to be addressed. The interview can always be completed by trained investigators at a later time.

Physical examination

Prior to commencing the examination the doctor must ensure that the parents and, where appropriate, the child are informed of the nature and extent of the examination and that valid consent has been given. In addition it is ideal to have spent some time with the child, to gain their confidence and thus increase the chances of keeping their co-operation during the examination.

Consent from the parent or legal guardian is necessary to conduct a physical examination, to perform investigations (including photographs) and to release clinical information in the form of a report to a third party. If consent is refused the protective agency or police must seek a court order. If there is an urgent medical problem that needs intervention and such intervention is clearly in the best interests of the child, then the examination and treatment should proceed and not be delayed by the lack of consent.

An adolescent may be able to give consent for their own examination as long as they are capable of understanding what the examination entails, what the results will be used for, and the implications that this may have for them.

A thorough physical examination of the child should be performed, with observation and palpation of skin, soft tissues, bones and joints, and giving specific attention to the eyes, ears and mouth. The examination should look for the following physical findings:

Bruising of the skin Bruises are extremely common in children. In the absence of a documented bleeding tendency they are evidence of blunt trauma and may provide some information on the site, the implement or force of an impact. Accidental bruises are commonly found in children once they have learnt to crawl, occurring over bony prominences, usually on the front of the body and are directly related to a child's increasing motor activity. Babies who are not yet crawling rarely have accidental bruising.

Bruises caused by abuse may occur anywhere on a child's body. Specifically, look in places where accidental bruises are uncommon such as the mouth, behind the ears, on the inner aspect of the upper arm and around the buttocks. Observe the shape and pattern of bruises, looking for features that may suggest a blow from an open hand or a single or multiple blows from an implement. Look for a pattern within the bruise that may suggest contact with a specific surface.

Whilst it is important to describe the appearance and colour of the bruising, it is not possible to be accurate about the age of a bruise. If a bruise is yellowing in colour then it is likely to be more than 18 hours old.

Laceration and abrasion of the skin

Lacerations are the tearing of tissues caused by a blow from a blunt object. Abrasions are the disruption of the outer layers of the skin caused when the skin contacts a surface at an angle. They occur at or close to the site of impact and may occur after a blow with an object or after a fall on to a surface. They are frequently associated with bruising.

Examine the wound for neurovascular and tendon injury and for foreign bodies. The presence of foreign material such as glass, dirt or gravel should be noted as they may be important in evaluating the injury.

Burns or scalds The appearance of a burn on a child is influenced by many factors: the temperature, size and shape of the causative agent, the depth of skin at the contact site, the length of time of contact and the application of first aid measures all have the potential to modify its characteristics. Whilst information on all of these factors should be sought from the caregivers it is often difficult to draw accurate conclusions from examination of the wound itself. Associated injuries such as bruises or fractures may help. Although classically described as associated with non-accidental injury, cigarette burns are rare. These appear as small, deep, round burns, usually on the limbs or back.

Healing burns can sometimes be especially difficult to diagnose and interpret. Inflammation can extend beyond the margins of the burn, obscuring the shape and increasing the size of the lesion. The healing area may become flaking or exudative, causing confusion with skin conditions such as impetigo.

Scalds are a common form of accidental injury in infants, often caused by a hot liquid being tipped over the upper torso, arms or hands: some features of a scald may suggest an intentional cause. Look at the position, shape and depth of the burn. Circumferential scalds of the hands or feet may be caused by forced immersion. Small round bruises above the burn may represent forcible gripping by a hand. Scalds of the buttocks extending on to the lower back or upper thighs with sparing of the natal cleft may indicate the child has been lowered into hot water.

Fractures   Fractures of long bones, ribs and skull may occur when a child is intentionally struck, pushed, squeezed or dropped. While any fracture may be caused by non-accidental injury, certain fractures have an association with abuse that should alert the ED clinician and prompt further action. Specifically, fractures in children under the age of 18 months, rib fractures, metaphyseal fractures, multiple fractures and fractures of differing ages should be carefully evaluated.

A bone scan and skeletal survey may be extremely useful in gathering evidence of multiple injuries when a child under the age of 2 years presents with suspicious bruising or other features of abuse.

Eye injuries   Direct blows to the face may cause subconjunctival haemorrhages or intraocular injuries such as retinal haemorrhages. A careful examination including visual acuity and funduscopy is necessary.

Ear injuries   Blows to the side of the face may cause bruising of and behind the pinna.

The ear drum may rupture due to the air pressure changes.

Head injuries   Head injuries are a major source of mortality and morbidity in non-accidental injury. Young children have a large head to body size ratio, relatively weak neck musculature and compliant skull bones that predispose them to intracranial injuries. The child may be struck, dropped, thrown or shaken, producing an open or closed head wound.

Skull fractures, cerebral contusion, intracerebral haemorrhages, extradural haematoma and subdural haematoma are all possible sequelae.

Intra-abdominal injury   Blows to the abdomen may cause laceration or rupture of either solid abdominal organs, such as the liver or spleen, or of the hollow organs, such as the duodenum. There may or may not be accompanying bruising of the abdominal skin to alert you to this possibility. Liver function tests and amylase may be helpful if this is suspected.

Investigations   Primarily, the findings of the clinical examination dictate the extent and type of investigations necessary. As would be the case in the investigation of any injured child, plain X-rays, computerised tomography scans, magnetic resonance imaging, ultrasound and other imaging should be directed at areas where there is clinical suspicion of injury.

Other investigations, such as a skeletal survey and bone scan, are used in an attempt to detect injuries that may not be clinically apparent but which will assist in establishing the likelihood of non-accidental injury. These are especially useful in children under the age of 2.

In a child with multiple bruises, the possibility of a bleeding disorder such as idiopathic thrombocytopenic purpura should be considered. A full blood examination and coagulation profile may be necessary in these circumstances.

Emotional abuse

Emotional or psychological abuse is difficult to define and even harder to detect, particularly in the ED, when frequently the child presents to a particular health worker on a single occasion. Five possible components

of emotional abuse have been described. These are the following behaviours:

- rejecting;
- isolating;
- terrorising;
- ignoring;
- corrupting.

The incidence of emotional abuse is unknown but it is likely to be common and under-diagnosed.

History and examination

Presentation is subtle and depends upon the age of the child. An infant may present with sleep or feeding problems, irritability or apathy. Older children may present with attention deficit, attention seeking, aggression, school failure, truancy, anxiety, depression and psychosomatic disease. It is likely that emotional abuse accompanies other forms of abuse, such as physical and sexual abuse. Consideration of its possible role is important in all assessments of a child at risk.

Detection by all health workers looking after children, including emergency staff, requires a high index of suspicion and vigilance. Diagnosis is suggested by the consequences in the child, as above.

Assessment should include that of behavioural, emotional and physical signs and the child–parent interaction. This will usually require time not available to emergency staff and therefore, when emotional abuse is suspected, referral is necessary. This may be to the hospital child protection/abuse unit and/or community social services.

Neglect

Neglect may also cause the child to be at risk and can be difficult to define and diagnose. A broad definition is anything that individuals, institutions or processes fail to do, which directly or indirectly harms children or damages their prospects of a safe and healthy development into adulthood. Other definitions have tended to be narrower and therefore target more severe or persistent neglect. It is important to differentiate neglect from poverty or ignorance, as these will require a different intervention.

The true incidence of neglect is unknown and it is probably the most common reason for the child to be at risk. Its diagnosis usually only occurs when harm has occurred, but consideration should be made of potential for harm and long-term effects. Types of neglect include medical neglect, safety neglect, educational neglect, physical neglect and emotional neglect. Non-organic failure to thrive is likely to be due to a combination of a lack of calories and affection.

History and examination

Some possible features to look out for are frequent presentation and admission to hospital with accidents or illness, delay or failure to access health care, malnutrition, failure to immunise, poor physical presentation, poor compliance, behaviour disorders, developmental delay and, very importantly, failure to thrive. The assessment of growth and development is clearly an essential part of child health assessment, even in the emergency setting. Measurement of height, weight and head circumference and their plotting on standardised growth charts can be very useful in assessment and follow up. Emotional and behavioural assessment is difficult in the emergency setting.

Treatment

The diagnosis of non-organic failure to thrive usually requires admission to hospital to assess the child's ability to grow with adequate nutrition and an interdisciplinary approach. Other forms of neglect may require admission or, if not, referral to child protection/abuse unit or community social services.

Münchausen's syndrome by proxy

Münchausen's syndrome by proxy (MSBP) is an unusual presentation of the child at risk that may present to an ED. This condition occurs when an adult, usually the mother, presents a false history to the physician regarding a child who is not truly suffering from any of the reported symptoms. This history may cause the emergency physician to perform unnecessary diagnostic and therapeutic procedures that do not result in any specific diagnosis.

In 1995, the *Diagnostic and Statistical Manual of Mental Disorders*, 4th edition-included a definition for factitious disorder by proxy, which is now the accepted psychiatric category for MSBP. The definition includes the following:

❶ Intentional production or feigning of physical or psychological signs or symptoms in another person who is under the individual's care.

❷ The motivation for the perpetrator's behaviour is to assume the sick role by proxy.

❸ External incentives for the behaviour, such as economic gain, avoiding legal responsibility, or improving physical well-being, are absent.

Children at risk for MSBP abuse are aged 15 months to 6 years. The emergency physician is often confronted with baffling symptoms. Frequently, the child has been taken to many care providers before the diagnosis is finally established. Warning signs that are suggestive of MSBP include the following:

- illness is multisystemic, prolonged, unusual, or rare;
- symptoms are inappropriate or incongruent;
- patient has multiple allergies;
- symptoms disappear when parent or caretaker is absent;
- in children, one parent, usually the father, is absent during hospitalisation;
- history of sudden infant death syndrome in siblings is noted;
- parent is overly attached to patient;
- patient has poor tolerance of treatment (e.g. frequent vomiting, rash, problems with intravenous lines);
- general health of patient clashes with results of laboratory tests;
- parent shows inordinate concern for feelings of the medical staff;
- seizure activity is unresponsive to anticonvulsants and is witnessed only by parent or caretaker.

The community response to the child at risk

Responsibilities to report

For medical practitioners working in acute medicine, often the first point of contact with a child at risk is when they present for treatment. Statistics suggest that doctors only diagnose cases in about 2% of notifications.

Mandatory reporting legislation brought in across all states of Australia has made it compulsory to report cases of non-accidental injury and suspected cases of neglect to the State Child Protection Agency. For example, in New South Wales under Section 22 of the Children (Care and Protection) Act 1987, medical practitioners were required to report physical and/or sexual abuse of children under the age of 16 years. Mandatory notifiers who failed to notify under Section 22 of the Act were guilty of an offence.

All healthcare staff are now mandatory reporters under the Children and Young Persons (Care and Protection) Act 1998. It is a criminal offence not to report.

Notification involves contacting the child protection authority relevant to the state. The Children (Care and Protection) Amendment (Disclosure of Information) Act 1996 extends voluntary reporting to any person who believes on reasonable grounds that a child who is aged 16 or 17 years has been, or is, in danger of being abused.

Once notification is made a process of risk management is commenced.

What to do as the medical practitioner, in suspected cases

❶ Take a concise history of events and physical examination.

❷ Document injuries and order appropriate investigations.

❸ Manage injuries as usual practice.

❹ Notify relevant child protection agency. (Clients consent is not required in child protection notification.)

This may be facilitated by social worker, nurses and paediatric specialists.

Legal responsibilities

❶ By law, health services staff must provide all relevant information that they have available when asked (in writing) to do so by the child protection authority.

❷ Staff do not have to get permission of the client in order to forward the relevant information.

❸ Protection for notifier. The Children (Care and Protection) Act 1987 made provision for the safeguarding of the identity of the person who makes the report.

❹ Neither the report nor its contents are admissible as evidence in any proceedings against the person who made the report.

❺ If, as a result of making a report, a person is threatened or fears personal violence, this should be reported to the police, who may apply for, and pursue on their behalf, an apprehended violence order.

What happens after notification?

❶ The Child Protection Agency must respond when someone reports that they think a child or young person under the age of 16 years has been, or is being, injured or neglected.

❷ When the agency receives information about non-accidental injury, it makes decisions about how to go ahead with investigating the claims and how others may be able to help. For example, it may contact the child's teacher, child-care worker, relatives or the police.

❸ The police will be contacted and may become involved if the agency thinks the law has been broken.

Actions based on risk assessment

❶ If the child is in immediate danger, steps will be taken to reduce the level of risk or move the child to a safe place. This may mean admission to hospital or foster care.

❷ In many cases, this might mean giving the family practical help, such as organising child care, emergency finance, providing a referral for counselling or information on health or other services.

❸ In some cases, the child protection agency takes the matter to the Children's Court. The court can order a child be placed in agency care for a period of time. The court can also order counselling and other types of support services including health services.

Further reading

Browne K, Hanks H, Stratton P, Hamilton C. *Early prediction and prevention of child abuse: A handbook.* Chichester: John Wiley & Sons; 2002.

Gabarino J, Guttman E, Seeley J. *The psychologically battered child.* San Francisco: Jossey-Bass; 1988.

Hobbs C, Hanks G, Wynne J. *Child abuse and neglect: A clinician's handbook.* London: Churchill Livingstone; 1999.

Oates KR. *The spectrum of child abuse: assessment, treatment and prevention.* New York: Brunner/Mazel; 1996.

ADMINISTRATION AND EMS

Section editor **Gary Browne**

19.1 Managing the death of a child in the ED: Bereavement issues

Paul Tait • Roger Barkin • Pat Clements

ESSENTIALS

1 The death of a child under any circumstances is likely to lead to a significant crisis and grief response in parents.

2 Emergency physicians should be prepared for parental presence in the resuscitation room, anticipate their high level of distress, and ensure that they are kept informed.

3 It is important that the family knows that everything that could have been done was done.

4 Parental questions should be answered honestly and directly, allowing humanity and empathy to show.

5 Personal, compassionate and individualised support should be provided for families, respecting their cultural, religious and social values.

6 Family members are likely to have impaired decision making and communication abilities, and this needs to be taken into consideration around informed consent issues.

7 The needs of the grieving family must be balanced with the legislative requirements of the Coroner's Act when this is relevant.

8 Relatives should be allowed to spend time with the deceased child if they want to, preferably in a quiet suite.

9 It is important to be available in the weeks following the death to clarify and answer any further questions from the family.

10 Team members need to be aware of their own likely emotional responses to the death of a child.

of self, the grief response of parents may be very painful and prolonged. The death of a child must be viewed as a tragedy for the entire continuum of family and friends. Additionally, paediatric deaths are frequently personalised by ED staff, and hence have broad implications for the whole ED clinical team.

In large hospital EDs, particularly in urban areas, there is rarely a pre-existing relationship between the health professionals and the patient/family. While this facilitates the professional detachment needed for ED staff to function effectively, it creates inherent voids in the ability to support grieving relatives and friends. In smaller hospitals like those found in rural and regional communities, a pre-existing relationship may exist, potentially lowering communication barriers but bringing out other stresses and strains for ED staff.

Good communication with family members must be established early and maintained throughout. This is best left to an experienced member of the staff. There is evidence to suggest that junior medical staff do not feel adequately trained in talking with parents in regards to end-of-life care matters.[4] Due consideration for the comfort of the family should be at the forefront of the minds of clinical staff at all times.

Introduction

Deaths occurring in the emergency department (ED) present unique challenges for the clinician, particularly if the patient is a child.[1,2]

The unexpected death of a child undoubtedly brings about the most severe and shattering grief response for the child's parents.[3] Because the loss is unexpected and involves someone so young and so intrinsically a part

The resuscitation process

Parents usually benefit from being present during the resuscitation process.[5] It is therefore unacceptable to discourage their presence unless they are interfering with, and compromising, the resuscitation itself. Family members watching monitors and seeing the trace 'go flat' experience much alarm and distress, but this should not be seen as a reason to exclude them.[6]

The resuscitation process can be traumatic for parents and family members, requiring ongoing communication and interpretation of events. It should be expected that parents will be visibly upset and distressed during this period. A staff member, often a social worker, should be assigned to support the family, to answer any questions about the procedures and responses, and to prevent distraught family members from impeding the resuscitation.[7] The ED medical officer in charge must communicate with this staff member and family members about the progress of the resuscitation. Viewing the resuscitation efforts allows the family to see a caring and competent staff, in control of their emotions, doing their best to save the child's life.

Where parents choose not, or feel unable, to be in the resuscitation room, it is essential that they be kept informed of progress. Panic, fear and a sense of isolation have been noted as the main responses of relatives who remain outside the resuscitation room.[6] Small, dull rooms with no windows or natural light were seen as heightening the sense of isolation, disconnectedness and fear for those family members unable to bring themselves to view the resuscitation.

It is important to be skilled in early recognition of the signs of trauma responses by parents, such as dissociation, as this can affect long-term adjustment. A social worker or other designated professional should ideally be available to provide support for parents and act as an advocate during what is likely to be an overwhelming and bewildering process. The social worker is also likely to be the main staff member to have an ongoing role after death has occurred and the family has left the hospital.

Talking to parents and families

When talking with the family about the child's deteriorating condition, give details in a simple, straightforward and accurate manner. Provide the information using appropriate language. Answer questions and be responsive to needs and concerns.

When death has occurred, or is imminent, it is essential to have identified the relevant family members so that discussions are with the appropriate individuals. At the point of death, the medical officer in charge of the resuscitation should advise those family members present in the resuscitation room or in a private, quiet location. Research has indicated that families appreciated a high level of physician involvement.[8]

Clear, distinct and accurate information is essential, and medical jargon should be avoided. It is very important to state initially that the child has died. This is the piece of information that the parents will most want clarified. It is then desirable to provide a brief chronology of events, while reassuring the family that everything was done and that the child did not suffer pain.

Sometimes family members are not present at the time of death. If practicable it is best to delay notification of death until it can be done in person.[9] If the family cannot readily access the ED, telephone notification may be necessary. A survey of survivors suggested that if delay in personal notification was greater than 1 hour, telephone notification may be appropriate.[10] However, it is obviously difficult to be sensitive to the family's response via a telephone, and there may be limited ability to provide immediate support. Ensure that the family is safe to transport themselves and that ongoing support options have been explored for those family members unable to make it to hospital.

If family members were not present at the hospital it is likely that they will have many questions related to the process, potential suffering, and any awareness by the child of the event. These may be asked either over the telephone or upon arrival. If parents arrive 'too late', this can create a further burden of guilt because they were not present.

Family members experiencing significant grief are likely to struggle with the integration of the information that they are being given and with the communication of any questions that they might have. They may need to revisit the same questions and information repeatedly in order to try to make sense of the event.[6]

It is important to allow parents and family members time to examine the implications of the loss, and to begin the process of searching for some answers and meaning in the midst of the event. It is also important to assist them to mobilise resources from their social, cultural and religious communities to help them to deal with their grief.

There can be a temptation to offer sedation to grief-stricken parents. This is often requested by relatives distressed by observing the parents' pain. Grief is a normal process, which is rarely helped by pharmacological intervention.

Junior medical staff are often involved in resuscitations, and it is essential that they have received some training/education to help them handle the unexpected death of a child. A number of programs have been described, which have been found to be useful in preparing staff to deal with loss in an effective manner, from the perspective of both the family and staff members.[11–14]

Laying out of the child

Where parents want to 'view' or spend time with their deceased child, it is important to facilitate their wishes (having due regard to the possibility that the death may need to be referred to the coroner and hence care not to interfere with evidence). All tubes inserted during the resuscitation process (endotracheal tubes, intravenous cannulae, drains, etc.) should be removed, unless the medical officer in charge considers that the placement of a tube may have been associated with an adverse event. All wounds and cannula sites should be dressed to avoid leakage of bodily fluids. The child's face and exposed areas should be bathed/cleaned and any soiling removed.

The impact of the death can often cause an overwhelming sense of numbness and helplessness, diminishing the ability to self advocate. Therefore, it is important to be proactive with family members and ask how much they want to be involved with the bathing and laying out of the child, and about any specific cultural or religious practices that they would like observed.

It can often be useful to obtain mementos of the child. Photographs, a lock of hair, or a foot/hand print may become important mementos along the grieving journey. It is recommended that hospital EDs have access to such items as a camera, memento books and bereavement packs to give to families.

There are specific requirements in place for deaths that must be referred to the coroner. These may limit the process of 'laying out' the body, and require that family members may not be left unsupervised with the child. ED staff need to balance the needs of grieving family members with their legal responsibilities to the coroner.

Viewing the body – quiet suite

Most available evidence strongly suggests that seeing the body of the deceased is an important part of accepting the reality of death.[15,16] This includes not only seeing, but also being able to touch and hold the loved one. It is helpful to describe to relatives what they are going to see prior to viewing the body, especially if there are trauma-related injuries.[6] Viewing the body can also relieve anxieties about mutilation, signs of trauma, or that the person was in pain when they died.[16] A parent or family member's preference not to spend time with the child should also be respected.

Most large paediatric hospitals have a 'quiet suite' or 'family room' to facilitate parents spending time with their deceased child. This can allow a private 'good bye' and time to reflect. It can also allow time to create an image of the child as dead, altered from the image of the living child.[16] The importance of the family/relatives' room cannot be overemphasised – privacy and basic facilities are essential.

Subsequently, additional relatives/ friends may arrive at the hospital. This can often lead to heightened distress for parents as they try to explain the events that have led to the child's death, hence taking them back to the initial traumatic stages. It can also be a useful process. By reviewing events, parents may build a clearer picture and 'fill in the blanks' as they retell their story.

The grief response

Grief is a normal reaction accompanying death. The severity of the grief response parallels the severity of the loss.

Perhaps the most well-known model of describing the process of grief is the 'stages' model with its clearly defined stages of shock, denial and isolation, anger and envy, bargaining, depression and acceptance.[17] These stages should not be seen as linear or rigid. Individuals can move back and forth between the stages or may appear 'stuck' in a stage. Although the 'stages' model is the most well known and can be a useful guide, there are a number of other models of grieving including psychodynamic,[18] attachment,[19,20] social constructionist,[21] cognitive/behavioural,[22,23] and personal construct.[24] Good practice requires being open and flexible, adapting to the needs of the grieving family as opposed to trying to fit the family into any particular model. It is important not to pathologise individuals whose grief response does not fit neatly into a particular model of grief.[25]

The death of a child provokes the most intense form of bereavement. It is certain to alter the course of the parents' lives, their relationship with each other and with others. Losing a child is more than losing a relationship. For a parent it is losing part of their self, their present and their future. Many parents experience a loss of meaning in their lives and may never fully recover from the impact of their child's death.[20] A child's death is not a singular loss, but produces a ripple effect overwhelming all aspects of the family and environment. Parents, and even the extended family, may feel that they have failed, irrespective of the nature of the death and level of love, nurturing and caring that existed during the child's life.[16,26,27]

The parental relationship faces severe stress following the death of a child. It can pull a dysfunctional relationship further apart, or glue a functional one closer together. Adverse impacts on the relationship can occur through the real or perceived apportioning of blame by one parent to the other. This can occur where a child died while under the specific supervision of one parent, or one parent was simply not present when a critical event occurred.

Siblings of the deceased child will also experience a significant grief reaction. Not only must they manage the actual loss of their deceased sibling, but they must also cope with the loss of their normal family environment. Their parents will be struggling to cope with their own grief, and thus

will be less emotionally available. The cognitive developmental level of a sibling has a significant bearing on their capacity to understand concepts of death like permanent, irreversible, inevitable, universal.[28] Regardless of how siblings understand and express their grief, it is critically important to remember that they are part of the social context in which the death has occurred. Their needs for explanation and support are just as important as the needs of their parents.

The death of a child does not occur in isolation, but rather it occurs in a social context that includes many variables. The main ones are parental coping capacity and skills, family and relationship functionality, social networks, parental physical and mental health issues, education, socioeconomic status, and, importantly, any real or perceived parental responsibility in the death of the child. Thus the broader social context will have relevance to how parents and extended family members manage the impact of the child's death.[26] Any available psychosocial assessment or information, such as that provided by the ED social worker, should be factored into the management of the family.

Support of the family

Generally, parents are completely unprepared for the impact of their child's death as they have no prior knowledge or experience to draw on.[29] Arranging support is essential, and early social worker involvement is highly desirable. Parents and other family members must be provided with information about 'normal' grieving, and should be linked to appropriate resources. This can take the form of written information packs that parents can take away, and which they may choose to read at a later time.[30,31] Referral information should be readily available for support groups with particular expertise relating to the death of a child such as Sids & Kids,[32] SANDS Australia,[33] Compassionate Friends,[34] and other relevant organisations. The extent of involvement of support by ministers of religion will depend on the wishes of and the religious commitment of the family. Ideally there should be a protocol that facilitates ready access to this material.

Practical assistance with arrangements at the time of the child's death, including organising family support, funeral and financial assistance, should be offered to families as appropriate, while being sensitive to the social and cultural environment of the family.

Cultural implications

Many cultures have specific rituals and practices concerning death. It is critical to listen to the family members and be guided as much as possible by their requests. Some of these rituals may require modification when the death of a child has been referred to the coroner's office. Sensitivity is essential.

It is difficult to make broad statements about the cultural practices related to death and dying in indigenous (Aboriginal and Torres Strait Islander) communities, because across Australia there are different practices and rituals. Examples of the kinds of cultural practices and rituals to be aware of include:

- When a child is dying many families will want any extended family present to be in attendance.
- During the grieving process pre- and post-death, loud crying/wailing may need to occur as part of the community's customs. Privacy in these circumstances is desirable.
- Senior female or male figures may wish to take a lead role in mourning rituals after death has occurred. This can include ceremonial cleansing (washing the child's body), dressing and handling.
- Funeral arrangements may have to be organised by a specific extended family member or a senior member of the community.
- 'House smoking' (burning leaves in order to prevent the spirit from 'rising up') may need to occur relatively quickly after death has occurred. This can mean that the family will want to return to their community quickly.
- Many communities forbid the use of the deceased person's name after death (for up to one year). Nicknames or aliases may be used after death has occurred. A family member with the same name as the deceased may use their second name during the mourning period.

- After a year, there may be some ritual (i.e. tombstone opening) associated with the end of the mourning process, which requires community members to return home even if in hospital themselves.

The Maori culture of New Zealand traditionally has family members present with the body from the time of death through interment. This maintains the harmony of the child, assisting the decedent to join their ancestors. Family members will want to be part of the 'laying out' of the body, washing, dressing, etc.

Other practices reflecting different cultural belief systems that may need to be considered include parents needing to remain with the body 24 hours after the death, caring of the body by staff of the same gender as the deceased child, laying the body to face a certain direction (Mecca), special roles for specific religious/spiritual leaders, and the burning of incense/candles.

When working with families from different cultures following the death of a child, it is important to be guided by custom, ritual, experience, and the family's cultural environment.

Legal issues

Each state and territory will have subtle variations as to the legal requirements for the documentation and handling of the body of a deceased. An up to date protocol should be available to ensure that proper procedures are followed.

A life extinct form will need to be completed by one of the attending ED medical staff. However, it will also be necessary to decide whether or not a death certificate can be completed. If the patient was known to the hospital and the death was not unexpected, the child's usual physician may be prepared to sign a death certificate. This physician may also discuss with the parents the option of performing a hospital-based autopsy.

Usually the death of a child in the ED is not anticipated, and hence becomes a coroner's case (see Chapter 19.2 on Forensic paediatrics and the law). For a coroner's case, only a life extinct form can be completed, laying out of the body will be restricted to spot cleaning, the local police must be notified, and parents must not be left

unsupervised with the body. It is desirable for the family to formally identify the child's body in the presence of the police. Otherwise identification will have to be performed later and probably at the morgue, a process likely to increase family distress. All medical notes, investigations, observation sheets, etc., should be provided to the police when they depart with the child's body for the morgue. Full and accurate documentation of all events in the patient's hospital chart is essential. This should include the date and time of death, the observations that specify that the child is clinically deceased, any relevant history surrounding the circumstances of the child's death and any relevant conversations held with the parents or family members. There are potentially legal consequences following any death and the forensic issues need to be considered. For example, child abuse remains an important cause of deaths in infancy.

Organ and tissue donation and collection

Organ donation (e.g. heart, lungs, liver, kidneys) requires intact cardiorespiratory function but brain death. Because of the preconditions required by Transplant Acts before brain death can be declared, organ donation discussions are commonly deferred until admission to the intensive care unit.[35]

Tissue donation (e.g. corneas, heart valves) can occur from cadavers, and hence theoretically this issue could arise for children who die in the ED. However, deaths of children in the ED are usually coroner's cases. For parents faced with the extreme distress of the sudden death of a child and the need for coroner's-case status, it may be potentially too distressing to parents for ED staff to raise the further issue of tissue donation in this setting. This can come a little later at the Forensic Pathology Institute level, when parents have had a little time to regain some degree of composure and hence may be better able to give informed consent. On the rare occasion when the issue of tissue donation is spontaneously brought up by parents in the ED setting, contact with the transplant coordinator can be initiated if there are no potential medical contraindications to tissue donation. Consent by the coroner must be obtained prior to tissue removal.

When children die suddenly and unexpectedly there may be merit in considering collecting perimortem samples in order to obtain as much information as possible. This might include urine and blood for metabolic profiling, genetics screening and other possible investigations such as liver of other tissues samples that may contribute to the understanding of cause of death. This will depend on location and is more likely to be valuable in a major centre where appropriate pathology facilities are immediately available.

Debriefing and support for ED staff

Much of what is written about the family grief reactions applies equally to the ED staff and due consideration of staff reactions is very important. A healthy approach is to factor the reality of day to day exposure of grief and loss into the culture of a busy ED. There is a paucity of literature on the reactions of staff and grief management among ED staff members.

Identifying abnormal psychological symptomatology in ED staff (flashbacks, sleep disturbance, bad dreams, absenteeism, detachment, intensified emotions, etc.) and making ongoing psychological counselling available to affected staff is clearly important. Such symptomatology may occur as a result of either a single exposure or cumulative exposures to traumatic situations. It is important for senior ED staff to promote the concept of self-care, to guarantee confidentiality to staff experiencing problems, and to ensure staff are made aware of counselling options available to them should they experience problems.[36]

Performing an operational debriefing of the resuscitative process with a view to clarifying events for attending staff and identifying areas for potential improvement is essential.

The same cannot be said for psychological debriefing sessions. It has become a popular and widespread practice to conduct single session psychological counselling for personnel attending traumatic critical incidents. ED staff in attendance at an unsuccessful resuscitation fit into this situation. A recent Cochrane Review concluded that single session psychological debriefings have not only

failed to reduce the incidence of post-traumatic stress disorder but actually increased the risk of developing it.[37] In addition, there was no evidence of reduction in general psychological disturbance, depression or anxiety. This is an area where more research is required.

Conclusion

The death of a child has the most profound effect on parents, family and friends. It can also have a profound effect on staff involved in the resuscitation process. It requires the sensitivity and strength of clinical staff to help relatives through this difficult time and to assist in the initiation of a healthy grieving process. A thoughtful and sensitive approach is likely to have profound and positive long-term implications for all those impacted upon by the death of a child.

Acknowledgements

The authors gratefully acknowledge the assistance of the Indigenous Liaison Service, Herston Hospitals Complex, Brisbane.

Controversies

❶ There remains some controversy about actively encouraging parents to be in the resuscitation room.

❷ There is little evidence to support the widespread practice of mandatory single-session psychological counselling of distressed staff who attended the child.

❸ Raising the issue of tissue donation with parents in the ED setting is difficult.

References

1. ACEP. Death of a child in the emergency department: A joint statement by the American Academy of Pediatrics and the American College of Emergency Physicians. Ann Emerg Med 2002;40:409–10.
2. Olsen JC, Buenefe ML, Falco WE. Death in the emergency department. Ann Emerg Med 1998;31:758–65.
3. Seecharan GA, Andersen EM, Norris K, Toce SS. Parents' assessment of quality of care and grief following a child's death. Arch Pediatr Adolesc Med 2004;158:515–20.
4. McCabe ME, Hunt EA, Serwent JR. Pediatric residents' clinical and educational experiences with end-of-life care. Pediatrics 2008;121(4):e731–7.
5. Doyle CJ, Post H, Burney RE, et al. Family participation during resuscitation: An option. Ann Emerg Med 1987;16(6):673–5.
6. Wright B. Sudden death: Intervention skills for the caring professions. New York: Churchill Livingstone; 1996.
7. Tsai E. Should family members be present during cardiopulmonary resuscitation? N Engl J Med 2002;346:1019–21.
8. Scott JL, Sanford SM, Strong L, Gable K. Survivor notification of sudden death in the emergency department. Acad Emerg Med 1995;2:408–9.
9. Stewart AE. Complicated bereavement and post-traumatic stress disorder following fatal car crashes: Recommendations for death notification practice. Death Stud 1999;23:289–321.
10. Leash RM. Death notification: Practical guidelines for health care professionals. Crit Care Nurs Q 1996;19:21–34.
11. Schmidt TA, Norton RL, Tolle SW. Sudden death in the ED: Educating residents to compassionately inform families. J Emerg Med 1992;10:643–7.
12. Bagatell R, Meyer R, Derron S, et al. When children die: A seminar series for paediatric residents. Pediatrics 2002;110:348–53.
13. Swisher LA, Nieman LZ, Nilsen GJ, Spivey WH. Death notification in the emergency department: A survey of residents and attending physician. Ann Emerg Med 1993;22:1319–23.
14. Rutkowski A. Death notification in the emergency department. Ann Emerg Med 2002;40:521–3.
15. Jones WH, Buttery M. Sudden death. Survivors perceptions of their emergency department experience. J Emerg Nurs 1981;1:7.
16. Raphael R. The anatomy of bereavement: A handbook for the caring professions. London: Hutchinson; 1984.
17. Kubler-Ross E. On Death and Dying. London: Tavistock; 1970.
18. Freud S. Mourning and melancholia. Standard Edition XIV. London: Hogarth Press; 1917.
19. Bowlby J. Attachment and loss. Vol. 1. Attachment. London: Hogarth Press; 1969.
20. Parkes CM. Bereavement: Studies of grief in adult life. London: Tavistock; 1972.
21. Glick IO, Weiss RS, Parkes CM. The first year of bereavement. New York: John Wiley & Sons; 1974.
22. Attig T. The importance of conceiving of grief as an active process. Death Stud 1994;15(4):585–647.
23. Worden JW. Grief counselling and grief therapy: A handbook for the mental health professional. London: Routledge; 1983.
24. Neimeyer RA, Neimeyer GJ. Advances in personal construct psychology. Science & Technology Books. New York: Jai Press; 1997.
25. Dubin WR, Sarnoff JR. Sudden unexpected death: Intervention with the survivors. Ann Emerg Med 1986;15:54–7.
26. Murray J. Loss as a universal concept: A review of literature to identify common aspects of loss in diverse situations. J Loss Trauma 2001;6:219–41.
27. Murray J. Children, adolescents and loss. Loss and Grief Unit. Brisbane: University of Queensland; 2002.
28. Murray J. Understanding loss in the lives of children and adolescents: A contribution to the promotion of well being among the young. Aust J Guid Counsel 2000;10(1):95–109.
29. Heiney S, Hasan L, Price K. Developing and implementing a bereavement program for a children's hospital. J Pediatr Nurs 1993;876:385–91.
30. Johnson L, Rincon C, Gober C, Rexin D. The development of a comprehensive bereavement program to assist families experiencing paediatric loss. J Pediatr Nurs 1993;8:3.
31. Murray J. An ache in their hearts. Brisbane: University of Queensland Press; 1993.
32. SIDS and Kids – www.sidsandkids.org.
33. SANDS Australia – www.sands.org.au.
34. Compassionate Friends – www.thecompassionatefriends.org.au.
35. Rivers EP, Buse SM, Bivins BA, et al. Organ and tissue procurement in the acute care setting: Principles and practice, part 1. Ann Emerg Med 1990;19:78–85.
36. Everly GS, Flannery RB, Mitchell JT. Critical incident stress management: A review of the literature. Aggr Violent Behav 1999;5(1):23–40.
37. Rose S, Bisson J, Wessely S. Psychological debriefing for preventing post traumatic stress disorder (PTSD). Cochrane Database Syst Rev 2002;(2):CD000560.

19.2 Forensic paediatrics and the law

Maree Crawford • Natalie Phillips

ESSENTIALS

1 Emergency physicians will frequently be involved in the area of forensic medicine and hence require skills and knowledge of their responsibilities with regard to the legal system.

2 Thorough history, examination and documentation provide the basis for well-prepared legal reports. This, in turn, greatly assists in the presentation of evidence to courts.

3 Emergency physicians who deal with children must be aware of their legal obligations with regards to reporting of child abuse, reporting of criminal matters and management of deaths.

4 Doctors providing evidence in court must be seen to be independent, and competent within their level of expertise.

Introduction

The emergency department (ED) is the initial point of contact for many children presenting with acute injuries. While the majority of injuries are accidental, within this large group will be a number of children with inflicted injury or with findings resulting from abuse or neglect, on whose behalf legal proceedings may be initiated in a variety of legal jurisdictions. Hence ED staff require some expertise in forensic medicine or medicine as it relates to the law.

The role of medical staff in the ED is to carefully assess and treat children with such injuries. A number will present with a clear history or findings to indicate that injury or abuse has been inflicted. Many others will present with non-specific injuries or findings that will not be flagged as abusive, but at a later date may evolve to require legal involvement. It is therefore essential that doctors in the front line adopt high standards of history, examination and documentation for all cases of injury, both to allow detection of abuse and also to meet the standards required should a matter progress into the legal system.

Medical staff have a number of legal obligations in such matters. These include mandatory notification of suspected abuse or neglect, a need to advise the police of a potential criminal matter and to assist police in their investigation of such an event. There are also obligations with regard to the management and notification of deaths to the state coroner.

By virtue of this front-line contact, emergency physicians will at times be required to provide evidence in a variety of legal jurisdictions. Familiarity with these systems, good preparation, and a neutral unbiased approach will allow doctors to discharge their duty to provide the courts with accurate representation of facts and balanced expert opinion.

Forensic medical assessment

Forensic medicine, also known as medical jurisprudence, deals with the interaction of medicine and the law. All specialities or areas of medicine will have overlap with forensic matters at some time, and this is particularly so in paediatric emergency medicine. The aims of a forensic medical assessment are diagnosis and management that incorporates the requirements of the legal system. The qualities required include precision and thoroughness, objectivity, neutrality, clarity of thought and expression, and logical formulation of opinion.

Forensic paediatric medicine largely revolves around the assessment of trauma to develop an understanding of the mechanism of an injury, and the nature of the forces required. This then allows consideration and evaluation of the provided history to determine whether it adequately and plausibly accounts for the injuries seen. An opinion can then be formulated that an injury is truly accidental, resulting from an unpredictable or unavoidable event; that it has been inflicted or imposed on the child; or that it is accidental but involves caregiver neglect, or failure to protect from harm.

As in all areas of medicine, a forensic medical opinion must be based on the information available to the clinician. This is obtained using standard clinical tools of history, examination and investigation, but also incorporates additional standards and procedures and may require more expansive investigations to consider all differential diagnoses.

Accurate history and examination and appropriate investigation

The following points may assist in forensic matters.

Physical injuries

❶ Key questions that should be asked and recorded in all cases of injury include:
- Who was present at the time of injury?
- When and where did it occur?
- How did it occur?
- What happened after the injury?

❷ It is important to document from whom each part of the history is obtained and any differing accounts. Any explanation that the child gives for the injury should be recorded.

❸ A *child's developmental abilities* should be evaluated to ensure that any actions the child has allegedly taken are within their developmental ability, e.g. standing and turning on hot-water taps.

❹ Any injury must be accurately described including site, colour, size and pattern.

❺ Accurate terminology for injuries should be used e.g.:
- Abrasion – superficial denuding of the skin confined to the epidermis, often called a graze or scratch

- Bruise or contusion – extravasation of blood into surrounding tissue caused by blunt trauma
- Laceration – tearing wound through the full thickness of the skin, or through other tissues and organs caused by blunt trauma
- Incised wounds – sharply cut injuries from any object with a cutting edge, e.g. stab or slash wounds.

❻ If an injury or injuries are present, there must be careful examination for other abnormalities that might not be immediately obvious, e.g. a child with facial bruising should have careful examination of mouth and ears.

❼ In addition to a child's injuries, notice should also be taken of their general presentation, appearance and demeanour, and of any non-concerning injuries or skin markings.

❽ When ED medical staff encounter injuries or findings that are suspicious of abuse or neglect they should, in the first instance, involve more senior staff, either a senior paediatric emergency physician, or a child protection paediatrician, for guidance.

❾ In consultation with senior staff, *further testing for occult injury* may be required when injuries or findings are suspicious for abuse or neglect e.g. skeletal survey in infants with bruising to look for occult fractures, or funduscopy with dilated pupils in infants with rib fractures, looking for retinal haemorrhages (Table 19.2.1).

❿ *Additional testing* may also be indicated to exclude differential diagnoses and to assess for other factors that may impact on the extent of any injuries for a given history e.g. testing for bleeding tendency (see Table 19.2.1).

⓫ Specific forensic sampling may be required in some instances, e.g. toxicology, swabbing for DNA in suspected bites, or specimen collection in sexual abuse. Child protection or forensic physicians should be involved, and a clear 'chain of evidence' must be maintained from clinician to police to forensic pathologist.

Other circumstances

❶ *Sexual abuse allegations* should be discussed with a child protection paediatrician as soon as possible and generally prior to any further assessment and physical examination.

❷ *Child protection concerns not specifically related to injury* may arise in an ED context. These may include concerns of suspected emotional/psychological abuse, factitious illness and neglect e.g. non-organic failure to thrive, significant hygiene concerns, failure to attend to medical needs, concerning parent–child interactions.

Documentation

Both history and examination findings should be recorded clearly, and in detail. Accurate printed diagrams of body parts

are an excellent aid and should be used. Any injury thought to be suspicious of being inflicted or of being caused by abuse should be photographed. This can be done using hospital photographic services or ED photographic equipment if available. However, if there are suspicions of abuse, staff will be notifying child protection agencies and the resources of the police may be used for photography. These are usually of higher quality, and police involvement overcomes problems of confirming a chain of evidence if the material is later used in a legal setting.

Notes made at the time of consultation will provide the doctor with information from which to prepare a statement or report for a court if this is required at a later time (sometimes years later). They also will assist the doctor in providing evidence if asked to appear in court proceedings. For this reason documentation must be detailed and accurate.

Opinion formulation

The next step is to infer the mechanism of the injury, if possible, from the clinical findings, e.g. a patterned bruise is due to blunt trauma from contact with a specific object, and posterior rib fractures are due to chest compression. Frequently there are no discriminating features to assist with determining the mechanism, e.g. a child with multiple non-specific bruises. In all cases the adequacy of the parent or carer's explanation of the injury must be considered.

Any opinions as to causation and mechanism must be based on the medical findings and their compatibility with the history, and not on extraneous factors, e.g. adverse psychosocial history. Additional information

---

Table 19.2.1 Further investigations

I. For occult injury

Skeletal survey: to examine for occult fractures. Generally indicated in any child under 2 years of age where inflicted physical injury is suspected. This may be done at older ages in specific cases. A second skeletal survey, 11–14 days after the original, may be helpful in detecting healing fractures not easily visible in the very acute phase.

Funduscopy with dilated pupils: to examine for retinal haemorrhage and define nature and extent. Generally indicated if suspected shaking, or concerns for inflicted head and neck trauma.

Neuroimaging: CT is generally indicated in the acute and hyperacute settings, with MRI preferred in the subacute and chronic phases, after suspected injury. MRI is increasingly sensitive for intraparenchymal injury and often allows more accurate delineation of subacute and chronic haemorrhage.

Bone scan: may be indicated to examine for acute fractures (prior to callus formation). Any positive findings still require confirmatory X-rays at a later date.

II. For underlying medical conditions:

Full blood count and film, coagulation screen
Extended coagulation screen: may include von Willebrand's factor testing, factor assays, platelet function tests. These tests should be discussed with a haematologist prior to collection.
Further testing as advised and according to injury e.g. calcium, phosphate, PTH, vitamin D, urine metabolic screen including organic acids, copper, ceruloplasmin, bone mineral density imaging, skull X-ray for wormian bones.

CT, computerised tomography; MRI, magnetic resonance imaging; PTH, parathyroid hormone.

from site visits may be provided by Police investigators and should be incorporated in formulating an opinion. Opinions must be logical and not based on speculation. An attempt should be made to differentiate whether injuries are truly accidental, accidental but with a component of neglect, or inflicted. In many cases, no definite conclusion can be drawn.

Legal obligations

Mandatory reporting of child abuse

Medical practitioners in all states and territories of Australia are now mandated to notify suspicions of abuse and/or neglect to the relevant statutory authority in their state, although the forms of abuse/neglect to which mandatory reporting applies vary between states e.g. only sexual abuse in Western Australia, sexual/emotional/physical abuse and neglect in New South Wales (Table 19.2.2). Definitions of abuse commonly relate to the concept of harm, which, for example, under the Queensland Child Protection Act 1999, is defined as 'any detrimental effect of a significant nature on the child's physical, psychological or emotional

wellbeing'. In many states, it is mandatory to report not only *actual* suspected harm but also significant *risk* of harm. Practitioners should be familiar with the requirements and mechanisms for notification within their state and locality. Doctors are free of any liability if such reports are made in good faith.

Notification of suspected criminal matters

If a medical officer considers that an injury is not accidentally caused or that a crime has been attempted or completed, there is also an obligation to notify the police. All involved individuals, including medical practitioners, are required to assist police in their investigations.

Notification to the coroner of deaths under certain circumstances

Medical practitioners are required to notify the coroner's office of deaths that occur in a variety of circumstances. These include, in broad terms, situations of any sudden, unexplained death, situations where cause of death is unknown, and situations where there are any suspicious circumstances

surrounding the death. The coroner has the responsibility to investigate and report on these matters.

Legal jurisdictions

At times, emergency physicians will be involved with children whose injuries or other findings will result from physical assault or abuse, sexual assault or abuse, or emotional abuse or neglect. Some of these cases will end with involvement in the legal system in various jurisdictions.

Inflicted injury in which there is a single alleged offender may lead to criminal charges of assault or of torture. The child protection statutory agency may look to provide safety for a child and their siblings via a range of orders in the Children's Court or information may be sought regarding a child's well-being by the Family Law Court in matters of contested custody or residency between parents.

To assist medical practitioners in their interaction with the legal system a brief outline of the different court systems follows.

Table 19.2.2   Mandatory reporting requirements for medical professionals (2009) in children and young people by state

State	Maltreatment types for which mandatory reporting applies	Legislation	Statutory agency
Australian Capital Territory	P, S	Section 356 of Children & Young People Act 2008 (ACT)	Office for Children, Youth & Family Support-Dept of Disability, Housing and Community Services
New South Wales	P, S, E, Neglect, Exposure to family violence	Section 23 & 27 of Children & Young Person Act 1998 (NSW)	Department of Community Services
Northern Territory	P, S, E, Neglect, Exposure to family violence	Section 15 & 26 of Care &Protection of Children Act 2007 (NT)	Children, Youth and Families- Department of Health and Families
Queensland	P, S, E, Neglect, Sexual exploitation	Section 191-192 & 158, Public Health Act 2005 (QLD)	Child Safety Services - Department of Communities
South Australia	P, S, E, Neglect	Section 11 of Children's Protection Act 1993 (SA)	Families SA- Department of Families & Communities
Tasmania	P, S, E, Neglect, Exposure to family violence	Section 13 & 12 of Children, Young persons and their Families Act 1997 (Tas)	Child Protection Services– Department of Health and Human Services
Victoria	P, S	Section 182 (1) a-e, 184 and 162 c-d of the Children, Youth and Families Act 2005 (Vic)	Child Protection and Family Services- Department of Human Services
Western Australia	S	Section 124 B of Children & Community Services Act 2004	Department for Child Protection

Notes:
Mandatory reporting requirements apply to all individuals under 18 years of age, except in New South Wales where they apply to individuals under 16 years old.
States vary on whether it is mandatory to report only actual suspected harm, or also significant future risk of harm.
Key: P, physical abuse, S, sexual abuse, E, emotional/psychological abuse.
Source: Adapted from Higgins et al. 2009. National Child Protection Clearinghouse Resource Sheet No 3. Mandatory reporting of Child Abuse and Neglect. Australian Institute of Family Studies, Australian Government.

Criminal court

In a criminal matter, a person is charged with committing an offence under the criminal code of the state in which the offence occurred. Criminal courts are adversarial systems where the Crown must prove that the accused is guilty of the offence with which they have been charged. The level of proof required is *beyond reasonable doubt*.

Police are responsible for investigating any alleged crime and for laying charges against an individual if grounds exist. They are also responsible for assisting the Director of Prosecutions in obtaining witness statements. Initial evidence is heard in a committal proceeding before a magistrate. In this court, the evidence is tested to ensure that there is sufficient for the matter to proceed to a higher court.

Whether the matter is heard in a higher court is determined by the nature of the offence. *Summary offences* (usually relatively minor offences, e.g. traffic offences, some assaults) are dealt with solely in the Magistrate's Court. *Indictable offences* proceed to a higher court before judge and jury in either District or Supreme Courts.

Doctors may be called to provide evidence either as a professional witness providing factual evidence of something that occurred in the clinical setting, or as an expert witness, that is, a specialist or senior doctor who can provide expert opinion on certain facts.

The first involvement that a doctor may have with the proceedings is via a request from police for a statement of witness. This statement, which must be in a format acceptable to the court, will provide the basis for oral evidence to be provided. The report must be clear, truthful and unambiguous, should avoid the use of medical jargon and should clearly describe terminology in such a way that it may be understood by a lay person.

The statement should include details of professional qualifications and experience, a brief history provided to the doctor, and an accurate description of clinical findings. Reference should be made to any other documentation or investigation, e.g. photographs, so that they can be admitted as evidence. It is important to address whether the injuries found could produce effects consistent with the definition of the charges (Table 19.2.3). This usually requires comments as to effects on the child with regards to pain and suffering, and prognosis assuming medical intervention had not occurred. It is not appropriate to describe injuries as, for example, constituting 'grievous bodily harm' as this is for the court to determine.

Table 19.2.3   Terminology of criminal charges

- *Bodily harm* – an injury which interferes with health or comfort (e.g. causes moderate pain or discomfort) but does not endanger life or cause permanent disability
- *Grievous bodily harm* – any bodily injury of such a nature as to endanger or be likely to endanger life, or to cause or be likely to cause permanent injury to health if left untreated
- *Unlawful wounding* – an injury in which the true skin has been broken, e.g. laceration or incised wound
- *Torture* – an intentional infliction of severe pain or suffering on a person by an act or series of acts done on one or more than one occasion

Source: Derived from Queensland Criminal Code Act 1899.

Children's court – child protection proceedings

Children's courts deal with criminal charges brought against children up to 17 or 18 years. They also handle matters related to children's welfare.

An ED medical officer who provides assessment and treatment of a child with inflicted injury or abuse may be required to provide information and expertise to assist this court in making decisions regarding a child's need for care and protection by the state or the need for other protective orders. This court is conducted before a magistrate and is adversarial; however, it requires a lower standard of proof than criminal court, i.e. *on the balance of probability*. The nature of evidence that can be admitted is more lenient than in criminal proceedings, allowing hearsay (second hand) information. As in criminal proceedings, a sworn report or affidavit will often be sought prior to appearance in court, and should follow the general principles for statements for criminal court.

Family law court

This is a federal court created to administer the Family Law Act 1975. In this jurisdiction, medical practitioners may be required to provide evidence on behalf of children in contested matters between parents, related to guardianship and residency of involved children. Again, the system is adversarial, with legal representatives for both parental parties, and often an independent representative for the child or children, outlining a case before a judge for ruling. Proof is on the basis of the *balance of probability*.

Coroner's inquest

The coroner's role is to investigate and report on the circumstances surrounding a person's death. The coroner's powers are defined by state or territory legislation. This legislation also defines a medical practitioner's obligations to notify reportable deaths and to co-operate in any inquiry. The precise definition of reportable death varies between states but, in general, includes any death for which the cause is unknown or where the cause of death appears to be by violent, unnatural or accidental means, or where there are suspicious circumstances.

Emergency physicians will sometimes encounter children dying or presenting dead to the ED and must be familiar with their state or territory requirements. The death should be notified to the coroner's office and also to the police. Police will assist the coroner in the investigation, and a forensic pathologist will conduct an autopsy and report back to the coroner.

At times doctors will be called to provide a statement and may be required to give evidence at a coronial inquest. This is not a trial but a fact-finding inquiry. A mix of inquisitorial and adversarial procedures is used and hearsay evidence can be accepted.

The coroner will make public the findings of the inquest and may comment on inadequacies in systems and management. The coroner does not directly recommend criminal proceedings.

Providing evidence in court

Doctors may be called to give evidence in any of the courts outlined. This will be either as a professional witness providing evidence in fact, related to what they saw or did as part of their work, or, alternatively, to provide an expert opinion on a matter.

Prior to attendance at court, the doctor may have been requested to provide a statement of witness, affidavit, or medical report that is composed from the doctor's notes. The statement must include professional qualifications and, in the case of an expert witness, must establish that they have specialised skills and knowledge in their area of expertise.

The report should include a brief history of the reasons for seeing the child, the date, time and place the child was seen, and the person accompanying the child. Any spontaneous disclosures that the child has made to the doctor should be included. The general state and demeanour of the child, and detailed specific findings are important. Lastly, an opinion regarding the mechanism of any injury, and the effects on the child of that injury with regards to pain and disability, are important.

Court appearances can be stressful for doctors. However, it is important to remember that an individual's evidence is but a small part of any case. The doctor is there

to assist the court in its deliberations and is not personally on trial. The doctor must adopt an independent neutral role and be prepared to consider objectively any statements put to them. Doctors are not there to support a particular 'side'.

When appearing as an expert witness, a doctor will be asked initially to describe their qualifications and expertise. They will then be questioned by one counsel and cross-examined by the other. They should listen carefully to all questions and answer as accurately as possible. They should have their notes of the consultation available and ask leave of the court to refer to them. It is important to remain calm and professional in all ways and never be tempted to outsmart the lawyers in their domain. Careful preparation and a sound knowledge of the relevant medical problems will assist the doctor greatly in this whole process. If questioned about a matter outside their level of experience or expertise, a doctor should indicate that this is the case and not attempt to speculate.

Doctors providing evidence to a coronial inquest will normally be independent parties. However, if there are issues of possible

medical negligence involved, prior contact with their medical indemnity organisation should be made.

Further reading

Breen K, Plueckhahn V, Cordner S. *Ethics, law and medical practice.* Allen & Unwin, St. Leonards: NSW; 1997.

Dix A, Errington M, Nicholson K, Powe R. *Law for the medical profession in Australia.* 2nd ed. Port Melbourne: Butterworth-Heinemann; 1996.

Higgins D, Bromfield L, Richardson N, et al. *National Child Protection Clearinghouse(NCPC) Resource Sheet No 3. Mandatory reporting of Child Abuse and Neglect.* Australian Institute of Family Studies, Australian Government; 2009.

Queensland Child Protection Act. 1999.

Queensland Criminal Code Act. 1899.

Royal College of Paediatrics & Child Health (RCPCH). *Child Protection Companion.* 2006.

Royal College of Paediatrics & Child Health (RCPCH). *Child Protection Reader.* 2007.

Royal College of Paediatrics & Child Health (RCPCH). *Standards for Radiological Investigation in Suspected Non-Accidental Injury.* Intercollegiate Guideline RCPCH and Royal College of Pathologists; 2008.

Shepherd R. *Simpson's forensic medicine.* 12th ed. London & Baltimore MD, USA: Hodder Arnold; 2003.

References available online (2010)

RCPCH guidelines http://www.rcpch.ac.uk/Publications/Publications-list-by-title.

NCPC resource sheet http://www.aifs.gov.au/nch/pubs/sheets/rs3/rs3.pdf.

Table 20.1.3   Pain scoring

FLACC scale

The FLACC Scale is a behavioural scale for scoring pain in children between the ages of 2 months and 7 years or in persons unable to communicate. Each of the 5 categories is scored from 0-2 and the scores are added to get a total score from 0 to 10.

	0	1	2
Face	No particular expression or smile	Occasional grimace or frown, withdrawn, disinterested	Frequent to constant frown, clenched jaw, quivering chin
Legs	Normal position or relaxed	Uneasy, restless, tense	Kicking, or legs drawn up
Activity	Lying quietly, normal position, moves easily	Squirming, shifting back and forth, tense	Arched, rigid, or jerking
Cry	No cry (awake or asleep)	Moans or whimpers, occasional complaint	Crying steadily, screams or sobs, frequent complaints
Consolability	Content, relaxed	Reassured by occasional touching, hugging or 'talking to', distractible	Difficult to console or comfort

The FLACC behavioural pain assessment scale © University of Michigan Health System can be reproduced for clinical or research use.

Faces rating scales (FRS)

These scales can be used with young children (as young as 4 years of age). They also work well for older children and adolescents, including those who speak a different language.
Ask the patient to choose the face that best describes how they feel. The far left face indicates 'no hurt' and the far right face indicates 'hurts worst'.

The Faces Pain Scale – Revised (FPS-R) can be downloaded (including instructions in multiple languages) from the *Pediatric Pain Sourcebook* at www.painsourcebook.ca.

Numerical rating score (NRS)

This tool may be used for children over the age of 6-8 years. Instruct the patient to rate their pain intensity on a scale of 0 ('no pain') to 10 ('the worst pain imaginable').

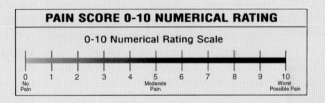

Table 20.1.4   Patient factors to consider in procedural sedation

- Current illness – URTI, active asthma, altered conscious state, haemodynamic compromise
- Age under 12 months (especially <3 months)
- Airway abnormalities – craniofacial deformities, tracheomalacia, predicted difficult airway
- Cardiac conditions – congenital heart disease, arrhythmias, cardiac failure
- Neurological conditions – seizure disorders, raised intracranial pressure
- Respiratory conditions – active asthma, upper or lower respiratory tract infections, respiratory failure
- Hepatic and renal disorders
- Prior history of failure of sedation
- Prior adverse event due to sedation, analgesia or anaesthesia

is likely to be significantly lower than that associated with general anaesthesia and the requirement for fasting remains a subject of debate. Fasting requirements should be adjusted for individual cases, following consideration of an individual patient's risks of aspiration and the nature and urgency of the sedation.[23]

Physical examination should include patient weight, baseline vital signs including oxygen saturation, assessment of conscious state, evaluation of the airway and examination of the cardiovascular and respiratory systems.

The ASA physical status categories developed for general anaesthesia are not generally used for ED procedural sedation as it is unclear how they extrapolate to this setting.[24] Following risk assessment and generation of a sedation plan, this plan should be discussed with the child's parent or carer to obtain informed consent. A clear explanation of the sedation plan and what is to happen for the older child is often useful in an effort to allay anxiety and optimise co-operation.

The expected effects on the child, risks, benefits, alternatives and need for monitoring and observation during and after the procedure prior to safe discharge must be discussed with the parent or guardian. As the expected effects, risks and recovery times prior to discharge will vary greatly between different agents, the use of a standardised procedural sedation consent form for all sedative drugs is suboptimal. It is recommended that drug or drug combination-specific consent forms should be generated that reflect the individual features of the different agents, to clearly identify that these issues have been discussed with the child's parent. An alternative to this involves standard documentation in the medical record that agent-specific issues were discussed with the parent(s)/carer(s).

In most EDs there is a policy that informed consent for procedural sedation is obtained in written form unless it is employed in a life- or limb-threatening situation.

Medications

A medication order containing all sedative drugs to be used should be recorded on the appropriate medication chart or sedation record, and the doses, route and time of administration should also be recorded.

Reversal drugs and life-support drugs should also be available (Table 20.1.5).

Environment

Paediatric procedural sedation must be performed in a facility that is adequate in size and has equipment available for drug administration, clinical monitoring, airway management, vascular access and cardio-respiratory resuscitation.

Sedation in environments where the area does not meet these requirements is associated with an increased level of serious adverse events.[6]

Equipment

Equipment must be suitable for children of all the ages and sizes being treated. The ability to recognise respiratory or circulatory compromise early with the use of monitoring equipment is essential. Devices for airway management and techniques of advanced life support are recommended, along with sedative drug-reversal agents and life-support drugs.

Intravenous access

In patients receiving intravenous (IV) sedation, the IV access should be retained until the patient's conscious state has improved. Patients receiving sedation by a non-IV route may benefit from the safety of having an IV line placed, particularly when the level of sedation is deep or if there is a higher than usual probability of complications as a consequence of current illness or injury or comorbidities. Where an IV line is not established prior to sedation, a practitioner with skills in establishing vascular access in children must be readily available.

Recommended equipment and drugs are listed in Table 20.1.5.

Personnel

There must always be at least two clinical staff involved in procedural sedation, with at least one doctor.

One acts as the 'sedationist' and is responsible for giving drugs and monitoring the patient – particularly from a respiratory and circulatory perspective. The sedationist should have no other responsibilities in the procedure thus enabling that person to be able to respond as rapidly as necessary to changes in the patient's vital signs or clinical state. If another staff member is not present, the sedationist should also be responsible for documenting observations, times and doses of drugs administered and recording specific interventions.

Staff providing and monitoring sedation must be knowledgeable about the drugs being used and be trained to identify and rapidly manage complications – particularly airway and respiratory adverse events – and be proficient in paediatric resuscitation. The role of sedationist may be filled by a nurse or doctor with appropriate knowledge and training.

The second staff member ('the proceduralist') is responsible for performing the procedure, e.g. fracture reduction or suturing.

When performing deep sedation (e.g.: propofol, thiopentone or other intravenous anaesthetic agents), three staff members should be present – a trained sedationist with paediatric resuscitation skills, a proceduralist and another staff member to record observations, assist the other staff as needed and liaise with the child's parent or carer, who may often be present during the procedure.

Finally, it is recommended that there is a supervising senior doctor – generally at specialist or advanced trainee level, that has specific experience and competence in paediatric airway management and resuscitation. This person may be taking the role of sedationist but if not directly involved in the procedure it is appropriate that he or she is aware that the procedure is occurring and has guaranteed that they will be in the department and available to assist rapidly should complications arise.

Management during the procedure

A number of recommendations and statements from clinical authorities have been published detailing particular aspects of required personnel, monitoring equipment, patient preparation for procedural sedation in children both inside and outside of the operating theatre.[25–27]

It is essential that the team administering procedural sedation is aware that it is impossible to reliably predict in advance the level of sedation that will occur in an individual patient given a sedative drug or combination of drugs. Regardless of the intended level of sedation or route of administration, the sedation of a patient represents a continuum, and may result in the loss of the patient's protective reflexes – a patient may move easily from a light level of sedation to deep sedation. As a consequence, it is imperative to plan for situations where the child becomes sedated to a far greater level than intended or experiences significant cardio-respiratory complications of sedation.

Table 20.1.5 List of drugs and equipment recommended for safe procedural sedation

Equipment[a]
- Oxygen source, masks and tubing
- Suction source and suction devices
- Self-inflating bag–mask device
- Oral and nasal airways
- Endotracheal tubes and difficult airway management devices
- Laryngoscopes
- Defibrillator with paediatric paddles
- ECG monitor
- Non-invasive blood pressure measurement device
  Intravenous cannulation equipment
- Oxygen saturation monitor
- Delivery system and scavenger device for continuous nitrous oxide administration
- End-tidal carbon dioxide monitor (ETCO$_2$)

Drugs[b]
- Epinephrine (adrenaline)
- Atropine
- Lidocaine
- Dextrose 10%
- Reversal agents – naloxone and flumazenil
- Hydrocortisone

[a]All equipment must be available in varying sizes appropriate to patient population.
[b]Correct weight-based dose information should be readily available.

Table 20.1.6 Elements of safe procedural sedation management

1. Personnel
2. Environment
3. Medications
4. Risk assessment
5. Patient preparation and consent
6. Monitoring
7. Recovery
8. Documentation
9. Discharge criteria

Accordingly, well-understood policies and procedures detailing the requirements for procedure management should be developed by EDs providing procedural sedation to children. Table 20.1.6 details the important elements of the conduct of procedural sedation management.

Monitoring, observations and recording

The most important element of monitoring during sedation is close, continuous observation of the patient.

Recommended monitoring equipment includes electrocardiogram (ECG), non-invasive blood pressure measurements, oxygen saturations and end-tidal carbon dioxide monitoring (ETCO$_2$) (Table 20.1.5).

Continuous oxygen saturation monitoring is recommended in all forms of procedural sedation as is continuous observation of colour, airway and rate and depth of ventilation.

It is recommended that intermittent heart rate and blood pressure monitoring is used when the level of sedation is deep.

Capnography

Capnography provides a more sensitive means of identifying respiratory depression or airway complications resulting from sedative agents than conventional monitoring and observation, but has been underutilised.[28]

With abnormalities in ventilation that are detectable by capnography and then only later evolve into the typical clinical manifestations of respiratory depression, apnoea, or airway obstruction.[29–33] Oxygen desaturation is often the last sign of the complication, particularly when supplemental oxygen has been administered.[29]

Observation and recording of heart rate, blood pressure, respiratory rate, conscious level or sedation score, O$_2$ saturation and ETCO$_2$ should be recorded prior to the procedure, after sedative drug administration and at 5–10-minute intervals during the procedure, depending on the level of sedation achieved. Times of administration, drugs given, dosages and routes of administration of drugs should be clearly recorded on a time-based observation chart.

Interventions performed, such as provision of supplemental oxygen or basic airway management should also be recorded.

Supplemental oxygen

The use of supplemental oxygen is largely unstudied in children undergoing procedural sedation in the emergency department.[32,34,35]

The addition of supplemental oxygen has the potential to mask respiratory depression as hypoxia may not manifest even in the presence of significant hypoventilation. Use of ETCO$_2$ monitoring is recommended when supplemental oxygen is administered as changes in ETCO$_2$ associated with respiratory depression are detectable before the onset of hypoxia.[34]

Many physicians use supplemental oxygen coupled with ETCO$_2$ monitoring with patients who are undergoing deep sedation.

Sedation scores

There is no universally validated and accepted score for recording the depth of sedation in patients undergoing procedural sedation in the emergency department.

Benefits of the use of a valid scoring method include the monitoring and recording of depth of sedation during episodes of procedural sedation along with assisting in standardisation of terminology and classification of sedation depth, particularly in clinical audit and research, looking at the effectiveness and adverse event profiles of different drugs at different doses.

These scores are observational in nature and are recorded during the episode of sedation.

A commonly used sedation score is the Children's Hospital of Wisconsin Sedation Scale.[9]

The scale has seven levels of sedation ranging from 6 to 0:

6: anxious, agitated or in pain;
5: spontaneously awake without stimulus;
4: drowsy, eyes open or closed, but easily arouses to consciousness with verbal stimulus;
3: arouses to consciousness with moderate tactile or loud verbal stimulus;
2: arouses slowly to consciousness with sustained painful stimulus;
1: arouses, but not to consciousness, with painful stimulus;
0: unresponsive to painful stimulus.

Deep sedation is commonly defined as a score of 0–2 and moderate sedation as a score of 3.

The Modified Ramsay Sedation Score[36] is also commonly used and ranges from a score of 1: awake and alert, through to a maximum score of 8: unresponsive to external stimuli, including pain.

Bispectral index monitoring

The advent of bispectral index (BIS) monitoring to measure the depth of anaesthesia in patients in the operating room may potentially be a useful adjunct in procedural sedation in the ED.[29,37–39]

Further studies using this index will better define what role an objective measure of sedation level may play in reduced complications of oversedation along with avoidance of inadequate sedation during procedures.

Post-procedure management

It is imperative that children are closely observed and monitored in an appropriate environment following procedural sedation. Children vary greatly in their speed of recovery from sedation. This is also influenced by the drug(s) used, the route of administration and the total dosage given.

The period immediately following the completion of the procedure – with cessation of the painful or unpleasant stimulus – is a period during which cardiorespiratory depressant effects of the sedation drugs may be most apparent and it is during this time that there is an increased risk of complications.[40]

If the child is moved to another area following the completion of the procedure, they should continue to be closely observed and monitored by a suitably experienced nurse and resuscitation equipment should still be immediately available if needed. The frequency of vital signs observation can gradually lessen as the child awakens and the risk of cardiorespiratory complications

Table 20.1.7 Discharge criteria post-procedural sedation

- Normal age-specific vital signs
- Child has regained pre-sedation conscious state and communication skills
- Child is able to ambulate independently (relative to age and pre-sedation ability)
- Child is able to tolerate oral food or fluids
- Post-procedure analgesia is satisfactory
- Parent or carer has been provided with post-discharge instructions, understands them and is capable of following them

diminishes. Generally, the frequency of vital signs observation will lessen from 5-minutely to 30-minutely as the child returns to their pre-sedation state.

Post-procedural observations should be recorded on the same time-based observation sheet as used during the procedure and evidence of improvement in conscious level and activity should also be recorded.

It is important to have standard discharge criteria, which must be met by the child prior to leaving the ED, and nursing staff caring for the child must be familiar with these. Suggested discharge criteria are listed in Table 20.1.7.

Development of a standard post-procedural sedation discharge instruction sheet, which includes advice regarding diet, activities, observation, and sleeping in the 24 hours after discharge, along with specific signs to watch for and a direct ED contact number, is also valuable. The adult taking responsibility for the child after discharge should receive a copy prior to leaving and staff should both check that they understand it clearly and answer any questions about it that they may have.

Finally, follow-up arrangements relating to the procedure performed (e.g. review of wound, suture removal) should also be provided before discharge.

Complications of paediatric procedural sedation

Paediatric procedural sedation can be hazardous and both mortality and significant morbidity have been reported in the literature.[41-43]

Studies of procedural sedation in EDs with adherence to published guidelines and involvement of staff trained in sedation and paediatric resuscitation techniques have yielded variable rates of complications

of 2.3–25%, with the incidence of serious complications such as laryngospasm, pulmonary aspiration or cardio-respiratory arrest being extremely low.[43-45]

Establishing accurate adverse event and complications rates of different agents from the available literature has been difficult because of the difficulty in aggregating results from previous studies that have used varied terminology to describe the same adverse events and outcomes.[46,47]

In 2009, a Consensus Panel on Sedation[46] proposed a standardised terminology and reporting methodology for adverse events in EDPS in children. Moving away from the traditional event- and threshold-based definitions of an adverse event (e.g. oxygen saturation <92%), the Panel proposed reporting based on whether a particular event required an intervention to be performed by the clinician, i.e. whether the event was clinically relevant rather than simply transient, self-limiting and without clinical sequelae. Adoption of such standardised reporting guidelines by researchers will provide data that may be readily compared and aggregated across a variety of drugs, drug combinations, sedation providers and sedation locations.

A number of recent studies have reported on large cohorts of children undergoing procedural sedation.

The Paediatric Sedation Research Consortium reported on the nature and frequency of adverse events in 30 000 children receiving sedation and/or anaesthesia for diagnostic and therapeutic procedures outside of the operating room.[43] The overall reported adverse event rate was 1 in 29 cases (3.4%) and the rate of unplanned treatments was 1 in 89 cases (1.1%) Serious adverse events were rare and there were no deaths. One case of cardiac arrest and one case of pulmonary aspiration were reported. Conversely, more minor but potentially serious adverse events were not rare. Oxygen desaturation below 90% was the most common adverse event reported, with an incidence of 1.5%. Vomiting was common and occurred in 1 in 200 sedations (0.5%). Approximately 1 in 400 procedures were associated with stridor, laryngospasm, wheezing or apnoea and 1 in 200 sedations required airway and ventilation interventions ranging from bag–mask ventilation (0.6%), to oral airway placement (0.3%) to emergency intubation (0.1%). The same research group has also reported

the incidence and nature of paediatric sedation with propofol outside the operating room using a large database of 49 836 propofol sedation encounters.[44] There were no deaths reported. Cardiopulmonary resuscitation was required twice and there were four episodes of pulmonary aspiration. Less serious events were reasonably common, with oxygen desaturation below 90% for more than 30 s having an incidence of 1.5% and apnoea, airway obstruction, wheezing, stridor or laryngospasm occurring at a rate of 1.6%, with a reported rate of unplanned airway interventions (from simple airway manoeuvres to emergency intubation) of 1.5%, which equates to 1 in 70 propofol sedations requiring airway and ventilation interventions.

Metanalyses of predictors of adverse events in procedural sedation with ketamine in children have reported an overall incidence of airway and respiratory adverse events of 3.9% from 8282 episodes of ketamine sedation. The rate of unplanned airway interventions was not reported and many of these observed adverse events required no intervention. The overall incidence of emesis, any recovery agitation, and clinically important recovery agitation was 8.4%, 7.6%, and 1.4%, respectively.[45,48]

The majority of significant adverse events in paediatric procedural sedation are related to airway obstruction, hypoventilation requiring stimulation, supplemental oxygenation and/or a short period of assisted ventilation by bag–mask device. Paradoxical excitation (benzodiazepines) or clinically significant recovery agitation (ketamine) may require specific management.

Table 20.1.8 lists adverse events and complications associated with paediatric procedural sedation.

Adherence to published guidelines recommending minimum requirements for personnel, patient monitoring and assessment for safe discharge has been shown to reduce adverse events associated with procedural sedation in children.[9]

In particular, the generation of an individual sedation plan comprising an individual risk assessment with documentation of variables such as fasting status, quantitative sedation scoring, time-based recording of vital signs and pulse oximetry combined with standardised recovery and discharge criteria and use of a standardised record has been shown to progressively reduce

Table 20.1.8 Adverse events and complications in procedural sedation
• Sedation failure • Paradoxical excitation • Recovery agitation • Vomiting • Airway obstruction requiring suction, repositioning or use of an airway adjunct. • Hypoxia • Hypercarbia • Apnoea • Hypoventilation requiring supplemental oxygenation and/or assisted ventilation • Laryngospasm • Bronchospasm • Pulmonary aspiration • Hypotension • Bradycardia/tachycardia/cardiac arrhythmias • Cardiorespiratory arrest • Allergic reactions • Over sedation • Seizures

risk in procedural sedation, particularly in those children requiring a deep level of sedation.[9]

Non-pharmacological methods

A balanced multidisciplinary approach using pharmacological and non-pharmacological strategies is essential to providing optimal analgesia and sedation for the child. Non-pharmacological techniques can be particularly useful in pain management (whether or not medications are used as well) as they are free of side effects and may be utilised before, during and after painful procedures. The planning of procedures for children in the ED should include age-appropriate psychological interventions, such as distraction techniques. Distraction reduced self-reported pain following needle-related procedural pain.[49] Age-appropriate distraction techniques reduced situational anxiety in older children and lowered parental perception of distress in younger children undergoing laceration repair.[50] A child's anxiety and co-operation are affected by age, anxiety of the parent and previous medical experiences. Toddlers are very distractible and storytelling and guided imagery are very effective methods. Some useful non-pharmacological strategies are outlined in Table 20.1.9.

Pharmacological methods

Some of the most commonly used agents are listed in Table 20.1.10.

Table 20.1.9 Supportive and distractive techniques
Environment • Calm friendly non-clinical atmosphere • Toys, mobiles, pictures and videos
Psychological • Parental presence • Age-appropriate communication • Clear confident instructions
Cognitive–behavioural • Distraction techniques • Hypnosis and biofeedback • Art/stories • Music/video/TV • Interactive computer games • Guided imagery • Muscle relaxation and deep breathing techniques • Reinforcement of coping behaviours
Physical • Massage/rubbing • Comfort swaddling (infants) • Heat/cold techniques • Immobilisation and elevation (injured part)
Breast-feeding • Comforter (favourite blanket/soft toy)

Pure sedative agents

Sedative agents relieve anxiety but not pain. They may reduce the child's ability to communicate pain and discomfort and a common side effect is paradoxical hyperexcitability. They are useful for painless diagnostic studies and, when used in combination with opioids or nitrous oxide, can produce a state of deep sedation.

Oral analgesic agents

Paracetamol is usually the first line of therapy for mild to moderate painful conditions. It can be given orally and rectally. Non-steroidal anti-inflammatory drugs (NSAIDs), such as ibuprofen, are usually second-line therapy and have excellent analgesic and anti-inflammatory properties, which may enhance the effects of paracetamol.

Oxycodone and codeine

Oral codeine has traditionally been used for moderate to severe pain; however, evidence from recent work shows that oral oxycodone produces greater pain relief compared with codeine.[51] Oxycodone also has a better side effect profile with less itching, less nausea, and fewer allergic reactions. Codeine is a

prodrug of morphine and nine percent of children do not have the liver enzyme CYP2D6 to convert the inactive codeine and therefore in this group it provides no analgesia.

Oral sucrose for infant analgesia

Oral sucrose (25%) has been shown to be a simple, safe and effective means of providing analgesia for young infants (up to 2 months of age) for short painful events (e.g. venepuncture, lumbar puncture).[52–54] It stimulates endogenous opioid and non-opioid pathways in the brain. Up to 2 mL may be administered via oral syringe or on a pacifier approximately 2 minutes prior to the painful event.

Parenteral opioid analgesics

Opioid analgesics are the mainstay of treatment of severe pain. Infants and neonates require lower doses of opioid medication. Opioids are ideally administered IV in a dilute solution, e.g. morphine (1 mg mL^{-1}) given slowly over a few minutes and titrated against response. A further dose may be given after 5–10 minutes. Fentanyl is a potent rapid-acting analgesic with a shorter duration of action and used in combination with midazolam produces a state of dissociation and deep sedation.

Intranasal fentanyl

Intranasal fentanyl provides safe and effective analgesia equivalent to parenteral morphine in children as young as 1 year of age.[55–58] It offers a quicker onset, is less invasive, and its duration of action, although short, allows time for topical anaesthetic application prior to intravenous cannulation for ongoing analgesia. It is particularly useful for analgesia for fractures or burns dressings but its utilisation is spreading into other areas.

Nitrous oxide

Nitrous oxide mixed with oxygen has a potent analgesic action with rapid onset and offset. It is an excellent analgesic sedative for gaining rapid IV access, injecting local anaesthetics, performing a nerve block or splinting a fractured limb.[59–61]

Entonox® (50% nitrous oxide, 50% oxygen) is usually delivered via a demand-valve system. This limits its use in younger or unco-operative children. Machines that

Table 20.1.10 Commonly-used agents for sedation and analgesia

Classification	Doses	Comments
Pure analgesics		
Paracetamol	15–30 mg kg^{-1} PO/PR (<3 months 10 mg kg^{-1})	30 mg kg^{-1} stat. only as a single dose (check no recent doses of paracetamol)
Ibuprofen (NSAID)	5–10 mg kg^{-1} PO	
Liquegesic Co paracetamol/ codeine mixture (e.g. Painstop®)	Dose based on paracetamol content	
Oxycodone	0.1 mg kg^{-1} PO	Better analgesia and fewer side effects than codeine
Pure sedatives		
Midazolam	0.05–0.15 mg kg^{-1} IV/IM; 0.5–0.75 mg kg^{-1} PO; 0.3–0.5 mg kg^{-1} IN	Paradoxical excitement reaction in 10% of children when used PO or IN
Sedative/analgesics		
Morphine	0.1–0.2 mg kg^{-1} per dose (>3 months) IV, IM 0.05–0.1 mg kg^{-1} per dose (<3 months) IV, IM Infusion (>3 months) 0.01–0.04 mg kg^{-1} hr^{-1}	Cardio-respiratory depression with IV/IM doses IV dose preferred
Fentanyl	1.5 mcg kg^{-1} per dose	
Nitrous oxide	50:50 mix inhalation agent (ENTONOX®); N$_2$O continuous flow variable mix 30–70% with oxygen	Rapid onset; continuous flow delivery system allows use in young children/short duration of action. Vomiting can occur; contraindicated with pneumothorax/chest injuries
Dissociative agent		
Ketamine	1–2 mg kg^{-1} IV; 2.5–4.0 mg kg^{-1} IM; 5–10 mg kg^{-1} PO	Excellent safety profile in selected patients undergoing painful procedures; contraindicated in head injury, seizure disorders, ocular injuries
Sedative/hypnotic agent		
Propofol	0.5–3.0 mg kg^{-1} induction dose (titrate slowly to achieve desired sedation depth), halve the induction dose for top-up dosing	Median dose 0.75 mg kg^{-1} when used with adjunctive analgesia. Respiratory depression is the most common adverse effect
Local anaesthetic agents		
Injectable		
Lidocaine	1% or 2%; 3 mg kg^{-1} maximum dose without adrenaline (epinephrine); 7 mg kg^{-1} maximum dose with adrenaline	Pain of injection can be minimised by using small needles (e.g. 31G), slow infiltration, infiltrating through wound edges, pre-treatment with topical LA, buffering and warming
Levobupivicaine or bupivacaine	3 mg kg^{-1} (maximum dose)	Slower onset, longer duration of action compared with lidocaine; useful for nerve blocks
Prilocaine	0.5% solution common; 2.5–3.0 mg kg^{-1}	Safe agent for intravenous regional anaesthesia (Bier's blocks)
Topical		
Surface EMLA®	Eutectic mix of lidocaine 2.5% and prilocaine 2.5%	Requires 60 minutes post-application to achieve satisfactory dermal anaesthesia
AnGel®/Ametop®	Amethocaine 4%	Requires 30–45 minutes post-application to achieve satisfactory dermal anaesthesia
Laceraine®	Laceraine® solution is a mixture of 4% lidocaine, 0.5% tetracaine and adrenaline 1:1000	Contains adrenaline so cannot be used in end arteriole regions, e.g. digits, penis; requires > 20 minutes of good contact with wound to provide anaesthesia; may require supplementation with small doses infiltrated LA
Reversal agents		
Naloxone	10 mcg kg^{-1} IV	May need to repeat doses
Flumazenil	0.02 mg kg^{-1} IV	

LA, local anaesthetic; IM, intramuscular; IN, intranasal; IV, intravenous; PO, per oram; PR, per rectum.

deliver variable concentration (30–70%) nitrous oxide via a continuous flow system allow the use of this agent down to age 1 year, where it has been shown to be safe when embedded in a comprehensive sedation programme.[61]

Nitrous oxide alone is effective in achieving moderate levels of procedural sedation for a high percentage of children with painful conditions but may require the use of adjunctive analgesics for very painful procedures.[61,62]

Oxygen should be administered for 3–5 minutes after cessation of nitrous oxide to prevent diffusion hypoxia. Nitrous oxide is contraindicated in conditions involving closed air spaces (e.g. pneumothorax, bowel obstruction).

Ketamine

Ketamine is a unique analgesic dissociative agent. Its action produces a near ideal state of sedation, amnesia, analgesia and motion control with few side effects. It has been extensively studied, with safety and efficiency documented in several large paediatric studies. It is particularly suitable for laceration repair and orthopaedic procedures in the emergency department. Emergence reactions, common in adults during the recovery phase, are rare in children. Co-administration of midazolam has not been shown to reduce the rate of emergence phenomena but may be associated with less post-procedure emesis. Intravenous ondansetron significantly reduces the incidence of vomiting associated with ketamine sedation.[63]

Airway complications (including stridor, laryngospasm, respiratory depression, and apnoea) very rarely occur and have been reported as being associated with high intravenous dosing (initial dose >2.5 mg kg^{-1} or total dose ≥5.0 mg kg^{-1}), administration to children younger than 2 years or aged 13 years or older, and the use of co-administered anticholinergics or benzodiazepines.[45] There are few data on EDPS in relation to infants under the age of 3 months and the traditional contraindication to ketamine in this age group should continue until there is evidence of safety in this group.

Multiple routes of administration are available but IV and IM routes are preferred.

Both routes display similar risk of airway and respiratory adverse events, and of clinically important recovery agitation. The IM route is associated with a higher rate of vomiting.[45,48]

Comprehensive ketamine clinical practice guidelines were published in 2004.[64,65]

Methoxyflurane

A recent review has shown that the inhalational agent Methoxyflurane, long used by ambulance services, is also safe and effective in the ED setting.[66] The commonly-used 'Penthrox' inhaler is now available with an activated charcoal scavenging chamber to reduce environmental contamination.

Propofol

Propofol is an excellent ultra-short acting sedative/hypnotic agent, very useful for EDPS. It provides deep sedation and has anti-emetic and euphoric properties. Propofol has no analgesic properties and therefore needs adjunctive analgesic agents, e.g. fentanyl or ketamine when used for procedural analgesia and sedation (PSA) for short painful procedures. Used alone, it is effective in producing co-operation for painless diagnostic studies in emergency department patients. When combined with opiate agents, it has been used effectively for

painful procedures in children (e.g. fracture reduction). It is associated with a significantly higher rate of adverse airway events (oxygen desaturation and need for airway repositioning) when compared to ketamine,[67] emphasising the importance of having skilled and experienced practitioners available when it is being used.

It does offer quick recovery to pre-sedation state, allowing more rapid discharge. It may be delivered in a variety of manners from repeated boluses to continuous infusion. Despite initial barriers to the use of propofol in the ED, a large number of studies have produced evidence that propofol can be given in a safe and effective manner in ED for children.[68–72] Titrating and optimising the dose will enhance control of depth of sedation and recovery time.[73] Predictable cardiovascular and respiratory events respond to repositioning the airway, increasing oxygen delivery or limited BVM-assisted ventilation without adverse sequelae.[73] Capnography is now considered essential for early detection of hypopnoea and apnoea.[31]

An evidence-based Clinical Practice Advisory describing propofol use in EDPS was published in 2007.[74]

Ketafol

Ketafol refers to a mixture of ketamine/propofol in a 1:1 ratio (i.e. 1 mg ketamine: 1 mg propofol). A median dose of 0.75 mg kg^{-1} of each drug (range 0.2–2.0) has been shown to be safe and effective for procedural sedation in children.[75] Fentanyl is usually used as adjunctive analgesia but a study looking at combining propofol with a sub-dissociative dose of ketamine (0.3 mg kg^{-1} IV) compared with fentanyl suggested that the ketamine/propofol combination was safer.[76] Further research is required to determine if combining the two agents together is associated with fewer cardiovascular and respiratory adverse effects than using propofol alone.[77]

Local and topical anaesthetic agents

The expanded use of topical anaesthetics has revolutionised the management of simple lacerations in the ED and has also greatly improved conditions for intravenous cannulation and lumbar puncture. These agents provide a non-invasive means of producing local anaesthesia and can be applied at triage to facilitate timely management in the ED.[78]

EMLA® (2.5% lidocaine, 2.5% prilocaine) is a well-established topical anaesthetic for use on intact skin prior to venepuncture, intravenous cannulation or lumbar puncture. Its use in the ED is, however, limited, due to its long onset to peak effect (at least one hour) and its vasoconstrictive effect, which may make cannulation more difficult. EMLA® has a theoretical risk of methaemoglobinaemia and is not recommended in infants less than 3 months of age.[79]

Amethocaine (e.g. AnGel® – 4% amethocaine) has a quicker onset of action (30–45 minutes) than EMLA® and its vasodilating effect may facilitate cannulation. Tetracaine is superior to EMLA® in terms of lessening pain associated with intravenous cannulation and is more effective than EMLA® when application time is less than 60 minutes.[80]

Itching and erythema are side effects of tetracaine, whilst skin blanching is seen with EMLA® as a consequence of vasoconstriction.[80]

Topical wound anaesthetics, e.g. Laceraine® (adrenaline [epinephrine] 1:1000, lidocaine 4%, tetracaine 0.5%) and Adrenaline Cocaine Gel (adrenaline 1:1000, cocaine 12%) permit wound management with minimal to no discomfort.[81,82]

Cocaine-containing topical wound anaesthetics (e.g. TAC – tetracaine, adrenaline, cocaine) were originally found to be very effective in providing good wound anaesthesia but non-cocaine-containing topical wound anaesthetics have now been shown to be equivalent or superior to cocaine-containing preparations, Such preparations are significantly cheaper, are not associated with the requirement for secure storage and avoid the potentially serious systemic side effects that have been reported with cocaine-containing preparations.[83–85]

There are no commercially available cocaine-based wound anaesthetics available in Australia currently.

Local anaesthetic combination solutions such as Laceraine® instilled in a wound for 20–30 minutes provide sufficient anaesthesia for suturing 75–90% of scalp and facial lacerations[82,86] and 40–60% of extremity wounds. Its vasoconstrictive effect is also useful prior to application of cyanoacrylate tissue adhesive.

Wound infiltration with injectable local anaesthetics can be carried out with lessened pain by buffering the local anaesthetic, warming the solution to body temperature, using fine-bore needles and slow administration techniques through the wound edges rather than through intact skin.[87-91] Nitrous oxide and distraction techniques during the process of injection often provide good analgesia. Safe dosage regimes must be adhered to by the clinician.

Regional anaesthetic techniques

Regional nerve blocks may be used for either pain relief (e.g. femoral nerve block for femur fracture) or to facilitate suturing, fracture or dislocation reduction (e.g. digital or metacarpal blocks).[79,92] Nerve blocks have traditionally been performed using anatomical landmarks, with variable results. The use of ultrasound has been shown to increase the success of regional anaesthetic techniques. Intravenous regional anaesthesia (Bier's block) is useful and effective for some older children. Tired children, reluctant children, parental concern, or the lack of ED resources may make deep sedation or a general anaesthetic the preferred approach.

Discharge analgesia

Lack of appropriate or inadequate dosing of discharge analgesia is an ongoing problem. Pain experienced at home post acute injury or PSA in the ED can place considerable extra burden on family physicians for pain-related issues. It is essential to include adequate discharge analgesia in ED pain management guidelines. Ibuprofen was found to be preferable to paracetamol and codeine for outpatient management for children with uncomplicated arm fractures.[93]

Selection of agents by procedure and age

Pain management can be simplified by dividing pain into mild, moderate and severe categories and matching this with the appropriate analgesic agent(s) (Table 20.1.11). It is best to minimise the number of agents used and to be familiar with doses, duration of action, adverse effects and contraindications. Choice of agent should be individualised for the child's level of pain and the procedure. Dissociative techniques using various combinations of agents are useful for very painful procedures or in infants and toddlers.

Table 20.1.11 Analgesia options										
Wong–Baker faces score			2		3		4		5	
Pain score	1	2	3	4	5	6	7	8	9	10
Mild pain			Moderate pain					Severe pain		
Paracetamol			Ibuprofen Paracetamol-Codeine mix Oxycodone					Morphine Nitrous oxide IN Fentanyl		

Table 20.1.12 Balanced analgesia and sedation

The four components
1. Sedation
2. Analgesia
3. Amnesia
4. Motion control

Ideally, routes of administration should be non-invasive. Extensive knowledge and experience of the synergistic effects of analgesics and sedative agents can produce a 'balanced' state of sedation and analgesia (Table 20.1.12).

Recommendations for some common procedures

Painless diagnostic study

Motion control for imaging procedures, such as CT scan or even plain X-ray, can be a challenge. Oral anxiolytics given prior may be useful. It is important to apply topical local anaesthetic (AnGel® or EMLA®) 45–60 minutes prior to the procedure to facilitate intravenous cannula placement if adjunctive intravenous sedation becomes necessary.

Venepuncture and IV cannulation

Topical local anaesthetic agents are useful for semi-urgent IV access. Rapid access is best gained using nitrous oxide analgesia/sedation and distraction techniques. Oral sucrose is useful in young infants.

Nasogastric tube insertion

Although nebulised lidocaine has been shown to be a useful analgesic method for this distressing procedure in adults, it has been shown to be ineffective in children.[94] Oral sucrose may be useful in neonates requiring nasogastric tubes. Topical Cophenylcaine Forte® may help alleviate pain,

lessen epistaxis and assist passage of the tube by decreasing swelling.

Suprapubic aspiration

Topical application of EMLA® prior to the procedure will help alleviate pain. As this procedure is usually only performed on young infants, oral sucrose should be offered.

Urinary catheterisation

Oral sucrose may be useful in young infants and nitrous oxide in older children. Lignocaine gel should be used as lubricant.

Lumbar puncture

EMLA® should be applied in any child for whom a lumbar puncture may be considered but the procedure should not be delayed while waiting for it to work. Instillation of 1% lidocaine (using a small needle e.g. 27G) into the skin overlying the interspace will reduce the pain of the procedure. Oral sucrose on a pacifier should be offered to young infants and inhaled nitrous oxide may be offered to older children.

Small laceration

A pre-emptive approach using a combination of oral anxiolytics/analgesic medication will improve co-operation during the procedure. Topical wound anaesthetics allow wound cleaning and closure with minimal or no pain. Tissue adhesives are helpful for smaller wounds. Nitrous oxide and distraction are again useful.

Complex wound management

Infants and toddlers may require dissociative methods using a choice of ketamine IM or IV, fentanyl and midazolam IV, or nitrous oxide. With appropriate premedication older children can be managed with local or regional anaesthetic blocks.

Foreign body removal

Anxiolytic pre-medication may be all that is needed for the older child; however, younger children usually require dissociative techniques.

Fracture, joint dislocation, splinting and manipulation

Severe pain associated with these injuries is best managed initially with nitrous oxide or intranasal fentanyl while IV access is gained for ongoing opioid analgesia. Regional local anaesthetic blocks, e.g. femoral nerve block, are useful to enable splints and traction to be applied. Intravenous regional anaesthesia (IVRA) is a useful technique for fracture manipulation in older children. Many children under the age of 10 years are referred for general anaesthesia.

Multi-trauma

Children with severe multiple injuries often require many painful procedures during the initial assessment phase. A team approach is needed, with special attention to analgesia and sedation. Rapid sequence intubation (RSI) is often the most humane option. This allows a more rapid approach to investigation and management. Other alternatives for managing ongoing pain relief include continuous opioid infusion during the initial phases of resuscitation and stabilisation and patient-controlled analgesia once the patient is stable.

Controversies and Future Directions

❶ The future for clinical practice in the area of analgesia and sedation for children will focus on making our practices safer, more time efficient for the ED and less distressing for the child. Consensus-based recommendations for standardising the terminology used for reporting adverse events related to paediatric emergency department procedural sedation have recently been published.[46] These should help to create a uniform reporting mechanism for future studies in this area.

❷ Development of guidelines with greater attention paid to selection of appropriate patients, provision of adequate facilities and training of staff

(as outlined earlier in this chapter) will further improve the safety profile of our practices. Clinical audit of sedation/analgesia practice should be routine. Our practices will be made more efficient by future research to help define the optimal agent(s) and route of administration for particular procedures and patient age groups.

❸ Alternative routes of drug administration have already had a great impact on paediatric sedation and analgesia practices. The delivery of established drugs by innovative, less-invasive methods is an exciting area for future research.

References

1. Maurice SC, O'Donnell JJ, Beattie TF. Emergency analgesia in the pediatric population. Part 1, Current practice and perspectives. *J Emerg Med* 2002;19:4–7.
2. American Academy of Pediatrics, Society, A. P. The assessment and management of acute pain in infants, children and adolescents. *Pediatrics* 2001;108:793–7.
3. Zempsky WT, Cravero JP, Committee on Pediatric Emergency Medicine, and Section on Anesthesiology and Pain Medicine. Relief of pain and anxiety in pediatric patients in emergency medical systems. *Pediatrics* 2004;114:1348–56.
4. Wilson GA, Doyle E. Validation of three paediatric pain scores for use by parents. *Anaesthesia* 1996;51:1005–7.
5. Kelly AM, Powell CV, Williams A. Parent visual analogue scale ratings of children's pain do not reliably reflect pain reported by child. *Pediatr Emerg Care* 2002;18:159–62.
6. Cote CJ, Notterman DA, Karl HW, et al. Adverse sedation events in pediatrics: A critical incident analysis of contributing factors. *Pediatrics* 2000;105:804–14.
7. Priestley S, Babl F, Krieser D, et al. Evaluation of the impact of a paediatric procedural sedation credentialing programme on quality of care. *Emerg Med Australas* 2006;18:498–504.
8. Nicol MF. Risk management audit: Are we complying with the national guidelines for sedation by non-anaesthetists? *J Accid Emerg Med* 1999;16:120–2.
9. Hoffman GM, Nowakowski R, Troshynski TJ, et al. Risk reduction in pediatric procedural sedation by application of an American Academy of Pediatrics/American Society of Anesthesiologists Process Model. *Pediatrics* 2002;109:236–43.
10. Schneeweiss S, Ratnapalan S. Impact of a multifaceted pediatric sedation course: self-directed learning versus a formal continuing medical education course to improve knowledge of sedation guidelines. *Can J Emerg Med Care* 2007;9:93–100.
11. Shavit I, Steiner IP, Idelman S, et al. Comparison of adverse events during procedural sedation between specially trained pediatric residents and pediatric emergency physicians in Israel. *Acad Emerg Med* 2008;15:617–22.
12. Ratnapalan S, Schneeweiss S. Guidelines to practice: the process of planning and implementing a pediatric sedation program. *Pediatr Emerg Care* 2007;23:262–4.
13. Babl F, Priestley S, Kreiser D, et al. Development and implementation of an education and credentialing programme to provide safe paediatric procedural sedation in emergency departments. *Emerg Med Australas* 2006;18.
14. Shavit I, Keidan I, Hoffmann Y, et al. Enhancing patient safety during paediatric sedation: The impact of

15. Borland M, Esson A, Babl F, Krieser D. Procedural sedation in children in the emergency department: A PREDICT study. *Emerg Med Australas* 2009;21:71–9.
16. Everitt I, Younge P, Barnett P. Paediatric sedation in EDs: What is our practice? *Emerg Med Australas* 2002;14:62–6.
17. Olsson GL, Hallen B. Laryngospasm during anaesthesia - a computer-aided incidence study in 136,929 patients. *Acta Anaesthesiol Scand* 1984;28:567–75.
18. American Academy of Pediatrics, American Academy of Pediatric Dentistry, Cote CJ, Wilson S, the Workgroup on Sedation. Guidelines for monitoring and management of pediatric patients during and after sedation for diagnostic and therapeutic procedures: an update. *Pediatrics* 2006;118:2587–602.
19. American Society of Anesthesiologists Task Force on Sedation and Analgesia by Non-Anesthesiologists. Practice guidelines for sedation and analgesia by non-anesthesiologists. *Anesthesiology* 2002;96:1004–17.
20. Green SM, Krauss B. Pulmonary aspiration risk during ED procedural sedation – An examination of the role of fasting and sedation depth. *Acad Emerg Med* 2002;9:35–42.
21. Agrawal D, Manzi SF, Gupta R, Krauss B. Preprocedural fasting state and adverse events in children undergoing procedural sedation and analgesia in a pediatric emergency department. *Ann Emerg Med* 2003;42:636–46.
22. Roback MG, Bajaj L, Wathen JE, Bothner J. Preprocedural fasting and adverse events in procedural sedation and analgesia in a pediatric emergency department: Are they related? *Ann Emerg Med* 2004;44:454–9.
23. Green SM, Roback MG, Miner JR, et al. Fasting and emergency department procedural sedation and analgesia: a consensus-based clinical practice advisory. *Ann Emerg Med* 2007;49:454–61.
24. American Society of Anaesthesiologists. *Manual for Anaesthesia Department Organization and Management.* 2001.
25. Australian and New Zealand College of Anaesthetists Policy Statement 9 (Review). *Guidelines on Sedation and/or Analgesia for Diagnostic and Interventional Medical or Surgical Procedures.* 2008. http://www.anzca.edu.au/resources/professional-documents/pdf/PS9-2010.pdf [accessed 08.03.11].
26. Mace SE, Brown LA, Francis L, et al. Clinical policy: critical issues in the sedation of pediatric patients in the emergency department. *Ann Emerg Med* 2008;51:378–99.
27. Steven A, Godwin MD, David A, et al. Clinical policy: Procedural sedation and analgesia in the emergency department. *Ann Emerg Med* 2005;45:177–96.
28. Langhan ML, Chen L. Current utilization of continuous end-tidal carbon dioxide monitoring in pediatric emergency departments. *Pediatr Emerg Care* 2008;24:211–3.
29. Green SM. Research Advances in Procedural Sedation and Analgesia. *Ann Emerg Med* 2007;49:31–6.
30. Burton JH, Harrah JD, Germann CA, et al. Does end-tidal carbon dioxide monitoring detects respiratory events prior to current sedation monitoring practices? *Acad Emerg Med* 2006;13:500–504.
31. Anderson JL, Junkins E, Pribble C, Guenther E. Capnography and depth of sedation during propofol sedation in children. *Ann Emerg Med* 2007;49:9–13.
32. Krauss B, Hess DR. Capnography for procedural sedation in the emergency department. *Ann Emerg Med* 2007;50:172–81.
33. Miner J, Heegaard W, Plummer D. End–tidal carbon dioxide monitoring during procedural sedation. *Acad Emerg Med* 2002;9:275–80.
34. Deitch K, Chudnofsky CR, Dominici P. The utility of supplemental oxygen during emergency department procedural sedation and analgesia with midazolam and fentanyl: a randomized, controlled trial. *Ann Emerg Med* 2007;49:1–9.
35. Deitch K, Chudnofsky CR, Dominici P. The utility of supplemental oxygen during emergency department procedural sedation with propofol: a randomized, controlled trial. *Ann Emerg Med* 2008;52:1–8.

simulation-based training of non-anaesthesiologists. *Arch Pediatr Adolesc Med* 2007;161:740–3.

36. Gill M, Green SM, Krauss B. A study of the bispectral index monitor during procedural sedation and analgesia in the emergency department. *Ann Emerg Med* 2003;**41**:234–41.

37. Agrawal D, Feldman HA, Krauss B, Waltzman ML. Bispectral index monitoring quantifies depth of sedation during emergency department procedural sedation and analgesia in children. *Ann Emerg Med* 2004;**43**:247–55.

38. Fatovich DM, Gope M, Paech MJ. A pilot trial of BIS monitoring for procedural sedation in the emergency department. *Emerg Med Australas* 2004;**16**:103–7.

39. Dominguez TE, Helfaer MA. Review of bispectral index monitoring in the emergency department and pediatric intensive care unit. *Pediatr Emerg Care* 2006;**22**:815–21.

40. Krauss B, Green SM. Primary care: Sedation and analgesia for procedures in children. *N Engl J Med* 2000;**342**:938–45.

41. Yaster M, Nichols DG, Deshpande JK, et al. Midazolam-fentanyl intravenous sedation: Case report of respiratory arrest. *Pediatrics* 1990;**86**:463–7.

42. Jastak JT, Pallasch T. Death after chloral hydrate sedation: Report of case. *J Am Dent Assoc* 1988;**116**:345–8.

43. Cravero JP, Blike GT, Beach M, et al. Incidence and nature of adverse events during paediatric sedation/anesthesia for procedures outside the operating room: Report From the Paediatric Sedation Research Consortium. *Pediatrics* 2006;**118**:1087–96.

44. Cravero JP, Beach M, Blike GT, et al. Incidence and nature of adverse events during paediatric sedation/anesthesia with propofol for procedures outside the operating room: A Report From the Paediatric Sedation Research Consortium. *Anesth Analg* 2009;**108**:795–804.

45. Green SM, Roback MG, Krauss B, et al. Predictors of airway and respiratory adverse events with ketamine sedation in the emergency department: an individual-patient data meta-analysis of 8282 children. *Ann Emerg Med* 2009;**54**:158–68.

46. Bhatt M, Kennedy RM, Osmond MH, et al. Consensus-based recommendations for standardizing terminology and reporting adverse events for emergency department procedural sedation and analgesia in children. *Ann Emerg Med* 2009;**53**:426–35.

47. Green SM, Yealy DM. Procedural sedation goes Utstein: the Quebec guidelines. *Ann Emerg Med* 2009;**53**:436–68.

48. Green SM, Roback MG, Krauss B, et al. Predictors of emesis and recovery agitation with emergency department ketamine sedation: an individual-patient data meta-analysis of 8,282 children. *Ann Emerg Med* 2009;**54**:171–80.

49. Uman LS, Christine T, Chambers P, et al. Systematic review of randomized controlled trials examining psychological interventions for needle related procedural pain and distress in children and adolescents: An Abbreviated Cochrane Review. *J Pediatr Psychol* 2008;**33**:842–54.

50. Sinha M, Christopher NC, Fenn R, Reeves L. Evaluation of nonpharmacologic methods of pain and anxiety management for laceration repair in the pediatric emergency department. *Pediatrics* 2006;**117**:1162–8.

51. Charney RL, Yan Y, Schootman M, et al. Oxycodone versus codeine for children with suspected forearm fracture: a randomized controlled trial. *Pediatr Emerg Care* 2008;**9**:595–600.

52. Stevens B, Yamada J, Ohlsson A. Sucrose for analgesia in newborn infants undergoing painful procedures. *Cochrane Database Syst Rev* 4:CD001069.

53. Le Frak L, Knoerlein N, Duncan J, et al. Sucrose analgesia: Identifying potentially better practices. *Paediatrician* 2006;**118**:197–202.

54. Carbajal R, Verapen S, Coudere S. Analgesic effect of breast feeding In term neonates: randomised controlled trial. *Br Med J* 2003;**326**:13.

55. Cole J, Shepherd M, Young P. Intranasal fentanyl in 1-3-year-olds: a prospective study of the effectiveness of intranasal fentanyl as acute analgesia. *Emerg Med Australas* 2009;**21**:395–400.

56. Borland M, Jacobs I, King B, O'Brien D. A randomized controlled trial comparing intranasal fentanyl to intravenous morphine for managing acute pain in children in the emergency department. *Ann Emerg Med* 2007;**49**:335–40.

57. Borland ML, Bergesio R, Pascoe EM, et al. Intranasal fentanyl is an equivalent analgesic to oral morphine in paediatric burns patients for dressing changes: a randomised double blind crossover study. *Burns* 2005;**31**:831–7.

58. Borland ML, Jacobs I, Geelhoed G. Intranasal fentanyl reduces acute pain in children in the emergency department: a safety and efficacy study. *Emerg Med Australas* 2002;**14**:275–80.

59. Kanagasundaram SA, Lane LJ, Cavalletto BP, et al. Efficacy and safety of nitrous oxide in alleviating pain and anxiety during painful procedures. *Arch Dis Child* 2001;**84**:492–5.

60. Gall O, Annequin D, Benoit G, et al. Adverse events of premixed nitrous oxide and oxygen for procedural sedation in children. *Lancet* 2001;**358**:1514–5.

61. Babl FE, Oakley E, Seaman C, et al. High-concentration nitrous oxide for procedural sedation in children: adverse events and depth of sedation. *Pediatrics* 2008;**121**:528–32.

62. Babl FE, Oakley E, Puspitadewi A, et al. Limited analgesic efficacy of nitrous oxide for painful procedures in children. *Emerg Med J* 2008;**25**:717–21.

63. Langston WT, Wathen JE, Roback MG, Bajaj L. Effect of ondansetron on the incidence of vomiting associated with ketamine sedation in children: a double-blind randomized placebo-controlled trial. *Ann Emerg Med* 2008;**52**:30–4.

64. Mace SE, Barata IA, Cravero JP, et al. Evidence-based approach to pharmacologic agents used in pediatric sedation and analgesia in the emergency department. *Ann Emerg Med* 2004;**44**(342):377.

65. Green SM, Krauss B. Clinical practice guideline for emergency department ketamine dissociative sedation in children. *Ann Emerg Med* 2004;**44**:460–71.

66. Grindley J, Babl FE. Review article: Efficacy and safety of methoxyflurane analgesia in the emergency department and prehospital setting. *Emerg Med Australas* 2009;**2**:4–11.

67. Migita RT, Klein EJ, Garrison MM. Sedation and analgesia for pediatric fracture reduction in the emergency department: a systematic review. *Arch Pediatr Adolesc Med* 2006;**160**:46–51.

68. Bell A, Treston G, Cardwell R, et al. Optimization of propofol dose shortens procedural sedation time, prevents resedation and removes the requirement for post-procedure physiologic monitoring. *Emerg Med Australas* 2007;**19**:411–7.

69. Burton JH, Miner JR, Shipley TD, et al. Propofol for emergency department procedural sedation and analgesia: a tale of three centers. *Acad Emerg Med* 2006;**13**:24–30.

70. Green SM. Propofol in emergency medicine: further evidence of safety. *Emerg Med Australas* 2007;**19**:389–93.

71. Patel DK, Keeling PA, Newman GB, Radford P. Induction dose of propofol in children. *Anaesthesia* 2007;**43**:949–52.

72. Hohl CM, Mohsen S, Nosyk B, et al. Safety and clinical effectiveness of midazolam versus propofol for procedural sedation in the emergency department: a systematic review. *Acad Emerg Med* 2008;**15**:1–8.

73. Bell A, Treston G, McNabb C, et al. Profiling adverse respiratory events and vomiting when using propofol for emergency department procedural sedation. *Emerg Med Australas* 2007;**19**:405–10.

74. Miner JR, Burton JH. Clinical practice advisory: Emergency department sedation with propofol. *Ann Emerg Med* 2007;**50**:182–7.

75. Willman EV, Andolfatto G. A prospective evaluation of 'kefofol (ketamine/propofol combination) for procedural sedation & analgesia in the emergency department. *Ann Emerg Med* 2007;**49**:23–30.

76. Messenger DW, Murray HE, Dungey PE, et al. Subdissociative-dose ketamine versus fentanyl for analgesia during propofol procedural sedation: a randomized clinical trial. *Acad Emerg Med* 2008;**16**:877–886.

77. Arora S. Combining ketamine and propofol ("Ketofol") for emergency department procedural sedation and analgesia: a review. *West J Emerg Med* 2008;**9**:20–23.

78. Priestley SJ, Kelly AM, Chow L, et al. Application of topical local anesthetic at triage reduces treatment time for children with laceration: A randomized controlled trial. *Ann Emerg Med* 2003;**42**:34–40.

79. Barnett P. Alternatives to sedation for painful procedures. *Pediatr Emerg Care* 2009;**25**:415–9.

80. Lander JA, Welman BJ, So SS. EMLA and amethocaine for reduction of children's pain associated with needle insertion. *Cochrane Database Syst Rev* 2006; Art. No.: CD004236. DOI:10.1002/14651858.CD004236.pub2.

81. Dart C. Comparison of lignocaine 1% injection and adrenaline-cocaine gel for local anaesthesia in repair of lacerations. *Emerg Med Australas* 1998;**10**:38–44.

82. Schilling CG, Bank DE, Borchert BA, et al. Tetracaine, epinephrine (adrenalin), and cocaine (TAC) versus lidocaine, epinephrine and tetracaine (LET) for anesthesia of laceration in children. *Ann Emerg Med* 1995;**2**(5):203–8.

83. Eidelman A, Weiss JM, Enu IK, et al. Comparative efficacy and costs of various topical anaesthetics for repair of dermal lacerations: a systematic review of randomized, controlled trials. *J Clin Anesth* 2005;**17**:106–16.

84. Barnett P. Cocaine toxicity following dermal application of adrenaline-cocaine preparation. *Pediatr Emerg Care* 1998;**14**:280–1.

85. Daya MR, Burton BT, Schleiss MR, et al. Recurrent seizures following mucosal application of TAC. *Ann Emerg Med* 1988;**17**:646–8.

86. Ernst AA, Marvez E, Nick TG, et al. Lidocaine adrenaline tetracaine gel versus tetracaine adrenaline cocaine gel for topical anesthesia in linear scalp and facial laceration in children aged 5 to 17 years. *Pediatrics* 1995;**95**:255–8.

87. Mader TJ, Playe SJ, Garb JL. Reducing the pain of local anesthetic infiltration: Warming and buffering have a synergistic effect. *Ann Emerg Med* 1994;**23**:550–4.

88. Bartfield JM, Gennis P, Barbera J, et al. Buffered versus plain lidocaine as a local anesthetic for simple laceration repair. *Ann Emerg Med* 1990;**19**:1387–90.

89. Scarfone RJ. Pain of local anesthetics: Rate of administration and buffering. *Ann Emerg Med* 1998;**31**:36–40.

90. Kelly AM, Cohen M, Richards D. Minimizing the pain of local infiltration anesthesia for wounds by injection into the wound edges. *J Emerg Med* 1994;**12**:593–5.

91. Davies RJ. Buffering the pain of local anaesthetics: A systematic review. *Emerg Med Australas* 2003;**15**:81–8.

92. Peutrell JM, Mather SJ. *Regional Anaesthesia in Babies & Children.* Oxford: Oxford University Press; 1997.

93. Drendel AL, Gorelick MH, Weisman SJ, et al. A randomized clinical trial of ibuprofen versus acetaminophen with codeine for acute pediatric arm fracture pain. *Ann Emerg Med* 2009;**54**:553–60.

94. Babl FE, Goldfinch C, Mandrawa C, et al. Does nebulized lidocaine reduce the pain and distress of nasogastric tube insertion in young children? A randomized, double-blind, placebo-controlled trial. *Pediatrics* 2009;**123**:1548–55.

Further reading

Cote CJ, Notterman DA, Karl HW, et al. Adverse sedation events in pediatrics: A critical incident analysis of contributing factors. *Paediatrics* 2000;**105**:804–14.

Green SM. Research advances in procedural sedation and analgesia. *Ann Emerg Med* 2007;**49**:31–6.

Green SM, Krauss B. Pulmonary aspiration risk during ED procedural sedation – An examination of the role of fasting and sedation depth. *Acad Emerg Med* 2002;**9**:35–42.

Mace SE, Brown LA, Francis L, et al. Clinical policy: Critical issues in the sedation of pediatric patients in the emergency department. *Ann Emerg Med* 2008;**51**:378–99.

Paediatrics & Child Health Division, The Royal Australasian College of Physicians. Guideline Statement: Management of procedure-related pain in children and adolescents. *J Paediatr Child Health* 2006;**42**:S1–S29.

POISONING

Section editor **Gary Browne**

21.1   General approach to poisoning

Naren Gunja

ESSENTIALS

1 Poisoning in children is usually accidental, particularly in the under-6 age group. Deliberate self poisoning may become apparent as they mature into teenage years.

2 Poisoning in most children runs an uneventful course and emergency department (ED) observation is often the only management needed.

3 The potential for non-accidental poisoning (either deliberate or due to neglect) should be considered, particularly in children under the age of 1 year. Where non-accidental poisoning is suspected, the child should be referred to the relevant child protection authorities.

4 A focused history and examination should lead to a risk assessment on the likely outcome, and worst-case scenario.

5 Advice regarding management of poisoned children can be sought from Australasian Poisons Information Centres (Australia: 13 11 26; New Zealand: 0800 764 766).

6 Poisoning in children manifests clinically in a similar manner to adults. The management of poisoning in children is also similar.

7 Gastrointestinal decontamination is not necessary in the majority of cases.

8 Parents and carers should be advised to keep medicines and chemicals away from the reach of children – medicines should be stored in locked containers or cupboards at a height of at least 1.5 metres.

Introduction and epidemiology

In 2009, the NSW Poisons Information Centre received in excess of 50 000 calls from around Australia regarding paediatric exposures to pharmaceuticals, chemicals, plants and animals. There is a bimodal distribution in the frequency of exposures, with the larger peak occurring in the toddler age group (ages 1–3 years) and a much smaller peak in the mid to late teens. The latter peak relates to deliberate self-poisoning in adolescents. Over eighty percent of poisons centre calls relating to childhood exposures are advised to stay at home as no acute management is necessary. Pharmaceuticals are by far the commonest exposure in children as per American Poison Control Center data. The top ten unintentional exposures in children (under the age of 18 years) reported to Australian Poisons Information Centres are listed in Table 21.1.1. It is important to note that paracetamol is present in many preparations as well as in combination products (e.g. with codeine, pseudoephedrine, doxylamine, dextromethorphan).

Diagnosis

As opposed to overdose in the adult population, exposures in children are nearly always accidental or unintentional. The circumstances around the exposure or ingestion are often unknown or difficult to elucidate. Parents and carers are usually uncertain about time of exposure or dosage of drug ingested. As such, the clear history required to make an accurate risk assessment is difficult or sometimes impossible. Regardless of whether the entire history and circumstances surrounding the exposure are available, it is prudent to plan for a 'worst-case scenario', assuming maximal exposure.

Important elements of the focused history include:

- age and gender of child;
- agent involved – drug, chemical or plant;
- approximate time of exposure;
- dose ingested, including maximum possible ingestion;
- circumstances around exposure;
- symptoms, in particular vomiting;
- first aid and pre-hospital management.

Deliberate self-poisoning in adolescents warrants further enquiry into previous ingestions, pre-existing psychiatric illness and management, drug use and social circumstances. In cases of unknown drug exposure, it is important to explore the availability of

Table 21.1.1 Top 10 exposures in children

No.	Agent
1	Paracetamol
2	Detergents
3	Household cleaning agents
4	Dessicants (e.g. silica gel)
5	Ibuprofen
6	Cough & cold preparations
7	Rodenticides
8	Light sticks/glow toys
9	Zinc-containing barrier creams
10	Bleach (containing hypochlorite)

Table 21.1.2 Common toxidromes

Toxidrome	Agents	Clinical features
Sympathomimetic	Amphetamines Pseudoephedrine Caffeine	Tachycardia Hypertension Mydriasis Sweating Agitation Delirium Fever
Anticholinergic	Atropine Hyoscine Antihistamines Plants Mushrooms	Tachycardia Mydriasis Loss of visual accommodation Flushed skin Dry skin/mouth/eyes Fever Delirium
Opiate	Opiates Tramadol Clonidine	Sedation Respiratory depression Hypotension Miosis
Cholinergic	Organophosphates Carbamates	Delirium Coma Seizures Excess secretions (DUMBELS) Weakness Fasciculations
Serotonergic	SSRIs Cyclic antidepressants Opiates Tramadol Lithium MDMA (ecstasy)	Delirium/agitation Hyperreflexia Hypertonia Tremor Clonus Diaphoresis Fever

SSRI, selective serotonin reuptake inhibitor.

pharmaceuticals and/or chemicals to which the child may have had access. Plant and mushroom ingestion is common in children and needs to be considered in the acutely unwell child who has been outdoors.

Non-accidental (or deliberate) poisoning of a child requires mandatory reporting to child protection authorities in all jurisdictions within Australia. The index of suspicion is higher in children under the age of 1 year, or where the circumstances of the exposure do not fit the capabilities of the child in question. Rare cases of Munchausen's syndrome by proxy are also reported in the literature, involving deliberate poisoning of children by their parent/carer.

Physical examination of the potentially poisoned child is usually unremarkable, particularly in asymptomatic children or in the early stage of ED presentation. However, in children presenting with symptoms or patients with altered level of consciousness, a thorough physical examination is vital. Key elements of the toxicological examination include:

- vital signs: heart rate, blood pressure, temperature, respiratory rate, oxygen saturation;
- odour suggesting intoxication or poisoning;
- airway patency and adequacy of ventilation;
- cardiovascular status and end-organ perfusion;
- level of consciousness or altered mental status, presence of delirium or psychosis (including blood glucose level);

- neurological signs: abnormal tone, reflexes, clonus, seizures;
- external signs of trauma, bruising, bite marks;
- saliva or vomitus, pill fragments.

Children may also present with a cluster of symptoms and signs suggestive of poisoning, i.e. a toxidrome. Although most cases do not manifest the full spectrum of signs and symptoms, pattern recognition amongst clinicians may provide a clue to diagnosis. Toxidromes and corresponding causative agents commonly seen in children are listed in Table 21.1.2.

Risk assessment

Following the history and examination of the potentially poisoned child, the clinician must undertake a risk assessment of the likely exposure and probable course of toxicity, if any. This requires knowledge of the toxicodynamics and kinetics of the agents, an understanding of potential complications and experience with previous similar cases. At this stage, it is prudent to obtain advice

from expert clinicians in paediatric toxicology, such as through the Australasian Poisons Information Centres (Australia: 13 11 26; New Zealand: 0800 764 766). These centres are available 24/7 and provide expert advice on the assessment and management of poisoning in children. The majority of paediatric exposures do not present to hospital, and even those that do, require observation only. However, there are a few highly toxic pharmaceuticals and chemicals that, even in small doses, can cause severe toxicity. Patients exposed to these select few agents may require close monitoring and potentially aggressive resuscitation – these are discussed in Chapter 21.2.

Investigations

The vast majority of children exposed to a substance require no investigations at all. There are some instances where a specific agent is ingested and a specific investigation may aid diagnosis and/or management. Screening tests in the poisoned child should be performed based on the risk assessment.

Table 21.1.3 Investigation of the poisoned child

Investigation	Potential toxicological indication(s)
Screening tests	
Blood glucose level	Altered mental status Deliberate self-poisoning All exposures to insulin or oral hypoglycaemic agents
β-HCG pregnancy test	Female patients of childbearing age presenting with overdose
Paracetamol level	Deliberate self-poisoning (of any substance)
Urine drug screen	Known or suspected exposure to illicit substances/drugs of abuse Altered mental status (delirium, psychosis, coma)

ECG	Heart rate outside normal parameters for age
	Haemodynamic instability or shock
	Poisoning with specific agents:
	    Cardiovascular drugs
	    Sedatives
	    Neuroleptics
	    Antidepressants
	    Amphetamines and sympathomimetics
	    Clonidine and baclofen
	    Metals (e.g. potassium, lithium, iron)

Blood gas measurement	Known or suspected acid–base abnormality
	Poisoning with specific agents:
	    Salicylates
	    Tricyclic antidepressants
	    Ethanol
	    Toxic alcohols
	    Iron
	    Isoniazid
	    Carbon monoxide
	    Cyanide
	    Metformin
	    Methaemoglobinaemia

Specific investigations	
Chest/abdominal X-ray	Radio-opaque tablet or foreign body ingestion Known or suspected aspiration pneumonitis Tube (e.g. endotracheal, gastric) placement
Liver function tests	Known or suspected paracetamol poisoning Suspected hepatotoxicity from any systemic poisoning

Coagulation panel	Snake bite
	Suspected coagulopathy from poisoning/envenoming
	Poisoning with specific agents:
	    Paracetamol
	    Anticoagulants (e.g. warfarin, rodenticides)
	    Salicylates
	    Iron and heavy metals

Paracetamol level	In all cases of paracetamol ingestion (incl. deliberate self-poisoning, accidental, supratherapeutic, chronic)

Specific drug levels	Known or suspected poisoning from:
	    Anticonvulsants (carbamazepine, valproic acid, phenytoin)
	    Aspirin/salicylates
	    Digoxin
	    Metals (potassium, lithium, iron)
	    Ethanol
	    Toxic alcohols (ethylene glycol, methanol)
	    Methotrexate
	    Theophylline
	    Phenobarbital

Notes:
Salicylate levels should not be routinely ordered as their screening value is negligible
Tricyclic antidepressant levels are not useful in the management of poisoning from these agents, nor are they a useful screening test
Rarely performed investigations for specific toxins include cholinesterase levels, carboxyhaemoglobin and methaemoglobin amongst others.
Computerised tomography of brain is not routinely required in the comatose child with a reliable history of poisoning; it may be warranted when the history is unclear, or there is suspicion of trauma or non-accidental injury.
HCG, human chorionic gonadotrophin.

Specific investigations, which may be invasive or time-consuming to return a result, should be discussed with an expert toxicologist prior to embarking on these tests. Table 21.1.3 summarises the potential indications for screening and specific investigations in paediatric poisoning. Baseline blood investigations (blood counts, electrolytes, renal function test) should be performed if any of the screening or specific laboratory investigations are ordered.

Resuscitation

In the severely poisoned child, timely and effective resuscitation is the key to better outcomes. Thankfully, this scenario is uncommon in Australasia. Resuscitation of the poisoned child should follow standard advanced paediatric guidelines with regards to promoting haemodynamic stability, preventing secondary brain injury and best practice supportive care.

The majority of cases require no more than oxygen therapy and intravenous fluid boluses. In the presence of coma or cardiovascular collapse, resuscitation involves airway protection and ventilatory support as well as the potential use of agent-specific antidotes. In cases where early decontamination is required, such as exposure or ingestion of chemicals, decontamination should occur concurrently with, and not to the detriment of, active resuscitation.

Decontamination

Decontamination involves the removal of a toxic substance to which a child has been exposed in order to minimise its absorption into the systemic circulation. In a child with dermal, eye or mucosal exposure to a substance, decontamination simply involves removal of the toxic substance and irrigation or washing of the contaminated skin, eye or mucosa. Inhalational injury to toxic fumes or gases should include the removal of the patient from the source of exposure and, if necessary, administration of supplemental oxygen. In extreme situations, these patients may need advanced airway and ventilatory support. The use of universal precautions (gown, gloves, goggles) by staff during the process of decontamination is sufficient for the vast majority of poisoning situations, including hydrocarbons and organophosphate insecticides.

Oral exposure to pharmaceuticals, chemicals or plants requires a risk assessment-based approach as to whether decontamination is deemed worthwhile. The need for active oral decontamination in paediatric poisoning is rare. Clinicians are advised to seek expert advice prior to decontamination in children with oral exposures.

Syrup of ipecacuanha (derived from the root of a South American plant) is no longer

Table 21.1.4 Antidotes

Antidote or specific therapy	Dose	Potential indications
Atropine	0.02–0.05 mg kg^{-1}, repeat every 5–10 minutes (use doubling regimen)	Known or suspected cholinergic toxidrome from organophosphate or carbamate pesticide poisoning. Titrate to pupil size, heart rate, blood pressure and drying of chest secretions.
Calcium	Calcium gluconate 10%, 0.6 mL kg^{-1} Calcium chloride 10%, 0.2 mL kg^{-1}	Calcium-channel blockers: Bradycardia or heart block Hypotension
Desferrioxamine	15 mg kg^{-1} hr^{-1}	Iron toxicity: Serum iron >90 μmol L^{-1} Clinically severe systemic toxicity
Digoxin Fab antibodies	Empiric dose: Acute poisoning - 5 vials Chronic poisoning - 1–2 vials	Digoxin toxicity: Life-threatening arrhythmias Clinical signs of severe digitoxicity
Ethanol	PO/NG route preferred Loading dose: 750 mg kg^{-1} Infusion: 80–150 mg kg^{-1} hr^{-1}	Known or suspected poisoning from toxic alcohols (ethylene glycol, methanol): Elevated osmolar gap Metabolic acidosis Maintain blood ethanol at 100 mg dL^{-1}
Flumazenil	0.005–0.01 mg kg^{-1} (max 2 mg)	Benzodiazepine poisoning: Reduced level of consciousness Bradypnoea N.B. Titrate to respiratory rate
Glucagon	0.05–0.1 mg kg^{-1}	β-Blockers Bradycardia Hypotension
Insulin (high dose + dextrose)	Initial dose: 1 unit kg^{-1} Infusion: 1–2 units kg^{-1} hr^{-1}	β-Blockers Calcium channel blockers Bradycardia or heart block Hypotension
N-Acetylcysteine	1st: 150 mg kg^{-1} over 15–30 min, 2nd: 50 mg kg^{-1} over 4 hours, 3rd: 100 mg kg^{-1} over 16 hours	Paracetamol poisoning: Patients at risk of, or with established, hepatotoxicity
Naloxone	Bolus: 0.005-0.01 mg kg^{-1} (max 2 mg); Infusion: 0.01 mg kg^{-1} hr^{-1}	Known or suspected opiate toxidrome. Titrate to respiratory rate
Octreotide	Bolus: 1 mcg kg^{-1} IV or SC Infusion: 0.5 mcg kg^{-1} hr^{-1} IV	Sulfonylurea poisoning with recurrent hypoglycaemia
Physostigmine	0.02 mg kg^{-1} (max 0.5 mg)	Anticholinergic poisoning with delirium
Sodium bicarbonate	1–2 mmol kg^{-1} IV bolus (serum alkalinisation)	Cyclic antidepressants (and other cardiac sodium channel blocking agents): Cardiac arrest Wide-complex tachyarrhythmias Hypotension Seizures
Vitamin K	5–10 mg, PO 1–2 mg, IV or IM	Poisoning from warfarin (or other coumadin anticoagulants) with established, or risk of, coagulopathy

IM, intramuscular; IV, intravenous; PO, per oram; SC, subcutaneous.

recommended in the management of poisoning. The induced emesis does little to prevent drug absorption and potentially can cause a myriad of complications including protracted vomiting, aspiration and oesophageal tears and haemorrhage. Gastric lavage ('stomach pumping'), involving the injection of fluid into the stomach via a tube and aspirating gastric contents, is also a discontinued practice which has little or no role in the management of poisoned children. Whole bowel irrigation involves the administration of a polyethylene glycol solution through the gastrointestinal tract for the purpose of promoting tablet residue in effluent and thus preventing drug absorption. It is reserved for specific ingestions such as sustained-release preparations or metals; expert advice should be sought prior to instituting whole bowel irrigation.

Activated charcoal is a colloidal suspension of charcoal particles able to bind to most pharmaceuticals. Charcoal does not adsorb metals, hydrocarbons, corrosives or alcohols. Although the need for activated charcoal in children is uncommon, it is potentially indicated when a child ingests a highly toxic substance, which is bound by charcoal, and the charcoal can be administered within an hour post-ingestion to an alert child (or in the case of intubated children, via a gastric tube). Clinicians should avoid inserting a gastric tube for the purpose of administering charcoal to a patient with altered level of consciousness. The presence of bowel sounds should always be confirmed prior to the administration of oral charcoal. When indicated, the activated charcoal dose is 1 g kg^{-1}. Expert advice should be sought regarding the use of charcoal in situations beyond an hour post-ingestion or multi-dose activated charcoal (discussed below). Common side effects of charcoal administration include vomiting and the passage of black stools. Aspiration of charcoal can lead to chemical pneumonitis and potentially acute respiratory distress syndrome.

Antidotes

The need for agent-specific antidotes in children is uncommon. Knowledge of antidotes and their potential utility may, in rare cases, be life-saving. Table 21.1.4 lists select antidotes used in paediatric poisoning and their indications. The use of these agents should be discussed with a toxicologist.

Enhanced elimination

Techniques used to promote drug elimination from the body are employed in a limited number of poisonings. These methods include haemodialysis, multidose activated charcoal and alkaline diuresis. Various forms of haemodialysis methods are utilised in paediatric poisoning after insertion of a temporary vascular catheter. Agents that are potentially dialysable include potassium, salicylates, toxic alcohols, theophylline and carbamazepine, amongst others. Multidose activated charcoal is rarely used when promoting charcoal adsorption and elimination of poisons that undergo enterohepatic circulation, such as carbamazepine. Urinary alkalinisation with sodium bicarbonate is indicated in salicylate poisoning to promote the renal excretion of salicylate ions. These techniques are seldom used in childhood poisonings and expert advice should be sought prior to their institution.

Supportive care

Active resuscitation of the severely poisoned child is paramount and should be followed by meticulous attention to supportive care in a high dependency or intensive care environment. Although specific poisoning scenarios are dealt with in the next chapter, the guiding principles of excellent supportive management of the poisoned child are likely to be more crucial.

All children with altered level of consciousness should have close glucose monitoring. Coma from drug overdose should be managed with advanced airway and ventilatory manoeuvres. In general, non-invasive ventilation does not have a role in the poisoned child. Drug-induced seizures from all causes should be treated with parenteral benzodiazepines as the first-line agents of choice. Phenytoin should be avoided as its sodium channel blocking properties may exacerbate the problem.

Cardiovascular collapse and asystole in the poisoned child should be managed as per standard advanced paediatric life support guidelines. Drug-induced arrhythmias may warrant agent-specific strategies, such as antidotes. Wide QRS complex tachyarrhythmias, usually due to sodium channel blocking agent poisoning, should in the first instance be treated with boluses of sodium bicarbonate ($1–2 \text{ mmol kg}^{-1}$).

Close monitoring and maintenance of normothermia, euglycaemia, acid–base balance and electrolyte levels are vital in the severely poisoned child. Other potential complications in this group of patients include rhabdomyolysis (seen in snake bite, prolonged coma), aspiration pneumonitis, and persistent delirium (commonly due to anti-cholinergic drugs or plants).

Consultation and disposition

Poisoning in children, as in adults, is a symptom of an underlying issue, be it psychological, parental neglect or accidental access to harmful substances. The mainstay of management involves observation in the ED. Occasionally the child is exposed to an unusual substance or develops severe toxicity that requires input from clinical toxicologists. Clinicians should seek advice from local experts in the field and/or their local Poisons Information Centre.

The underlying issue or disease process also requires attention, such as mental health assessment or counselling. Children who are overdosed with analgesics or antipyretics may warrant investigation into the cause of pain or fever. In the case of neglect or deliberate poisoning the child is likely to need referral to relevant child protection authorities. All carers involved in accidental poisoning should have counselling with regards to safe storage of medicines and chemicals in the home.

Further reading

Bronstein AC, Spyker DA, Cantilena LR Jr, et al. 2008 Annual report of the American Association of Poison Control Centers' National Poison Data System (NDPS): 26th Annual Report. *Clin Toxicol* 2009;47(10):911–1084.

Including beta-blockers, calcium channel blockers, clonidine, chloroquine, salicylates, phenothiazines, sulfonylureas, opiates and others. *J Emerg Med* series on paediatric exposures of 1–2 pills 2004;**26**.

NSW Poisons Information Centre Annual Report. Westmead, NSW Australia: The Children's Hospital; 2009. www.poisonsinfo.nsw.gov.au.

21.2 Specific poisons

Naren Gunja • Helen Mead • Nicholas Cheng

ESSENTIALS

1 Medically-important paediatric poisoning usually falls into two categories: common ingestions, and rare or dangerous toxins.

2 The Emergency Physician plays a crucial role in forming an appropriate management strategy based on the risk and knowledge of the relevant drug(s)' toxicity.

3 The management of common ingestions is essentially supportive, with the potential utility of a specific antidote. Gastrointestinal decontamination is rarely indicated in these cases.

4 Although most substances are harmless to children in small amounts, a few pharmaceuticals and chemicals are extremely toxic in minute quantities – these substances are potentially lethal in a toddler even if only one to two pills or one to two mouthfuls are ingested.

Common poisons

Paracetamol

Paracetamol is by far the commonest paediatric poisoning presentation to the Emergency Department (ED), but the large majority will have no toxic effects. Absorption from the gastrointestinal (GI) tract is rapid, particularly with the liquid formulation (approx. 30 minutes). Most of the paracetamol is conjugated by the hepatic pathways of sulfation and glucuronidation to inactive metabolites, which are excreted in the urine. Children under the age of 9–12 years have a more active sulfation pathway. Less than 5% is excreted unchanged by the kidney and 5–15% is oxidised by the hepatic cytochrome P450 enzyme system to form a highly reactive intermediate metabolite – NAPQI (*N*-acetyl-*p*-benzoquinone imine), which binds to hepatocytes and leads to oxidative stress and cell death. With therapeutic dosing, NAPQI is metabolized to a non-toxic metabolite with glutathione as a sulfhydryl donor. In overdose, when glutathione reserves are depleted, NAPQI accumulates and causes hepatotoxicity. Acute toxicity from accidental ingestion is extremely rare in children. Paracetamol toxicity is more likely to be problematic in children taking standard doses of paracetamol chronically or in repeated supratherapeutic doses, rather than after a single ingestion.

Children appear less sensitive to the hepatotoxic effects of acute paracetamol overdose than adults. This may be related to metabolic differences, age-related clearance rates and to the increased propensity for children to vomit after acute paracetamol ingestion. The peak serum concentration is reached in <2 hours in the majority of children having a single ingestion of paracetamol elixir.

In the early phase, <24 hours, a child may be totally asymptomatic or complain only of mild abdominal pain, nausea and vomiting. Following a period of latency, hepatoxicity progresses to multiorgan failure. Paracetamol can directly cause renal impairment and coagulopathy with prolonged prothrombin time. The hepatorenal syndrome can also complicate severe hepatotoxicity. Finally, fulminant hepatic failure may occur or the patient may enter the recovery phase with return to normal hepatic function within 4 weeks. Rare consequences of paracetamol toxicity include myocardial necrosis, haemolytic anaemia, methaemoglobinaemia, skin rashes and pancreatitis.

In acute overdose, a serum level should be obtained 4 hours post-ingestion in all children with potential paracetamol ingestions of greater than 200 mg kg^{-1}. Children with acute single ingestions of liquid paracetamol preparations are likely to have reliable post-peak levels earlier than 4 hours post-

ingestion – in these children, a 2-hour level above 1500 μmol L^{-1} suggests risk of hepatotoxicity. Other relevant investigations include electrolytes, renal function, liver function tests and coagulation panel.

The paracetamol nomogram (Fig. 21.2.1), based on adult toxicity profiles, is extrapolated to children and predicts the potential for significant hepatotoxicity. The nomogram is applicable when a paracetamol level is taken between 4 and 16 hours post-acute ingestion. The nomogram cannot be utilised when the time of ingestion is unknown or in the case of staggered or chronic ingestions. Paracetamol treatment guidelines were reviewed by a representative panel of Clinical Toxicologists to the Australasian Poisons Information Centres and published in 2008. A major shift in management was the amalgamation of the high- and low-risk nomogram treatment lines into a single curve for both adults and children. This current line commences at 1000 μmol L^{-1} at 4 hours post-ingestion and has a half-life of 4 hours.

N-acetylcysteine (NAC), a glutathione precursor, is the antidote of choice in paracetamol poisoning. NAC is indicated in the setting of acute paracetamol ingestion, where the measured paracetamol level falls above the nomogram treatment line. The full course involves a loading dose of 150 mg kg^{-1} in dextrose over 15–60 minutes, followed by a second infusion of 50 mg kg^{-1} over 4 hours, and finally a 100 mg kg^{-1} infusion over 16 hours. NAC is preferably commenced within 8 hours of ingestion, but has been documented to be effective in adult patients when given up to 48 hours after a serious ingestion, and can even be considered later when hepatic failure is established. Anaphylactoid reactions, including rash, bronchospasm, pruritus, hypotension and tachycardia, occur in up to 15% of cases, and are most common during the second infusion. These reactions are managed similarly to other hypersensitivity reactions; the NAC infusion should be temporarily ceased and recommenced at half the rate.

As children usually ingest the elixir formulation rather than tablets, rapid absorption

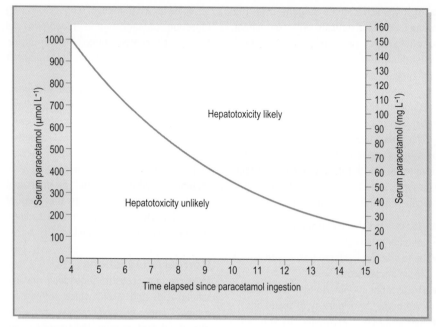

Fig. 21.2.1 Paracetamol nomogram.

precludes the utility of oral activated charcoal. Activated charcoal can be administered for potentially toxic doses of the tablet formulation, if given within 1 hour. Children who present with established hepatic failure must receive prompt resuscitation and stabilisation. NAC is still indicated when hepatotoxicity is established. Coagulopathy and encephalopathy should be managed as from other causes of liver failure. These children are managed in the intensive care and should be assessed for potential liver transplantation.

Chronic over-dosing or repeated supratherapeutic ingestion is a significant problem. The treatment nomogram is not applicable to these situations and cases should be discussed with a toxicologist. Children with paracetamol levels below the nomogram treatment line after acute single ingestions can be cleared from a toxicological point of view. Parents or carers should be educated on correct paracetamol dosing and safe storage. Children with deliberate self-poisoning should be assessed by the mental health team.

NSAIDs

Of the many non-steroidal anti-inflammatory drugs (NSAIDs) available, some obtainable as over-the-counter medicines without prescription, ibuprofen is the most significant NSAID ingested by children. As a group NSAIDs are generally of low toxicity, producing gastrointestinal upset, headache, dizziness, tinnitus, and visual disturbance. Hypotension, tachycardia, and hypothermia and coagulopathy have been reported when NSAIDs were consumed in large amounts. In massive overdose, electrolyte disturbances, metabolic acidosis, central nervous system depression, and respiratory failure can occur.

Asymptomatic children can be discharged at 4 hours post-ingestion. Symptomatic children require hospital admission. Oral fluids should be encouraged and dehydration corrected. Electrolytes, blood sugar level, renal function and acid–base status should be monitored. Activated charcoal may be indicated in massive ingestions that present early. Methods of enhanced elimination are not usually beneficial.

Benzodiazepines

Benzodiazepine overdose is commonly seen in toddlers who ingest 1–2 tablets, or as part of a mixed overdose in adolescents. Benzodiazepines bind predominantly to the γ-aminobutyric acid (GABA) type-A receptor complex in the central nervous system (CNS) and enhance GABA activity to produce sedative, anxiolytic and anticonvulsant activity. The duration of sedation ranges from 4–36 hours, depending on the agent. Flumazenil is a competitive antagonist at benzodiazepine receptors. Drowsiness, slurred speech and ataxia are the most common manifestations. This may progress to coma and hypotension, hypothermia and respiratory depression in more significant ingestions. Death is rare unless other CNS depressants have been co-ingested.

Management is entirely supportive. Hypotension usually responds to fluid administration. GI decontamination is not indicated in pure benzodiazepine poisoning. A blood sugar level should be checked in all children with an altered level of consciousness. Other laboratory investigations are not routinely indicated. Chest radiography is only indicated if aspiration is suspected. A qualitative urine test for benzodiazepines may provide reassurance as to the aetiology of drowsiness in the setting of an unconscious patient without a clear history of ingestion. In some clinical scenarios, flumazenil may avert the need for intubation and mechanical support but its use should be discussed with a toxicologist. Flumazenil should be administered in boluses of 5–10 mcg kg^{-1} and titrated to clinical effect (respiratory rate and effort).

Most children can be discharged after 4–6 hours if vital signs are satisfactory and the child can walk unaided.

Opioids

Opioids are frequently available where family members suffer chronic pain, abuse drugs or are on drug-rehabilitation programmes. Iatrogenic intravenous overdosing of children is commonly a result of 10-fold errors in dose calculation.

Morphine and codeine are natural opium alkaloids. Other opioids are synthetic or semisynthetic analogues. The opioids act on various receptors on the brain, spinal cord and gastrointestinal tract as full or partial agonists or antagonists. Opioids are well absorbed by all routes except skin, are metabolised by the liver and are renally excreted. Some opioids (e.g. pethidine and diphenoxylate) have potent metabolites. Opioids vary in their duration of action and some are available as sustained release preparations (e.g. morphine). Toxicity is enhanced by co-ingestion of other sedative medications, which may be found in some cough remedies or analgesic preparations. Children are especially sensitive to the depressive effects of opioids.

Paediatric overdose of a parent's methadone (long-acting opioid) syrup requires overnight admission for extended observation and monitoring. Antidiarrhoeal preparations contain diphenoxylate (with atropine) and produce delayed onset of symptoms, with numerous paediatric deaths reported. A major metabolite of diphenoxylate is more potent than the parent compound and undergoes enterohepatic circulation. Dextropropoxyphene has a membrane-stabilising effect on cardiac conducting tissue and may induce ventricular arrhythmias and heart block.

The classic features are of nausea and vomiting, drowsiness, pinpoint pupils, respiratory depression, and occasionally bradycardia and hypotension. Respiratory depression may lead to hypoxia and respiratory arrest. The histamine-releasing effects of some opioids may cause urticaria and hypotension.

Management of the opioid toxidrome is essentially supportive, with attention to airway and ventilation. All children with altered level of consciousness should have a blood sugar level checked. Activated charcoal may be considered for massive ingestions or long-acting preparations. Insertion of gastric tubes for charcoal administration is not recommended unless the child is intubated for other indications.

Naloxone, the antidote for opiate toxicity, is a competitive antagonist at opioid receptors. Naloxone (intravenously (IV) 0.01 mg kg^{-1}, maximum 2 mg, as a bolus, repeated every few minutes till appropriate response) may be useful to reverse the neurological and respiratory depression, and should be titrated to respiratory rate and effort. Naloxone's short therapeutic half-life of 30–60 minutes may necessitate a continuous infusion, in order to maintain the reversal and obviate the need for mechanical ventilation, particularly for ingestions of long-acting opiates.

All patients should be observed for a minimum of 6 hours. Methadone, dextropropoxyphene and sustained-release morphine sulfate may cause symptoms persisting for 24–48 hours so prolonged observation is necessary after ingestion of these agents.

Anticholinergics and antihistamines

Anticholinergic (antimuscarinic) poisoning can result from a diverse range of therapeutic substances, plants and natural remedies, many of which can be bought over the counter. Pharmaceuticals with prominent anticholinergic properties include first-generation antihistamines, antipsychotics and tricyclic antidepressants. Some plants, e.g. Jimsonweed, angel's trumpet, and mushrooms contain alkaloids with potent anticholinergic effects.

The anticholinergic toxidrome is caused by competitive inhibition of the muscarinic receptor in the autonomic nervous system. The classic anticholinergic toxidrome is well described by the following rhyme:

- Hot as a hare – hyperthermia from inability to sweat.
- Blind as a bat – dilated pupils with loss of accommodation.
- Dry as a bone – hot, dry skin and mucous membranes with paucity of secretions.
- Red as a beet – erythematous skin.
- Mad as a hatter – central anticholinergic delirium manifest by agitation, confusion, hallucinations (often visual), dystonic movements and seizures.

Other anticholinergic effects include tachycardia, gastrointestinal ileus and urinary retention.

The management of anticholinergic poisoning includes attention to the ABCs with appropriate supportive therapy and monitoring of vital signs and mental state. Symptomatic patients should have IV access, a 12-lead electrocardiogram (ECG) and continuous cardiac monitoring. Benzodiazepines are useful in managing agitation or seizures. Physostigmine is a cholinesterase inhibitor which enters the CNS and is effective at reversing central anticholinergic delirium. Due to concerns regarding adverse cardiac side effects, the use of physostigmine should be discussed with a toxicologist. The initial dose in children is 0.02 mg kg^{-1} (maximum 0.5 mg) by slow IV push; doses may be repeated every 15 minutes.

Aggressive cooling measures may be required in severe hyperthermia. Urinary catheterisation is required for patients with urinary retention. Asymptomatic patients may be discharged after 6 hours. Patients with moderate or severe toxicity should be admitted to an intensive-care facility.

Antihistamine poisoning in children is of concern only for first-generation agents (e.g. promethazine), which have significant anticholinergic effects. Children should be observed for a minimum of 6 hours following ingestion. Management is supportive and the anticholinergic effects of antihistamines, while unpleasant, are generally not life threatening.

Hypotension should be treated with intravenous fluids. Convulsions and anticholinergic delirium are best managed with benzodiazepines. Continuous ECG monitoring is advised for symptomatic children and those with persistent tachycardia. Ventricular arrhythmias should be managed with sodium bicarbonate as the drug of choice for QRS prolongation with sodium-channel blocking antihistamines.

Corrosive ingestions

Most serious caustic ingestions involve strong acids and alkalis which account for a high number of presentations to the ED. The initial presentation and treatment are similar to other burns. Domestic bleaches and ammonia products generally cause minor injuries. Serious injuries result most often from the ingestion of drain and oven cleaners (NaOH, KOH). Dishwashing powder residue left in the dispenser of machines is a commonly accessed alkali that may cause serious injury.

The severity of burn depends on the nature, volume, pH and concentration of the agent and the duration of contact. Stomach contents may afford some protection from injury, but pylorospasm, oesophageal reflux and vomiting may exacerbate injury. Liquids may cause a circumferential injury and powders/granules or tablets may cause prolonged contact with a mucosal surface, with potential for linear burns, deep erosion and penetration. Acids cause superficial corrosion and a coagulative necrosis, and the extent of tissue penetration is limited by eschar formation. Alkalis start to burn immediately on contact and cause a liquefaction necrosis of fat and protein, penetrating deeply into tissues. Acids typically injure the stomach while alkalis damage the oropharynx and oesophagus.

Many children will be asymptomatic, especially if low-concentration household products are involved. Pain, drooling, dysphagia, vomiting and abdominal pain and haematemesis may occur. Airway compromise with laryngeal oedema, cough and bronchospasm may be seen after ingestion of high-concentration agents. Endoscopy provides the best guide to prognosis and management. The extent of injury is graded by the depth of ulceration and the presence of necrosis. Typically, after ingestion the mouth or oesophagus is red and ulceration follows within 24 hours. One-third of patients with oral burns have associated oesophageal lesions, whereas 10–15% of patients with oesophageal lesions have no oropharyngeal burns. Asymptomatic patients with no oral burns may have significant oesophageal injuries. Drooling and dysphagia persisting beyond 12–24 hours are reliable predictors for oesophageal scar formation and suggest the need for upper GI endoscopy.

Oesophageal perforation and mediastinitis may be suspected by chest pain, fever, pleural rub, dyspnoea. Abdominal pain, fever, peritonism and ileus may indicate gastric or abdominal oesophageal perforation. These signs may progress to septic shock, multiorgan failure and death. Large acid ingestions may be associated with hypotension, metabolic acidosis, haemolysis, nephrotoxicity and pulmonary oedema.

Late complications are infection, achlorhydria and stricture formation in 1–3%. All patients with full-thickness and 70% with deep ulceration will develop strictures. Eighty percent of all strictures occur within 2 months of ingestion and 99% within 1 year.

The management of caustic ingestions is aimed at limiting the extent of injury and preventing strictures and other complications. Immediate management consists of rinsing the skin with water or drinking water unless respiratory distress is notable or visceral perforation is suspected. Acids and alkalis do not bind to charcoal. Attempts to neutralise the substance are contraindicated, but dilution with water may possibly be helpful for acids and may reduce mucosal contact time in ingestion with particulate alkalis. Early treatment focuses on ensuring an adequate airway, intravenous fluid replacement, monitoring fluid balance, avoiding vomiting and adequate analgesia. Oesophagoscopy in the symptomatic patient guides further management. Patients with deep, especially circumferential burns of the oesophagus should be admitted to an intensive care unit and may require prolonged parenteral feeding and repeated endoscopic stricture dilatations. Early surgical intervention and prophylactic

antibiotics are required if perforation or penetration is suspected clinically, on endoscopy or contrast radiography. Steroids have no proven benefit and may possibly increase the risk of perforation.

Asymptomatic patients should be advised to return if they develop respiratory difficulty, pain or dysphagia. All symptomatic children should be admitted for observation and potential endoscopy.

Ethanol

Ethanol is available in numerous household medicinals, mouthwashes and perfumery products as well as alcoholic drinks. All products marketed in Australia as 'methylated spirits' contain ethanol. Although frequently ingested by children, serious toxicity is uncommon.

Ethanol is well absorbed across gastrointestinal mucosa and respiratory tract, most within 30–60 minutes, and distributes to total body water. Children metabolise alcohol faster than adults. Only very small amounts are excreted unchanged in the urine and the breath. Hypoglycaemia is caused by depressed gluconeogenesis. The potentially fatal dose of alcohol for children is 4 mL kg^{-1} of absolute alcohol (e.g. 10 mL kg^{-1} for a 40% alcohol spirit), about half the dose required for adults. Quite low serum levels (>10 mmol L^{-1}, >0.05% or >500 mg L^{-1}) may produce clinically significant effects in children.

Ethanol acts on the reticular activating system to cause CNS depression. Low concentrations result in alterations of mood and thought processes, whereas higher concentrations affect cerebellar function, causing ataxia and slurred speech. Higher levels still depress all cortical function and brainstem activity, depressing respiratory drive and protective airway reflexes. Respiratory arrest or aspiration is a frequent cause of death. Facial flushing, excessive sweating and vomiting are common.

Management depends on the time elapsed since ingestion. Assess and secure the ABCs and correct electrolyte abnormalities and dehydration. Patients with severe CNS depression are at risk of aspiration and require airway protection. Blood glucose should be monitored. A blood alcohol level may be taken at least 1 hour post-ingestion if symptoms are present, although management is generally determined by

the clinical state. Hypoglycaemia should be corrected with 5 mL kg^{-1} 10% dextrose. Hypotension will usually respond to intravenous fluids and acidosis usually responds to correction of hypovolaemia and hypoglycaemia. Hypothermia should be corrected. Activated charcoal does not bind ethanol but may be considered if co-ingestants are suspected, provided the airway is protected. Gastric lavage is likely to be ineffective due to the rapid absorption from the stomach. Haemodialysis may be indicated in the extremely intoxicated child who is haemodynamically unstable, but this is uncommon. Admit all children who are clinically intoxicated until asymptomatic.

Rare and dangerous poisons

Although most substances are harmless to children in small amounts, a few pharmaceuticals and chemicals are extremely toxic in minute quantities. Table 21.2.1 lists drugs where 'one pill can kill' and chemicals where a sip or mouthful is potentially lethal.

Salicylates

The incidence of acute salicylate poisoning has declined due to improvements in medication packaging, removal of aspirin from oral paediatric formulations and due to paracetamol now being the favoured over-the-counter analgesic. Methylsalicylate and salicylic acid are common in many topical preparations. Oil of Wintergreen containing methylsalicylate can be significantly toxic when ingested. Choline salicylate is a constituent of many teething gels.

Aspirin is rapidly absorbed from the upper gastrointestinal tract, with peak plasma concentrations at 1–3 hours after therapeutic doses. An ingestion of 150–300 mg kg^{-1} may result in mild to moderate toxicity. Ingestions over 500 mg kg^{-1} are potentially lethal. Oil of Wintergreen is 100% methylsalicylate and extremely small amounts may be lethal.

Aspirin is hydrolysed to form salicylic acid (salicylate). In large overdoses, the potential for pharmacobezoar formation in the gut may alter absorption kinetics. In therapeutic doses, salicylate is 85–95% plasma bound, but in overdose, free salicylate concentration rises as plasma protein

Table 21.2.1   Potentially lethal ingestions in small amounts for a toddler

Pharmaceuticals	Chemicals
CCBs (diltiazem & verapamil)	Organophosphate & carbamate pesticides
Chloroquine & hydroxychloroquine	Paraquat
Clonidine	Camphor
Tricyclic antidepressants	Naphthalene
Sulfonylureas	Toxic alcohols
Amphetamines & ecstasy	Essential oils

binding is saturated. As metabolic pathways in the liver become saturated, the kidney becomes the main route of elimination. Clearance is markedly enhanced by an alkaline urinary pH.

Salicylate poisoning leads to the uncoupling of oxidative phosphorylation and anaerobic metabolism. The resulting lactic acidosis is more prominent in young children. Early signs of salicylism include a respiratory alkalosis from centrally driven hyperventilation and tinnitus. With increasing toxicity, confusion, hallucinations and seizures are reported. Metabolic derangements include temperature dysregulation, impaired glucose metabolism and transport as well as electrolyte abnormalities. Mixed picture acid–base derangement is a hallmark of severe salicylate poisoning, with serum pH below 7.3 being a late and ominous sign. Coagulopathy may result from competitive inhibition of synthesis of vitamin-K dependent factors. Non-cardiogenic pulmonary oedema has been reported, but the mechanism is unclear.

Investigations include baseline blood sugar level, electrolyte and renal function, acid–base status, coagulation panel and 6-hour salicylate level. Decontamination with activated charcoal is indicated in early presentations and may be considered in late presentations of enteric-coated preparations. Meticulous monitoring of fluid balance, temperature, glucose and electrolyte levels is recommended. In particular, potassium replacement is often required, along with maintenance of urine output.

Methods of enhancing elimination should be instituted following consultation with a toxicologist. Urinary alkalinisation with intravenous sodium bicarbonate infusion is known to enhance renal excretion of salicylate ions. The target urinary pH is at least 7.5 with maintenance bicarbonate doses ranging from $1–2 \ mmol \ kg^{-1} \ hr^{-1}$. Haemodialysis is indicated in severe toxicity with acidaemia, cardiorespiratory failure, renal impairment or CNS manifestations (coma, seizures). Complications of salicylate poisoning require aggressive supportive management. The development of non-cardiogenic pulmonary oedema often signals the need for invasive ventilation and haemodialysis. Seizures warrant benzodiazepine therapy and correction of any glucose or electrolyte derangement.

Observe all symptomatic children and those with ingestions of greater than $150 \ mg \ kg^{-1}$. Most patients will require admission for 6–12 hours for observation of clinical state and serum salicylate level.

Digoxin

Digoxin is a cardiac glycoside used for management of heart failure and supraventricular arrhythmias. Many plants contain digitalis glycosides (e.g. foxglove, oleander) and poisoning from these plants should be managed in a similar manner to digitoxicity. Acute digoxin poisoning in children is more often seen in the context of toddlers who obtain access to grandparents' medication. Rarely, children with underlying cardiac disease on maintenance digoxin therapy can develop chronic toxicity and therapeutic drug monitoring is crucial. Chronic overdosing or renal impairment can lead to chronic digitoxicity.

Digoxin is well absorbed from the gastrointestinal tract and has a relatively large volume of distribution. Digoxin is predominantly excreted unchanged by the kidney, with an elimination half-life of about 36 hours. Digoxin inhibits the action of the cardiac Na/K ATPase pump and accumulation of sodium and calcium ions leads to intracellular depletion of potassium and hyperkalaemia. The slowing of conduction, as well as increased refractory period, through the AV node, enhanced automaticity of the Purkinje fibres and enhanced vagal tone leads to a multitude of arrhythmias including sinus bradycardia, sinoatrial arrest, conduction blocks, ventricular tachycardia and fibrillation.

Early signs of chronic toxicity include nausea, vomiting and diarrhoea. The child is often asymptomatic in acute poisoning, until haemodynamic instability from cardiac toxicity becomes clinically apparent. Patients can deteriorate suddenly and digitoxicity can produce a myriad of both brady- and tachyarrhythmias. Assess ABCs, secure IV access and continuously monitor blood pressure (BP) and ECG. Although digoxin is well bound by activated charcoal, repeated vomiting may reduce its effectiveness. Obtain a serum digoxin concentration and electrolytes. Serum potassium concentration should be monitored every 4 hours. Hyperkalaemia should be corrected to within upper limits of normal with sodium bicarbonate and insulin/dextrose. Calcium is relatively contraindicated due to potential for myocardial destabilisation.

Digoxin Fab antibodies are a specific and highly effective antidote in digoxin poisoning. Intravenous Fab fragments of digoxin-specific antibodies are first-line therapy for patients with cardiac arrhythmias with haemodynamic instability. The dosage is based on total body load, estimated from the serum digoxin concentration or from the ingested dose. Alternatively, a dose estimation can be made on the presumption that one vial of 40 mg will bind 0.6 mg of digoxin. A clinical response is seen in 20–30 minutes, with maximum effect at 2–4 hours. An empiric dose of 5 vials of digoxin Fab may be given IV over 20 minutes in severe life-threatening toxicity. It is important to note that subsequent digoxin levels post-treatment with antibodies are not interpretable and should not be performed.

Acute overdoses should be observed for a minimum of 12 hours or overnight. Symptomatic patients should be monitored in an intensive care unit or coronary care facility. Patients treated with Fab fragments should be monitored for subsequent hypokalaemia and for deterioration of pre-existing cardiac disease.

Calcium-channel blockers

Calcium-channel blockers (CCBs) are widely used in the treatment of hypertension, coronary artery disease and supraventricular tachyarrhythmias.

CCBs are rapidly absorbed from the gastrointestinal tract and have peak plasma concentrations ranging from 30 minutes (nifedipine) to 90 minutes (verapamil), but sustained-release preparations are associated with longer times to peak concentration and prolonged clinical effect. These agents inhibit the entry of calcium into the cells of cardiac and smooth muscle, decreasing the activity of the calcium-dependent actin-myosin ATPase. Dihydropyridines (represented by the prototype agent nifedipine) are more potent at peripheral vascular calcium channels and have little cardiac toxicity. Verapamil and diltiazem are highly toxic drugs where a single large dose tablet can cause profound cardiogenic shock in a toddler. Dihydropyridine CCBs are unlikely to cause hypotension or cardiac conduction abnormalities in small doses.

The features of cardiotoxicity include brady-arrhythmias, such as sinus bradycardia, varying degrees of AV block, and asystole. Myocardial depression may cause congestive failure or cardiogenic shock. Dose-dependent peripheral vasodilatation with hypotension may occur. Other manifestations include nausea and vomiting, lethargy, coma, seizures, hyperglycaemia and lactic acidosis.

Good supportive management is essential. Intravenous access should be secured, and blood glucose and electrolytes measured. ECG and BP should be continuously monitored. Activated charcoal is worth considering in patients that present early with a significant ingestion. Whole bowel irrigation with polyethylene glycol should be considered for large ingestions of sustained-release preparations.

Calcium is the initial antidote for hypotension and bradycardia (bolus: 10% calcium chloride 0.2 mL kg^{-1} or 10% calcium gluconate 0.6 mL kg^{-1}). Atropine is likely to be ineffective. Catecholamine infusions (e.g. adrenaline (epinephrine) commencing at 1 mcg kg^{-1} min^{-1}) may be required. Other inotropes that do not require calcium influx are potentially useful in managing intractable shock from CCBs. These include high-dose insulin (1–2 units kg^{-1} IV bolus; 1–2 units kg^{-1} hr^{-1} infusion) and glucagon (0.05–0.1 mg kg^{-1} IV bolus). Rarely, more extraordinary measures may be necessary such as transvenous pacing, cardiopulmonary bypass or aortic balloon pumps. Prolonged resuscitation and aggressive supportive care may allow the peak toxicity to pass and improve survival.

Symptomatic children should be monitored in an intensive-care setting. Observation for 24 hours is warranted for ingestion of sustained-release formulations.

β-Blockers

β-Blockers have wide clinical use in the treatment of cardiac conditions, hypertension, thyrotoxicosis and prophylaxis for migraine.

β-Blockers are class II antiarrhythmics, which act by competing with catecholamines at β-receptor sites. Different β-blockers have differing cardioselectivity, membrane-stabilising activity, partial agonist activity and lipid solubility. They are well absorbed from small intestine, with peak serum levels within 1–4 hours. The elimination half-life is less than 12 hours. They have a moderate to large volume of distribution. Highly lipid soluble drugs, such as propranolol, cross the blood–brain barrier and thus have more potent CNS effects. Propranolol is also known for its cardiac sodium channel blocking properties, which cause prolongation of the QRS complex.

The major clinical effects are the cardiovascular effects. Bradycardia may be sinus, junctional or ventricular and may progress to cardiac arrest. Hypotension results from bradycardia, myocardial depression and vasodilatation. Deterioration can be sudden and precipitous, particularly with propranolol, which can cause seizures, coma and wide complex arrhythmias. Hypoglycaemia may occur due to impaired gluconeogenesis and glycogenolysis. Bronchospasm is more likely in atopic subjects, and more prominent with non-selective agents.

Good supportive management is essential. Activated charcoal is the decontamination method of choice. Intravenous access should be secured, and blood glucose and electrolytes measured. ECG and BP should be continuously monitored. Cardiovascular effects should be treated with atropine, volume expansion and catecholamines. High-dose insulin enhances heart rate and myocardial contractility independently of β-receptor activation and is currently the preferred inotrope over glucagon. Doses are similar to those above in calcium channel blocker poisoning. Extreme measures such as transvenous pacing and cardiopulmonary bypass may be required in cases of intractable hypotension. Importantly, prolonged resuscitation and aggressive supportive care may allow the peak toxicity to pass and improve survival. Hypoglycaemia should be treated in the usual manner with 2.5–5 mL kg^{-1} 10% dextrose. Seizures may respond to IV dextrose, even if blood glucose is normal. Benzodiazepines are the preferred anticonvulsant. Bronchoconstriction should be treated with inhaled β$_2$-agonists. Symptomatic children should be monitored in an intensive-care setting.

Clonidine

Until recently clonidine was used primarily as an anti-hypertensive agent and accessibility to children was limited. The drug is now widely prescribed in the treatment of attention deficit hyperactivity disorder, conduct disorders, Tourette's syndrome and for narcotic and alcohol withdrawal symptoms. Clonidine overdose is commonly seen in children with behavioural disorders, and their siblings who have access to clonidine.

Clonidine is a central α$_2$-adrenoceptor agonist that acts on brainstem receptors, causing inhibition of sympathetic outflow. Its stimulation of peripheral α$_2$-receptors on vascular smooth muscle may cause transient hypertension, but hypotension usually occurs subsequently. Clonidine also has opiate-like effects which may be mediated through mu receptors. It is rapidly absorbed and distributed, with peak plasma concentrations 60–80 minutes post-ingestion. The elimination half-life is 6–24 hours.

Clinical effects are seen 30–60 minutes after ingestion. Depression of the CNS with lethargy and impaired conscious state is the most frequent manifestation. Miosis and hypothermia may be observed. Symptoms are minimal with ingestions of under 10 mcg kg^{-1}, but cardiovascular compromise with hypotension and bradycardia may occur after ingestion of 10–20 mcg kg^{-1}. Respiratory depression and apnoea may be seen after ingestions of 20 mcg kg^{-1}. There have been no reports of in-hospital paediatric deaths.

Treatment is largely supportive. Activated charcoal is only useful if given under 1 hour post-exposure. Hypotension should be treated with volume expansion and vasopressors. Hypertension is usually transient and, if treatment is required, a short-acting agent such as nitroprusside should be used. Atropine may be useful in the treatment of bradycardia. Naloxone therapy in clonidine poisoning is controversial and unreliable. There may be inconsistent reversal of the neurological, cardiovascular and respiratory effects after administration of naloxone.

Maximal toxicity is expected in the first 6 hours and children who show no symptoms at that stage can be discharged. Children with significant respiratory and cardiovascular compromise may require admission to an intensive-care unit for up to 24 hours.

Tricyclic antidepressants

Despite the declining prescription of tricyclic antidepressants (TCAs), the low therapeutic index and potential for lethal toxicity remain a concerning cause of paediatric morbidity and mortality.

TCAs are rapidly absorbed. TCAs have a high degree of protein binding and a large volume of distribution. Although different TCAs have different pharmacokinetic parameters, the effects in overdose are similar. Dothiepin is associated with the greatest lethality. Minor TCA toxicity is generally manifest by central and peripheral anticholinergic signs and the antiadrenergic effect of vasodilatation. More serious toxicity results from fast sodium-channel blockade in the myocardium, causing a wide variety of atrial and ventricular dysrhythmias, impaired contractility and impaired conduction with ECG changes of prolonged QT interval and widened QRS complexes.

Tricyclic ingestions of <5 mg kg^{-1} result in minimal toxicity and no treatment is required. Ingestions of 5–10 mg kg^{-1} may cause mild anticholinergic symptoms of drowsiness, ataxia, dilated pupils, ileus and urinary retention but life-threatening toxicity is unlikely. Ingestions over 10 mg kg^{-1} may cause life-threatening coma, seizures and cardiac dysrhythmias. There may be acidosis, hypokalaemia and inappropriate antidiuretic hormone secretion. Onset of symptoms is usually within 2 hours and persists for less than 12–24 hours.

The management of TCA poisoning includes attention to the ABCs, good supportive therapy and GI decontamination for potentially serious ingestions. Continuous cardiac monitoring, serial 12-lead ECGs and close observation of vital signs and mental state are required for all ingestions of >5 mg kg^{-1}. Secure IV access. Airway protection should precede administration of charcoal if the patient is less than fully conscious.

Depressed conscious state is the best predictor of serious toxic complications (seizures, ventricular arrhythmias, hypotension and the need for mechanical ventilation) and the ECG limb lead QRS duration of 100 ms or greater is associated with an increased incidence of seizures and cardiotoxicity. Early intubation and hyperventilation to a serum pH of 7.45–7.55 may attenuate or prevent seizures and ventricular dysrhythmias. Intubate and mechanically ventilate all patients with rapidly decreasing conscious state, seizures and ventricular dysrhythmias. Hypotension should be treated with volume replacement and adrenaline (epinephrine) or noradrenaline (norepinephrine) infusion if required.

Sodium bicarbonate is regarded as a specific antidote in the treatment of the cardiovascular effects of TCA toxicity. It competitively overcomes sodium-channel blockade and its effect on serum pH appears to improve sodium-channel function. Ventricular dysrhythmias will usually respond to treatment with sodium bicarbonate (1–2 mEq kg^{-1} IV bolus, repeated till the QRS narrows or serum pH reaches 7.45–7.55). Refractory ventricular arrhythmias should be treated according to standard ACLS protocols avoiding type 1a and 1c antiarrhythmics. Lidocaine is safe. There is no documented evidence to support the use of phenytoin, which may aggravate hypotension and conduction problems due to its effect on fast sodium channels.

Seizures may be averted or attenuated by bicarbonate therapy. Benzodiazepines are the preferred agents to treat seizures but barbiturates may be required to treat refractory seizures. TCAs are not amenable to removal by extracorporeal methods due to their large volume of distribution. Quantitative analysis of TCA levels does not aid management but screening for other drugs should be considered in deliberate self-harm.

Patients who ingest >5 mg kg^{-1} TCA should be admitted for observation for at least 6 hours, but may be discharged at that time if the ECG remains normal and the child is well. TCA ingestions with significant CNS depression, seizures or significant cardiotoxicity should be admitted to an intensive-care facility.

Iron

Iron tablets are commonly available in the homes of toddlers but severe poisoning is uncommon.

The amount of elemental iron varies according to the formulation. Initial toxicity is due to the corrosive effects on the gastrointestinal tract. Iron is absorbed in the ferrous state and after oxidation to the ferric state becomes bound to ferritin. Toxicity occurs when ferritin and transferrin are saturated and serum iron exceeds the total iron-binding capacity (TIBC). High concentrations of intracellular iron cause mitochondrial dysfunction, interfering with mitochondrial processes, causing lactic acidosis and cell death.

Ingestions of less than 20 mg kg^{-1} elemental iron usually remain asymptomatic. Significant symptoms usually only occur in ingestions above 60 mg kg^{-1}. Potentially lethal systemic toxicity may follow ingestions of greater than 100 mg kg^{-1} elemental iron. Serum iron peaks at 4–6 hours. Serum iron levels should be considered in conjunction with the clinical state.

Although four stages of iron poisoning are classically described, distinct phases may not be apparent with severe poisoning. In the initial 6 hours the gastric irritant effects predominate, with vomiting, diarrhoea and haematemesis or melaena. Circulating free iron may damage blood vessels and cause a transudate of fluid and hypotension. There may be a quiescent phase when the patient may appear to be improving, but about 12–24 hours after ingestion the physiological processes of cells are disrupted, leading to metabolic acidosis, gastrointestinal haemorrhage, altered mental state, pulmonary oedema, cardiovascular, hepatic and renal failure. The liver is particularly vulnerable and fulminant hepatic failure may cause hypoglycaemia, coagulopathy and death. At 4–6 weeks there may be stricture formation in the gastrointestinal tract due to scarring.

Symptomatic patients and those with ingestions greater than 60 mg kg^{-1} of elemental iron require laboratory investigations and an abdominal X-ray. Baseline electrolytes, renal function and a 4–6 hour iron level is recommended. Iron does not bind well to activated charcoal. Patients with ingestions potentially in excess of 60 mg kg^{-1} of elemental iron should have IV access and a blood glucose level. IV fluid resuscitation may be required and electrolytes and glucose should be monitored. Whole bowel irrigation with polyethylene glycol at 20 mL kg^{-1} hr^{-1} via a nasogastric tube is reserved for massive ingestions. A venous bicarbonate level should be performed and serum iron concentration is indicated at 4–6 hours after ingestion. The peripheral blood white cell count greater than 15×10 L^{-1} and hyperglycaemia are suggestive of systemic toxicity.

Desferrioxamine (desferoxamine) binds unbound iron in the intravascular and extracellular space and the chelated complex is eliminated in the urine, imparting a pink-brown colour (vin-rose urine). The decision to use chelation therapy should be based on the combination of the patient's clinical condition and serum iron concentration. IV desferrioxamine (15 mg kg^{-1} hr^{-1} to a maximum of 80 mg kg^{-1} per 24 hours) is indicated in patients with hypotension, shock, coma, convulsions or potentially if serum iron concentration is greater than 90 µmol L^{-1}. Desferrioxamine infusion is usually required for 6–12 hours. The endpoints of chelation therapy are clinical improvement and a reduction in free iron levels. Acid–base and electrolyte balance should be maintained and hepatic and renal function monitored. The chelated complex can be removed with haemodialysis should renal function be significantly impaired.

Asymptomatic children with ingestions of under 60 mg kg^{-1} may be observed at home. Symptomatic patients, or those with ingestions greater than 60 mg kg^{-1} of elemental iron, require further evaluation in hospital and an admission of 12–24 hours.

Warfarin and rodenticides

Domestic rodenticides are widely available in almost every household. The majority of products available use superwarfarins, long-acting anticoagulants, as their base (e.g. brodifacoum). A limited number of rodenticides have a combination of short-acting warfarin and long-acting superwarfarin – these pose a management challenge.

Short-acting warfarin ingestion in children is of concern at doses greater than 0.5 mg kg^{-1}. Prolongation of the prothrombin time usually occurs at 12–36 hours. Treatment with vitamin K is dependent on dose ingested, prothrombin time and presence of bleeding.

Acute ingestion of a few pellets of superwarfarin is usually not a problem. Coagulopathy is likely to occur in repeated or chronic ingestions of rodenticides. In these cases, prothrombin time should be measured and, if prolonged, treatment with vitamin K instituted; follow up with serial coagulation tests is usually necessary.

Toxic alcohols

Ethylene glycol is encountered in antifreeze compounds and radiator additives. Methanol is found in model aeroplane fuel and in home brewing concoctions. Toxic alcohols are rapidly absorbed from the GI tract and distribute to total body water.

Methanol is oxidised to formaldehyde by the rate-limiting enzyme alcohol dehydrogenase, and then aldehyde dehydrogenase converts the formaldehyde to formic acid (formate). Approximately 2% of methanol is excreted unchanged by the kidneys and a small amount is excreted via the lungs. The optic nerve is particularly susceptible to the toxic effects of formic acid. Lactate is produced from anaerobic glycolysis as a result of tissue hypoxia and a formate-induced inhibition of mitochondrial respiration. Ingestion of 1.5 mL of 100% methanol in a child weighing 10 kg would produce a potential peak plasma level of 6 mmol L^{-1} (0.02%, 20 mg dL^{-1}), so a single mouthful is potentially lethal. Symptoms of methanol poisoning may be delayed with a 12–24 hour latent period because of the slow metabolism to formate. The most common presentation of intoxication consists of a triad of findings related to the GI tract, eyes and metabolic acidosis. Nausea and vomiting, epigastric abdominal pain, pancreatitis and GI bleeding may occur. Visual disturbance including blurred vision, central scotoma, yellow spots and complete blindness offer an important diagnostic clue.

Ethylene glycol depresses the CNS, but the hepatic metabolites glycoaldehyde, glycolic acid, glyoxylate and oxalate are responsible for toxicity. Formation of glycolic acid and some lactic acid is the primary cause of the delayed metabolic acidosis, which can occur 4–12 hours after ingestion. Oxalate is highly toxic, causing myocardial depression and acute renal tubular acidosis. Calcium oxalate crystals may be noted on examination of the urine. Ethanol has a 100-fold greater affinity for alcohol dehydrogenase than ethylene glycol, hence it is used to prevent metabolism of ethylene glycol into toxic metabolites. The initial symptoms of an acute ethylene glycol poisoning include those of alcohol intoxication with lethargy, slurred speech, nystagmus, ataxia and vomiting. Papilloedema occurs less frequently than with methanol poisoning. An elevated anion osmol gap acidosis may occur. Seizures, myoclonic jerks and tetanic contractions reflect hypocalcaemia. At 12–36 hours post-ingestion, progressive pulmonary oedema and congestive heart failure occur and may be followed by death due to cardiovascular collapse. If the child survives, renal insufficiency may ensue over the next 2–3 days.

Fomepizole and ethanol block alcohol dehydrogenase, which is involved in the metabolism of the parent compounds of methanol and ethylene glycol to their toxic metabolites. These antidotes do not prevent the toxic effects of the acid metabolites and are only useful if an osmolar gap exists. Fomepizole, which is difficult to source in Australasia, is expensive but easier to administer and monitor than IV ethanol, without the complications of profound hypoglycaemia, hepatotoxicity and inebriation that may occur with ethanol infusions.

The target serum ethanol concentration of 20 mmol L^{-1} (100 mg dL^{-1}, 0.1%) will fully inhibit alcohol dehydrogenase. This can be difficult to achieve in children without advanced support of airway and ventilation. Ethanol is preferably administered orally or via gastric tube. The loading dose is 7.5 mL kg^{-1} of 10% ethanol in 5% glucose water over 30 minutes, followed by a maintenance dose of 0.8–1.5 mL kg^{-1} hr^{-1} of 10% ethanol. Serum ethanol and glucose levels should be monitored after the loading dose and frequently thereafter. Haemodialysis enhances elimination and is indicated for renal failure, visual impairment or severe metabolic acidosis. Asymptomatic children should have blood taken for determination of acid–base status, presence of osmolar gap and electrolytes. Admit all children who are clinically intoxicated until asymptomatic.

Essential oils

Essential oils are complex aromatic mixtures of alcohols, esters, aldehydes, ketones and turpenes widely used in perfumery, food flavourings, massage and alternative remedies. Eucalyptus oil is an essential oil commonly implicated in hospitalisations for childhood poisoning. Incidents usually involve vaporiser solutions, eucalyptus oil preparations and other medicinal preparations, which are freely available over the counter. Citronella oil is used as an insect repellent. Oil of turpentine has been largely replaced by white spirit and turpentine substitutes, which are less toxic.

Essential oils are complex mixtures of substances distilled from plant species, including oil of cloves, eucalyptus, citronella, lavender, peppermint, melaleuca (tea tree) and turpentine. The oils probably differ in the degree of toxicity but comparative data are lacking. The irritant effects are manifest by vomiting after ingestion and aspiration causing a chemical pneumonitis.

Essential oils are potentially very toxic. The breath, vomitus, urine and faeces smell strongly of the oil. Skin irritation may occur. Oil of turpentine has been reported to cause gastrointestinal irritation, central nervous system toxicity, hepatic and renal failure and metabolic acidosis. Eucalyptus oil toxicity has been reported to involve all major body systems and death has been reported in an adult after ingestion of 4 mL. CNS depression, seizures and gastrointestinal effects generally occur within 1 hour after ingestion and respiratory complications including respiratory depression, bronchospasm, aspiration pneumonitis and pulmonary oedema have been reported. In a retrospective hospital-based series of 41 paediatric cases of eucalyptus ingestion, 80% remained asymptomatic, eight children had transient symptoms prior to attendance at ED (vomiting in seven patients, respiratory distress in one patient) but only two children remained symptomatic on presentation to ED (one with drowsiness, hypertonia and hyper-reflexia and another with drowsiness and rash). Both children were discharged the following day.

As management is entirely supportive, assess and secure the ABCs. Benefit from oral activated charcoal or gastric lavage is dubious and not routinely recommended. A chest X-ray is indicated only if respiratory symptoms are apparent. Aspiration pneumonia is treated with respiratory support if required. Benzodiazepines are preferred for managing seizures.

With regards to eucalyptus oil, asymptomatic children can be discharged after 2 hours' observation. Patients with impaired conscious state or respiratory distress on presentation should be admitted to an intensive-care unit.

Organophosphates and carbamates

Pesticide poisoning in children is a rare event in Australasia. Organophosphates and carbamates inactivate the enzyme acetylcholinesterase at cholinergic nerve terminals and neuromuscular junctions, resulting in the cholinergic toxidrome. Plasma (butyl) cholinesterase and red blood cell cholinesterase levels are surrogate markers for exposure and toxicity.

The cholinergic toxidrome involves excess secretions from muscarinic overstimulation, neuromuscular dysfunction and paralysis from nicotinic over-stimulation and central effects including delirium, seizures and eventually, coma. The onset, peak and duration of toxicity varies with each organophosphate.

In children, lethargy, coma and hypotonia are common early features of organophosphate toxicity. Excess secretions can be absent in children. Severe cases can progress rapidly to generalised weakness, coma, convulsions and respiratory failure. Organophosphates do not off-gas, unlike nerve agents, and do not cause secondary respiratory contamination of treating staff. They do, however, warrant the use of universal precautions including gown, gloves and goggles. Pesticides are often dissolved in hydrocarbon solvents and these chemicals give the characteristic odour, as well as causing symptoms in clinicians such as headaches and dyspnoea. Staff should be rotated regularly and the patient should be placed in a well ventilated resuscitation area.

Resuscitation and decontamination should be carried out concurrently. Vomitus and secretions should be washed off the skin with soap and water. Contaminated clothing should be removed and disposed into biohazard bins. The main treatment for organophosphate and carbamate poisoning is anticholinergic therapy with atropine. Charcoal decontamination or gastric lavage has not been proven to be effective. Atropine is indicated for the muscarinic symptoms of bradycardia and excess secretions. Bolus doses of atropine (0.05 mg kg^{-1}, max 1–2 mg) should be repeated every 2–3 minutes until the end-points of normal heart rate, blood pressure and drying of secretions are reached. An atropine infusion may be necessary and should be discussed with a toxicologist. Tachycardia and dilated pupils following atropine therapy may indicate atropine toxicity. Oxime therapy in organophosphate poisoning is controversial and unproven. Pralidoxime, a cholinesterase reactivator at the neuromuscular junction, may be effective in re-establishing respiratory muscle and diaphragmatic function in some types of organophosphate poisoning. The loading dose is 25–50 mg kg^{-1} (maximum 2 g) infused IV over 30 minutes, followed by an infusion at 10–20 mg kg^{-1} hr^{-1} for up to 48 hours.

All children with possible or potential organophosphate or carbamate ingestion should be admitted for prolonged observation. Patients who remain asymptomatic in the ED after 12 hours, or overnight, may be discharged home for observation.

Oral hypoglycaemics

Sulfonylurea poisoning is uncommon in children, but even ingestions of a single tablet have led to significant morbidity and mortality, and the onset of symptoms may be delayed and prolonged. Children may access the tablets in the home of diabetic relatives. In Australasia, gliclazide, glipizide and glibenclamide are responsible for the majority of poisonings. Ingestion of the newer sustained release preparations of gliclazide warrant prolonged monitoring of blood glucose levels.

Sulfonylureas induce hypoglycaemia by stimulating endogenous insulin secretion. In contrast, biguanides do not cause hypoglycaemia, but can induce severe lactic acidosis. Children are more susceptible to hypoglycaemia than adults because of their increased metabolic rate and limited ability for gluconeogenesis.

Hypoglycaemic manifestations occur with palpitations, shaking, hunger, sweating, weakness and with increasing neuroglycopenia, confusion, coma and seizures occur. Long-term neurological disability and death may occur.

Following assessment and management of the ABCs, a blood glucose level should be performed immediately and checked hourly. An initial serum insulin level may be helpful in guiding subsequent management. Gastric decontamination with activated charcoal is not routinely warranted. Hypoglycaemia should be treated with dextrose 10% 5 mL kg^{-1} IV bolus. Glucagon is not recommended for sulfonylurea-induced hypoglycaemia.

Octreotide, a long-acting synthetic somatostatin analogue, inhibits secretion of insulin from the pancreas and may be the most appropriate method of stabilising blood glucose levels. Patients with persistent or recurrent hypoglycaemia requiring repeat bolus of dextrose should be given octreotide (1 mcg kg^{-1} IV bolus), followed by an octreotide infusion (250 mcg in 250 mL 5% dextrose at 1 mcg kg^{-1} hr^{-1}, to maximum of 25 mcg hr^{-1}). If octreotide is not available, a dextrose 10% infusion should be commenced at 1–2 mL kg^{-1} hr^{-1}. Hourly blood glucose measurements are required until octreotide and/or dextrose infusions are ceased. Serum insulin levels may have a role in ongoing management.

Asymptomatic children should be observed for at least 8 hours, longer for sustained release preparations. Symptomatic children require intensive monitoring of blood sugar and clinical condition.

House fires

From a toxicological point of view, the main exposures relate to carbon monoxide (CO) and cyanide, derived from combustion products of nitrogen-containing polymers, both natural (wool and silk) and synthetic (polyurethane and polyacrylonitrile), which are used extensively in domestic furnishings. In children, carbon monoxide poisoning is often associated with other injuries, such as burns or smoke inhalation. The affinity of haemoglobin for carbon monoxide is 210-times its affinity for oxygen. Carbon monoxide dissolved in the plasma acts as a direct cellular poison reacting with other

haem proteins, such as mitochondrial cytochromes, to disrupt cellular metabolism.

Although carboxyhaemoglobin (COHb) levels poorly correlate with symptoms or prognosis, patients with up to 20% of haemoglobin affected complain of headaches and nausea. At 20–40%, patients tire and become confused. COHb greater than 40% can result in ataxia, collapse, and coma. Death is preceded by cardiac arrhythmias, cerebral oedema, and severe metabolic acidosis. Standard oxygen saturation monitors are unreliable in the presence of COHb, with saturations of 100% occurring in the presence of significant hypoxia. Accurate oxyhaemoglobin saturation requires measurement with a co-oximeter. Conventional blood gas analysers can also be misleading.

Cyanide binds to ferric iron (Fe^{3+}) in the cytochrome a-a$_3$ complex, inhibiting its action and blocking the final step in oxidative phosphorylation. Aerobic metabolism is halted and carbohydrate metabolism is diverted to the production of lactic acid.

The diagnosis of cyanide poisoning requires a high index of suspicion as clinical signs are limited and made even more difficult with co-existing CO poisoning. Cardinal features are the presence of cyanosis with severe high anion gap metabolic acidosis and elevated lactate. Complications include coma, seizures and myocardial ischaemia. Treatment usually cannot wait until definitive diagnosis is made with cyanohaemoglobin levels.

Management of CO and cyanide poisoning involves high flow oxygen, supportive care and the potential use of cyanide antidotes. Unconscious patients require airway and ventilatory support and may warrant cerebral imaging in the event of trauma. Current evidence suggests that hydroxocobalamin is the most effective cyanide antidote with the fewest side effects.

Psychostimulants

Amphetamines and cocaine are psychomotor stimulants that promote central and peripheral sympathetic outflow. Ecstasy, 3,4-methylenedioxymethamfetamine (MDMA), is an amfetamine derivative and common drug of abuse. It produces typical amfetamine effects, such as locomotor stimulation, euphoria, excitement and stereotyped behaviour. Ecstasy has additional

psychoactive effects that alter perception and mood.

Complications of amphetamine and ecstasy ingestion include coma, convulsions, arrhythmias, malignant hyperthermia, rhabdomyolysis, hypertension, and multiorgan failure. Cocaine also has sodium-channel blocking properties which can induce ventricular tachyarrhythmias. Hyponatraemia can be seen in ecstasy ingestion, leading to intractable seizures.

Patients who are asymptomatic should receive activated charcoal if ingestion has occurred within 1 hour. Blood pressure, temperature, and ECG monitoring should be instituted. Symptomatic patients and those with persistent tachycardia should be admitted to a monitored environment. Asymptomatic children may be discharged after 24 hours.

Patients with signs of cardiac or central nervous system toxicity require admission to the paediatric intensive care unit. Careful monitoring of haematological and biochemical parameters is essential. Hyperthermia may respond to fluid resuscitation and simple cooling measures; however, intractable cases should receive muscle paralysis and be ventilated in an intensive-care setting. Convulsions and agitation should be treated with benzodiazepines; phenytoin and neuroleptics should be avoided. Ventricular tachyarrhythmias are managed with sodium bicarbonate and benzodiazepines.

Further reading

Daly FFS, Fountain JS, Murray L, et al. Guidelines for the management of paracetamol poisoning in Australia and New Zealand – explanation and elaboration. *Med J Aust* 2008;**188**:296–301.

Erickson SJ, Duncan A. Clonidine poisoning - an emerging problem: Epidemiology, clinical features, management and preventative strategies. *J Paediatr Child Health* 1998;**134**:280–2.

Kerns W, Kline J, Ford MD, et al. Beta-blocker and calcium channel blocker toxicity. *Emerg Med Clin N Am* 1994;**12**(2):365–90.

Lifshitz M, Shahak E, Sofer S, et al. Carbamate and organophosphate poisoning in young children. *Pediatr Emerg Care* 1999;**15**:102–3.

Nuutinen M, Uhari M, Karvali T, et al. Consequences of caustic ingestions in children. *Acta Paediatr* 1994;**83**:1200–5.

Quadrani DA, Spiller HA, Widder P. Five-year retrospective evaluation of sulphonylurea ingestion in children. *Clin Toxicol* 1996;**34**:267–70.

Riordan M, Rylance G, Berry K. Poisoning in children 1-5. *Arch Dis Child* 2002;**87**:392–410.

Tibballs J. Clinical effects and management of eucalyptus oil ingestion in infants and young children. *Med J Aus* 1995;**163**:177–80.

Woolf AD, Wenger TL, Smith TW, Lovejoy FH Jr, et al. The use of digoxin-specific Fab fragments for severe digitalis intoxication in children. *N Engl J Med* 1992;**26**:1739–44.

ENVIRONMENTAL

Section editor **Gary Browne**

22.1 Envenomation

Julian White

ESSENTIALS

1 Snakebite is the most important form of envenoming globally, causing significant morbidity and mortality.

2 Envenoming can cause rapid and severe medical problems in children, such as shock, collapse, convulsions, bleeding and respiratory failure due to either neurotoxic paralysis or neuroexcitatory pulmonary oedema.

3 Stabilisation of vital systems takes priority, followed by specific antidote therapy (usually antivenom) when indicated and appropriate fluid management.

4 Not all patients bitten/stung by venomous animals develop major envenoming, so antidote (antivenom) therapy is only appropriate where significant envenoming occurs.

5 In most cases antivenom, if required, should be given IV, but always with adrenaline and resuscitation facilities immediately to hand.

6 Assessment of degree of envenoming is critical in determining the need for antivenom.

7 Observe all patients for long enough to exclude late-developing envenoming; duration of observation varies dependent on the type of venomous animal.

Introduction

Envenoming is a significant global problem, particularly in the rural tropics, but more temperate and urban environments are not immune. Children represent 25% or less of all cases, but because of their lower body mass, are disproportionately represented in cases of severe envenoming. In general, early diagnosis and treatment is required to optimise outcomes, but diagnosis is not always easy and specific treatments frequently unavailable. With estimates as high as several million cases of envenoming worldwide each year, it is not surprising that deaths may exceed 100 000 per year. For most major causes of envenoming, antivenom remains the definitive treatment, when available. Dosage is based on extent of envenoming, not patient size, so there is no paediatric dosage – children receive the same dose as adults.

Snakebite

Introduction

Snakebite is the single most important cause of envenoming. Some experts have estimated more than 2.5 million venomous snakebites per year, with more than 125 000 deaths. Accurate data to confirm such estimates are unavailable, but small regional studies point to the broad veracity of such statements. It is not just the number of fatalities that are of concern in snakebite; many survivors are left with permanent physical impairment, sometimes severe. Paediatric cases represent 20–25% of the total, but a higher proportion of fatalities.

Snakes are ectothermic ('coldblooded') reptiles, comprising around 3000 species. Venomous snakes are restricted to just four families: Colubridae, Elapidae, Atractaspididae, Viperidae (Table 22.1.1 and Figs 22.1.1–22.1.4). Fang structures and venom types vary between families, but the common theme is a bite resulting in injection or inoculation of venom through a break in the victim's skin. In most cases, venom is injected by fangs, paired teeth evolved to deliver venom, usually through a venom groove or enclosed channel, exiting near the tip. The act of biting can leave a variety of bite marks, which may be highly visible or almost invisible. Venom need not be injected ('dry bites').

Venom varies between snake families, within families, between genera, within genera, between species, within species, between individual snakes, and even over time for a particular snake. It follows that while broad patterns of envenoming can be stated, there is always the possibility of an atypical pattern of effects occurring, because of venom variability. This is just

Table 22.1.1 Families of venomous snakes and their principal characteristics

Family	Fang type	Common names of selected medically important species	Geographic range of Family
Colubridae (colubrids)	Back-fanged (opisthoglyphs) (see Fig. 22.1.1) OR No fangs (aglyphs)[a]	Boomslang (Africa) Vine snakes (Africa) Yamakagashi and red-necked keelbacks (Asia)	Global
Elapidae (elapids)	Front-fanged (proteroglyphs) (see Fig. 22.1.2) Fangs fixed or with minimal rotation	Cobras (Africa, Middle East, Asia) Coral snakes (Americas, Asia) Kraits (Asia) Mambas (Africa) Tiger snakes (Australia) Brown snakes (Australia and New Guinea) Taipans (Australia and New Guinea) Death adders (Australia, New Guinea, and eastern Indonesia) Mulga and black snakes (Australia and New Guinea) Small-eyed snake (New Guinea) Sea snakes (Pacific and Indian Oceans)	Global
Atractaspididae (atractaspids)	Front-fanged (proteroglyphs) (see Fig. 22.1.3) Fang placed to exit mouth through side ('side-fanged')	Side-fanged and mole vipers	Africa and Middle East
Viperidae Subfamily Viperinae (viperids) Subfamily Crotalinae (crotalids)	Front-fanged (solenoglyphs) (see Fig. 22.1.4) Fangs on mobile maxilla, with considerable rotation possible	Common vipers and asps (Europe) Puff adders and Gaboon vipers Night adders (Africa) Carpet or saw-scaled vipers (Africa, Middle East, and western Asia) Russell's vipers (Asia) Rattlesnakes (Americas) Lance-headed vipers (Americas) Bushmasters (Americas) Green tree vipers (Asia) Mamushis (Asia)	Global, except New Guinea and Australia

[a]The absence of fangs in most colubrids does not exclude the possibility of at least local envenoming from toxic salivary secretions inoculated into the wound in the act of biting.

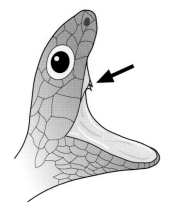

Fig. 22.1.1 Diagramatic representation of the head of an opisthoglyph (back fanged) snake. Reproduced with permission of Dr Julian White.

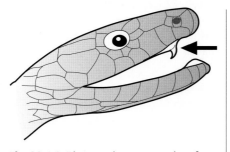

Fig. 22.1.2 Diagramatic representation of the head of a proteroglyph (front fanged) snake of the cobra type. Reproduced with permission of Dr Julian White.

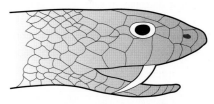

Fig. 22.1.3 Diagramatic representation of the head of a side 'fanged' atractaspid snake. Reproduced with permission of Dr Julian White.

one aspect of the potential difficulties in diagnosing and treating snakebite.

Venom has evolved from digestive juices. It has a variety of functions, which vary between species, but, in broad terms, venom has evolved to fulfil one or more of the following:

- assist prey capture by promoting immobilisation;
- assist prey death, to avoid injury to the snake;
- assist prey digestion;
- act as a deterrent to predators, by causing rapid, unpleasant effects.

As humans, we tend to focus on the last function, but it is the other three functions that cause major medical problems.

Venom actions are diverse. Some major actions are listed in Table 22.1.2. From a clinical perspective, venom effects can be divided into three major groups:

❶ Local effects.
❷ Non-specific general effects.
❸ Specific systemic effects.

For many snakebites, in most regions of the world, local effects are a major, often the principal, medical problem. In these cases there may be local pain, swelling, which may be severe, involving much or all of the bitten limb, resulting in fluid shifts,

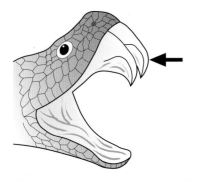

Fig. 22.1.4 Diagramatic representation of the head of a solenoglyph (front fanged) snake of the viper type, with maxillary rotation to allow folding of the fang against the mouth.
Reproduced with permission of Dr Julian White.

secondary hypovolaemic shock and the risk of compartment syndrome. There may be local blistering, bruising or development of skin necrosis. Systemic coagulopathy may manifest locally as persistent oozing or bleeding from the bite or damaged areas of the affected limb. The extent of local necrosis may be significant, with potential, often realised, for long-term tissue injury and dysfunction. Secondary infection may develop in the injured limb. For some species (e.g. lance-headed vipers, such as *Bothrops* spp. in South America) there may be local abscess formation. Long-term disability is a frequent outcome. In some cases, amputation is required. In cases with ongoing skin damage, never fully healed, skin tumours can develop after some years. This range

of major local effects and secondary systemic effects can be seen following bites by many, but not all, species of viper and atractaspids but not colubrids and only selected African and Asian cobras amongst the elapids. Such severe local effects are generally absent from snakebite in New Guinea and Australia, where the only medically important venomous snakes are all elapids.

The non-specific general effects of envenoming vary between species, but usually include one or more of the following:

- nausea or vomiting;
- abdominal pain or cramps;
- headache;
- dizziness;
- non-paralytic blurred vision;
- tender or enlarged draining lymph nodes;
- brief period of collapse;
- hypertension (occasionally hypotension).

As most of these can be the result of anxiety as well as envenoming, they may not be reliable indicators of systemic envenoming.

The specific systemic effects of snake venoms are the most intensely studied, partly because they can usually be ascribed to particular venom components that can be isolated and studied in detail. An overview of these components is listed in Table 22.1.2. Specific clinical findings for the effects of these components will be discussed in the sections on 'history', 'examination' and 'investigations'.

History

There may be a clear history of snakebite, or an encounter with a snake, where an actual bite is uncertain, or no history of a snake or bite. Particularly in young children, there may be no possibility of obtaining a history. Listen carefully to the story from young children, because relevant information may be disguised by rudimentary language. Some key points are listed in Table 22.1.3.

The environment and circumstances can be of great importance in deciding if a snakebite is likely. Do not assume that bites are unlikely indoors; snakes do enter houses, commonly in the rural tropics, but even in temperate urban areas such as Australian cities.

If there is a history of an encounter with a snake, note if the snake struck, how many times, if bites were through clothing, as well as noting the apparent length and colouration of the snake. For selected cobra attacks in Africa and Asia, the snake may spit first, particularly aiming for the eyes, before either retreating or pressing home an attack with actual bites. A chewing bite, where the snake hangs on is also important, as there is more opportunity for venom injection. Similarly, multiple bites are associated with higher rates of major envenoming.

A description of the snake and geographical location may help narrow the range of possible culprit species. This can be

Type of venom action	General site of action	Type of venom component	Clinical effects
Local toxins	Bite site and bitten limb	Necrotoxins, cytotoxins, etc.	Local effects; may include pain, swelling, blistering, bruising, necrosis
Paralytic toxins	Specific systemic (neuromuscular junction)	Neurotoxins (presynaptic, postsynaptic, dendrotoxins, fasciculins)	Progressive flaccid paralysis of skeletal muscle and diaphragm
Myolytic toxins	Specific systemic (skeletal muscle)	Myotoxins	Destruction of skeletal muscle throughout body (or locally in bitten limb only for some crotalids)
Haematological toxins	Specific systemic (interfere with haemostasis in a variety of ways, or may damage vessel walls, promote bleeding)	Procoagulants Fibrino(geno)lytics Anticoagulants Haemorrhagins Various other toxins affecting haemostasis	Varies, depending on type of toxin; may cause consumption coagulopathy, complete defibrination, active haemorrhage promoting, or even thrombosis and infarction or embolism (Martinique vipers only)
Nephrotoxic toxins	Specific systemic (kidneys)	Nephrotoxins	Renal damage, failure, or necrosis
Cardiotoxic toxins	Specific systemic (heart)	Cardiotoxins	Cardiac arrhythmias, failure or arrest

Table 22.1.2 Broad overview of major clinical actions of snake venoms

Table 22.1.3 Summary of principal points in history for snakebite

Broad category	Question	Significance
Details of bite	Was snake seen?	Increases likelihood of snakebite
	Description of snake?	May assist identifying type of snake, so possible problems can be anticipated
	Size of snake?	May indicate potential for severe bite if large specimen, but beware, even juvenile snakes can inflict a severe bite
	Geographical location?	May limit types of snake to be considered
	Environment?	May indicate likelihood of snake encounter, if no clear history of snake being seen
	Number of bites?	Multiple bites increase the likelihood of severe effects
	Was bite through clothing?	Clothing may soak up some venom, reduce the chance of an effective bite. This may also be a source for venom detection (Australia)
Details of first aid	Was first aid used?	If no first aid then nothing to impair development of effects of venom
	What type of first aid?	Some types of first aid (e.g. tourniquets, cut and suck, suction devices, snake stones, electric shock/stun guns) may make matters worse or be ineffective
		Effective first aid (e.g. immobilisation of the bitten limb, or full pressure immobilisation bandage) may delay onset of envenoming, thus the patient may present well, yet deteriorate after removal of first aid
	When was first aid applied?	If applied promptly, it may be effective, delaying envenoming
		If applied late or after physical activity (e.g. chasing snake, running for help) it may be ineffective
Local effects of bite	Were any bite marks, etc. noted prior to application of first aid?	If bite marks present, snakebite more likely, but absence of visible bites does not exclude snakebite (especially for some Australian elapids, notably brown snakes)
	Is there any local pain, swelling, bleeding, blistering, skin discolouration or other local effect?	May indicate likelihood of effective bite and possibly even type of bite
General symptoms	Headache, nausea, vomiting, abdominal pain?	Non-specific indicators of possible systemic envenoming (or anxiety)
	Collapse?	If in association with a definite bite, is suggestive of systemic envenoming
	Convulsion?	If in association with a definite bite is strongly suggestive of major systemic envenoming
	Blurred or double vision experienced within a few minutes of the bite?	Common effect, not likely to indicate developing paralysis
Specific systemic effects Paralytic effects	Presence and time of onset of paralytic symptoms? (Early ptosis may be described as heavy or sleepy eyes/eyelids)	Cranial nerves affected first, usually ptosis. Important to pick this up, before paralysis advances too far. May also help indicate the most likely type of snake
Myolytic effects	Presence and time of onset of myolytic symptoms? (muscle pain, tenderness, weakness; urine becoming pink, red, brown or black)	Usually takes several hours to manifest. May indicate most likely type of snake
Coagulopathic and haemorrhagic effects	Presence of coagulopathy effects, such as persistent bleeding from bite site or cuts, gums, or bruising, haemoptysis, haematemesis, haematuria?	Indicates coagulopathy likely and probably significant. May indicate most likely type of snake
Renal effects	Presence of anuria or oliguria or polyuria	Indicates likely significant renal damage
General history Medications	Anticoagulants or NSAIDS?	May affect coagulation test results or increase likelihood of a major bleed if coagulopathy present
	Antihypertensives?	Though not proven for antivenoms, it is suspected that β-blockers and ACE inhibitors may increase the chance of and severity of anaphylactic reactions to antivenom
Past history	Past bites requiring antivenom?	Past exposure to antivenom may increase the likelihood of reactions to subsequent antivenom therapy
	Past renal problems?	May increase the likelihood of envenoming causing renal damage
	Other past medical history?	Evaluate as appropriate

combined with clinical features to assist in identifying the most likely culprits using diagnostic algorithms (Figs 22.1.5 and 22.1.6).

It is important to ask about any local, general or specific symptoms that might indicate developing significant envenoming (see Table 22.1.3).

In children it may prove difficult, even impossible, to obtain any history from the child; however, parents, siblings or bystanders may have useful information. For instance, a small child seeking a parent because they are upset, then collapsing, having a convulsion, then recovering, but remaining miserable is a classic presentation for significant snakebite in some regions (e.g. Australia).

Examination

While examination must be thorough, time is of the essence in major envenoming. Therefore, if snakebite is suspected, examination should be directed initially to determine if there is evidence for snakebite and the extent of any envenoming.

It is clearly important to look at the bite site, or look for a bite, if no site is indicated from the history. Snakebites may result in single or paired fang punctures, multiple teeth punctures or even scratches, as fangs are dragged through the skin during release (Figs 22.1.7–22.1.10). If there is a bandage over the bite site, as first aid, cut a window only to inspect. Keep the removed bandage portion, if in Australia, for possible venom detection later. If venom detection is available (Australia, New Guinea), swab

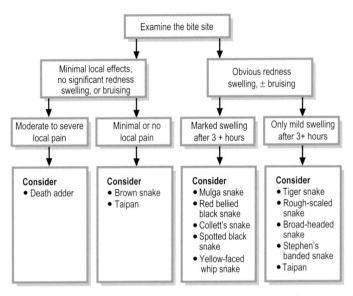

Fig. 22.1.5 Diagnostic algorithm for Australian snakes using the bite site effects. Reproduced with permission of Dr Julian White.

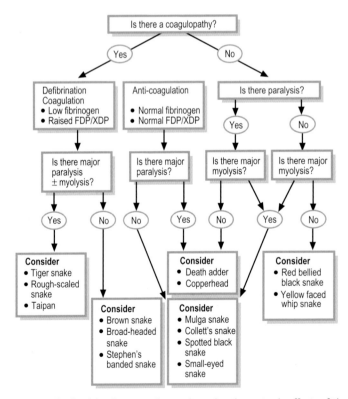

Fig. 22.1.6 Diagnostic algorithm for Australian snakes using the systemic effects of the bite. Reproduced with permission of Dr Julian White.

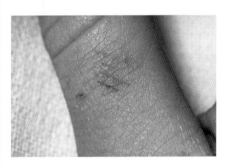

Fig. 22.1.7 Brown snake bite. Note scratches rather than punctures and lack of local reaction. Reproduced with permission of Dr Julian White.

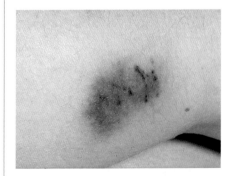

Fig. 22.1.8 Tiger snake bite. Multiple bite with two sets of marks and local bruising. Reproduced with permission of Dr Julian White.

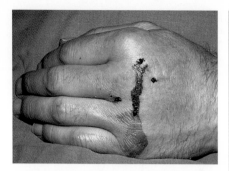

Fig. 22.1.9 Persistent bleeding from bite site, a sign of coagulopathy. Reproduced with permission of Dr Julian White.

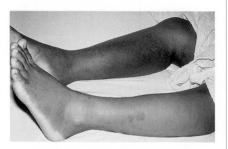

Fig. 22.1.10 Extensive bruising of bitten limb. Typical of viper bites causing coagulopathy (green pit viper bite). Reproduced with permission of Dr Julian White.

the bite site with the stick provided in the test kit. Do not allow anyone to clean the bite area until it has been swabbed for venom. Look for bite marks and particularly for multiple bites. Observe for local bruising, bleeding, blistering, swelling or necrosis. If there is significant local tissue injury or swelling, check pulses, etc., to exclude compartment syndrome in affected compartments. Compartment syndrome, if suspected clinically, must be confirmed by measuring intracompartmental pressure, before any consideration of surgical intervention.

Check draining lymph nodes; if they are tender or swollen it may indicate venom absorption and movement.

Examine for specific effects, notably neurotoxicity (flaccid paralysis; check for cranial nerve paralysis first, starting with ptosis; Figs 22.1.11, 22.1.12), myolysis (muscle tenderness and weakness), coagulopathy (persistent bleeding from bite site, needle punctures, etc.; Fig. 22.1.13) or deep vein thrombosis (DVT, pulmonary embolism; Martinique crotalids only), cardiotoxicity

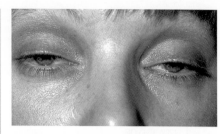

Fig. 22.1.11 Early stage flaccid neurotoxic paralysis with mild ptosis. An important early sign, easily missed (tiger snake bite). Reproduced with permission of Dr Julian White.

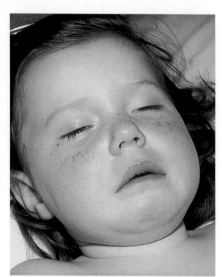

Fig. 22.1.12 Flat facial appearance. Caused by progressive involvement of cranial nerves in flaccid neurotoxic paralysis. Ptosis is also present (tiger snake bite). Reproduced with permission of Dr Julian White.

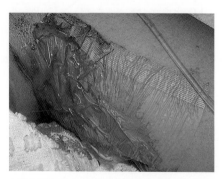

Fig. 22.1.13 Persistent blood ooze from IV site indicative of coagulopathy (taipan bite). Reproduced with permission of Dr Julian White.

(arrhythmias), 'allergy' (angioneurotic oedema; particularly European vipers).

Investigations

The most specific investigation is venom detection, but currently this is only routinely

available in Australia (most reliable sample is bite site swab; urine can be tested if there is systemic envenoming; blood is unreliable). However, venom detection will not always provide a useful answer, even if available, so it is important to be aware of other diagnostic tools in determining the type of bite and clinical effects. These are discussed further under 'differential diagnosis'.

Laboratory or similar investigations are often crucial to the management of snakebite. The key areas are coagulation, renal function and muscle integrity.

Many snakes, especially vipers but also some colubrids and many Australian elapids, can cause coagulopathy, which in many cases is potentially lethal. Coagulopathy can develop early or gradually over many hours. The type of coagulopathy is determined by the type of venom components, but just a few tests are adequate in most situations to determine the extent of pathology. For rural areas or hospitals without laboratory facilities, including outback Australia, the whole blood clotting test (WBCT) is the only practical test. 5–10 mL of venous blood is placed in a glass test tube or similar and allowed to clot. If possible, the time to clot is measured. Normal blood should clot in under 10 minutes. If there is minimal or no clot at 20 minutes, this strongly suggests a coagulopathy. If possible, perform a parallel test on blood from a normal control (e.g. relative or staff member). If laboratory facilities are available, the key tests are prothrombin time (PT) or international normalised ratio (INR), activated partial thromboplastin time (aPTT), fibrinogen titre, fibrin (ogen) degradation products (or d-dimer) titre, and platelet count.

Renal function tests are usually urea and creatinine levels. In the absence of a laboratory, monitoring renal output is all that is practical.

Muscle integrity relates to myolytic-venoms, the best measure being creatine phosphokinase level (CK, CPK). In the absence of a laboratory, the presence of red, brown or black urine is suggestive of myolysis and myoglobinuria. However, red urine can also be caused by haematuria. If in doubt, spin down the urine and examine under a microscope, looking for evidence of red cell casts. Both haemoglobin and myoglobin test positive for blood with dipstix testing of urine.

ENVIRONMENTAL

If there is evidence of infection around the bitten area, culture and sensitivity should be performed on wound swabs.

In cases where there is clinical evidence of cardiovascular effects of envenoming, primary or secondary, or for bites by snakes known to be cardiotoxic, ECG monitoring is appropriate, but in other cases it may be unnecessary.

Chest X-ray (CXR) is only required if there are clinical grounds to suspect respiratory pathology. Similarly, arterial blood gas examination is not routinely required, but could be considered if there is respiratory impairment, particularly if there is respiratory paralysis developing. In the later stages, after extensive intravenous (IV) fluid therapy, secondary pulmonary oedema is a risk, especially in young children; if suspected, a CXR may be diagnostic.

Envenoming does not always manifest early. It is therefore appropriate to retest for coagulopathy, renal impairment and elevated CK, if the initial tests are normal. In general, a useful protocol is to retest 2–3 hours and 5–6 hours after the initial test, or earlier if symptoms or signs of envenoming develop and at 12 hours or later post bite, prior to any decision to discharge.

Differential diagnosis

A full discussion of all possible differential diagnoses for snakebite is beyond the scope of this chapter. It is important to include snakebite in the differential diagnosis for patients with unexplained collapse, convulsions, bleeding, coagulopathy, thrombosis (in Martinique, specifically), myolysis, flaccid paralysis, muscle fasciculation (mamba bites in Africa), renal failure or impairment, or local tissue injury.

Differential diagnosis can also be applied within snakebite, in determining the type of snake most likely to have caused the bite. Diagnostic algorithms have been developed for Australia (see Figs 22.1.5 and 22.1.6) and South-East Asia (Figure 22.1.14). These are based on cases with significant envenoming and will not function if the patient is not envenomed, though this hardly matters, as such a patient will not require antivenom therapy. In some regions, notably Australia, it is important to know the type of snake involved, because antivenom therapy

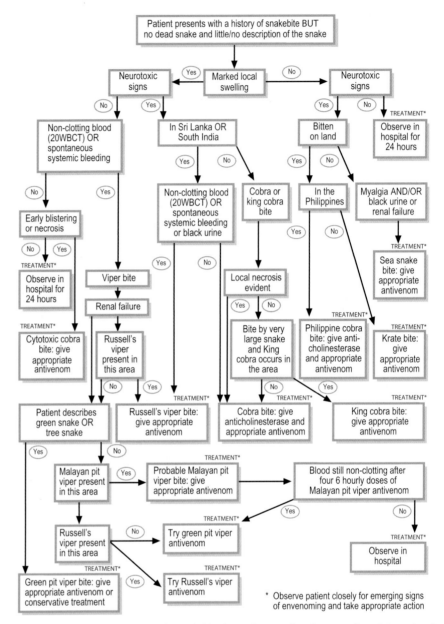

Fig. 22.1.14 Diagnostic algorithm for snakebite in southeast Asia. After Warrell et al. Reproduced with permission of Dr Julian White.

can be targeted appropriately. A similar situation applies in some other regions, where specific antivenoms are available. In regions such as North America, this is less important, because there is only one polyvalent antivenom covering all venomous species, except coral snakes.

Treatment

Snakebite treatment can be divided into several areas: first aid; diagnosis; and treatment, the latter further divided into specific (antivenom) and non-specific treatment.

First aid for snakebite is controversial. Many techniques have been advocated and are in use throughout the world. Almost none meet the critical criteria of safety and effectiveness. For snakes not likely to cause major tissue injury in the bitten area, the Australian-developed 'pressure immobilisation' method is appropriate. A broad bandage is applied over the bite site, then the rest of the bitten limb, at the same pressure as used for a sprain, that is firm but not occlusive. The limb is then immobilised using a splint. Correctly and promptly applied, this method is both safe and effective. However, for snakes likely to cause local tissue injury, even the pressure of this technique may cause further tissue damage, at least theoretically. For this reason, the pressure immobilisation method has not been recommended for all snakebites. The theoretical danger from this method has been challenged by recent research and it may be that extension of this research will show that the pressure immobilisation method is safe and effective for all snakebites.

Other popular first aid methods enjoy no such success and are either unsafe or ineffective, or both, and should never be used. Amongst these are tourniquets, 'cut & suck', patent venom extraction devices (suction), electric shock ('stun guns' etc), application of chemicals to the bite, snake stones and 'witch doctor' treatments. The application of certain plant extracts is still undergoing evaluation.

Diagnosis of snakebite has been discussed earlier.

Definitive treatment for snakebite will vary depending on the type of snake, but some general principles apply.

First, not every bite will result in envenoming, but the extent of envenoming, if any, may not be immediately apparent, therefore all bites should be treated with caution.

Second, in many regions, the bulk of snake fauna is non-venomous, so many snake bites may be trivial. However, it is necessary to be sure of the snake's identity as non-venomous, before dismissing the case and identification is rarely easy, especially in paediatric cases where history is scant. An exception is Australia, where almost all snakes causing bites are potentially lethal.

Third, if significant envenoming has occurred, with few exceptions, antivenom, if available, is the treatment of choice and should always be given IV. Choice of antivenom will be determined by the type of snake and the availability of methods to determine snake identity. Thus, in Australia, specific antivenoms are available, together with venom detection and diagnostic algorithms, so polyvalent antivenom is often not required. In contrast, in North America

the only available snake antivenom is polyvalent, covering all endemic pit-viper species, so identifying the snake is less important. In general, antivenom will be more effective than any other therapeutic agent at reversing envenoming. Used appropriately it is life saving and the old 'wisdom' that 'the antivenom is more dangerous than the venom' is outdated, inappropriate and dangerous.

Fourth, antivenom is generally disappointing as therapy for local effects of envenoming, but is still better than other therapies in most cases. Equally, do not overlook adjunctive therapies, in particular adequate IV hydration if there is massive local or limb swelling following the bite, as untreated hypovolaemic shock secondary to such fluid shifts is potentially lethal, especially in children.

Fifth, for coagulopathy caused by venom, antivenom is the best treatment to reverse effects, and factor replacement therapy, including even whole blood, is best reserved for those cases with catastrophic bleeding, or no available antivenom, or where sufficient antivenom has already been given to neutralise all venom. Giving factor replacement therapy while active venom is still circulating is to invite worsening of the coagulopathy. Heparin is generally ineffective in these cases and should be avoided.

Finally, for cases with flaccid paralysis, consider anticholinesterase therapy as an adjunct to antivenom, if a Tensilon test has shown benefit (there is likely benefit for cobra bite causing paralysis, also death adders (but only some cases), possibly some kraits, sea snakes, possibly some coral snakes). Venoms with presynaptic neurotoxins will not show response to anticholinesterase therapy (most Australian snakes causing paralysis; exception is the death adder, which sometimes has only postsynaptic neurotoxins).

From the above it will be clear that antivenom is the key treatment for snakebite, when available. The latter is a real issue, because for many species and substantial areas of the rural tropics, antivenom is not available.

Prognosis

The majority of all snakebites globally prove non-fatal, but with an estimated global

fatality of more than 100 000 per year, death is clearly a significant risk. This is especially true for children. Their lower body mass and often delayed application of appropriate first aid puts them at greater risk. With such a wide variety of snake species, it is beyond the scope of this chapter to define prognosis for all snakes. However, some general principles apply.

The more rapid and severe the onset of envenoming, the more grave the prognosis, but this is not absolute. For instance, in Australia, a small child (under 5 years) may show early irritability, collapse, even convulsions following a snakebite (especially bites by brown snakes, tiger snakes, taipans), yet will usually spontaneously recover consciousness. Such a presentation is indicative of major envenoming, but with correct treatment, is survivable. Thus prognosis is determined by several factors, not just the type and toxicity of the snake, but also the treatment response. It is likely that if high standard treatment were universally available, the global toll from snakebite would be far lower.

For local effects of envenoming, after bites by snakes causing local tissue injury (most vipers, many African and Asian cobras), the more rapid the swelling, the more extensive blistering, the more serious the bite. Similarly, development of discolouration of the skin with a well-demarcated edge often indicates an area of impending necrosis.

For general systemic effects, the more severe the symptoms, such as vomiting, abdominal pain, headache, often, though not universally, the more severe the envenoming.

For specific systemic effects, rapid onset often indicates severity. Early development of progressive flaccid paralysis is usually indicative of severe envenoming, while paralysis of very limited extent after 6 hours is often indicative of a less severe bite. However, this may not always be the case. Occasionally flaccid paralysis may not be evident; even a patient with just ptosis, until 24 hours post bite, yet may progress to severe paralysis without treatment. This may occur with many snakes causing paralysis, but notably Australian death adders. This is an important reason why early discharge of an apparently well patient is ill advised. Once flaccid paralysis is extensive, with respiratory failure, the patient can still survive if ventilation is supported. However, for snakes with presynaptic neurotoxins, reversal of paralysis will not occur until the damaged terminal axons at neuromuscular junctions have recovered, which may take days to weeks. Antivenom will not reverse such paralysis. In contrast, paralysis caused by snakes with purely postsynaptic neurotoxins will usually reverse with adequate antivenom therapy. The Tensilon test will generally predict such responses.

For coagulopathy, rapidity of onset and presence of signs such as persistent oozing from the bite site and bleeding gums indicate significant coagulopathy. With appropriate treatment, this does not imply a poor prognosis, but is a warning that more critical haemorrhaging is possible. Any bleeding into a vital organ, most commonly the brain, indicates a poor prognosis, with a fatal outcome most likely with intracranial bleeds. For Russell's viper in Myanmar (Burma) and southern India, there may be haemorrhagic infarction of the anterior pituitary gland, with resulting Sheehan's syndrome developing, though this may not be rapidly apparent.

Myolysis is most often measured as profoundly elevated CK levels, and may progress to secondary renal failure and hyperkalaemia, the latter indicating a poor prognosis, as cardiac complications may ensue. In general, the more rapid the rise in CK levels, the more severe is the myolysis, but this is not always the case. In some cases the CK rise may initially be slight, but become more significant after 24 hours, rising to high levels over several days. Early muscle pain and myoglobinuria is also suggestive of more severe myolysis.

Renal damage may be primary or secondary and can prove lethal if untreated. Rapid development of anuric renal failure indicates a poor prognosis, unless dialysis can be instituted. A slower rise in creatinine levels, without anuria, usually indicates less severe renal damage, but still may take a week or more for return of normal renal function. In most cases, even acute renal failure after snakebite is reversible, over days to weeks. A small minority of cases will develop more lasting renal failure, generally because bilateral

renal cortical necrosis has occurred. This severe complication with a poor prognosis is not easily predicted and is generally only discovered at renal biopsy in patients who have failed to recover from early renal failure. It has been reported after bites by only a few species, such as the Australian taipan and South American lance-headed pit vipers (jararacusu, jararaca), but other species could potentially cause this outcome.

Prevention

Prevention of snakebite can be considered in two ways. First, there is prevention of bites, by educating the population about ways to avoid contact. These will vary from region to region and are beyond the scope of this chapter. Second, there is prevention of the more severe effects or complications of envenoming, by prompt diagnosis and appropriate treatment. This commences with early application of appropriate first aid pre-hospital, to minimise the chance of severe envenoming developing before treatment can be instituted. Once in hospital, urgent triage and assessment will permit prompt IV rehydration, for cases where there is a major fluid shift into the bitten limb, or rapid commencement of IV antivenom, if indicated, before more delayed forms of envenoming (e.g. flaccid paralysis, myolysis) have progressed too far, as well as instituting any life-support measures required.

Many deaths or cases with long-term morbidity after snakebite are the result of either delays in commencing treatment, or inadequate or inappropriate treatment. The latter may be the result of poor training of health personnel. It follows, therefore, that adequate training of staff will be preventative.

Controversies

❶ First aid – Possibly the most controversial aspect of snakebite management is the recommended type of first aid. Many types of first aid have been advocated and remain in widespread use, but only immobilisation, or pressure bandaging and immobilisation have consistently enjoyed both scientific and

medical expert support (see earlier discussion on first aid).

❷ Type of antivenom – The role of antivenom in treatment should no longer be considered controversial, as where available, if of reasonable quality, it is the treatment of choice. Less certain is the role of antivenom in treating purely local effects of envenoming, especially in preventing necrosis. Recent clinical experience suggests that high-quality antivenoms, particularly Fab' antivenoms, are at least able to lessen the extent of local tissue injury, if used promptly. No antivenom can be expected to reverse established local necrosis. However, debate continues on the relative merits of different types of antivenom. The most recent Fab' antivenoms have proven clinically effective, but are rapidly cleared, requiring higher and repeat doses. $F(ab')_2$ antivenoms are less rapidly cleared and are effective. Whole IgG antivenoms have the highest rate of adverse reactions, but are cheaper and may be the most potent. New methods of producing whole IgG antivenoms are proving cost effective and appear to significantly reduce the adverse effect profile, so there is a likely resurgence of safe, effective IgG antivenoms. The choice of animal is also contested. Horses, while traditional and easy to use in most regions, produce an antivenom with higher rates of adverse reactions than sheep, but sheep can only be used safely if raised in regions free from prion diseases, essentially limiting them to Australia and New Zealand. IgY antivenoms from egg yolk, produced by immunising chickens, are potentially easy and cheap to produce, but their safety and effectiveness is not yet established and recent research indicates both limits on effectiveness and a likely unacceptable adverse effects profile.

❸ Premedication – There remains debate on the value of premedication prior to antivenom therapy to reduce the likelihood of acute adverse reactions, especially 'anaphylaxis'. Antihistamines have been shown to be ineffective at preventing such reactions. They have adverse side effects (drowsiness and occasionally hyperexcitability) and should not be used. Hydrocortisone carries no proven benefit, but no great risk. Adrenaline (epinephrine) remains the most controversial, as it can reduce the incidence of reactions for poor-quality antivenoms, but has a significant risk profile, so for most antivenoms its use is not recommended. It is particularly dangerous for bites likely to cause coagulopathy (e.g. many Australian snakebites, most viper bites). The practice of pre-testing for allergy to antivenom, using a small subcutaneous dose of the antivenom is to be discouraged. It has been shown to have no reliable predictive value, but carries a significant risk, without benefit, and will delay commencement of antivenom therapy.

❹ Coagulopathy – The treatment of coagulopathy remains contentious, though most experts agree antivenom is the best therapeutic choice, if available. Factor replacement therapy is often the only option if no antivenom is available, as for some colubrid snakes, but is not without hazard. Heparin has been advocated, but most evidence suggests that it is both ineffective and dangerous in this setting.

❺ Local necrosis – The treatment of local swelling should be standard, with fasciotomy reserved for those few cases with proven compartment syndrome (intracompartmental pressure measurement). Fasciotomy should be avoided, if possible, in cases with active coagulopathy. However, early fasciotomy is still practised in some areas, often with distressing and unacceptable functional and cosmetic sequelae.

Future directions

❶ Even for many common species of venomous snakes, known to cause significant numbers of bites, reliable clinical studies of envenoming are scant or lacking. The medical literature on snakebite is replete with epidemiological studies that fail to relate bite effects to particular species of snakes, rendering these studies almost useless. It is essential that accurate profiles of the clinical spectrum of envenoming be documented for every species biting humans, preferably in controlled prospective studies.

❷ Controlled studies to establish antivenom effectiveness and dosage are required. Use of modern techniques to measure venom and component levels in serial patient blood samples should greatly assist in such research. Antivenoms need to become safer, more effective and much more widely available, particularly in the rural tropics.

Scorpion stings

Introduction

Scorpion stings are the second most important form of terrestrial envenoming, after snakebite, with global cases probably exceeding one million per year, and deaths numbered in the many hundreds, to possibly as high as 5000 per year, nearly all in children. Scorpion envenoming is unpleasant for adults and occasionally is severe enough to threaten life. In children, however, it can be a rapidly severe and lethal disease, with some centres still reporting paediatric fatality rates in excess of 10%.

Scorpions vary in size, with over 1600 species known. All have a sting in the 'tail' (telson) with associated venom glands. Most scorpions either rarely sting humans, or are too small to cause envenoming, or have venom of little potency in humans. Unfortunately, a small number of scorpions do possess potent venoms and these species predominate in parts of the world where humans exist in large numbers, often in less than affluent conditions. The combination of warm to hot evenings, sandy soils, a tendency to walk around barefoot and dwellings that do not exclude scorpions leads to the large number of stings. Major risk areas include South and Central America, particularly Brazil (*Tityus* spp.), Mexico and adjacent USA (*Centruroides* spp.), North Africa and the Middle East (*Leiurus* quinquestriatus, *Androctonus* spp., *Buthus* spp.), Western Asia and India (*Buthus* spp., *Mesobuthus* spp.) and in Iran, the unique *Hemiscorpius lepturus*.

In general, it is not the larger scorpions with robust front 'pincers' that are most concerning, but the smaller, more delicate species with unimpressive front 'pincers', because they rely on the toxicity of their venom.

Scorpion venoms contain a wide array of ion-channel toxins of great potency, causing an excitatory neurotoxic reaction (not paralysis), not dissimilar to an autonomic storm. Only a matter of minutes, not hours, may elapse from the time of the sting to major systemic envenoming. Once the systemic toxicity is established, antivenom therapy has less chance of success, though it may still save lives. In Mexico, with >280 000 cases per year, death rates in children following scorpion sting have fallen from thousands per year to a handful following the introduction of antivenom.

Scorpion venoms do not contain paralytic neurotoxins, myolysins, components affecting coagulation or renal function, nor do they contain local necrotic toxins (except for one species in the Middle East; *Hemiscorpius lepturus* in Iran).

History

Often a scorpion will have been seen. There will usually be a clear history of an immediately painful sting (except *Hemiscorpius lepturus*), followed by development of systemic envenoming with effects that may include some of the following:

- tingling of the lips;
- nausea, vomiting;
- abdominal pain;
- collapse;
- convulsions;
- hypertension or labile blood pressure;
- increased sweating, salivation or lacrimation;
- piloerection;
- dyspnoea;
- pulmonary oedema;
- cardiac collapse;
- multiple organ failure.

Symptoms appropriate to each of these effects may be described. It is important to note the time of onset for symptoms – a rapid onset and escalation in severity indicates a severe sting.

Examination

The local effects of the sting are not generally impressive, though there may be local sweating and piloerection. It is the systemic effects that will be most important, so particularly check blood pressure, look for signs of neuroexcitation, pulmonary oedema and cardiac collapse. In small children there may be a nystagmus. The exception is *Hemiscorpius lepturus* in part of Iran. This species causes severe local effects, plus systemic effects including multiorgan failure and shock. Stings by this scorpion particularly affect children with a significant fatality rate.

Investigations

There are no specific tests for scorpion venom, nor specific indicators of envenoming, but in severe cases it is important to exclude secondary effects of envenoming and multiple organ failure.

Differential diagnosis

Full differential diagnosis of scorpion sting is beyond the scope of this chapter. The 'autonomic storm' clinical picture seen in severe scorpion envenoming can also be caused by some other venomous animals, particularly funnel web spiders (in Australia, where major scorpion stings do not occur), banana spiders (in Brazil; typically also cause priapism in boys), and some jellyfish (irukandji type). Accidental or deliberate exposure to certain pesticides and pharmaceuticals should also be considered.

Treatment

Treatment of major scorpion envenoming is controversial, particularly centring around the role of antivenom. Most evidence suggests that antivenom use has resulted in greatly reduced fatality rates in children, but a few doctors argue that pharmacotherapy is more effective than antivenom, particularly focusing on the cardiac failure seen in fatal cases. Prazosin, in particular, has enjoyed success and should be considered, both as an adjunct to antivenom and as first-line therapy in the absence of antivenom (i.e. in India). If antivenom is available it should be used IV without delay. Dose will vary depending on product.

Prognosis

The prognosis in scorpion envenoming depends on several factors. More severe envenoming is likely in smaller children, with more rapid development of effects and a shorter window for effective antivenom therapy. If multiple organ failure develops then prognosis is generally poor.

Controversies and future directions

❶ The major controversy in management of scorpion sting is the issue of antivenom effectiveness, as discussed earlier. Of the various types of antivenom, animal studies have indicated that Fab' antivenoms are not more effective than F(ab)2 or IgG antivenoms.

❷ Among non-antivenom therapies, the most controversy has surrounded the proposal to use insulin, suggested by an Indian doctor (where no antivenom is available). This technique is not favoured by most experts, considering it both highly risky and of most uncertain theoretical and practical benefit.

❸ Despite the frequency of scorpion stings, there are still few published studies of series of stings by particular species and few trials of various methods of treatment. There is a need for more intensive systematic study of scorpion envenoming and controlled trials of treatment alternatives.

Prevention

Most scorpion stings occur because of the patterns of human living, and thus are theoretically avoidable. It is possible to 'scorpion-proof' houses, by use of tiles around the lower walls, preventing scorpion entry. Use of enclosed footwear and avoidance of sitting down or lying down outside after dusk can also reduce sting incidence.

Spiderbite

Introduction

Spiderbite is probably very common, but most bites are trivial, with only a few species likely to cause major harm to humans (Table 22.1.4). For these species, morbidity can be significant, but mortality is low, with global deaths directly related to spiderbite probably measuring 20 or less per year. Even the world's most dangerous spiders, the Australian funnel web spiders, have only caused one known fatality in the last 20 years. As with other venomous animals,

Table 22.1.4 Medically important spider groups				
Family	Genera	Common name	Distribution	Clinical effects
Hexathelidae	Atrax Hadronyche	Australian funnel web spiders	Eastern Australia, from Cape York to Tasmania	Severe neuroexcitatory ('autonomic storm') envenoming; about 10% of cases develop major envenoming, which untreated, carries a significant risk of fatality
Theriidae	Latrodectus Steatoda	Red back or widow spiders	Global	Moderate, generally non-lethal neuroexcitatory envenoming
Ctenidae	Phoneutria	Banana spiders	Central and South America, especially Brazil	Moderate to severe neuroexcitatory envenoming, rarely lethal
Loxoscelidae	Loxosceles	Recluse or fiddleback spiders	Global, particularly the Americas	Severe local tissue injury, with occasional major, potentially lethal systemic effects

spiderbite is more likely to be severe in small children.

History

Spiderbite is not always initially painful, and spiders are small and easily misidentified, so most commonly there will be no certainty from the history about the species involved. However, particular spiders cause quite specific envenoming syndromes, making diagnosis possible even without a spider being available. The common presentations for the medically important spiders are listed below. In general, however, it is important to note the circumstances of definite or possible exposure to spiderbite, a description of the spider, if seen, and the timing of onset for any symptoms that develop.

Australian funnel web spiders

These large mygalomorph spiders are robust in appearance (Fig. 22.1.15), generally ground dwelling (there are tree-dwelling species) and are found only in eastern Australia (Fig. 22.1.16). Their large fangs and acidic venom generally cause immediate local pain on biting and they may hang on, being difficult to dislodge. Apart from pain, other local effects are not prominent. In about 10% of cases, systemic envenoming will develop, often rapidly, and can be lethal in less than 60 minutes in children. First symptoms are tingling of the lips and twitching of the tongue, followed by non-specific symptoms, which may include headache, nausea, vomiting and abdominal pain. There is frequently evidence of neuroexcitation, with sweating, salivation, lacrimation and piloerection. Hypertension is usual and dyspnoea secondary to pulmonary oedema can develop rapidly. Without

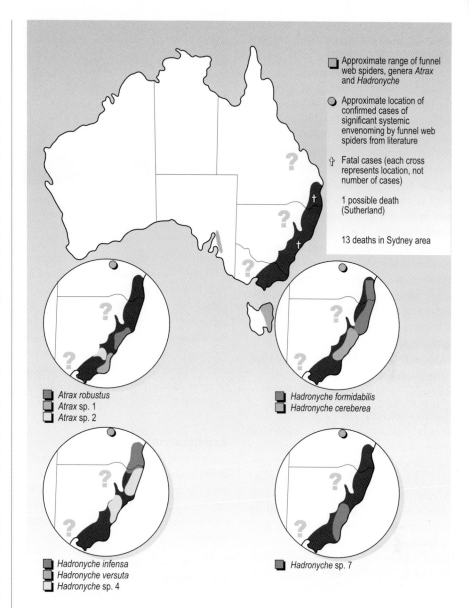

Fig. 22.1.16 Distribution of Australian funnel web spiders (*Atrax* spp. and *Hadronyche* spp.). Reproduced with permission of Dr Julian White.

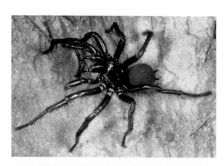

Fig. 22.1.15 Male Sydney funnel web spider (*Atrax robustus*). Reproduced with permission of Dr Julian White.

treatment this can progress to hypoxia, coma and death.

Widow spiders including Australian redback spiders

Widow spiders have a classic appearance (Fig. 22.1.17) with a globular abdomen, comparatively small cephalothorax and long thin legs. They utilise a drop-line web structure to capture prey. Humans most often receive bites when they either come in contact with the web or occasionally when touching a wandering spider (i.e. caught in footwear, clothing or similar). Widow spider

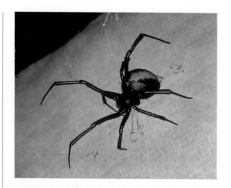

Fig. 22.1.17 Female widow (redback) spider. Reproduced with permission of Dr Julian White.

447

venom, though neuroexcitatory, is rarely lethal in humans. A typical significant bite causes local pain, becoming more severe, sometimes with local sweating, then progressive proximal movement of pain and sweating, ultimately becoming severe regional or generalised pain, sweating, plus hypertension, nausea and malaise. Envenoming can mimic acute abdomen and cardiac chest pain. Untreated, pain may take days or weeks to resolve and often gravitates to the lower limbs, causing burning pain in the feet and legs, often with associated sweating. Rarely, severe systemic envenoming can cause pulmonary oedema or a secondary rise in creatine kinase. In infants, a generalised rash is common, the infant presenting as highly distressed and irritable, not consolable, erythematous, but with no obvious cause apparent. A widow spider may be found in the bedding or underneath the bed. Less than 20% of bites cause major envenoming.

Banana spiders

Banana spiders are large aggressive spiders, well known within their range. They are active hunters and invade houses, with bites occurring year round, but especially in autumn. They are a common cause of bites in Brazil, accounting for 20% of all presentations in some hospitals. The neuroexcitatory venom has effects similar to widow spider bites in many ways, with pain being a predominant feature, as is sweating, hypertension and nausea. However, unlike widow spiders, there is often local swelling of the bite area and priapism is a classic feature of envenoming in boys. Death is a rare outcome, but severe cases can develop pulmonary oedema or cardiac arrhythmias.

Recluse or fiddleback spiders

These small, delicate spiders are generally brown with long spindly legs and a darker brown pattern on the cephalothorax in the rough shape of a violin (Fig. 22.1.18). They have a venom that is predominantly dermonecrotic. The most common effect of bites is 'cutaneous loxoscelism'. The bite is rarely noticed and often occurs in bed at night. However, hours later the area becomes red, painful, may blister or bruise and darken

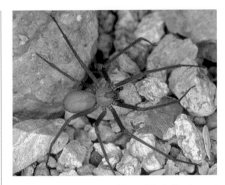

Fig. 22.1.18 Recluse spider, with violin-shaped marking on the cephalothorax. Reproduced with permission of Dr Julian White.

as necrosis develops over the following 4–7 days. The area finally involved can be local to extensive, with skip lesions, and is usually painful. There is commonly an associated non-specific, self-limited, systemic illness. In a few cases, a more severe systemic illness can occur, potentially lethal, with haemolysis, shock, coagulopathy, or renal failure. This is 'viscerocutaneous loxoscelism'.

Examination

Initial examination may show little locally at the bite site, depending on the type of envenoming involved. For those spiders causing predominantly regional or systemic effects, these will dominate examination findings.

Investigations

There are no clinical diagnostic tests specific for spiderbite. Most bites will result in leucocytosis. For suspected loxoscelism, it is important to look for haemolysis, disseminated intravascular coagulation and renal failure, especially in children.

Differential diagnosis

Detailed differential diagnosis is beyond the scope of this chapter, but the geographical location and pattern of local and systemic effects makes differentiation between these types of spiderbite straightforward. For severe neuroexcitatory envenoming, as seen with Australian funnel web spiders, consider pesticide or pharmaceutical poisoning in the differential. Widow spiderbite should be considered in the differential for selected cases of apparent

unexplained acute abdomen or chest pain, before laparotomy is scheduled.

Treatment

Treatment for Australian funnel web spiderbite is principally the use of specific IV antivenom, available in Australia only. Initially 2–4 vials are needed, but severe cases require more. All cases with any evidence of venom spread require antivenom urgently, before life-threatening envenoming develops, which may occur rapidly in children.

Widow spiderbite only requires treatment in those cases with significant local, regional or systemic envenoming, which is a minority of cases. Antivenom is the most effective treatment and may be given intramuscularly (IM, in Australia), but is more rapidly effective if used IV (even in Australia). Experience has shown that only antivenom reliably reverses envenoming and is more effective than narcotic analgesics in treating pain. It can be effective for up to days post-bite. It is usually given as single vials (2 vials in Australia), waiting 2+ hours before giving a further dose, if symptoms warrant. Some recent research in Australia has questioned the effectiveness of antivenom, but this is in contrast to decades of positive experience using this antivenom.

Banana spiderbite is most often managed without use of antivenom, the latter reserved for severe cases, where it should be given IV, most of these cases being children under 7 years of age. In the less severe cases, local anaesthetic block is usually adequate.

Loxoscelism is difficult to treat. Specific antivenom is only available in Brazil and its place in management is controversial, though it is widely used in Brazil and considered effective. In general, patients present late, after tissue injury has commenced, requiring good wound care. Secondary infection requires appropriate antibiotic therapy. Early surgical debridement can extend the area of injury and should be avoided. Steroids have not been shown to be effective. Dapsone, given early, can reduce injury, but is toxic and not widely favoured as therapy. Hyperbaric oxygen therapy is controversial. It may benefit some patients, but is unsuitable for most children.

Prognosis

Prognosis varies depending on the type of spider, but only for Australian funnel web spiders is death a likely outcome unless specific treatment is urgently instituted.

Prevention

Spiders are ubiquitous and it is not practical to avoid human contact. In areas where the potentially deadly funnel web spiders are common, such as parts of Sydney, residents should avoid walking barefoot, leaving clothes on the ground or putting on footwear without first checking for spiders.

Controversies and future directions

❶ Major controversies for spiderbite centre around adequate treatment, particularly the role of antivenom, with attendant risks, in envenoming unlikely to prove lethal. This concern has held sway in North America for widow spiderbites, with few cases offered antivenom therapy. As a result countless patients probably suffer prolonged periods of eminently treatable major discomfort. The opposite situation occurs in Australia where widow (redback) spiderbites routinely receive antivenom, with apparently good results and little risk.

❷ Bites by most spiders remain poorly documented and, even for major species, treatment is controversial. For these latter, controlled trials are required to establish best treatment practice.

Tick bite paralysis

Introduction

Tick bite is probably common in some regions, but rarely causes major harm to humans. However, a few species of ticks have toxic saliva, containing paralytic neurotoxins, which can cause potentially lethal

flaccid paralysis, especially in children. In Australia, for instance, paralysis ticks (*Ixodes* spp.) have caused more deaths than funnel web spiders.

History

There may be a clear history of a tick being found, but often in children presentation is as an unexplained progressive flaccid paralysis, first manifesting as an ataxic gait. Occasionally the paralysis may be purely local, notably a Bell's palsy. Without treatment, the envenoming may cause complete respiratory paralysis. For Australian paralysis ticks only, the paralysis may worsen for up to 48 hours after removal of all ticks. It is important to ascertain if the patient had exposure to ticks, such as walking in scrubland in eastern Australia.

Examination

Examination is crucial, both to document the extent of paralysis and to locate every attached tick. These may be hiding in the scalp, behind or in the ears or in body skin folds.

Investigations

There are no specific investigations for tick envenoming.

Differential diagnosis

Apart from ticks, at least in Australia, flaccid paralysis can be caused by snakebite. Ataxia only can also be caused by exposure to pesticides or some pharmaceuticals.

Treatment

The principal treatment for tick envenoming is prompt removal of all ticks. Care must be taken to lever the tick off, including mouthparts, and not squeeze it between fingers, which forces in more saliva and often leaves the head embedded, when secondary infection can ensue. The previously available tick antivenom (Australia) is no longer produced. The paralysis resolves after several days, during which time ventilatory support may be needed.

Prognosis

With removal of all ticks and respiratory support, the prognosis should be optimistic.

The more rapid the onset of paralytic features, the more likely is major paralysis.

Prevention

If visiting tick-infested areas, it may be difficult to exclude all tick contact risk, so routine checking for ticks after departure and their removal is advisable.

Controversies and future directions

The major controversy in the past was the value of tick antivenom. This antivenom is no longer available.

Jellyfish stings

Introduction

Jellyfish are numerous in all seas and oceans and stings, mostly trivial, are common. A few jellyfish can cause more severe stings and an even smaller number can cause potentially lethal envenoming. Of the many species that cause some effects, only the three groups of most medical significance will be discussed here. All jellyfish have a common mechanism of envenoming, using individual sting organelles (nematocysts) that both produce and inject the venom. This can result in some venom directly entering small blood vessels in the skin, causing rapid envenoming. In the case of large jellyfish, like the box jellyfish, with millions of nematocysts discharging simultaneously through the skin, very rapid and severe envenoming can develop.

Box jellyfish

The Australian box jellyfish, *Chironex fleckeri,* is found in northern Australian marine waters and areas to the north, including Borneo. It is the most dangerous of all jellyfish and can even kill an adult human in less than 5 minutes, from cardiac arrhythmia and arrest. Most stings are minor, not a threat to life, and cause local pain only. In cases with extensive and severe stings, there is immediate excruciating pain, with a ladder mark present, often with adherent tentacles. Collapse may follow rapidly, either due to the pain or to cardiac effects. Respiratory failure can develop, but it is cardiac toxicity that is most likely to prove lethal.

Irukandji syndrome

This is caused by envenoming by a variety of jellyfish, including *Carukia barnesii*, some of which are very small. The initial sting may be trivial and may be from the bell rather than tentacles. However, 20–40 minutes later systemic envenoming develops, with muscle and back pain, often severe, hypertension and malaise and pulmonary oedema, consistent with an 'autonomic storm'. While death is very rare, it has been recorded as a result of intracranial haemorrhage associated with severe hypertension, though the actual contribution of envenoming is controversial.

Portuguese-man-o-war

Blue bottles or Portuguese-man-o-war are global oceanic 'jellyfish' (actually hydrozoan colony organisms), which swarm and can cause stings from their tentacles. In most cases the stings are minor, with local pain and wheal formation, but rarely more severe envenoming is reported, with a very few cases of vascular injury locally. More common is an allergic reaction to stings, occasionally resulting in lethal anaphylaxis.

History

For most jellyfish there will be a clear history of being stung while in the sea and tentacles may still be adherent. These may still be active, so caution is advisable on removal. For box jellyfish only, the first aid application of copious amounts of vinegar may inactivate the tentacles, so they may be removed safely. The geographical location is important, as is the time of day and season, as this affects the likely local jellyfish fauna.

For stings by Irukandji-type jellyfish, the presentation may be one of unexplained severe pain following a swim in the sea, at any time of the year (but only in northern Australian waters and adjacent areas). It is important to note pre-existing medical conditions and medications that might increase the risk from envenoming.

Examination

The sting area should be examined and the extent determined. For box jellyfish, stings covering half or more of one limb or an equivalent area on the trunk should be considered as potentially lethal. Such a sting area is easily achieved in small children, who are those most often involved in fatal envenoming. Evidence of systemic effects should be sought.

Investigations

There are no specific tests for jellyfish envenoming.

Differential diagnosis

Except for Irukandji syndrome, which can be confused with non-envenoming illness, jellyfish stings are usually easily diagnosed, the major differential diagnosis being other types of marine envenoming, particularly stings from venomous fish, but these usually show only a few spine penetration points, not the widespread tentacle tracks of jellyfish.

Treatment

Most jellyfish stings require either no treatment or simple symptomatic relief of pain. Hot water (45°C, usually as a hot shower) has proved the most effective first aid for reducing local pain from jellyfish stings, though its applicability to box jellyfish stings remains untested, so for these stings a cold pack is preferred. For box jellyfish stings, where either an extensive area has been stung or systemic envenoming is evident, then box jellyfish antivenom is required urgently, either IM if pre-hospital, or preferably IV in hospital, 1–3 vials. In addition full cardiorespiratory support should be instituted, where needed. Local infection of the tentacle tracks can occur, requiring antibiotic therapy. Many cases develop delayed 'allergic' reactions locally, responding to antihistamines and topical corticosteroids.

Irukandji envenoming cannot be treated with antivenom (there is none suitable), so treatment should be supportive and symptomatic. Narcotic analgesia (excluding pethidine) is often required, with hypertension most often treated with glyceryl trinitrate (beware hypotension) and pulmonary oedema managed with oxygen, dopamine, adrenaline (epinephrine) and positive pressure ventilation.

Bluebottle envenoming is treated with supportive and symptomatic care only.

Prognosis

For box jellyfish envenoming, the larger the area of sting, the more severe the envenoming, with half or more of one limb involved being potentially lethal. For Irukandji, the prognostic indicators are less clear.

Prevention

The only sure way of preventing jellyfish stings is to avoid using the sea. Stinger suits can greatly reduce the chance of contact and will prevent potentially lethal box jellyfish stings, by limiting the area stung, but since only a small contact area is required for Irukandji jellyfish, exposed face, hands or feet may permit major envenoming. Similarly, stinger exclusion nets on beaches will prevent large box jellyfish from entering, so preventing major stings, but do nothing to prevent Irukandji stings.

Controversies and future directions

❶ There are a number of current controversies for jellyfish sting management. For box jellyfish, while vinegar is widely accepted as first aid to inactivate unfired nematocysts, the use of pressure immobilisation bandages in severe cases has been questioned, research showing that this technique may actually increase envenoming. As a consequence, most authorities now do not recommend using pressure immobilisation bandages for any jellyfish stings.

❷ The role of antivenom for box jellyfish stings remains clouded in uncertainty, but most authorities still recommend its use. Verapamil, once suggested for treating severe cardiotoxic box jellyfish envenoming, is no longer recommended by most authorities and has never undergone clinical testing in this setting.

❸ Irukandji envenoming remains problematic. There are still calls for antivenom development, but the delayed nature of envenoming and the increasing and varied range of the species of jellyfish involved make development of an effective antivenom problematic and economically unviable.

❹ Research is required into the mechanisms of major jellyfish envenoming in humans, as these are still not fully understood, mirroring the difficulties in collecting and studying jellyfish venom.

❺ Research is required to determine most effective treatment strategies for jellyfish envenoming. Irukandji syndrome, in particular, requires more research at all levels, starting with a concerted effort to identify and describe all likely culprit species.

❻ The shift from cold pack to a hot shower as first aid for most jellyfish stings, though supported by evidence (unlike cold packs), is still questioned by a few 'authorities'.

Venomous fish stings

Introduction

There are numerous species of fish, in both marine and freshwater environments, both bony and cartilaginous, capable of inflicting venomous stings, but envenoming, though often distressing, is rarely likely to be lethal, even in children. More concerning, in the case of cartilaginous fish, specifically stingrays, is the potential for major, even lethal, mechanical injury during the act of stinging. Stingray spines on the muscular tail can inflict major trauma, with cases of transection of

vessels, nerves, tendons and direct penetration of the chest and abdomen, including direct cardiac puncture. Such mechanical wounds can pose a great threat to life, but are beyond the scope of this chapter, as envenoming is not the significant problem in such cases.

Venomous fish exist in many families, representing hundreds of species, with venomous spines in a number of different locations, depending on species, including on the back (dorsal as in stonefish), pectoral, behind the head (particularly catfish) and even on the tail. A primitive venom gland surrounds the spine and as the spine is forced into the skin by mechanical pressure (such as by stepping on a stonefish or handling a fish) the gland is compressed, forcing venom up groves in the spine and into the victim.

Most venomous fish species have never had their venom studied. For those few that have been investigated, notably the stonefish, while the venom may contain a variety of components, in the clinical setting it is toxins causing pain and swelling that predominate. There is no evidence that the neurotoxin found in stonefish venom has any clinical effect in humans.

History

There is always a history of definite or likely exposure to a stinging fish, in a marine or freshwater environment, or of handling a fish out of water. This includes sudden pain in a foot after walking in water, such as reef walking, usually indicative of stepping on a fish, notably stonefish. The pain may be very severe, sufficient to cause collapse, but systemic symptoms are related principally to local pain, not general toxicity. There are very rare reports of pulmonary oedema following stonefish stings (in Madagascar). Portions of the sting may have been seen in the wound.

Examination

For venomous fish stings, there may be sting present in the wound(s). The number of wounds can be significant (i.e. for stonefish, as it determines antivenom dose). For stingray wounds, apart from residual sting left in the wound, careful examination to

determine the extent of any mechanical trauma is essential.

Investigations

There are no specific investigations for fish sting envenoming.

Differential diagnosis

The sharp and localised pain of a fish sting is distinctive and can be separated from jellyfish stings due to the tentacle tracks caused by the latter.

Treatment

With the exception of stonefish, for which there is an antivenom, fish stings must be treated symptomatically and supportively. Both for first aid and in-hospital care, hot water immersion appears effective at reducing pain in the short term. The contralateral limb should first be immersed in water that is hot, but not so hot that thermal injury might occur. The affected limb is then immersed, usually bringing rapid relief of pain. Unfortunately, pain may recur on removal from the water and if this persists, other analgesia must be considered, often a local or regional anaesthetic block in more severe cases. The wound must be examined for remnants of stings, which should be removed. The wound should be allowed to heal by secondary intention and the temptation to surgically close the wound resisted. For any wound that is extensive (i.e. many stingray injuries) a course of antibiotics should be considered. For stingray injuries with extensive trauma, surgical input on managing this injury should be paramount.

For stonefish, there is a specific antivenom in Australia, which can be given IM or IV, the dose depending on the number of stings. It is effective at reducing the severe pain and should be considered in all cases of stonefish sting with more than trivial symptoms.

Prognosis

With the exception of severe mechanical trauma from stingray injuries, the prognosis for fish stings is generally optimistic, with recovery likely. The greater the number of stings, the more likely that symptoms will be severe and possibly prolonged.

Prevention

Avoidance of contact with stinging fish is the obvious preventative measure. When reef walking or on sandy bottoms where stingrays may hide, avoid sudden movements, running into water, wear strong-soled reef shoes and observe and choose carefully when placing feet. Despite all such precautions, stings may occur, particularly if reef walking, by stepping on larger stonefish.

Controversies and future directions

❶ There are no major controversies for fish stings. There is uncertainty if stonefish antivenom is useful for stings by other types of fish. There is no formal study to validate such non-specific use, but anecdotal clinical experience suggests that this antivenom may work for some related species, including the bullrout.

❷ There is great scope for studies on fish sting venoms and for research into more targeted treatment strategies.

Venomous marine molluscs

Introduction

There are two groups of marine molluscs (snails) that are able to inflict major, even lethal, envenoming on humans. These are the blue-ringed octopus, from Australian and adjacent waters and selected cone snails, found widely in the Indo-Pacific area. Neither are a common cause of envenoming, surprisingly, since both groups are common – the blue-ringed octopus particularly, with its various species common all around the Australian coast.

The blue-ringed octopus has a potent paralysing neurotoxin, tetrodotoxin, in its saliva. Bites, which usually occur when the octopus is removed from the water and placed in contact with skin, are often painless and may go unnoticed until 5–20 minutes or so later, when paralytic features start to develop. These may rapidly progress to respiratory paralysis and collapse, with death possible in under an hour. The paralysis is a general flaccid paralysis.

Cone snails fire poisoned 'darts' at their prey, or human victims, the venom being both complex and incredibly potent, immobilising fish prey in a few seconds. In humans the sting may be painless or quite painful. Systemic envenoming, with collapse and flaccid paralysis, rapidly follows.

History

There is usually a clear history of picking up and handling a blue ringed octopus or cone snail. In significant cases, which are rare, envenoming is rapid, with neurotoxic symptoms quickly evident. The earliest feature of envenoming is often tingling of the lips.

Examination

The sting or bite site may not be readily evident. The key effects to exclude are those of progressive flaccid paralysis and cardiovascular collapse, notably hypotension.

Investigations

There are no investigations specific to envenoming by molluscs.

Differential diagnosis

The onset of progressive flaccid paralysis after a marine sting or bite is uncommon and apart from mollusc envenoming, the likely differential is sea snake bite, which may manifest as either paralysis and/or myolysis. However, the development of paralysis is much less acute than with mollusc envenoming.

Treatment

There are no antivenoms for venomous molluscs, so both first aid and treatment are supportive and symptomatic. Pressure immobilisation bandaging may reduce the rate of development of systemic envenoming, if applied early enough. The key requirement is to support respiratory function and blood pressure. The latter may require pressor therapy. The former may require intubation and mechanical ventilation, but this may not be for a prolonged period, often only for 6–12 hours, unlike snakebite, where ventilation may be needed for days, weeks, even months.

Prognosis

If respiratory support is instituted early, before irreversible hypoxic organ injury occurs, ultimate prognosis is good. Cases without evidence of significant systemic envenoming 6 hours post-exposure are unlikely to develop envenoming.

Prevention

The principal preventative measure is abstinence from contact with and certainly handling these molluscs. This may require local education programmes, particularly directed at children, who will find these small and attractive animals tempting to pick up.

Controversies

There are no major controversies in managing marine mollusc envenoming, in part reflecting the rarity of this clinical problem.

Further reading

While there are numerous papers on various aspects of envenoming, covering different regions, there are few texts giving a detailed overview of snakebite or other types of specific envenoming or clinical toxinology. Some recent key texts are noted here. A major source of information is the Clinical Toxinology Resources Website (www.toxinology.com), a detailed site, initially developed with public funds, global in scope.

Chippaux J-P. *Venins de Serpent et Envenimations*. IRD ed. Paris: 2002. p. 288 [French handbook on global snakebite].

Covacevich J, Davie P, Pearn J. *Toxic plants and animals: A guide for Australia*. Brisbane: Queensland Museum; 1987. p. 501 [a comprehensive textbook with a clinical focus].

Gopalakrishnakone P, Chou LM. *Snakes of medical importance (Asia-Pacific Region)*. Singapore: National University of Singapore; 1990. p. 670 [covers snakes in the designate region].

Goyffon M, Heurtault J. *La Fonction Venimeuse*. Paris: Masson; 1995. p. 284 [French handbook covering many aspects of toxinology].

Junghanss J, Bodio M. *Notfall-Handbuch Gifttiere: Diagnose, Therapie, Biologie*. Stuttgart: Georg Thieme Verlag; 1996. p. 646 [this German textbook covers a global spectrum of envenoming with a focus on management in EDs].

Mebs D. *Venomous and poisonous animals*. Boca Raton, FL: Medpharm/CRC Press; 2002. p. 339 [this textbook, beautifully illustrated in colour, covers the broad scope of venoms, the animals that produce them and their clinical effects and treatment – the focus is more on toxinology than detailed medical advice, but it is a valuable source of information].

Meier J, White J, editors. *Handbook of clinical toxinology of animal venoms and poisons*. Boca Raton, FL: CRC Press; 1995. p. 752 [this is the standard textbook for clinical toxinology and contains chapters covering all aspects of envenoming, especially snakebite, scorpion stings, spiderbite, tick envenoming and marine envenoming – the coverage is global, but with considerable detail for most regions and animal types].

Sutherland SK, Tibballs J. *Australian animal toxins.*
    Melbourne: Oxford University Press; 2001. p. 856 [a major
    work covering the Australian venomous fauna].
Warrell DA. WHO/SEARO guidelines for the clinical
    management of snake bites in the Southeast Asian region.
    SE Asian Journal of Tropical Medicine and Public Hygiene
    1999;**30**(Suppl 1):1–85.

Warrell DA, et al. *Oxford textbook of medicine.* Oxford: Oxford
    University Press; 1996 [this standard medical text includes
    an extensive chapter on envenoming].
White J. *CSL Antivenom handbook.* Melbourne: CSL; 2002. p.
    69 [a concise handbook on the diagnosis and
    treatment of envenoming by Australian fauna, which

is available in its entirety on the toxinology website:
    www.toxinology.com].
Williamson JA, Fenner PJ, Burnett JW, Rifkin JF. *Venomous and
    poisonous marine animals: A medical and biological
    handbook.* Sydney: University of NSW Press; 1996. p. 504
    [this is the major textbook covering marine toxinology].

22.2 Drowning

Simon Wood

ESSENTIALS

1 Drowning is defined as the process of experiencing respiratory impairment from immersion in liquid, regardless of the outcome.

2 Drowning is a leading cause of accidental death in Australian children. Children aged 0–4 years are the most vulnerable. The most common site of drowning in this age group is the domestic swimming pool.

3 There is no clinical or therapeutic difference between submersion in fresh or salt water.

4 The major pathophysiological consequence of submersion is hypoxic brain injury.

5 Pulmonary injury due to aspiration of water is an important clinical consideration in all submersion victims.

6 The mainstay of treatment is early effective oxygenation.

7 Whilst hypothermia may be protective in small children who suffer a submersion event, it does not reliably predict good outcome.

8 Response to resuscitation is the single most important predictor of outcome in children who have suffered submersion.

9 Isolation pool-fencing with a self-locking gate has been shown to effectively reduce submersion incidents in pre-school-age children.

Introduction

Definition

Traditionally *drowning* has been defined as death due to suffocation within 24 hours of submersion in a liquid medium and *near-drowning* as survival for 24 hours or more following such an incident.[1] Considerable confusion has surrounded the use of these terms. In part this is because the distinction between drowning and near-drowning often cannot be made before 24 hours, making the terms clinically irrelevant. In addition it has been suggested that the

use of a time limit for survival is not a scientific concept and is not in accordance with outcome parameters as used in the internationally accepted Utstein style.[1]

To address this issue the Utstein Taskforce on Drowning was convened in Amsterdam as part of the 2002 World Congress on Drowning. The International Liaison Committee on Resuscitation (ILCOR) has since endorsed a review of the terminology and defines drowning in the following way:

Drowning. Drowning is a process resulting in primary respiratory impairment from

submersion/immersion in a liquid medium. Implicit in this definition is that a liquid/air interface is present at the entrance of the victim's airway, preventing the victim from breathing air. The victim may live or die after this process, but whatever the outcome, he or she has been involved in a drowning incident.[2]

The term *submersion* is generally accepted to indicate an incident in which the victim's body is totally covered by water, while the term *immersion* refers to an incident in which the victim is only partially covered by water, although for drowning to occur the face and airway must at least be covered.[2]

ILCOR recommends that other terms such as *dry drowning* versus *wet drowning*, *active* versus *passive* versus *silent drowning*, *secondary drowning* and *near drowning* be abandoned.[2]

Epidemiology

In Australia drowning is a leading cause of accidental death in children. Its incidence peaks in early childhood and again in adolescence. Males outnumber females in both groups. Children under 5 years of age are the most vulnerable to drowning in Australia.[3] In the period between 1 July 2008 and 30 June 2009 there were 302 drowning deaths in Australian waterways. Children aged 0-4 years accounted for 11% of deaths overall and 74% of deaths under the age of 14 years. 59% of drowning deaths in the 0–4 years age group occurred in swimming pools, with around 84% of cases occurring from wandering or falling in.[4]

Risk groups for childhood drowning are children aged 0–4 years, children living in cities with high swimming pool to population ratios, children living in hot climates, children living in areas with lack of isolation pool fencing, and Indigenous children.[5] More toddlers drown in swimming pools than from any other cause.[6] Most children who drown in pools are out of sight for less than 5 minutes and are in the care of one or both parents.[7] Around the home small children can also drown in baths, buckets, and garden ponds. Up to 8% of cases of drowning in small children in the domestic setting may be secondary to non-accidental injury.[8]

While pool-fencing legislation has proven to be effective in reducing the incidence of drowning in small children it has had little impact on rates of drowning in older children and adolescents. In this group alcohol, suicide, and risk-taking behaviours are important factors that lead to increased risk of drowning.[8]

Aetiology

Drowning is most commonly a primary event. In children it most often occurs when the victim is unable to rescue him or herself after entering the water, as in the case of a toddler falling into a swimming pool, or an infant drowning in a bath whilst unattended. In older children and adolescents fatigue while swimming may play a role, but drowning in these age groups is more likely to be secondary to other causes.

Drowning can occur secondarily to a number of underlying causes. These should be considered during assessment of the submersion victim. Individuals with seizure disorders have up to 19-times higher risk for drowning accidents, regardless of age.[3,8,9] Prolonged QT-syndrome leading to dysrhythmia has been implicated as a significant cause of drowning, although the true incidence of this condition in drowned children is unknown. Ethanol is an important risk factor for drowning injury, particularly in adolescents. Elevated serum ethanol levels are documented in 10–50% of adolescent drownings.[8] Head and cervical trauma from diving and boating-related accidents may also lead to drowning as a secondary event. Non-accidental injury is an important cause

of drowning in infants and smaller children, particularly in events that occur in the home, such as in baths and buckets. Up to 8% of drownings presenting to tertiary paediatric centres may be attributed to child abuse.[8]

The immersion syndrome is sudden loss of consciousness secondary to a bradycardia, or tachyarrhythmia induced by contact with water at a temperature of at least 5°C below body temperature. This can lead secondarily to drowning. The immersion syndrome can occur in water with temperatures as warm as 31°C, although it is more likely to occur in much colder water. Wetting the face before entering the water may reduce its incidence.[1]

Pathophysiology

The two most significant pathophysiological consequences of submersion are hypoxia from asphyxiation during the submersion itself, and aspiration of water into the lungs. It is the severity of the initial hypoxic insult that is the major determinant of outcome. If the initial hypoxic event is survived, the degree of hypoxic organ injury and pulmonary injury secondary to aspiration become the clinically important factors.

Much that is known about the sequence of events following submersion has come from animal models. Aspiration of water initially causes breath-holding or laryngospasm and the resultant asphyxiation leads to progressive hypoxia. Active and passive swallowing of water follows and, as hypoxia worsens, breath-holding and laryngospasm are terminated, resulting in aspiration of water into the lungs.[1]

Anoxia lasting 1–3 minutes can shut down both the brain and the heart, causing loss of consciousness and hypoxic cardiac arrest. Rescue and early institution of cardiopulmonary resuscitation can salvage myocardial function, but the brain is more sensitive to hypoxic injury and it is the severity of this injury that determines outcome. Effects of hypoxia on other organ systems are delayed. Profound hypoxia can cause an acute respiratory distress syndrome, which develops within hours and further worsens hypoxic injury. Posthypoxic cerebral oedema is a major complication and can develop 6–12 hours following successful initial resuscitation from a serious submersion

event. Most paediatric drowning deaths in hospital are due to hypoxic cerebral injury rather than pulmonary complications.[8]

The average volume of water aspirated in human drownings is 10–15 mL kg^{-1}. Aspiration of volumes as little as 1–3 mL kg^{-1} of water can cause profound alterations in gas exchange and subsequent ventilatory abnormalities.[10] Laryngospasm is thought to occur in 10–15% of drowning victims and a subset of patients who drown without evidence of significant aspiration of water at post-mortem, so-called *dry-drowning*, has been described. This concept has recently been questioned and it has been suggested that in these cases death has occurred prior to submersion.[1] Regardless of whether dry-drowning is a true clinical entity, or whether laryngospasm has occurred at the time of submersion, aspiration of water into the lungs remains a clinically important consideration in the management of all drowning victims.

Despite the large literature dedicated to the subject, there are no clinically or therapeutically important differences between drowning in fresh or salt water.[1,8] Pulmonary injury is related more to the amount of water aspirated than to the composition of the water itself. Both fresh and salt water cause loss of pulmonary surfactant, non-cardiogenic pulmonary oedema, impaired alveolar-capillary gas exchange, and increased intrapulmonary shunting with the potential for profound hypoxia.[1] Aspiration of water that is contaminated with particulate matter or bacteria can lead to complications from obstruction of small airways or increased risk of pulmonary infection, although neither is seen in the majority of patients.[11] If present, evidence of significant pulmonary injury due to aspiration will usually manifest or progress within hours of rescue. Delayed onset of respiratory distress and hypoxia, the so-called 'delayed immersion syndrome' or 'secondary drowning' has been refuted by recent evidence.[8]

Clinically significant electrolyte and fluid volume abnormalities are rarely seen in cases of drowning in humans despite being demonstrated in animal models.[1,3,8,11] Occasionally a mild hyponatraemia, which self-corrects without specific therapy, is observed.[8] Theoretical exceptions are drownings occurring in hypertonic solutions, such as the Dead Sea, or water contaminated with industrial waste.

Hypothermia is an important issue following drowning, particularly in small children who have a large body surface area to weight ratio. Cooling can occur at the time of submersion, but can also continue following rescue and during attempted resuscitation due to heat loss through evaporation. Hypothermia can confer some degree of protection from cerebral hypoxia, particularly in small children. Multiple case reports in the literature attest to intact survival of both children and adults following prolonged (>15 minutes) drownings in icy water (water temperature <10°C).[12] Profound hypothermia and subsequent intact survival has also been documented in children suffering drowning in non-icy water and in temperate climates.

The mechanisms of temperature drop and cerebral protection remain unclear. Surface cooling at the time of submersion is thought to be insufficient on its own to provide central cooling of a degree that confers cerebral protection. Other mechanisms of heat loss, such as via ingestion and/or aspiration of cold water, are not supported by quantitative evidence. Some authors suggest that core temperature drop is insufficient on its own to explain the cerebral protection afforded by hypothermia.[13] The diving reflex, in which blood is shunted from the limbs and splanchnic circulation to the brain and heart alongside slowing of the heart rate and reduction of the basal metabolic rate, has been suggested as being an important mechanism for cerebral protection in children.[13] There is little clinical evidence to indicate that the diving reflex is sufficiently active in humans, even small children, to confer any benefit on its own.[1,8] It is most likely that a combination of the effects of the diving reflex initially, followed by rapid and continued cooling, is what underlies the cerebral preservation that is sometimes seen in small children who suffer submersion and who are profoundly hypothermic.

By whatever mechanism cooling occurs, and whether the diving reflex plays a significant role in cerebral protection or not, hypothermia in the drowning victim, particularly if the victim is an infant or young child, should be considered to be an indication for aggressive and prolonged resuscitation efforts. This issue is discussed further in Chapter 22.4 on cold injuries.

History

Key points in history are summarised in Table 22.2.1. Broad areas in history include details of the drowning event itself, details of rescue and resuscitation, response to resuscitative efforts, possible underlying causal factors, and medical conditions that may influence recovery. Features of history that alert to the possibility of non-accidental injury should be recognised. These include a history that is inconsistent or a history that is incompatible with the victim's developmental level.

Examination

Examination is dictated by the clinical condition of the victim on arrival in the emergency department (ED) and is mainly directed at assessing the degree of neurological impairment due to hypoxic cerebral injury, the severity of respiratory embarrassment due to aspiration, and cardiovascular instability due to a combination of the initial insult and/or ongoing hypoxia. In broad terms drowning victims arriving in the ED will fall into two categories: (1) those who respond to minimal resuscitation and who will generally do well with minimal complications; and (2) those 'high risk' patients who fail to respond to resuscitation and who will require ongoing resuscitation and/or monitoring.[8]

Vital signs, including oxygen saturation, a bedside blood glucose estimate, and a temperature should be recorded on all

Table 22.2.1 Key points in history
The circumstances leading to the submersion
The location of the submersion
Water and environmental temperatures
Duration of submersion
Time from when the victim was last seen to the time when found (if the submersion was unwitnessed)
Time from rescue to effective CPR
Time to first gasp or return of spontaneous circulation
Elements of basic and advanced life support employed
Symptomatology following successful resuscitation
Medical history particularly with regard to possible predisposing factors (i.e. neurological disorders, such as epilepsy)
Factors that may complicate recovery (i.e. respiratory illness, such as asthma)

patients. It is important to detect hypothermia, particularly in patients who have failed to respond to resuscitation efforts. Small children may rapidly become hypothermic due to evaporative heat loss during resuscitation efforts and transfer to the hospital. Apparent lifelessness and severe bradycardia due to profound hypothermia need to be distinguished from asystole and brain death. Assessment of cardiac rhythm requires observation of the continuous electrocardiograph (ECG) monitor for up to a minute to detect very slow heart rates that can occur in profound hypothermia. Similarly, lack of response to painful stimulus, along with fixed and dilated pupils should not be interpreted as brain death in the presence of profound hypothermia.

Depending on the clinical condition of the victim at arrival, neurological evaluation may range from an assessment of level of responsiveness as graded by the AVPU or Glasgow coma score (GCS) and pupillary reaction, to a focused neurological examination looking for focal deficit or spinal-cord injury. An assessment should always be made for the possibility of cranial or cervical spine trauma, particularly in diving-related accidents. Trauma to other areas of the body should also be sought.

In the awake child, examination of the respiratory system can establish a clinical baseline against which subsequent deterioration can be measured. Work of breathing should be assessed, and abnormalities found on auscultation, such as crackles and wheezes, should be noted. The finding of signs on an initial examination indicates the possibility of significant aspiration and dictates close observation to identify deterioration. A clear chest initially does not exclude aspiration and a period of observation and re-examination is necessary in all children who have been symptomatic following drowning.

Investigations

Investigations will also be dictated by the clinical condition of the patient on arrival in the ED. A child who has suffered a drowning injury and who is alert and asymptomatic on arrival requires little in the way of laboratory or radiological evaluation. The more symptomatic or seriously unwell child may benefit from further evaluation with laboratory and radiological investigations.

Useful investigations include arterial blood gas (ABG) analysis, serum glucose, and chest radiography. ABG analysis may demonstrate a metabolic acidosis, which confirms a significant drowning injury.[8] The severity of the acidosis reflects the severity of the hypoxic insult as well as ongoing hypoxic injury. Profound acidosis (pH <7.10) implies a poorer prognosis but needs to be interpreted in the clinical context.[14] ABG analysis can be used to guide decisions regarding oxygenation and ventilation, and serial determinations may be useful in monitoring and quantifying deterioration of pulmonary function due to non-cardiogenic pulmonary oedema secondary to hypoxia or aspiration. Determination of the blood glucose level is important in any critically ill child as hypoglycaemia can complicate physiological stress and should be actively treated. Hyperglycaemia in a comatose child, although not requiring treatment, implies a poor prognosis.[8] Initially the chest X-ray (CXR) may be normal, may demonstrate pulmonary infiltrates, or may display frank pulmonary oedema. Abnormalities detected on an early CXR mandate close observation and the patient should be monitored for clinical deterioration. Repeated CXR may be required but should be dictated by the patient's clinical condition.

Other investigations that may be helpful include baseline electrolytes and full blood count, although rarely are any clinically or therapeutically significant abnormalities found on initial determinations. Blood ethanol levels may be relevant, depending on the age of the patient. A 12-lead ECG may be helpful in excluding prolonged QT syndrome as a cause for the drowning event.[10] Cervical spine films should be considered if cervical injury is suspected or the drowning is secondary to a diving accident.

Differential diagnosis

The major issues in differential diagnosis relate to the cause of the drowning event. Underlying medical conditions, such as epilepsy, should be considered. Trauma, either leading to or as a consequence of the drowning, should be recognised. Non-accidental injury should be suspected when there are inconsistencies in the history.

Severe hypothermia (core temperature less than 29°C) can mimic irretrievable cardiorespiratory arrest and brain death. The profound bradycardia associated with very low core body temperature can easily be confused with brady-asystole secondary to hypoxic injury and will not respond to usual resuscitation measures until hypothermia is corrected. Similarly, severe hypothermia can cause depression of cerebral function leading to unresponsiveness and fixed, dilated pupils, indistinguishable from irreversible hypoxic cerebral injury.[15] Failure of the core temperature to rise despite aggressive, active rewarming may be the only indication that death has occurred.

Treatment

Treatment of the drowning victim occurs in three major phases: (1) rescue and resuscitation at the scene; (2) initial assessment and stabilisation in the emergency department; and (3) subsequent observation and supportive care in the hospital ward, intensive-care unit (ICU), or after discharge.

Early institution of effective cardiopulmonary resuscitation with an emphasis on providing adequate ventilation is the key task in pre-hospital management. Manoeuvres to drain the lungs of water have not been shown to be clinically effective and may increase the risk of aspiration of gastric contents. The Heimlich manoeuvre should be reserved for cases in which repeated attempts to position the airway and provide ventilation have been unsuccessful or when foreign body aspiration and obstruction is suspected.[1] Emesis is common in drowning victims, both spontaneously and as a complication of resuscitation, and aspiration of gastric contents is a major potential complication following rescue. Spontaneously breathing patients should be managed and transported in the right lateral decubitus position. Cricoid pressure may reduce the risk of gastric distension and aspiration during cardiopulmonary resuscitation but requires an additional rescuer.[1]

Hypothermia can be exacerbated by ongoing evaporative heat loss during resuscitation efforts following rescue. Wet clothing should be removed and the patient should be dried if possible. Exposure during cardiopulmonary resuscitation (CPR) should be minimised as much as is practicable. If hypothermia is severe at the scene (<30°C), rewarming should probably be delayed until adequate ventilation and oxygenation has been instituted.[15] Invasive rewarming techniques should be reserved for the hospital phase of management.

Treatment in the ED involves provision of adequate oxygenation, stabilisation of the body temperature, prevention of complications such as aspiration, and assessment of the patient's clinical status in order to make decisions regarding ongoing management and disposition.

Supplemental oxygen should be administered at concentrations and via delivery systems appropriate to the patient's oxygen requirement. Continuous pulse oximetry and serial estimations of respiratory rate and work of breathing should be undertaken during observation in the ED to determine worsening or improvement of the patient's respiratory status. If available, non-invasive ventilation techniques, although not extensively evaluated in paediatric drowning victims, may be considered if the oxygen requirement outstrips conventional mechanisms of oxygen delivery. Intubation to isolate the airway and provide ventilation with positive end-expiratory pressure (PEEP) may be required in patients with depressed neurological status or if respiratory compromise progresses despite supplemental oxygen therapy. Failure to maintain an SaO_2 of greater than 90% with an FiO_2 of 0.50 or higher, a $PaCO_2$ of more than 35 mmHg, an abnormally high respiratory rate (>50 bpm) or inadequate spontaneous ventilation, are all indications that mechanical ventilation is likely to be required.[1,10] Passage of a nasogastric or orogastric tube, if cranial trauma is suspected, should be performed following intubation to decompress the stomach and facilitate mechanical ventilation.

Diuretics are not recommended in the management of non-cardiogenic pulmonary oedema.[1,8,10] Steroids have not been shown to be useful in the management of aspiration pneumonitis and the role of antibiotics in this setting remains controversial.[1,8,10] Prophylactic antibiotics are generally not recommended, although they are sometimes used when there is a history of drowning in heavily contaminated or polluted water. In general, antibiotics should be reserved for patients who develop signs of pulmonary infection, such as fever or leukocytosis.[1] Fluid therapy should be judicious and should be aimed at maintaining adequate circulatory status and euglycaemia without overloading the patient.

Hypothermic patients should be warmed once adequate ventilation and oxygenation has been assured. Awake and spontaneously breathing patients with mild to moderate hypothermia (core temperature >32°C) require passive or external active rewarming techniques only. Patients with severe hypothermia (core temperature <32°C) who are obtunded or in cardiorespiratory arrest will require invasive active rewarming techniques. These are discussed fully elsewhere in this text (see Chapter 22.4 on cold injuries). Whilst there is increasing support for the use of therapeutic hypothermia (cooling to a core temperature of 33°C) following cardiac arrest in adults, and the technique has been used in adults following drowning, its role in the management of children remains to be established and may, in fact, be associated with harm.[16]

In the setting of cardiorespiratory arrest and severe hypothermia, resuscitation efforts should be continued until the core temperature has risen to around 32°C before a decision to cease resuscitation is made. Although there are no clear guidelines to determine how long efforts at rewarming should be continued, failure to effect rewarming despite maximal invasive efforts may be an indication that continuing resuscitation is futile. The decision to cease resuscitative efforts in the presence of persistent severe hypothermia should follow a multidisciplinary approach involving the emergency physician, paediatrician and/or paediatric intensivist and other members of the resuscitation team, together with the parents and family. Cardiorespiratory arrest on arrival in the ED in a patient with a core temperature above 32°C carries a uniformly poor prognosis and prolonged efforts at resuscitation are generally not indicated.

Treatment in the ICU involves provision of ventilatory support to ensure adequate oxygenation, maintenance of cardiovascular stability, minimisation of secondary brain injury due to cerebral oedema, management of hypoxic organ injury, and management of the complications of pulmonary aspiration. The use of PEEP in drowning victims ventilated in the ICU is controversial. Although PEEP may be necessary to maintain adequate oxygenation, some authorities express concern regarding the potential reduction in cerebral venous outflow and subsequent increase in intracerebral pressure associated with its use. PEEP may have unfavourable effects on cardiovascular status and may increase the risk of barotrauma in already insulted lungs.[8] Other ventilation strategies to minimise non-cardiogenic pulmonary oedema and barotrauma, such as pressure-control ventilation with low-peak airway pressure and prolonged expiratory time, and permissive hypercapnia have been suggested, although again the trade-off is the risk in adversely influencing intracerebral pressure.[8] Various measures to provide cerebral resuscitation and control intracranial pressure have been evaluated in the literature and have generally been found to be not helpful in influencing outcome.[1] In general, the aim should be to maintain adequate cerebral oxygenation and to minimise causes of secondary cerebral injury such as hypotension, hypercapnia, and hypo/hyperglycaemia.

Disposition

Disposition is dictated by the clinical condition of the patient in the ED, the nature of the drowning event, the need for resuscitation, and the presence or absence of other factors, such as trauma, suspicion of non-accidental injury, and underlying or complicating medical conditions. In general, all victims of drowning will require some period of observation.

The alert, otherwise healthy, patient who is asymptomatic or who has suffered only mild, transient symptoms following a brief drowning can be safely discharged if they remain well after 6–8 hours of observation.[8] Patients with a history of drowning for longer than 1 minute, a period of cyanosis or apnoea, or who required pulmonary resuscitation, should be admitted for observation for 24 hours, or at least overnight, even if they are well in the ED. Although recent evidence discredits the idea of the 'delayed immersion syndrome', cases of fulminant pulmonary oedema up to 12 hours after drowning have been reported as occurring in patients who appear well and display normal chest radiography in the ED.[1] Any child discharged from the ED following a drowning event should be in the care of a reliable and responsible adult. Instructions should be given to re-present for further medical assessment in the event of any change in the child's respiratory status.

Patients who have suffered trauma may require admission for the management of their injuries. Children with underlying cardiac or respiratory disorders, those who suffer drowning secondary to a pre-existing illness, and victims of suspected non-accidental injury also warrant inpatient evaluation.

Asymptomatic children and children with mild symptoms who are admitted for observation can be managed in a general ward environment, provided that there is the facility to increase the level of monitoring and care should it be required. Children who have required CPR, who have abnormal chest radiography or ABGs on arrival in the ED, or who have required ventilatory support, should be admitted to a high-dependency unit or ICU for observation and management.[1] Transfer to a facility that provides paediatric ICU should be considered for all such patients prior to clinical deterioration.

Prognosis

Most children who suffer drowning injury will either survive intact or die. Death occurs in 30–50% of drowning victims, most of these not surviving to treatment in the ED. A small proportion of victims will be left with severe neurological deficit, either persistent vegetative state or spastic quadriplegia. Mild learning deficits may occur in apparently intact survivors, although the extent of these and the impact on subsequent function have not been clearly quantified.[8] In general, however, the prognosis of children who suffer drowning events and survive to hospital admission is excellent.[17]

Despite a large body of literature dedicated to the subject, the factors that predict prognosis in the ED following childhood drowning injury remain poorly defined. There are no prospectively validated scoring systems and most of the literature is based on retrospective data. Individual case reports of children surviving prolonged resuscitative efforts with good outcome continue to arise in the popular press and medical literature.

Factors elicited in history that influence prognosis are duration of submersion, time to institution of effective CPR, and time to first spontaneous gasp, all three reflecting the duration of the hypoxic cerebral insult. Duration of submersion can often be difficult to determine but submersion for longer than 5 minutes is associated with a poorer prognosis.[14] Although time to institution of effective CPR can be similarly difficult to ascertain accurately, delays of longer than 10–20 minutes are also associated with poorer outcomes, while early effective CPR has been shown to be an important factor in improving survival after rescue.[14]

As already discussed, hypothermia may be protective in small children who suffer drowning, particularly, but not exclusively, if the drowning has occurred in cold or icy water. However, neither hypothermia nor water temperature can be reliably used to predict outcome.[18,19]

Response to resuscitation following rescue and prior to arrival in the ED is the single most important indicator of outcome in children who have suffered drowning. Children who arrive conscious in the ED after successful resuscitation have almost universally excellent outcomes. Similarly, lack of response to early resuscitation efforts and coma on arrival in the ED are associated with a poor outcome.[10] In a classification system based on the neurological status of the patient on arrival in the ED, it was discovered that less than 15% of patients who were unresponsive and flaccid to painful stimulation had intact survival. This is supported by the findings of other investigators that a GCS of 5 or less on arrival in the ED is associated with a dismal outcome, either death or severe neurological disability.[1,20] Lack of pupillary response in the ED has similarly been identified as a predictor of dismal outcome.[21] The caveat concerning the use of level of responsiveness and pupillary reaction to predict poor prognosis and withdraw treatment applies to the child who presents with severe hypothermia, which may mimic brain death. In these

patients lack of response to aggressive rewarming and resuscitation becomes a surrogate indicator of poor outcome. In non-hypothermic patients who are in cardio-respiratory arrest, a lack of response to 25 minutes of effective advanced life support measures is almost universally associated with poor outcome.[8] It should be noted, however, that studies of outcome following out-of-hospital cardiac arrest in children indicate that children who suffer cardiac arrest secondary to drowning have significantly better outcomes than those who suffer cardiac arrest from other causes.

Prevention

Drowning remains a leading cause of accidental death in toddlers and adolescents in Australia. Most drowning-prevention strategies are aimed at the small child who drowns after falling into the domestic swimming pool, with few or none aimed at older children and adolescents.

Although programmes to prevent drowning by teaching children under the age of 4 to swim remain unproven, there is increasing evidence that such programmes may be effective and at least are not associated with an increased risk of drowning. One recently reported case–control study demonstrated an 88% reduction in the risk of drowning in children aged 1 to 4 years, although the 95% confidence intervals were wide (3–99%).[22]

Public-education programmes outlining the need to provide adult supervision when children are near water may be helpful. Pool alarms, pool covers, and fencing that does not isolate the pool from the home are probably not effective, although evidence is lacking. Isolation or four-sided fencing with a self-locking or dynamic gate, on the other hand, has been shown to effectively reduce drowning incidents by up to 50%, in both Australia and New Zealand, and in the United States.[8] Pool-fencing legislation exists in Australia, but is not uniform across states. Compliance with legislation remains incomplete. Further research is required to aid in establishing uniform pool-fencing requirements based on Standards Australia specifications.[6]

Controversies and future directions

❶ The role of therapeutic hypothermia following cardiac arrest due to drowning in children is controversial.

❷ Prospective collection of data on drowning victims is needed to generate more useful information regarding prognosis. Scoring systems for prognosis should also be prospectively validated.

❸ Further research regarding preventative strategies is required. Areas of interest would be the relationship between swimming lessons and drowning and the development of standardised and uniform legislation pertaining to pool fencing in Australia.

❹ Preventive educational programmes aimed at older children and adolescents are lacking, and are an area of possible future development in public health.

References

1. Orlowski JP, Spilzman D. Drowning: Rescue, resuscitation, reanimation. *Pediatr Clin North Am* 2001;**48**(3):627–46.
2. Idris AH, Berg RA, Bierens J, et al. Recommended guidelines for uniform reporting of data from drowning. The 'Utstein' style. ILCOR Advisory Statement. *Circulation* 2003;**108**:2565–74.
3. Mackie IJ. Patterns of drowning in Australia, 1992–1997. *Med J Aust* 1999;**171**:587–90.
4. Royal Life Saving Society Australia. The National Drowning Report. Sydney: RLSSA. Available from http://www.royallifesaving.com.au; 2009 [accessed 26.10.10].
5. Edmond KM, Attia JR, D'Este CA, Condon JT. Drowning and near-drowning in Northern Territory children. *Med J Aust* 2001;**175**:605–8.
6. Pitt WR, Cass DT. Preventing children drowning in Australia. *Med J Aust* 2001;**175**:603–4.
7. Moon RE, Long RJ. Drowning and near-drowning. *Emerg Med* 2002;**14**:377–86.
8. Quan L. Near-drowning. *Pediatr Rev* 1999;**20**(8):255–60.
9. Bell GS, Gaitatzis A, Bell CL, et al. Drowning in people with epilepsy. How great is the risk? *Neurology* 2008;**71**:578–82.
10. Sachdeva RC. Environmental emergencies. Near drowning. *Crit Care Clin* 1999;**15**(2):81–96.
11. Modell JH. Drowning. *N Engl J Med* 1993;**328**(4):253–6.
12. Orlowski JP. Drowning, near-drowning, and ice-water submersions. *Pediatr Clin North Am* 1987;**34**(1):75–92.
13. Gooden BA. Why some people do not drown. Hypothermia versus the diving response. *Med J Aust* 1992;**157**:629–32.
14. Orlowski JP. Prognostic factors in pediatric cases of drowning and near-drowning. *J Am Coll Emerg Phys* 1979;**8**(5):176–9.
15. Theilade D. The danger of fatal misjudgement in hypothermia after immersion. Successful resuscitation following immersion for 25 minutes. *Anaesthesia* 1977;**32**:889–92.
16. Williamson JP, Illing R, Gertler P, Braude S. Near-drowning treated with therapeutic hypothermia. *Med J Aust* 2004;**181**(9):500–1.

17. Pearn J. Neurological and psychometric studies in children surviving freshwater immersion accidents. *Lancet* 1977;1(8001):7–9.
18. Suominen PK, Korpela RE, Silfvast TGO, Olkkola KT. Does water temperature affect outcome of nearly drowned children? *Resuscitation* 1997;35: 111–5.
19. Conn AW, Montes JE, Barker GA, Edmonds JF. Cerebral salvage in near-drowning following neurological classification by triage. *Can Anaesth Soc J* 1980;27 (3):201–9.
20. Dean JM, Kaufman ND. Prognostic indicators in pediatric near-drowning: the Glasgow coma scale. *Crit Care Med* 1981;9(7):536–9.
21. Graf WD, Cummings P, Quan L, Brutaco D. Predicting outcome in pediatric submersion victims. *Ann Emerg Med* 1995;26(3):312–9.
22. Brenner RA, Saluja Taneja G, Haynie DL, et al. Association between swimming lessons and drowning in childhood. A case-control study. *Arch Pediatr Adolesc Med* 2009;163(3):203–10.

22.3 Heat-induced illness

Michael Ragg

ESSENTIALS

1 Most heat-induced illness in children is due to overheating from exogenous sources.

2 Children are particularly susceptible to heat-related illness due to their unique physiology.

3 Certain genetic and dermatological disorders in children put them at high risk of heat-related illness.

4 Genuine heat stroke is a true medical emergency. It is characterised by a core body temperature above 40.5 Celsius in association with acute mental state changes.

5 Immediate aggressive cooling methods should be instituted for heat stroke.

6 Children account for almost one-fifth of all cases of malignant hyperthermia. Dantrolene should be given early for suspected cases. Approximately 50% of cases have a gene defect of the ryanodine receptor.

Introduction

Hyperthermia in the paediatric patient differs physiologically from fever. Fever is caused by an elevation of body temperature secondary to regulation by the hypothalamus. High body temperature not caused by hypothalamic thermoregulatory mechanisms is usually caused in children by one of the following: prolonged exposure to high ambient temperature (overheating), increased heat production or reduced heat loss. In the neonate and small infant, overheating is almost always the cause.

In children, heat-related illness is the second most common cause of non-traumatic death after heart disease.[1] Children are particularly at risk because of the following:

- Children have a greater body surface area relative to mass and therefore are more susceptible to radiant heat.

- Children have fewer cardiovascular compensatory mechanisms to deal with heat insult.
- Young children, particularly, produce less sweat, which limits their ability to lose heat through evaporation.
- Children depend on parents or adult caregivers to protect them from exogenous heat sources and cannot manipulate their environment to cool themselves.[2]

Certain genetic disorders such as ectodermal dysplasia and Fabry's disease also put children at risk of heat-related illness.[3] In these conditions, there is an impaired ability to dissipate heat through sweating.

Rising temperatures and more extreme weather events due to climate change have the potential to increase the incidence of heat-related illness in children.

Causes of heat-related illness

❶ Overheating
Usually seen in the setting of high ambient temperature and humidity. Examples are athletics, summertime sporting events and during heat waves. Young children left in cars are also particularly at risk. A review of 171 cases of heat-related car deaths found that in approximately 25% of cases the child gained access to an unlocked vehicle and in 75% of cases the child was left by an adult.[4]

❷ Increased heat production:
Metabolic (e.g. hyperthyroidism)
Drugs (e.g. anticholinergics such as atropine, sympathomimetics, aspirin, neuroleptic agents, selective serotonin reuptake inhibitor drugs)
Seizures.

❸ Decreased heat loss:
Over-wrapped babies
Excess clothing on hot/humid days
Disease states (e.g. cystic fibrosis)
Heart disease
Drugs (e.g. phenothiazines, anticholinergics).

Clinical syndromes
The neonate/infant

Overheating is the most common cause in the neonate and infant. It is important to distinguish the healthy infant who is overheated from the febrile infant (Table 22.3.1).[5]

Mild overheating is usually not dangerous to infants though there may be some association with apnoeic episodes in premature babies.[5] Hyperthermia from overheating, however, is dangerous and has been linked

Table 22.3.1 The overheated and febrile infant

Overheated infant	Febrile infant
High rectal temp	High rectal temperature
Warm hands and feet	Cool hands and feet
Pink skin	Pale skin
Extended posture	Lethargic
Healthy appearance	Looks unwell
Abdomen temperature > hand temperature by <2 degrees	Abdomen exceeds hand skin temperature by >3 degrees

with sudden death,[6] particularly in families with a history of malignant hyperthermia.

Babies with heat-related illness may present like any seriously ill infant. Hewson's work has summarised this as A,B,C, fluids in and out approach.[7]

Heat syncope

Heat syncope commonly involves children who have been standing for prolonged periods in hot/humid weather or who have undergone strenuous exertion.

Heat cramps

Heat cramps occur in the setting of strenuous exercise in hot/humid conditions. A relative lack of body salt plays a part. Heat cramps can be very painful; however, most last for less than 1 minute. Abdominal muscle cramps have been known to simulate an acute abdomen.[8]

Heat exhaustion

Heat exhaustion in children presents as hyperpyrexia, vomiting, headache, lethargy and weakness with a normal mental state. The major problem is body water depletion; however, in some paediatric patients (e.g. cystic fibrosis where greater amounts of salt are lost in their sweat), heat exhaustion may occur predominantly due to salt depletion.[8]

Heat stroke

Heat stroke is defined as a core body temperature >40.5°C + acute mental state changes. There are two types: exertional and classical. In the paediatric population, exertional heat stroke is most likely to occur in the adolescent who is exercising vigorously in a hot and humid environment. Sweating is usually present in this group. Classical heat stroke, however, may be seen during heat waves or when children are left in cars in hot weather.

Irritability, confusion, ataxia are common. Seizures may be seen, particularly during cooling. Coma may be the most common presentation; however, the child's conscious state may improve in the pre-hospital environment.

Other serious complications of heat stroke include cerebral oedema, liver injury, renal failure secondary to rhabdomyolysis, non-cardiogenic pulmonary oedema and disseminated intravascular coagulation.

See Table 22.3.2 for comparison of signs and symptoms of heat-induced syndromes.

Other heat-related syndromes

Malignant hyperthermia (MH) is usually seen in the paediatric patient after general anaesthesia. 75% of victims have no family history and 20.9% have had a previous 'normal' anaesthetic.[9] Mutations in the gene that programmes the ryanodine receptor, which is a tetrameric calcium release channel in the sarcoplasmic reticulum, are associated with malignant hyperthermia.[10] This gene defect of the ryanodine receptor is present in 50% of cases. Approximately 18% of all cases of malignant hyperthermia occur in children, and their mortality rate is lower as compared to adults.[11]

Initially, an increase in heart rate is followed by an elevation of blood pressure. Because these children are often paralysed, tachypnoea may not be seen. Elevation of the end tidal CO_2 is also an early sign. Muscle rigidity or increased tone may become apparent and the body temperature rises at a rate of 1–2 degrees Celsius every 5 minutes. When succinylcholine is used, however, an acceleration of the syndrome may occur. Hyperkalaemia, hypercalcaemia, metabolic acidaemia and myoglobinuria follow.

The condition of masseter muscle rigidity (MMR) is said to be associated with malignant hyperthermia. The peak age group is 8–12 years. It occurs after administration of succinylcholine. In approximately 50% of patients MH occurs after MMR is first seen. The rigidity can usually be overcome with effort and resolves after 2–3 minutes. Repeat doses of succinylcholine do not help.

The association between MH and skeletal abnormalities such as osteogenesis imperfecta is unclear.[9]

Serotonin syndrome, neuroleptic malignant syndrome (NMS) and anticholinergic syndrome: Serotonin syndrome is the clinical syndrome seen in the setting of excessive serotonin neurotransmission as a result of the ingestion of serotonergic agents. The triad of clinical features of the serotonin syndrome can be grouped under the headings of: central nervous system (CNS), autonomic and neuromuscular. NMS is a rare but potentially lethal syndrome, the exact aetiology of which is unclear. It is seen in children and adolescents taking antipsychotic medication. It has been suggested that the duration of NMS was one-third shorter in children taking atypical antipsychotics when compared with older, more

Table 22.3.2 Comparative table of the signs and symptoms of heat-induced syndromes

Condition	Symptoms	Signs
Heat syncope	Dizziness, feeling faint, may have brief loss of consciousness	Pallor, sweating, moist and cool skin, normal body temperature
Heat cramps	Painful, brief muscle cramps during or after strenuous exercise	Spasm of affected muscle group, body temperature usually normal
Heat exhaustion	Vomiting, headache, lethargy, weakness, normal mental state	Signs of dehydration, tachycardia, orthostatic hypotension, core temperature <40°C
Heat stroke	Episode of loss of consciousness common, neurological symptoms, irritability, confusion	Core temperature >40.5°C, acute change in mental state, sweating often present if exertional heat stroke

typical agents.[12] Methylphenidate (Ritalin) has been implicated in NMS. The anticholinergic syndrome is usually seen in the setting of deliberate self-poisoning with potent anticholinergic agents.[13] Clinically there are both central and peripheral features. The latter are an extension of the physiological effects of blocking cholinergic receptors.

Drug-related: amphetamine use (e.g. ecstasy at rave parties) and other drugs (e.g. salicylates, anticholinergics) can cause heat-related emergencies in the adolescent group. Vigorous activity, high ambient temperatures and ingestion of amphetamine compounds contribute to the risk of hyperthermia at rave parties.[14]

Investigations

Heat-related illness in children is diagnosed on clinical criteria and rectal temperature. Investigations are directed at the complications of heat-related illness in the paediatric patient.

Children who present with heat syncope or heat cramps usually do not require any investigations. Those children with more severe heat-related illness, however, require further work up. In heat exhaustion, basic bloods including full blood examination, urea and electrolytes, as well as serum creatinine kinase and glucose should be performed. Urinalysis would also be indicated.

The paediatric patient with heat stroke or other life-threatening hyperpyrexial illness requires full investigation: full blood examination, electrolytes, liver function tests, total creatine kinase, coagulation studies, urinalysis, arterial blood gases and 12-lead electrocardiogram.

Management

Heat syncope and heat cramps

For children with heat syncope and heat cramps, external cooling and oral fluids (e.g. gastrolyte) is usually sufficient. These patients usually do not require admission.

Heat exhaustion

The child with heat exhaustion needs fluids (oral if able to tolerate, otherwise intravenous) and rest in a cool environment. The decision to admit will depend on a number of factors.

Heat stroke

Heat stroke in children is a medical emergency. The ABC approach is important and all children with heat stroke should be triaged to a resuscitation environment. Rapid external cooling is the next immediate goal. Evaporative methods are probably best. Initial cooling should aim for a core temperature of 38.5°C. Removing the child's clothes, spraying with water and fanning ('wet and windy approach') and applying ice packs to the neck, groin and axillae are all indicated. It is important to prevent shivering, which can generate heat, by the administration of diazepam or chlorpromazine. Antipyretics such as paracetamol or ibuprofen have no role.

All children with genuine heat stroke require intravenous fluids, an indwelling urinary catheter and admission to the intensive care unit. Standard treatment of shock, non-cardiogenic pulmonary oedema and cerebral oedema, disseminated intravascular coagulation and renal/hepatic failure should be given, should these life-threatening complications occur.

Malignant hyperthermia

The principles of treatment of malignant hyperthermia are similar to those of heat stroke. The antidote is dantrolene which inhibits the release of calcium into muscles. Several regimes have been suggested. Shann suggests an initial dose of 1 mg kg^{-1} min^{-1} until improvement, with a maximum dose of 10 mg kg^{-1} total.[15] Another regime suggests giving 2.5 mg kg^{-1} intravenously and repeating every 10 minutes to a maximum of 10 mg kg^{-1}.[9] If the MH has been caused by an inhalational anaesthetic, the agent should be stopped immediately. Other manoeuvres include hyperventilation with 100% oxygen, bicarbonate in fulminant cases (2–4 mEq kg^{-1}), lidocaine to treat arrhythmias and aggressive cooling of the child.

Serotonin syndrome, NMS and anticholinergic syndrome

These conditions are rare in children. The serotonin syndrome is usually seen when drug combinations are used, whereas NMS is most commonly an idiosyncratic reaction to a single agent. In patients with the serotonin syndrome, most resolve within 24–48 hours with supportive management and stopping the serotonergic agent/s. In severe cases, attention to ABCs, continuous core temperature monitoring and titrated intravenous benzodiazepines are often necessary.[13,16] Specific serotonin antagonists have also been used such as cyproheptadine (0.1 mg kg^{-1} per dose) or chlorpromazine (0.25–1.0 mg kg^{-1} per dose). In NMS, benzodiazepines are useful in mild cases. In more severe cases, bromocriptine and dantrolene may have a role. The treatment of the anticholinergic syndrome is similar. Physostigmine (0.02 mg kg^{-1} per dose up to a maximum of 0.1 mg kg^{-1}) is a centrally acting acetylcholinesterase inhibitor. Its exact role is controversial, but one review has suggested that in confirmed cases of anticholinergic poisoning in children, physostigmine might be more effective than benzodiazepines.[17]

Prognosis and disposition

Apart from children with mild heat-related illness (i.e. heat syncope, heat cramps and mild heat exhaustion), who can be managed in the emergency department, all others should be admitted to hospital. Any child with suspected heat stroke should be admitted to intensive care.

Prognosis in heat-related illness is related both to the absolute temperature level and the duration of the elevation.[18] Persisting coma and multiorgan failure are poor prognostic signs. As prognosis correlates with duration of hyperthermia, immediate cooling is critical. The mortality rate for heat stroke is approximately 10% and malignant hyperthermia, 7%.

Prevention, particularly in babies and infants, centres around educating new parents about the risks of sun exposure, clothing and leaving children in cars in hot weather even for brief periods. Sports medicine guidelines regarding older children taking part in sporting activities in hot, humid weather need to be in place.

Controversies

Controversies relevant to heat-related illness in children include:

❶ The likely effects of climate change on environmental heat-related illness in the future.

❷ Cooling techniques used in children.

❸ The association between malignant hyperthermia and masseter muscle rigidity (MMR).

❹ Neuroleptic malignant syndrome (NMS) occurring with methyphenidate (Ritalin) use.

❺ Lack of public education about the susceptibility of infants and young children to heat-related illness compared to adults.

References

1. Behrma RE, Kliegman RM, Arvin AM, et al., editors. *Nelson Textbook of Pediatrics*. Philadelphia: W.B. Saunders Company; 1996. p. 2106.
2. Kristie LE, Paulson JA. Climate change and children. *Pediatr Clin North Am* 2007;(54):213–26.
3. Dann EJ, Berkman N. Chronic idiopathic anhydrosis- a rare cause of heat stroke. *Postgrad Med J* 1992;**68**:750–2.
4. Guard A, Gallagher S. Heat related deaths to young children in parked cars: an analysis of 171 fatalities in the United States, 1995–2002. *Inj Prev* 2005;**11**:33–7.
5. Robertson NRC. Temperature control and its disorders. In: *Textbook of Neonatology*. Edinburgh: Churchill Livingstone; p. 299 [chapter 12].
6. Denborough MA, Galloway GJ, Hopkinson KC. Malignant hyperpyrexia and sudden infant death. *Lancet* 1982;**11**:1068–9.
7. Hewson P, Oberklaid F. Recognition of serious illness in infants. *Mod Med* 1994;89–96.
8. Thompson A. Environmental emergencies. In: Fleisher GR, et al., editor. *Synopsis of Pediatric Emergency Medicine*. Baltimore: Williams & Wilkins; 1996. p. 452–6.
9. Rosenberg H, Bramdom BW, Nyamkhishig S, Fletcher JE. Malignant hyperthermia and other pharmacogenetic disorders. In: Barash PG, Cullen BF, Stoelting RK, editors. *Clinical Anaesthesia Textbook*. Baltimore: Lippincott Williams & Wilkins; 2001 [chapter 20].
10. Neuromuscular disorders. In: *Nelson Textbook of Pediatrics*. 18th ed. Saunders Elsevier; 2007. p. 2552.
11. Rosero EB, Adesanya AO, Timaran CH, Joshi GP. Trends and outcomes of malignant hyperthermia in the United States, 2000 to 2005. *Anaesthesiology* 2009;**110**(1):89–94.
12. Neuhut R, Lindenmayer JP, Silva R. Neuroleptic malignant syndrome in children and adolescents on atypical antipsychotic medication: a review. *J Child Adolesc Psychopharmacol* 2009;**19**(4):415–422.
13. Murray L, Daly F, Little M, Cadogan M. *Toxicology Handbook*. Edinburgh: Churchill Livingstone Elsevier; 2007. p. 47–65.
14. Rieder MJ. Some light from the heat: implications of rave parties for clinicians. *Can Med Assoc J* 2000;**162**(13):1829–30.
15. Shann F. *Drug doses*. 14th ed. Melbourne: Intensive Care Unit, Royal Children's Hospital; 2008. p. 22.
16. Gillman P. Successful treatment of serotonin syndrome with chlorpromazine. *Med J Aust* 1996;**165**:345.
17. Frascogna N. Physostigmine: is there a role for this antidote in pediatric poisoning? *Curr Opin Pediatr* 2007;**19**(2):201–5.
18. Rogers IR, Williams A. Heat-related illness. In: Cameron P, Jelinek G, Kelly A-M, Murray L, Heyworth J, editors. *Textbook of Adult Emergency Medicine*. Edinburgh: Churchill Livingstone; 2000. p. 607–10.

22.4 Cold injuries

Simon Chu • Nicholas Cheng

ESSENTIALS

1 Hypothermia is defined as a core body temperature less than 35°C.

2 Cold injury is uncommon in Australia, but when cold injuries do occur they are more significant in children than in adults.

3 The major complications of hypothermia are altered mentation and arrhythmias.

4 Hypothermia is treated with passive external, active external, active internal, and/or extracorporeal rewarming, depending on severity. In addition, hypothermia should be rigorously prevented in any patient with a severe illness.

5 The major complications of rewarming are an 'after-drop' in temperature and vasodilatory shock.

6 Severe local cold injuries are treated with rapid immersion rewarming, then care given as for burns.

7 In Australia patients are almost always dead, then cold. Situations where patients become cold enough to apply 'warm and dead' criteria are very rare.

Introduction

Cold injury is uncommon in Australia due to its warm climates. However, its significance is more important in children, as they have:

- a larger surface area:weight ratio;[1]
- underdeveloped behaviour responses to cope with extreme cold (young children can't put on more clothes).

When cold injuries do occur, they can be subdivided into generalised injury (namely accidental or environmental hypothermia) and localised injury. Cold injury is also a common problem potentially complicating any other severe illness (especially trauma) and must be prevented.[2]

Normal physiology: a review

Heat production is derived from basal metabolism, digestion, and muscular activity, which may be voluntary (exercise) or involuntary (shivering). Emotional factors and hormonal fluctuations influence heat production. The main mechanisms by which the body compensates for low core body temperature are by increasing its metabolic rate, primarily through shivering, and by shunting blood away from non-essential organs to preserve vital organs. The capacity to shiver is dependent on local glycogen stores and the rate of change of core and external temperature.[1,3]

Neonates are the patients most prone to hypothermia. They are unable to shiver and have limited stores of energy. Because of this, newborn children utilise catabolism of brown fat to generate heat. This is an inefficient process that consumes oxygen, thus exacerbating hypoxia. In addition, the large surface area to weight ratio, due to a relatively large head, contributes to heat loss. At birth, neonates are covered in amniotic fluid, and evaporative losses are significant. An overhead radiant heater is not adequate to compensate for this evaporative loss.[4,5]

Heat loss from the human body is by four methods:

- radiation;
- conduction;
- convection;
- evaporation.[1]

Radiation occurs when heat energy leaves the skin at the speed of light. Patients with more fat become more hypothermic than thinner patients, due to the former's larger surface area for radiation heat loss. In children, who have a higher surface area to weight ratio, it accounts for up to 50% of all heat loss; indeed, up to 75% in neonates. This higher number in neonates is due to a proportionally larger head increasing the surface area:weight ratio.[1,4] Radiation losses decrease when a patient is clothed.

Conduction of heat is poor in air and therefore does not contribute much to hypothermia in normal circumstances. However, water-conductive heat loss is 24 times more than that of air. It is this method by which patients suffering from water immersion become profoundly hypothermic, and how patients in wet clothes become hypothermic quickly. The surface on which the patient is lying also contributes to conduction heat loss. For instance, a patient lying on snow is likely to become more hypothermic than a person lying on sand.

Convection occurs as warm air next to the skin is replaced by cool air. This can contribute to 25% of total body heat loss in still air. In a wind of 63 km hr^{-1}, this increases by 14 times. This is described as the 'wind chill factor'.

Evaporation from the skin accounts for only 7% of heat loss at rest. This may be increased in cold, dry conditions and by sweating. Evaporation from the respiratory tract removes another 7%. This can increase by breathing faster (such as at high altitude or during exercise).

Temperature is perceived through central and peripheral mechanisms. Heat sensors in the central hypothalamus receive input from the skin, central arteries, and viscera. It is this central thermostat that is reset, which causes fever. Skin receptors respond to a change in skin temperature but do not themselves indicate the patient's core temperature. A result of all this input is that the body responds by those autonomic reflexes listed below to increase or decrease core body temperature.[3]

Hypothermia

This is defined as a core temperature of <35°C.[1] Hypothermia is classified on the basis of severity. The reason for this classification is that it influences the rewarming mechanisms that are most often deployed. It is also related to the physiological ability of the patient to compensate for hypothermia. An easy way to remember these temperature ranges is:

- acceptable low temperature: 2°C below 37°C (>35°C);
- true mild hypothermia: 3°C below that (32–35°C);
- moderate hypothermia: 4°C below that (28–32°C);
- severe hypothermia: anything below that (<28°C).

Tables 22.4.1 and 22.4.2 show the main consequences of hypothermia at a given temperature.[1,3,6] Much of our understanding of this pathophysiology comes from controlled hypothermia in cardiac surgery. Note that there is a huge variation of the onset of certain clinical signs based on temperature level. For instance, some patients may exhibit confusion at higher temperatures compared with others. Note that in children clinical manifestations of altered consciousness may be subtle.

Note that only during severe hypothermia does protection from hypoxia occur, due to decreased demand for oxygen by tissues, and even then only at extremely low temperatures (patients <20°C can tolerate anoxia for up to 60 minutes). Metabolic processes slow by approximately 6% for each 1°C drop in body temperature.[1] Thus at 28°C the basal metabolic rate is about 50% of normal. This leads to hypoventilation and hypoxia. However, at this temperature the decreased cellular metabolism affords some protection against hypoxia.

Cold diuresis is an initial brisk diuresis; this is due to decreased tubular reabsorption and also a decreased production of antidiuretic hormone. There is also an increased central blood circulating volume as blood is shunted away from the periphery, thus presenting the kidneys with an apparent increased blood volume for filtration.[1]

History

Important points in history are:

- approximate time of exposure, if known;
- environment in which patient was found;
- resuscitation at the scene, including duration of time with no cardiac output ('downtime');
- pre-existent illnesses (e.g. thyroid disease);
- drugs, medications, allergies, and immunisation status.

Table 22.4.1 Compensatory mechanisms at different severities of hypothermia		
Mild (32–35°C)	*Moderate (28–32°C)*	*Severe (<28°C)*
Increased basal metabolic rate by shivering Vasoconstriction peripherally, leading to fluid shift Mild tachycardia Cold diuresis (see text) Apathy, ataxia, amnesia, dysarthria	Limits of increasing basal metabolic rate reached Shivering stops Decreasing cerebral blood flow, causing delirium and gradual decreased level of consciousness Decreased rate of neural impulse transmission, causing clumsiness and numbness Muscle rigidity due to increasing acidosis	Complete loss of thermoregulation Stupor, coma Pulseless Fixed dilated pupils Absent reflexes Dysrhythmias, initially slow atrial fibrillation then ventricular fibrillation Appearance of death at < 25°C with asystole Falling blood pressure See text for more specific changes

Table 22.4.2 Findings at low body temperatures

Temperature (°C)	Findings
27	Reflexes absent, no response to pain, comatose
25	Cerebral blood flow one-third of normal, cardiac output one-half of normal
23	No corneal reflex, ventricular fibrillation risk is maximal
19	Asystole, flat EEG
15	Lowest temperature survived from accidental hypothermia

Examination

- Full primary and secondary assessment of patient.
- Accurate measurement of core body temperature.

Diagnosis

This requires only two essentials:[1]

- a thermometer able to record low core temperatures accurately;
- a high index of suspicion.

Core temperatures can be measured best with oesophageal or rectal probes. The most direct method of measurement is with a cardiac catheter such as a Swan–Ganz, but this is impractical in the emergency setting. Rectal probes are often used,[7] but care must be taken when using these. The probe must be at least 10 cm into the rectum in older children (more than 8 years old) and 5 cm in younger children. Inaccuracies may occur due to the presence of faecal material,[1] and the probe must be left in until the temperature equilibrates. Tympanic measurements are well known to be unreliable in the very young,[7] but they are a good indicator of therapy progression in the older child. Oral and axillary temperature probes are unreliable and impractical in the setting of true hypothermia.

Treatment

Pre-hospital treatment

This is mainly the realm of passive external rewarming methods (see below). Patients should be carefully removed from the precipitant cold environment to a dry, sheltered area. If clothes are wet, they should be removed, and the patient dried and covered with a warm dry blanket. All patients should be gently handled, especially during transport, as there is evidence that sudden movements to a body in severe hypothermia can precipitate arrhythmias, particularly ventricular fibrillation.[6] While this is occurring, one should attend to the patient's airway, breathing, and circulation, as per any resuscitation.

Active rewarming should be avoided until the patient reaches the emergency department. This is because of the complications of rewarming, namely 'after-drop' and shock.[1,6,8]

Treatment in the emergency department

Once in the emergency department, the patient should be triaged to an appropriate area, which is warm. In the very young, a radiant warmer bed and heating lamps should be available when the patient presents.[4,9] Patients should have their airway, breathing, and circulation reassessed and appropriate resuscitation commenced. Appropriate monitoring should be instituted, including electrocardiogram (ECG), and core temperature, either by rectal or oesophageal means. Oxygen saturation monitoring should be attempted, whilst understanding that initial vasoconstriction will give inadequate readings. Urine output should be monitored. Gentle handling should be continued to avoid precipitation of arrhythmias.[6] Patients should continue 100% oxygen on arrival in emergency.

Blood tests taken should include arterial blood gas (ABG); full blood count; electrolyte, urea, creatinine (EUC); liver function tests; amylase; comprehensive metabolic panel (CMP); glucose; thyroid function tests (TFTs); coagulations; tests for infection; and, if suspected, a screen for sedative drugs and ethanol. Hypothermia causes measured pH to fall and pO_2 and pCO_2 to be higher. It is recommended that these ABG values should not be corrected for temperature to better reflect the physiological state of the patient.[6]

A 12-lead ECG should be taken. Classic changes include the presence of a J (Osborn) wave, interval (PR, QRS, QT) prolongation, atrial dysrhythmias, and ventricular dysrhythmias.[10] Other less well-known changes include abnormalities similar to myocardial infarction. Hypothermia can also blunt the ECG changes with hyperkalaemia.[6] Note that all these are not present in all hypothermic patients.

Once temperature is measured, the severity of hypothermia determines the methods of rewarming. Specific methods of rewarming are classically divided into four categories:[6,8,11]

- passive external rewarming;
- active external rewarming;
- active internal (core) rewarming;
- extracorporeal rewarming.

Passive external rewarming These are methods used to prevent excessive endogenous heat loss and promote the patient to self-warm to normal core temperature. They include placing the patient in a warm room to prevent excessive convection, evaporation, and conduction heat losses. Sheets of foil (foil space blankets) are placed over the patient to decrease loss of heat through radiation.

Active external rewarming These are methods used to transfer heat energy to the patient from the external environment. They include:

- warmed blankets;
- chemical hot packs and warm water bottles;
- forced warm air blankets;
- radiant heaters and lights;
- warm-water body immersion.

Active internal rewarming These are methods used to transfer heat energy to the patient that deliver heat internally. They can be subdivided into simple methods (the first two methods below) and invasive methods. They include:

- warmed intravenous (IV) fluids (normal saline 40°C);
- inhalation of humidified warm oxygen (40°C);
- gastric lavage;
- bladder lavage;
- colonic lavage;
- pleural and peritoneal lavage ($10–20$ mL kg^{-1} of 40°C saline).

Extracorporeal rewarming These are methods by which the patient's blood is removed, rewarmed outside the body, and replaced. They include:

- haemodialysis;
- venovenous transfer of blood;
- extracorporeal (coronary bypass) circulation.

Due to the child's larger surface area to weight ratio,[1,5] emergency physicians should start to institute limited active external rewarming methods, such as radiant light warmers and forced warm air blankets, even in mild hypothermia.[11] If the child is unable to produce extra heat, then the institution of simple active internal rewarming methods (warm humidified oxygen and warmed IV fluids) is appropriate.

In older children, asking them to drink some warm liquids (hot chocolate or soup) will in effect give them the effects of a warm gastric lavage. However, patients should only have warmed fluids if they are fully conscious, can protect their airway, and have no evidence of gastroparesis.

Moderate hypothermia (28–32°C) should have all active external rewarming techniques instituted except immersion in warm bath therapy, which is limited to localised cold injury in the emergency setting (see frostbite below). It is almost impossible to adequately monitor patients while they are in an immersion bath. Forced air warming blankets can increase core temperature by up to 1.5°C hr⁻¹. Patients should also have warmed IV fluids and heated humidified oxygen for inhalation. Together, they can increase core temperature by 1–2°C hr⁻¹. Normal saline bags can be safely warmed in a microwave oven. The optimum operating system for warming 500-mL bags of crystalloid is 400-W microwave for 100 seconds or 800-W microwave for 50 seconds.[12] Alternatively, if a heat infusion pump is available, this should be used. Intravenous infusion tubing should be as short as possible, as longer tubing loses more heat to the atmosphere.

Severe hypothermia requires institution of invasive core-rewarming techniques. All can raise core temperature by 2°C every 5 minutes.[6] In cardiac arrest, cardiopulmonary resuscitation (CPR) should be commenced until core temperature has reached 35°C, and then a further assessment of the patient

done (see Controversies). Note that, according to criteria for diagnosing brain death as quoted from the Australian and New Zealand Intensive Care Society,[13] the patient must have a core temperature above 35°C, whereas other sources say 32°C.[14]

The decision of who to rewarm continues to evolve. There is a case report of a 26-month-old patient with a core temperature of 15°C who, after rewarming, recovered neurologically intact.[15] For patients without submersion, extreme duration of exposure is not incompatible with life. In immersion patients, successful recovery is very rarely seen unless patients are immersed in ice-cold water (< 10°C) for long periods of time (see Chapter 22.2). However, further attempts to resuscitate after failure to restore a circulating cardiac rhythm within 30 minutes of rewarming to above 32°C are likely to be ineffective.[14] In most Australian cases, however, the adage 'you're not dead till you're warm and dead' does not apply. The above only relates to patients that are 'snap frozen' in snowy weather.

With the recent evidence of inducing hypothermia for out-of-hospital arrests, it would make sense for patients who present hypothermic due to out-of-hospital arrests to be warmed to 34°C. In this way, hypothermia has been treated, whilst giving the patient admitted to the paediatric intensive care unit an opportunity to recover with the best possible neurological outcome.[16]

Neonatal resuscitation

In neonatal resuscitation, a warm ambient environment for the newborn child is prepared. A heated room with an overhead warmer is required. Warmed towels and blankets are used to rapidly dry the newborn to prevent evaporative heat loss. Unwell neonates should be admitted to special care nurseries or neonatal intensive care within humidicribs or transport cribs with radiant heat. If ventilated, humidified warm gases should be used.[4,5]

There is now increasing evidence that in neonates suffering hypoxic ischaemic encephalopathy a period of hypothermia may be beneficial (see Controversies). Some centres in Australia have already changed their practice to cool such neonates. The reader is advised to consult local guidelines and their referring neonatal intensive care unit for more information, and the latest

resuscitation guidelines of their country which were released following the latest ILCOR guidelines released in late 2010.

Complications

Complications can be classified as due to the hypothermia itself and complications as a result of rewarming.

Complications from hypothermia include:[1,3]

- cardiac: arrhythmia;
- haematological: platelet dysfunction, thrombocytopenia and disseminated intravascular coagulopathy;
- pulmonary: pneumonia, pulmonary oedema and (adult) acute respiratory distress syndrome;
- infection: immune complex suppression;
- renal: acute tubular necrosis and rhabdomyolysis;
- neurological: cerebral oedema, prolonged coma and slow neurological recovery (up to 6 months);
- gastrointestinal: pancreatitis;
- biochemical and metabolic derangements (including glucose, sodium and potassium).

There are two main complications that result directly from the rewarming of patients: after-drop and shock.[1,6,8] After-drop is a drop in core temperature after rewarming therapies have commenced. There are two proposed mechanisms for after-drop:

❶ Cold peripheral blood re-enters the circulation once peripheral vasodilatation occurs with rewarming.

❷ After-drop is due to ongoing conduction of heat from the warmer core into colder peripheries and surface layers of the body.

In reality, after-drop is most probably a combination of the two mechanisms described. This can be minimised by ensuring that rewarming only occurs over the core of the body, while the peripheries of the body are not actively rewarmed. For instance, a forced warm air blanket is placed over the patient's body, but their hands and feet are left outside the blanket.

Shock occurs from the same mechanism, where peripheral vasodilatation increases the intravascular space to be filled, causing a consequent drop in blood pressure and rise in heart rate. In addition, the cold diuresis experienced has already decreased the circulating blood volume (up to 35%). In immersion patients, there is also a hydrostatic squeeze effect, which further decreases blood volume. Rewarming should therefore occur only once vascular access is established and warmed normal saline is instituted if active rewarming occurs, starting with usual shock doses of 20 mL kg^{-1}. Insertion of a central venous pressure (CVP) line would be useful; however, this needs to be balanced against the increased rough handling of the body during insertion.

Medications in hypothermia behave unpredictably. Metabolism of most drugs will be slowed due to hypothermia. Some drugs have decreased effectiveness; others, such as morphine, have increased effects. Drugs not used in treatment include sodium bicarbonate, insulin, corticosteroids, empirical antibiotics, and ethanol (contrary to popular belief).[3,6]

Electrical defibrillation and antiarrhythmics may be administered at any temperature, but most efforts do not succeed until the temperature reaches above 28–30°C.[3]

·Disposition

A patient with mild hypothermia, once treated, may be observed in the emergency department for a few hours before discharge if the patient is well. Moderate and severe hypothermia are an indication for ward or intensive care unit admission, depending on if cardiac abnormalities are present during assessment. Discharge should include education to patients on prevention of further occurrences, for example the proper use of clothing, checking weather reports, etc.[1]

Localised cold injuries

Frostbite is the most severe of the injuries, but others include chilblain (perniosis), cold-induced fat necrosis (panniculitis), frost nip, and trench foot.[17,18]

Frost nip is transient blanching and numbness of peripheries that resolves with rewarming. Only the skin surface is damaged. No ice crystals form within tissues, as opposed to frostbite (see below).

Trench foot, also known as immersion foot, is historically the most interesting, with the most famous cases occurring at Napoleon's failed invasion of Russia in the winter of 1812. It is due to prolonged exposure to wet and cold, most common in the feet when poorly ventilated cold shoes are worn. There is peripheral neurovascular damage, but no ice crystal formation within tissues.

Perniosis or chilblain is injury due to repeated exposure to dry cold. Bullae form 12 hours post injury. These bullae burst to form ulcers, which are painful and pruritic. It is possibly due to repeated vasoconstriction. Common areas involved are the feet, lower legs and face.

Panniculitis consists of red lesions due to cold. Treatment is with non-steroidal anti-inflammatory drugs (NSAIDs), and the lesions resolve in 10–21 days.

Frostbite

Frostbite is the most dangerous of the local cold injuries. It is caused by freezing and ice crystal formation within the interstitial and cellular spaces due to prolonged exposure to freezing temperatures. It tends to occur more if the skin is directly exposed to temperatures less than −10°C. Several pathogenic phases evolve, called the frostbite injury cascade:[8,18]

❶ Prefreeze phase. Superficial tissue cooling occurs, which leads to increased blood viscosity, microvascular constriction, and endothelial plasma leakage.

❷ Freeze phase. Ice crystals form in the extracellular space, leading to disruption of endothelium, disruption of cell anatomy, and hyperosmolality within cells due to crystals osmotically drawing water out of cells. This leads to protein denaturation and DNA synthesis inhibition.

❸ Vascular stasis. There is arteriovenous shunting within damaged tissue, leading to stasis coagulopathy and thrombus formation.

❹ Late progressive ischaemic phase. The thrombus induces inflammation, distal hypoxia, and anaerobic metabolism, which eventually leads to tissue necrosis.

Clinical features and diagnosis

Symptomatically, frostbite begins as an initial coldness of the skin. It then progresses to a stinging or burning pain, then to an anaesthetic limb, loss of fine motor function, loss of gross motor function, and finally severe joint pain. Examination of the affected limb will reveal varying degrees of frostbite.[18] In the past, they have been classified similarly to burns, from first-degree to fourth-degree injury. It is much easier to classify them as superficial or deep.[8] Superficial injuries go only to the skin and subcutaneous tissues, whereas deep frostbite also affects bones, joints, and tendons.

Most investigations are unhelpful. However, a full blood work up with full blood count, EUC, liver function tests, glucose, and creatine kinase to look for rhabdomyolysis should be done. Urinary myoglobin should be checked. Imaging is unhelpful initially; however, there is some evidence that a bone scan will help surgeons later determine how much limb is still viable, and whether superimposed osteomyelitis has developed.[8,18,19]

Treatment

Premedical treatment involves preventing further hypothermia and initiating resuscitation. As for hypothermia, removing the patient from the cold environment is paramount. Rubbing the limb to try to warm it should be avoided, as this increases tissue damage.[8,18]

Once in emergency, the mainstay of treatment is rapid immersion rewarming.[8,18] The affected limb should be placed in a whirlpool of water about 40°C for 20–40 minutes for superficial frostbite, 1 hour for deep frostbite. This procedure will be painful, sometimes exceedingly so, hence narcotic and NSAID analgesia should be started before treatment is commenced. Rewarming is complete when the distal area of the limb is flushed, soft, and pliable. The patient should start to move the limb during rewarming to encourage blood flow in the limb. The main reason for suboptimal results is premature cessation of rewarming. After rewarming, the limb is dried and placed in a splint and elevated, and dressings applied four times a day.

Blistering of the limb will occur. The blisters are usually clear in superficial frostbite, and haemorrhagic blisters in deep frostbite. Controversy exists as to whether to aspirate these blisters. Haemorrhagic blisters should not be aspirated, as this increases trauma to the wound. The treatment of clear blisters is not as well defined.

All patients should have their tetanus status updated and, as 30% of wounds become infected, IV prophylactic antibiotics may be of use. IV penicillin G is most commonly used.[18]

Disposition

All patients should be admitted under a specialised (burns) unit.[8,18] Patients are observed for up to 6 weeks, which is usually the time the gangrenous parts of the limb are fully delineated so that safe amputation, if necessary, will occur. Good prognostic factors are patients with superficial injuries only, clear blisters, and sensation still present after rewarming.[18]

Hypothermia not due to environmental causes

There are many other causes of hypothermia,[1,3] as seen in Table 22.4.3.

Once the hypothermia is treated, then non-environmental causes should be investigated and, if found, appropriate treatment instituted. Iatrogenic causes need to be prevented. Always prevent hypothermia in trauma patients after full assessment, as hypothermia worsens the diagnosis.

Controversies

❶ In certain countries, active rewarming is commenced prior to arrival in the emergency department.[8] This is due to well-organised emergency medical systems catering for such emergencies, like in Canada. In Australia, this is more of a contentious issue, as we don't see hypothermia as often.

❷ Controversy exists regarding CPR causing arrhythmias when a patient loses spontaneous circulation.[1] However, the evidence that CPR causes ventricular fibrillation in hypothermic patients is at best circumstantial, and therefore the

general consensus is that, to promote brain perfusion, CPR should be continued till the core body temperature reaches 35°C.[13]

❸ Continuing CPR in the absence of cardiac output in a hypothermic patient has traditionally been mandatory. However, as survival occurs only in patients who have been immersed in water <5°C prior to cardiac arrest,[1] it is more likely that patients arrest in Australia before they become hypothermic. Therefore when to stop cardiac resuscitation is an issue.

❹ The use of hypothermia in treatment, particularly in trauma and head injury, has always been of some debate.[11] Hypothermia causes a reduction in oxygen consumption and is theoretically cerebroprotective. This contradicts the results that trauma patients presenting with hypothermia have a worse prognosis.[2]

❺ In neonates with hypoxic–ischaemic injury, cooling of the head is now accepted in many centres as best-practice treatment, ahead of changes in the ILCOR guidelines. However, the means to do so is not fully determined. This is an area in which there are rapid developments and the recent ILCOR guidelines in 2010 are likely to reflect this new evidence.

Table 22.4.3	Hypothermia not due to environmental causes
Cause	*Details*
Metabolic or endocrine	Hypoglycaemia Diabetic ketoacidosis Hypopituitarism Hypothyroidism Addison's disease Uraemia Malnutrition
Toxicological	Alcohol Barbiturates Anaesthetic agents Carbon monoxide Cyclic antidepressants Narcotics Phenothiazines
CNS disorders	Head trauma Spinal trauma Subarachnoid haemorrhage Degenerative diseases Cerebrovascular accidents Intracranial neoplasm
Infections	Sepsis Meningitis Encephalitis Pneumonia
Vascular or skin	Shock Gastrointestinal tract haemorrhage Pulmonary embolism Burns Erythrodermas
Iatrogenic	Cold fluid infusion Exposure during treatment Prolonged extrications Exposure during transport Exposure post birth

References

1. Corneli HM. Accidental hypothermia. *J Pediatr* 1992;**120**(5):671–9.
2. Kirkpatrick AW, Chun R, Brown R, et al. Hypothermia and the trauma patient. *Can J Surg* 1999;**42**(5):333–43.
3. Strange G, Cooper M. Cold illness. In: Strange G, Ahrenf W, Lelyveld S, et al., editors. *Pediatric Emergency Medicine, A Comprehensive Study Guide*. 1st ed. New York: McGraw-Hill; 1996. p. 616–22.
4. Australian Resuscitation Council, 2010. The New Australian Resuscitation Guidelines. Website http://resus.org.au/ [accessed 10.03.10].
5. Bissinger RL. *Neonatal resuscitation. eMedicine Journal* 2001;**2**(11). Online. Available from http://author.emedicine.com/ped/topic2598.htm; [accessed 27.10.10].
6. Danzl DF, Pozos RS. Accidental hypothermia. *N Engl J Med* 1994;**331**(26):1756–60.
7. Riddell A, Eppich W. Should tympanic temperature measurement be trusted? *Arch Dis Child* 2001;**85**(5):431–4.
8. Biem J, Koehncke N, Classen D, et al. Out of the cold: Management of hypothermia and frostbite. *Can Med Assoc J* 2003;**168**(3):305–11.
9. Day SE. Intra-transport stabilization and management of the pediatric patient. *Pediatr Clin North Am* 1993;**40**(2):263–74.

10. Mattu A, Brady WJ, Perron AD. Electrocardiographic manifestations of hypothermia. *Am J Emerg Med* 2002;**20**(4):314–26.
11. Bernardo LM, Henker R, O'Connor J. Treatment of trauma-associated hypothermia in children: Evidence-based practice. *Am J Crit Care* 2000;**9**(4):227–34.
12. Lindhoff GA, Mac G, Palmer JH. An assessment of the thermal safety of microwave warming of crystalloid fluids. *Anaesthesia* 2000;**55**(3):251–4.
13. Australian and New Zealand Intensive Care Society. *Recommendations on brain death and organ donation.* 3rd ed. Melbourne: Australian and New Zealand Intensive Care Society; 1998. Available from *http://www.anzics.com.au/downloads/cat_view/12-death-and-organ-donation* [accessed 27.10.10].
14. Wijdicks EFM. The diagnosis of brain death. *N Engl J Med* 2001;**344**:1215–21.
15. Kelly K, Glaeser P, Rice T, et al. Profound accidental hypothermia and freeze injury of the extremities in a child. *Crit Care Med* 1990;**18**(6):679–80.
16. Soar J, Deakin CD, Nolan JP, et al. European Resuscitation Council Guidelines for Resuscitation 2005. Section 7.

Cardiac arrest in special circumstances. *Resuscitation* 2005;**67S1**:S135–S170.
17. Herrin J, Antoon A. Cold injuries. In: Behrman R, Kliegman R, Arvin A, editors. *Nelson's Textbook of Pediatrics.* 15th ed. Philadelphia: Saunders; 1996. p. 277–8.
18. Cheng D, Hackshaw D. *Frostbite. eMedicine Journal* Jan 2003. Available from http://www.emedicine.com/ped/topic803.htm; [accessed 27.10.10].
19. Cauchy E, Chetaille E, Lefevre M, et al. The role of bone scanning in severe frostbite of the extremities: A retrospective study of 88 cases. *Eur J Nucl Med* 2000;**27**(5):497–502.

Further reading

Adnot J, Lewis CW. Immersion foot syndromes. In: James WD, editor. *Textbook of Military Medicine: Military Dermatology.* Washington: United States Government Printing Office;

1994, 55-68. Online. Available http://www.vnh.org/MilitaryDerm/Ch14.pdf 11 Sep 2003 – a comprehensive text on military dermatology, part of a large tome on military medicine; unlikely to be specifically useful in a paediatric sense, but this chapter is useful to round out understanding of localised cold injury.

Douwens R. *Hypothermia prevention, recognition and treatment.* Available from http://www.hypothermia.org; 2003 [accessed 27.10.10] – an excellent web site with up-to-date insight on hypothermia and future directions in management.

Meteorological Service of Canada. *Wind chill charts and tables.* Ottawa: Meteorological Service of Canada; 2002. Online. Available: http://www.msc.ec.gc.ca/education/windchill/charts_tables_e.cfm 11 Sep 2003 – an excellent article with excellent graphical depictions of wind chill effects; the reader should also peruse the rest of the website.

22.5 Anaphylaxis

Andrew Stewart Kemp

ESSENTIALS

1 Adrenaline (epinephrine) is the treatment of choice and should be administered if there are any respiratory symptoms.

2 Biphasic reactions occur, with relapse 4–10 hours after initial successful treatment.

3 A full history should be obtained with the aim of identifying the triggering factor.

4 If repeated exposure is considered possible, consider provision of an anaphylaxis action plan and instruction in use of adrenaline injector.

5 An allergy referral is indicated for definitive diagnosis of precipitating factors.

Introduction

Acute allergic reactions resulting from the degranulation of mast cells present as a continuum of responses from mild cutaneous erythema and urticaria to severe hypotension, collapse, and death. Different authorities include varying components of this continuum in the definition of anaphylaxis.[1] Anaphylaxis may be defined as a severe acute allergic reaction that involves the respiratory tract and/or results in circulatory compromise with hypotension.

Along with the increasing incidence of allergic diseases, anaphylaxis admissions to Australian, USA and UK hospitals have increased. Australian studies reported a 2- to

4-fold rise in anaphylaxis hospital admissions over an 11-year period from 1994.[2,3] The most dramatic rise was reported in children less than 5 years of age, with an almost 7-fold increase in hospital admissions from anaphylaxis. The increasing reactions are predominately due to foods. Despite the increase in admissions, death from anaphylaxis in childhood remains rare (the Australian mortality rate has remained stable at 1 per million population per year over an 11-year time period).[3] Thus there is a paradox that although anaphylaxis admissions are increasing, particularly in children less than 5 years of age, death from anaphylaxis remains rare, with the majority of deaths occurring in teenage or adult years rather than in early childhood.

Pathophysiology

Anaphylaxis is due to mast cell mediator release. Those mediators with vasoactive and/or bronchoconstrictive activities (histamine and the sulfidopeptide leukotrienes) are principal factors in the development of anaphylaxis. An increase in vascular permeability causes loss of fluid from the circulation into the interstitial space. The relative contributions of the mediators to the various clinical features are not completely defined. Mediators may directly compromise cardiac muscle function, and the intravascular volume depletion and haemoconcentration further compromises the cardiac output. Secondary cardiac arrhythmias can occur. Both upper and lower airways are affected. Laryngeal oedema results in a variable degree of upper airway obstruction, and bronchospasm and increased mucus secretion compromise the lower airways. Bronchospasm is more marked in asthmatic patients or in those taking beta-blockers.

Aetiology

The triggering agent can be identified in about three-quarters of patients presenting to emergency departments.[4]

In one childhood series the triggers were:[5]

- food: 50%;
- medications: 25%;
- insect bites: 10%;
- immunotherapy: 1%;
- immunisations: 1%.

In a more recent series, food anaphylaxis comprised 85% of presentations to a tertiary paediatric hospital emergency department.[6]

Clinical features

Symptoms occur along a continuum, from reactions that are primarily cutaneous in nature, through mild to moderate anaphylactic reactions that may have respiratory symptoms but without tachypnoea or hypotension, to severe life-threatening anaphylaxis with hypotension and hypoxia.

In children, cutaneous (90% of cases) and respiratory (80% of cases) manifestations occur earlier and are more common than gastrointestinal and cardiovascular manifestations. In 'food' anaphylaxis, gastrointestinal symptoms are more frequent, whereas cardiovascular symptoms are rare. Gastrointestinal symptoms include abdominal discomfort and vomiting. Gastrointestinal features are associated with cardiovascular rather than respiratory manifestations. The cutaneous features of pruritus, erythema, urticaria, and angio-oedema occur in nearly all children. These are commonly the first symptoms experienced, occurring within minutes following allergen exposure. Life-threatening symptoms and signs include loss of consciousness, syncope, dizziness, light-headedness, cerebral dysfunction, hypotension, hypoxia, stridor, cyanosis, and laryngeal oedema.

Table 22.5.1 lists the frequency of the presenting symptoms and signs in children admitted to hospital for anaphylaxis.

Biphasic anaphylactic reactions are defined as worsening of symptoms, requiring new therapy, after the resolution of anaphylaxis, and occur in 3–20% of anaphylactic presentations.[5,6] The reaction usually occurs 4–10 hours after the initial event; however, it has been described up to 48 hours later. Biphasic reactions are not accurately predicted from the initial clinical features. The more severe the initial anaphylactic event and/or its inadequate treatment with adrenaline, the more likely a biphasic reaction will occur.[6]

Investigations

Anaphylaxis is a clinical diagnosis, and investigations do not have a role in the acute management. On occasions, it may be difficult to differentiate anaphylaxis from other cardiac, respiratory, or neurological episodes. In this situation, determination of plasma levels of mast cell mediators (histamine and mast cell tryptase) may provide additional diagnostic help.[7] Mast cell tryptase occurs in an alpha form that is constitutively released and a beta form that is released only following mast cell activation. In anaphylaxis, mediators are elevated in approximately 50% of patients presenting to emergency departments and in approximately 80% of fatal cases. Histamine elevation is better correlated than tryptase with the severity of the symptoms. However, histamine and tryptase may also be elevated in milder cases of acute allergic reactions with cutaneous reaction alone.

It is necessary to collect blood for histamine within 10 minutes to 1 hour following the reaction, as histamine levels peak at 5–10 minutes and decline rapidly to baseline by 15–60 minutes. Tryptase should be collected not later than 6 hours after the initial reaction. Peak levels of beta-tryptase occur at 1–2 hours and decline with a half-life of approximately 2 hours. If blood is collected in the initial 30 minutes after a reaction, tryptase elevation may not be detected. Tryptase is stable and can be identified in plasma or serum stored at room temperature for several days. Interpretation of tryptase levels is often difficult and is improved if baseline levels are available; however, in the majority of cases this is unlikely to be present. Comparison with a baseline may be helpful in cases with recurrent presentation where the diagnosis is uncertain.

The reliability of measuring mast cell tryptase post mortem has been questioned, because elevation of tryptase may be seen in control cases where death has occurred from other causes. Constitutionally raised levels of mast cell tryptase in the non-acute phase have been associated with an increased incidence of severe reactions following insect stings, suggesting that the patients most likely to develop anaphylaxis may have either an increased mast cell mass or an increased mast cell releasability.

The investigation of allergic triggers requires referral to a consultant allergist for performance of appropriate skin prick and blood tests to determine the presence of specific IgE antibodies. Serum allergen specific IgE levels determined via UniCAP® above which patients have a >95% chance of having an immediate IgE-mediated reaction[8] have been determined for some foods (e.g. cow's milk, egg, peanut, wheat). It is not possible to predict the severity of a future allergic reaction based on the skin prick test size or allergen specific IgE levels.

Treatment

Adrenaline (epinephrine)

Adrenaline should be given via the intramuscular rather than the subcutaneous route, due to better absorption from muscle.[9] In children, peak adrenaline levels were reached 8 minutes after intramuscular and 34 minutes after subcutaneous injection. Peak levels were 20% higher after intramuscular injection. The preferred injection site for intramuscular administration is the

Table 22.5.1 Presenting features of children with anaphylaxis[5]

Presenting feature	Per cent
Cutaneous (urticaria, angio-oedema, flushing, or warmth	90
Upper airway (throat tightness or itchiness, drooling, stridor, oropharyngeal swelling)	80
Lower airway (chest tightness, wheezing)	60
Gastrointestinal (abdominal discomfort, vomiting)	40
Cardiovascular (arrhythmias, hypotension, poor capillary refill, weak pulses)	30
Neurological (confusion, decreased conscious state)	25
Generalised (diaphoresis, tingling, an impending sense of doom)	15

upper outer side of the thigh, which gives significantly better absorption as compared with the deltoid muscle.

- The dose of adrenaline is 0.01 mL kg^{-1} of 1 in 1000 intramuscular injection. Improvement should be seen within minutes. The dose should be repeated after 5–15 minutes if the effect is incomplete. Approximately one-third of patients will require more than one dose of adrenaline.
- In situations where there is severe circulatory compromise, adrenaline 1 in 10000 0.1 mL kg^{-1} should be given by slow intravenous injection over 10 minutes. Patients given intravenous adrenaline require cardiac, respiratory, and blood pressure monitoring.
- If there is an inadequate response, administer continuous intravenous adrenaline using a 1:100 000 (0.01 mg mL^{-1}) dilution at a rate of 0.1 mcg kg^{-1} per minute, to a maximum of 1 mcg kg^{-1} per minute, titrated according to the response.
- For refractory cardiorespiratory arrest, the initial intravenous dose is 10 mcg (0.01 mg) per kg body weight of a 1 in 10 000 (wt/vol) dilution. Subsequent doses are 100 mcg kg^{-1}. (1 mL of 1 in 10 000) (wt/vol) every 3–5 minutes and, if still refractory, the dose may be increased to 200 mcg kg^{-1}.
- Adverse effects of adrenaline include transient pallor, tremor, anxiety, palpitations, cardiac arrhythmias, headache, and nausea.

Airway and breathing
- Give high-flow oxygen by mask.
- For bronchospasm, give continuous nebulised salbutamol (0.5%).
- Nebulised adrenaline (epinephrine) 0.5 mL of 1% may be used in conjunction with systemic administration or alone for isolated mild upper airway obstruction.
- Intubate if obstruction is severe.

Circulation
- Achieve intravascular access with large-bore cannula.
- Treat hypotension with normal saline 20 mL kg^{-1}.
- If hypotension continues, give further colloid boluses of 10 mL kg^{-1} and repeat adrenaline (epinephrine) dose.

- In unrelenting hypotension, pressors such as dopamine or isoproterenol may be indicated.

Supplemental treatment
- The rationales for supplementary treatment with steroid and antihistamines are less well defined.
- If steroid is used, give methylprednisolone 1 mg kg^{-1} intravenously.
- Antihistamine: promethazine 1.0 mg kg^{-1} per dose (maximum 25 mg) orally or intravenously (slow) is given for symptomatic relief of urticaria.

Duration of treatment
Duration of treatment is determined by clinical response. Repeated doses of adrenaline (epinephrine) are often required.

Admission
Admit or observe for at least 12 hours all patients with significant anaphylaxis, as a biphasic reaction with deterioration may occur following the initial episode.

The role of H$_1$ and H$_2$ blockers
The role of antihistamines is unclear. Addition of H$_2$ to H$_1$ antagonists produces no differences in blood pressure and symptoms; however, there is less urticaria at 2 hours in patients treated with combined H$_1$ and H$_2$ blockers. Antihistamine is not a substitute for adrenaline.

Patients on beta-blockers
Glucagon 0.02 mg kg^{-1} intravenously has been used in an attempt to reverse beta blockade.

Diagnosis

It is important to determine the cause of the anaphylactic reaction whenever possible.

Types of anaphylaxis
Common

Foods Severe life-threatening reactions are predominantly due to peanut and tree nuts. In pre-school-age children, they may be due to egg and cow's milk proteins.

Drugs Many reactions, in particular those due to antibiotics, are IgE-mediated.

Non–IgE-mediated anaphylactoid reactions are clinically indistinguishable from anaphylaxis. Drugs that can cause anaphylactoid reactions include opiates, muscle relaxants, radiocontrast media, non-steroidal anti-inflammatory drugs and quinolone and vancomycin antibiotics.

Stings Stings are most commonly due to bees and less often wasps. In Australia, jumper ant *(Myrmecia* spp.) stings are a common cause of anaphylaxis in endemic areas.

Latex Sensitisation occurs particularly in children with multiple exposure to latex-containing items during medical procedures. Children with spina bifida are particularly at risk due to multiple exposures following surgery and urinary tract catheterisation.

Less common

Idiopathic No triggers are identified, despite full investigation. Cases may present with laryngeal oedema as the only manifestation. The episodes can usually be controlled by regular antihistamine and, if necessary, the addition of alternate day steroids.[10] Psychogenic anaphylaxis has been classified as a variant of idiopathic anaphylaxis and should be considered in the differential diagnosis.

Uncommon

Exercise-induced Symptoms of urticaria, angio-oedema, and stridor plus or minus hypotension develop during or soon after cessation of vigorous exercise.

Food-dependent exercise-induced In this situation, exercise induces symptoms only following ingestion of the relevant foodstuff, which has included wheat, celery, shellfish, oranges, and peaches. In some but not all cases, IgE sensitisation to the relevant food can be demonstrated.

Recurrent anaphylaxis
Anaphylaxis is frequently multiple, and in one series two-thirds of patients had three or more anaphylactic episodes. Efforts should be made to identify unrecognised triggers. In children, this is often due to foods (generally peanut or tree nut products) contained in manufactured or processed foods. Some cases without an identifiable cause are due to idiopathic anaphylaxis.

Differential diagnosis

Anaphylaxis should be distinguished from other presentations that may cause confusion. These include:

- acute asthma;
- vasovagal syncope;
- urticaria or angio-oedema;
- psychogenic stridor;
- cardiovascular events;
- seizure disorders;
- mast cell mediator release in mastocytosis;
- hereditary angio-oedema.

Prevention

Advice concerning the avoidance of the triggering allergen is critical. This will usually require referral to a consultant allergist.

The provision of self-injectable or carer-administered adrenaline should be considered for all children with anaphylaxis. Inadvertent re-exposure is most likely in the case of insect stings and foods, and least likely for drugs. The prescription of a self-injectable adrenaline also requires instruction in the indications for and demonstration of use and the provision of a clear and simple written anaphylaxis action plan.

Self-injectable adrenaline is available in two fixed-dosages: (0.15 mg of adrenaline) for children 15–30 kg and (0.3 mg of adrenaline) for children greater than 30 kg. The American Academy of Asthma Allergy and Immunology recommends the 0.3 mg dose for children >20 kg.[11]

In venom-induced anaphylaxis referral to an allergist for desensitisation should be considered for life-threatening reactions with respiratory or cardiovascular involvement if there is an appropriate reagent available, such as honey bee (Apis mellifera), paper wasp (Polistes spp.) or European wasp (Vespula spp.). This will involve a series of injections with venom for a duration of 3 or more years. In general, venom desensitisation is not recommended for children with generalised cutaneous reactions in the absence of respiratory or cardiovascular involvement.

Controversies

Currently, there are no clear guidelines on which children should be prescribed an EpiPen. The great majority of fatalities are recorded in children over 5 years of age, despite the fact that food-allergic reactions are more common in pre-school children and frequently lessen with time. As the prescription of an EpiPen is primarily concerned with risk management, it is necessary to consider the factors that point to the likelihood of developing a severe life-threatening reaction.[12] These are:

- age over 5 years;
- a history of respiratory tract involvement with the initial or subsequent reactions;
- a history of asthma requiring preventive medication;
- peanut or tree nut sensitivity;
- reactions induced by traces or small amounts of allergen;
- a strongly positive skin prick test (>8 mm).

Each factor should be considered, and the greater the number that are positive, the lower the threshold for prescribing an EpiPen. In addition, these factors need to be weighed in the light of the parental wishes and environmental circumstances. Providing the parents with a rational perspective on the remote risk of death is essential.

Future directions and research

❶ Humanised monoclonal anti-IgE antibodies increase the threshold dose of food required to trigger symptoms in food-induced anaphylaxis. Regular administration is required. Unlike desensitisation, the treatment is not allergen-specific, and therefore offers promise to individuals with life-threatening reactions to multiple allergens.

❷ Characterisation of the molecular structure of allergenic epitopes may allow the construction of peptides for immunotherapy that trigger T-cell responses without binding IgE, thus significantly reducing the risks and increasing the efficacy of immunotherapy.

❸ The promotion of desensitisation or tolerance in food allergy by graded oral administration of food allergens such as peanut or egg.

Acknowledgement

The contribution of David Singh as author in the first edition is hereby acknowledged.

References

1. Sampson HA, Munoz-Furlong A, Campbell RL, et al. Second symposium on the definition and management of anaphylaxis: summary report–Second National Institute of Allergy and Infectious Disease/Food Allergy and Anaphylaxis Network symposium. J Allergy Clin Immunol 2006;117(2):391–7.
2. Poulos LM, Waters AM, Correll PK, et al. Trends in hospitalizations for anaphylaxis, angioedema, and urticaria in Australia, 1993–1994 to 2004–2005. J Allergy Clin Immunol 2007;120(4):878–84.
3. Liew WK, Williamson E, Tang ML. Anaphylaxis fatalities and admissions in Australia. J Allergy Clin Immunol 2009;123(2):434–42.
4. Kemp SF, Lockey RF. Anaphylaxis: A review of causes and mechanisms. J Allergy Clin Immunol 2002;1103: 341–8.
5. Lee JM, Greenes DS. Biphasic anaphylactic reactions in pediatrics. Pediatrics 2000;1064:762–6.
6. Mehr S, Liew WK, Tey D, Tang ML. Clinical predictors for biphasic reactions in children presenting with anaphylaxis. Clin Exp Allergy 2009;39(9):1390–6.
7. Lin RY, Schwartz LB, Curry A, et al. Histamine and tryptase levels in patients with acute allergic reactions: An emergency department-based study. J Allergy Clin Immunol 2000;106(1 Part 1):65–71.
8. Sampson HA. Utility of food-specific IgE concentrations in predicting symptomatic food allergy. J Allergy Clin Immunol 2001;107(5):891–6.
9. Simons FE, Roberts JR, Gu X, et al. Epinephrine absorption in children with a history of anaphylaxis. J Allergy Clin Immunol 1998;101(1 Part 1):33–7.
10. Ditto AM, Krasnick J, Greenberger PA, et al. Pediatric idiopathic anaphylaxis: Experience with 22 patients. J Allergy Clin Immunol 1997;1003:320–6.
11. AAAI Board of Directors. The use of epinephrine in the treatment of anaphylaxis. J All Clin Immunol 1994;944:666–8.
12. Kemp AS. EpiPen epidemic: suggestions for rational prescribing in childhood food allergy. J Paediatr Child Health 2003;39(5):372–5.

Further reading

Brown SG. Anaphylaxis: clinical concepts and research priorities. Emerg Med Australas. 2006;18(2):155–69.
Joint Task Force on Practice Parameters, American Academy of Allergy, Asthma and Immunology, American College of Allergy, Asthma and Immunology, and the Joint Council of Allergy, Asthma and Immunology. The diagnosis and management of anaphylaxis. J Allergy Clin Immunol 1998;101(6 Part 2):S465–528.
Muraro A, Roberts G, Clark A, et al. EAACI Task Force on Anaphylaxis in Children. The management of anaphylaxis in childhood: position paper of the European academy of allergology and clinical immunology. Allergy. 2007;62 (8):857–71.

23.1 Length-based paediatric drug dosing and equipment sizing

Ronald A. Dieckmann

Background

Emergency treatment of infants and children is sometimes difficult because children of different ages require different sizes of equipment, doses of medications, and volumes of fluids. Errors are common when selecting appropriate equipment and medications in critical paediatric emergencies, and mistakes are especially frequent with doses of drugs that are powerful cardiovascular agents, such as adrenaline (epinephrine).

Length-based drug dosing and equipment sizing is an effective method for rapid selection of emergency treatments. Using length as a basis for ordering drugs and equipment is at least as accurate as weight, and length may be more accurate than weight for equipment sizing. It is also less likely to cause error in high-stress circumstances.

There are two methods of rapid drug dosing and equipment sizing: (1) a software paediatric decision support program; (2) a length-based resuscitation tape. Software decision support programs for desktop, or laptop computers or PDA are now available: by imprinting a child's length, the programs provide exact drug doses or equipment sizes for a vast range of medications and equipment.

The paediatric resuscitation tape or length-based resuscitation tape is a simple visual tool to measure lengths and to approximate weights in children. There are several commercial products available. One type of tape utilises colour zones to cluster closely matched sizes of children into categories that have the same drug and equipment requirements. A disadvantage of the resuscitation tape is that only a few drugs are listed on the tape. Hence, a current additional comprehensive drug reference is imperative to address the multiple pharmacological needs of children.

Indication

Children requiring equipment, medication, or fluids, weighing 3–34 kg body weight (about age 10–12 years).

Contraindications

- Premature infant weighing less than 3 kg.
- Child older than 10–12 years of age or weighing more than 34 kg body weight (use adult equipment and drug dosages).

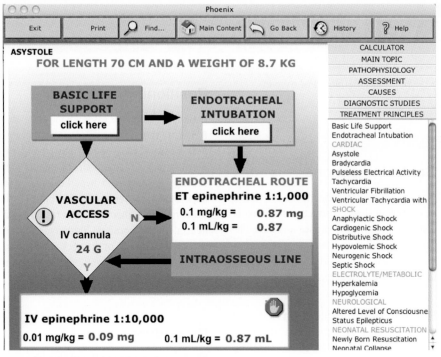

Fig. 23.1.1 Decision support software allows instantaneous calculations of drug doses and equipment sizes, based upon patient length.

Equipment

❶ Computer or PDA based paediatric decision support software (Fig. 23.1.1).

❷ Colour-coded paediatric resuscitation tape (Fig. 23.1.2). Store the tape in a place that is easily accessible, such as in the paediatric equipment kit, on the paediatric code cart, or on a wall hook. Lamination of the tape may preserve longevity. There are several different brands of length-based paediatric resuscitation tapes, and these have not been compared for speed, accuracy, or safety.

Preparation

❶ Place the patient in a supine position.
❷ Extend the patient's legs.
❸ Measure the child in centimetres.

Procedure decision support software

After measuring the child's length, input into computer program and read drug doses and equipment sizes (see Fig. 23.1.1).

Tape

❶ Measure child's length – from head to heel – with the tape. Note and say

weight in kilograms that corresponds to the child's measured length at the heel.

❷ If the child is longer than the tape, use adult equipment and medication doses.

❸ From the tape, identify appropriate equipment sizes (see Fig. 23.1.2).

❹ From the tape, identify appropriate medication doses (see Fig. 23.1.2).

Complications

None.

Tips

- Use the decision support software or resuscitation tape instead of attempting to estimate weight or calculate equipment sizes or drug doses.
- Measuring to the child's toes (instead of heel) will add a number of kilograms to the estimated weight and may result in over-sized equipment and over-large drug doses.

Further reading

Black K, Barnett P, Wolfe R, Young S. Are methods used to estimate weight in children accurate? *Emerg Med (Fremantle)* 2002;**14**(2):160–5.

Davis D, Barbee L, Ririe D. Paediatric endotracheal tube selection: A comparison of age-based and height-based criteria. *Am Ass Nurse Anesth J* 1998;**66**(3):299–303.

Hofer CK, Ganter M, Tucci M, et al. How reliable is length-based determination of body weight and tracheal tube size in the paediatric age group? The Broselow tape reconsidered. *Br J Anaesth* 2002;**88**(2):283–5.

Lubitz DS, Seidel JS, Chameides L, et al. A rapid method for estimating weight and resuscitation drug dosages from length in the paediatric age group. *Ann Emerg Med* 1988;**17**(6):576–81.

Luten RC, Wears RL, Broselow J, et al. Related articles, links abstract length-based endotracheal tube and emergency equipment in paediatrics. *Ann Emerg Med* 1992;**21**:1454–60.

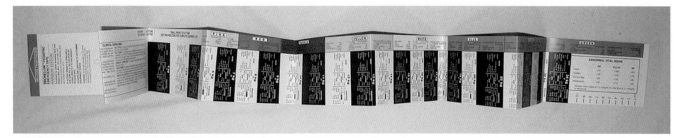

Fig. 23.1.2 Colour-coded paediatric resuscitation tape.

23.2 Bag–mask ventilation

Michelle Lin

Background

Bag–mask (BM) ventilation is the most important skill in paediatric airway management. This non-invasive manoeuvre for assisted, positive-pressure ventilation is effective treatment for most children with hypoventilation and hypoxia. A child with respiratory insufficiency may require only temporary assisted ventilation with BM. Some children in respiratory failure who require prolonged ventilation or airway protection may need tracheal intubation (Chapter 23.3).

In the BM setup, oxygen flows into a bag reservoir, through a pop-off valve, and into a mask, which forms a tight seal around the child's nose and mouth. Squeezing the bag administers oxygen under positive pressure to the lungs. While this manoeuvre does not fully protect the airway, as tracheal intubation does, BM ventilation adequately provides emergent airway support during the acute decompensation period (Table 23.2.1). Additionally, Gausche et al demonstrated that BM ventilation is as effective as tracheal intubation in the pre-hospital setting for airway management, regardless of the underlying aetiology.[1] Thus, both pre-hospital and in-hospital practitioners must be comfortable and proficient in performing BM ventilation.

Indications

- Hypoventilation or apnoea.
- Respiratory failure.

- Hypoxia despite high-flow oxygen administration via a non-rebreather mask.

Contraindications

Do not perform BM ventilation in the setting of a complete airway obstruction. If this exists, first perform airway clearance and basic life-support manoeuvres. Then attempt foreign-body removal of the obstruction, if necessary, under direct laryngoscopy with Magill forceps.

Relative contraindication

In the presence of a congenital diaphragmatic hernia or a tracheo-oesophageal fistula, BM can cause insufflation of the stomach and subsequent extrapulmonary compression of the lungs. This may compromise adequate oxygenation and ventilation.

Equipment

❶ Appropriately-sized mask (Fig. 23.2.1).
❷ Self-inflating bag reservoir (Fig. 23.2.2).
❸ Oxygen saturation monitor.

Preparation

❶ Select an appropriately-sized mask and ventilation bag.
❷ Connect the oxygen tubing to the ventilation bag, and attach to the face mask.
❸ Begin 15 litres of oxygen per minute.

Positioning

Patient positioning is essential for successful BM ventilation. Maintain a supine, neutral neck position to keep the airway patent. Because of their large occiputs, infants and toddlers are prone to hyperflexion of the neck and consequently benefit from a small towel roll under their shoulders to achieve a neutral 'sniffing' position. Both hyperflexion and hyperextension of the neck may worsen airway obstruction, compromise ventilation, and increase risk of spinal injury.

Procedure

❶ Perform the head-tilt and chin-lift manoeuvre to open the airway and lift the tongue away from the soft palate of the oropharynx. Proper positioning and suctioning of excess secretions will often relieve the respiratory compromise without BM ventilation.
❷ In the setting of trauma where spinal injury is a consideration, do not perform the head-tilt/chin-lift manoeuvre. Instead, provide in-line spinal immobilisation and perform a jaw-thrust manoeuvre to create a patent airway.
❸ If airway patency is still suboptimal, reposition and suction the patient. If still inadequate, insert an oropharyngeal or nasopharyngeal airway underneath the mask to lift the tongue from the posterior oropharynx (Chapter 23.3).
❹ In the *one-person BM technique* place the mask on the patient's face and achieve an airtight seal over the mouth and nose. Using the non-dominant hand, place the thumb and index finger on the superior and inferior parts of the face mask, respectively. Cradle the tips of the other three fingers along the mandible and lift the jaw up toward the mask to create the seal. This is the 'E–C clamp' manoeuvre, based on the E-shape of the three fingers along the jaw and the C-shape of the thumb and index finger along the face mask (Fig. 23.2.3). In creating the seal, pull

Table 23.2.1 Choosing BM ventilation versus tracheal intubation		
Sample patient case	**BM**	**Intubation**
Hypoventilation during procedural sedation	+	
Hypoventilation during post-ictal stage	+	
Hypoxia during asthma exacerbation despite non-rebreather oxygen mask	+	
Persistent hypoxia or hypoventilation despite BM		+
Partial airway obstruction (laryngeal burn, angio-oedema)		+
Cardiopulmonary arrest	+	+

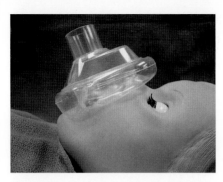

Fig. 23.2.1 Choosing the appropriately sized bag–mask. Variously-sized, clear masks are available for all ages, ranging from neonates to adults. These masks have an inflated circumferential rim, which provides a tight seal to the patient's lower face. With an appropriately-sized mask, the superior aspect of the mask should rest over the patient's nasal bridge and the inferior aspect should rest over the cleft of the chin. Too large a mask may compress the patient's eyes, and too small a mask may occlude the nostrils and impede adequate oxygenation and ventilation.

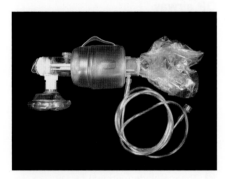

Fig. 23.2.2 Paediatric oxygen bag. Supplemental, high-flow oxygen flowing into a bag serves as the oxygen reservoir for BM ventilation. A paediatric bag, which has a volume of 450–750 mL, is adequate to oxygenate and ventilate a small child. Alternatively, if a paediatric bag is not readily available, an adult bag, which has a volume of about 1200 mL, can also provide adequate oxygenation and ventilation. Be careful not to administer excessive tidal volumes with this larger bag.

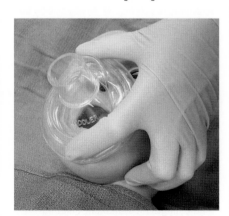

Fig. 23.2.3 E–C clamp BM technique.

the jaw anteriorly rather than push the mask posteriorly into the patient's face. To ventilate, squeeze the oxygen reservoir bag using the dominant hand. For prolonged BM ventilation, use the little finger of your non-dominant hand (used for the E–C clamp) and apply cricoid pressure to reduce gastric air insufflation.

❺ In the *two-person technique* place the mask on the patient's face and achieve an airtight seal over the mouth and nose. For operator #1, place the thumb and index finger of both hands on the superior and inferior parts of the face mask, respectively. Cradle the tips of the other three fingers of both hands along either side of the mandible and symmetrically lift the jaw up toward the mask to create a seal. This is a double 'E–C clamp' manoeuvre (Fig. 23.2.4). Again, pull the jaw anteriorly rather than push the mask posteriorly into the patient's face. Operator #2 ventilates the patient by squeezing the oxygen reservoir bag, and applies cricoid pressure for prolonged BM ventilation to reduce gastric air insufflation.

❻ Provide BM ventilation at a rate of 20, 30, and 40 inspirations per minute for the child, infant, and neonate, respectively. Squeeze and release the bag at an inspiratory-to-expiratory ratio of 1:2. A common error is to over-ventilate the patient with too rapid a rate.

❼ Provide a BM tidal volume of 8 mL kg^{-1} to oxygenate and ventilate the patient. As an equally effective alternative measure of appropriate ventilation volume, watch for bilateral chest rise and fall.

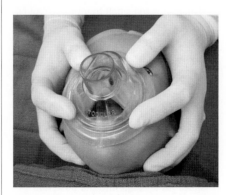

Fig. 23.2.4 Double E–C clamp BM technique.

❽ In addition to visualisation, auscultation of bilateral breath sounds in the mid-axilla and improvement of the oxygen saturation both corroborate with adequate ventilation.

❾ With prolonged BM ventilation, decompress the likely over-distended stomach with an orogastric (OG) or nasogastric (NG) tube. This reduces the risk of emesis and consequent aspiration.

Complications

- Incorrect mask sizing causing inadequate ventilation or trauma to the eyes.
- Gastric insufflation and distension.
- Aspiration from emesis.
- Pneumothorax from poor lung compliance or excessive tidal volumes.
- Hypoxia.

Tips

- In paediatric trauma cases requiring in-line spinal immobilisation, perform BM ventilation with the two-person technique. One operator focuses on providing an adequate mask seal, while the other operator focuses on squeezing the bag and maintaining spinal alignment. In comparison, a one-person BM technique often inadvertently extends the patient's neck while trying to achieve an adequate mask seal.
- When elevating the jaw anteriorly to form a mask seal with the third, fourth and fifth fingers, be sure to lift up along the bony mandible rather than the submandibular soft tissue. In addition to trauma, compressing the submandibular soft tissue may inadvertently occlude the airway.
- Some BM reservoir bags have a pop-off valve to prevent excessive positive pressure ventilation. This may inadequately ventilate a patient with low lung compliance. Occlude this valve to allow higher positive pressures during inspiration, while watching for chest rise.

- For the neonate and infant, assessing chest rise and fall for adequate BM tidal volume is subtle. The optimal viewing angle is from the patient's side at the level of his or her bed.
- In order to prevent the common complication of over-ventilating a patient, say aloud 'squeeze – release – release' repeatedly while correspondingly squeezing and releasing the bag.

This approximates the correct ventilatory rate and inspiratory-to-expiratory ratio for the patient.

Reference

1. Gausche M, Lewis RJ, Stratton SJ, et al. Effect of out-of-hospital paediatric endotracheal intubation on survival and neurological outcome: A controlled clinical trial. *JAMA* 2000;**283**(6):783–90.

Further reading

Brown RE. Bag and mask ventilation. In: Dieckmann RA, et al., editors. *Paediatric emergency and critical care procedures*. St Louis, MO: Mosby; 1997.

Chameides L, Hazinski MF, editors. *Paediatric advanced life support*. Dallas, Texas: American Heart Association; 1997.

Dieckmann RA, Brownstein DR, Gausche-Hill M, editors. *Paediatric Education for Prehospital Professionals*. Sudbury, MA: Jones & Bartlett Publishers; 2000.

Lee BS, Gausche-Hill M. Paediatric airway management. *Clin Paediatr Emerg Med* 2001;**2**(2):91–106.

Zideman D, et al. Airways in paediatric and newborn resuscitation. *Ann Emerg Med* 2001;**37**(4 Suppl):S126–36.

23.3 Nasopharyngeal, oropharyngeal airways and the laryngeal mask airway

Michelle Lin • Conor Deasy

Background

Children have relatively large tongues, which may fall back and cause airway obstruction when there is loss of nasopharyngeal muscle tone, for instance, in patients who are post-ictal or overly sedated by drugs. Hypoxia and hypercarbia may develop. Non-invasive airway adjuncts, such as nasopharyngeal (NP) and oropharyngeal (OP) airways, can maintain a patent airway even when the tongue falls back against the posterior pharyngeal wall. The laryngeal mask airway (LMA) is designed to provide a seal around the laryngeal inlet when inserted and the cuff inflated, and is used in situations involving a difficult bag–valve–mask fit in an unconscious patient and as a back-up device where tracheal intubation is not successful.

Structurally, an NP airway is hollow, made of latex or a latex-like substance, and has a slight curvature to approximate the curvature of the nasopharynx. The distal end has a bevel, which helps to tunnel through the nasopharyngeal soft tissue, but which may also cause inadvertent shearing trauma to the nasal septum. The proximal end of the NP airway has a wide flange to anchor the tube in place at the nostril orifice. Patients tolerate this airway adjunct better than an OP airway because it does not trigger the gag reflex.

The OP airway is hollow, made of plastic, and has a slight curvature to approximate the curvature of the oropharynx. The distal end rests along the posterior tongue, which would trigger the gag reflex in an awake patient, and the proximal end has a wide flange to anchor the tube in place at the lips.

Airway adjuncts may allow adequate spontaneous ventilation and avert the need for bag–valve–mask ventilation or the more invasive technique of tracheal intubation.

Indications for OP or NP

- Airway obstruction.
- Respiratory decompensation.
- Seizures.

Contraindications

NP airway

- Age less than 1 year old – the nares diameter is too small to introduce an NP airway.
- Nasal obstruction – attempting to introduce an NP airway into a nasal passage that is obstructed will be unsuccessful and may cause traumatic epistaxis.
- Severe facial injury or suspicion for basilar skull fracture – a fractured cribriform plate may allow an NP airway to traverse incorrectly into the intracranial space rather than into the posterior oropharynx.

OP airway

Intact gag reflex – because the OP airway tip rests on the posterior tongue, a patient with an intact gag reflex will likely vomit and aspirate gastric contents.

Equipment

❶ Lubricating jelly (for NP airway).
❷ Tongue blade (optional for OP airway).
❸ NP airway (Fig. 23.3.1).
❹ OP airway (Fig. 23.3.2).

Preparation

NP airway

Determine the correct NP airway size by one of three methods:

❶ Follow the recommendations on a length-based resuscitation tape.
❷ Choose an NP airway the length of which is equivalent to the distance from the patient's nasal tip to the tragus of the ear (Fig. 23.3.3).
❸ Choose an NP airway the outer diameter of which is equivalent to the nostril's inner diameter. Cut the length of the tube according to the length-measurement guide in Method 2.

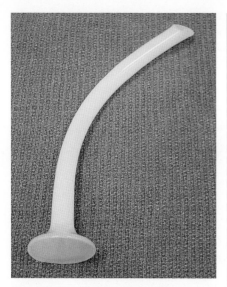

Fig. 23.3.1 Nasopharyngeal airway.

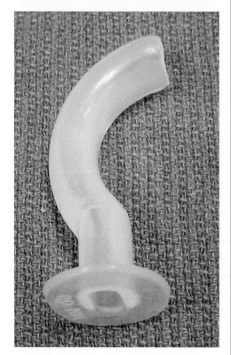

Fig. 23.3.2 Oropharyngeal airway.

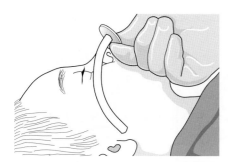

Fig. 23.3.3 Sizing the NP airway: nasal tip to tragus of ear.

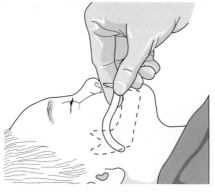

Fig. 23.3.4 Sizing the OP airway: corner of mouth to mandibular angle.

OP airway

Determine the correct OP airway size by one of two methods:

❶ Follow the recommendations on a length-based resuscitation tape.

❷ Choose an OP airway the length of which is equivalent to the distance from the patient's incisors to the mandibular angle, as measured from the side of the patient's face (Fig. 23.3.4).

Positioning

❶ Place the patient in a supine, neutral 'sniffing' position.

❷ To prevent the patient's tongue from worsening the airway obstruction, perform a chin-lift manoeuvre. Use a jaw-thrust manoeuvre for the trauma patient in whom spinal immobilisation is crucial.

Procedure

NP airway

❶ Prelubricate the NP airway before insertion.

❷ When inserting the NP airway in the *right nostril*, the bevel already points toward the septum and is of minimal risk for nasal septal trauma. Gently introduce the NP airway directly posteriorly into the patient's nostril until the flange rests just external to the nostril orifice.

❸ When inserting the NP airway in the *left nostril*, the bevel is pointed away from the septum. To avoid septal trauma, rotate the NP airway 180 degrees so that the bevel now points towards the septum. Insert the airway approximately 2 cm so

that the tip passes the septal border. When resistance is felt, re-rotate the NP airway 180 degrees into its original, correct orientation. Finish inserting the NP posteriorly into the nostril until it rests just external to the nostril orifice.

OP airway

The most common mistake in OP airway insertion is causing damage to the soft palate or pushing the tongue further back while inserting it and thus worsening airway obstruction. Two methods will prevent this:

❶ With tongue blade – after pushing the tongue inferiorly with a tongue blade, slide the OP airway directly over it concave down, i.e. with the tip pointed inferiorly. Continue until the flange gently rests against the lips.

❷ Without tongue blade – rotate the OP airway 180 degrees such that the tip points superiorly and insert it into the mouth. When it contacts the hard palate, depress the tongue with the OP airway curvature. Insert the OP airway completely until the flange reaches the lips. Then re-rotate the airway 180 degrees so that the tip correctly points inferiorly and rests along the posterior tongue.

Complications

- Emesis and aspiration.
- Laryngospasm.
- Local trauma and bleeding.
- Worsening airway obstruction – when the OP airway is inappropriately long, it may directly occlude the posterior oropharynx; when it is inappropriately short, it may push the tongue further back, causing more airway obstruction.
- NP airway plug – the relatively small diameter of the NP airway makes it easily prone to occlusion with mucus, secretions, and blood.
- Intracranial placement of the NP airway.

Tips

❶ Insert the NP airway directly posteriorly along the floor of the nose and not superiorly.

❷ Do not select too wide an NP tube, which may cause pressure necrosis to the nasal ala.

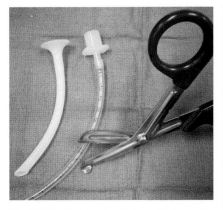

Fig. 23.3.5 Endotracheal tube cut into an NP airway.

Table 23.3.1 Recommended weight-based sizing and inflation volumes

Weight of patient	Recommended size guidelines	Maximum air in cuff (mL)
5 kg	Size 1	4
5–10 kg	Size 1.5	7
10–20 kg	Size 2	10
20–30 kg	Size 2.5	14
30 kg–small adult	Size 3	20
Adult	Size 4	30
Large adult	Size 5	40

❸ If an NP airway is not immediately available, an alternative is to use a endotracheal tube, normally used for intubations. First, choose the tube where the outer diameter is equivalent to the inner diameter of the patient's nostril. Second, trim the tube from the proximal end to the appropriate length as measured from the patient's nasal tip to the tragus of the ear. Leave the proximal ventilator adapter on the endotracheal tube in place so that the tube is anchored at the nasal tip and does not accidentally slip beyond the nares (Fig. 23.3.5).

❹ Be sure the patient does not have a gag reflex before placing an OP airway.

Indications for laryngeal mask airway

- Situations involving a difficult mask (bag–valve–mask) fit.
- May be used as a back-up device where tracheal intubation is not successful.
- May be used as a 'second-last-ditch' airway where a surgical airway is the only remaining option.

Equipment

- Appropriate size LMA.
- Syringe with appropriate volume for LMA cuff inflation.
- Water soluble lubricant.
- Bag–valve–mask to ventilate.
- Stethoscope to check for adequate air entry into both lungs once in place.
- Tape or other device(s) to secure LMA.

Preparation

- Select correct size (Table 23.3.1).
- Check the LMA testing inflation and deflation of the cuff.
- Lubricate the back of the LMA thoroughly using a water soluble lubricant; however, avoid excessive amounts as inhalation of the lubricant result in coughing or obstruction.

Positioning

Extend the head and flex the neck if possible.

Procedure (Fig. 23.3.6)

- The mask is held like a pen and inserted while pressing against the palate and posterior pharyngeal wall using the index finger until resistance is felt when the mask tip reaches the triangular base of the oropharynx.
- The lumen of the LMA should be facing the patient's tongue and not the hard palate.
- Inflate the mask with the recommended volume of air (see Table 23.3.1), avoiding over inflation.
- Normally the mask should be allowed to rise up slightly out of the hypopharynx as it is inflated to find its correct position.

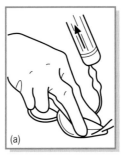
(a)
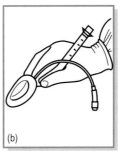
(b)
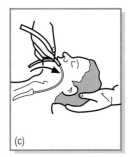
(c)
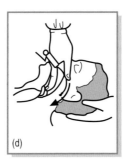
(d)
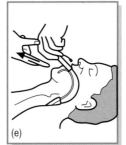
(e)
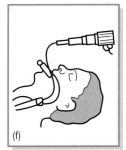
(f)

Fig. 23.3.6 Placing a laryngeal mask airway.

- Connect the LMA to a bag–valve–mask device or low pressure ventilator.
- Ventilate the patient while confirming equal breath sounds over both lungs in all fields and the absence of ventilatory sounds over the epigastrium.
- Secure the LMA in position using the same techniques as for an endotracheal tube.

Complications

Inadequate lubrication or lack of pressure on the deflated mask up against the hard palate on placement can cause the mask tip to fold back on itself. This may progress, pushing the epiglottis into its down-folded position, causing mechanical obstruction.

Tips

- The insertion of the LMA by the standard technique is not always easy owing to the anatomy of the paediatric airway. Some advocate a rotational technique: with a partially inflated cuff, the mask is inserted with its lumen facing backwards and then rotated through 180 degrees, when the resistance of the posterior pharyngeal wall is felt, and then passed downwards into position behind the larynx.

- Insert a bite-block or roll of gauze to prevent occlusion of the tube should the patient bite down.

Further reading

Chameides L, Hazinski MF, editors. *Paediatric advanced life support*. Dallas, TX: American Heart Association; 1997.
Dieckmann RA, et al., editors. *Paediatric education for prehospital professionals*. Sudbury, MA: Jones & Bartlett Publishers; 2000.
Greenberg RS. Facemask, nasal and oral airway devices. *Anesthesiol Clin N Am* 2002;**20**(4):833–61.
Shifrm SW. Insertion of oral and nasal airways. In: Dieckmann RA, et al., editors. *Paediatric emergency and critical care procedures*. St Louis, MO: Mosby; 1997.

23.4 Endotracheal tube and tracheal intubation

Michelle Lin

Background

Tracheal intubation (TI) provides a definitive airway. Insertion of a tube between the vocal cords and into the trachea allows optimal management of the patient's oxygenation and ventilation, while also protecting the airway from aspiration. Depending on the preparation and skill of the practitioner, this procedure can be either life saving or life compromising. TI is the standard rescue procedure when bag–mask (BM) ventilation is ineffective or insufficient.

The anatomy of the paediatric airway creates unique considerations during intubation as compared to adult intubation. Specifically, the differences are as follows:

❶ A paediatric patient has a relatively larger tongue, making visualisation of the vocal cords more difficult. Hence, preintubation positioning of the patient plays a crucial role in TI success.

❷ A paediatric patient has a wider and floppier epiglottis. Thus, in neonates and infants, use a straight laryngoscopic blade to achieve the best visualisation of the vocal cords. The blade moves the posteriorly-hanging epiglottis anteriorly, exposing the vocal cords.

❸ A paediatric patient has more anterior and cephalad vocal cords. A straight laryngoscopic blade provides the best direct line-of-sight to the anteriorly-positioned cords.

❹ The cricoid ring is the narrowest part of the airway in patients less than 8 years old. This anatomical narrowing naturally secures the endotracheal tube in place at the cricoid ring level without an air leak. Endotracheal tubes therefore do not need to be cuffed. In contrast, adolescents and adults have a cylindrical-shaped rather than a funnel-shaped airway, and they do require cuffed endotracheal tubes to help secure the tube and prevent an air leak.

❺ A paediatric patient has large adenoidal tissue and relatively small nares. Consequently, nasotracheal intubation in the paediatric population is technically difficult and has a high complication rate from traumatic bleeding, aspiration, and oesophageal intubation. These intubations also generally take a longer time to perform and require a patient who is awake and co-operative. The orotracheal route is the preferred approach.

In addition to proper positioning and equipment selection, successful emergent intubation often requires the administration of rapid sequence induction (RSI) medications. These medications provide transient sedation and neuromuscular relaxation during the procedure. Induction agents include ketamine, fentanyl, and midazolam, and neuromuscular paralysing agents include succinylcholine, rocuronium, and vecuronium. The advantages of RSI are twofold. First, the patient will not instinctually struggle against noxious stimuli, such as the laryngoscopic blade and endotracheal tube insertion. This optimises the chances of visualising the vocal cords. Second, the induction agents affect the following autonomic responses.

❶ Bradycardia – patients less than 5 years old have a higher risk for bradyarrhythmias with direct laryngoscopy because of vagal nerve stimulation. Consequently, they may require atropine prophylactically in their RSI drug regimen.

❷ Tachycardia and hypertension – induction medications attenuate this catecholamine response to laryngoscopy and intubation.

❸ Gag reflex – patients requiring emergency intubation benefit from RSI medications because patients are assumed to have a full stomach, the contents of which may regurgitate during intubation. By blunting the gag reflex using RSI, the risk of oesophageal reflux and pulmonary aspiration decreases. The process of RSI includes cricoid pressure, which also limits regurgitation and aspiration.

The advantages of RSI agents, however, must be balanced against the primary disadvantage of persistent apnoea after a failed intubation. The practitioner must be aware that when patients receive these drugs, unsuccessful intubations may cause the patient to drop their oxygen saturation precipitously.

Indications

- Cardiopulmonary arrest.
- Respiratory failure or obstruction.
- Excessive work of breathing refractory to BM ventilation.
- Loss of the gag reflex.
- Need for prolonged ventilation or hyperventilation.

Contraindications

- Adequate response to bag mask (BM) ventilation with anticipated short requirement for assisted ventilation.
- Structural abnormalities, such as a large tongue haematoma, or massive facial injuries that require a tracheostomy or cricothyrotomy.
- Functioning tracheostomy.

Equipment

❶ Cardiopulmonary and oxygen saturation monitor.
❷ Rigid-tip suction catheter.
❸ BM and self-inflating bag.
❹ Laryngoscope (Figs 23.4.1, 23.4.2).
❺ Endotracheal tube (Fig. 23.4.3).
❻ Endotracheal tube stylet.
❼ Syringe for cuffed endotracheal tube.
❽ Device for confirmation of intubation (Chapter 23.5).

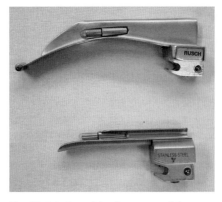

Fig. 23.4.1 Curved (top) versus straight (bottom) laryngoscopic blades.

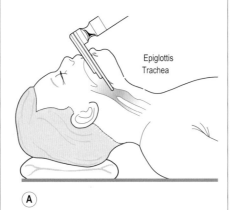

Ⓐ

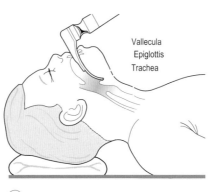

Ⓑ

Fig. 23.4.2 Insertion of laryngoscopic blades.
Laryngoscopes are available with either a straight blade end (A) or a curved blade end (B). The straight laryngoscopic blade should slide just 'under' or posterior to the epiglottis and elevate the tongue and epiglottis as a unit to visualise the vocal cords. Because of their floppy and large epiglottis, neonates and infants less than 5 years old require this straight blade for better visualisation of the cords. For older patients, both straight and curved blades are acceptable. When the curved laryngoscopic blade is used, the blade should rest in the vallecular space just anterior to the epiglottis and posterior to the base of the tongue. Lifting the laryngoscope up towards the ceiling elevates the vallecular space and the tongue as a unit, which indirectly lifts the epiglottis anteriorly to allow visualisation of the vocal cords.

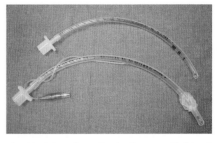

Fig. 23.4.3 Endotracheal tubes, uncuffed (top) and cuffed (bottom).

❾ Strong adhesive tape for securing the endotracheal tube.
❿ Bite block or oropharyngeal (OP) airway.

Preparation

Because many pieces of equipment require preparation, the 'SOAP ME' mnemonic is a helpful checklist reminder for the provider (Table 23.4.1).

Laryngoscope There are two types of blades to visualise the vocal cords – straight and curved. For the neonate or infant, use a straight blade to more easily visualise the anteriorly located vocal cords. For older patients, whose anatomy more resembles that of adults, use either a straight or a curved laryngoscopic blade.

Additionally, the laryngoscopic blades come in different sizes. To determine the correct size to use for a specific patient, either (1) use the length-based resuscitation tape

Table 23.4.1 Preparing the equipment – 'SOAP ME' mnemonic
1. Suction – turn the suction apparatus on and test the suction catheter.
2. Oxygenation equipment – test the self-inflating reservoir bag and bag mask (BM) setup.
3. Airway equipment – select the appropriately sized endotracheal tube and insert a stylet. Check the endotracheal tube cuff integrity with a syringe, if applicable. Also obtain tube sizes slightly larger and smaller than expected, in case of unexpected anatomy. Obtain laryngoscopic blades slightly larger and smaller than anticipated, and test the blade lights. Finally, check the rescue airway devices in case of a failed intubation.
4. Pharmacological agents – prepare rapid sequence intubation drugs.
5. Monitoring equipment – turn on the cardiopulmonary monitor, oxygen saturation monitor, and tracheal confirmation device.

Table 23.4.2 Laryngoscope size selection	
Age	Blade type and size
Premature infant	Straight blade 0
Newborn to 2 years	Straight blade 1
2–6 years	Straight blade 2
6–12 years	Straight blade 2, Curved blade 2
Adolescent	Straight blade 2 or 3, Curved blade 3

(Chapter 23.1) or (2) use an age-based table (Table 23.4.2).

Endotracheal tube Cuffed endotracheal tubes serve to prevent an air leak around the tube. Because of the relatively funnel-shaped airway in patients less than 8 years old, an uncuffed tube should be used. Conversely, for older patients and adults, cuffed tubes are essential because of their cylindrical-shaped airway. Without a balloon cuff, this airway shape is susceptible to significant air leaks. After choosing a cuffed or uncuffed endotracheal tube, select the appropriate size of the tube for the patient (Table 23.4.3). The tube sizes range from 1.0 to 9.0, representing the tube inner diameter in millimetres.

Positioning

The patient should be placed in a supine, neutral 'sniffing' position. For infants and small children, placing a small towel roll under the shoulders prevents the occiput from hyperflexing the neck and occluding the airway.

Procedure

❶ Provide in-line spinal immobilisation, if necessary. Have an assistant stand at the side of the bed, and maintain the neutral position of the head and neck by cupping the patient's ears with both hands (Fig. 23.4.4).

❷ Pre-oxygenate the patient by BM ventilation with 100% oxygen for 1–2 minutes. Be aware that the smaller the child, the faster the rate of oxygen desaturation during the intubation procedure. If time permits, fully pre-oxygenate the patient.

❸ During preoxygenation and intubation, have an assistant apply gentle posterior pressure to the cricoid cartilage. This reduces oesophageal reflux of gastric contents and the risk of aspiration.

❹ Administer RSI medications and continue BM ventilation until neuromuscular paralysis occurs.

❺ Grasp the laryngoscopic handle with the left hand and engage the blade so that the attached light bulb illuminates.

❻ Gently insert the laryngoscope, starting from the patient's right side of the mouth and 'sweep' the tongue towards the left.

❼ Continue inserting the blade deep while lifting the laryngoscope anteriorly and inferiorly, trying to visualise the vocal cords.

❽ Suction any excessive secretions or gastric contents that are obscuring adequate visualisation of the epiglottis and vocal cords.

❾ Once the vocal cords are identified, use the right hand to insert the endotracheal tube into the right side of the mouth, aiming between the vocal cords.

❿ Watch the tube actually pass between the vocal cords and enter the trachea. The best way to determine whether a TI is successful (i.e. not an oesophageal intubation) is by direct visualisation. Other confirmatory modalities may provide false and misleading information.

⓫ Insert the tube to the appropriate length (Table 23.4.4).

⓬ Inflate the cuff, if applicable.

⓭ Attach the oxygen bag to the endotracheal tube and ventilate the patient, watching for equal chest rise with each bag insufflation.

⓮ Listen for equal breath sounds in bilateral axilla and the absence of breath sounds in the epigastrium.

⓯ Check for successful placement of the endotracheal tube by a confirmatory device (see Chapter 23.5).

⓰ Obtain a postintubation chest radiograph to check for successful tube placement and adequate depth of tube insertion. The tube should end 1–2 cm above the carina.

⓱ Secure the tube in place with adhesive tape.

⓲ Insert a bite block or OP airway to prevent the patient from chewing off the endotracheal tube.

Table 23.4.3 Endotracheal tube size selection
• Option 1 – use a length-based resuscitation tape.
• Option 2 – the inner diameter of the endotracheal tube should equal the patient's fifth fingernail.
• Option 3 – the tube size should equal the sum of the patient's age in years divided by four and added to four. For instance, an 8-year-old child requires a $(\frac{8}{4}) + 4$ tube, or a 6.0 tube.

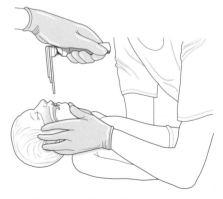

Fig. 23.4.4 Spinal immobilisation by assistant.

Table 23.4.4 Determining the correct endotracheal tube insertion depth
• Option 1 – insert the endotracheal tube (3× endotracheal tube size) centimetres as marked at the patient's teeth. For instance, a 5.0 tube correlates with a 15 cm insertion depth.
• Option 2 – there exists a black double line drawn circumferentially about 2–5 cm from the tube's distal tip. Insert the endotracheal tube until this double line rests at the level of the vocal cords.

Complications

- Traumatic injury to lips, teeth, oropharynx, larynx, vocal cords and oesophagus
- Incorrect insertion of tube into oesophagus or intracranially
- Emesis and aspiration
- Increased intracranial, intraocular, and intragastric pressures
- Cervical spinal injury
- Dysrhythmia
- Hypertension or hypotension
- Hypoxia and/or hypercarbia
- Pain and anxiety
- Dislodgement of endotracheal tube during movement

Tips

- Equipment failure is an unnecessary complication with potentially devastating consequences. Be sure to test the functionality of the suction apparatus, the brightness of the laryngoscope light bulb, and the integrity of the endotracheal tube cuff prior to intubation.
- Anticipating a failed initial intubation reduces the complication rate in tracheal intubation. Prepare variously-sized laryngoscopes, slightly larger and smaller endotracheal tubes, and failed-airway alternatives at the bedside.

- During preoxygenation and intubation, applying cricoid pressure too aggressively may not only occlude the oesophagus but also the airway.
- While looking for the vocal cords with the laryngoscope, a common mistake is to use the patient's teeth as a fulcrum for the blade. Beware of fracturing the patient's teeth.
- To help visualise a patient's vocal cords, which are being obscured by a floppy epiglottis, use the BURP manoeuvre (Fig. 23.4.5).
- Because of the short trachea in the paediatric population, a common mistake

during intubation is inserting the endotracheal tube too deep, resulting in a right mainstem intubation.
- Also, because of the short trachea in the paediatric population, the endotracheal tube may easily dislodge from its position in the airway. Be vigilant about securing the tube at all times, but especially during transport or with any movements. Frequently recheck its position.

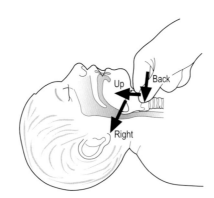

Fig. 23.4.5 Improving vocal cord visualisation – BURP manoeuvre. Using your right hand (non-laryngoscope hand), manipulate the external cricoid cartilage with Back (posterior), Up (superior), and Rightward Pressure. This essentially moves the vocal cords towards the right and out from 'under' the overhanging epiglottis.

Further reading

Chameides L, Hazinski MF, editors. *Paediatric advanced life support.* Dallas, TX: American Heart Association; 1997.

Dieckmann RA, Brownstein DR, Gausche-Hill M, editors. *Paediatric education for prehospital professionals.* Sudbury, MA: Jones & Bartlett Publishers; 2000.

Gnauck K, et al. Emergency intubation of the paediatric medical patient: Use of anesthetic agents in the ED. *Ann Emerg Med* 1994;**23**(6):1242–7.

Knill RL. Difficult laryngoscopy made easy with a BURP. *Can J Anaesth* 1993;**40**(3):279–82.

Lee BS, Gausche-Hill M. Paediatric airway management. *Clin Paediatr Emerg Med* 2001;**2**(2):91–106.

McAllister JD, Gnauck KA. Rapid sequence intubation of the paediatric patient. Fundamentals of practice. *Paediatr Clin N Am* 1999;**46**(6):1249–84.

Moynihan RJ, Brock-Utne JG, Archer JH, et al. The effect of cricoid pressure on preventing gastric insufflation in infants and children. *Anesthesiology* 1993;**78**(4):652–6.

Stoelting RK. Circulatory changes during direct laryngoscopy and tracheal intubation: Influence of duration of laryngoscopy with or without prior lidocaine. *Anesthesiology* 1977;**47**(4):381–4.

Thompson A. Paediatric emergency airway management. In: Dieckmann RA, et al., editors. *Paediatric emergency and critical care procedures.* St Louis, MO: Mosby; 1997.

Tintinalli JE, Claffey J. Complications of nasotracheal intubation. *Ann Emerg Med* 1981;**10**(3):142–4.

23.5 Confirmation of intubation

Michelle Lin

Background

Confirming correct placement of the endotracheal tube is crucial because of the high morbidity and mortality of an inadvertent and unrecognised oesophageal intubation. The most accurate means of assuring success is by visualising the endotracheal tube between the vocal cords and into the trachea. A successful tracheal intubation (TI) is also highly likely when condensation appears in the plastic endotracheal tube during assisted ventilation, when breath sounds are heard in both axillae but not in the epigastrium, when the pulse oximetry is 100%, and when the chest cavity rises and falls with positive-pressure ventilation. At times, however, these findings can be equivocal, especially in children. The clinical exam is notoriously deceptive in determining correct endotracheal tube placement, and it is imperative to use at least one of the following techniques for every intubated patient.

❶ Oesophageal aspiration. An oesophageal aspirator is a large syringe or a self-inflating bulb (Fig. 23.5.1), which attaches to the proximal end of the endotracheal tube. The aspirator differentiates between an oesophageal versus a tracheal placement because the oesophagus is a collapsible structure under negative pressure, while the trachea is not. Successful air aspiration is highly associated with trachea placement. It has been determined that the oesophageal aspiration modality has a sensitivity of 99% and specificity of 100% in confirming endotracheal tube placement in patients weighing more than 20 kg.

- Oesophageal intubation. When air is aspirated from the endotracheal tube,

significant airflow resistance suggests an oesophageal intubation, because of oesophageal wall collapse. The large syringe or self-inflating bulb will not fill with air to full capacity.

- Tracheal intubation. When air is aspirated from the endotracheal tube, there will be no resistance to 30–40 mL of airflow if the tube indeed lies in the trachea.

❷ End-tidal colorimetric capnometry (Fig. 23.5.2). The capnometer attaches to the proximal end of the endotracheal tube and detects the presence of CO_2 within the tube. The capnometer will display a yellow (CO_2 present) or purple (CO_2 absent) colour in the indicator window, which generally correlates with a tracheal or oesophageal intubation, respectively. Multiple studies find that a yellow colour change has a 100% positive predictive value for correct endotracheal tube placement. When used for a poorly perfused patient (e.g. cardiac arrest), however, there will often be no yellow colour change because of expected low CO_2 levels. This is the primary limitation when using this modality. Colorimetric capnometry is not commonly used in hospital. Table 23.5.1 provides a mnemonic to help remember the colour scheme.

❸ Digital capnography (Fig. 23.5.3). This latest technology continuously detects and displays the partial pressure of CO_2 at the proximal end of the endotracheal tube. In adult cardiac arrest patients, a $pCO_2 < 5$ mmHg correlates with an extremely poor prognosis. Digital capnography is the standard for confirmation of intubations.

- Tracheal intubation. With each exhalation and inhalation, a characteristic waveform, showing the rise, plateau, and fall of CO_2 levels, confirms correct positioning of the tube in the trachea.

- Oesophageal intubation. With each exhalation and inhalation, an unchanging, flat waveform demonstrates the absence of CO_2 and thus the misplacement of the endotracheal tube into the oesophagus.

Indications

All intubated patients.

Contraindications

- Do not use an adult-sized colorimetric capnometry device on intubated patients weighing less than 15 kg, because the device adds a significant dead-space volume for the neonate to rebreathe CO_2. Instead, attach a paediatric-sized capnometer for these patients.

- Use caution with oesophageal aspiration on patients weighing less than 20 kg. Several studies, however, suggest that

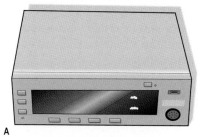
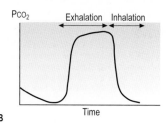

Fig. 23.5.3 Digital capnography instrument (A) and typical waveform reading (B).

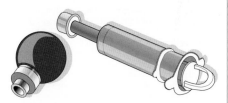

Fig. 23.5.1 Oesophageal bulb (left) and aspirator (right).

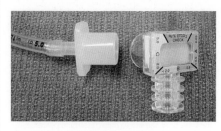

Fig. 23.5.2 Colorimetric capnometer.

oesophageal aspiration may still be safe at a lower weight limit of 4 kg, because the resting lung volume is still greater than 50 cm^3, which is the typical volume in an oesophageal aspirator.

Equipment

❶ Oesophageal aspiration syringe or bulb (see Fig. 23.5.1).
❷ End-tidal colorimetric capnometer (see Fig. 23.5.2).
❸ Digital capnography (see Fig. 23.5.3).

Preparation and positioning

- Prepare at least one confirmation device for bedside use before the patient is intubated so that immediate confirmation is available.
- Specific for the colorimetric capnometer, open the packaging for this disposable device. Check that the unit is dry and initially displays a purple colour in the indicator window to ensure proper functioning.
- Specific for digital capnography, be sure that the device is plugged in and turned on. Blowing across the capnography tubing tests the monitoring and sensing function.

Procedure

Oesophageal aspiration

❶ Expel all the air out of the oesophageal syringe or bulb, and attach it to the proximal end of the endotracheal tube just after intubation. Inadvertently instilling air into the endotracheal tube with the syringe or bulb may cause a falsely reassuring aspiration result.
❷ Slowly aspirate air over 5 seconds.
❸ If the endotracheal tube is correctly positioned in the trachea, there will be no resistance during aspiration.

❹ If the endotracheal tube is incorrectly positioned in the oesophagus, there will be resistance during aspiration. Reposition the tube under direct laryngoscopy.

End-tidal colorimetric capnometer

❶ Attach the capnometer in series with the entire ventilation system between the endotracheal tube and the bag–valve device. Ventilation can continue through the capnometer.
❷ After ventilating the patient over six times, check the colour of the capnometer indicator window during the exhalation phase. Initially purple in colour when attached, exhalation phases correlate with a yellow colour change.
❸ Recall that a yellow colour confirms correct TI because it indicates the presence of CO_2.
❹ Secure the capnometer in place for continuous monitoring while the patient transfers to the intensive-care unit.

Digital capnography

❶ Connect the digital capnography tubing to the distal end of the bag–valve device. The air in the endotracheal tube is now contiguous with the air in this tubing.
❷ Ventilate the patient and observe the live-time waveforms of CO_2 return during exhalation. The absence of CO_2 indicates a failed intubation.

Complications

There are no direct complications to the patient by using these devices. Indirectly, however, the misinterpretation of their findings may cause the practitioner to incorrectly change patient management.

Tips

❶ Check tube placement after every intubation and after any patient movement, such as during transport, because the endotracheal tube can easily shift into the oesophagus.
❷ Use a paediatric-sized colorimetric capnometer for patients less than 15 kg to decrease the volume of dead space in the ventilatory circuit.
❸ When intubating a poorly perfused patient, using an oesophageal aspirator is more accurate than the end-tidal colorimetry capnometer or digital capnography, because the endotracheal tube's CO_2 level is extremely low. In this case, the latter instruments, which rely on CO_2 levels, may only give equivocal confirm of endotracheal tube placement. The oesophageal aspirator, however, relies on the anatomical differences between the collapsible oesophagus and the semi-rigid trachea, independent of expired CO_2 levels. Thus, with low perfusion states, the aspirator provides a more accurate confirmation of correct endotracheal tube placement.

Further reading

Anderson KH, Schultz-Leban T. Oesophageal intubation can be undetected by auscultation of the chest. *Acta Anaesthesiol Scand* 1994;**38**:580–2.

Bhende MS, Thompson AE, Orr RA. Utility of an end-tidal carbon dioxide detector during stabilization and transport of critically ill children. *Paediatrics* 1992;**89**: 1042–4.

Bhende MS, Thompson AE, Orr RA. Validity of a disposable end-tidal CO_2 detector in verifying endotracheal tube placement in infants and children. *Ann Emerg Med* 1992;**21**:142–5.

Burnett YL, et al. Efficacy of the self-inflating bulb in verifying tracheal tube placement in children. *Anesth Analg* 1995;**80**:S63 [abstract].

Dieckmann RA, Brownstein D, Gausche-Hill M, editors. *Paediatric education for prehospital professionals.* Sudbury, MA: Jones & Bartlett Publishers; 2000.

Marley CD Jr, et al. Evaluation of a prototype oesophageal detection device. *Acad Emerg Med* 1995;**2**(6):503–7.

Sharieff GQ, et al. The self-inflating bulb as an oesophageal detector device in children weighing more than twenty kilograms: A comparison between two techniques. *Acad Emerg Med* 2003;**41**(5):623–9.

Ward KR, Yealy DM. End-tidal carbon dioxide monitoring in emergency medicine. Part 1. Basic principles. *Acad Emerg Med* 1998;**5**(6):628–36.

Wee MYK. The oesophageal detector device: Assessment of a new method to distinguish oesophageal from tracheal intubation. *Anaesthesia* 1998;**43**(1):27–9.

Zideman D, et al. Airways in paediatric and newborn resuscitation. *Ann Emerg Med* 2001;**37**(4 Suppl): S126–36.

Table 23.5.1   End-tidal colour capnometer – interpreting the colour

- If you see Yellow, then 'Yes' – there is CO_2 return. At least 20 mmHg of CO_2 is detectable. Several studies show a 100% positive predictive value of a yellow indicator colour with a tracheal space intubation (rather than an oesophageal).
- If you see Purple, then there is a 'Problem' - there is no CO_2 return. A TI is unlikely, unless the patient has extremely poor perfusion, such as during asystole. If a purple colour is displayed, less than 4 mmHg of CO_2 is detectable.
- If you see an intermediate 'Tan' colour, then 'Think about it', because the tube could be sitting in the trachea or the oesophagus. The capnometer is sensing between 4–15 mmHg of CO_2. This equivocal finding requires direct laryngoscopy re-visualisation of the tube's placement to help determine placement.

23.6 The surgical airway

Judith Klein

Background

The paediatric airway is distinct from that of the adult. The epiglottis is floppy and the larynx is shorter, more anterior, and more cephalad. The larynx is narrower and therefore more prone to obstruction by oedema, scarring, fluids, or foreign bodies. The cartilage of the larynx is also softer, which makes palpation of landmarks on the skin more difficult. The cricoid ring is the only spot where cartilage encircles the paediatric trachea, and it is also the narrowest portion of the airway (Fig. 23.6.1).

The vast majority of paediatric airway emergencies can be readily managed with bag–valve–mask (BVM) ventilation and/or tracheal intubation (TI). Rarely, a child presents with complete airway obstruction or anatomic abnormalities, and ventilation with BVM or TI is impossible. In these situations, a surgical airway may be necessary to provide life-saving oxygenation and ventilation to avoid anoxic brain injury. Surgical airways in children include: needle cricothyroidotomy; surgical cricothyroidotomy; and, rarely, tracheostomy. Placing a needle, catheter or tube directly into the trachea through the neck will temporarily relieve airway obstruction or bypass anatomic abnormalities.

In children under the age of 5 years, the membrane between the thyroid cartilage and the cricoid cartilage, the cricothyroid membrane (see Fig. 23.6.1), is extremely

small. For this group, needle cricothyroidotomy is easier than surgical cricothyroidotomy. While the needle technique will provide emergency oxygenation, it may not provide adequate ventilation, especially over time. Even a jet 'ventilator', a rescue device that attaches to the needle and provides intermittent bursts of high-pressure oxygen to simulate the normal respiratory cycle, may not allow for adequate ventilation and clearance of CO_2.

In children 5 years and over, surgical cricothyroidotomy is easier and more effective, because it creates a larger conduit and allows both immediate oxygenation and ventilation via a bag–valve device. Tracheotomy in a young child is extremely difficult to perform emergently and is rarely indicated in the emergency derpartment.

Indications

- Failure to ventilate with BVM and/or TI.
- Obstructed or disrupted larynx.

Table 23.6.1 lists situations in which these indications occur. The most common circumstances in which intubations fail are the

presence of massive nasopharyngeal haemorrhage, large tongue haematoma, laryngeal spasm, laryngeal stenosis, or obstruction of the airway by a foreign body that cannot be removed.

Contraindications

- Presence of a secure airway.
- Traumatic destruction of the cricothyroid membrane.
- Transection of the trachea with retraction of the distal segment.
- Surgical cricothyroidotomy is relatively contraindicated in children under the age of 5 years. In this group, perform needle cricothyroidotomy.

Needle cricothyroidotomy

Equipment

Table 23.6.2 lists the equipment for this procedure, which can be divided into three categories:

❶ Oxygen source. A transtracheal jet ventilator device is ideal. It provides high-pressure 100% oxygen (50 psi) in intermittent bursts, which allows *more* time for passive CO_2 exhalation (Fig. 23.6.2). Alternatively, use a bag–valve device connected to 15 L min⁻¹ of wall oxygen.

❷ Adaptors. The jet ventilator device connects directly to the catheter at the neck. To use the bag–valve system,

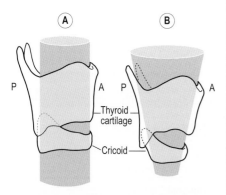

Fig. 23.6.1 Locating the cricoid membrane. Comparison of adult (A) and paediatric (B) airways. Note funnel shape of paediatric airway with narrowest portion at cricoid ring.

Table 23.6.1 Situations requiring cricothyroidotomy
Trauma   • Laryngeal fracture   • Airway burns   • Massive haemorrhage   • Foreign body   • Subglottic stenosis (late)   • Burn contractures (late)
Congenital abnormalities   • Laryngeal atresia/stenosis/clefts   • Tracheoesophageal fistula   • Pierre–Robin syndrome   • Treacher–Collins syndrome
Cervical spine abnormalities   • Trisomy 21 syndrome   • Klippel–Feil malformation   • Torticollis
Inflammatory/infectious   • Severe croup   • Epiglottis   • Bacterial tracheitis   • Retropharyngeal abscess   • Cricoarytenoid arthritis
Laryngeal spasm

Table 23.6.2 Equipment for needle cricothyroidotomy
Oxygen source   • Jet ventilator (50 psi)   • Bag–valve–mask device attached to 15 L min⁻¹ wall oxygen
Adaptor   • 3 mm endotracheal tube adaptor   • 3 cm³ syringe barrel and 8.0 mm endotracheal tube
Catheter   • 14-gauge catheter over a needle   • 3 cm³ syringe

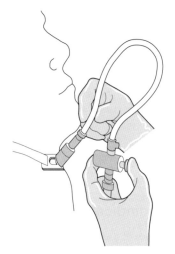

Fig. 23.6.2 Transtracheal jet ventilator device.

attach a 3-mm paediatric tracheal tube adapter with one end connected to the bag–valve device and the other to the end of the cricothyroidotomy catheter. Alternatively, set up a ventilation system with a 3-mL syringe and an 8-mm tracheal tube that attaches to the bag–valve device (Fig. 23.6.3).

❸ Needle/cannula. A 14G over-the-needle catheter.

Preparation

❶ Since children have relatively large occiputs, place a shoulder roll transversely to prevent hyperflexion of the neck and improve visualisation of the anterior neck anatomy.

❷ If time allows, prepare the skin with povidone-iodine solution.

Procedure

❶ Palpate the hyoid bone high in the neck and move caudally to identify the thyroid and cricoid cartilages (Fig. 23.6.4A).

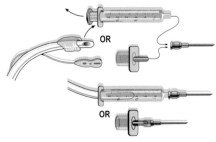

Fig. 23.6.3 Using a 3.0-mm tracheal tube or an 8-mm tracheal tube into a 3-mL syringe hub as a connector.

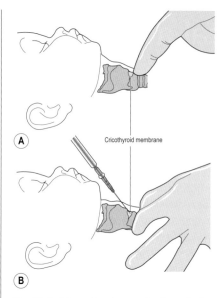

Cricothyroid membrane

Fig. 23.6.4 Inserting the needle through the membrane.

❷ Stabilise the cartilage using the thumb and index finger of the non-dominant hand.

❸ Insert a 14G over-the-needle catheter attached to a 3-cm³ syringe just superior to the cricoid cartilage (Fig. 23.6.4B). Angle the catheter caudally at about a 45° angle to the skin.

❹ Apply continuous backpressure to the syringe barrel. A rush of air into the syringe confirms entry into the trachea. Alternatively, fill the syringe with saline to use as an indicator. The marker of entry into the trachea is the presence of air bubbles in the syringe.

❺ Advance the catheter into the trachea and remove the needle and syringe. Do not let go of the catheter until it is secured or an alternative airway is obtained.

❻ If a jet ventilator device is available, attach it directly to the catheter. If this device is not available, attach a bag–valve system to high-flow (15 L min⁻¹) wall oxygen. Place an adaptor between the catheter and the bag–valve device. Either attach a 3-mm endotracheal tube adaptor directly onto the catheter or attach an 8-mm endotracheal tube in a 3-mL syringe barrel.

❼ With a jet ventilator, administer 100% oxygen at 20 bursts per minute with an approximate I:E ratio of 1:4 to allow for passive exhalation. If a bag–valve device is used, provide 20 'breaths' per minute with the same I:E ratio.

Complications
- Bleeding, but it is rarely massive.
- Inappropriate placement of a needle can cause injury to:
  - the larynx and vocal cords
  - great vessels of the neck
  - nerves
  - oesophagus.
- High-pressure oxygen can also cause significant barotrauma resulting in extensive subcutaneous emphysema, pneumothorax, and pneumomediastinum.

Tips
- Needle cricothyroidotomy is a temporising measure that may provide enough ventilation for about 30 minutes. Immediately consider other airway options.
- Remember to allow adequate time for passive exhalation to prevent barotrauma.
- Do *not* let go of the catheter until an alternative airway is established.

Surgical cricothyroidotomy

Equipment

Table 23.6.3 lists the equipment for surgical cricothyroidotomy.

Several commercial kits contain all equipment for a cricothyroidotomy tube using the guidewire or Seldinger technique. Other useful instruments include a tracheal hook and a tracheal dilator.

Table 23.6.3 Equipment for surgical cricothyroidotomy

- Frazier tip suction
- Scalpel
- Haemostat
- Tracheostomy or endotracheal tube
- Oxygen delivery system
- Tracheostomy suction

Optional
- Povidone-iodine solution
- Lidocaine with adrenaline (epinephrine)
- Tracheal hook
- Tracheal dilator

Preparation

❶ Expose the thyroid and cricoid cartilage by placing a roll under the child's shoulders.

❷ If time permits, prepare the skin with povidone-iodine solution and infiltrate the skin with lidocaine with adrenaline (epinephrine) to provide local anaesthesia and haemostasis.

Procedure

❶ Palpate the hyoid bone high in the neck and move caudally to identify the thyroid and cricoid cartilages (see Fig. 23.6.4A).

❷ Stabilise the larynx by placing thumb and forefinger of the non-dominant hand on either side of the thyroid cartilage.

❸ Make a midline vertical incision in the skin from thyroid cartilage to cricoid cartilage (Fig. 23.6.5). Expose the cricothyroid membrane via blunt dissection with haemostats.

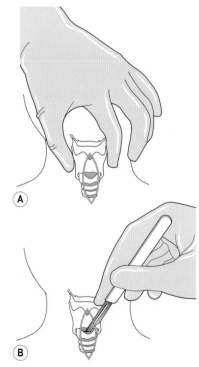

Fig. 23.6.5 Making the surgical incision in the skin.

❹ Make a horizontal incision in the cricothyroid membrane, carefully avoiding inserting the scalpel too far and lacerating the posterior aspect of the larynx.

❺ Insert the haemostat into the airway next to the scalpel to hold the space and widen the opening.

❻ Use a tracheal hook, if available, to maintain the opening and provide traction cranially while inserting the tube caudally (Fig. 23.6.6).

❼ If a tracheostomy tube of the appropriate size is not available, use an endotracheal tube of the same calibre. Trim the length of the tube to 3/2 of its diameter in centimetres (e.g. 4.0 ETT (cut to $3/2 \times 4 = 6$ cm).

❽ Attach a bag–valve device and ventilate the patient. Do not let go of the tube until it has been secured to the patient's neck.

The guidewire or Seldinger technique is an alternative to surgical placement of a cricothyroidotomy tube.

❶ Position the patient for surgical cricothyroidotomy.

❷ Identify the cricothyroid membrane and prepare the skin with povidone-iodine solution.

❸ Insert the needle mounted on a syringe through the cricothyroid membrane.

❹ Angle caudally at 45 degrees to the skin with the bevel of the needle up.

❺ Once air rushes into the syringe, pass the J-tipped guidewire through the needle and remove the needle.

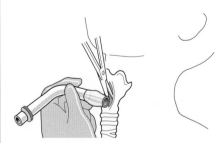

Fig. 23.6.6 Inserting the cricothyroidotomy tube.

❻ Make a stab incision over the needle through the skin and membrane.

❼ Insert the catheter and dilator over the guidewire into the trachea and remove both the wire and the dilator.

❽ Provide ventilation via a bag–valve device.

Complications

- Bleeding.
- Tube misplacement, resulting in hypoxia and subcutaneous emphysema.
- Laryngeal, oesophageal, or neurovascular injury.
- Barotrauma, which can result in pneumothorax or pneumomediastinum.
- Significant late complications include voice change due to vocal cord damage and subglottic stenosis.

Tips

- If the cricothyroid membrane is not visible with the initial vertical incision, extend it.
- Do not cut into the larynx blindly as this will increase the rate of complications.
- Have suction readily available for any bleeding into the trachea.
- Avoid using too large a tube. This can lead to laryngeal fracture.
- Size the catheter by using a length-based resuscitation tape.
- If a child requires prolonged ventilation, establish a definitive airway (tracheal intubation or tracheostomy) as soon as possible.

Further reading

Bower CM. The surgical airway. In: Dieckmann RA, Fiser DH, Selbst SM, editors. *Paediatric emergency and critical care procedures*. St Louis, MO: Mosby; 1997. p. 116–22.

Granholm T, Farmer DL. The surgical airway. *Resp Care Clin N Am* 2001;**7**(1):13–23.

Mace SE. Cricothyrotomy and translaryngeal jet ventilation. In: Roberts JR, Hedges JR, editors. *Clinical procedures in emergency medicine*. 3rd edn. Philadelphia, PA: WB Saunders; 1998. p. 57–74.

Peak DA, Roy S. Needle cricothyroidotomy revisited. *Paediatr Emerg Care* 1999;**15**(3):224–6.

Yealy DM, Plewa MC, Steward RD. An evaluation of cannulae and oxygen sources for paediatric jet ventilation. *Am J Emerg Med* 1991;**9**(1):20–3.

23.7 Needle thoracostomy

Judith Klein

Background

Normally, the visceral and parietal pleura are closely adherent to one another. However, if either surface is violated, air enters into the potential space between visceral and parietal pleura, creating a simple pneumothorax (Fig. 23.7.1). This typically occurs in the setting of blunt or penetrating trauma. Occasionally, spontaneous pneumothorax occurs, as with excessive air trapping in an asthmatic child. If enough air collects, a tension pneumothorax can develop in which pressure in the space shifts the mediastinum, impedes venous return to the heart, and decreases cardiac output (Fig. 23.7.2). Another pathophysiological mechanism for tension pneumothorax occurs when a patient with a simple pneumothorax is intubated – positive pressure ventilation will force air into the pleural space resulting in a tension pneumothorax. Tension pneumothorax can progress to shock and cardiopulmonary arrest.

The typical clinical scenario for tension pneumothorax is the child who experiences a penetrating injury to the chest wall or back. A sucking chest wound (open pneumothorax) may be present. The classic adult clinical findings of unilateral decreased air movement and trachea shift may not be readily detectable in children. More commonly, the clinical signs are tachypnea, oxygen desaturation, retractions, flaring, grunting and shock. Once tension pneumothorax develops, progression to shock and cardiopulmonary arrest can be rapid.

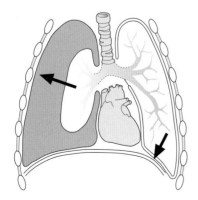

Fig. 23.7.1 Simple pneumothorax.

Needle evacuation of the air between the visceral and parietal pleura and conversion of the tension pneumothorax to an open pneumothorax will re-expand the lung and improve venous return and cardiac output. Needle thoracostomy is a temporising procedure. Immediately after needle thoracostomy, insert a chest tube to provide ongoing drainage in a closed system (Chapter 23.8). The risk of not performing needle thoracostomy in a child spiralling towards death from a tension pneumothorax is far greater than the risk of performing the procedure in a child without a pneumothorax.

Indications

- Blunt or penetrating trauma with signs of tension pneumothorax.
- Chest X-ray evidence of a tension pneumothorax in a child in respiratory distress for any reason.

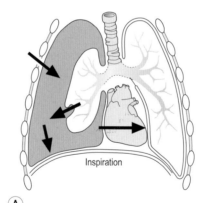
Inspiration
(A)

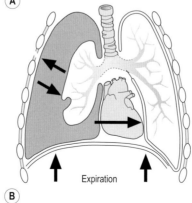
Expiration
(B)

Fig. 23.7.2 Tension pneumothorax. (A) Inspiration, (B) Expiration.

- Suspected tension pneumothorax in an intubated patient who is rapidly deteriorating (e.g. hypotension, hypoxia).
- Pulseless electrical activity (PEA) in the setting of trauma or asthma.

Contraindications

- A stable child with a simple pneumothorax, not under tension.
- There is no absolute contraindication to needle thoracostomy in a child with possible tension pneumothorax and shock. While preparing for open thoracotomy in the emergency department, placing a needle in the pleural space will not cause further deterioration.
- If a skin infection is present at the preferred needle site, select an alternative location.

Equipment

❶ 14-gauge catheter over a needle.
❷ 30-mL syringe.
❸ Povidone-iodine solution.

Preparation

❶ Inspect the anatomy of the ribs and select an entry site above the rib that avoids injuring the intercostal neurovascular bundle (Fig. 23.7.3).
❷ Identify a site to insert the needle over the rib.
❸ Position the child supine with the head of the bed angled up at 30 degrees. Have an assistant gently restrain the conscious child.
❹ Use a local and/or intravenous analgesic if time allows and if the child is conscious.
❺ Identify the 2nd intercostal space (above the 3rd rib) at the midclavicular line. This space is ideal since air in the pleural space rises and typically collects toward the top

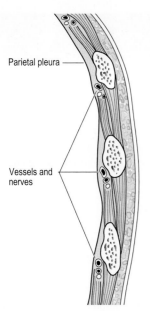

Fig. 23.7.3 Anatomy of the ribs and intercostal neurovascular bundle.

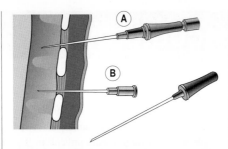

Fig. 23.7.4 Inserting the thoracostomy needle.

❹ Remove the syringe and the needle, and leave the catheter in place (Fig. 23.7.4B).

❺ Place a chest tube immediately.

If there is an open connection between the chest wall and the pleural space from a penetrating injury – an open pneumothorax or sucking chest wound – cover with a petrolatum gauze, extending 6–8 cm from the wound edges on all sides and taped on three sides, to stop further air entry during inspiration (Fig. 23.7.5). Leave one side free to allow for the ongoing egress of air from the pleural space.

Complications

- Performing needle thoracostomy in a patient without a pneumothorax who is subsequently intubated can cause a pneumothorax or injury to the lung parenchyma. Under positive pressure ventilation, this pleural penetration can result in an ongoing air leak, which can then lead to a tension pneumothorax. Always place a chest tube after needle thoracostomy to prevent this complication.
- Placing the needle below the rib can cause laceration of an intercostal artery and, subsequently, a haemothorax.
- Placing the catheter lower in the chest or closer to the mediastinum can result in

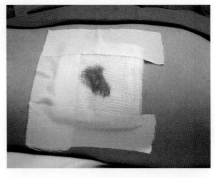

Fig. 23.7.5 Treating a sucking chest wound.

diaphragm penetration, bowel penetration, haemopericardium or coronary vessel.
- If the catheter becomes occluded and fails to drain air, the tension pneumothorax can reoccur.

Tips

- Perform tube thoracostomy as soon as possible in the setting of suspected tension pneumothorax. This relieves tension and creates an open pneumothorax.
- Always perform tube thoracostomy after needle thoracostomy to prevent tension pneumothorax from developing.

Further reading

Barton ED, Epperson M, Hoyt DB, Rosen P. Prehospital needle aspiration and tube thoracostomy in trauma victims: A six-year experience with aero medical crews. *J Emerg Med* 1995;**13**(2):155–63.

Bliss D, Silen M. Paediatric thoracic trauma. *Crit Care Med* 2002;**30**(11 Suppl):S409–15.

Wright SW. Tube thoracostomy. In: Roberts JR, Hedges JR, editors. *Clinical procedures in emergency medicine*. 3rd ed. Philadelphia, PA: WB Saunders; 1998.

Zimmerman KR. Needle thoracostomy. In: Dieckmann RA, Fiser DH, Selbst SM, editors. *Paediatric emergency and critical care procedures*. St Louis, MO: Mosby; 1997.

of the lungs. A lateral approach is an alternative, but may have more complications, including lung penetration and subsequent adhesions.

❻ Prepare the skin of the entry site with povidone-iodine solution.

Procedure

❶ Attach the catheter over the needle to the 30-mL syringe.

❷ Insert the catheter into the chest wall at a 90 degree angle above the 3rd rib (2nd intercostal space) at the midclavicular line (Fig. 23.7.4A).

❸ Provide back pressure on the syringe. Once there is a free flow of air in the syringe, continue to pull back on the plunger to evacuate the air.

23.8 Tube thoracostomy

Ronald A. Dieckmann

Background

Traumatic pneumothorax and haemothorax are the most frequent paediatric indications for tube thoracostomy. Pneumothorax is a serious sequela of major chest trauma in children and may occur as a result of blunt injury without rib fractures or chest penetration. Sometimes, spontaneous pneumothorax occurs without trauma, from rapid increase in intraluminal pressure, especially with patients who have pre-existing bronchopulmonary disease. Air or fluid in the pleural space can cause significant impediments to oxygenation/ventilation and drastically reduce cardiac output, usually when the haemothorax is large or the pneumothorax is under tension. Tension pneumothorax and large haemothorax are potentially lethal emergencies that require immediate chest decompression. Rarely, large pleural fluid collections from non-traumatic aetiologies, such as empyemas, that are causing respiratory distress, require tube thoracostomy for drainage.

The typical clinical presentation for tension pneumothorax and/or large haemothorax is the child who experiences a penetrating injury to the chest wall or back. A sucking chest wound may be present. Sometimes, these conditions result from penetrations below the nipple line or tip of the scapula that may also involve penetration into the abdomen, or from remote penetrations with gunshots that traverse multiple anatomic regions. Less frequently, blunt trauma is the mechanism. The classic adult clinical findings of unilateral decreased air movement and trachea shift are rarely present in children. More commonly, the clinical signs are tachypnoea, oxygen desaturation, retractions, flaring, grunting and shock.

Tube thoracostomy is the insertion of an intrapleural tube to evacuate air and/or fluid from the pleural space. The procedure is a time-honoured evacuation technique for all age patients, and it may be life saving. The technique is effective for removal of most pleural air or fluid collections and has a good safety record in children. The main differences in the procedure between adults and children are the need for more meticulous patient preparation and smaller catheters in children. Sometimes, detection of pleural air or fluid is more difficult in children, requiring computerised tomography (CT) imaging to localise and quantify.

In the setting of tension pneumothorax, needle thoracostomy (Chapter 23.7) may precede tube thoracostomy, but tube thoracostomy must always follow needle thoracostomy. Stable, small pneumothoraces not under tension (e.g. <20%), are usually managed with observation alone, without a chest tube. There is an increasing tendency to manage even moderate sized pneumothoraces without tension with observation only. Massive haemothorax occurs when a large vascular structure under systemic pressure bleeds into the pleural space. This is usually the internal mammary artery or an intercostal artery. In this setting, tube thoracostomy is the only treatment likely to salvage the child. Occasionally, recirculation or autotransfusion of evacuated blood from the pleural space is indicated to treat massive haemothorax. In the overwhelming majority of children with significant chest-wall penetrations, tube thoracostomy is the only treatment indicated.

Indications

- Tension pneumothorax.
- Haemothorax.
- Rapid pleural fluid accumulation with respiratory distress.

Contraindications

Need for immediate open thoracotomy.

Equipment

❶ Chest tube tray (Table 23.8.1).
❷ Chest tube sizes French 12–36.
❸ Pigtail chest tubes.
❹ Chest tube drainage device.
❺ Wall suction.

Preparation

❶ Identify the presence of pneumothorax/haemothorax and the affected side by clinical examination and/or chest X-ray.
❷ Establish secure vascular access and apply cardiac monitor and pulse oximetry.
❸ If the child is conscious, provide parenteral sedation/analgesia.
❹ If the child is stable, consider an intercostal nerve block.
❺ Explain the procedure to the verbal child.
❻ Place a nasogastric tube to decompress the stomach, when there is abdominal distension.
❼ Place the child in the supine or upright position with the arm raised on the affected side.
❽ Identify the entry site (Fig. 23.8.1), on the middle–anterior axillary line between the fourth and fifth rib, at the nipple level.
❾ Drape the area and prepare the area widely between the fourth and sixth ribs with povidone-iodine solution.
❿ Infiltrate the entry site above the sixth rib generously with lidocaine in conscious patients, and also infiltrate along the insertion site superiorly to the fourth interspace.
⓫ Select a properly-sized standard chest tube or pigtail catheter (Table 23.8.2).

Table 23.8.1 Chest tube tray
• Kelly clamps (2)
• Mayo scissors
• Suture scissors
• Needle holder
• Scalpel
• Forceps
• Silk suture
• 10 mL syringe
• 25-gauge needle
• 20-gauge needle
• Sterile towels
• 4 × 4 sterile gauze
• Vacuum device
• Drainage apparatus with water seal
• Plastic connectors (straight and Y type)
• Chest tubes
• Petrolatum
• Lidocaine or bupivacaine for local injection
• Antiseptic prep solution
• Wide cloth tap

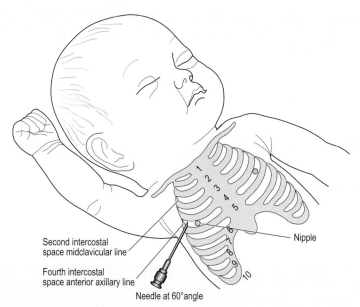

Second intercostal space midclavicular line

Fourth intercostal space anterior axillary line

Needle at 60°angle

Nipple

Fig. 23.8.1 Entry site for chest tube.

Procedure

Inserting the tube

❶ Incise the skin above the sixth rib 1–3 cm horizontally.

❷ Insert a curved Kelly into the incision, with tips away from the chest, and dissect the track superiorly to the fourth interspace (Fig. 23.8.2).

❸ Rotate the Kelly and puncture through the chest wall.

❹ Enter over the rib to avoid the neurovascular bundle.

❺ Widen the hole with the Kelly then insert a gloved finger into the hole to assure the track is clear to the pleura.

❻ Insert the appropriately-sized thoracostomy tube into the hole and direct the tube posteriorly.

❼ Facilitate tube entry by grasping the tube with the Kelly to guide tube entry

into the pleural space. Assure the tube is inserted beyond the last hole.

❽ Attach the tube to the drainage system.

Securing the tube

❶ Use 2–0 silk to secure the tube.

❷ Employ a purse string suture, and wrap the suture material around the tube (Fig. 23.8.3). This will allow removal of the tube and closing of the incision without additional suturing.

❸ Place a gauze, slit in half and coated with petrolatum jelly over the tube and entry site.

❹ Secure all tube connections with tape.

❺ Obtain an X-ray to confirm tube placement and decompression of air or fluid.

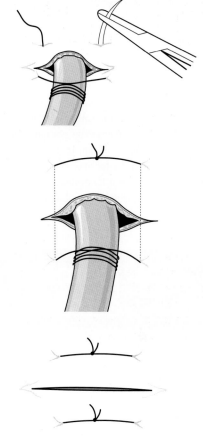

Fig. 23.8.3 Securing the chest tube.

Complications

● Haemopericardium.
● Tension pneumothorax.
● Haemothorax.
● Myocardial injury.
● Diaphragm perforation.
● Solid organ injury.
● Viscus injury.
● Cardiopulmonary arrest.

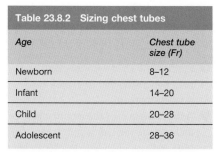

Table 23.8.2	Sizing chest tubes
Age	*Chest tube size (Fr)*
Newborn	8–12
Infant	14–20
Child	20–28
Adolescent	28–36

Formula: chest tube size (in Fr) = 4 × endotracheal tube size (mm).
Use larger tube size for haemothorax.

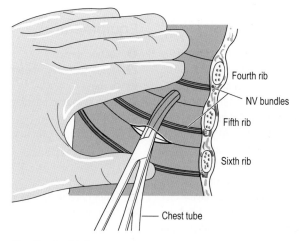

Fourth rib

NV bundles

Fifth rib

Sixth rib

Chest tube

Fig. 23.8.2 Inserting the chest tube.

Tips

- Sizing a chest tube involves estimation of the size of the child. If an exact size is not known, use the following formula: chest tube size = 2 x nasogastric tube size or 4 x endotracheal tube size.
- Use a smaller pigtail catheter if the pneumothorax needs to be evacuated but is not causing significant tension.
- Use a larger tube for haemothorax.
- Monitor for air leak for evidence of system air leak or tracheobronchial injury.

- Avoid trocars, to minimise lung lacerations.
- If a child with a penetrating chest injury is in shock or respiratory failure, do not wait for a chest X-ray before performing tube thoracostomy.
- Use of CT or video imaging may assist chest-tube placement.

Further reading

Cullen ML. Pulmonary and respiratory complications of paediatric trauma. *Respir Care Clin N Am* 2001;7(1):59–77.

Dieckmann RA, Fiser D, Selbst S. *Illustrated textbook of paediatric emergency and critical care procedures.* St Louis, MO: Mosby; 1997, 579–83.

Dull KE, Fleisher GR. Pigtail catheters versus large-bore chest tubes for pneumothoraces in children treated in the ED. *Paediatr Emerg Care* 2002;18(4):265–7.

Genc A, Ozcan C, Erdener A, Mutaf O. Management of pneumothorax in children. *J Cardiovasc Surg (Torino)* 1998;39(6):849–51.

Sarihan H, Cay A, Aynaci M, et al. Empyema in children. *J Cardiovasc Surg (Torino)* 1998;39(1):113–6.

Wilcox DT, Glick PL, Karamanoukian HL, et al. Spontaneous pneumothorax: A single-institution, 12-year experience in patients under 16 years of age. *J Paediatr Surg* 1995;10:1452–4.

23.9 Removing and replacing a tracheostomy tube

Ronald A. Dieckmann

Background

Children with tracheostomy tubes are increasingly common in out-of-hospital and emergency department settings. Laryngeal trauma, cervical cord injury, subglottic stenosis, and conditions requiring prolonged ventilation often need short- or long-term tracheostomy-tube placement. Most of these children live at home and have trained caregivers, often parents. Because the tracheostomy tube may be the primary airway for the child, if the tube comes out (decannulation) or becomes obstructed (mucus plugging), immediate action is necessary to secure the airway and preserve gas exchange.

Treatment of most tracheostomy problems requires only simple techniques to establish a patent airway, such as suctioning of the existing tube, or removal of the old tracheostomy tube and replacement with a new tube. The child's major ongoing risk is airway obstruction from clogging of the old tube with secretions or foreign bodies. Occasionally, it is impossible to ventilate a child through an existing tracheostomy tube because of frank decannulation or complete tube obstruction. Under these conditions, ventilating through the nose and mouth with a bag–valve–mask (BVM) device, or inserting a new tracheostomy tube or another temporary airway will save the child's life.

Indications for emergent replacement

Respiratory distress or failure in the presence of:

- decannulation;
- tube obstruction.

Contraindications

Inadequately sized tract or stoma for insertion of a new tracheostomy tube. In this case, insert an endotracheal tube or replacement tracheostomy tube that is smaller in diameter than the original tracheostomy tube.

Equipment

1. Suction device.
2. Sterile suction catheters.
3. Oxygen.
4. BVM, standard paediatric and adult mask sizes.
5. Tracheostomy cannulas, appropriately sized for patient (Fig. 23.9.1).
6. Endotracheal tubes, standard paediatric and adult sizes.
7. Laryngoscope handle with blades.
8. Tape or tracheostomy ties.
9. Gauze pads.
10. Syringes, 5 mL or 10 mL.
11. Water-soluble lubricant.
12. Scissors.
13. Sterile saline.
14. Stethoscope.

Preparation

1. Ask the caregiver if there are any special problems with the child's trachea or special requirements involving the child's tracheostomy.
2. If the child has an obstruction of the airway as a reason for tracheostomy placement, rescue breathing with a BVM may be difficult or impossible.
3. Ask the caregiver if a replacement tracheostomy tube is available.
4. Speak directly to the child about what to expect and attempt to enlist co-operation.

Procedure

Removing an old tracheostomy tube:

1. Position the child with the head and neck hyperextended to expose the tracheostomy site.
2. Apply oxygen over the mouth and nose, and occlude the stoma or tracheostomy tube. Most children with tracheostomies have an intact airway from the mouth and nose to the trachea.

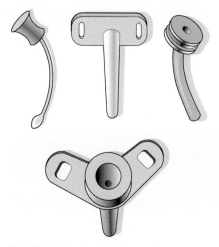

Fig. 23.9.1 Tracheostomy cannulas.

❸ If the existing tube has a cuff, deflate it:
  • Connect a 5–10-mL syringe to the valve on the pilot balloon.
  • Draw air out until the balloon collapses.
  • Cutting the balloon will not deflate the cuff.
❹ Cut or untie the cloth ties that hold the tracheostomy tube in place.
❺ Withdraw the tracheostomy tube using a slow, steady, outward and downward motion.
❻ Assess airway for patency and adequate ventilation.
❼ Provide oxygen and ventilation through the stoma as needed.

Replacing the tracheostomy tube
Option 1. Using a new tracheostomy tube
Insert a tracheostomy tube of the same size and model whenever possible. If the tube uses an insertion obturator, place this in the tube. If the tube has an inner and outer cannula, use the *outer* cannula and obturator for insertion.

❶ Moisten or lubricate the tip of the tube (and obturator) with water, sterile saline, or a water-soluble lubricant.
❷ Hold the device by the flange (wings) or hold the actual tube like a pencil.
❸ Gently insert the tube with an arching motion (follow the curvature of the tube) posteriorly then downward. Slight traction on the skin above or below the stoma may help (Fig. 23.9.2).
❹ Once the tube is in place, remove the obturator, attach the bag, and attempt to ventilate. If the tube has an inner

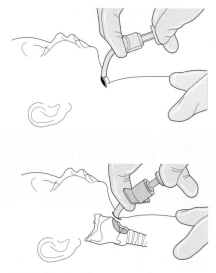

Fig. 23.9.2 Inserting a new tracheostomy tube.

cannula, insert to allow mechanical ventilation with a BVM device.
❺ Check for proper placement by watching for bilateral chest rise, listening for equal breath sounds, and observing the patient. Signs of improper placement include lack of chest rise, resistance to assisted ventilation, air in the surrounding tissues, and patient agitation.
❻ If the tube cannot be inserted, withdraw the tube, administer oxygen, and ventilate as needed.
❼ Use a smaller size tracheostomy tube for the second attempt.

Option 2. Using an endotracheal tube
If a replacement tracheostomy tube is not available, use an endotracheal tube of the same outer diameter as the tracheostomy tube.

Check the length of the original tracheostomy tube, note the markings on the endotracheal tube, and advance it to the same depth as the original tube.

  • The inserted portion of the endotracheal tube will be approximately half the distance needed for oral insertion.
  • Do not advance the tube too far, or it may go into the right main-stem bronchus.

Option 3. Using a suction catheter as a guidewire
If unsuccessful with the initial replacement attempt, use a suction catheter as a guide:

❶ Insert a small, sterile suction catheter through the tracheostomy tube.

❷ Without applying suction, insert the suction catheter into the stoma.
❸ Slide the tracheostomy tube along the suction catheter and into the stoma, until it is in the proper position.
❹ Remove the suction catheter.
❺ Assess ventilation through the tracheostomy tube.

Option 4. Endotracheal intubation
❶ If still unsuccessful, consider either orotracheal intubation or ventilation through the stoma, using a stoma mask or newborn mask.
❷ Alternatively, do BVM over the nose and mouth while covering the stoma with a sterile gauze.

Securing the tracheostomy tube
After proper placement, cut the ends of the tracheostomy ties or tape diagonally (allows for easy insertion), pass through eyelets (openings) on the flanges, and tie around the patient's neck, so that only a little finger can pass between the ties and the neck.

Complications

  • Creation of a false lumen.
  • Subcutaneous air.
  • Pneumomediastinum.
  • Pneumothorax.
  • Bleeding at insertion site.
  • Bleeding through tube.
  • Right main-stem intubation with endotracheal tube.

Tips

  • Talk to the caregiver about the size and type of tracheostomy tube and about known problems with the stoma, trachea or tube before proceeding.
  • Most children who have lost a tracheostomy tube can be ventilated by BVM over the nose and mouth, with the stoma occluded.
  • If unable to reinsert a tracheostomy tube, use a similarly sized endotracheal tube.
  • Do not force a large tracheostomy tube through a new stoma site.
  • Do not advance an endotracheal tube too far through the stoma, or it may intubate the right main-stem bronchus.

Further reading

Bahng SC, VanHala S, Nelson VS, et al. Parental report of paediatric tracheostomy care. *Archives Physiology of Medical Rehabilitation* 1998;**79**(11):1367–9.

Bosch JD, Cuyler JP. Home care of the paediatric tracheostomy: Our experience. *J Otolaryngol* 1987;**16**(2):120–2.

Dieckmann RA, Fiser D, Selbst S. *Illustrated textbook of paediatric emergency and critical care procedures.* St Louis, MO: Mosby; 1997. p. 121–2.

Dieckmann RA, Brownstein D, Gausche M. *Textbook for paediatric education for prehospital professionals.* Sudbury, MA: Jones & Bartlett; 2001. p. 300–2.

23.10 Central and peripheral intravenous lines

Judith Klein

Background

Most children who present to an emergency department do not need vascular access for drug or fluid therapy. Medications can usually be administered orally, transmucosally, intramuscularly or by inhalation. Even fluid administration in dehydrated children does not ordinarily require vascular access. Oral rehydration, performed slowly and methodically, is often successful in children with vomiting and/or diarrhoea. However, when oral rehydration is unsuccessful or when a child presents critically ill or injured, intravenous (IV) or intraosseous (IO) access (Chapter 23.11) becomes essential.

Finding veins to cannulate in infants and small children can be quite a challenge. The higher ratio of subcutaneous fat and smaller vessel size in young patients pose significant barriers to rapid venous cannulation. A peripheral venous site, rather than a central site, offers the highest benefit:risk ratio of any vascular access option. Fig. 23.10.1 illustrates common sites for peripheral IV line insertion.

When a peripheral site is unavailable, an IO site provides a second option (Chapter 23.11). When peripheral venous and IO access cannot be obtained or if central venous pressure monitoring is required, consider cannulating central veins, such as the femoral vein, subclavian vein, or internal jugular vein. Avoid saphenous vein cutdowns in children, because they are technically difficult to perform and the technique is time consuming in infants and young children, even for experienced operators. Make every effort to provide the least invasive form of access required by the degree of the child's illness.

Indications

- Peripheral IV access is indicated if oral, transmucosal, intramuscular or inhalation routes are not adequate to meet the patient's needs for fluids and/or medications.
- Use a central IV for:
  Central venous pressure monitoring.
  Administration of hypertonic solutions.
  Essential access when peripheral and IO attempts have failed.

Contraindications

- Peripheral IV catheters are contraindicated if other, non-invasive, routes can meet the child's needs.
- Central venous catheters are contraindicated if peripheral venous access sites are available and there are no special indications for central venous catheter placement.
- If possible, do not pass peripheral IV catheters:
  Through cellulitic skin.
  In an extremity that has a wound, e.g. burn or laceration.
  Distal to unstable fractures or injured veins.
- Avoid placing central lines in non-compressible sites in patients with bleeding diatheses.

Peripheral venous line placement

Equipment

Table 23.10.1 lists peripheral IV equipment. Determine appropriate sizing of IV catheters by consulting a length-based resuscitation tape.

❶ If time permits, consider anaesthetising the skin with an anaesthetic drug or by iontophoresis. To anaesthetise skin, apply a topical anaesthetic, such as the eutectic mixture of local anaesthetics (EMLA™) cream, under an occlusive dressing at the selected entry site at least 45 minutes prior to any IV attempt. The alternative technique of iontophoresis requires specialised equipment for delivery of a low amperage, painless electrical charge to the skin. The technique is safe, non-invasive and usually quite effective. Iontophoresis takes 10–20 minutes to numb skin for peripheral IV insertion.

❷ Use over-the-needle catheters whenever possible. Butterfly needles are far less stable but are acceptable for short-term infusions. Use armboards/legboards and a plastic container to cover the IV to avoid unintentional (or deliberate!) dislodgement of the catheter. Prime the tubing, and set up the IV fluid chamber with microdrip and an infusion pump in advance. Carefully monitor infusions in infants and small children to prevent over-administration of fluids. Select the smallest-sized catheter that will meet the patient's needs for drug and fluid administration.

Preparation

❶ Prepare all equipment and place near the child. Avoid using the bed as an equipment table as the equipment may find its way quickly to the floor with an active child.

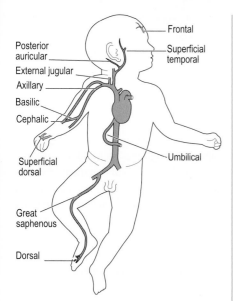

Fig. 23.10.1 Common peripheral IV sites.

Table 23.10.1 Equipment for peripheral IV insertion
• Gloves • Arm or leg board • Tourniquet • Alcohol pads • Gauze pads • 22–24-gauge venous catheters • Saline flush • IV tubing, solution and pump • Protective covering for IV (small plastic cup, roller gauze) • Tape

❷ Flush the catheter with saline solution if diagnostic blood samples are not necessary during IV insertion. This will reduce the risk of air embolisation.

❸ Remove any topical anaesthetic at the IV site or the apparatus for iontophoresis.

❹ Have an assistant restrain an infant or toddler with a sheet (Figs 23.10.2 and 23.10.3).

❺ Attempt to talk an older child through the procedure with a parent or caregiver present.

❻ Have the assistant gently restrain the extremity/body part selected for IV access. Use padded boards to stabilise arm or leg access sites in infants and young children.

❼ Locate landmarks and determine insertion sites first with an ungloved hand that is more sensitive in detecting surface veins and palpating landmarks than the gloved hand.

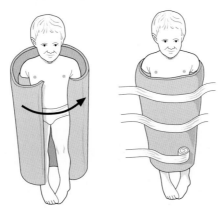

Fig. 23.10.2 Restraining an infant.

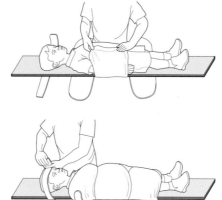

Fig. 23.10.3 Restraining a child.

Procedure

There are a number of possible sites for placement of peripheral IV lines in infants and children. The easiest sites are the dorsum of the hands and feet, the antecubital fossa and, in infants less than 1 year, the scalp. In non-emergent situations, start distally and move proximally when initial attempts fail. Consider using a warm compress to dilate constricted veins and make them more visible. In emergent situations, cannulate the largest vein available and consider less commonly used peripheral sites, such as the external jugular vein and deep brachial vein.

❶ Make sure that the child is well immobilised.

❷ Don gloves and clean the insertion site with isopropyl alcohol or povidone-iodine solution.

❸ Apply a tourniquet just proximal to the insertion site. Use a rubber band around the scalp caudad of the insertion site to cannulate scalp veins.

❹ Locate a straight segment of the vein and provide in-line traction away from the direction of catheter insertion.

❺ Insert the catheter at about a 10–20 degree angle to the skin. Once there is a flash of blood in the hub of the catheter, advance the catheter with the needle in place another 1–2 mm. Then advance the catheter over the needle into the vein.

❻ Draw any blood samples needed, remove the tourniquet, and connect the IV line.

❼ Secure the catheter and IV line to the patient with tape and a plastic container over the IV (Fig. 23.10.4).

If insertion is unsuccessful at traditional peripheral IV, consider two alternative sites prior to moving to a central line: the external jugular vein and the deep brachial vein. To cannulate the external jugular vein, place the patient in Trendelenburg position to dilate the vein. Restrain the patient well and turn his/her head slightly away from the cannulation site (Fig. 23.10.5). Do not use a tourniquet for placement of an IV at this site. Clean the area with isopropyl alcohol or povidone-iodine solution and use an 18G needle to make a nick in the skin at the catheter site. This will facilitate passage of the catheter through the skin. Use the peripheral insertion technique but apply firm counter-traction at the entry site to help stabilise the vessel. Secure the needle carefully to avoid dislodgement.

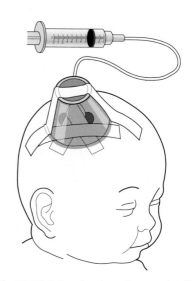

Fig. 23.10.4 Securing the catheter to the skin.

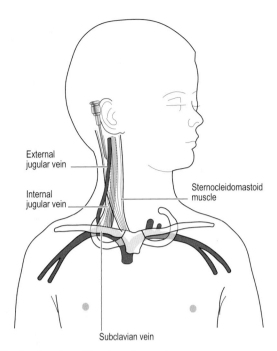

Fig. 23.10.5 Positioning for external jugular vein puncture.

The second alternative site is the deep brachial vein. In contrast to the other sites, identify the likely location of the deep brachial vein by anatomic landmarks, not by visualisation or by palpation. Ultrasound can assist in localisation of the vein. Consider this option in older children. Palpate the brachial artery medial to the biceps just proximal to the antecubital fossa (Fig. 23.10.6). Place a tourniquet and prepare the skin with isopropyl alcohol or povidone-iodine solution. Insert the catheter at a 30 degree angle approximately the patient's finger breath medial to the brachial artery. Angle the catheter parallel to the course of the brachial artery and slowly advance the catheter. If arterial blood appears or the patient complains of hand paraesthesiae (median nerve irritation), remove the catheter and hold pressure at the site. There is anatomic variability in the position of the vein, so try marginally different slightly medial insertion sites if initial attempts are unsuccessful.

Complications

Local complications
- Phlebitis.
- Site infection.
- Infiltration.
- Bleeding.
- Pressure necrosis due to IV stabilisation methods.

To avoid these complications, clean insertion sites well prior to passing the needle through the skin. Make sure blood can be easily withdrawn from and fluids easily infused through the IV. Avoid infusing irritant or hyperosmolar solutions through peripheral lines. Tape IV lines securely but do not create a tourniquet with tape and remember to pad all joints. Replace peripheral lines every 48–72 hours.

Systemic complications
- Thrombosis.
- Air embolism.
- Catheter tip embolisation.

Flush catheters regularly but not forcefully. Do not re-insert the needle stylet into the catheter once it has been removed. Doing this can shear the catheter and cause catheter fragment embolisation.

Tips

- Whenever possible, use a topical anaesthetic at several possible IV sites at least 45 minutes prior to line placement, or consider iontophoresis.
- Avoid joint surfaces and the patient's dominant hand. If a large-bore catheter is required, use more proximal sites, such as those at the antecubital fossa or external jugular vein.
- Do not let go of recently-placed IV catheters until they are well secured.
- Monitor newly-placed IVs closely, particularly in infants and small children with persistent crying. A swollen extremity may be the only marker of an infiltrated catheter.

Central venous line placement

Equipment
The equipment for placement of a central venous line is usually in a prepackaged kit. The simplest and most straightforward technique for central-line placement is the guidewire or Seldinger technique. Pre-packaged

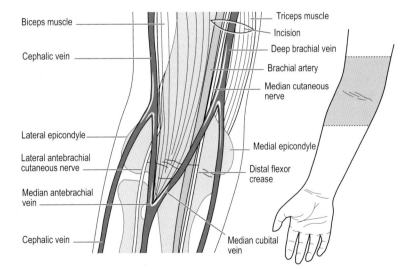

Fig. 23.10.6 Cannulating the deep brachial vein.

Table 23.10.2 Sizing central IV catheters		
Weight (kg)	Age	Catheter size (French)
<5	Newborn to 6 months	3, 4
5–15	6 months to 5 years	5, 7
15	>5 years	5–11

kits will contain, among other things, a needle, syringe, J-wire, scalpel, dilator and catheter. Determine appropriate catheter sizes by measuring the child next to a length-based resuscitation tape or by consulting Table 23.10.2. Estimate insertion distance by measuring from the insertion site externally to the desired tip position.

Preparation

❶ If time allows, sedate the child prior to insertion of a central venous catheter and/or use a topical anaesthetic such as EMLA™ cream. If the situation is emergent, use a sheet wrapped around the child and an assistant to restrain the child. Excessive patient movement will increase the rate of complication and decrease the likelihood of procedure success.

❷ Prepare all equipment on the tray so that items can be easily located. Do not use the child's bed as an instrument table as the instruments will soon find their way to the floor.

❸ Flush the catheter with saline solution in advance unless diagnostic blood specimens are required.

Procedure

Sites for central venous line placement in children include: the femoral vein, the internal jugular vein, and the subclavian vein. The external jugular vein is also a possible central venous insertion site. Passage of the catheter centrally via the external jugular vein is difficult because of the acute angle of entry of the external jugular into the subclavian vein. It is, therefore, the least desirable site.

Fig. 23.10.7 illustrates the essential anatomy for placement of a femoral venous catheter.

❶ Place the patient supine in a mild reverse Trendelenburg position. Maintain the hip in slight external rotation and abduction.

❷ Palpate the femoral artery at the inguinal ligament. The insertion site is about a patient's finger breadth medial to the artery and 2–3 cm distal to the inguinal ligament. The right side is easier for a right-handed operator.

❸ Measure from insertion site to the umbilicus to estimate catheter insertion distance.

To cannulate the internal jugular vein, place the patient in Trendelenburg position with

the neck extended and the head turned slightly away from the insertion site. A roll placed under the ipsilateral shoulder will facilitate neck extension, particularly in infants. Fig. 23.10.8 illustrates the relevant anatomy and landmarks.

❶ Identify the triangle formed by the sternal and clavicular heads of the sternocleidomastoid muscle and the clavicle.

❷ Palpate the carotid artery just medial to the triangle.

❸ The insertion site is either at the apex of the triangle or halfway (from mastoid to sternum) along the medial border of the sternal head. In either case, aim towards the ipsilateral nipple and away from the carotid artery. The right side is preferable because of the straighter course to the superior vena cava, the lower pleural dome, and the absence of the thoracic duct.

❹ Place the catheter tip at the junction of the superior vena cava and the right atrium.

Positioning and anatomy relevant for placement of a subclavian central venous line is similar to that for placement of an internal jugular venous line (Fig. 23.10.9).

❶ Sedate conscious patients before attempting a subclavian line, as patient movement can result in a high rate of complications. Place the patient in Trendelenburg position with a towel roll underneath the ipsilateral shoulder to help keep the neck in extension.

❷ Mentally divide the clavicle into thirds.

❸ The insertion site is just inferior to the junction of the middle and medial thirds of the clavicle aiming towards the sternal notch. Aim the J curve of the guidewire caudally during insertion. Also, turn the patient's head toward the site of insertion while advancing the wire to avoid passage of the wire up the internal jugular vein.

❹ Place the catheter tip at the junction of the superior vena cava and the right atrium.

The general procedure for placement of a central venous catheter is the same regardless of location.

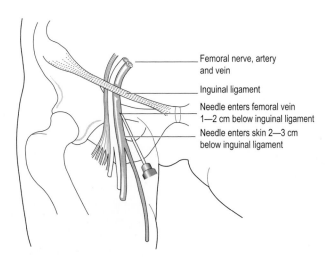

Femoral nerve, artery and vein

Inguinal ligament

Needle enters femoral vein 1—2 cm below inguinal ligament

Needle enters skin 2—3 cm below inguinal ligament

Fig. 23.10.7 Essential anatomy for placement of a femoral venous catheter.

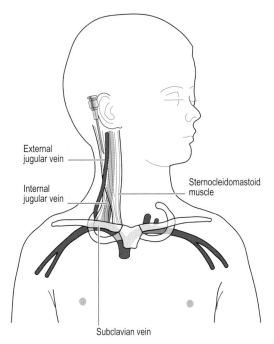

Fig. 23.10.8 Cannulating the internal jugular vein.

❶ Clean the skin with a povidone-iodine or chlorhexidine solution.

❷ Anaesthetise the site with 1% lidocaine.

❸ Attach a syringe to the insertion needle so that the bevel lines up with the numbers on the syringe. This allows for identification of bevel direction even when the needle is inside the patient.

❹ Insert the needle at the selected insertion site with the bevel pointed anteriorly (femoral), medially (internal jugular), or caudally (subclavian).

❺ Angle the needle at approximately 30 degrees to the skin, except when placing a subclavian line. With subclavian line placement, use the shallowest angle possible that allows insertion of the needle underneath the clavicle aiming towards the sternal notch.

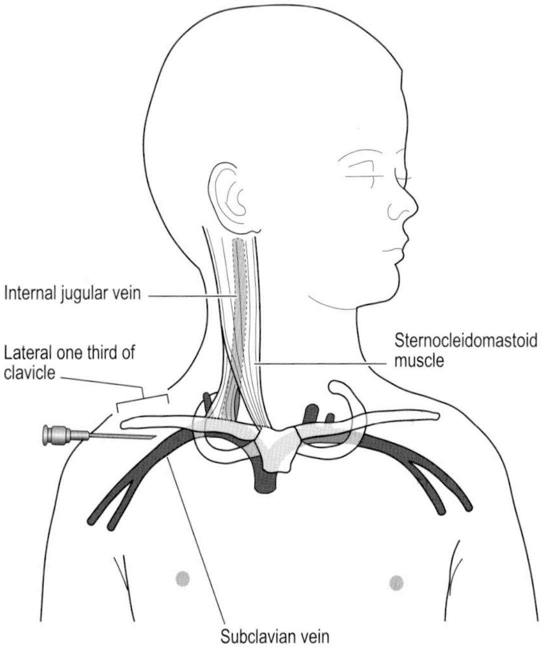

Maintain constant negative pressure on the syringe while inserting or withdrawing the needle as vessel entry may occur during withdrawal. Once blood flows freely into the syringe, stabilise the needle with a hand resting on the patient. Remove the syringe carefully, trying not to alter the position of the needle. Insert the J-wire through the needle, J end first (Fig. 23.10.10). Point the J of the guidewire in the direction the catheter is intended to go. The wire should pass easily. Do not force it if it does not. Removing the wire and repositioning the needle can often resolve gentle resistance. If strong resistance is met, remove the needle and wire together to avoid shearing off the wire into the vein.

Once the wire is passed to the pre-marked distance, remove the needle. Never let go of the wire. Make a small stab incision with a scalpel over the wire. Insert a dilator over the wire, once again, remembering to hold onto the wire at all times. Remove the dilator and insert the catheter over the wire to the pre-measured distance (Fig. 23.10.11). Remove the wire. Draw off any diagnostic blood specimens. If the catheter has not been flushed in advance, withdraw blood

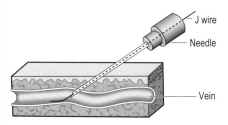

Fig. 23.10.10 Inserting the J-wire through the needle.

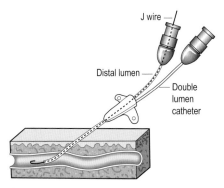

Fig. 23.10.11 Inserting the catheter over the wire to the pre-measured distance.

Fig. 23.10.9 Cannulating the subclavian vein.

from all lumens of the catheter prior to infusing any fluids or medications to avoid air embolisation. Suture the catheter in place and apply a sterile dressing. Verify location of the catheter tip with an X-ray.

Complications

Table 23.10.3 lists the most common complications of central venous line placement.

- Bleeding can occur during traumatic line placement or after arterial puncture. Patients with bleeding diatheses are at great risk for bleeding complications. Compress bleeding sites from femoral or internal jugular sites. These sites are safer than the subclavian route where the internal bleeding site is non-compressible. Avoid subclavian catheterisation in patients who are moving around or who have clotting problems.
- Pneumothorax can occur with internal jugular or subclavian line insertion.

Table 23.10.3 Complications of central venous line placement

- Bleeding
- Arterial puncture/cannulation/laceration
- Infection
- Catheter thrombosis
- Pneumothorax
- Haemothorax
- Thoracic duct laceration

A shallow angle of insertion with subclavian lines can help prevent this complication. Obtain an X-ray after all line placements, not only to verify catheter position but also to detect a pneumothorax.

- Suspect catheter thrombosis if withdrawal of blood or infusion of fluids becomes difficult. Eventually pain and swelling of the extremity will tip the clinician off to the presence of the clot. Manage thromboses expeditiously with catheter removal.
- Infection is equally likely to occur at any of the central venous sites. Remove infected catheters as soon as possible and treat with antibiotics. If possible, avoid insertion of a new central catheter for 24–48 hours.

Tips

- In the awake patient, restraint and proper sedation and analgesia will improve procedural success and avoid complications.
- Use ultrasound, if possible, to identify vessels prior to line placement.
- If the patient is moving and there is no time for sedation, the femoral site is the safest and most easily compressible vein if bleeding occurs.

- If central venous pressure monitoring is required, use an access site above the diaphragm. While the internal jugular vein is larger, the subclavian site is more comfortable for the patient in the long term.
- If the patient is pulseless, the subclavian vein is the preferred site for central venous catheterisation as it does not require a pulse for localisation and can be used for central venous pressure monitoring.

Further reading

Bagwell CE, Salzberg AM, Sonnino RE, Haynes JH. Potentially lethal complications of central venous catheter placement. *J Paediatr Surg* 2000;**35**(5):709–13.

Chiang VW, Baskin MN. Uses and complications of central venous catheters inserted in a paediatric emergency department. *Paediatr Emerg Care* 2000;**16**(4):230–2.

Cunningham FJ, Engle WA. Paediatric vascular access and blood sampling techniques. In: Roberts JR, Hedges JR, editors. *Clinical procedures in emergency medicine*. 3rd ed. Philadelphia, PA: WB Saunders; 1998.

Fernandez EG, Sweeney MF, Green TP. Central venous catheters. In: Dieckmann RA, Fiser DH, Selbst SM, editors. *Paediatric emergency and critical care procedures*. St Louis, MO: Mosby; 1997.

King D, Conway EE Jr. Vascular access. *Paediatr Ann* 1996;**25**(12):693–8.

Macnab AJ, Macnab M. Teaching paediatric procedures: The Vancouver model for instructing Seldinger's technique of central venous access via the femoral vein. *Paediatrics* 1999;**103**(1):E8.

Stoyroff M, Teague WG. Intravenous access in infants and children. *Paediatr Clin N Am* 1998;**45**(6):1373–93.

Webster PA, Salassi-Scotter MR. Peripheral vascular access. In: Dieckmann RA, Fiser DH, Selbst SM, editors. *Paediatric emergency and critical care procedures*. St Louis, MO: Mosby; 1997.

23.11 Intraosseous infusions

Lindsay Bridgford • Ronald A. Dieckmann

Background

Peripheral intravenous cannulation in a critically ill or injured child can be difficult, time consuming, and sometimes impossible. Small veins collapse or disappear during shock, and increased body fat may camouflage superficial skin veins. Central venous access and surgical cut-down are also technically difficult procedures that may be risky or impossible in critical situations. Although the endotracheal route is an alternative to vascular access in cardiopulmonary arrest, endotracheal intubation may be delayed, drug absorption may not be reliable, and large fluid administration is contraindicated by this route.

The intraosseous (IO) or intramedullary route for the delivery of resuscitation fluids and medications has been used for over 50 years in children and adults. Many studies have confirmed that the highly vascularised IO space is an excellent route for medications and fluids. The only technical problem is successfully piercing the bony cortex in older children. The bones of neonates and infants are usually soft and the IO space is relatively large, so needle insertion is easy in children of youngest age. Good equipment, preparation, and effective technique are especially important for success in IO needle insertion. While IO access is easy, quick, and safe, it is painful in a conscious child and therefore is only practical in a critically ill or injured child.

The IO space functions as a non-collapsible vein. There are several possible sites for insertion; but the easiest location in children is the proximal tibia. The emissary veins of the IO space absorb all parenteral medications, crystalloid fluids, or blood products – which move quickly into the central circulation. Complications are minor and infrequent. Out-of-hospital emergency-care professionals have also employed the IO technique with a high rate of success.

Indications

- Cardiopulmonary arrest.
- Any critical emergency when a peripheral cannulation site is unavailable and oral, transmucosal, intramuscular or inhalation routes are not adequate to meet the patient's needs for fluids and/or medications.

Contraindications

- Do not use an IO infusion if the child is stable.
- Do not place an IO needle below a fracture site. Use the other side.
- Avoid placement of an IO below any open injury on an extremity. Use the other side.

Relative contraindications

- Avoid IO needle insertion in children with osteoporosis and osteogenesis imperfecta, due to the high fracture potential.
- Recent prior use of the same bone for IO infusion, due to the potential for extravasation from previous IO sites.

Equipment

❶ The EZ IO or intraosseous gun is an excellent alternative to the manual needle.
❷ A variety of needles will work. Butterfly needles and spinal needles may be effective, especially in neonates and infants, but these needles bend too easily in the more calcified bones of children and adolescents.
❸ Commercially available IO needles have more durable parts intended for penetration of bone. There are several styles (Fig. 23.11.1). A central stylet is universal. There are short, 2.5-cm, needles for neonates and infants and longer, 3.0 and 3.5-cm, needles for older children. Some needles have stylets with multifaceted cutting edges intended for a rotary insertion, others have bevels, and others can be screwed in place. The shaft may have side ports.
❹ 10-mL syringe.
❺ Normal saline.
❻ Stopcock (optional).

Preparation

Identification of the entry site

The best site in children is the anteromedial aspect of the proximal tibia lateral to the tibial tuberosity. Alternative sites are the distal end of the femur 2–3 cm above the patella in the midline, and the medial malleolus at the ankle (Fig. 23.11.2). The sternum is not recommended in children. In adults, the medial malleolus may be the best site, although studies are lacking.

Positioning the child

Place the child supine with the knee slightly flexed and a small towel roll or other bulky material under the popliteal fossa. Make sure the conscious child is well immobilised.

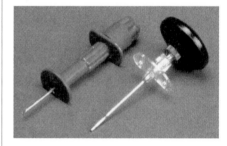

Fig. 23.11.1 IO needles.

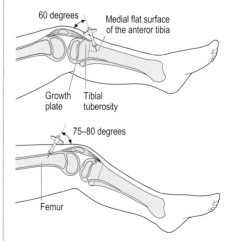

Fig. 23.11.2 IO needle entry sites.

Selecting the correct side

A right-handed operator will more easily insert the needle in the child's right leg, and vice-versa for the left-handed operator.

Procedure

❶ Introduce the IO needle in the skin, directed slightly away from the growth plate. Grasping the limb with the non-dominant hand beside the insertion site (e.g. behind the knee for proximal tibia insertion) helps to steady the bone during placement.

❷ Pierce the bony cortex with a firm, twisting motion from a position directly above the entry site. A 'pop' may be felt as the needle passes through the bony cortex and into the marrow cavity. Do not push too hard on the needle. Too much force may push the needle all the way through the bone and into the soft tissues.

❸ Remove the stylet and aspirate marrow contents with a 10-mL syringe. Keep any bone marrow aspirate for glucose check or for other tests in the emergency department. Sometimes, marrow cannot be aspirated.

❹ Confirm correct placement by infusing 10 mL of normal saline without resistance. Once the IO needle has been placed, attach a stopcock (if available) to the end of the needle before attaching the intravenous (IV) line.

❺ Attach IV line to the hub and infuse fluids or drugs directly into IO space. Pushing the fluids too hard may force the fluids out of the IO space. The rate of fluid infusion may be limited by the small marrow space.

❻ Secure the needle to the overlying skin with tape.

❼ Monitor the calf to ensure that there is no swelling to indicate leakage of fluid.

Complications

- Compartment syndrome.
- Failed infusion.

- Growth-plate injury.
- Bone infection.
- Skin infection.
- Skin necrosis.
- Bony fracture.

Tips

- Be extremely careful using an EZ IO in a young infant, because it is quite easy to penetrate through the bone into the soft tissues and cause a compartment syndrome.
- If the child is conscious, provide generous local anaesthesia at the entry site.
- In addition to serving as a route for drug and fluid administration, blood samples drawn from the site can be used for culture, haematological, and biochemical analysis, but there are limitations. Emergency type and crossmatch is reliable with an adequate sample. A complete blood cell count may not be reliable, as it reflects the marrow cell count rather than the cell count in the peripheral circulation, and also because blood aspirated from the marrow usually clots rapidly, even if it is placed in a tube that contains heparin. Blood chemistry determinations are possible, but they may not correlate with blood samples taken from central veins.
- All commonly used intravenous fluids and drugs can be administered via the IO route.
- The rate of infection from IO needle placement is low and comparable to IV cannulation.
- A slow infusion rate does not mean the IO needle is misplaced, and pressure infusion may be necessary to maintain flow.

The EZ-IO

Mechanical devices such as the EZ-IO have simplified the insertion of an IO needle as they are not dependent on the manual process. The EZ-IO (Vidacare, San Antonio, TX, USA) is a reusable battery-powered device

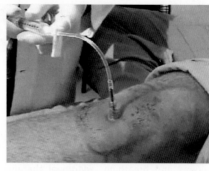

Fig. 23.11.3 EZ-IO.

that operates like a small drill. The driver itself is a sealed unit that is good for about 700 insertions. The EZ-IO uses a bevelled drill tip that rotates into the IO space at a preset depth (Fig. 23.11.3).

The procedures for insertion of the EZ-IO needle are similar to those described above for the manual device. The difference is in the preparation of the EZ-IO driver and paediatric needle set, with a 15-gauge, 15-mm long needle generally used for children weighing between 3 kg and 39 kg, a 15-gauge, 25-mm long needle for children weighing greater than 40 kg and a new 45-mm length needle is available for larger children with significant tissue or oedema overlying bone.

Further reading

Brunette DD, Fischer R. Intravascular access in paediatric cardiac arrest. *Ann Emerg Med* 1988;**6**:577.

Fiser DH. Intraosseous infusion. *N Engl J Med* 1990;**322**:1579.

Johnson L, Kissoon N, Fiallos M, et al. Use of intraosseous blood to assess blood chemistries and haemoglobin during cardiopulmonary resuscitation with drug infusions. *Crit Care Med* 1999;**27**:1147–52.

Phillips B, Zideman D, Garcia-Castrillo L, et al. European Resuscitation Council guidelines 2000 for advanced paediatric life support. *Resuscitation* 2001;**48**:231–324.

Vidal R, Kissoon N, Gaylor M. Compartment syndrome following intraosseous infusion. *Paediatrics* 1993;**91**:1201–2.

Wenzel V, Lindner KH, Augenstein S, et al. Intraosseous vasopressin improves coronary perfusion pressure rapidly during cardiopulmonary resuscitation in pigs. *Crit Care Med* 1999;**27**:1565–9.

Tobias JD, Ross AK. Intraosseous infusions: a review for the anesthesiologist with a focus on pediatric use. *Anesth Analg* 2010;**110**(2):391–401.

23.12 Rectal drug administration

Ronald A. Dieckmann

Background

Status epilepticus is a major paediatric medical emergency that requires emergency treatment. Although the first priority is airway and breathing, additional therapy includes termination of the seizure. Cannulating a peripheral vein in a child in status epilepticus limits timely delivery of essential advanced life support (ALS) drugs, especially in infants and toddlers. However, intravenous (IV), intramuscular (IM), or intraosseous drug administration is not necessary because rectal benzodiazepine administration is probably as effective and has no added complications. Rectal drug administration is a time-honoured drug-delivery technique in children and is useful for many medications, including antipyretics and anticonvulsants. The rectum is highly vascularised, and lipid-soluble drugs are rapidly absorbed when correctly administered (Fig. 23.12.1). Diazepam is a lipid-soluble benzodiazepine that is reliably absorbed through the rectum and will terminate most seizures without further treatment. Lorazepam is an effective alternative drug choice.

Rectal drug administration is a technique that allows delivery of an absorbable benzodiazepine in the setting of status epilepticus. The relative effectiveness and safety of rectal diazepam versus IM midazolam, lorazepam or other benzodiazepines for treatment of status epilepticus are not known. Rectal diazepam or lorazepam administration may take a few minutes longer to stop the seizure, compared to IV administration, and drug levels may be more variable. Occasionally, as with the IV diazepam preparation, more than one dose of rectal diazepam is necessary.

Indications

- Repetitive seizures.
- Status epilepticus.

Contraindications

- Newborn age (a month or less).
- Recent prior rectal surgery (e.g. for Hirschsprung's disease, imperforate anus).

Equipment

❶ Diazepam gel preparation or IV solution of diazepam or lorazepam.
❷ Lubricant.
❸ Tuberculin syringe, or 14–20-gauge over-the-needle catheter with 3–5-mL syringe.
❹ Tape (optional).

Preparation

Determine the weight of the child using a decision support software program or paediatric resuscitation tape or other accurate estimate of size. Or obtain the patient's weight from the caregiver.

Option 1. Diazepam gel preparation
❶ Remove the rubber-tipped gel container from the sterile package.

Option 2. IV diazepam preparation
❶ Draw up the calculated dose of IV medication into a disposable

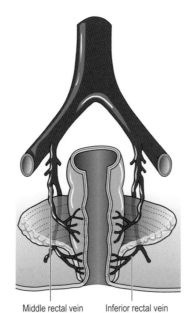

Middle rectal vein   Inferior rectal vein

Fig. 23.12.1 Anatomy of the rectum.

tuberculin syringe or into a 3–5-mL syringe.
❷ Lubricate the syringe or catheter:
   a. If using the tuberculin syringe as the administration device, remove needle and apply lubricant to the tip of the syringe.
   b. If using a 3–5-mL syringe, remove needle, attach over-the-needle catheter (plastic portion only), and lubricate catheter.

Procedure

❶ Position the patient in the decubitus position, knee–chest position, or supine position (Fig. 23.12.2) and have a second person hold the legs apart.
❷ Carefully introduce the rubber tip of the gel container, or the syringe or over-the-needle catheter approximately 5 cm (2 inches) into the rectum.
❸ Inject the gel or solution into the rectum. Remove the syringe.
❹ Hold buttocks closed for 10 seconds.
❺ Tape buttocks closed (optional).

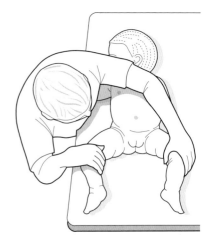

Fig. 23.12.2 Administering rectal drugs.

Complications

- The most serious potential complication of rectal diazepam is respiratory depression, which is usually from the drug, but may be from the prolonged seizure, or the underlying cause of the seizure.
- Administration of diazepam too high or too proximal into the rectum may decrease its anticonvulsant effect. When the drug is delivered too proximal in the rectum, absorption may occur into the superior haemorrhoidal veins, which drain into the portal system instead of the middle and inferior haemorrhoidal veins, which drain into the systemic venous system. The drug will then undergo hepatic metabolism, which will significantly reduce brain concentrations.
- Rectal tearing.

Tips

- The rectal dose of diazepam is 0.5 mg kg^{-1}, or five-times the IV dose, to a maximum dose of 10 mg. Onset of action for rectal diazepam is slower.
- Do not give additional rectal diazepam until approximately 5 minutes after the first dose, to avoid 'stacking' doses and increasing the risk of respiratory depression.
- Rectal lorazepam may be at least as effective as rectal diazepam in status epilepticus.
- Do not perform endotracheal intubation on every child with diminished breathing after rectal diazepam. Most will not need it if bag–valve–mask is effectively performed for a few minutes until the child begins breathing again spontaneously.
- Do not use the benzodiazepine reversal agent flumazenil when respiratory depression occurs after diazepam administration. The drug may precipitate seizures by interfering with the effect of the diazepam in the brain.

Further reading

Appleton R, Martland T, Phillips B. Drug management for acute tonic-clonic convulsions including convulsive status epilepticus in children. *Cochrane Database Syst Rev* 2002;**4**:CD001905.

Dieckmann RA, Brownstein D, Gausche M. *Textbook for paediatric education for prehospital professionals.* Sudbury, MA: Jones & Bartlett; 2001. p. 291–2.

Dieckmann RA, Fiser D, Selbst S. *Illustrated textbook of paediatric emergency and critical care procedures.* St Louis, MO: Mosby; 1997. p. 274–8.

Dieckmann RA. Rectal diazepam for prehospital paediatric status epilepticus. *Ann Emerg Med* 1994;**23**(2):216–24.

Fitzgerald BJ, Okos AJ, Miller JW. Treatment of out-of-hospital status epilepticus with diazepam rectal gel. *Seizure* 2003;**12**(1):52–5.

Mitchell WG, Conry JA, Crumrine PK, et al. An open-label study of repeated use of diazepam rectal gel (Diastat) for episodes of acute breakthrough seizures and clusters: Safety, efficacy, and tolerance. North American Diastat Group. *Epilepsia* 1999;**40**(11):1610–7.

23.13 Umbilical vessel cannulation

Judith Klein

Background

During fetal life, two umbilical arteries transport nutrients and oxygen from the placenta and one umbilical vein helps dispose of fetal waste. During delivery, these vessels are cut and clamped and the newborn is separated from the placenta. However, the umbilical vessels can be recannulated and utilised for emergent vascular access in ill neonates for up to 7 days after birth. This is an excellent method of central drug and fluid delivery, because peripheral venous access in infants in the first week of life is quite difficult, particularly in the ill or intravascularly depleted neonate. The other alternative for emergency vascular access in newborns is the insertion of an intraosseous needle (Chapter 23.11).

While either of the umbilical arteries and the umbilical vein is available for vascular access, the umbilical vein is technically easier to cannulate. Therefore, use the vein in an emergent situation. Cannulate one of the umbilical arteries if blood pressure monitoring and arterial blood gas sampling are important for patient management.

Indications

- Emergent vascular access for resuscitation.
- Central access for delivery of fluids, medications, or exchange transfusion.
- Frequent blood gas sampling.
- Haemodynamic monitoring.

Contraindications

Do not place an umbilical vessel line if a peripheral intravenous line is available and adequate for the infant's needs.

Equipment

Table 23.13.1 lists the equipment for cannulation of either the umbilical artery or vein.

Preparation

❶ Prepare all equipment in advance.
❷ Flush the umbilical catheter with saline or heparin flush and attach the stopcock.
❸ Place the infant supine under a radiant warmer with all extremities restrained.

Table 23.13.1   Equipment for cannulation of the umbilical artery or vein

- Sterile gown, gloves and mask
- Povidone-iodine solution
- Sterile gauze
- Sterile drapes
- Umbilical tape
- 3.0 Silk suture with needle
- Scalpel
- Haemostats
- Smooth, curved iris forceps
- Iris scissors
- Needle holder
- Umbilical catheter (3.5 or 5.0F)
- Heparinised saline/syringes
- Three-way stopcock

❹ Utilise cardiorespiratory and pulse oximetry monitors for the duration of the procedure.

❺ Don a mask, sterile gown and sterile gloves.

Procedure

Umbilical vein catheterisation

❶ Have an assistant to hold the umbilical stump up, scrub the umbilicus with povidone-iodine solution from xiphoid to pubis.

❷ Apply a sterile drape.

❸ To provide haemostasis, loosely tie umbilical tape at the base of the umbilical cord at the junction with the skin and cut the cord approximately 1–2 cm from the skin.

❹ Identify the two thick-walled arteries and the larger, thin-walled umbilical vein (Fig. 23.13.1).

❺ Holding the umbilical cord with a haemostat, insert the flushed 3.5F (preterm) or 5F (term) catheter into the umbilical vein (Fig. 23.13.2).

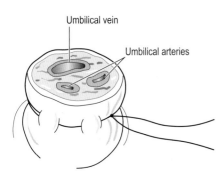

Fig. 23.13.1 Identifying the umbilical arteries and vein.

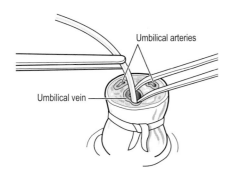

Fig. 23.13.2 Inserting the catheter into the umbilical vein.

❻ Use gentle, but steady, pressure while inserting the catheter and provide gentle traction on the cord if resistance is met. Insert the catheter so that the tip is in the inferior vena cava below the diaphragm at a depth of approximately 4–5 cm or above the diaphragm (via the portal system) at a depth of 8–12 cm (Fig. 23.13.3).

❼ The deeper line allows for administration of higher concentration fluids as well as central venous pressure monitoring. Confirm that blood returns freely through the catheter prior to infusion of any fluids or medications.

Umbilical artery catheterisation

❶ Prepare and drape the umbilical cord as with umbilical vein catheterisation.

❷ Loosely tie umbilical tape at the base of the umbilical cord at the junction with the skin and cut the cord approximately 1–2 cm from the skin.

❸ Identify the two thick-walled arteries and attach two haemostats to either side of the umbilical cord to stabilise the vessels (Fig. 23.13.4).

❹ Do not place the haemostats on the arteries.

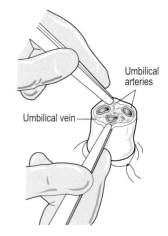

Fig. 23.13.4 Stabilising the vessels.

❺ Insert the smooth-curved iris forceps into the artery selected, and gently dilate the artery (Fig. 23.13.5).

❻ Continue dilating until the forceps can be inserted about 1 cm. Gently introduce and advance the preflushed catheter (3.5 preterm; 5.0 term) towards the patient's feet with gentle cephalad traction on the cord (Fig. 23.13.6).

❼ Overcome any resistance with gentle steady pressure, but do not force the catheter. Place the catheter either 'low' at the level of the L3 vertebra or 'high' between the T6 and T9 vertebrae

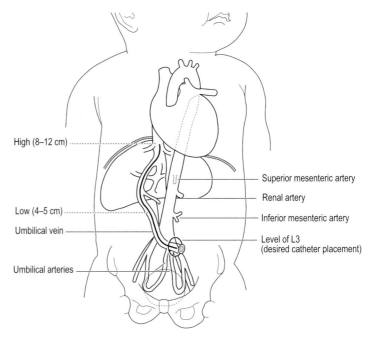

Fig. 23.13.3 Location of tip of catheter.

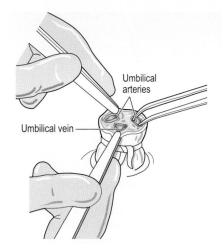

Fig. 23.13.5 Inserting the iris forceps into the artery.

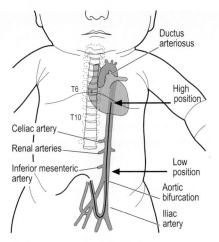

Fig. 23.13.7 Placing the catheter.

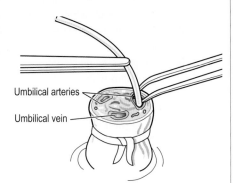

Fig. 23.13.6 Advancing the catheter.

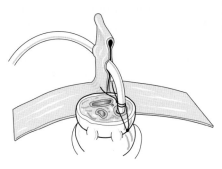

Fig. 23.13.8 Anchoring the catheter to the umbilical cord.

(Fig. 23.13.7). Low catheter insertion distances are based on patient weight and are available on graphs. High catheter insertion distance is approximately 60% of the distance between the infant's umbilicus and either shoulder.

❽ Anchor the catheter to the umbilical cord with a purse-string suture then secure the catheter to the abdomen with tape (Fig. 23.13.8).

❾ Verify placement of the radio-opaque catheter by thoracoabdominal X-ray.

Complications

- Haemorrhage.
- Infection.
- Air embolism.
- Vessel dissection.
- Perforation.
- If umbilical venous catheters are left in the liver, sclerosing substances injected via the catheter can cause hepatic damage.
- Thromboembolic events, particularly to kidneys, intestines and the lower

extremities. If blanching or cyanosis of the lower extremities occurs, remove the catheter immediately.

Tips

- Always advance catheters slowly and use only gentle pressure if resistance is encountered.
- Aggressive catheter insertion can result in creation of a false lumen or perforation of a vessel.
- Always confirm catheter position radiographically.
- If an umbilical venous catheter is needed emergently prior to radiographic confirmation of position, place it 'low' to avoid accidental injection of sclerosing medications directly into the liver. However, if time allows for radiographic confirmation of catheter position, place the umbilical artery catheter 'high' since that position appears to be associated with fewer complications.

Further reading

Barrington KJ. Umbilical artery catheters in the newborn: Effects of catheter materials. *Cochrane Database Syst Rev* 2000;**2**:CD000949.
Barrington KJ. Umbilical artery catheters in the newborn: Effects of position of the catheter tip. *Cochrane Database Syst Rev* 2000;**2**:CD000505.
Cohen RS, Ramachandran P, Kim EH, Glasscock GF. Retrospective analysis of risks associated with an umbilical artery catheter system for continuous monitoring of arterial oxygen tension. *J Perinatol* 1995;**15**(3):195–8.
Cunningham FJ, Engle WA, Rescorla FJ. Paediatric vascular access and blood sampling techniques. In: Roberts JR, Hedges JR, editors. *Clinical procedures in emergency medicine*. 3rd ed. Philadelphia, PA: WB Saunders; 1998. p. 281–308.
Green C, Yohannan MD. Umbilical arterial and venous catheters: Placement, use, and complications. *Neonatal Netw* 1998;**17**(6):23–8.
Kim JH, Lee YS, Km SH, et al. Does umbilical vein catheterisation lead to portal venous thrombosis? Prospective US evaluation in 100 neonates. *Radiology* 2001;**219**(3):645–50.
McAneney C. Umbilical vessel catheterisation. In: Dieckmann RA, Fiser DH, Selbst SM, editors. *Paediatric emergency and critical care procedures*. St Louis, MO: Mosby; 1997.
Weber HS. Transumbilical artery interventions in the neonate. *J Invas Cardiol* 2001;**13**(1):39–43.

COMMON PROCEDURES

23.14 Electrical countershock

Ronald A. Dieckmann • Conor Deasy

Background

When a child's heart deteriorates into ventricular fibrillation (VF) or pulseless ventricular tachycardia (VT), there is usually a severe systemic insult, such as profound hypoxia, ischaemia, acidosis, electrocution, or myocarditis. Sometimes the child has a congenital heart defect such as idiopathic hypertrophic subaortic stenosis or long QT syndrome. Any detectable ventricular rhythm, even fibrillation, suggests that there is still some perfusion of the heart – therefore VF or pulseless VT is a survivable presenting rhythm. This is in distinction to the clinical circumstances with asystole or bradyasystole, the most common paediatric cardiopulmonary arrest rhythms. In these rhythm presentations, the degree of hypoxia is usually so severe that treatment of any kind is less to work. Ventricular dysrhythmias represent approximately 5–10% of presenting paediatric cardiopulmonary arrest rhythms. SVT represents <1%. Resuscitation from such pulseless rhythms also includes ventilation, oxygenation, and effective chest compressions.

Electrical countershock for tachydysrhythmias is a common life-saving procedure in adult emergency cardiac care and is the most effective treatment for sudden cardiac arrest from ventricular dysrhythmias in all age groups. The concept behind electrical countershock is that if a properly delivered electrical dose is applied to the heart in a magnitude that does not damage the myocardium, all electrical activity will be momentarily ablated through depolarisation, and the intrinsic pacemaker of the heart will resume rhythm control (automaticity). When the child is pulseless and has a ventricular dysrhythmia the most effective treatment is immediate electrical asynchronised countershock (defibrillation) performed as quickly as possible with the appropriate technique. In contrast, if a child has a pulse, and the rhythm is either SVT or VT, use synchronised countershock.

Electrical countershock is frequently effective in children with ventricular dysrhythmias but it will not provide benefit in asystole, bradyasystole or pulseless electrical activity (PEA). Essential treatments for VF, such as cardiopulmonary resuscitation (CPR), improved gas exchange, correction of acidosis and vasopressor support of perfusion may change the type of VF from fine, low amplitude VF to coarse, high amplitude VF. Coarse, high amplitude VF is more responsive to electrical countershock than fine, low amplitude VF. After electrical countershock for a ventricular dysrhythmia, administer amiodarone to reduce recurrence. In addition, in children with *torsades de pointes* VT, give magnesium.

In certain clinical scenarios, other interventions in addition to countershock may also improve survival, e.g. fluids for hypovolaemia, potassium-lowering treatment for hyperkalaemia, calcium for hypocalcaemia, pericardiocentesis for pericardial tamponade and needle thoracostomy for tension pneumothorax.

Indications for asynchronous countershock (defibrillation)

- VF.
- Pulseless VT.

Indications for synchronous countershock

- SVT with shock and pulse but no vascular access rapidly available.
- VT with shock and pulse present.
- Atrial fibrillation or atrial flutter with shock.
- Stable VT or SVT in collaboration with specialist.

Contraindications

Conscious patient with good perfusion.

Equipment

❶ Standard defibrillator (monophasic or biphasic).
❷ Automated external defibrillator (AED).
❸ Newer models feature lower power outputs to deliver lower energy countershocks.

Standard preparation

❶ Open airway. Look listen and feel for no more than 10 seconds. If the child is not breathing or is not breathing normally then deliver 5 rescue breaths. Take no more than 10 seconds to assess for signs of life or a pulse. If there are no signs of life, no pulse, or a pulse rate less than 60 beats per minute commence chest compressions.
❷ If child is pulseless, begin closed chest compressions without delay, delivering 100 chest compressions per minute. For lone rescuers with victims of all ages the chest compression to ventilation rate is 30:2. For healthcare providers performing 2-rescuer CPR for infants and children: 15:2 (and 3:1 for neonates).
❸ Turn *on* the defibrillator but do *not* activate the synchronised mode.
❹ Select the proper paddles size. Use the 8-cm adult paddles if these will fit on the chest wall; otherwise, use the 4.5-cm paediatric paddles. Self-adhesive electrode pads are simpler, safer and more efficient than the conventional paddles when defibrillating or cardioverting. Paediatric pads are usually recommended for any child under 10–15 kg.
❺ Prep paddles with electrode jelly, paste, or saline-soaked gauze pads, or use self-adhesive defibrillator pads. Do not let jelly or paste from one site touch the other and form an 'electrical bridge' between sites, which could result in ineffective defibrillation or skin burns.
❻ Establish appropriate electrical charge which is 4 J kg^{-1} asynchronous for VF/pulseless VT (Table 23.14.1).
❼ Charge the defibrillator while another rescuer continues chest compressions. Stop CPR, verify rhythm and if shockable

Table 23.14.1	Appropriate electrical charge for countershock	
Dysrhythmia	Mode	Charge
VF Pulseless tachycardia	Asynchronised (defibrillation)	Initial shock 2 J kg^{-1}, subsequent shocks 4 J kg^{-1}
VT with pulse SVT Atrial fibrillation and atrial flutter with shock	Synchronised	0.5–1.0 J kg^{-1}

deliver 4 J kg^{-1} asynchronous and immediately resume chest compressions without pulse or rhythm check.

Standard procedure

❶ Apply the paddles or self-adhesive electrode pads directly to the skin of the chest wall with firm pressure, placing one defibrillator pad or paddle on the chest wall just below the right clavicle, and one in the left anterior axillary line, under the left nipple (Fig. 23.14.1).

❷ As another option, use the anterior–posterior position (Fig. 23.14.2) however it is not then possible to continue CPR easily.

❸ Clear the nearby area of personnel except the person delivering chesty compressions so that no-one is in contact with the patient, gurney or

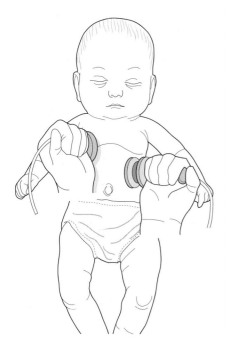

Fig. 23.14.1 Placement of paddles on the child's chest.

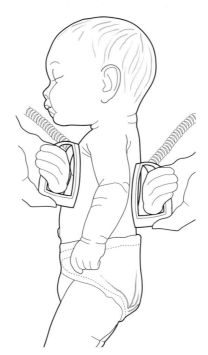

Fig. 23.14.2 Placement of paddles on the child's chest and back.

equipment. Charge the defibrillator while chest compressions are ongoing. Then stop chest compressions, if the patient is in a shockable rhythm (VF/pulseless VT) then deliver the asynchronous shocks. If not in a shockable rhythm press disarm on the defibrillator which will dump the charge. Another way of dumping the charge is by turning the defibrillator off. Immediately resume CPR.

❹ This is followed by immediate uninterrupted cardiopulmonary resuscitation (15:2) for 2 minutes then rhythm is assessed.

❺ If there has been no rhythm response, immediately recommence chest compressions and administer adrenaline (epinephrine) 10 mcg kg^{-1}. Adrenaline (epinephrine) 10 mcg kg^{-1} should be given every 3–5 minutes during CPR.

❻ If still VF/VT, give a second shock at 4 J kg^{-1}.

❼ After 2 minutes, if no response with an additional shock, administer amiodarone (5 mg kg^{-1}) for defibrillation resistant rhythms.

❽ Treat reversible causes, remembering the 'Hs' and the 'Ts': Hypoxia, Hypovolaemia, Hypo/hyperkalaemia, Hypothermia, Tension pneumothorax, Tamponade (cardiac), Toxins, Thromboembolism.

❾ Treat other rhythms that develop such as PEA or asystole.

❿ Therapeutic hypothermia is recommended if the victim fails to resume consciousness after resuscitation.

AED procedure

❶ A standard AED can be used in children over 1 year. If it is likely that the AED will be used for children the purchaser should check that the performance of the particular model has been tested against paediatric arrhythmias. Purpose-made paediatric pads, or programs which attenuate the energy output of an AED, are recommended for children 1–8 years. However, if this is not available an unmodified adult AED may be used in children over 1 year. In children less than 1 year there is little evidence beyond case reports so the decision may be taken on a risk or benefit ratio which in this setting will probably be in favour of using whatever is available. Several AEDs that are currently on the market have paediatric attenuating devices to reduce the electrical dose delivered to children younger than 8 years, including infants; whilst these are the preferred AED, if not available the responder should use a standard AED rather than delay the delivery of a potentially life-saving intervention.

Open airway ventilate while preparing equipment.

If child is pulseless, begin chest compression.

❷ Turn AED on.

❸ Attach AED electrodes to chest wall (right clavicle, and one in the left anterior axillary line, under the left nipple.).

❹ Allow the device to analyse rhythm.

❺ If countershock indicated, clear the area and deliver electricity.

❻ Do CPR and check airway, breathing and circulation for 2 minutes, then re-analyse rhythm and deliver additional countershocks as indicated.

Complications

- Ineffective delivery of countershock because of failure to charge, improper positioning on the chest, incorrect paddle size, or improper conduction medium (e.g. alcohol swabs).
- Burns on the chest wall.
- Failure to 'clear' before voltage discharge, leading to electrical shock of a team member or bystanders.
- Tachydysrhythmias.
- Bradycardia.
- Myocardial damage or necrosis.
- Cardiogenic shock.
- Embolic phenomena.

TIPS

- Biphasic defibrillators have better speed and efficiency on the first shock than older monophasic defibrillators.
- Minimize the interval between stopping compressions and delivering shocks and always resume CPR immediately after shock delivery.
- The correct energy dose for defibrillation (with either a monophasic or biphasic device) in infants and children is

unknown. When shocks are indicated for VF or pulseless VT, use an initial energy dose of 2 to 4 J kg^{-1} of either waveform; doses higher than 4 J kg^{-1}, especially if delivered with a biphasic defibrillator, may also be safe and effective.

- When performing chest compressions push hard, push fast, and minimise interruptions of chest compression; allow full chest recoil, and don't provide excessive ventilation.
- Take no more than 10 seconds for the pulse check. It is often difficult to detect a pulse in an infant or child; the carotid pulse in the neck in the case of a child, the brachial pulse on the inner aspect of the upper arm in the case of an infant are the sites where pulse should be checked.
- For a child with VF or pulseless VT, use the asynchronised mode – the defibrillator will not discharge in the synchronised mode.
- Failure to apply paddles firmly to the chest wall, using too small paddles or too low energy will decrease effectiveness.
- Self-adhesive electrode pads are simpler, safer and more efficient than the conventional paddles when defibrillating or cardioverting.
- Either uncuffed or cuffed tracheal tubes may be used in infants and children.
- Endotracheal tube placement should be confirmed with the use of carbon dioxide detection.
- If the child has SVT or VT *and* is in shock and unresponsive, give electrical countershock at 0.5–1.0 J kg^{-1}.

Use sedation with analgesia for conscious children receiving countershocks.

Assure the device is in the synchronised mode (SYNC) before every countershock.

Further reading

Biarent D, Bingham R, Eich C, et al. European Resuscitation Council Guidelines for Resuscitation 2010 Section 6. Paediatric life support. *Resuscitation* 2010;**81**(10):1364–88.

Kleinman ME, de Caen AR, Chameides L, et al. Part 10: Pediatric basic and advanced life support: International Consensus on Cardiopulmonary Resuscitation and Emergency Cardiovascular Care Science With Treatment Recommendations. *Circulation* 2010;**122**(16 Suppl 2): S466–515.

American Heart Association Guidelines for Cardiopulmonary Resuscitation and Emergency Cardiovascular Care. *Circulation* 2005;**112**(24 Suppl):IV1–203.

APLS: *Student Manual: The Pediatric Emergency Medicine Course by The American Academy of Pediatrics.* 4th ed.

PALS Provider Manual (Paperback) American Heart Association.

Markenson D, Pyles L, Neish S; American Academy of Pediatrics Committee on Pediatric Emergency Medicine; American Academy of Pediatrics Section on Cardiology and Cardiac Surgery. Ventricular fibrillation and the use of automated external defibrillators on children. *Pediatrics* 2007;**120**(5):e1368–79. Epub 2007 Oct 29. Review. PubMed PMID: 17967922.

Cecchin F, Jorgenson DB, Berul CI, et al. Is arrhythmia detection by automatic external defibrillator accurate for children? Sensitivity and specificity of an automatic external defibrillator algorithm in 696 paediatric arrhythmias. *Circulation* 2001;**103**(20):2483–8.

Deboer S, Sicilia MR, Seaver M, et al. Paediatric defibrillation: Concerns and opportunities. *Paediatr Emerg Care* 2002;**18** (6):466–8.

Dieckmann RA, Brownstein D, Gausche M. *Textbook for paediatric education for prehospital professionals.* Sudbury, MA: Jones & Bartlett; 2001. p. 283–5.

Dieckmann RA, Fiser D, Selbst S. *Illustrated textbook of paediatric emergency and critical care procedures.* St Louis, MO: Mosby; 1997. p. 323–36.

Silka MJ, Kron J, Walance CG, et al. Assessment and follow-up of paediatric survivors of sudden cardiac death. *Circulation* 1990;**82**(2):341–9.

Field JM, Hazinski MF, Sayr MR, et al. American Heart Association Guidelines for Cardiopulmonary Resuscitation and Emergency Cardiovascular Care Science. *Circulation* 2010;**122**:S640–56.

23.15 Pericardiocentesis

Ronald A. Dieckmann

Background

The pumping heart is extremely sensitive to rapid accumulation of pericardial fluid. Small amounts of fluid acutely increase intrapericardial pressure and may significantly impede venous return and cardiac output. Haemopericardium is the most common fluid collection – blood collects between the visceral and parietal pericardium after

a penetrating injury in the high-risk zone formed by the triangle of the two nipples and the sternal notch. The risk of death from a penetrating injury to the heart is higher from the haemopericardium than from direct injury to the myocardium, coronary arteries or cardiac valves.

The classical presentation of paediatric cardiac tamponade is a child with a penetrating anterior chest-wall injury who has

distant heart sounds, neck vein distension and hypotension (Beck's triad). However, because other blood loss may concurrently reduce central venous pressures, and because audible intensity of heart sounds may be difficult to distinguish in children, suspect tamponade in any child with a high-risk chest-wall penetration in the triangle, even tiny, with signs of a possible perfusion deficiency – tachycardia, poor skin colour or temperature, delayed capillary refill or diminished pulses.

In contrast to haemopericardium, slow fluid accumulation in the pericardium from other aetiologies, such as viral, bacterial or myco-bacterial infection, or from immunological/collagen vascular disease or malignancy, has a minimal effect on cardiac function. The distensible pericardium readily accommodates slow fluid collections and the presentation of such patients often does not involve perfusion abnormalities. In this setting, needle pericardiocentesis is best accomplished with echocardiographic guidance.

Pericardiocentesis is a needle procedure for either life-saving decompression of acute cardiac tamponade, or for diagnostic evaluation of a non-emergent pericardial effusion. Rapid removal of acute haemopericardial fluid by needle pericardiocentesis is sometimes life saving. The decompression of the pericardium will temporarily restore myocardial performance in a perfusing patient, until reaccumulation occurs. Hence, needle pericardiocentesis is a temporising measure that precedes open surgical decompression. Sometimes, it is a heroic intervention in cardiopulmonary arrest. In non-emergent settings, an indwelling catheter may be necessary to prevent fluid reaccumulation. The procedure can be done with or without electrocardiographic or echocardiographic guidance, depending on the urgency of the clinical situation. Because the majority of needle pericardiocentesis procedures are performed on children in cardiopulmonary arrest, who have low probability of survival, the efficacy and safety of the procedure are poorly understood.

Indications

- Cardiac tamponade.
- Pericardial effusion of unknown aetiology.

Contraindications

- There are no contraindications in the child presenting emergently with shock or cardiopulmonary arrest and evidence of acute tamponade. If equipment and appropriate personnel are present, open thoracotomy may be preferred over needle pericardiocentesis.

- In the non-emergent situation, an uncorrected bleeding diathesis is a contraindication.

Equipment

Emergent procedure
1. Povidone-iodine solution.
2. 30–50-mL syringe.
3. 2.5 or 3.5-inch 18–20-gauge spinal needle.
4. Ultrasound machine.

Non-emergent procedure
1. 1% lidocaine.
2. 25-gauge needle.
3. Two 5-mL syringes.
4. Two 6–8-cm (2.5 or 3.5-inch) 18–20-gauge spinal needles.
5. Three-way stopcock.
6. 30–50-mL syringe.
7. 18 and 20-gauge over-the-needle catheters.
8. Cable with alligator clip at each end.
9. Sample containers.
10. Electrocardiograph (ECG) machine.
11. Echocardiograph (desirable).
12. Ultrasound machine.

Indwelling catheter
1. Flexible guidewire or J-wire.
2. Plastic over-the-wire catheter.

Standard preparation
1. Place the child in a semi-reclining position (30–45 degrees).
2. Establish secure vascular access and apply cardiac monitor.
3. Secure the airway if necessary.
4. If the procedure is non-emergent, administer sedation.
5. Identify the subxiphoid entry site (Fig. 23.15.1), below and to the left of the xiphoid process.
6. Prepare the area widely with povidone-iodine solution.
7. Infiltrate the entry site with lidocaine in conscious patients.

Non-emergent procedure
In addition to the preparation:
1. Attach the correctly-sized spinal needle to a stop cock and 30-mL syringe.
2. Attach one clip of the cable to the hub of the spinal needle and one clip to the V-lead of the ECG machine (Fig. 23.15.2).
3. Turn the ECG to the V-lead position.

Procedure
1. Establish location of effusion with ultrasound (Fig. 23.15.3).
2. Under constant ultrasound guidance, aim the needle to the left shoulder and

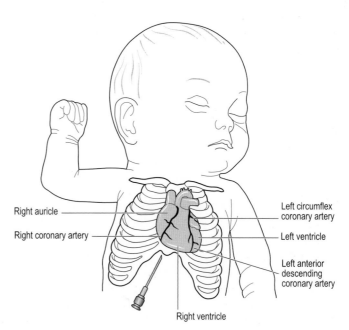

Fig. 23.15.1 Subxiphoid entry site.

Right auricle

Right coronary artery

Left circumflex coronary artery

Left ventricle

Left anterior descending coronary artery

Right ventricle

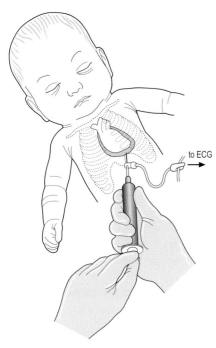

Fig. 23.15.2 Using the ECG for guidance.

enter at a 30–45 degree angle (Fig. 23.15.2) toward the anatomic location of the effusion.

❸ Apply continuous negative pressure and advance the needle until there is a 'pop' as the needle enters the pericardium.

❹ When blood flows into the syringe, place a haemostat at the skin surface to prevent further advancement of the needle.

❺ Aspirate until blood is evacuated from the pericardium.

❻ If prolonged drainage is necessary, advance the guidewire or J-wire through the needle, remove the spinal needle,

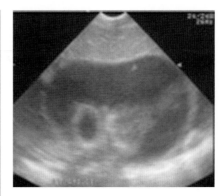

Fig. 23.15.3 Pericardial effusion. Image courtesy of Dr. Ronald Dieckmann.

and place the larger catheter with side holes over the wire.

Non-emergent procedure
After the preparation:

❶ Do constant ECG monitoring.
❷ If the needle punctures the ventricular epicardium, ST segment elevation or a dysrhythmia may occur (Fig. 23.15.4).
❸ If an injury pattern develops, withdraw the needle slightly or reposition more medially.
❹ Always use the ultrasound to guide the needle to the area of largest fluid accumulation.

Complications

- Ventricular puncture.
- Atrial puncture.
- Coronary artery laceration.
- Cardiac dysrhythmia.
- Haemopericardium.
- Pneumothorax.

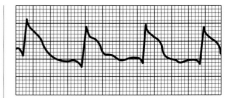

Fig. 23.15.4 Injury current with needle in myocardium.

- Haemothorax.
- Diaphragm perforation.
- Bowel or stomach perforation.
- Infection.
- Cardiac arrest.

Tips

- If the effusion is not causing tamponade, identify the size and location of the effusion with echocardiography, computerised tomography or magnetic resonance imaging before doing pericardiocentesis.
- Always use ultrasound guidance.
- If there is a large volume of aspirated blood, the needle may be in the ventricle. The presence or absence of clotting does not reliably indicate needle location.

Further reading

Dieckmann RA, Fiser D, Selbst S. *Illustrated textbook of paediatric emergency and critical care procedures*. St Louis, MO: Mosby; 1997. p. 592–5.

Lee C, Mason LJ. Paediatric cardiac emergencies. *Anesthesiol Clin N Am* 2001;**19**(2):287–308.

Tsang TS, El-Najdawi EK, Seward JB, et al. Percutaneous echocardiographically guided pericardiocentesis in paediatric patients: Evaluation of safety and efficacy. *J Am Soc Echocardiogr* 1998;**11**(11):1072–7.

23.16 Transurethral catheterisation and suprapubic bladder aspiration

Conor Deasy • Judith Klein

Background

Obtaining an uncontaminated specimen of urine is essential to diagnose urinary tract infection (UTI). UTIs are a common aetiology of fever and serious bacterial infection in infants. In children who cannot provide clean-catch urine specimens, the diagnosis of UTI involves obtaining a urine sample directly from the bladder. Urine specimens obtained via bags attached temporarily on to the perineum are frequently contaminated samples, particularly with infant girls. Waiting for bagged urine specimens is also time-consuming and frustrating in the emergency department (ED) setting. Hence, urinary bag specimens frequently confuse diagnosis of UTI, and often result in false positive specimens and unnecessary treatment.

Obtaining an appropriate urine specimen requires either transurethral catheterisation or suprapubic aspiration. Unfortunately, in very young females and circumcised males with small foreskins, the urethra can be difficult to find and even more difficult to cannulate. In these cases, perform suprapubic aspiration of urine directly from the bladder, whenever possible under ultrasound guidance. This is an easy procedure that requires minimal equipment. Suprapubic aspiration provides a sterile urine specimen with less trauma to the infant than repeated, failed attempts at urethral catheterisation.

Transurethral catheterisation and placement of an indwelling bladder catheter is also useful in the management of critically ill and injured children, to monitor urine output in the setting of shock or trauma. Urine output is one of the best measures of core perfusion and can help guide fluid resuscitation of a child in shock. The combination of heart rate and urinary bladder output are two excellent measurements of intravascular volume and response to treatment.

Indications

Indications for transurethral catheterisation

- Collection of a diagnostic urine specimen.
- Intermittent bladder decompression for neurogenic bladder.
- Urological study.
- Measurement of urine output in critically ill or injured child.
- Acute urinary retention.

Indications for suprapubic bladder aspiration

Collection of a clean diagnostic urine specimen when transurethral catheterisation is impossible or unsuccessful.

Contraindications

Urethral catheterisation

- Obvious pelvic trauma.
- Blood at the urethral meatus.
- Upward displacement of the prostate in males following trauma.
- Perineal haematoma.

In these circumstances, perform a retrograde urethrogram prior to cannulation of the urethra. Placement of a catheter without such a study could convert a partial urethral tear into a complete transection. Urethral injuries are uncommon in females because of the relatively short distance between the urethral meatus and the bladder. Bladder injuries, however, are more common in females and children in general because of the higher abdominal location of the organ in children versus adults. If blood appears following urethral catheterisation in trauma, perform a retrograde cystogram to search for bladder injury.

Suprapubic aspiration

- Coagulopathy.
- Thrombocytopenia.
- Significant abdominal distension.
- Recent abdominal surgery.

In addition, if ultrasound is available, do not perform suprapubic aspiration if the bladder diameter is less than 3.5 cm or if a volumetric scan demonstrates less than 10 mL of urine (Fig. 23.16.1). Under these circumstances, delay the procedure because it is unlikely to be successful.

Transurethral catheterisation

Equipment

The equipment required for transurethral catheterisation is often available in prepackaged trays to which only the appropriately sized catheter need be added. Determine the appropriate catheter size either by using a length-based resuscitation tape, by using the formula $2 \times$ (endotracheal tube size), or by using a table listing equipment sizes by age (Table 23.16.1). Remember to use lidocaine jelly in a syringe, particularly when catheterising the male urethra.

Preparation

❶ Review the male and female anatomy of the perineum.

❷ Have all equipment readily near the child.

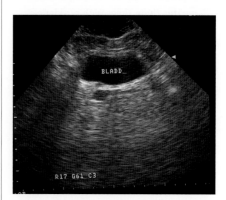

Fig. 23.16.1 Using ultrasound for suprapubic aspiration.

Table 23.16.1 Catheter sizing for children			
	Male (French)	*Girl (French)*	*Type*
Newborn	3	3-5	Straight
1–2 years	5	5 or 8	Straight
3–5 years	8	8	Balloon-tipped
6–10 years	8 or 10	8 or 10	Balloon
10–12 years	10 or 12	12	Balloon
13 years and older	12	12 or 14	Balloon

❸ Place the appropriately sized catheter and the syringe with lidocaine jelly (Lidojet) on to the sterile field.

❹ Have an assistant gently restrain the child in a frog-leg position to prevent disruption of the sterile field and unnecessary trauma due to patient movement.

❺ If the child is older, discuss the procedure, clearly relate the steps of the procedure to the child, and move slowly.

Procedure

❶ Use sterile procedure.

❷ With a male patient, use the non-dominant hand and a gauze to retract the foreskin and expose the meatus. In the circumcised male, the gauze is still useful to maintain a firm grasp on the penis during catheterisation.

❸ With a female patient, use the thumb and forefinger of the non-dominant hand to spread the labia majora and expose the urethra. Clean the urethral meatus three times with povidone-iodine solution, making sure to swab from front to back in females to avoid contamination.

❹ Insert a few millilitres of lidocaine jelly using a syringe device to provide topical anaesthesia, particularly in male patients.

❺ Lubricate the catheter with the same jelly and insert the catheter into the urethra. Do not force the catheter against resistance. Once urine flows through the catheter, stop advancing.

❻ Discard the first 1 mL of urine, which may be contaminated, and collect a specimen.

❼ If the catheter is being left in, inflate the balloon, if there is one, and pull back until resistance is met. Inflate the balloon with the amount of fluid listed on the catheter itself.

❽ Connect the catheter to a sterile closed drainage system. With a balloon-tipped catheter, secure the catheter or tubing to the inner thigh with tape. With non-balloon catheters, tape the tube to the shaft of the penis in a spiral fashion or to the proximal inner thigh next to the labia majora in females.

❾ Remember to return the foreskin to its original position in uncircumcised males to prevent paraphimosis and penile constriction.

Complications

Table 23.16.2 lists the complications of urethral catheterisation.

- The most common complication of urethral catheterisation is infection, particularly if a catheter is left indwelling for a prolonged period of time. Single urethral catheterisations for collection of diagnostic specimens are rarely complicated by infections.

- Urethral or bladder trauma can also occur with urethral catheterisation, particularly with oversized catheters or when a

Table 23.16.2 Complications of urethral catheterisation
- Urinary tract infection - Urethral or bladder trauma - Haematuria - Paraphimosis - Vaginal catheterisation - Urethral strictures

catheter is placed in a child with urethral trauma.

- Urethral strictures can also occur if catheters are left indwelling for a prolonged period of time.

Tips

- There are circumstances in which urine specimens can be obtained non-invasively using urinary bags.

- For example, in the setting of trauma, microscopic haematuria (urinalysis >10–25 red blood cells (RBC) per high-powered field) can help detect occult intra-abdominal and genitourinary trauma in children.

- In uninjured children, a bag urine specimen is acceptable if the intent of diagnostic specimen collection is not the detection of infection.

Suprapubic aspiration

Equipment

Fig. 23.16.2 illustrates the equipment required for suprapubic aspiration. Use an ultrasound to improve the likelihood of success.

Preparation

❶ Review the anatomy of the lower abdomen (Fig. 23.16.3).

❷ Restrain the child in a frog-leg position using an assistant who can help soothe the child.

❸ Have all equipment near the patient's abdomen including the ultrasound.

Procedure

❶ Locate a spot approximately 1 cm cephalad of the pubic symphysis in the midline.

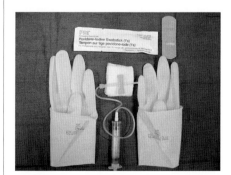

Fig. 23.16.2 Equipment for suprapubic aspiration.

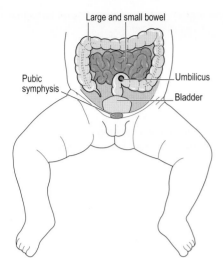

Fig. 23.16.3 Anatomy of the lower abdomen.

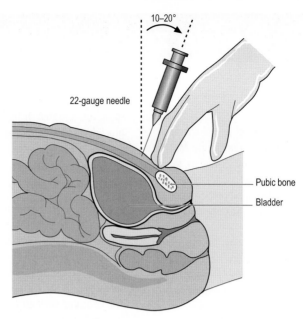

Fig. 23.16.4 Inserting the suprapubic needle.

❷ Use ultrasound to determine if the bladder is full enough. If the bladder diameter is 3.5 cm or if 10 cm³ of urine is present on a volumetric bladder scanner, the procedure is likely to be successful.

❸ Prepare the skin at this spot with povidone-iodine solution.

❹ In males, provide gentle penile compression prior to skin cleansing to prevent voiding prior to the procedure.

❺ Using a 3-cm³ syringe attached to either a 23-gauge butterfly or 22-gauge 3.5-cm (1.5-inch) needle, insert the needle at an angle approximately 10–20 degrees cranially (Fig. 23.16.4). Remember that the bladder lies higher in the abdomen in children than in adults.

❻ Provide constant backpressure on the syringe.

❼ Aspirate the urine specimen, remove the needle, and place a small bandage on the site.

Complications

- Bowel perforation. This is a rare complication. The only reports of bowel penetration are in children with markedly distended abdomens. Even if needle penetration of the bowel occurs, there is no treatment and infection is extremely unusual.

- Infections around the puncture site can occur, but are unusual with a sterile technique.

- Microscopic haematuria (<10 RBC per high powered field) can occur transiently following aspiration.

Tips

- Suprapubic aspiration is not often required in the ED. However, when urethral catheterisation is unsuccessful, it is a straightforward and safe procedure that provides diagnostic specimens with a contamination rate approximately half that of transurethral catheterisation.

- Ultrasound guidance of suprabubic aspiration improves the success rate of the procedure considerably, from 36% to 90%. The ultrasound is performed to determine whether there is enough urine present for a suprapubic tap to be successful, not to direct needle placement. The ultrasound is performed using gel placed on the ultrasound probe head to improve the quality of the image. If the bladder contains greater than 20 mL of urine the suprapubic aspiration should be successful. If the volume is less than this, or the bladder diameter is less than 3.5 cm then give fluids and wait for more urinary volume to be present.

- It is a good tip to always have a container at the ready to collect a clean catch of urine as pressure with the probe in the suprapubic area may stimulate urination.

Further reading

Bell LM. Transurethral bladder catheterization. In: Dieckmann RA, Fiser DH, Selbst SM, editors. *Paediatric emergency and critical care procedures*. St Louis, MO: Mosby; 1997. p. 533.

Bell LM. Suprapubic bladder aspiration. In: Dieckmann RA, Fiser DH, Selbst SM, editors. *Paediatric emergency and critical care procedures*. St Louis, MO: Mosby; 1997.

Garcia-Nieto V, Navarro JF, Sanchez-Almeida E, Garcia-Garcia M. Standards for ultrasound guidance of suprapubic bladder aspiration. *Paediatr Nephrol* 1997;11 (5):607–9.

Liso JC, Churchill BM. Paediatric urine testing. *Paediatr Clin N Am* 2001;48(6):425–40.

Pollack CV, Pollack ES, Andrew ME. Suprapubic bladder aspiration versus urethral catheterization in ill infants: Success, efficiency and complication rates. *Ann Emerg Med* 1994;23(2):225–30.

Schneider RE. Urologic procedures. In: Roberts JR, Hedges JR, editors. *Clinical procedures in emergency medicine*. 3rd ed. Philadelphia, PA: WB Saunders; 1998. pp. 45–57.

23.17 Penile zipper injury

Michelle Lin

Background

The most common cause of penile entrapment is an unintentional zipper injury. Most commonly seen in boys aged 2–6 years, this injury occurs while the child is zipping up his pants. In addition to being painful, this condition is a tremendously anxiety-inducing injury for the child.

The patient usually presents for medical attention only after failed attempts at self-extrication. There are two patterns of entrapment for the often-macerated and oedematous soft tissue. First, the movable zipper head may 'catch onto' the external genitalia tissue. Second, the interlocking teeth along the zipper path may entrap some soft tissue. In order to disassemble a zipper, one must understand its anatomy. Specifically, a thin median bar is the only structure separating the two tracks on the zipper-sliding device, interlocking them.

Indications

Soft-tissue entrapment in a zipper.

Contraindications

None.

Equipment

❶ Bone or wire cutters.
❷ Mineral oil.
❸ Local anaesthesia (1% lidocaine without adrenaline (epinephrine), syringe, 30-gauge needle).

Preparation and positioning

❶ Carefully position the patient supine or semisupine in the caregiver's lap, being careful not to jostle the pants or zipper.

❷ In a child whom you anticipate is going to be too agitated or fearful of the procedure, consider procedural sedation.

Procedure

❶ Soak the exposed external genitalia in mineral oil for 10 minutes to lubricate the contact points. Occasionally, this manoeuvre alone will allow the zipper to easily retract so that the tissue is freed.
❷ Anaesthetise the entrapped tissue using 1% lidocaine without adrenaline (epinephrine).
❸ For the external genitalia entrapped *in the zipper sliding device*, use the bone or wire cutter to break the thin median bar that separates the two sliding tracks. The front and back plates will fall apart, releasing the entrapped skin (Fig. 23.17.1).
❹ For the external genitalia entrapped *in the interlocking teeth*, cut the zipper just inferiorly to the entrapment site. The two interlocking rows of teeth will, with gentle manipulation, slowly separate from one another and release the skin.

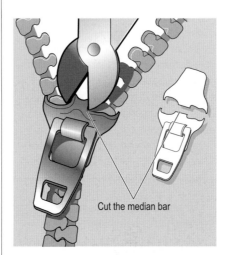

Cut the median bar

Fig. 23.17.1 Diagram of zipper separation after cutting median bar.

❺ Provide supportive wound care to the injury site using warm soaks and apply a dressing. In severe soft tissue injuries, however, suture repair and/or debridement of the wound may be necessary under the guidance of a consulting urologist.

Complications

The primary complication in penile zipper removal is pain. This occurs most commonly during the positioning and preparation of the patient. Gentle manipulation and positioning are essential for this procedure.

Tips

- Cutting off the pant legs (and possibly even the rest of the pants around the zipper) can provide significant pain relief.
- Because pain is a significant fear in these patients, a compromise between local anaesthesia and procedural sedation is a regional block. A dorsal penile block will anaesthetise the entire penis.

Further reading

Kanegaye JT, Shonfeld N. Penile zipper entrapment: A simple and less threatening approach using mineral oil. *Paediatr Emerg Care* 1993;**9**(2):90–1.

Lundquist ST, Stack LB. Diseases of the foreskin, penis, and urethra. *Emerg Med Clin N Am* 2001;**19**(3):529–46.

Nolan JF, et al. Acute management of the zipper-entrapped penis. *J Emerg Med* 1990;**8**(3):305–7.

Woodward GA. Penile zipper injuries. In: Dieckmann RA, et al., editors. *Paediatric emergency and critical care procedures.* St Louis, MO: Mosby; 1997. p. 425–6.

Wyatt JP, Scobie WG. The management of penile zip entrapment in children. *Injury* 1994;**25**(1):59–60.

23.18 Lumbar puncture

Ronald A. Dieckmann

Background

Lumbar puncture (LP) is a time-honoured method for obtaining cerebrospinal fluid (CSF) for diagnostic evaluation of suspected central nervous system (CNS) abnormalities. LP is an essential procedure in children with suspected meningitis, and represents the only simple method of obtaining fluid for rapid diagnosis and appropriate pathogen analysis for specific treatment. While LP is most commonly performed to diagnose meningitis, it is also a useful procedure to help identify encephalitis, CNS haemorrhage, malignancy, and other rare metabolic and degenerative conditions of childhood. Occasionally, LP is a therapeutic procedure in treatment of such conditions as pseudotumour cerebri, or for administration of intrathecal antibiotics or chemotherapeutic agents.

LP is a relatively simple procedure in infants and children but has a known complication rate, with both minor and major sequelae. Appropriate patient selection, preparation and patient positioning, and aseptic technique will avoid most complications. Do not perform LP immediately on haemodynamically unstable patients, who first require meticulous management of airway, breathing and circulation, or on patients with clinical signs of focal CNS processes or significantly elevated intracranial pressure. In such patients, obtain blood cultures and administer antibiotics first, then perform LP after stabilisation and brain imaging, when indicated.

Indications

- Clinical symptoms and signs of meningitis or encephalitis in neonate, infant or child.
- Evaluation of sepsis in infant <3 months of age.
- Seizure with fever in child <12 months of age.
- Intrathecal drug administration.

Contraindications

- Haemodynamic instability.
- Active seizure activity.

- Focal neurological signs.
- Significant intracranial pressure elevation (hypertension, bradycardia, and apnoea).

In children with possible significant intracranial pressure elevation from oedema or space-occupying brain lesions, brain herniation after LP is an important consideration. Obtain a computerised axial tomography (CT) brain scan before the LP.

Equipment

Pre-packaged LP trays are available in most hospitals.

❶ 18-, 20- or 22-gauge styleted spinal needles:
  3.5-cm (1.5-inch) for neonates, infants, young children
  6-cm (2.5-inch) for older children and adolescents
  9-cm (3.5-inch) for large patients.
❷ Povidone-iodine solution.
❸ 1% lidocaine.
❹ 25-gauge needle.
❺ 20-gauge needle.
❻ 3–5-mL syringe.
❼ Four capped sterile specimen tubes.
❽ Manometer (for children aged 2 years).
❾ Stopcock.

Preparation and positioning

❶ In most patients, establish secure vascular access, obtain blood cultures ×2 and appropriate blood tests,

administer oxygen and begin cardiac monitoring and pulse oximetry.
❷ Secure the airway if necessary.
❸ Place the child in a lateral recumbent (Fig. 23.18.1) or sitting position (Fig. 23.18.2) at the edge of the gurney.
❹ If the child is conscious, consider sedation.
❺ Identify the entry site at the L3–L4 interspace.
❻ Don sterile gloves and prepare the area widely with povidone-iodine solution.
❼ If the child is conscious, infiltrate the entry site with 1% lidocaine and a 25-gauge needle, then the deeper tissue to the level of the paraspinous ligaments with a 20-gauge needle.

Lateral decubitus position

❶ Flex the child's knees and torso, but do not over-flex the neck and compress the airway.
❷ Have an assistant hold the child firmly in the decubitus position.

Sitting position

❶ Have an assistant hold the child upright with the hips flexed. Hold the child's right elbow and knee with the left hand and the left elbow and knee with the right hand.
❷ Put the thighs against the abdomen and flex the trunk.
❸ Keep the craniospinal axis perpendicular to the transverse plane of the line connecting the iliac crests.

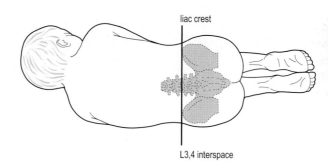

liac crest

L3,4 interspace

Fig. 23.18.1 Lateral decubitus position.

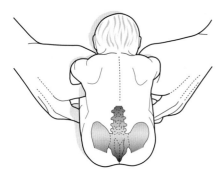

Fig. 23.18.2 Sitting position.

Procedure

❶ Drape the area.

❷ Grasp the needle with the thumbs and index fingers.

❸ Position the needle with the bevel up (if in the lateral position).

❹ Aim the needle into the interspace at 90 degrees, just above the L4 spinous process and advance slowly until there is resistance at the paraspinous ligaments.

❺ Advance the needle until there is a 'pop' as the needle enters through the dura, into the subarachnoid space.

❻ Remove the stylet.

❼ If CSF does not appear at the hub, replace the stylet and advance further.

❽ If the child is over 2 years old, attach a three-way stopcock and manometer to the hub, and measure opening pressure. Normal opening pressure for a child in the lateral decubitus position is 5–20 cm, but a struggling child may artificially elevate this number. Do not attempt an opening pressure in a sitting child, because it is unreliable.

❾ Limit CSF withdrawal to 2 mL in neonates, or 3–6 mL in infants and older children. Put the CSF in 3–4 separate tubes, labelled #1, #2, #3, and #4.

❿ Replace the stylet and remove the needle.

⓫ Bandage the entry site and encourage the child to remain prone for 3–4 hours to minimise CSF leak.

⓬ Send CSF for white blood cell (WBC) count and differential, glucose, protein, Gram stain, other pathogen studies (e.g. viral, AFB or fungal cultures, antigen studies, VDRL). If the CSF is bloody, ask for a cell count on both tubes #1 and #4. Clearing of blood suggests a traumatic tap, whereas no clearing suggests subarachnoid haemorrhage.

⓭ Interpret CSF findings (Table 23.18.1).

Complications

Local

- Puncture-site pain.
- Backache.
- Headache (uncommon <10 years of age).
- Vomiting.

- Temporary paralysis.
- Epidermoid tumours.
- Discitis.
- Epidural haematoma.
- Epidural abscess.
- Osteomyelitis.
- Traumatic LP.

CNS

- Subarachnoid haemorrhage.
- Subdural haemorrhage.
- Brainstem herniation.
- Cardiopulmonary arrest.

Tips

- Positioning and restraining the infant or child properly greatly facilitates the procedure.
- If no CSF appears in the hub after initial penetration, rotate the needle 90 degrees and withdraw the stylet.
- If there is no success with multiple attempts, try a paramedian approach a few millimetres off the midline.
- Use latex agglutination or another bacterial antigen test for partially treated or Gram-stain negative CSF.
- If the child appears ill, administer empiric antibiotics after blood cultures are obtained.
- If the LP is traumatic and CSF is bloody, calculate a WBC:red blood cell (RBC)

Table 23.18.1	Interpretation of CSF				
Condition	WBC mm⁻³	Protein (mg dL⁻¹)	Glucose (mg dL⁻¹)	Gram stain	Opening pressure (cmH₂O)
Normal	<6	<45	60–70% peripheral	Negative	5–20
Bacterial meningitis	100–10 000 (PMN predominance)	50–100	<50% peripheral	Positive (80% of cases)	Elevated
Partially treated	10–100 (PMNs or lymphs)	50–100	<50% peripheral	Negative or positive	Elevated
Viral meningitis	20–100 (early PMNs, late lymphs)	<100	Normal	Negative	Normal or slightly elevated
TB meningitis	20–500 (usually lymphs)	50–200	<40%	Negative	Elevated
Crypto meningitis	Few–100s	100s	<40%	Negative	Elevated
Brain abscess	10–100s	50–100s	Normal	Negative	Elevated

PMN, polymorphonuclear.

ratio and 'Observed: Predicted' (O:P) CSF WBC to help predict probability of bacterial infection. The WBC:RBC ratio is calculated as a simple ratio on CSF fluid. The Predicted CSF WBC is calculated using the formula Predicted CSF WBC = CSF RBC × blood WBC/blood RBC. A WBC:RBC ratio <0.01 (1:100) and an O:P ratio <0.01 makes bacterial infection unlikely.

Further reading

Al-Eissa YA. Lumbar puncture in the clinical evaluation of children with seizures associated with fever. *Paediatr Emerg Care* 1995;**11**(6):347–50.

Barnett ED, Bauchner H, Teele DW, Klein JO. Serious bacterial infections in febrile infants and children selected for lumbar puncture. *Paediatr Infect Dis J* 1994;**13**(11):950–3.

Dieckmann RA, Fiser D, Selbst S. *Illustrated textbook of paediatric emergency and critical care procedures.* St Louis, MO: Mosby; 1997. p. 533–7.

Grant T. Paediatric meningitis. *Ann Emerg Med* 1994;**24**(1):118.

Ward E, Gushurst CA. Uses and technique of pediatric lumbar puncture. *Am J Dis Child* 1992;**146**(10):1160–5.

COMMON PROCEDURES

23

24.1 Orthopaedics and rheumatology

Robyn Brady • Navid Adib

ESSENTIALS

1 Painful dysfunction of limb, posture, or gait may be caused by trauma, infection, or less commonly, inflammatory or neoplastic developments.

2 Hip, knee, abdominal, pelvic, and spinal pathology must be considered with each presentation. In particular, isolated knee pain may be the only presenting feature of serious hip pathology.

3 Careful attention to history and close assessment of posture and response to palpation are required to delineate focal pathology.

Introduction

The child who has pathology of the bones and joints may present in a variety of ways. Acute paediatric musculoskeletal conditions range from the many infective, inflammatory and other causes of limp and limb pains, to the isolated acute limb fracture as a result of moderate trauma, which is among the top ten paediatric emergency department (ED) presentations in Australia.[1] An awareness of the range of possible conditions and their clinical appearance, and skilled physical examination and clinical reasoning, are essential for optimal outcomes.

THE CHILD WITH ACUTE MUSCULOSKELETAL PAIN OR DYSFUNCTION

General approach

The spectrum of musculoskeletal pathology occurring in the paediatric population, with the exception of some fractures and adolescent injury, is very different from that seen in the adult population.

Infant and child development have extensive influence on the musculoskeletal pathology seen and its manifestations,

as well as the techniques used in assessment. These differences are outlined in Table 24.1.1.

The limping child

The wide spectrum of causes of limp in children is illustrated in Table 24.1.2. In terms of frequency, common causes in different age groups are outlined in Table 24.1.3.

Diagnoses that require specific treatment to avoid further damage or danger are primarily displaced or unstable fractures (including slipped upper femoral epiphysis), abusive injury (as a presenting feature or incidental finding), bone or joint infection, and neoplastic processes, principally bone tumours and leukaemia.

Assessment

The most important characteristics of a child with an acute limp or painful limb dysfunction are the following:

- age;
- trauma history;
- well-being;
- pain magnitude;
- pain localisation.

Age

The neonate or infant with focal pain or dysfunction should not be discharged without a specific diagnosis, (most of

Table 24.1.1　How children differ: impact of development on musculoskeletal pathology

Body proportions
- Large, heavy head: higher fulcrum for spinal disruption
- Low centre of gravity
- Relatively short legs

Physiology of developing bone
- Zone of calcification: weakest point of muscle/tendon/ligamentous/bony continuum
- Increased plasticity means increased susceptibility to plastic deformation, e.g. torus, bowing fractures
- Physeal vulnerability predisposes to specific pathological responses to subacute or chronic microtrauma, e.g. avascular necrosis of ossification centres, slipped upper femoral epiphysis
- Physeal damage from fracture or ischaemia produces long-term complications
- High blood flow to physeal zones increases risk of vascular dissemination of bacterial disease, e.g. osteomyelitis

Joints and ligaments
- Increased flexibility means less brittleness and fewer fractures in response to arcuate deformation, e.g. carpal, tarsal, rib, vertebral fractures less common
- Ligaments generally stronger than bones: sprains uncommon and complete ligamentous tears rare

Exposure to mechanisms
- Infant-abuse mechanisms especially shearing/shaking forces
- Pre-school children fall on average four times a day (same-level falls)
- Highly active pre- and school-age children have frequent, relatively low-force impactions from falls (monkeybars, trees)
- Pedestrian vs. car causes classical femoral or tibial/fibula injuries from fender, plus head injury from secondary impact
- High-force MVA/MBA/high energy sports injuries increase from adolescence

Immunology
- Increased incidence of bacterial and viral infection
- More rapid dissemination of, and destruction from, bacterial infection

Psychology
- Fear and pain make young children difficult to examine and increase importance of observation and gentle handling
- Immature intellectual development means poor verbalisation of symptoms, incomplete self-other differentiation, and other blocks to symptom communication
- Medical management of traumatic experiences, such as injuries, may influence future psychological responses to trauma
- Altered body perception increases susceptibility of adolescents (particularly females) to unconsciously exaggerated dysfunction in response to minor injuries

Healing
- Rapid healing of most fractures (e.g. femoral fractures: infants 3 weeks!)
- Enormous remodelling potential of deformation within arc of use
- Great ability to compensate, physically and psychologically, for loss of function
- Minimal stiffness after immobilisation

MBA, motorbike accident; MVA, motor vehicle accident.

which, with the specific exception of pulled elbow, warrant admission), and should generally be assessed by someone experienced in this area. Adolescents with a limp or knee or hip pain must have slipped upper femoral epiphysis (SUFE) specifically ruled out.

Trauma history

The history is less sensitive or specific than in adult medicine because:

- children are often poor historians;
- minor injuries are very frequent;

- there is always a possibility of abusive injury and inadequate or erroneous history.

However, a clear history of completely normal function prior to a specific event that precipitated crying and subsequent pain and dysfunction should prompt a search for a fracture.

Well-being

The following key points should be sought:

- history of fever/malaise;

- eating and activity level, which are usually abnormal in sepsis;
- minor illnesses are also common and can co-exist with injury.

Pain magnitude

- Septic arthritis is painful to the slightest movement.
- Subacute arthritides and Perthes' disease present fluctuating disability and pain.
- Disruption of night sleep needs further assessment.

Pain localisation

This is the foundation of acute orthopaedic diagnosis and efficient investigation use. A suggested sequence of examination for young children with musculoskeletal pain is shown in Table 24.1.4.

Other useful features in assessment include:

History

- Details of onset.
- Whether symptoms are constant or intermittent.
- Exacerbations.
- Daily pattern, particularly the presence or absence of night pain.
- History of previous limp or similar pains.
- Physical activities, such as elite sport.
- Bullying or school/home problems.

Observation and examination

- Gait if ambulant.
- Posture and symmetry.
- Activity level.
- Well-being – fever, heart rate.
- Bones, joints, soft tissues.
- Skin integrity.
- Abdomen and spine.
- Lymphadenopathy and lymphadenitis.
- Focal pathology, e.g. warts, bites, and callosities.

Lower limb joint examination should occur with the patient lying supine on the couch. Take note of the resting position of the joints and any asymmetry, redness, swelling, or wasting. Joints should be compared in symmetrical posture as position influences external appearance. Isolate joints (e.g. knee)

Table 24.1.2 Causes of acute limp in children

Trauma
- Fractures – accidental and non-accidental

Infection (point focus)
- Septic arthritis
- Osteomyelitis
- Inguinal lymphadenitis
- Muscle abscess, e.g. psoas

Post-infective
- Rheumatic fever/post-streptococcal arthritis
- Post-infectious arthritis, e.g. Salmonella, Shigella, or Campylobacter enteritis
- Serum sickness
- Post-immunisation inflammation

Inflammatory
- Transient synovitis
- Vasculitis, e.g. Henoch–Schönlein purpura or Kawasaki disease
- Inflammatory arthritis in lower limbs or axial skeleton, e.g. oligoarthritis
- Enthesitis in pelvis or lower limbs, e.g. enthesitis related arthritis
- Associated with, e.g. systemic lupus erythematosus, dermatomyositis, or inflammatory bowel disease

Primary bone disorders
- Slipped upper femoral epiphysis (SUFE)
- Avascular necrosis, e.g. Perthes' disease (hip), Freiberg's disease (metatarsal heads)
- Osteochondroses, e.g. Osgood–Schlatter disease (patellar tendon insertion), Sever's disease (Achilles tendon insertion)
- Unicameral bone cyst/aneurysmal bone cyst/fibrocystic disease/eosinophilic granuloma
- Blount disease (asymmetrical tibial physis closure)
- Tarsal coalitions

Neoplastic
- Leukaemia
- Neuroblastoma
- Bony tumours, e.g. Ewing's sarcoma, osteosarcoma
- Non-malignant tumours, e.g. osteoid osteoma, enchondroma

Haematological
- Haemarthrosis, e.g. Haemophilia A
- Sickle cell disease arthropathy

Physical
- Splinter/foreign body
- Compensatory, e.g. footwear
- Soft-tissue and overuse injury
- Joint hypermobility syndrome
- Plantar warts/calcaneal spurs
- Bites and envenomation

Psychological and idiopathic pain syndromes
- Pain amplification syndromes, conversion disorders
- Complex regional pain syndrome (CRPS, previously known as reflex sympathetic dystrophy)

Abdominal
- Appendix
- Infective and inflammatory bowel disease

Spine
- Scoliosis
- Discitis
- Transverse myelitis
- Spondylolisthesis
- Scheurman's disease
- Guillain–Barré syndrome

child lifting the buttock off the couch. In the normal hip this adduction should allow the ipsilateral knee to be positioned over the opposite leg whereas an inability to adduct past the midline is common in the irritable hip or other causes of hip joint pathology.

At the conclusion of the history and examination the emergency physician should have established the overall well-being of the child, the site and severity of musculoskeletal pain, practical precipitants, and the likelihood of traumatic, infective, or other processes. In patients with minimal physical findings, or findings out of keeping with other aspects of history and examination, the environmental and psychological context of the limp should be explored further. Clues to possible neoplastic illness are discussed later in this chapter.

The child whose examination findings suggest an isolated irritable hip is likely to have one of the pathologies outlined in Table 24.1.5. A suggested pathway for investigation is shown in the algorithm in Fig. 24.1.1. This algorithm incorporates the findings of a number of studies of the prognostic significance of various features of the limping child with respect to septic arthritis, which are further discussed below.

Investigations
A number of recent research findings have allowed for more selective and meaningful investigation of the limping child.

Inflammatory markers
Traditional blood investigations for inflammatory markers include full blood count (FBC), erythrocyte sedimentation rate (ESR) and C-reactive protein (CRP).

FBC is useful primarily to flag bone marrow dysfunction. Each cell line (haemoglobin, white cells and platelets) should be individually assessed. The sensitivity of a raised white cell count (WCC) ($>12 \times 10^9$ L^{-1}) for the identification of septic arthritis is variable (20–75%).[3,4] The absence of an elevated white cell response should never be used to rule out septic arthritis. ESR has shown higher sensitivity (90–95%) in identifying the subgroup with septic arthritis; however, this may miss early infection.[3] CRP has shown superior sensitivity (up to 80%)[4] and specificity in the early identification of invasive

when assessing range of motion so that incidental movement of another joint (e.g. hip) does not cause misleading results.

When assessing hip range of motion, the 'flexion adduction' test[2] may be helpful:

with buttocks flat on the bed, flex the hip (first the unaffected and then the affected) to 90 degrees while supporting the lower leg. Then gently attempt to fold the knee over the contralateral leg without

Table 24.1.3 Common causes of acute limp/single-limb dysfunction in children of various ages presenting to the ED with no specific history of trauma

Infants	Young children	Primary school - age children	Adolescents
Occult fracture[a]	Occult fracture[b]	Transient synovitis	Septic arthritis/ osteomyelitis
Septic arthritis/ osteomyelitis Inflammatory arthritis	Transient synovitis Inflammatory arthritis	Septic arthritis/ osteomyelitis Inflammatory arthritis	SUFE Inflammatory arthritis
	Septic arthritis/ osteomyelitis Perthes' disease	Perthes' disease Psychogenic pain	Osteochondroses Tumour

[a]Includes pulled elbow, accidental and non-accidental injury.
[b]Includes pulled elbow, toddler fracture.

Table 24.1.4 Tips for assessing young children

- The foundation of acute musculoskeletal diagnosis is precise localisation of pain and dysfunction
- The foundation of a productive paediatric examination is a relaxed, non-fearful child
- Personality and parental factors aside, a gentle, slow-moving, highly observant examiner whom the child senses has the trust of the parent, will be most successful in gaining meaningful information

1. Be friendly and establish rapport with the parent
2. Ask parents for clues about site of pain, e.g. is it worse during nappy changes or being picked up under arm, crying associated with going over bumps in car ride, etc. If the child is old enough, ask them to tell or show you exactly where it hurts
3. Where possible, observe child at free play before attempting palpation
4. Visually assess child for alterations of posture, symmetry, or function
5. Record any other clues, such as temperature, dysmorphic features, bruising, psychological state
6. Examine the infant or child in parent's arms (under 6 months and over 5 years they may often be assessed on the couch without concern)
7. Introduce a washable or disposable toy, such as light, name-badge, or 'funny face'
8. Make your first touch very gentle and at a site distant from the target limb! Keep some touch continuous so the rhythm is reassuring. Verbal soothing, such as a hum, may settle anxiety
9. Palpate the limb in question from one end to the other, watching the child's face continuously
10. The first sign of discomfort may be an eyebrow flicker (i.e. a pre-frown) or a flinch
11. If discomfort is sensed, move touch to another area immediately and slowly move back in even more gently for confirmation and further information
12. Put all joints through their full range of movement unless discomfort is noted
13. Examine the spine, groin, and abdomen of all lower limb or gait-disturbed children
14. Areas of focal tenderness or limited range of motion can be further assessed by radiology or ultrasound

bacterial infection in general and of septic arthritis in particular. CRP rises within 24 hours of acute illness, and also falls rapidly and can be used to monitor effectiveness of treatment.[5]

Radiology

X-ray

X-rays are usually non-contributory in children under 10 years of age with acute onset limp (<1 week) without a specific trauma history. Radiological findings in osteomyelitis are usually not present for up to 10 days from the onset of illness, at which time there may be periosteal elevation outlined by new bone formation and/ or lucent areas.[6] Due to the higher burden of pelvic or gonadal irradiation, non-selective or routine pelvic/lower limb radiology should not be encouraged. An effusion is better diagnosed by ultrasound, and deep soft tissue infection such as osteomyelitis, by magnetic resonance imaging (MRI). X-rays are required in trauma with focal tenderness or non-weight-bearing, to rule out SUFE (see below) in the adolescent child with hip pain/dysfunction with or without a trauma history, and in cases of persistent unexplained pain or limb dysfunction.

Ultrasound

Ultrasound is a sensitive, non-invasive assessment tool for evaluation of the irritable hip. It will detect even small hip effusions, may show a subperiosteal pus collection in some cases of osteomyelitis, and may be diagnostic for Perthes' disease and SUFE,[7] although it is not usually the first-line investigation

for these pathologies. Disadvantages of ultrasound include variations in quality from different operators, and difficulty in after-hours access. An ultrasound cannot distinguish between reactive and infective effusions; however, the presence of an effusion confirms organic pathology and its absence in a clinically abnormal presentation should prompt a search for an extrasynovial focus. There is controversy over the place of ultrasound-guided hip aspiration in the evaluation of the irritable hip with an effusion.[8] The majority of Australian paediatric orthapaedic units favour orthopaedic evaluation of irritable hips with selective aspiration and arthrotomy/washout under general anaesthesia. However, ultrasound-guided diagnostic hip aspiration has a role in some units.[9-11]

Bone scan

Isotope bone scans with three-phase technetium-99m MDP are sensitive early, and well tolerated by children, but lack specificity. Confusion may arise particularly in relation to physeal sites, where uptake is already above base-line. 'Hot' scans indicate increased osteoblastic uptake and generally relate to a response to infection or injury. A 'cold' scan suggests infarction, which in severe cases may be a consequence of osteomyelitis. Bone scan is of particular value in children in whom multifocal disease is suspected e.g. neonatal osteomyelitis or chronic recurrent multifocal osteomyelitis (CRMO).[6]

MRI

MRI is excellent for detailed delineation of soft-tissue and bony pathology, particularly when surgery is planned.[12] It is the investigative modality of choice to delineate the site of possible bacterial infection in a child with localised musculoskeletal pain and a septic picture in whom septic arthritis has been ruled out by clinical assessment, ultrasound or arthrocentesis.[13] Limitations include cost, access limitations, and the need to remain still for a longer time period, necessitating general anaesthetic in most small children.

Clinical decision making in a child with a limp

Relative weightings of various symptoms and signs in the various acute paediatric hip pathologies are expressed in Table 24.1.5 and Fig. 24.1.1. However, spinal, abdominal, and pelvic pathology can present as a

Table 24.1.5 Comparative features of paediatric hip-joint pathology

Diagnosis	Transient synovitis	Septic arthritis	Femoral neck osteomyelitis	Perthes'	SUFE	Inflammatory arthritis	Bone tumour
Age	3–6	Any	Any	3–12	9–15	Any	Any
Joint	Hip	Hip, knee	Hip	Hip	Hip	Any	Not joint
Pain (0–3)	1	3	1	0–1 early	1–3	0–2	= 1
Illness (0–3)	0	1–3	1–3	0	0	0–2	Variable
ROM	>80%	<50%	<80%	60–80%	Flexes into external rotation	Usually some movement possible	Normal unless spasm
Inflammatory markers	Normal	Elevated	Elevated	Normal	Normal	Variable	Variable
Ultrasound	Effusion	Effusion	?Reactive effusion, ?subperiosteal collection	Diagnostic changes	Diagnostic changes	?Effusion	n/a
Plain X-ray	?HTDD up	?HTDD up	Bony changes delayed	Diagnostic changes eventually	Diagnostic changes, e.g. widened physis in preslip; Trethowan's sign	May be normal	May be diagnostic

ROM, range of movement; HTDD, head-teardrop distance.

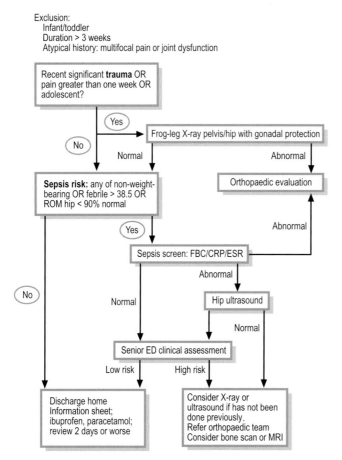

Fig. 24.1.1 Algorithm for management of children >2 years presenting with acute irritable hip.

limp, and must be considered prior to this narrowed focus. The infant or toddler, because of their increased risk for invasive bacterial illness, also represents a special circumstance and the ill child under 2 with an abnormal acute musculoskeletal assessment is best admitted for combined paediatric and orthopaedic assessment and investigation.

The child over 2 with acute atraumatic localised knee or hip pain and an abnormal hip examination is most likely to have an irritable hip (transient synovitis), and the main issue is to exclude septic arthritis. An ultrasound assessment should confirm the suspicion of a hip effusion as suggested by examination, but does not differentiate between transudate and exudate. Table 24.1.6 lists conditions at higher risk of septic arthritis which must be flagged; however, the majority of infections occur in children without underlying pathology. Various attempts have been made to create a valid decision rule with a high sensitivity and specificity for bacterial infection,[4,14–16] however none have demonstrated sustained power prospectively. The four most important variables to give a predicted probability of septic arthritis in a given child with an acutely irritable hip are shown in Table 24.1.7. Degree of pain and range of motion of the joint are auxiliary clinically important variables in the differentiation.

Table 24.1.6   Risk factors for septic arthritis

Relative immune deficit
- Neonates
- Malnourished
- HIV infection
- Immunosuppressive therapy
- Corticosteroid therapy

Injury mechanism
- Penetrating trauma

Joint disease
- Chronic arthritis
- Sickle cell disease

Table 24.1.7   Features suggestive of deep bacterial infection in a child with an acutely irritable hip

Non-weight-bearing
Febrile >38.5°C
WCC > 12×10^9 L^{-1}
ESR > 40 mm hr^{-1}
CRP > 20 mg L^{-1}

Specific syndromes

Transient synovitis

Transient synovitis is a self-limited inflammatory disorder of uncertain aetiology, occurring particularly in boys (70%) in the age group 3–10 years. The onset of lower limb pain is generally gradual and initially may be localised to hip, knee, groin or thigh. The child may be mildly unwell or have had a recent non-specific upper respiratory tract illness, although this is not uniformly present. Range of movement at the hip joint is usually mildly diminished, with discomfort at the end-points of the range. A hip effusion is present. Transient synovitis is a diagnosis of exclusion, the major differential being septic arthritis. Children with localised hip pain should be managed according to the algorithm in Fig. 24.1.1, and non-weight-bearing children with a hip effusion who do not have needle aspiration to rule out septic arthritis should be admitted under the close observation of the orthopaedic team. Weight-bearing children without unusual or high risk features can be managed with parental instruction, ibuprofen, and ED follow up in 2 days.[17,18]

Prognosis

Taylor et al showed a 15% recurrence rate in transient synovitis,[19] and there is some concern about occult Perthes' being an underlying diagnosis, especially in those with delayed bone age at the first imaging.[20] All children discharged with this presumptive diagnosis should have orthopaedic follow up if pain or limp persists or recurs.

ESSENTIALS

1 Diagnosis of septic arthritis is suspected on clinical features, and confirmed by blood and synovial cell count and fluid culture. Isotope scans and MRI have an important role in localising osteomyelitis.

2 Delayed or inadequate treatment of septic arthritis can lead to irreversible joint damage and/or septicaemia.

3 *Staphylococcus aureus* and *Streptococcus* species are the most frequent pathogens, via haematogenous spread or direct extension from infected joint to bone. Community-acquired methicillin resistant *Staph. aureus* (CAMRSA) is increasingly common worldwide and mandates alternative antibiotic treatment.

4 Successful treatment requires parenteral antibiotics and complete drainage of pus from the joint, or surgical clearance of necrotic bone, with long-term follow up.

Septic arthritis and osteomyelitis

Introduction

Septic arthritis is infection of the synovial lining and fluid of a joint. Bacteria are the usual pathogens through haematogenous spread from other, sometimes occult, sites. Direct spread from adjacent bone infection may also occur, particularly where the metaphysis is intracapsular, as in the proximal femur. Phagocytic and neutrophil responses to the bacteria result in proteolytic enzyme release and cytokine production, with synovial abscess formation and cartilage necrosis.[21] Pus under pressure may also reduce epiphyseal blood flow.

Most infections in children are community acquired and occur in normal joints. Infants and children under 3 are at particular risk of septic arthritis, comprising one-third and one-half, respectively, of a large paediatric series.[22] As well as focal clinical inflammation, children may present with occult infection, pseudo-paralysis or generalised sepsis. Comorbidity or deficient host defences, such as those shown in Table 24.1.6, predispose to infection that may be more rapidly progressive or occur in the older child.

Joints of the lower limb, especially hip and knee, account for two-thirds of the infections in children.

In osteomyelitis, bacteria enter the vascular metaphyseal bone initially, then typically extend to the sub-periosteal space forming an abscess. New bone deposition results, with later necrosis of cortical bone. Classically, bone fragments or sequestra are formed over time, which harbour bacteria. Successful treatment must combine eradication of the bacteria and complete removal of any necrotic infected bone. However, in the developed world, earlier diagnosis and aggressive antibiotic therapy have limited the degree of bone destruction present.

The disorder of CRMO has been recognised in infants and children. This is an inflammatory process of unknown origin, which demonstrates culture-negative bony inflammation with histological evidence of necrosis and chronic inflammatory cell infiltrates. Biopsy and culture are mandatory to diagnose the disorder, but antibiotics may be discontinued if pathology is consistent with CRMO. In mild cases, treatment of symptoms may be possible with non-steroidal anti-inflammatory drugs (NSAIDs); however, in more severe cases systemic steroids or treatment with intravenous bisphosphonates, and long-term follow up will be required.[23–27]

Presentation

History

Cardinal features of septic arthritis are recent onset of a painful, red or swollen joint or limb, limp or refusal to bear weight. Pseudoparalysis or refusal to move a limb may occur in neonates and young infants. Infants may present with non-specific symptoms such as poor feeding, vomiting, lethargy or fever. Infrequently, a vertebral or pelvic infection will be the cause of an abnormal gait or abdominal pain. Relevant past history includes trauma, past history of recurrent staphylococcal infection such as boils, and immunisation status in respect to *Haemophilus influenzae* and *Pneumococcus*.

Examination

Typical findings in septic arthritis include a warm tender joint with marked limitation of passive and active movement due to pain. Children with a painful hip will usually maintain the joint in slight (20 degrees) flexion and external rotation. In most distal joints, an effusion is usually clinically evident. In general, fever is low grade and most patients will not appear 'toxic' or unwell. Osteomyelitis may be suggested by an area of maximal tenderness next to a joint, with a greater range of movement of that joint than would be expected with septic arthritis. Deep or partially treated infections may be clinically subtle, with minimal specific examination findings. Careful examination of the skin may reveal areas of infection or trauma as an entry point for haematogenous seeding.

Differential diagnosis

The differential diagnosis of single focus septic arthritis and osteomyelitis is discussed in detail in the section on the limping child. The child presenting with polyarthralgia/polyarthritis is considered in the section on acute arthritides.

Microbiology

Synovial fluid examination and culture Aspiration of affected joints should be performed promptly to confirm the diagnosis and obtain culture specimens. Most young children will require general anaesthesia or conscious sedation for these procedures, and in the majority of units in Australia, arthrotomy with washout performed by the orthopaedic team is the procedure of choice in probable septic arthritis of the hip. The overriding principles are early accurate diagnosis, and minimal delay or exposure of the joint to the chondrolytic enzymes of bacterial joint infection.[28]

A cell count of greater than 50 000 per microlitre of synovial fluid aspirate suggests a bacterial cause, although positive cultures can occur with lower counts, and higher counts may occasionally occur in inflammatory conditions.[29] Synovial fluid should also be inoculated directly into culture medium to avoid loss of fastidious organisms such

Table 24.1.8 Organisms cultured in paediatric invasive bone and joint infection in Australia
Most common (80% of most isolates)
Staphylococcus aureus
Streptococcus species
Other organisms
Pneumococcus
Kingella kingae
Fusobacterium
Meningococcus
Pseudomonas
Salmonella

as *Kingella*.[30] Initial Gram stain results and clinical history will guide empiric antibiotic therapy, with definitive therapy based on final cultures.

Organisms implicated in two recent series involving Australian children[4,31] are shown in Table 24.1.8. An algorithm for initial intravenous therapy of paediatric septic arthritis and osteomyelitis is shown in Fig. 24.1.2.

Negative cultures of blood, synovium, or infected bone occur in 40–80% of cases

of paediatric septic- and osteomyelitis worldwide.[4,29–31] Increasing availability of polymerase chain reaction (PCR) may increase specific bacteriological identification.[32] Despite increasing CAMRSA and a high negative culture rate, the Australian experience has also been of a low rate in treatment failure, presumably due to early case identification and susceptible organisms. However, the increased prevalence of CAMRSA in the US has been associated with an increase in severity of osteomyelitis.[33,34] Tuberculosis is still a cause of chronic bone and spine infection in South-East Asia, Papua New Guinea, and the Torres Strait Islands and should be considered in atypical cases.[35,36]

Management

Joint drainage and empiric parenteral antibiotic therapy are the mainstays of treatment for septic arthritis and should take place without delay. Suggested antibiotic regimes for bone and joint infection are

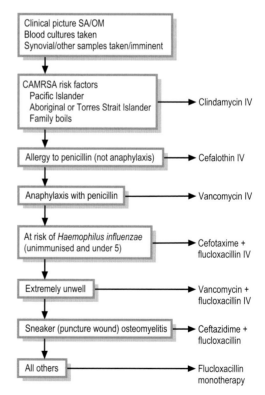

Fig. 24.1.2 Antibiotic therapy for septic arthritis (SA)/osteomyelitis (OM) in Australia.

shown in Fig. 24.1.2, and should be further guided by Gram stain and culture/sensitivity results.

Community-acquired methicillin resistance is becoming an increasing problem world-wide. Specific populations at high risk of CAMRSA include Aboriginal and Torres Strait Islanders in Western and Northern Australia, and Pacific Islanders in Eastern Australia and parts of New Zealand.[37] Children with a personal or family history of recurrent treatment for boils are also at risk.[38]

Neonatal septic arthritis requires special consideration in view of the destructive potential and broader microbiological differential.[39] These children should be reviewed by a team of orthopaedic, neonatal, and infectious-disease specialists.

Because of earlier diagnosis and other aspects of modern care, in most cases beyond the neonatal period combined in-patient/outpatient treatment can occur with length of treatment guided by clinical and inflammatory markers.[4]

Prognosis

This depends upon the organism, patient comorbidity, age of patient and the adequacy and rapidity of treatment. Remarkable remodelling of bony deformity can occur in the young child providing treatment has been adequate. Out of a 30-year series of 332 infants and children with osteomyelitis, with documented follow up of 170 cases, complications were described in 19%.[22] These related largely to joint complications, but some 8% demonstrated epiphyseal damage. However, more recent series showed many fewer complication rates.[40] Patients at highest risk of complication include neonates, septic arthritis in which diagnosis has been delayed, complicated osteomyelitis (involucrae, sequestrum or sinus formation) or epiphyseal involvement, which may cause subsequent limb length discrepancy or deformity. All cases should have close orthopaedic follow up.

Prevention

Primary prevention involves minimising skin or muscular trauma or sepsis (e.g. boils, infected scabies), since damaged tissue predisposes to haematogenous bacterial spread of skin micro-organisms. Secondary prevention can be provided by thorough debridement, wound cleansing and antibiotics in the management of open bone trauma.

Controversies

❶ The role of ultrasound-guided hip aspiration: most orthopaedic surgeons prefer open arthrotomy on selected patients.

❷ Extent and timing of surgery in suspected osteomyelitis.

❸ Duration and route of antimicrobial therapy for bone and joint infections.

Perthes' disease

ESSENTIALS

1 Perthes' disease is a chronic disorder of the femoral head in children, causing limp and usually low-grade pain. While most children outgrow their disease, a proportion have permanent structural changes requiring orthopaedic correction.

2 Clinical findings are of decreased range of hip motion, particularly internal rotation and adduction, with low-grade discomfort.

3 X-ray changes of established disease include joint effusion, loss of femoral head height, fragmentation of epiphysis.

4 Early X-ray changes may be subtle and children with persisting undiagnosed limp should have MRI examination of their hip and, if necessary, orthopaedic follow up.

Pathophysiology

Legg–Calve–Perthes' disease is a disorder of unknown aetiology principally affecting boys (M:F 5:1), commonly in the 4–8-year age group. It is bilateral in approximately 10%. The pathophysiology affects articular cartilage, where synovitis results in oedema, hypermetabolism, hypertrophy, and deterioration of the cartilaginous mechanical properties. Cartilaginous ischaemia is thought to be the active mechanism. It is more prevalent in malnourished children,[41] those with delayed bone age, and those exposed to passive smoking.[20,42,43] The end result may be subchondral fracturing, anterolateral deformation and joint incongruence, although the majority of children have spontaneous gradual remission of their disease process. Four stages are recognised:[44]

❶ Initial – ischaemia causes cartilage hypertrophy and synovitis; X-ray smaller femoral head, increased joint space.

❷ Fragmentation – X-ray shows fragmented epiphysis and subchondral radiolucency ('Caffey's crescent line').

❸ Reossification – altered shape of femoral head with increased radiopacity.

❹ Healing – resolution or persistence of deformity.

ED presentations

When hip pain is present in Perthes' disease it is usually mild, chronic and dull, increasing with physical activity, often with a history of pain for weeks to months. There are no systemic symptoms. Because of the gradual onset of Perthes' disease, acute presentations to the ED usually represent either an early (stage 1) Perthes' and fall within the 'irritable hip' differential, as discussed previously, or a flare-up in a child with known Perthes' disease in whom coincidental comorbidity must be excluded. Remember Perthes' can present as a painless limp.

Examination

Children with Perthes' disease have limited range of hip movement, particularly in adduction and internal rotation, from synovial thickening and adductor muscle spasm. Those with long-standing disease may have muscle atrophy, leg-length discrepancy, and a positive Trendelenburg test on the affected side.

Differential diagnosis

In the early stages of disease, X-ray changes will mimic those of transient synovitis, and children should be managed according to the irritable hip outline suggested earlier.

Children with more minor hip discomfort and non-specific X-ray or ultrasound evaluations should be referred for MRI examination of hip for detection of early stages of avascular necrosis[45–48] and orthopaedic evaluation if symptoms persist longer than 3 weeks.

Investigation and disposition

The plain hip X-ray is diagnostic in established Perthes' disease, although findings may be subtle in early disease. Extensive head involvement, loss of the femoral head 'lateral pillars', subluxation of head beyond the acetabular margin, and late age at presentation are all poor prognostic indicators. MRI examination of the hip joint may be necessary to provide early diagnosis and prognosis (references from above). Orthopaedic management goals are restoration of range of hip movement and containment of the hip within the acetabulum. These goals are sought through a variety of methods including traction, surgery, orthotics and physiotherapy. In general, the younger the child the better the outcome; girls do worse than boys of the same age as they are skeletally more mature. Some three-quarters of patients with Perthes' disease are pain-free and active in 10–20-year follow-up studies.[44]

Slipped upper femoral epiphysis (SUFE)

Epidemiology and pathophysiology

SUFE is more common in males, with a peak age of 10–16 years in males and 9–15 years in females, although it has been reported in children as young as 8 years. SUFE is usually related to puberty (80% occurring during the adolescent growth spurt), and obesity (two-thirds are >90th centile weight-for-height), with genetic and endocrine factors playing a role.[44] Mechanical failure occurs at a widened zone of hypertrophy within the physeal plate. It is important to note that although traditional Salter–Harris proximal femoral physeal fractures can occasionally occur in adolescence from high-energy injuries, these differ from classical SUFE both in the amount of force involved and in the histological plane of cleavage, i.e. the SUFE can be thought of as a 'pathological Salter–Harris type 1 fracture' occurring as a result of minor torsional or low-energy injury in a weakened physeal plate with a high-shear stress load.[44]

Clinical presentation

The classic child with SUFE will be an obese adolescent with pain either in the groin or referred to knee (femoral) or medial thigh (obturator nerve). They may have some leg-length discrepancy and hold the leg in external rotation. Range of motion depends on degree of slip and chronicity. A classical feature of the chronic slip is that passive flexion is accompanied by external rotation.

Initial presentation of SUFE may take one of four patterns:

❶ Preslip. This is usually a retrospective diagnosis, relating to an episode of intermittent pain and evidence of synovitis with widening of the growth plate but without radiological evidence of epiphyseal shift.

❷ Chronic slip. Pain longer than 3 weeks in an ambulant child suffering mild to moderate pain, with decreased range of motion. X-ray shows SUFE ± evidence of remodelling.

❸ Acute-on-chronic slip. Increased pain and radiological evidence of slip following a period of lower-grade symptoms. Acute slip and evidence of remodelling are present on X-ray.

❹ Acute slip (≈10%). Acute, severe hip pain and diminished range of movement

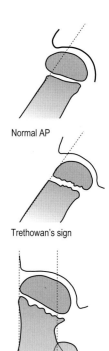

Fig. 24.1.3 Slipped upper femoral epiphysis (SUFE). In the normal pelvic AP, (top) a Klein line (a continuation of the superior border of the femoral neck) should INTERSECT a portion of the femoral head. Trethowan's sign, (middle) in which the Klein line fails to intersect the head in the AP view, is abnormal and represents Grade 1 SUFE. Note the frog-leg view (shown above as in a normal hip) is a better view for diagnosing SUFE in the ambulant child with hip pain, since the posterior slip is usually more clearly shown. However the hip must not be manipulated into frog-leg position in an unstable (non-weight-bearing) child with possible SUFE, as inadvertent reduction may occur and potentially increase risk of avascular necrosis.

with less than 3 weeks' prodrome and no radiological evidence of remodelling.

SUFE is also graded as Stable or Unstable depending on the ability to weight-bear at the time of presentation, and as mild, moderate or severe depending on the percentage of epiphyseal translation. This grading is important, as unstable slips have a high incidence (∼50%) of complications such as avascular necrosis.

The radiological findings in SUFE are outlined in Fig. 24.1.3. It is essential that the emergency physician be aware of the clinical and radiological features of SUFE so that they can recognise at-risk presentations, and actively seek Klein's line (a line extending from the superior border of the femoral neck which should intersect the lateral femoral head in the AP view of normal hip/pelvis).

Although the slip is usually radiologically more evident in the frog-leg lateral, manipulation into this position should be avoided in unstable (non-weight-bearing) children with possible SUFE, in case the process of obtaining it may precipitate further shear.

Ultrasound by experienced operators has also been shown to have high sensitivity and specificity for epiphyseal displacement, even in the early stages.[7]

Differential diagnosis

The differential diagnosis of SUFE has been discussed in the section on limp. A normal frog-leg pelvic X-ray in the ambulant child rules out all but the preslip phase of SUFE. In high-risk clinical situations (e.g. past or family history of contralateral SUFE), MRI may be helpful.

Treatment

Once an unstable SUFE has been diagnosed, patients should be treated as at risk of avascular necrosis. Admission under the orthopaedic team pending surgical fixation should be expedited. Bed-rest with toilet privileges is usual, with pain relief as required. The acutely slipped femoral head is usually fixed by percutaneous or minimal-incision internal fixation.

Complications

Avascular necrosis may occur in up to 50% of unstable slips, with an overall incidence in SUFE of ≈5%. Other complications include chondrolysis and leg-length discrepancy.

Controversies/ developments

❶ The necessity or danger of attempted reduction (which may precipitate avascular necrosis) prior to fixation.

❷ The value of pinning the contralateral hip (asymptomatic bilateral SUFE evolves in up to 40% of children).

Delays in diagnosis and referral are common and avoidable.[49] Causes of delay include:

- Failure to X-ray (particularly with low-grade and/or referred pain).
- Failure to recognise knee pain as a presenting symptom of hip pathology.
- Failure to interpret X-ray correctly, particularly in Grade 1 (ED training should include the X-ray appearance of the normal femoral head).
- Failure to refer appropriately (immediate telephone contact with orthopaedic team).

GENERALISED OR MULTIFOCAL BONE/ JOINT PAIN

Introduction

The child presenting with generalised or multifocal acute musculoskeletal disturbance represents a different diagnostic spectrum. This is outlined in Table 24.1.9. As might be expected, infective and inflammatory disorders predominate and the 'risk profile' relates to the possible consequences of the generalised disease process, such as rheumatic fever, nephritis in association with Henoch–Schönlein purpura (HSP), leukaemia, or juvenile arthritis.

In assessing the child with multifocal joint or bone pain, or with arthralgia or arthritis in a setting of a febrile illness, the following features should be explored:

History

- Antigen exposure – drugs, infections, insects, animals.
- Previous infection or autoimmune dysfunction.
- Features suggestive of infection – fever and its pattern and duration, other symptoms.
- Features suggestive of metabolic drain – lethargy, weight loss, anorexia, night sweats.

Examination

- Skin and mucosae.
- Eyes (visual acuity mandatory).
- Bones (including spine), joints, and surrounding soft tissues.

Table 24.1.9 Causes of acute multifocal limb or joint pain in children presenting to the ED

Infection
- Acute viral illness[†]
- Streptococcal disease
- Other bacterial illness, e.g. *Neisseria*
- Kawasaki disease

Post-infectious (immune-mediated)
- Serum sickness[†]
- Reactive arthritis[†]
- Rheumatic fever

Inflammatory/vasculitic
- Henoch–Schönlein purpura[†]
- Juvenile idiopathic arthritis (JIA)
- Associated with SLE/IBD/other systemic inflammatory disorders

Neoplastic
- Leukaemia[†]
- Neuroblastoma

Haematological
- Sickle cell
- Haemophilia

IBD, inflammatory bowel disease; SLE, systemic lupus erythematosus.
[†]Common causes.

- Lymph nodes.
- Liver and spleen.
- Heart and lungs.
- Kidneys and urine.

Investigations

- Urinalysis and microscopy for casts.
- Inflammatory markers – FBC and film, CRP, ESR.
- Serology, for recent infection due to e.g. streptococcus (antistreptolysin O test (ASOT), antiDNAse), Epstein–Barr virus (EBV), cytomegalovirus (CMV), parvovirus, mycoplasma, Barmah Forest Virus, Ross River fever virus, *Yersinia*.
- Rheumatological investigations – antinuclear antibodies, rheumatoid factor, HLA-B27 antigen.

Juvenile idiopathic arthritis (JIA)

This spectrum of disorders is outlined in Table 24.1.10.[50] Whilst the course of these disorders can be chronic, the onset of arthritis may be sudden, although the affected child may not be as acutely unwell as seen in septic arthritis. Presentation with pain is variable and patients may present to their

Table 24.1.10   Juvenile idiopathic arthritis (JIA)

- Systemic arthritis: fever 2 weeks plus at least one of rash, enlarged lymph nodes, hepatosplenomegaly, serositis
- Oligoarthritis (<5 joints in first 6 months since onset):
  Persistent oligoarthritis: <5 joints involved after 6 months
  Extended oligoarthritis >4 joints after 6 months
- Polyarthritis: at least 5 joints in first 6 months since onset
  RF negative
  RF positive
- Enthesitis-related arthritis: arthritis and/or enthesitis, plus two of sacroiliac/spine inflammation, or HLA B27, or family history HLA-B27-associated disease in first- or second-degree relative, or anterior uveitis, or boy with arthritis onset over 6 years age
- Psoriatic arthritis: arthritis and psoriasis or two of dactylitis, nail abnormalities (dystrophy or pitting), family history of psoriasis in a first-degree relative
  Undifferentiated arthritis: fits into more than one category, or excluded from any category by exclusion criteria

RF, rheumatoid factor.

primary care services or ED. Associated symptoms may include reduced function (e.g. unwillingness to play) or gait abnormalities. Inflammatory symptoms (e.g. gelling) may be more pronounced after a period of inactivity e.g. early morning stiffness. For appropriate risk management, septic arthritis needs to be excluded. High fevers, refusal to allow examination of the joint, as well as important elevation in inflammatory markers and leucocyte count, may suggest septic arthritis. Multiple joint involvement usually suggests inflammatory arthropathy; however, the most common subtype of JIA is oligoarthritis, with the knee as the most frequent presenting joint.[51]

Presence of systemic features such as persistent fevers (more than 2 weeks), especially with quotidian pattern (regular spikes of temperature at a predictable time), evanescent rash, lymphadenopathy and organomegaly, with or without arthritis, should alert the attending clinician to the possibility of systemic arthritis. Serositis may manifest as pleural or pericardial effusion, requiring urgent treatment as cardiovascular emergency. Abdominal pain may be the result of peritoneal irritation by the intra-abdominal inflammatory fluid, or non-specific vasculitis affecting abdominal viscera.

Arthritis or arthralgia may be minimal or absent in the early stages of disease.[52]

Depending on the duration of fever at the time of ED presentation, and the clinical features present, differential diagnosis for these children may include acute viral or bacterial infection, Kawasaki disease and other vasculitides, malignancy (e.g. neuroblastoma), and other autoimmune disorders such as systemic lupus erythematosus. Investigations must include blood culture, full blood examination and inflammatory markers, viral serology, and coagulation studies. Investigations as appropriate to the clinical findings and differential diagnoses, e.g. chest X-ray, electrocardiogram (ECG), echocardiogram, and abdominal ultrasound may be warranted. Anaemia of chronic disease is usual, with elevated inflammatory markers and thrombocytosis, which may exceed 10^6 per cubic millimetre.[53] Liver enzymes may be elevated, whilst coagulation abnormalities may be present and correlate with disease activity.[54]

In order to optimise the outcomes of children with JIA, contact with a paediatric rheumatologist must be made. NSAIDs may be used to treat the symptoms; however, disease-modifying drugs such as systemic steroids, cytotoxics, and joint procedures may be required.

Macrophage activation syndrome (haemophagocytic lymphohistiocytosis)

This rare disorder may present as a complication of systemic arthritis and include coagulopathy and disseminated intravascular coagulation, encephalopathy, with liver and multiorgan failure.

Laboratory investigations reveal hepatic dysfunction, consumption coagulopathy with hypofibrinogenaemia, lowered haematological indices without classical leukaemic features, and a rapidly falling ESR usually inappropriate to the level of severity of the patient's condition. High-dose steroids, ciclosporin and other cytotoxics, with high-dependency support in an intensive care unit can be life-saving.[55]

Urticaria and serum sickness

The young child presenting with low-grade fever and urticarial rash may also have arthralgia or arthritis. Toddlers and pre-school children may present with dramatic skin signs of urticaria, with migratory wheals with or without target lesions, which are the hallmark of erythema multiforme. Low-grade temperature may be present and there may be significant soft-tissue swelling and arthralgias. Whilst up to 50% of cases may be idiopathic, the most common single trigger identified with this symptom complex in Australia is cephalosporin use.[56] Atypical features such as mucosal lesions, inability to weight-bear, high fevers and 'sick' appearance, haematuria or organomegaly, require more detailed investigations and exclusion of more serious aetiologies. If symptoms are mild, this condition may be managed expectantly with removal of any unnecessary medication and rest. Antihistamines and NSAIDs may be useful for itch and joint pains.

Henoch–Schönlein purpura

This leucocytoclastic vasculitic disorder of uncertain aetiology is among the more frequent diagnoses presenting as joint pain and rash in the paediatric population. Characteristically there are four potentially affected systems:

❶ Skin – extensor surface petechiae and maculopapules in lower limbs and buttocks.
❷ Joints –acral arthritis, but more commonly arthralgia and associated limb swelling.
❸ Kidney – micro-or macroscopic haematuria, with or without proteinuria, may be present or there may be frank nephritis.
❹ Gastrointestinal system – abdominal pain with submucosal vasculitis presenting as intussusception, per rectum bleed or melaena, or peritoneal irritation.

Risk management involves ruling out other causes of petechial illness, including leukaemia, idiopathic thrombocytopenic purpura and partially treated meningococcal illness, and watching for renal complications. Children must be followed-up with urinalysis for 6 months for delayed renal complications.[57]

Rheumatic fever

Rheumatic fever has become rare amongst Caucasians in Australia and New Zealand but still occurs and causes preventable morbidity and mortality in the Aboriginal and Pacific Islander populations of these countries, particularly in northern and central Australia and the Maori and Pacific Islander population of certain regions of New Zealand.[58] The incidence in indigenous children aged between 5 and 14 years in northern Australia is estimated to be 250–350/1000 children.[58] Infected skin lesions from scabies are more often a source of the *Streptococcus* than throat carriage in this group. Because of the disparity of likelihood in different populations, the Australian Heart Foundation recommends different diagnostic criteria in high- and low-risk Australian sub-populations. These revised, bi-level Modified Jones criteria are shown in Table 24.1.11.

Rheumatic fever in indigenous Australian children classically presents with an extremely painful polyarthritis, particularly affecting knees or ankles. Pain out of proportion to clinical effusion is the rule. The arthritis is slowly migratory but affected joints often overlap in time. Treatment with NSAIDs and/or aspirin (to which the joints in rheumatic arthritis are acutely sensitive), reduces the clinically apparent number of joints involved.

Rheumatic fever classically occurs up to a month after a skin infection, whereas other immune-mediated post-streptococcal disorders (reactive arthritis and glomerulonephritis) tend to occur earlier, e.g. 2 weeks post-infection.

Although rheumatic fever and rheumatic heart disease are discussed in more detail in another section (see Chapter 5.6), it is critically important to consider rheumatic fever in any indigenous or Pacific Islander child presenting with acute arthralgias and fever, in view of the serious sequelae and preventable nature of this disease.

Table 24.1.11 Diagnosing acute rheumatic fever in Australia[60]

	High-Risk Groups*	All Other Groups
Initial episode of ARF	2 major or 1 major and 2 minor manifestations plus evidence of a preceding GAS infection[†]	
Recurrent attack of ARF in a patient with known past ARF or RHD	2 major or 1 major and 2 minor or 3 minor manifestations plus evidence of a preceding GAS infection[†]	
Major manifestations	Carditis (including subclinical evidence of rheumatic valve disease on echocardiogram) Polyarthritis or aseptic monoarthritis or polyarthralgia[‡] Chorea[¥] Erythema marginatum[§] Subcutaneous nodules	Carditis (excluding subclinical evidence of rheumatic valve disease on echocardiogram) Polyarthritis[‡] Chorea[¥] Erythema marginatum[§] Subcutaneous nodules
Minor manifestations	Fever[ʜ] ESR ≥30mm/hr or CRP ≥30mg/L Prolonged P-R interval on ECG[Θ]	Fever[ʜ] Polyarthralgia or aseptic mono-arthritis[‡] ESR ≥30mm/hr or CRP ≥30mg/L Prolonged P-R interval on ECG[Θ]

All categories assume that other more likely diagnoses have been excluded.
Please see text for details about specific manifestations.
CRP, C-reactive protein; ECG, electrocardiogram; ESR, erythrocyte sedimentation rate; GAS, group A streptococcus.
*High-risk groups are those living in communities with high rates of ARF (incidence >30 per 100 000 per year in 5–14-year-olds) or RHD (all-age prevalence >2 per 1000). Aboriginal and Torres Strait Islander Australians living in rural or remote settings are known to be at high risk. Data are not available for other populations, but Aboriginal and Torres Strait Islander Australians living in urban settings, Maori and Pacific Islander people, and potentially immigrants from developing countries may also be at high risk.
[†]Elevated or rising anti-streptolysin O or other streptococcal antibody, or a positive throat culture or rapid antigen test for GAS.
[‡]A definite history of arthritis is sufficient to satisfy this manifestation. Other causes of arthritis/arthralgia should be carefully excluded, particularly in the case of monoarthritis (e.g. septic arthritis, including disseminated gonococcal infection), infective or reactive arthritis (e.g. Ross River virus, Barmah Forest virus, influenza, rubella, *Mycoplasma*, cytomegalovirus, Epstein–Barr virus, parvovirus, hepatitis and *Yersinia*), and auto-immune arthropathy (e.g. juvenile chronic arthritis, inflammatory bowel disease, systemic lupus erythematosus, systemic vasculitis, sarcoidosis). Note that if polyarthritis is present as a major manifestation, polyarthralgia or aseptic monoarthritis cannot be considered an additional minor manifestation in the same person.
[¥]Rheumatic (Sydenham's) chorea does not require other manifestations or evidence of preceding GAS infection, provided other causes of chorea are excluded.
[§]Erythema marginatum is a distinctive rash (see text). Care should be taken not to label other rashes, particularly non-specific viral exanthemas, as erythema marginatum.
[ʜ]Oral, tympanic or rectal temperature ≥38°C on admission or documented during the current illness.
[Θ]Note that, if carditis is present as a major manifestation, prolonged P-R interval cannot be considered an additional minor manifestation in the same person.

Post-streptococcal and other post-infective immune-mediated reactive arthritides

Post-streptococcal and other post-infective reactive arthritides (as distinct from the rheumatic fever complex) need to be considered in the differential diagnosis of any young child presenting with rash and joint swelling. These conditions may occur after viral or bacterial infections, alone or in immunogenic combination with antibiotics. These conditions have generally a favourable joint outcome, although occasionally other system manifestations may be observed.

Children may also have other clinical manifestations, including cutaneous vasculitis (e.g. erythema nodosum) or uveitis. The reactive arthritis pattern of post-streptococcal arthritis is more fixed than the migratory arthritis of classical rheumatic fever; tenosynovitis is often present; and there are no cardiac manifestations. Post-streptococcal arthritis also lacks the characteristic aspirin sensitivity of rheumatic fever.[59] However, the association mandates investigation of these children with FBC, ASOT and anti-DNAse, ECG, and referral for follow up by a paediatrician or rheumatologist. Other organisms implicated in immune-mediated arthritis include EBV, CMV, parvovirus, mycoplasma, and various gastrointestinal pathogens.[60]

The triad of urethritis, arthritis, and conjunctivitis associated with *Chlamydia* infection may present as Reiter's syndrome in the sexually active adolescent, whilst other arthritogenic bacteria (e.g. *Salmonella* or *Shigella*) may cause arthritis associated with gastroenteritis. In each case, attempt must be made to identify the causative organism and, if indicated, antimicrobial treatment implemented.

Neoplastic presentations

Bone or joint pain may be among the presenting symptoms in children with leukaemia, neuroblastoma and other bone marrow-related malignancies. Features characteristic of these children by comparison with other causes of limp or joint pain are shown in Table 24.1.12. This pain is generally more severe and unremitting, and the debility more extreme, than in children with juvenile idiopathic arthritis. Blood films must always be carefully analysed for the three cell lines (red cells, white cells and platelets). Minor degrees of anaemia, leucopenia, or thrombocytopenia are common early features: these must be flagged and followed closely.[61,62] ESR is traditionally elevated out of proportion to the degree of 'arthritic' manifestations.[55]

Plain radiography has been suggested as first-line radiological investigation to differentiate between acute lymphocytic leukaemia (ALL) and JIA, to aid establishment of a correct diagnosis in the child with persistent bone or joint pain.[63] Soft tissue swelling and osteopenia were characteristics of JIA cases, whilst radiolucent metaphyseal bands and coarse trabeculation were almost exclusive to ALL patients.

Malignancies presenting in this fashion include leukaemia and neuroblastoma.[61,62,64]

Table 24.1.12 Features suggestive of malignancy in infants/children presenting with bone/joint pain or limp
Non-weight-bearing or refusal to walk
Night time pain, waking from sleep
Non-articular bone pain or tenderness
Back pain
Abnormal bone swelling
Systemic illness (fever, rash, weight loss, anorexia, night sweats)
Bruising
Abdominal mass or organomegaly
Abnormal neurology
Low Hb, WCC, or platelet count
High ESR or CRP (out of proportion to joint findings)

Bone tumours

Osteosarcoma and osteogenic sarcoma are uncommon but serious causes of recent-onset limb pain or limp in the paediatric population. Characteristic features include:

- osteosarcoma – bone destruction and infiltration;
- osteogenic sarcoma (Ewing's tumour) – periosteal new bone formation, 'sunray' and 'onion-skin' appearance.

Differential diagnosis includes neuroblastoma and osteomyelitis. These children should be referred for urgent orthopaedic review and investigation.

Osteoid osteoma is an occasional cause of leg pain, particularly nocturnal. X-rays show an area of periosteal thickening and new bone formation around a central radiolucency.

Simple and aneurysmal bone cysts may also be seen, either as incidental findings or in the setting of pathological fracture. All of these can be referred to the orthopaedic unit for further evaluation.

Tip

Beware the child who is carried into the examination room.

OTHER IMPORTANT SUBACUTE PAEDIATRIC MUSCULOSKELETAL PRESENTATIONS

Apophysisitis: Osgood–Schlatter and Sever's diseases

These disorders are the result of chronic micro-avulsion injury at the apophyseal insertion sites of the major leg-muscle groups. Commonest sites are the tibial tuberosity (quadriceps via patellar tendon: Osgood–Schlatter disease) and the calcaneal apophysis (calf muscle via Achilles tendon: Sever's disease). In Osgood–Schlatter disease, the child or adolescent typically presents during the growth spurt with a story of pain getting up from sitting or going up stairs, and has tenderness localised to the tibial tuberosity and some localised swelling, with an otherwise normal joint examination. In Sever's disease there is pain on walking or running, and heel tenderness. X-ray may show fragmentation of the

apophysis and soft-tissue swelling. However, this is primarily a clinical diagnosis (and fragmentation may be a normal radiological variant in developing apophyses). Treatment includes rest, non-steroidal anti-inflammatory medication, and rheumatology or orthopaedic referral for persistent disability.

Torticollis

The infant presenting with torticollis, without specific trauma or abnormal neurology, is most likely to have congenital muscular torticollis ('sternomastoid tumour'). Theories of pathogenesis include in-utero crowding and compartment syndrome. Characteristic features include:

- onset from birth, often brought to parents' attention by new observer;
- 'cock-robin' appearance (head tilt on involved side with contralateral chin rotation) with range of motion limited by the affected sternomastoid tightness;
- normal neurology, behaviour, and occipitofrontal circumference;
- firm painless swelling or tightness palpable within the sternomastoid muscle opposite the chin;
- mild facial hemihypertrophy due to increased relative blood flow to the dependent side.

Hips should always be checked, as a significant proportion may have developmental dysplasia.[65] Infants with this characteristic constellation of features should be referred for physiotherapy and follow up.

Other causes of torticollis in the paediatric period include vertebral anomalies such as Klippel–Feil syndrome and neurological disorders including brain and spinal-cord tumours and ocular dysfunction. Wide based gait and frequent falls may be accompanied by cervical spine tumours. Children with JIA may present with abnormalities in head and neck posture caused by cervical spine arthritis as their initial presentation, although symmetrical reduced range of motion is the more common finding.

Causes of acute torticollis in children with previously normal neck posture and motion include atlantoaxial rotary subluxation (see Chapter 24.2), a reaction to other acute head or neck pathologies, such as lymphadenopathy or retropharyngeal abscess, and short-term muscle spasm in association with respiratory-tract disorders or minor trauma.

Features suggestive of significant underlying pathology and need for radiological and specialist referral include:

- other congenital or orthopaedic anomaly;
- abnormality of neurological or ophthalmological assessment;
- symptoms suggestive of intracranial pathology, e.g. headache, vomiting, irritability;
- atypical musculoskeletal examination, e.g. limited range of motion, visual disorder, or persistent or fixed torticollis.

Vertebrospinal inflammation

While uncommon, vertebrospinal inflammatory and infectious problems are characterised by delay in diagnosis and diagnostic confusion.[66] These children may present with back or abdominal pain, or with altered gait or neurological dysfunction. In discitis and vertebral osteomyelitis there will be point tenderness over a spinous process, particularly to percussion, and localised scoliosis or muscle spasm. Fever and constitutional symptoms are variable. Inflammatory markers are characteristically elevated. X-ray may show muscle spasm or soft-tissue oedema, or an abnormal intervertebral disc space. Bone scans are helpful to localise an abnormality where examination findings are equivocal. Definitive diagnosis and evaluation are best made by MRI. Treatment with bed-rest and intravenous antibiotics is usual, although isolated discitis may respond better to steroid treatment.

Conclusion

Musculoskeletal presentations of children and adolescents to emergency rooms have a wide range from acute illnesses requiring immediate treatment to the more indolent conditions with longer time since symptom onset. Such presentations are age dependent and their urgency may also be related to patient characteristics and their respective environment. Eliciting accurate medical history as well as a detailed medical examination are essential requirements before investigations and ultimately a rational management plan can be improvised. Early communication with relevant specialties will aid the efficient delivery of the above healthcare path.

Acknowledgement

The contribution of Trevor Jackson as author in the first edition is hereby acknowledged.

References

1. Top 10 Paediatric Emergency Department EDIS Discharge Diagnoses. Brisbane, Australia: Mater Children's Hospital South Brisbane; 1999.
2. Woods D, Macnicol M. The flexion-adduction test: an early sign of hip disease. J Pediatr Orthop B 2001 07;10 (3):180–5.
3. Kallio M, Unkila-Kallio L. Serum CRP, ESR and WCC in septic arthritis of children. Pediatr Infect Dis J 1997;16(4):411–3.
4. Jagodzinski NAM, Kanwar RM, Graham KMDFF, Bache CEF. Prospective evaluation of a shortened regimen of treatment for acute osteomyelitis and septic arthritis in children. J Pediatr Orthop 2009;29 (5):518–25.
5. Ng T. ESR, plasma viscosity and CRP in clinical practice. Br J Hosp Med 1997;58(10):521–3.
6. Kothari NA, Pelchovitz DJ, Meyer JS. Imaging of musculoskeletal infections. Radiol Clin North Am 2001 07;39(4):653–71.
7. Kallio P, Lequesne G, Paterson D, et al. Ultrasonography in slipped capital femoral epiphysis. Diagnosis and assessment of severity. J Bone Joint Surg 1991;73 (6):884–9.
8. Skinner J, Glancy S, Beattie T, Hendry G. Transient synovitis: Is there a need to aspirate hip joint effusions? Eur J Emerg Med 2002;9(1):15–8.
9. Jaramillo D, Treves S, Kasser J. Osteomyelitis and septic arthritis in children: Appropriate use of imaging to guide treatment. Aust J Rheumatol 1995;165: 399–403.
10. Fink A, Bermann L, Edwards D, Jacobson S. The irritable hip: Immediate ultrasound guided aspiration and prevention of hospital admission. Arch Dis Child 1995;72 (2):110–3.
11. Beach R. Minimally invasive approach to management of irritable hip in children. Lancet 2000;355:1202–3.
12. White P, Boyd J, Beattie T, et al. Magnetic resonance imaging as the primary imaging modality in children presenting with acute non-traumatic hip pain. Emerg Med J 2001;18(1):25–9.
13. McPhee EMD, Eskander JPAB, Eskander MSMD, et al. Imaging in pelvic osteomyelitis: support for early magnetic resonance imaging. J Pediatr Orthopaed 2007;27(8):903–9.
14. Kocher MS, Zurakowski D, Kasser JR. Differentiating between septic arthritis and transient synovitis of the hip in children: an evidence-based clinical prediction algorithm. J Bone Joint Surg Am 1999 12;81 (12):1662–70.
15. Luhmann SJ, Jones A, Schootman M, et al. Differentiation between septic arthritis and transient synovitis of the hip in children with clinical prediction algorithms. J Bone Joint Surg Am 2004 05;86-A(5):956–62.
16. Kocher MS, Mandiga R, Zurakowski D, et al. Validation of a clinical prediction rule for the differentiation between septic arthritis and transient synovitis of the hip in children. J Bone Joint Surg Am 2004 08;86-A (8):1629–35.
17. Mattick A, Turner A, Ferguson J, et al. Seven year follow up of children presenting to the accident and emergency department with irritable hip. J Acc Emerg Med 1999 09;16(5):345–7.
18. Kermond S, Fink M, Graham K, et al. A randomized clinical trial: should the child with transient synovitis of the hip be treated with nonsteroidal anti-inflammatory drugs? Ann Emerg Med 2002 09;40(3):294–9.
19. Taylor GR, Clarke NM. Recurrent irritable hip in childhood. J Bone Joint Surg Br 1995 09;77(5): 748–51.
20. Keenan WN, Clegg J. Perthes' disease after 'irritable hip': delayed bone age shows the hip is a 'marked man'. J Pediatr Orthop 1996 01;16(1):20–3.
21. Goldenberg D. Bacterial arthritis. In: Kelley W, Harris E, Ruddy S, Sledge C, editors. Textbook of rheumatology. 4th ed. Philadelphia, PA: WB Saunders; 1993. p. 1449–66.
22. Trobs R, Moritz R, Huppertz H. Changing pattern of osteomyelitis in infants and children. Leipzig Paediatr Surg Int 1999;15:363–72.
23. Duffy CM, Lam PY, Ditchfield M, et al. Chronic recurrent multifocal osteomyelitis: review of orthopaedic complications at maturity. 07J Pediatr Orthop 2002;22 (4):501–5.
24. Girschick HJ, Raab P, Surbaum S, et al. Chronic non-bacterial osteomyelitis in children. Ann Rheum Dis 2005 02;64(2):279–85.
25. Huber AM, Lam P-Y, Duffy CM, et al. Chronic recurrent multifocal osteomyelitis: clinical outcomes after more than five years of follow-up. J Pediatr 2002 08;141 (2):198–203.
26. Simm P, Allen R, Zacharin M. Bisphosphonate treatment in chronic recurrent multifocal osteomyelitis. J Pediatr Apr;:571-5 Epub 2007 Nov 5. 2008;152 (4):571–5.
27. Gleeson H, Wiltshire E, Briody J, et al. Childhood chronic recurrent multifocal osteomyelitis: pamidronate therapy decreases pain and improves vertebral shape. J Rheumatol 2008;35(4):707–12.
28. Graham H. Acute septic arthritis of the hip in children in northern Australia [commentary]. Aust N Z J Surg 2003;73:91.
29. Appleton S, Nourse C. Mater Health Service Brisbane: Septic arthritis: cell counts and cultures 2007-2009.
30. Moumile K, Merckx J, Glorion C, et al. Bacterial aetiology of acute osteoarticular infections in children. Acta Paediatr 2005 04;94(4):419–22.
31. Tilse M. Organisms cultured in paediatric septic arthritis 1998-2007. Unpublished data: South Brisbane, Australia: Mater Children's Hospital; 2007.
32. Ilharreborde B, Bidet P, Lorrot M, et al. New real-time PCR-based method for Kingella kingae DNA detection: application to samples collected from 89 children with acute arthritis. J Clin Microbiol 2009; 06/15/;47 (6):1837–41.
33. Arnold SR, Elias D, Buckingham SC, et al. Changing patterns of acute hematogenous osteomyelitis and septic arthritis: emergence of community-associated methicillin-resistant Staphylococcus aureus. J Pediatr Orthop 2006;26(6):703–8.
34. Saavedra-Lozano JM, Mejias A, Ahmad N, et al. Changing trends in acute osteomyelitis in children: impact of methicillin-resistant Staphylococcus aureus infections. J Pediatr Orthop 2008;28(5):569–75.
35. Report WHO. Global tuberculosis control: surveillance, planning, finance 2003. Geneva: World Health Organization; 2003.
36. Teo HEL, Peh WCG. Skeletal tuberculosis in children. Pediatr Radiol 2004 11/24/;34(11):853–60.
37. Turnidge J, Bell J. Methicillin-resistant Staphylococcus aureus evolution in Australia over 35 years. Microb Drug Resist 2000;6(3):223–9.
38. Lo W-T, Lin W-J, Tseng M-H, et al. Risk factors and molecular analysis of panton-valentine leukocidin-positive methicillin-resistant Staphylococcus aureus colonization in healthy children. Pediatr Infect Dis J 2008 08;27(8):713–8.
39. Aroojis AJ, Johari AN. Epiphyseal separations after neonatal osteomyelitis and septic arthritis. J Pediatr Orthop 2000;20(4):544–9.
40. Rasmont Q, Yombi J-C, Van der Linden D, Docquier P-L. Osteoarticular infections in Belgian children: a survey of clinical, biological, radiological and microbiological data. Acta Orthop Belg 2008 06;74(3):374–85.
41. Kealey W, Moore A, Cook S, Cosgrove A. Deprivation, urbanisation and Perthes' disease in Northern Ireland. J Bone Joint Surg 2000;82(2):167–71.

42. Vila-Verde V, da Silva K. Bone-age delay in Perthes disease and transient synovitis of the hip. *Clin Orthop Relat Res* 2001;**385**:118–23.

43. Mata S, Aicua E, Ovejero A, Grande M. Legg–Calve–Perthes disease and passive smoking. *J Pediatr Orthop* 2000;**20**(3):326–30.

44. Morrissey R, Weinstein S. *Lovell and Winter's paediatric orthopaedics.* 5th ed. Philadelphia: Lippincott Williams & Wilkins; 2001.

45. Dillman JR, Hernandez RJ. MRI of Legg–Calve–Perthes disease. *AJR Am J Roentgenol* 2009;**193**(5):1394–407 Review.

46. Gent E, Antapur P, Fairhurst J, et al. Perthes' disease in the very young child. *J Pediatr Orthop B* 2006;**15**(1):16–22.

47. Comte F, De Rosa V, Zekri H, et al. Confirmation of the early prognostic value of bone scanning and pinhole imaging of the hip in Legg-Calvé-Perthes disease. *J Nucl Med* 2003;**44**(11):1761–6.

48. Lamer S, Dorgeret S, Khairouni A, et al. Femoral head vascularisation in Legg–Calvé–Perthes disease: comparison of dynamic gadolinium-enhanced subtraction MRI with bone scintigraphy. *Pediatr Radiol* 2002;**32**(8):580–6 Epub 2002 Jun 14.

49. Ankarath S, Ng A, Giannoudis P, Scott B. Delay in diagnosis of slipped upper femoral epiphysis. *J Roy Soc Med* 2002;**95**(7):356–8.

50. Petty R, Southwood T, Manners P, et al. International League of Associations for Rheumatology classification of juvenile idiopathic arthritis: second revision. *J Rheumatol* 2004;**31**(2):390–2.

51. Cassidy J, Petty R. *Textbook of pediatric rheumatology.* 4th ed. Philadelphia; London: W.B. Saunders; 2001.

52. Wright D. Juvenile idiopathic arthritis. In: Morrissey R, Weinstein S, editors. *Lovell and Winter's paediatric orthopedics.* 5th ed. Philadelphia: Lippincott Williams & Wilkins; 2001. p. 427–57.

53. Schneider R, Laxer R. Systemic onset juvenile rheumatoid arthritis. *Baillières Clin Rheumatol* 1998;**12**:245.

54. Bloom B, Tucker L, Miller L. Fibrin D dimer as a marker of disease activity in systemic onset juvenile rheumatoid arthritis. *J Rheumatol* 1998;**25**:1620.

55. Stephan JL, Zeller J, Hubert P, et al. Macrophage activation syndrome and rheumatic disease in childhood: a report of four new cases. *Clin Exp Rheumatol* 1993 07;**11**(4):451–6.

56. Isaacs D. Serum sickness-like reaction to cefaclor. *J Paediatr Child Health* 2001;**37**(3):298–9.

57. Narchi H. Risk of long term renal impairment and duration of follow up recommended for Henoch–Schönlein purpura with normal or minimal urinary findings: a systematic review. *Arch Dis Child* 2005;**90**(9):916–20.

58. *Rheumatic Heart Disease.* Canberra: Australian Institute of Health and Welfare; August, 2004. Contract No.: Issue 6.

59. Carapetis JR, McDonald M, Wilson NJ. Acute rheumatic fever. *Lancet* 2005;**366**:155–68.

60. Diagnosis and management of acute rheumatic fever and rheumatic heart disease in Australia–an evidence-based review: National Heart Foundation of Australia (RF/RHD guideline development working group) and the Cardiac Society of Australia and New Zealand 2006.

61. Gupta D, Singh S, Suri D, et al. Arthritic presentation of acute leukemia in children: experience from a tertiary care centre in North India. *Rheumatol Int* [serial on the Internet] 2009.

62. Jones O, Spencer C, Bowyer S, et al. A multicenter case-control study on predictive factors distinguishing childhood leukemia from juvenile rheumatoid arthritis. *Pediatrics* 2006;**117**(5):e840–4.

63. Tafaghodi F, Aghighi Y, Rokni Yazdi H, et al. Predictive plain X-ray findings in distinguishing early stage acute lymphoblastic leukemia from juvenile idiopathic arthritis. *Clin Rheumatol* [serial on the Internet]. 2009;**28**(11).

64. Mohan A, Gossain SR. Neuroblastoma: a differential diagnosis of irritable hip. *Acta Orthop Belg* 2006 10;**72**(5):651–2.

65. Cheng J, Au A. Infantile torticollis: A review of 624 cases. *J Paediatr Orthop* 1994;**14**:802–8.

66. Fernandez M, Carrol C, Baker C. Discitis and vertebral osteomyelitis in children: An 18-year review. *Paediatrics* 2000;**105**(6):1299–304.

24.2 Fractures and dislocations

Robyn Brady • John Walsh

ESSENTIALS

1 Fractures are common in childhood, due to high-level motor activity, developing co-ordination, and the mechanical properties of the growing skeleton. However, compared to adult mechanisms, the majority are relatively low-force injuries.

2 The patterns of bony disruption are completely different from adult fracture patterns and include buckle and greenstick fractures and growth-plate injuries. Bony disruption/deformity is more common than ligamentous disruption: 'sprains' and ruptures are uncommon.

3 Displaced fractures are a common and highly traumatic event for children and rapid attention to physical and psychological distress can minimise the effects of this trauma.

4 Certain missed fractures have a high propensity for serious long-term functional morbidity and must be actively sought. These include elbow injuries, such as lateral condylar and Monteggia-type fractures.

Fracture patterns in childhood

In the previous chapter the impact of development (behavioural and physiological) on musculoskeletal pathology was broadly outlined (see Table 24.1.1). With respect to injury, this means different points of cleavage or deformation from a given injury mechanism, and an extra anatomical structure (the physis) to consider when analysing the effects of trauma and the future outcome of a given disruption.

Fig. 24.2.1 shows the frequency of common fractures presenting to a children's emergency department (ED). Within different age subgroups, the distribution varies thus:

- infants/toddlers – higher proportions of femur and skull fractures;
- primary school – higher proportion of elbow-region fractures, especially supracondylar;
- adolescents – complex ankle fractures; higher force sporting injuries; transition to adult pattern with increasing ligamentous injuries, e.g. elbow dislocations.

The majority of ED paediatric fracture presentations occur at the distal radius and ulna. This is one of the top ten ED diagnoses for children in Australia. Many displaced forearm fractures can be reduced under sedation by emergency staff with appropriate training and follow up, making this a most valuable area of expertise.

Paediatric limb fractures, depending on the angle of force to which they have been subjected, can occur to shaft, metaphysis, or physeal region. The different quality of developing bone means that even injuries to shaft and metaphysis tend to have

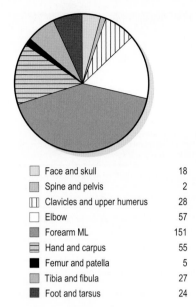

Face and skull	18
Spine and pelvis	2
Clavicles and upper humerus	28
Elbow	57
Forearm ML	151
Hand and carpus	55
Femur and patella	5
Tibia and fibula	27
Foot and tarsus	24

Fig. 24.2.1 Frequency of fracture types at Brisbane Mater Children's Hospital ED.

different patterns of deformation, including 'torus' or buckle injuries, bowing, and greenstick fractures. The importance of this awareness for the emergency physician is best illustrated by the Monteggia equivalent injury in which 'shortening' from proximal radial dislocation is 'matched' by ulnar bowing. The resultant injury has no radiologically obvious 'fracture' in the traditional sense but has serious consequences if not recognised and reduced (Fig. 24.2.2).

The Salter–Harris classification (Fig. 24.2.3) remains the most useful way of describing the pattern of cleavage with respect to the physis. In reality, types 1 and 5 represent mechanical force patterns (separation and compression) rather than a radiological pattern as, unless there is lateral translation or adjacent bony or soft-tissue deformation, the physis may appear radiologically normal in these injuries. An example of Salter–Harris type 1 injuries with lateral shift is the so-called 'slipped distal radial epiphysis' (Fig. 24.2.4). The disorder of slipped upper femoral epiphysis (SUFE) has been discussed in Chapter 24.1 as, although minor trauma may precipitate an acute slippage, the cleavage is due to an abnormal physeal predisposition and should not be looked upon as truly traumatic.

Salter–Harris type 2 injuries are the most common physeal injury pattern seen, the metaphyseal corner (the 'Thurston-Holland' fragment) ranging in size from a barely

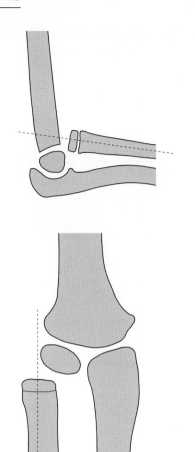

Fig. 24.2.2 Monteggia fracture-dislocation. Demonstration of the abnormal radio-capitellar relationship (see Fig. 24.2.8 for contrast). Drawing by Terry McGuire.

visible fragment to an extensive triangle. Injuries through the epiphysis itself, Salter–Harris types 3 and 4, are more worrying in their prognosis because they are intra-articular as well as involving the physis. The classic example of a Salter–Harris type 3 injury is the Tillaux fracture (Fig. 24.2.5), while lateral condylar fractures at the elbow are Salter–Harris 4 in type.

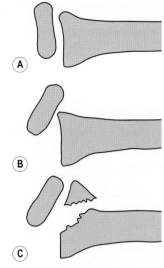

Fig. 24.2.4 Common distal radial epiphyseal fractures. (A) Partial slipped distal radial epiphysis (Salter–Harris 1) with 10% translation; (B) slipped distal radial epiphysis (Salter–Harris 1) with 50% translation and probable intact dorsal periosteal sleeve; (C) Salter–Harris 2 fracture of distal radius with metaphyseal fragment angulated to 45 degrees and 50% translation of epiphyseal plate. Drawing by Terry McGuire.

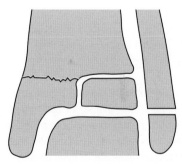

Fig. 24.2.5 Tillaux fracture (Salter–Harris 3). Early fusion of the medial distal tibial physis and relative superior strength of the distal tibiofibular ligament cause shearing force to separate the central physeal region and travel along the lateral distal tibial physis. Sometimes a metaphyseal fragment is also cleaved (Salter–Harris 4).

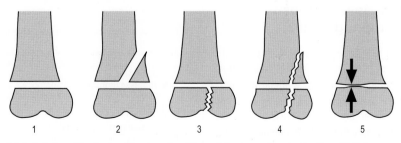

Fig. 24.2.3 Salter–Harris classification of epiphyseal fractures. Drawing by Terry McGuire.

Table 24.2.1 Examples of paediatric vs. adult outcomes of common fall mechanisms (different paediatric injuries occur at different ages depending on planes of weakness). The ligaments in children provide greater resistance to shear injury than the growing bone, so avulsion type injuries occur in place of ligamentous tears or dislocations.

Mechanism	Adult injury	Paediatric injury
Fall onto point of shoulder	AC separation	Lateral clavicular fracture
Shoulder extension/compression	Shoulder dislocation	Proximal humeral fracture
Fall on hand, elbow hyperextension	Elbow dislocation	Supracondylar/condylar fractures
Wrist hyperextension/compression	Scaphoid fracture	Distal forearm fracture
Fall onto hand	Colles' fracture	Midshaft, metaphyseal, or epiphyseal fracture
Thumb abduction 1	Bennet's fracture	Metaphyseal fracture base first metacarpal
Thumb abduction 2	Gamekeeper's thumb (UCL)	UCL avulsion fracture (Salter–Harris type 3 proximal phalanx thumb)
Rotation of knee on lower leg	ACL, cartilage tear	Tibial spine fracture
Valgus/varus knee stress	Ligament, cartilage tear	Distal femoral physeal separation
Forceful jump (quadriceps)	Ligament tear	Patellar tendon avulsion fracture (Tibial tubercle) fracture
Forceful jump (calf)	Achilles tendon tear	Calcaneal avulsion fracture
Rotation of tibia on calcaneus	Ankle sprains, Pott's fractures	Tibial spiral fracture, Tillaux fracture, triplane fracture
Inversion ankle	Talofibular ligament tear	Salter–Harris type 1 or 2 distal fibula

Table 24.2.1 shows some examples of the corresponding injury occurring in adults and children for a given mechanism. This table illustrates the maxim that children tend to fracture rather than 'sprain', as the physis is the weakest point of the musculoskeletal continuum, i.e. a ligament will avulse its bony origin or insertion rather than tearing. In some cases, this is to the child's advantage, as the cellular architects of bone development which contribute to its mechanical weakness contribute to rapid healing and extensive remodelling. A midshaft femoral fracture, for example, will heal in 2–3 weeks in an infant, whereas the same disruption will take 12 weeks to union in a teenager.

Initial assessment and management

The initial assessment of the paediatric isolated limb injury (fracture/dislocation) is shown in Table 24.2.2 and the neurovascular assessment in Table 24.2.3. Limb injury must always be considered in the broader context of trauma. Primary and secondary survey, however brief and targeted, should always be carried out bearing in mind the described injury mechanism and the child's complaints of pain, so that any associated injuries, e.g. to head, abdomen, or spine, may be recognised and evaluated early. An efficient early assessment should be able to establish mechanism, possible other sites of injury, probable fracture type, presence or absence of compound features or neurovascular impairment, and organise pain relief, fasting, radiology, splintage, and antibiotics if required, within a brief period.

Fracture descriptions to the orthopaedic team should start with the child's age, mechanism, and clinical findings, and proceed to the part of bone, type of fracture, and extent of angulation and/or displacement and

Table 24.2.2 Initial assessment and management of traumatic limb deformity

1. **Rapport:** establish rapport and explain procedures
2. **Mechanism and associated dangers:** rapidly ascertain mechanism and ensure primary survey stability and allergy potential
3. **Pain management:** where there is a greater than 90% likelihood of initial IV success, insert a small IV cannula into the opposite hand and titrate morphine 0.05 mg kg^{-1} until pain relieved (appropriate monitoring should be in place). When no parent is present the risks of medication must be weighed against the potential benefit and attempts made to contact someone familiar with serious allergies or other medical problems. Other means of rapid pain relief include inhaled Penthrane or NO$_2$, and or intranasal fentanyl
4. **Assess for site of anatomical disruption:** look at and gently palpate the injured limb to estimate probable anatomical site of disruption, e.g. lateral elbow, mid-shaft forearm, etc. (comparison with other limb is often helpful)
5. **Check for associated neurovascular dysfunction:** (see Table 24.2.3), document and notify deficits immediately
6. **Check for any evidence of an open wound:** if this is present, cover with a sterile dressing and commence appropriate antibiotics IV, e.g. cefalothin 50 mg kg^{-1} and notify orthopaedic team immediately
7. **Immobilise limb:** provide appropriate splintage (e.g. we use a POP slab for distal fractures, leaving radial artery palpable, and a fibreglass slab for elbow injuries, less radiological artefact-mouldable, re-usable, radiolucent slabs)
8. **Keep stomach empty:** identify time of last ingestion and inform patient and parent about fasting
9. **Organise appropriate radiology**
10. **Discuss clinical and radiological findings with orthopaedic team**

Table 24.2.3 Presence/absence of associated neurovascular injury

- Radial a:
  Pulse, cf. other side
  Hand perfusion/capillary refill, cf. other side
- Brachial a:
  Beware spasm or intimal shear in supracondylar injuries
- Radial n:
  Sensation dorsum hand, *action = dorsiflex wrist, extend fingers* (displaced humeral shaft injury)
- Median n:
  Sensation thenar eminence, *action = opposition, flexion IP thumb* (supracondylar # or elbow dislocation)
- Ulnar n:
  Sensation hypothenar eminence, *action = abduction, adduction fingers* (elbow dislocation, supracondylar #)
- Posterior interosseous n:
  Branch of radial n, *action = finger extension*, e.g. (Monteggia #/dislocation)

Table 24.2.4 Features suggestive of possible non-accidental injury

Fractures

- Proximal humeral or humeral shaft fractures under 3 years
- Fractures with a shearing or distracting mechanism
- Corner or 'bucket-handle' metaphyseal injuries
- Femoral fractures in infants
- Rib fractures
- Complex skull fractures
- Multiple fractures, especially different ages

Presentation features

- Delayed presentation
- Different care-giver
- Unwitnessed injury
- Recurrent fractures
- Unexplained soft-tissue markings
- Unexplained tension/anxiety

Assessment

- Draw diagram of injury history as described by witness
- Examine child all over and plot weight
- Ascertain any previous history of burns or fractures
- Is the developmental level compatible with the explanation?
- Is the history adequate to explain the injury?

Rule of thumb

- Infants within view, toddlers within earshot, unless asleep, i.e. injuries to pre-school children are usually seen or heard

Refer

- All fractures in children under 12 months, and all fractures in children under 4 years in which there is an inadequate or questionable mechanism, should be discussed with a child-protection specialist. In the interim, supportive and non-judgemental care for child and care-giver must be maintained

associated findings. Clinical findings must always be kept paramount. Skin breach must be actively sought and described, then photographed and covered with a sterile dressing. Prominently placed photographic displays of common paediatric fractures within the emergency department may aid accurate description.

Doctors share in the community responsibility for child safety. Within the ED setting this means getting a clear description of the setting and mechanism of injury, particularly with injuries to pre-verbal children. These data are important:

- to more clearly anticipate associated injuries (e.g. foreign bodies or distant possibility of abusive injury);
- to gather cumulative injury prevention data to support legislative change (e.g. road access); and
- to flag possible abusive injury, which is thought to have occurred in 1–2% of paediatric injury presentations, particularly in very young children.[1]

In general, fractures in pre-verbal children without a clear, developmentally appropriate mechanism/history or with other concerning features, will need further assessment. Features suggestive of non-accidental injury are shown in Table 24.2.4, and child abuse is discussed in more detail in Chapter 18.2. As a minimum, all fractures occurring in children under 12 months should be discussed with a paediatrician or child-protection specialist.

The following sections describe the mechanism, recognition, and ED treatment of individual fractures.

Upper limb and shoulder girdle injuries

Midshaft clavicular fractures

These may occur at any age from a fall onto the shoulder or outstretched hand, are usually greenstick in nature and heal well in a sling or figure-of-eight bandaging. A fall onto the point of the shoulder, such as would cause an acromioclavicular disruption in an adult, may cause a *lateral clavicular physeal fracture-separation.* If these are posteriorly displaced, operative treatment may be required. Treatment is by sling or shoulder immobilisation followed by graduated exercises.

The *neonatal shoulder* may come to medical attention due to asymmetrical arm movement or swelling. Causes include birth injury with clavicular fracture or brachial plexus injury, proximal humeral physeal separation, and joint or bone infection. Senior orthopaedic involvement is essential for the diagnosis, and non-accidental injury

must be considered. The prognosis for neonatal clavicular injuries is excellent.

Shoulder dislocation

This is uncommon under 10. The adolescent anterior dislocation can be reduced by traction in the prone position or by gentle arm traction to a seated child against counter-traction with a sheeted thorax.

Proximal humerus

These fractures vary from minor buckling at the proximal metaphysis, to proximal humeral epiphyseal Salter–Harris type 2 fracture-separations (Fig. 24.2.6). Because of the universal motion at the glenohumeral joint and the remodelling potential of children, a remarkable range of initial traumatic deformity is acceptable in children prior to physeal closure (age 14–16), including complete displacement and up to 60 degrees of angulation.[2] A collar and cuff is the usual treatment.

Midshaft humeral fractures

These are less common and sometimes the result of blunt or non-accidental trauma. Check and document radial nerve function, and immobilise with a U-slab.

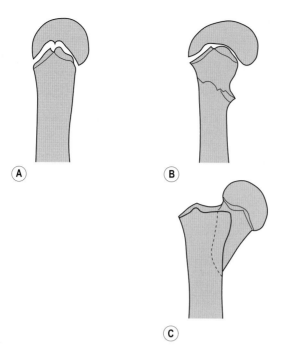

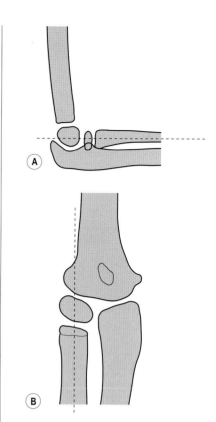

Fig. 24.2.6 Proximal humeral fractures. (A) Normal undulating physeal line (not a fracture); (B) greenstick metaphyseal fracture; (C) severely angulated and displaced Salter–Harris 2 fracture at the proximal humeral epiphysis. Due to the universal motion of the shoulder joint, this fracture will still unite and remodel completely with conservative treatment. Drawing by Terry McGuire.

Fig. 24.2.8 The normal capitello-radial head relationship. Drawing by Terry McGuire.

Injuries to the elbow region

The elbow region accounts for 10% of all paediatric fractures. Supracondylar fractures make up 75% of these, and lateral condylar fractures 17%.[3] Missed or inadequately treated paediatric elbow injuries figure prominently in orthopaedic litigation series.[4] Post-traumatic elbow effusion in childhood without a radiologically apparent fracture line most commonly represents a minimally displaced supracondylar fracture. These must be immobilised by collar and cuff to avoid any potential extension from further falls, and followed up in a fracture clinic for a repeat X-ray at 7–14 days. It is sometimes useful to start with the examination findings in the normal elbow, as outlined in Table 24.2.5 (Figs 24.2.7 and 24.2.8).

The first point in itself will define an anatomically intact elbow, while the other points help the physician to narrow down the type of abnormality where the first point is abnormal.

Supracondylar fracture

Supracondylar injuries occur in the young school-age child as a result of a fall on the outstretched hand, transmitted through elbow hyperextension to the narrow region between olecranon and coronoid fossae. Degrees of rotation of the distal region relative to the main axis of the humerus are common, depending on the degree of pronation/supination at the time of fall.

Gartland Type 1 – undisplaced supracondylar fracture This is the presumptive diagnosis with elbow effusions that are tender bilaterally and have no ulnar or radial dislocations or significant displacement/angulation. The fracture line through the bone between olecranon and coronoid fossae may be seen on the AP view or recognised as a disruption to the normal 'teardrop' between the opposing fossae on the lateral humeral view, but its absence should not prevent the immobilisation of these elbow effusions until early orthopaedic review.

Table 24.2.5 Requirements for 'elbow clearance'

The normal paediatric elbow must have
- Full extension, supination and pronation
- No swelling or significant focal bony tenderness
- No abnormal anterior or posterior fat-pad sign on radiographs
- Normally placed and age-appropriate ossification centres (see Fig. 24.2.7)
- An intact radio-capitellar relationship (see Fig. 24.2.8)

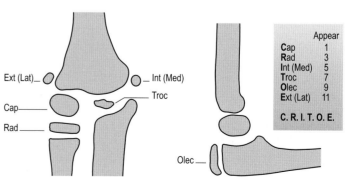

Fig. 24.2.7 CRITOE. The approximate order of appearance of the six elbow ossification centres according to the CRITOE mnemonic. Drawing by Terry McGuire.

Gartland Type 2 – posterior angulation with probable intact periosteal hinge (Fig. 24.2.9A)

In this situation it is important to check for associated rotation or varus/valgus injury. Use the 'anterior humeral line' as a guide to the degree of posterior angulation (Fig. 24.2.10), and consult orthopaedics about all injuries. Simple (2a) fractures with less than 20 degrees of angulation may be managed conservatively in a backslab and collar and cuff, with orthopaedic follow up. If there is varus/valgus angulation or rotation on the AP view (Gartland Type 2b), then orthopaedic consultation is required acutely as surgery may be indicated. Remember that remodelling may correct some loss of flexion or extension but will not correct rotation or varus/valgus deformity.

Gartland Type 3 – grossly displaced/rotated (Fig. 24.2.9B)

Check for open injury or neurovascular compromise. Brachial

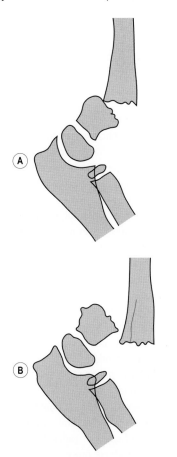

Fig. 24.2.9 Supracondylar fractures. (A) Grade Gartland Type 2, approximately 45 degrees dorsal angulation but probable intact dorsal periosteal 'hinge'; (B) grade Gartland Type 3, complete displacement, often co-existent rotation and/or neurovascular impairment. Drawing by Terry McGuire.

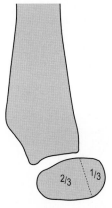

Fig. 24.2.10 The anterior humeral line rule for subtle supracondylar fractures. A line passed along the anterior humeral cortex on a lateral elbow radiograph should bisect the anterior and middle thirds of the capitellum. If it passes anterior to the capitellum, there is at least 20 degrees dorsal angulation of the distal humerus. Drawing by Terry McGuire.

artery spasm or kinking is common with this injury, and the gross associated swelling may predispose to compartment syndrome. Radial pulse and hand perfusion should be continuously reassessed. In cases with extreme swelling, extension may be safest. Immediate orthopaedic notification is required.

If orthopaedic help is not available within 1 hour of the onset of poor hand perfusion, attempt gentle traction and reduction under anaesthesia, e.g. ketamine, aiming for the position with best hand perfusion.

Median or radial nerve injury may also occur (usually as praxis), and require orthopaedic evaluation. Ulnar nerve injury is most commonly reported as an iatrogenic injury following internal fixation.

Supracondylar Gartland Types 2b and 3 fractures require admission for MUA and K-wiring and occasionally open reduction, and appropriate management of complications.

Intercondylar (T-condylar) fracture

This is a variant of the supracondylar fracture occurring in adolescents. It results from axial impaction and intra-articular separation of capitellum and trochlea, as well as proximal disruption of the medial and lateral distal humeral columns. Treatment is by internal fixation, with or without open reduction.

Lateral condyle

This fracture results from a varus force on the supinated forearm, avulsing the condyle (Figs 24.2.11 and 24.2.12). There is clinical swelling and tenderness, which is maximal over the lateral condyle. It is usually a Salter–Harris type 4 fracture, but the late

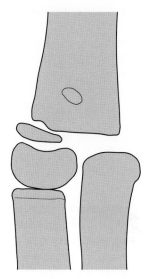

Fig. 24.2.11 Subtle lateral condylar fracture in a toddler. Note only two ossification centres (capitellum and radial head) and thin rim of metaphysis shorn away with capitellum. Greater angulation/displacement of metaphyseal fragment may be shown on lateral view. Gross clinical swelling is the key. Drawing by Terry McGuire.

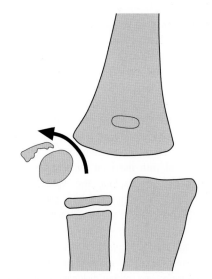

Fig. 24.2.12 Displaced and rotated lateral condylar fracture (Milch type I). Long-term complications may ensue if not surgically fixed. Drawing by Terry McGuire.

appearance of the trochlear and lateral epicondylar ossification centres means that the true structural disruption is not demonstrated by radiology, and therefore not appreciated by emergency staff, particularly in the younger child. The varus angulating force characteristically causes disruption commencing above the lateral condyle, passing to a varying extent along the physis, and in complete disruptions exiting either lateral (in the majority of cases; Milch type 1), or medial (Milch type 2) to the capitellar-trochlear groove. If uncorrected, the injury may result in valgus deformity, and possible delayed ulnar nerve palsy and degenerative elbow disease.

Bony displacement is often best seen on the lateral X-ray.

The clinical significance of this fracture means that:

❶ Any lateral condyle fracture with a greater than 2 mm separation of fracture segments is likely to require internal fixation, particularly if displacement is proximal.

❷ All young children with major elbow deformity/swelling as a result of injury should be assessed early by experienced orthopaedic personnel. Ultrasound, magnetic resonance imaging, and arthrography may all have a role to play in determining the line of injury and consequent best means of fixation. Within the ED, an internal oblique radiograph can be helpful.

The elbow may be supported in a radiolucent backslab while awaiting orthopaedic review, but X-rays in this radiologically complex region are best performed prior to plaster application.

In infants, lateral humeral condylar separation may occur as a Salter–Harris 1 type fracture and be difficult to diagnose radiologically, although the elbow will be grossly abnormal with maximal swelling laterally. History must explain the varus force, and abusive injury should be considered. Ultrasound may be useful diagnostically.

Medial epicondylar avulsion

This may occur in association with other disruptions, e.g. elbow dislocation, or as a discrete event (Fig. 24.2.13). The medial epicondyle is the origin of the common flexor tendon, and ossifies at approximately age

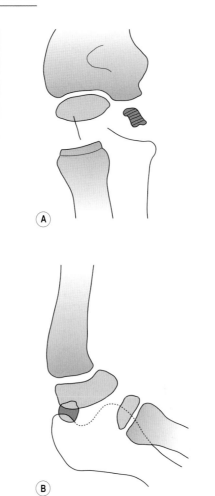

Fig. 24.2.13 Medial epicondylar avulsion. (A) The opacity below the humerus is the avulsed medial epicondyle, which should be sitting more proximal and medial. There should not be a trochlear opacity without a medial epicondylar ossification centre. Developmentally, there should not be an ossification centre in the trochlea position without one in the medial epicondylar position. (see Fig. 24.2.7). (B) Lateral view shows opacity 'between' capitellum and olecranon, possibly intra-articular. Drawing by Terry McGuire.

six. It will generally reunite readily with the humerus if it lies within 5 mm, unless there is interposing tissue. Occasionally, particularly when the avulsion has occurred in association with a posterior elbow dislocation, the epicondyle and its attachments may become lodged within the elbow joint and may block an attempt at closed reduction. Ulnar nerve injury is a common association. This circumstance is one of the main practical uses of knowledge of elbow ossification centres (see Fig. 24.2.7). These must be systematically reviewed on every elbow X-ray so that missing or misplaced opacities may be identified.

Pulled elbow (radial head subluxation, RHS)

Children from age 6 months presenting with acute disuse of one arm, which they hold in a semi-flexed and pronated posture, and a history of traction, can be presumed to have pulled elbow or RHS if there is point tenderness at the radial head and no palpable elbow effusion, i.e. no infilling of the soft tissue space medial and lateral to the olecranon in comparison with the unaffected arm.

Subluxation occurs because the oval shape of the radial head allows the head to sublux slightly through the annular ligament when the forearm is pulled in pronation. Part of the ligament is 'caught' in the radiocapitellar space, and in fact partial tears can occur.[5,6] In older children the ligament is thicker and more densely attached, and subluxation in a child over 5 is unusual.

X-ray and/or ultrasound, seeking alternative diagnoses, should be obtained in any child with other points of focal tenderness, an elbow effusion, a mechanism of greater trauma, an atypical history, e.g. fever, or a failure of the procedure detailed below.

Reduction of RHS

A recent prospective randomised trial has suggested that hyperpronation is more likely than supination to reduce the pulled elbow on the first occasion, and elicits less discomfort.[7]

After a brief parental explanation and oral or intranasal pain relief, these children should be held firmly by a parent while the forearm is hyperpronated. It is helpful for the doctor to cradle the elbow in the outer hand with the thumb over the radial head while their inner arm rotates. Success is usually denoted by a momentary pain, a palpable click, and a return to functional use. If the procedure is not successful, the procedure can be repeated, and if this fails, the traditional method of full, firm supination and flexion can be attempted. This combination of techniques should elicit success in >90% of cases of radial head subluxation.[7] If the above process is unsuccessful, the history and examination should be revisited and imaging sought. Interestingly, while radiographs should be normal (and should *not* show posterior fat pad elevation, which should suggest alternative diagnoses), the radiocapitellar distance is significantly increased in radial head subluxation on ultrasound due to the presence of the interposed ligament; a tear may sometimes be shown. If an alternative diagnosis is not suggested by imaging and careful re-assessment, RHS remains the most likely diagnosis: the child can be allowed home with the arm supported in a sling in a neutral position, and with review at 24-48 hours, at which time many will have spontaneously reduced. Persistent dysfunction beyond 48 hours requires orthopaedic evaluation. Although some children sustain recurrent RHS, it rarely requires operative intervention.[8]

Elbow dislocation

Appearing first in adolescence, this injury, the result of a fall on to the hand with partially flexed elbow, is uncommon in young children (who sustain supracondylar fractures instead). The majority dislocate posteriorly, tearing joint capsule, and stretching soft tissues. The displacement may cause fracture to the coronoid process of the ulna or radial neck, or the medial epicondyle may be avulsed. Neuropraxis of median or ulnar nerves may occur.

The dislocation should be suspected clinically. After assessing for associated injuries, it should be reduced in the ED, generally under ketamine anaesthesia (Fig. 24.2.14). Gentle downwards pressure can be applied to the supinated proximal forearm, with extension of the elbow to

about 135 degrees, against countertraction to distal humerus. Full extension should be avoided as it may cause further damage to the ulnar nerve. If there is difficulty in resiting the olecranon, there may be soft tissue inter-position and orthopaedic help should be sought, as a computerised tomography (CT) scan may be indicated. The reduced elbow should be held in flexion with a posterior splint, a check X-ray performed, and orthopaedic follow up arranged.

Proximal radial and ulnar fractures

Olecranon fractures

These may occur in older children as: (1) avulsion (flexion) fractures (generally requiring internal fixation); (2) extension fractures with intra-articular opening (may be stable in flexion); or (3) comminuted fractures from a direct blow to the elbow. Clinical correlation must be sought in diagnosing olecranon fractures, as the ossification centre, which appears around 10 years of age and may be bipartite or fragmentary in appearance, is easily mistaken for a fracture.

Radial neck fractures

These are relatively common injuries in the paediatric population. The radial head itself is largely cartilaginous and rarely injured. Injuries range from subtle torus type 'beaking' of the neck, which is best seen on the lateral side on the lateral projection, to displaced Salter–Harris type 1 or 2 fractures. Suspicion of an isolated injury may be made

by the presence of localised tenderness at the radial head. Neurovascular injury, particularly to posterior inter-osseous nerve (finger extension), should always be sought. Undisplaced fractures and those with up to 50–60% displacement do well with conservative treatment and may be immobilised in a collar and cuff with orthopaedic follow up.

Monteggia fracture dislocation

The peak incidence of this injury complex is in the 4–10 age group. Although, classically, radio-capitellar disruption accompanies an angulated or shortened ulnar fracture, the displacement may occur in association with any displacement to the radioulnar loop. Because of the significant complications of a missed radio-capitellar disruption, this lesion must be actively clinically and radiologically sought in any child with a forearm fracture and elbow swelling. Most units adopt a rule of always X-raying the elbow of any child with forearm or wrist injury, unless the elbow has been specifically clinically cleared (see Table 24.2.5).

The classical (Type 1) Monteggia lesion involves an angulated apex-volar ulnar shaft fracture and anterior displacement of the radial head (see Fig. 24.2.2). Variants include lateral radial head displacement, often in association with proximal ulnar/olecranon fractures (Type 3), 'Monteggia equivalent' fractures including proximal radial fracture/dislocation, and others. A bowing deformity may be the only evidence of fracture. Orthopaedic manipulation of the radial head into its articulation is the aim of the treatment.

Midshaft radial and ulnar fractures

These injuries fall into two broad groups: (1) common low-energy greenstick fractures as a common consequence of falls in childhood; and (2) higher-energy complete fractures, which may be difficult to reduce, requiring internal fixation in 5–10% of cases. In the former group, with the exception of bowing fractures (which generally require general anaesthetic/orthopaedic reduction, as prolonged corrective force is necessary), ED reduction may be possible thus:

- apex volar – pronate forearm and apply wrist traction and volar pressure;
- apex dorsum – supinate forearm and apply wrist traction and dorsal pressure.

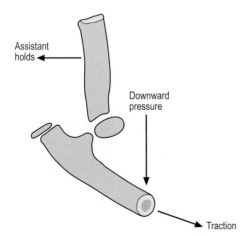

Assistant holds

Downward pressure

Traction

Fig. 24.2.14 Reduction of elbow dislocation. Assistant anchors humerus to avoid distal/anterior movement. Bring forearm in full supination to approximately 20 degrees from full extension, and provide simultaneous downwards traction and downwards pressure over the proximal forearm to lever the coronoid process back under the distal humerus. Drawing by Terry McGuire.

Although these fractures may be simple to relocate under anaesthesia, e.g. ketamine, their inherent instability makes expert three-point moulding essential. Therefore, manipulation should not be attempted unless such expertise and assistance is available, and follow up within 1 week is imperative in case of subsequent loss of position.

Distal radial and ulnar fractures

These common injuries may be metaphyseal or epiphyseal in nature. Dorsal angulation occurs in 80% of cases, but radial or volar angulation/displacement of the distal fragments may also occur. Regarding management, the following guidelines apply:

- Simple *torus (buckle) fractures* with no periosteal or cortical breach, which represent plastic deformation only, may be placed in a forearm splint or brace for comfort and referred for follow up in 1–2 weeks.[9]
- *Undisplaced greenstick fractures,* in which a cortex or periosteum has been breached, have inherent instability and the potential for further deformation. These should be managed in a well-moulded (three-point fixation) plaster in neutral position,[10] and reviewed within 1 week.
- *Angulated or displaced greenstick fractures* of the distal forearm generally require reduction if the angulation is greater than 20 degrees, although remodelling potential varies with the age of the child and the distance of the fracture from the physis. Closed reduction may be performed in the ED if staffing and expertise permit.

Again, attention must be paid to ensure that a well-moulded plaster will maintain reduction, and follow-up orthopaedic review should be early enough to detect this and remanipulate if necessary i.e. within 1 week. Early orthopaedic referral should occur for angulated isolated radial fractures and for fractures of radius and ulna with complete displacement and shortening, as a significant proportion of these manipulations will be problematic or require internal fixation.[11]

Distal radial epiphyseal fractures

These can generally be treated by manipulation and closed reduction in the same way as metaphyseal fractures. There is a very low incidence of subsequent premature physeal closure or other physeal disruption. This risk is greatest following multiple or delayed reduction attempts, or compressive injuries, or distal physeal separation of the ulna.[2] Following manipulation, referral to fracture clinic must be within a week as repeat manipulation of the physis is contraindicated after 7 days.

Carpal injuries: the scaphoid

Because of the flexibility of the paediatric wrist and the plastic properties of preossified bone, carpal injuries are very rare in children under 8 years. Scaphoid injuries are generally overdiagnosed in children in the ED setting. Of those fractures that do occur, 65% are distal pole and non-union is rare because of the different mechanical and vascular properties of immature bone. As children reach adolescence, their risk of adult-type scaphoid fractures increases. Scaphoid views (AP and oblique with attention to possible obliteration of the navicular fat pad) are suggested in older children if:[12–14]

- adolescent (10 years and over);
- high-velocity injury, especially kickback;
- single-point tenderness and swelling over scaphoid both dorsally (in anatomical snuffbox) and on volar surface under base of first metacarpal (more specific finding);
- Kirk–Watson test (pain/clunk in scaphoid/scapholunar ligament on passive radial deviation of wrist);
- pain to compression along first metacarpal ray.

Suspected fractures should be managed with scaphoid plaster and orthopaedic follow up as usual: conservative treatment usually allows resolution of true injuries but may take up to 6 months.

Metacarpal fractures

Crush injuries to metacarpal bones may occur, and adolescence sees an increase in fractures of the head of the fifth metacarpal, as in adults, although the intact distal metacarpal physis will allow some remodelling to correct flexion loss. Penetrating trauma, tendon damage, open injuries and neurovascular impairment must be identified and referred. Multiple fractures may create an unstable hand plate, and finger flexion should be observed for possible associated rotational malalignment, which is not acceptable. Isolated metacarpal fractures will not create malrotation. Isolated metacarpal neck fractures should be treated with neighbour strapping and mobilisation.

Phalangeal fractures

Common paediatric phalangeal fractures include Salter–Harris 2 fractures at the base of the first phalanx, which may cause radial/ulnar angulation and should be corrected by traction after a ring block.

These may be radiologically subtle and require careful clinical evaluation. All open, intra-articular or oblique (unstable) fractures should be referred for orthopaedic evaluation.

Thumb fractures

Forced thumb abduction, e.g. from fall onto the splayed hand, can cause avulsion of part of the proximal thumb physis (a Salter–Harris type 3 injury instead of the adult ulnar collateral ligament tear), or a metaphyseal fracture of the base of the first metacarpal. The intra-articular Salter–Harris type 3 avulsion injury should be internally fixed, so referral is essential. However, in the metaphyseal injury, because of the universal motion of the first carpometacarpal joint, significant angulation and displacement will remodel if the child is under 10 years, and the child may have the fracture immobilised in a scaphoid type plaster extending to the tip of the thumb, elevated, and be referred for early orthopaedic consultation.

Fingertip injuries

These injuries to young children are extremely common from inadvertent closure in doors or gates, especially in cooler climates. Injuries include partial or complete amputation, nail-plate injuries, and distal phalangeal fractures.

The classical crush injury includes a distal phalangeal tuft fracture and a partial amputation anteriorly through the nail bed, with intact volar soft tissue attachments and vascular integrity. Tip salvage is usual. However, without meticulous repair to the nail-bed laceration nail deformities are common, so referral to orthopaedics or plastic services is recommended.

Tip amputations distal to the terminal phalanx may often heal by secondary intent, because of the excellent vascular supply in childhood. More proximal injuries require assessment of nail-bed integrity, the possibility of soft-tissue (e.g. nail-bed) inter-position within an angulated/displaced fracture, or other indications for reconstruc-tive procedures. Simple procedures may be performed in the ED under ketamine anaes-thesia or sedation and ring block.

Lower limb and pelvis injuries

Pelvic fractures

These injuries are less common in paediatric than adult trauma. Avulsion injuries in ath-letic adolescents may occur. The implica-tions for blood loss and urogenital injury of unstable pelvic fractures in children are similar to those in adulthood. The bladder is an intra-abdominal organ in infants.

Hip dislocation

This is uncommon in childhood, occurring either with low force as a result of increased ligamentous laxity, or in the high-force mechanisms more typical of adult hip dislo-cation. The sequel of avascular necrosis is less common, occurring in only about 5% of cases.[2] Reduction, by gentle closed longi-tudinal traction against a fixed pelvis, should be performed within 6 hours. Particular care must be taken in the adolescent in whom an occult physeal injury may be displaced. Post manipulation X-rays ± CT are indicated.

Femoral fractures

Although comprising less than 5% of pae-diatric fracture presentations to the ED, the infant or child presenting with a femoral fracture presents particular challenges to the emergency physician because of:

- the frequent association with major trauma and other unstable injuries;
- the high level of pain and emotional distress for the child and the family, particularly in the setting of road trauma;
- the need for procedural skills, such as femoral nerve block, and the application of traction splinting, such as the Thomas splint;
- The possibility of non-accidental injury (possible incidence suggested at between 30 and 80% in children under 12 months[15,16]).

The simultaneous management of all these challenging priorities is a good test of the mature, multidimensional emergency physician.

As has been mentioned earlier, all limb fractures should be initially approached with rapid primary and secondary survey while the integrity of airways, breathing, circula-tion, conscious state and spinal column are assessed, mechanism ascertained, and areas of tenderness identified. An intravenous (IV) cannula should be inserted immediately, under nitrous oxide or intra-nasal fentanyl if necessary. Early attention to issues of pain and anxiety has been shown to reduce the stress and pain of later procedures. Femoral nerve block, preferably ultrasound guided, should be inserted early, with Thomas splint immobilisation following in a timely fashion.

Not all femoral fractures are the result of major trauma. In the newly ambulant child, the torsion resulting from a change of for-ward momentum with the foot fixed at an angle may produce a spiral midshaft frac-ture. Mechanisms in abusive injury include forced external rotation or abduction, e.g. from nappy change position, or direct blows.

Types of femoral fracture in children, and their orthopaedic implications, are as follows:

- Proximal femoral fractures include transepiphyseal, transcervical, basicervical, and intertrochanteric fractures. These are serious injuries. Avascular necrosis and physeal growth arrest are significant potential complications of higher fractures, and early notification and reduction are urgent.
- Slipped upper femoral epiphysis (masquerading as trauma) is discussed in Chapter 24.1.
- In femoral shaft fractures, definitive orthopaedic management depends on the degree of precipitating force, associated injuries, the age of the child, home circumstances, and the institution. Low-force injuries in young children may be treated by closed reduction and early hip spica casting. Options in older children usually involve internal or external fixation.

Injuries about the knee
Distal femoral physeal separation

These injuries result from high-force trauma to the knee. Any of the Salter–Harris pattern injuries may occur. Undisplaced injuries may

be managed by cast immobilisation. Ortho-paedic consultation is imperative because of:

- the possibility of co-existent intra-articular ligament disruption;
- the need for perfect articular surface realignment;
- the significant possibility of subsequent asymmetrical physeal arrest.

Tibial spine injury

Because of the mechanical properties of developing bone, twisting injuries to the paediatric knee result in avulsion of the tibial attachment of the anterior cruciate lig-ament (Fig. 24.2.15). The child presents non-weight-bearing, with a large effusion and joint-line tenderness. Although AP X-ray may be deceptive, lateral projections show a characteristic beak-like appear-ance of the superior surface of the tibial plateau, with posterior hinging. All children with large effusions should be referred for orthopaedic evaluation. Orthopaedic

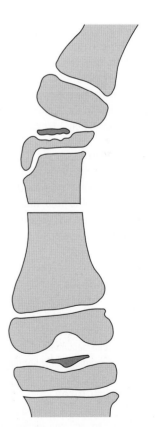

Fig. 24.2.15 Lateral and AP views of the paediatric knee with an avulsed tibial spine. Due to the intact anterior cruciate ligament, the tibial spine fracture (shaded) may be hinged posteriorly, opening anteriorly on knee flexion. Drawing by Terry McGuire.

management involves an assessment, generally under anaesthetic, of the reducibility of the avulsed spine and the likelihood of, e.g. meniscal interposition. Treatment options include immobilisation in extension or partial flexion, and internal fixation. Some degree of subsequent instability and loss of extension may follow.

Avulsion of tibial tubercle

This adolescent injury represents avulsion of the insertion site of the patellar tendon, usually as a result of forceful quadriceps contraction against resistance. Displaced injuries require internal fixation and immobilisation.

Patellar dislocation

This injury occurs most commonly in female adolescents with an excessive Q-angle (the complementary angle to the vastus lateralis/patellar tendon vectors), torsional anomalies, or hypermobility. The usual pattern is of lateral dislocation following a twist, e.g. during a fall. Most reduce spontaneously or during transport; extension of the knee may be facilitated in the prone position to relax hamstring muscles. A sky-line view should be obtained for best visualisation of osteochondral fragments from the medial patella. The knee should be placed in a Richards-type splint and the child referred for physiotherapy and orthopaedic follow up. Chronic dislocation occurs in approximately 1:6 cases.

Patellar fractures

These are less common in children than in adults. Osteochondral avulsions may occur with dislocation. Displaced fractures, with tense haemarthroses and lack of full knee extension, should be referred to the orthopaedic team. The patellar sleeve fracture may be radiographically occult as it represents separation of the cartilaginous distal patella from the ossification centre. Findings will include patella alta and excessive anterior tenderness and swelling.

Bipartite patella (secondary ossification centre) is a common radiographic normal variant.

Lower leg fractures

Lower leg fractures are common in childhood. Factors to be considered in their assessment include:

- age;
- mechanism (low- or high-force, type of injury, e.g. valgus/rotation);
- degree of angulation or displacement;
- associated soft-tissue damage or other injuries;
- involvement of physes;
- integrity of fibula.

Compound injuries and those with physeal involvement or significant angulation or displacement should be referred for inpatient orthopaedic evaluation. Proximal tibial epiphyseal injury may be complicated by vascular compromise, as with adult knee dislocation. Varus or valgus deformity, particularly at the proximal tibia, may progress. Stable, undisplaced or minimally displaced oblique or spiral shaft fractures of the tibia may be placed in a well-moulded above-knee cast with the knee flexed to 90 degrees and the ankle in 15 degrees of plantar flexion.[17] Admission is not required if swelling is minimal, mechanism is clear, and parents are sensible.

The so-called toddler fracture is an undisplaced tibial shaft fracture that occurs as a result of a rotational shearing force in the newly ambulant child. Presentation is with non-weight bearing or limp and the differential includes other pathologies, e.g. irritable or septic hip. Tenderness should be localised to the tibial shaft but initial radiology may be normal. If this diagnosis is suspected in a well child with normal joint examination, POP immobilisation and orthopaedic follow up with repeat X-ray at 10 days or nuclear bone scan may be helpful.

Controversies

❶ Controversy exists surrounding boundary issues between emergency medicine and orthopaedics. Who performs which reduction should be determined by consideration of safe, effective resource use between emergency and orthopaedic services. Structured opportunities for interdepartmental teamwork help reduce angst and improve systems and service quality.

❷ Length (SA vs LA POP) and type (circumferential vs 3/4 slab) of plaster for unstable forearm fractures post reduction is controversial; however, accuracy of moulding is probably more critical than either other variable.

Ankle fractures

As with adults, inversion, eversion and twisting mechanisms may cause a variety of injury patterns at the ankle depending on age, degree of force, and mechanism. Ankle injuries requiring same-day orthopaedic consultation include:

- open injuries;
- unstable injuries or ankles with extensive bilateral tenderness and swelling, suggesting possible mortice instability;
- displaced or angulated distal tibial fractures;
- Salter–Harris type 3 and 4 injuries;
- Triplane and Tillaux fractures.

Tillaux fracture

This is a Salter–Harris type 3 fracture at the distal tibial physis, occurring in adolescence after partial closure of the medial growth plate (see Fig. 24.2.5). External rotation of the foot and ankle causes avulsion of the anterolateral portion of the distal tibial physis by its attachment to the fibula (anterior tibiofibular ligament). The diagnosis should be suspected in a non-weight-bearing adolescent with significant anterolateral ankle swelling and tenderness. Oblique ankle views or CT assessment may be required to detail alignment.

Triplane fracture

This also occurs in the adolescent with external rotation injury, but the fracture line also tears off a section of posterior tibial metaphysis, which is clearly visible on the lateral radiograph.

Both of these transitional fractures may be complicated by subsequent joint incongruity or growth disturbance. Orthopaedic advice should always be sought.

Inversion injuries

Ligamentous rupture is rare in children. Carefully assess point of maximal tenderness. A point of maximal tenderness over the physis may represent a Salter–Harris type 1 separation of the distal fibular physis and should be cast immobilised for 2–3 weeks until stable. Bony injury may also occur at the base of the 5th metatarsal. Radiographically, this is shown by an avulsion fracture line at right angles to the metatarsal bones (the normal apophysis sits parallel and lateral). Although the

Ottawa ankle rules have not been specifically validated in children, the requirement for further assessment of an injury involving extensive swelling, bony tenderness, or inability to weight bear seems appropriate.

Controversies

Paediatric fracture management interfaces the emergency practitioner with orthopaedic and physiotherapy teams, amongst whom management of such issues as growth plate injuries (including SUFE), and early mobilisation, may be controversial.

Conclusions

Paediatric fracture patterns are completely different from adult fracture patterns and include buckle and greenstick fractures and growth-plate injuries.

Sprains are uncommon as the physis or ligamentous insertions are the 'weakest chains'

Despite a great propensity for remodelling, unrecognised displacement/angulation may have serious and long-term implications.

Future directions

The increasing trend to outpatient management of injuries will mean increasing numbers of paediatric fractures having definitive treatment in the emergency department. A thorough familiarity with paediatric fractures and their traps is essential, as is attention to quality assurance as discussed in Chapter 24.4.

Acknowledgement

The contribution of Terry McGuire as author in the first edition is hereby acknowledged.

References

1. Clark RC, Brady RM, Pitt WR, et al. Flagging possible abusive injury in young children: The role of the injury proforma. Abstract epublished in Emerg Med Australasia 2010 Feb.
2. Morrisey R, Weinstein S. *Lovell and Winter's pediatric orthopedics.* 5th ed. Philadelphia: Lippincott Williams & Wilkins; 2001.
3. Mater Children's Hospital B. *2002 Fractures in children by EDIS discharge diagnosis* Sep–Nov 2002.
4. United Medical Protection pc. Orthopaedic claims under 16 years over the period 1985-2002. In: RM B, ed. Brisbane: 2003.
5. Kim MC, Eckhardt BP, Craig C, Kuhns LR. Ultrasonography of the annular ligament partial tear and recurrent 'pulled elbow'. *Pediatr Radiol* 2004;12/27/;**34**(12):999–1004.
6. Kosuwon W, Mahaisavariya B, Saengnipanthkul S, et al. Ultrasonography of pulled elbow. *J Bone Joint Surg Br* 1993 05;**75**(3):421–2.
7. Bek D, Yildiz C, Kase O, et al. Pronation versus supination maneuvers for the reduction of 'pulled elbow': a randomized clinical trial. *Eur J Emerg Med* 2009 06;**16**(3):135–8.
8. Triantafyllou SJ, Wilson SC, Rychak JS. Irreducible 'pulled elbow' in a child. A case report. *Clin Orthop Relat Res* 1992;**11**(284):153–5.
9. Davidson J, Brown D, Barnes S. Simple treatment for torus fractures of the distal radius. *J Bone Joint Surg Br* 2002;**84**(7):1085.
10. Boyer B, Overton B, Scrader W, Riley P. Position of immobilisation for paediatric forearm fractures. *J Pediatr Orthop* 2002;**22**(2):185–7.
11. Gibbons C, Woods D, Pailthorpe C, et al. The management of isolated distal radius fractures in children. *J Pediatr Orthop* 1994;**14**(2):207–10.
12. Evenski AJ, Adamczyk MJ, Steiner RP, et al. Clinically suspected scaphoid fractures in children. *J Pediatr Orthop* 2009 06;**29**(4):352–5.
13. Hernandez JA, Swischuk LE, Bathurst GJ, Hendrick EP. Scaphoid (navicular) fractures of the wrist in children: attention to the impacted buckle fracture. *Emerg Radiol* 2002 12/09/;**9**(6):305–8.
14. Weber DM, Fricker R, Ramseier LE. Conservative treatment of scaphoid nonunion in children and adolescents. *J Bone Joint Surg Br* 2009 09;**91**(9):1213–6.
15. Thomas S, Rosenfield N, Leventhal J, Markowitz R. Long-bone fractures in young children: Distinguishing accidental injuries from child abuse. *Paediatrics* 1991;**88**(3):471–6.
16. Hui C, Joughin E, Goldstein S, et al. Femoral fractures in children younger than three years: the role of nonaccidental injury. *J Pediatr Orthop* 2008;**28**(3):297–302.
17. Yang J, Letts R. Isolated fractures of the tibia with intact fibula in children: A review of 95 patients. *J Pediatr Orthop* 1997;**17**:347–51.

ORTHOPAEDICS AND RHEUMATOLOGY

24.3 Spinal injury

Ed Oakley

ESSENTIALS

1 Spine injury is often associated with other severe injury.

2 Upper cervical spine injuries are more common in children. Thoracic and lumbar spine injury is strongly associated with spinal cord injury.

3 Adequate immobilisation of the entire spine is needed. Spinal immobilisation can cause complications, especially in the patient with spinal cord injury.

4 Clinical evaluation of the cervical spine can only occur in a child who is conscious, able to communicate and free from any other significant injuries. The cervical spine can be cleared on clinical findings alone in specific circumstances.

5 A good quality three-view series of the cervical spine (lateral, AP and odontoid view) is adequate to assess the bony structures. Clinical findings should be considered when clearing the cervical spine radiographically.

6 Patients with spinal injury have a high incidence of fractures at another level.

7 Spinal cord injury may cause hypotension and relative bradycardia.

8 Spinal cord injury may occur without radiographic abnormality.

Introduction

Injuries to the spine and spinal cord are less common in children than adults. The injuries have different distributions and frequency in different-aged children, dependent upon the developmental, anatomical and physiological differences with age. Children account for up to 10% of all spinal injuries, but the mortality among spine-injured children is higher than in adults, with estimates ranging from 25–30%, with death most often due to associated injuries to other organs, especially the brain.[1]

The incidence of spinal cord injury amongst spine-injured children is probably about 1%.[1,2] In neurologically impaired survivors the injuries are most commonly at the C1–C2 level, or in the lower cervical or thoracic spine.[1] The common causes of spine and spinal cord injuries in children are motor vehicle crashes, falls, diving accidents, sports injuries and, occasionally, non-accidental injury.[1,3,4]

The majority of injuries in children occur in the cervical spine. In children under 8, most (about 80%) occur in the C1–C3 region, whereas after 8 years of age the incidence is similar to that in adults, with the majority in the lower three cervical vertebrae.[2,5,6] The thoracolumbar junction is the most commonly injured area outside the cervical spine, with the thoracic and lumbar spines having roughly equal incidence of about 25%. There is an increased incidence of neurologic injury in fractures of the thoracolumbar junction. The relatively high incidence of injuries in this region is due to the large range of motion and the changing orientation of the facet joints.[1,7] Approximately 30% of patients with spinal cord injury have fractures at more than one spinal level. A majority of these are in contiguous vertebral segments, but 5–15% may be in different regions.[7]

Developmental anatomy and physiology

There are a number of injury patterns of the spine – and especially the cervical spine – that are unique to children. In order to understand the differences between adult and paediatric spine injuries knowledge of the developmental anatomy of the spine is essential.

The large amount of cartilage present in the paediatric cervical spine can make radiographic evaluation difficult. This is especially true in the first few years of life, and in the upper cervical vertebrae.

The *atlas* ossifies from three ossification centres: two ossification centres of the lateral masses and one ossification centre for the body. The ossification centre for the body does not ossify until about 1 year of age. The posterior arches fuse by 3 or 4 years of age, while the synchondrosis between the lateral masses and the body fuses at approximately 7 years of age.[3,5]

The *axis* ossifies from seven ossification centres. The five primary ossification centres are two for the lateral masses, two for the odontoid (which are usually fused at birth but occasionally persist as a dens bicornis), and one for the body. The odontoid is separated from the body by a synchondrosis, which fuses between 3 and 6 years old. The two secondary ossification centres are the tip of the odontoid process (which appears at about 3 years of age and is usually fused by 12 years of age), and the inferior ring apophysis (which, like other ring apophyses, generally ossifies after 8 years of age and fuses in the early 20s).[3,5]

The remainder of the cervical vertebrae each contain three primary ossification centres, one for the body and one for the two neural arches, and two secondary ossification centres, the ring apophyses. The neural arches fuse posteriorly by the age of 3, and anteriorly the three ossification centres fuse between 3 and 6 years of age. Importantly, the vertebral bodies are wedge-shaped until the age of 7 when they begin to square off.[3,4]

The thoracic and lumbar spines develop in a similar way, with secondary ossification centres for the spinous process and the transverse processes added. By the time the child is 8–10 years of age the spine has reached near-adult size.[3,4]

There are a number of other differences of importance for the spine. The fulcrum of movement of the neck is located at C2–C3 in the infant, at C3–C4 by the age of 6,

ORTHOPAEDICS AND RHEUMATOLOGY

and by the age of 8 the fulcrum is at C5–C6, as it is in the adult. There is a relatively large head and weak neck muscles; laxity of the ligaments and joint capsule; and relatively horizontal positioning of the facet joints with underdevelopment of the uncinate processes.[1,3,4] All these features increase the risk of injury to the child's spine.

Initial assessment

All patients with significant trauma should be assumed to have a spine or spinal cord injury and appropriate precautions must be taken to prevent further exacerbating any possible injury. The initial assessment of patients with potential spine or spinal cord injury should be directed at the airway, breathing and circulation, in line with trauma resuscitation guidelines (see Section 2). The patient should be stabilised and a thorough secondary survey performed. At this point all possible spine and spinal cord injuries should be identified. The lateral cervical spine X-ray will be done at this stage in patients with major trauma. Thorough radiological assessment of the injuries should be completed once resuscitation and stabilisation and the secondary survey have all been accomplished.

A thorough history of mechanism of injury, previous spinal injury, other illnesses, particularly respiratory illness (acute or chronic), cardiac illness, or bone disorders, medication and allergies is needed to determine the patient's premorbid physiological status.

Spinal immobilisation

Spinal immobilisation is currently a controversial issue, especially in young children. A balance must be found that will diminish the risk of further injury to the child's spine, but not interfere with the assessment, or the normal physiological functions, of the child. Traditionally the spine has been immobilised in a rigid cervical collar, on a spine board with a head immobiliser and straps, or with sandbags and tapes, thus providing adequate control of the entire spine (Table 24.3.1).[3,8,9]

There are a number of potential problems with this immobilisation (Table 24.3.2). Cervical collars are not made to fit infants

Table 24.3.1 Indications for initial immobilisation of the spine

- Level of consciousness
- Inability to give history of pain
- Neck or back pain
- Neurological signs or symptoms
- Multiple system trauma
- History of significant trauma
  Fall from height >3 metres
  Pedestrian or cyclist hit by car
  Unrestrained passenger in motor vehicle
  Crash diving accident
- History of spinal abnormality

Table 24.3.2 Problems associated with spinal immobilisation in children

- Incorrectly fitted cervical-spine collar causing distraction of the spine or allowing excessive movement
- Flexion of the spine in children under 8 years of age
- Reduction in tidal volume and limitation of respiratory effort
- Airway obstruction
- Increased intracranial pressure
- Discomfort
- Distress and anxiety
- Pressure sores

and alternative immobilisation is needed. An ill-fitting collar may cause the chin to become trapped under the chin support and may cause airway obstruction. The young child may become distressed from being rigidly immobilised, making further

assessment difficult, and potentially raising intracranial pressure. Rigid immobilisation in a collar and head immobiliser on a spinal board has also been shown to decrease tidal volume and respiratory excursion.[10] In addition, because the young child's head is disproportionately large, the neck is flexed when immobilised on a standard spinal board. This causes flexion of the cervical spine, which may cause movement at the site of injury. To prevent this, a spinal board with a recess for the head or padding that elevates the torso is needed for children less than 8 years old (Fig. 24.3.1).[11–13]

A number of different cervical collars are available and satisfactory to use. The clinician must be familiar with the method of sizing and applying the collar available, as an incorrect fit will allow too much movement of the collar if too small, or will produce a distraction of any existing injury if too large.

For children who have less major trauma but are at risk of spinal injury, a degree of judgement is needed by the clinician as to the level of immobilisation that is appropriate. However, in all patients with multiple or significant other injuries immobilisation is still recommended. If the child is not on a spine board, immobilisation solely in a cervical collar, maintaining alignment of the neck and the entire spine, is appropriate. Using sandbags and tape or other means to immobilise the head by fixing it to the bed risks

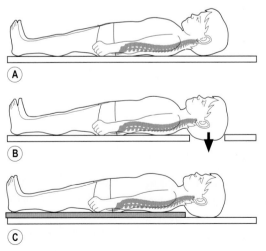

Fig. 24.3.1 Effects of spine-board on cervical spine position in children. Child immobilised on a standard backboard (A), and on backboards modified with an occipital recess (B) and a mattress pad (C). Modified from Herzenberg et al 1989 Emergency transport and positioning of young children who may have an injury of the cervical spine: The standard backboard may be hazardous. Journal of Bone & Joint Surgery 71(1): 15–22.

further complications, including airway compromise, and the risks are likely to outweigh the benefits.[14,15]

The back is examined by log rolling the child. This requires at least three people in the smallest of children, and up to five in larger patients. The child is freed from the head immobiliser and any strapping to the spinal board removed. One person must stabilise the cervical spine by supporting the head and neck in the neutral position throughout movement. No traction should be applied to the neck. The other team members control the shoulders, hips and legs, and one person must be free to inspect and palpate the back. The back is inspected for bruises, abrasions, wounds or deformity of the spine. The spinous processes are palpated for tenderness. The back of the neck and head and the buttocks and anus should be inspected. A rectal examination is not mandated in all children.

To limit discomfort and the likelihood of pressure sores a child should be kept on the spinal board for the shortest possible time. Once resuscitation and urgent procedures and investigations are completed the board should be removed. This is especially important in patients with suspected spinal cord injury.[16]

Cervical spine injuries

As the cervical spine is the most common region injured and accounts for the majority of spinal cord injuries, a thorough knowledge of injuries in this region and the appropriate assessment of the spine both clinically and radiographically is mandatory. In children younger than 8 years of age the majority (but not all) injuries occur above the fourth cervical vertebra. After 8, the pattern of injury is similar to that seen in adults (the majority of injuries below C4).[2,17]

Mechanisms of injury

The mechanism of injury is an important historical factor, as it will determine the type and possible instability of the underlying injury (Table 24.3.3).[15]

Flexion

The most common mechanism of injury seen is hyperflexion. This type of injury produces a compressive force on the anterior segment

Table 24.3.3 A classification of spine injuries	
Mechanism of injury	*Stability*
Flexion	
Flexion teardrop fracture	Very unstable
Bilateral facet joint dislocation	Unstable
Atlanto-occipital dislocation	Unstable
Displaced odontoid fracture	Unstable
Anterior subluxation	Unstable
Anterior wedge fracture	Stable
Clay shoveller's fracture	Very stable
Extension	
Atlantoaxial dislocation	Very unstable
Hangman's fracture C2	Unstable
Extension teardrop fracture	Unstable (in extension)
Rotation	
Rotary atlantoaxial dislocation	Unstable
Rotary atlantoaxial subluxation	Stable
Unilateral facet dislocation	Stable
Vertical compression	
Jefferson fracture (burst # C1)	Very unstable
Burst fracture vertebral body	Stable

Source: Modified from Rosen P et al 1997. Emergency Medicine, 4th edn. Mosby, St. Louis, MO, USA.

of the vertebra – leading to a compression fracture or teardrop fracture. The posterior elements of the spine are distracted with ligamentous injury, dislocations, or avulsion fractures of the spinous processes. These injuries can be stable (such as the anterior wedge compression fracture or the clay shoveller's fracture) or unstable (such as a bilateral facet joint dislocation).

Extension

Hyperextension injuries produce distracting forces anteriorly, while compressing the posterior vertebral structures. Most extension injuries are unstable, and buckling of the ligamentum flavum into the posterior of the spinal canal can cause a central or posterior spinal cord syndrome.

Rotation

In the cervical spine isolated rotary injuries are uncommon. Subluxation can be spontaneous or follow minor or major trauma. It is generally a stable injury. However, if there is dislocation of the facet joints of C1/C2 the lesion is unstable.

Vertical compression

These injuries are due to axial compression of the cervical spine. This can produce a burst fracture of any vertebra, with a lesion

at C1 being most unstable. Spinal cord involvement is from a retropulsed fragment of bone or intervertebral disc.

In many instances, not one but a combination of these mechanisms of injury is involved, producing more than one type of injury.

Clinical assessment

After immobilisation and resuscitation of the injured child and as part of the secondary survey the neck should be examined. This is done to look for neck abrasions and signs of injury to other structures in the neck as well as to examine the cervical spine. The decision to evaluate the cervical spine for injury should only be made in children who are conscious and alert, who are not drug or alcohol affected, and who do not have other injuries that are painful or distracting enough to make assessment of neck pain difficult.[2,17–19]

The cervical collar should be removed while another person holds the head inline. No traction should be applied to the neck. The cervical spine is palpated for tenderness over the spinous processes. If there is tenderness over a specific region the collar should be reapplied and the spine evaluated with X-ray. If there is no tenderness (or only soft tissue tenderness) the child should be allowed to gently move the head from side to side. If this produces pain posteriorly in the neck the collar should be reapplied and the spine X-rayed. If there is no pain on movement the collar and cervical spine protection can be removed.[2,17–19]

Young children represent a difficult subgroup. They are preverbal and cannot follow commands or communicate easily. If palpation of the posterior cervical spine does not cause distress the neck should be let free; if the child spontaneously moves the neck without discomfort the neck can be cleared. In this author's experience no young child with a neck fracture will spontaneously move its neck without discomfort.

Radiographic images

Radiological evaluation is required for all children who do not meet all the criteria for clinical clearance of the cervical spine. As part of the secondary survey in major trauma patients the cross-table lateral cervical spine X-ray would have been performed. This is a guide to the presence of serious cervical spine trauma only and cannot be used to exclude cervical spine injury.[2,17] All patients who require radiological evaluation require a full cervical spine series.

The cervical spine series consists of a lateral film, an anterior-posterior film and an odontoid view. Using these three views all abnormal cervical spines will be detected, allowing further investigation to fully delineate the individual injuries.[2,5] All seven vertebrae must be included in the lateral view, along with the cervicothoracic junction. If this is not visible gentle traction should be applied to the arms and the film repeated, or a swimmer's view (transaxillary) should be obtained. Oblique views of the cervical spine may also be of assistance, especially if the cervicothoracic junction is difficult to visualise. Oblique views, however, do not provide any more information regarding the likelihood of injury than the standard three views.[2,5,17]

In young children, getting co-operation for the odontoid (open mouth) view is difficult. It has been shown that this view can be excluded in children under 5 years of age with little likelihood of missing a fracture.[20,21]

Other specialised radiological investigations have been used to evaluate cervical spine injuries:

Flexion and extension

Lateral cervical spine radiographs have been used to assess the spine for ligamentous injury. The suggested indications have been symptomatic patients with normal plain X-rays, or the unconscious patient with normal X-rays and/or CT scans. These images have become popular in assessing adult patients but investigations to date have consistently failed to show a benefit over other imaging, with a significant number of studies limited by inadequate motion in the acute setting.[22] Most paediatric cervical-spine guidelines do not call for the routine use of these views.[23]

Computerised tomography (CT)

CT of the cervical spine is common. There have been a number of indications for routine CT suggested, with the most widely accepted being for further evaluation and elucidation of fractures identified, or to view areas not seen adequately on the initial cervical spine series.[17] Other suggested indications are for the assessment of the unconscious patient with normal initial radiographs, and for patients having a CT of the brain. Proponents of CT suggest scanning the entire spine in both of these instances and clearing the spine if scans are normal[19] (or progressing to flexion-extension views).[17,24] Another group suggests just scanning the upper cervical vertebrae in children under 8 as most injuries occur in this region.[25,26] There are no studies that have systematically evaluated the role of CT in the evaluation of paediatric cervical spine injuries. CT appears to be as good as any other modality in identifying injuries but the radiation exposure of young children needs to be considered.[23]

Magnetic resonance imaging (MRI)

MRI is the imaging method of choice for assessing ligamentous injuries and for spinal cord injuries. MRI will visualise most ligamentous injuries and all spinal cord injuries. In many instances MRI will alter the specifics of surgical management in those who require surgical stabilisation. MRI provides prognostic information in children with spinal cord injury.[17,27]

Radiographic evaluation

Once the X-rays have been obtained, care needs to be taken to interpret the images accurately and correlate the findings with the history and physical examination. Due to the physiological differences described above, a number of normal radiological findings in children are significantly different from those in adults. The common findings that cause concern are: pseudosubluxation of C2 on C3 (seen in up to 25% of children); exaggerated atlantodens distance (seen in 20% of children under 8 years of age); and radiolucent synchondrosis between the odontoid and C2 (seen in all children under 4 and in 50% of those under 10 years of age). Other normal findings that can be misinterpreted include a variable anterior soft tissue width – altering with head positioning and crying – the anterior ring apophyses of the vertebral bodies, and the anterior wedging of the vertebral bodies (especially C3).[17,28,29] All of these normal findings can be mistaken for acute traumatic injuries in children following trauma.

Evaluation of the lateral cervical spine radiograph begins with assessment of the four lines, corresponding to the anterior vertebral bodies, the posterior vertebral bodies, the spinolaminar line, and the tips of the spinous processes. All four of these lines should follow a smooth, even contour (Fig. 24.3.2). The articular facets should be parallel, the intervertebral disc spaces, at the posterior margin of the vertebral bodies, should be similar, and the distances between spinous processes should show no significant widening (fanning). Review of the soft tissue shadow should show a retropharyngeal space of not more than one half the AP diameter of the vertebral body at C2 and no wider than the full width of the vertebral body at C6. As mentioned, this may be difficult to interpret in the crying child.[1,3,17]

Assessment of these areas of possible abnormality has been made easier by the formulation of a series of normal measurements. For the atlantoaxial relationship (C1–C2), a measurement of the distance (on the lateral film) from the posterior border of the anterior arch of C1 to the anterior margin of the odontoid should be less than 5 mm in children under 8 years of age, and ≤3 mm in older children and adults. To assess the relationship of the basion of the skull to the atlas, the most reliable measurement in children is Harris's posterior axial line (Fig. 24.3.3), which should lie within 12 mm of the basion of the skull.

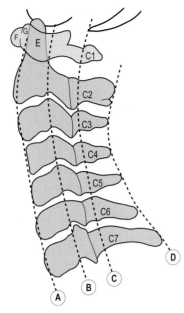

Fig. 24.3.2 Cervical spine lines. Lateral cervical spine. (A) Anterior vertebral bodies; (B) posterior vertebral bodies and anterior spinal canal; (C) spinolamial line and posterior spinal canal; (D) spinous process tips C2-C7; (E) odontoid process of dens of C2; (F) anterior arch of C1; (G) predental space between posterior surface of anterior arch of C1 and anterior surface of odontoid process. Modified from Barkin et al 1994 Emergency Pediatrics, 4th edn. Mosby, St. Louis, MO, USA.

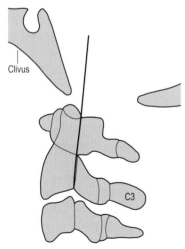

Fig. 24.3.3 Posterior axial line for identification of occipito-axial dislocation.

The subluxation of C2 on C3 and C3 on C4 consistently causes difficulty in interpretation of paediatric cervical spine films. Swischuk's line (posterior cervical line), which joins the spinolaminar line of C1 to that of C3, allows assessment of the

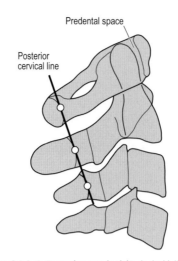

Fig. 24.3.4 Posterior cervical (Swischuk) line.

likelihood of the subluxation being physiological (Fig. 24.3.4). The spinolaminar junction of C2 should lie within 2 mm of this line. If the distance is greater than 2 mm a fracture or pathological subluxation is likely.

Cervical spine clearance guidelines

With the knowledge of mechanism of injury, immobilisation needed, clinical examination, and radiographic interpretation, it is possible to devise guidelines (Fig. 24.3.5) that allow safe and effective management of the potentially injured cervical spine while minimising the investigations needed. There is as yet no guideline that is well established for young children.[30,31] The guideline should include the following points:

- All patients with a significant mechanism of injury, altered conscious state, or neurological symptoms, or who cannot be assessed should be immobilised.
- If on assessment the patient is alert, not drug affected, has no other major injuries, has no posterior cervical tenderness, has no posterior cervical pain on movement, and has no neurological signs, the immobilisation can safely be removed and no further investigations are needed. If these criteria are not all satisfied or assessment is incomplete, immobilisation should be maintained and a three-view plain X-ray series performed.[18,19]
- If the X-rays are normal the patient should be re-examined. If the patient has a normal examination, the immobilisation

can be removed. If there is still significant pain or tenderness, a CT scan of the entire spine should be performed. If this is normal and the patient alert and co-operative, immobilisation should be kept in place and flexion and extension views performed 3–7 days later, once the muscle spasm has resolved. If the patient is significantly unwell, or has multiple trauma, CT or MRI scanning should be considered. Consultation with a paediatric orthopaedic surgeon or neurosurgeon is recommended.[19]

Atlantoaxial rotary subluxation

Fixed rotary subluxation at the atlantoaxial joint is more common during childhood than adulthood. It can present after minor trauma, in conjunction with an upper respiratory tract infection, and often no inciting cause is found. The clinical picture is that of the head turned to one side and held in the 'cock-robin' position. The child is unable to turn its head past the midline, and attempts to move the head often cause pain. The spasm of the sternocleidomastoid (SCM) muscle is on the side to which the head is turned (ipsilateral side), as the muscle is trying to right the head. In contrast, in a wry neck the SCM spasm is on the side opposite to which the head is turned (contralateral side), with the spasm causing the head turning.[1,15,17]

Plain radiographs may be diagnostic, revealing the lateral mass of C1 rotated anterior to the odontoid on the lateral view, or rotation of the spinous processes to the ipsilateral side on the AP view. If clinical examination and plain radiographs cannot confirm the diagnosis, CT imaging should be considered.[17]

Rotary subluxation of short duration will often spontaneously reduce; those that do not or that have been present for a longer duration (days) may need traction or manipulation to reduce. Post-reduction immobilisation is needed to maintain reduction and the duration of immobilisation should vary according to the duration of subluxation.[1,17,32]

Thoracic and lumbar spine injuries

Fractures of the thoracic spine account for 25–30% of spine injury in children, while lumbar fractures account for 20–25%.

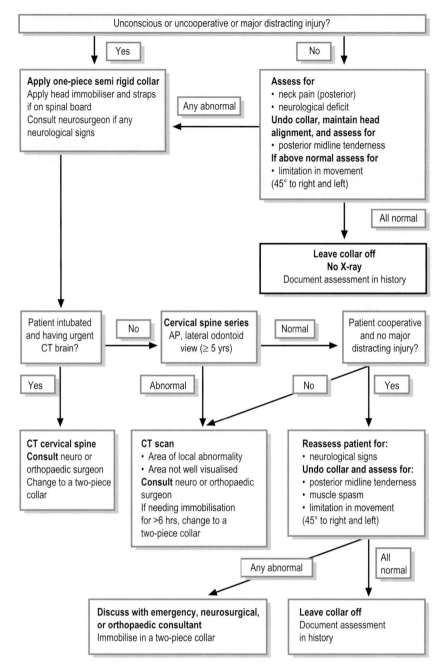

Fig. 24.3.5 Guide to management of the potentially injured cervical spine.

Injuries to the thoracic spine and the thoracolumbar junction have a higher incidence of spinal cord injury, with neurological deficit seen in up to 40% of cases.[1,7] The high incidence of cord injury is related to the relatively large size of the spinal cord in the thoracic region, the inherent stability of the thoracic spine requiring larger forces to cause bony injury. Multiple level injuries are seen in 30–40% of children with thoracic or lumbar spine fractures.[7] Fractures of the lower thoracic and upper lumbar spine have associated small bowel and visceral injury in up to 50% of cases.[1] Road traffic accidents and falls account for most of the injuries, but non-accidental injuries in these regions do occur.

Mechanism of injury

Injuries to the thoracic and lumbar spine are flexion/extension or vertical compression injuries; often a combination of these is present, and also a degree of distraction is not uncommon.

A number of bony injuries are caused by these mechanisms. Compression of the vertebral body with anterior wedging is the most common. However, a degree of anterior wedging is normal in children. Burst fractures occur where there is disruption of the endplates and herniation of the disc into the vertebral body. Retropulsed fragments can cause spinal cord injury. The 'seat-belt' fracture, associated with the lap-only seat belt, is a hyperflexion and distraction injury most commonly seen at the thoracolumbar junction, and is frequently associated with visceral or mesenteric injury. The posterior bony or ligamentous elements are disrupted and the fracture line extends horizontally into the vertebral body or through the intervertebral disc.[1,4,7,33]

Clinical assessment

As with all trauma patients, assessment of the spine should take place in the secondary survey after the airway, breathing and circulation have been assessed and stabilised. A history of mechanism of injury is important in identifying the risk of thoracic or lumbar spine injury. The presence of pain in the back makes injury more likely, but absence of pain does not exclude injury. Clinical examination should focus on tenderness and signs of bruising or deformity over the spine. This is assessed by log rolling the patient while spinal immobilisation is still in place. A search for signs of spinal cord or cauda equina lesions should also be made.

Any patient who has pain or tenderness over the spine should have the spine evaluated by radiography. Patients without pain or tenderness who have altered conscious state or other significant injuries are at risk of having thoracic or lumbar spine injuries missed (as they are for cervical spine injuries).[34] As multi-level injuries are common, any child with a proven cervical spine fracture or spinal cord injury should have the entire spine imaged with plain radiographs (see Fig. 24.3.5).

Radiographic evaluation

After clinical evaluation, radiographs should be taken on any child who is at risk of having a thoracic or lumbar spine injury (Table 24.3.4). The standard views for both areas are the anterior-posterior radiograph and the lateral film. In the thoracic region the radiographs need to be overexposed

ORTHOPAEDICS AND RHEUMATOLOGY

- Pain in the thoracic or lumbar region
- Tenderness of the spine in the thoracic or lumbar region
- Significant bruising or deformity of the spine
- Altered conscious state
- Proven fracture in another region of the spine

compared to a normal chest X-ray to allow adequate views of the spine. The shoulders often obscure the upper thoracic spine and a swimmer's view may be needed to visualise the first two thoracic vertebrae.

The films should be evaluated by following the anterior and posterior vertebral body lines and the spinolaminar line on the lateral view. These three lines should have a parallel course. The height of each vertebral body should be assessed anteriorly and posteriorly, and a difference of more than about 3 mm treated as pathological. On the AP view the paraspinal lines should be closely inspected to detect evidence of paraspinal haematoma. The posterior elements should be visible through the vertebral body and should be in alignment. Each vertebra should be inspected; an apparently empty or invisible vertebral body indicates a fracture dislocation with distraction.[1,33]

There are a number of features on the radiographs that indicate an unstable fracture: vertebral body collapse with widening of the pedicles; greater than 33% compromise of the spinal canal by retropulsed fragments of the lamina, pedicles or body; translocation of more than 2.5 mm between vertebral bodies in any direction; bilateral facet joint dislocation; or greater than 50% anterior compression of the vertebral body associated with widening of the interspinous space.[33]

While most thoracic and lumbar spine fractures are diagnosed on the initial plain radiographs, these films often do not provide enough information on the extent of the injury and a CT scan of the region is usually obtained to elucidate the full extent of the injury. MRI will be needed to visualise all ligamentous and spinal cord involvement.

Some fractures in the thoracic region can be difficult to see on plain films, especially if there were technical difficulties in obtaining the films in multiply-injured patients. A number of secondary signs of thoracic spine injury exist and can help make the diagnosis. A paravertebral haematoma can usually be seen at the site of injury, blood in the pleural space may be seen as a pleural cap, and widening of the mediastinum may be present. Unfortunately these signs cannot differentiate a thoracic spine injury from an aortic arch injury.[7]

Management

Management must start with care of the airway, breathing and circulation. Only once these areas have been stabilised should management of the spine proceed. However, while the patient is being stabilised the spine should be maintained in alignment and the patient moved by log rolling. A thorough assessment and investigation of the abdomen and chest is mandatory for all patients with significant thoracic and upper lumbar spine injuries, and injuries to the pelvis must not be forgotten with lumbar spine injuries. As many of these injuries are associated with intra-abdominal injuries an ileus is common and nasogastric or orogastric tube should be inserted. Consultation with a paediatric orthopaedic surgeon or neurosurgeon should be sought for the definitive care of the injury. Surgical stabilisation is usually required for unstable fractures and those fractures associated with neurological injury.[4,7,33]

Spinal cord injury

The goal of management of injury to the spinal cord or cauda equina is to minimise the resulting neurological deficit. This commences with adequate immobilisation of the spine and complete and thorough investigation to detail the anatomy of the injury.[35]

Spinal cord injury should be suspected in any child who has multisystem trauma, minor trauma associated with spinal pain, sensory or motor symptoms, and any patient with altered consciousness. The patient must be adequately immobilised, such as on a spinal board with a cervical collar and head immobiliser (see section on spinal immobilization, p. 545), and any assessment of the back or patient movement accomplished by log rolling. Up to 50% of patients with spinal cord injury will have at least moderate head injury.[35]

Spinal cord injury syndromes

A number of patterns of neurological deficit are seen in patients with spinal cord injury, with the deficit dependant on the portion of the spinal cord damaged. Neurogenic shock – the manifestations of loss of sympathetic output to the cardiovascular system – is seen immediately after complete cord injury at the level of T6 or above. This should not be confused with spinal shock, which is the reversible dysfunction of the spinal cord associated with injury. It is likened to a concussion of the cord without permanent damage. It may exist alone or in combination with permanent cord injury. Its resolution is responsible for the improvement in neurological function seen in the first few days post-injury.[15,35]

The distinction between a complete injury and a partial injury – with preservation of some motor or sensory function below the lesion – is vital for prognosis. Many patients with partial injury will regain much or all of the neurological function. A partial cord injury may occur at any region and with any mechanism of injury.

Complete cord injury is usually seen in injuries of the thoracic spine and thoracolumbar junction. The spinal cord is large in relation to the size of the spinal canal at this level. Complete cord injuries that remain at 24 hours rarely regain any significant function. Cauda equina lesions – injuries at or below L2 – involve the peripheral nerves rather than the spinal cord and can show significant recovery of lower limb and sphincter function even weeks after the injury.[15,35]

Central cord syndrome is usually seen in hyperextension injury resulting in herniation of the intervertebral disc into the spinal cord. The resulting injury causes a motor deficit that is greater in the arms than legs and most extensive in the small muscles of the hand. The sensory deficit is variable. Brown–Sequard syndrome – hemisection of the cord – causes a contralateral loss of pain and temperature sensation and an ipsilateral motor paralysis and loss of proprioception below the level of injury. Approximately two-thirds of those with central cord syndrome and one-third with Brown–Sequard syndrome will recover.[15,35]

Clinical assessment

Initial steps in the management of a patient with a suspected spinal cord lesion are the assessment and resuscitation of the airway, breathing and circulation. The most immediate threats to life and spinal cord function of patients with spinal cord injury remain hypoxia and hypotension. Spinal cord lesions in the upper cervical spine may impair respiratory function and require early intubation and mechanical ventilation. The unstable cervical spine must be maintained in alignment without traction during treatment of the airway. The loss of sympathetic vasomotor tone after cervical spinal cord injury will result in vasodilatation, venodilatation, and reduced venous return to the heart causing hypotension. There should be an associated relative bradycardia for age and existing blood pressure, which will help distinguish this response from haemorrhagic shock.[35]

Initial fluid resuscitation with 10–20 mL kg^{-1} should adequately replace the relative hypovolaemia. However, if hypotension persists, measurement of central venous pressure (CVP) may be needed to guide fluid replacement. Excessive fluid replacement that pushes central venous and pulmonary artery pressures above the normal range will result in pulmonary oedema. Treatment with a vasoconstrictor, such as metaraminol, may be useful for the patient who has adequate CVP and remains hypotensive. In patients who are also significantly bradycardic, inotropic agents, such as dopamine or adrenaline (epinephrine), may be useful. Patients requiring more than 40 mL kg^{-1} of fluid replacement and having a low CVP must be assumed to have other injuries causing blood loss.

Examination of the neurological impairment is done as part of the secondary survey. A thorough examination of the motor function of the limbs and assessment of reflexes should be performed and a level of sensory deficit sought. Knowledge of the dermatomes and myotomes will allow determination of the level of neurological injury.

Radiographic evaluation

In all patients with suspected spinal cord injury the spine should be X-rayed. The radiographs should include the entire spine, as multiple levels of injury are common. Once the patient is stabilised, further investigation of the lesion should follow. The bony injuries should be investigated as discussed above. Investigation of the cord itself will require MRI. MRI should be performed as soon as possible after identification of a spinal cord injury, as it will allow identification of remedial

intraspinal problems in patients with a partial neurological deficit. The appearance of the spinal cord on MRI also allows prediction of neurological outcome. Cord transection and major haemorrhage have a poor outcome, minor haemorrhage and oedema have a moderate to good outcome, and a normal MRI is associated with complete recovery.[1]

Treatment

Most of the treatment available for spinal cord injuries is supportive. The breathing and circulation must be supported as needed. As there will be a neurogenic bladder, catheterisation is necessary, and a nasogastric tube is needed to treat the gastric and bowel stasis that ensues. For transport, antiemetic is useful to prevent vomiting and spine movement or airway compromise. Subcutaneous low-molecular-weight heparin should be instigated once the patient is stable to prevent deep venous thrombosis.[36]

Specific treatment of the spinal cord lesion is controversial. Four substances have been studied in prospective, randomised trials – methylprednisolone, tirilazad, naloxone and GM-1 ganglioside. All studies to date have excluded children under 13 years of age. Tirilazad and naloxone have failed to show any benefit in trials to date. There is conflicting evidence regarding the benefits of methylprednisolone and documented evidence that its use increases the risk of bacterial infection. It is recommended that it be used with knowledge of the risks and possible benefits.[15,36] The current regimens for use are seen in Table 24.3.5. GM-1 ganglioside has yet to be shown to offer significant benefit in spinal cord injury, and is not recommended for routine use.

Once the patient has been stabilised and investigated, transfer to a spinal cord injury unit should be expedited. These units and associated intensive-care units are geared to manage the cardiorespiratory

compromise that may occur in the ensuing weeks, the psychosexual issues that accompany spinal cord injury, the urological problems, and the potential for skin breakdown, that are exaggerated in these patients.

SCIWORA

Spinal cord injury without radiographic abnormality (SCIWORA) is defined as objective signs of myelopathy as a result of trauma with no evidence of fracture or ligamentous instability on plain X-rays or tomography.[37] SCIWORA is most frequently seen in younger children (especially <8 years of age), and in injuries of the cervical spine. Postulated causes include ligamentous laxity and bony immaturity allowing excessive, transient movement during trauma, causing distraction or compression of the spinal cord, or cord ischaemia due to vascular injury or hypoperfusion. The incidence reported in children is 1–10% of all spinal cord injuries.[1,15,38,39]

Younger children tend to have more profound neurological injury, and hence less long-term improvement.[38,39] A number of children will present with minor neurological injury and progress to complete or partial spinal cord injury. The incidence of this delayed presentation of the serious symptoms is 5–50%. The delay to presentation of full symptoms has been as long as 4 days.[1,3] Because of these presentations, all children with history of neurological symptoms or any neurological deficit should be treated as patients with potential spinal cord injuries.

After the primary survey, resuscitation and secondary survey and radiographic evaluation, any patient with any neurological deficit should remain immobilised until all bony, ligamentous and spinal cord injury is

Table 24.3.5 Methylprednisolone administration in spinal cord injury			
	Time after injury		
	0–3 hours	3–8 hours	>8 hours
Initial IV dose	30 mg kg^{-1} (over 15 minutes)	30 mg kg^{-1} (over 15 minutes)	Not recommended
Maintenance IV dose	5.4 mg kg^{-1} hr^{-1}	5.4 mg kg^{-1} hr^{-1}	
Duration	24 hours	48 hours	

excluded or treated. Further investigation with a CT scan focused at the level of symptoms and MRI to view the cord should be performed. MRI provides the same prognostic information in SCIWORA injuries as in other spinal cord injuries.[15]

Controversies

❶ The clinical assessment of potential spinal injuries in the preverbal child can be very difficult.

❷ There is debate about how to adequately immobilise the cervical spine of a child less than 2 years of age.

❸ The use of flexion and extension films in the acute situation is controversial.

❹ The role of routine CT of the cervical spine in major trauma has been suggested, but needs to balanced against the radiation exposure to children.

❺ The timing of removal of spinal immobilisation in the unconscious child remains controversial.

❻ The role of methylprednisolone in spinal cord injury remains unproven despite one large study suggesting benefit.

References

1. Roche C, Carty H. Spinal trauma in children. *Pediatr Radiol* 2001;**31**(10):677–700.
2. Viccellio P, Simon H, Pressman BD, et al. A prospective multicentre study of cervical spine injury in children. *Paediatrics* 2001;**108**(2):e20.
3. Dormans JP. Evaluation of children with suspected cervical spine injury. *Instr Course Lect* 2002;**51**:401–10.
4. Reynolds R. Pediatric spinal injury. *Curr Opin Pediatr* 2000;**12**(1):67–71.
5. Jaffe DM, Binns H, Radkowski MA, et al. Developing a clinical algorithm for early management of cervical spine injury in child trauma victims. *Ann Emerg Med* 1987;**16**(3):270–6.
6. Platzer P, Jaindl M, Thalhammer G, et al. Cervical spine injuries in pediatric patients. *J Trauma-Injury Infect Crit Care* 2007;**62**(2):389–96; discussion 94–6.
7. Brandser EA, el-Khoury GY. Thoracic and lumbar spine trauma. *Radiol Clin North Am* 1997;**35**(3):533–57.
8. Jaffe DM. Evaluation of children for cervical spine injuries. In: Strange GR, editor. *Paediatric emergency medicine: a comprehensive study guide*. 2nd ed. New York: McGraw-Hill; 2002.
9. Woodward G. Neck trauma. In: Fleisher G, Ludwig S, editors. *Textbook of Paediatric Emergency Medicine*. 4th ed. Philadelphia: Lippincott Williams & Wilkins; 2000.
10. Schafermeyer RW, Ribbeck BM, Gaskins J, et al. Respiratory effects of spinal immobilisation in children. *Ann Emerg Med* 1991;**20**:1017–9.
11. Herzenberg JE, Hensinger RN, Dedrick DK, Phillips WA. Emergency transport and positioning of young children who have an injury of the cervical spine. The standard backboard may be hazardous. *J Bone Joint Surg Am* 1989;**71**(1):15–22.
12. Treloar DJ, Nypaver M. Angulation of the pediatric cervical spine with and without cervical collar. *Pediatr Emerg Care* 1997;**13**(1):5–8.
13. Curran C, Dietrich AM, Bowman MJ, et al. Pediatric cervical-spine immobilization: achieving neutral position? *J Trauma* 1995;**39**(4):729–32.
14. Anonymous. Cervical spine immobilization before admission to the hospital. *Neurosurgery* 2002;**50**(Suppl. 5):S7–17.
15. Mathison DJ, Kadom N, Krug SE. Spinal cord injury in the pediatric patient. *Clin Ped Emerg Med* 2008;**9**:106–23.
16. Quigley S, Curley M. Skin integrity in the pediatric population: preventing and managing pressure ulcers. *JSPN* 1996;**1**(1):7–18.
17. Anonymous. Management of pediatric cervical spine and spinal cord injuries. *Neurosurgery* 2002;**50**(Suppl. 3): S85–99.
18. Hoffman JR, Mower JR, Wolfson AB, et al. Validity of a set of clinical criteria to rule out injury to the cervical spine in patients with blunt trauma. *N Engl J Med* 2000;**343**:94–9.
19. Hutchings L, Willett K. Cervical spine clearance in pediatric trauma: a review of current literature. *J Trauma-Injury Infect Crit Care* 2009;**67**(4):687–91.
20. Buhs C, Cullen L, Klein M, Farmer D. The pediatric trauma C-spine: is the 'odontoid' view necessary? *J Pediatr Surg* 2000;**35**(6):994–7.
21. Swischuk LE, John SD, Hendrick EP. Is the open-mouth odontoid view necesary in children under 5 years? *Pediatr Radiol* 2000;**30**:186–9.
22. Insko E, Gracias V, Gupta R, et al. Utility of flexion and extension radiographs of the cervical spine in the acute evaluation of blunt trauma. *J Trauma* 2002;**53**:426–9.
23. Rana AR, Drongowski R, Breckner G, Ehrlich PF. Traumatic cervical spine injuries: characteristics of missed injuries. *J Pediatr Surg* 2009;**44**(1):151–5; discussion 55.
24. Berne JD, Velmahos GC, El-Tawil Q, et al. Value of complete cervical helical computed tomographic scanning in identifying cervical spine injury in the unevaluable blunt trauma patient with multiple injuries: a prospective study. *J Trauma-Injury Infect Crit Care* 1999;**47**(5):896–902; discussion 02-3.
25. Browne GJ, Cocks AJ, McCaskill ME. Current trends in the management of major paediatric trauma. *Emerg Med (Fremantle)* 2001;**13**(4):418–25.
26. Hutchings L, Atijosan O, Burgess C, Willett K. Developing a spinal clearance protocol for unconscious pediatric trauma patients. *J Trauma-Injury Infect Crit Care* 2009;**67**(4):681–6.
27. Holmes J, Mirvis S, Panacek E, et al. Variability in computed tomography and magnetic resonance imaging in patients with cervical spine injuries. *J Trauma* 2002;**53**:524–30.
28. Swischuk L. The cervical spine in childhood. *Curr Probl Diagn Radiol* 1984;**13**:1–26.
29. Kriss VM, Kriss TC. imaging of the cervical spine in infants. *Pediatr Emerg Care* 1996;**13**(1):44–9.
30. Ehrlich PF, Wee C, Drongowski R, Rana AR. Canadian C-spine Rule and the National Emergency X-Radiography Utilization Low-Risk Criteria for C-spine radiography in young trauma patients. *J Pediatr Surg* 2009; **44**(5):987–91.
31. Garton HJ, Hammer MR. Detection of pediatric cervical spine injury. *Neurosurgery* 2008;**62**(3):700–8; discussion 00-8.
32. Subach BR, McLaughlin MR, Albright AL, Pollack IF. Current management of pediatric atlantoaxial rotatory subluxation. *Spine* 1998;**23**(20):2174–9.
33. Clark P, Letts M. Trauma to the thoracic and lumbar spine in the adolescent. *Can J Surg* 2001; **44**(5):337–45.
34. Meek S. Lesson of the week: fractures of the thoracolumbar spine in major trauma patients. [comment]. *Br Med J* 1998;**317**(7170):1442–3.
35. Chiles BW, Cooper PR. Acute spinal injury. *N Engl J Med* 1996;**334**(8):514–20.
36. Anonymous. Pharmacological therapy after acute cervical spinal cord injury. *Neurosurgery* 2002; **50**(Suppl. 3):S63–72.
37. Pang D, Pollack I. Spinal cord injury without radiographic abnormality in children - The SCIWORA syndrome. *J Trauma* 1989;**29**(5):654–64.
38. Pang D, Wilberger J. Spinal cord injury without radiographic abnormalities in children. *J. Neurosurg.* 1982;**57**:114–29.
39. Anonymous. Spinal cord injury without radiographic abnormality. *Neurosurgery* 2002;**50**(Suppl. 3): S100–4.

24.4 Risk management in acute paediatric orthopaedics

Robyn Brady

ESSENTIALS

1 Inadequate identification and management of unstable or displaced injuries such as lateral condylar elbow fractures, Monteggia fracture dislocations, and slipped upper femoral epiphysis (SUFE), can cause serious long-term deformity and malfunction.

2 Immobilisation complications, from loss of position to skin ulceration or compartment syndromes, demand scrupulous departmental risk management protocols, as they often relate to 'weakest link' situations.

3 The importance of adequate initial clinical evaluation and follow up of patient or clinician concerns cannot be over-stressed.

4 A variety of departmental risk-management strategies provide a safety net for doctor and patient.

Introduction

Emergency medicine is an area of medical practice with a high rate of litigation, and orthopaedic conditions (especially missed fractures) make up a high proportion of successful claims. Many factors intrinsic to emergency medicine contribute to this danger, including high staff turnover, 24-hour practice with multiple hand-overs, wide-ranging procedural demands, and workload flux.

Just as many of the problems are systemic, so too are many of the solutions. Adverse outcomes can occur when the clinical problems discussed in this section are not recognised or dealt with adequately, and there are clear emergency department (ED) systemic interventions that can minimise their occurrence.

Adverse events in paediatric acute orthopaedics

Non-identification or delayed identification

'Missed fractures' are commonly associated with ED litigation, accounting for approximately half of ED negligence claims in the UK and Australia.[1] Articles auditing the correlation of ED doctor X-ray analysis with radiologist reporting in recent years show

that 1–2% of these reports have a discrepant concordance significant enough to alter management[2–6] although in many series there were no long-term adverse events detailed. Fractures can also be missed because of primary assessment failure (failure of thorough history or examination, therefore failure to X-ray). X-rays may be inadequate in coverage or resolution, the abnormality may be missed by the ED physician(s), or by radiologists; this too tends not to show in reported series, which presume radiology reports to be the gold standard, and there may be breakdown between radiologist reporting and ED physician notification and recall of patient. All such oversights have been specifically associated with adverse outcomes[7] and the physician responsibility for follow up and communication, which extends to ensuring that a booked follow up does actually occur, must not be overlooked.

Common or serious acute paediatric orthopaedic adverse events are shown in Table 24.4.1.

Regarding missed displaced fractures and dislocations, the following points should be considered:

❶ Anatomical distortions should be clinically apparent to patient and physician. In fact, in a series of 80 injuries with delayed identification,[5] there were

comments about pain, swelling or loss of function documented in more than 60% of cases, which had not been acted upon. In 20% of cases the doctor was alerted to the possible problem by the patient or his/her relatives.

❷ Fractures about the joint are at disproportionately high risk both for being missed and for adverse events. Although most series of fractures missed in the ED include a large array of different sites (45 fractures at 15 sites and 69 fractures at 27 sites[5] in two series not exclusively paediatric), knee injuries (tibial spine and plateau) were disproportionately represented in the former (nine fractures compared with

---

Table 24.4.1 Adverse events in acute paediatric orthopaedics

Missed displaced fracture/dislocations

- Elbow
  Supra-condylar fractures
  Lateral condyle fractures
  Monteggia fracture dislocations
  Medial epicondylar joint entrapment
- Knee
  Tibial spine
- Phalangeal fractures with angulation
- Hip
  Slipped upper femoral epiphysis (SUFE)
- Open injuries
- Fracture complications, e.g. compartment syndrome, neurovascular compromise
- High-risk patients
  Multitrauma, multiple disability

Missed undisplaced fractures

- Buckle fractures
  Proximal humerus
  Radial neck
  Distal radius and ulna
  Distal femur
- Toddler's fracture (tibial stress fracture)

Delayed identification of

- Septic arthritis
- Osteomyelitis
- Leukaemia/other neoplastic infiltration
- Congenital serious orthopaedic disorder, e.g. CDH, spinal problems

Procedural problems

- POP-related injuries
- Loss of position post-manipulation
- Mal-union
- Adverse events in association with procedural sedation

---

only one missed scaphoid fracture), and elbow injuries were disproportionately represented in paediatric adverse events. However, in all the significant paediatric elbow injuries listed as potentially missed (unstable supracondylar fracture, lateral condyle fracture, Monteggia fracture-dislocation and a trapped medial epicondyle, e.g. after elbow dislocation), elbow examination was grossly abnormal, including an effusion and a limitation of range of motion. Although the radiological Monteggia fracture-dislocation has often been missed by an untrained X-ray viewer, the clinical elbow abnormality should not be. A lack of clinical joint integrity (effusion, asymmetry cf. the other side, reduced range of movement) is an indication for early orthopaedic review even if the X-ray appears normal.

❸ Two special categories of high-risk patients deserve mention. The first is multitrauma patients,[7,8] due to several factors including urgency of other clinical problems, the possibility of an altered or distracted conscious state, and hand-over problems. The second group of note is children with complex medical conditions including autistic spectrum disorders, due to difficulties in patient communication, occasional pre-existing anatomical abnormalities, varying pain thresholds, and a need to establish base-line 'normal'. Both of these categories of patient require senior medical involvement, careful and often repeated systematic assessment and documentation.

Procedure-related problems

Problems relating to ED interventions fall into a separate category, and increase proportionally with the number and types of procedural activity undertaken in a department, which varies widely in Australia, particularly for the paediatric population. Strategies to minimise these problems are now so well described in the risk-management literature that any department planning to change procedural practice would do well to follow these guidelines (Table 24.4.2).

Table 24.4.2 Risk management strategies: acute paediatric orthopaedics

1. Training
   - Credentialing of staff for individual procedures, e.g. plastering, sedation
   - Independent learning multimedia programs, e.g. for plastering, fracture identification
   - Orthopaedic/fracture management tutorials as core resident/registrar training
2. Departmental information milieu
   - Textbooks, e.g. Keats, McRae, Gill, Swischuck, Rockwood
   - On-line 'point-of-care' clinical management guides, e.g. PEMsoft, MD consult, etc.
   - POP 'how-to' wall charts and templates
   - Paediatric fracture identification photo-chart
3. Computer-based CQI strategies
   - Computer-generated links to discharge advice, e.g. wound care, POP management, post-sedation advice
   - Automated prompt-sheets for particular presentations, e.g. injury under 2, multitrauma
   - Automated communications, e.g. faxed feedback to registered LMO
4. Procedural policies, flow-sheets, and credentialing for
   - Procedural sedation
   - Fracture/dislocation reduction
5. Departmental audits
   - X-ray results
   - Procedural sedation audit
   - Fracture reduction feedback system
   - POP quality audit/feedback system

Plaster of Paris (POP) immobilisation results in many complications: too soft; too tight; too cylindrical; inadequately immobilising; excessively immobilised; etc. At the serious end of the spectrum is the possibility of compartment syndrome. More frequent adverse outcomes include skin loss, due to internally protruding plaster shelves, or incompetent plaster saw use. Departments performing manipulations must be equipped and staffed to monitor their patients for anaesthetic adverse events, and must balance the need to avoid a tight POP with the need to maintain reduction through appropriately positioned moulding. The restriction of paediatric ED orthopaedic manipulations to experienced medical personnel, and next day follow up, may minimise problems.

References

1. Gwynne A, Barber P, Taverner F. A review of 105 negligence claims against accident and emergency departments. *J Accid Emerg Med* 1997;**14**:243–5.
2. Klein EJ, Koenig M, et al. Discordant radiograph interpretation between emergency physicians and radiologists in a paediatric emergency department. *Pediatr Emerg Care* 1999;**4**:245–8.
3. Walsh-Kelly CM, Hennes HM, Melzer-Lange MD. False-positive preliminary radiograph interpretations in a pediatric emergency department: Clinical and economic impact. *Am J Emerg Med* 1997;**15**(4):354–6.
4. Simon HK, Khan NS, Nordenberg DF, Wright JA. Paediatric emergency physician interpretation of plain radiographs: Is routine review by a radiologist necessary and cost-effective? *Ann Emerg Med* 1996;**27**(3):295–8.
5. Kremli MK. Missed musculoskeletal injuries in a university hospital in Riyadh: Types of missed injuries and responsible factors. *Injury* 1996;**27**(7):503–6.
6. Cameron MG. Missed fractures in the emergency department. *Emerg Med* 1994;**6**(1):37–9.
7. Alpers A. Key legal principles for hospitalists. *Disease Monitor* 2002;**48**(4):197–206.
8. Connors JM, Ruddy RM, McCall J, et al. Delayed diagnosis in paediatric blunt trauma. *Pediatr Emerg Care* 2001;**17**(1):1–4.

MALE GENITALIA

Section editor *Gary Browne*

25.1 Male genitalia

Colin S. Kikiros

ESSENTIALS

1 A paediatric surgeon or urologist should be contacted to assess an acute scrotum so as not to miss a testicular torsion.

2 The testicles must always be examined when boys present with abdominal pain.

3 Testicular torsion is a condition requiring urgent surgery.

4 Colour Doppler ultrasound examination and nuclear scans of the testicle may be helpful, but should not be relied upon, in the diagnosis of testicular torsion. When in doubt, exploration of the testicle is by far the safest treatment.

THE ACUTE SCROTUM

Introduction

The acute scrotum is defined as a painful and/or enlarged scrotum and may be acute or subacute in onset. The origin of the pathology may be from the testis, the groin or the scrotal skin. In a younger child, the pain will cause the child to be unsettled with crying, and it may be intractable. In an older child, the reluctance to ambulate may be a predominant feature. In addition, referred pain from a sore testis may present as abdominal pain. Therefore, in patients presenting with abdominal (especially lower-abdominal) pain one must examine the inguinal scrotal region so as not to overlook torsion of a testicle.

The diffuse vasculitis of Henoch–Schönlein purpura may affect the testis and/or scrotum. Usually other manifestations of the condition such as a skin rash or haematuria are present. A radionuclide scan may assist in differentiating this condition from torsion of the testicle.

Torsion of a testicular or epididymal appendage

Appendages of the testis and epididymis occur in 90% of testicles. Torsion of these appendages is the most common cause of testicular pain. The most common age of presentation is at the onset of puberty and this is thought to be due to the release of oestrogens and androgens from the male adrenal gland stimulating the appendages and causing them to enlarge. As the appendages are on a narrow stalk they have a tendency to twist.[1] Oedema of the appendages may also occur following trauma to the testis. Onset of the pain is usually gradual and the child is often able to ambulate without difficulty. Redness and swelling of the scrotum are also mild in the first 24 hours but may increase to an alarming degree in the following days and appearances can then be similar to those of testicular torsion. The scrotal swelling is often due to a small secondary hydrocele. The testis is usually normally aligned and in normal position in the scrotum. Tenderness is maximal at the upper pole of the testis (where the appendage is located) and a blue dot may be seen through the skin at the upper pole consistent with an infarcted appendage.

Torsion of the testis

This is an acute emergency and is due, in most situations, to medial rotation of the spermatic cord. However, in one-third of cases the testis rotates in a lateral direction.[2] The torsion usually occurs spontaneously. However, sometimes it can follow direct trauma to the testis. The pain is likely to be acute and severe and may be associated with nausea or vomiting. The older child is often reluctant to ambulate. Often there is a history of previous short-lived pain in a testis consistent with intermittent episodes of spontaneously resolving torsion. The testis is usually enlarged and in a high position in the scrotum or even in the groin. It is not usually in its normal lie and there is much redness and swelling of the scrotal skin. Usually a secondary hydrocele is present. The contralateral testicle may lie in a bell-clapper fashion owing to the insertion of the epididymis in the central part of the testicle and this in turn predisposes the testicle to undergo torsion. The child should be taken to the operating theatre urgently, even if the child is not adequately fasted, as prolonged obstruction of the testicular vessels may lead to partial or complete atrophy of the testicle. Therefore nuclear scans and colour Doppler ultrasound should be avoided if the diagnosis is clear, as these investigations may result in unnecessary delay and they are not reliable. False negatives and false positives have been reported with both modalities. Colour Doppler ultrasonography may be misleading as intratesticular flow may be seen even in testicles that have undergone torsion.[3] Visualisation of a twist in the cord is more reliable.[4] Survival of the testicle will depend on the number of twists that the spermatic cord has undergone, along with the length of time that the cord has been twisted, with the prognosis being excellent for those undergoing surgery within 6 hours of the onset of symptoms.[5,6]

Epididymo-orchitis

Infection or inflammation may affect the epididymis or the testis. Infections in the epididymis may arise from retrograde flow along the vas deferens or lymphatics from urinary tract infections, or from the bloodstream. Inflammation of the testis may arise from conditions such as mumps. The epididymis is tender and swollen and the testis also may be tender. The testis is of normal lie and in a normal position in the scrotum. A raised interleukin-6 level may be clinically helpful in assisting the diagnosis of epididymitis.[7] Once the diagnosis has been confirmed the child's urine should be sent for analysis and he should then be commenced on antibiotics. Enteric organisms are the usual cause of the urinary tract infection.[8] Once the condition has resolved renal ultrasound and micturating cystourethrogram should be performed as the urine infection may have resulted from an abnormality in the urinary tract, such as posterior urethral valves.[9]

Idiopathic scrotal oedema

The cause of this condition is unknown. The child presents with scrotal discomfort, oedema and erythema of one side of the scrotum, which may spread to affect the entire scrotum, the penis and inguinal and perineal regions. The testis is not swollen and is normally aligned and the tenderness arises from the palpably thickened scrotal wall. Occasionally, eosinophilia may occur and, characteristically, ultrasound examination shows marked thickening of the scrotal wall, increased peri-testicular blood flow and a mild reactive hydrocele.[10] The condition resolves in 1–4 days and no treatment, apart from pain relief, is required.

Testicular tumours

Primary or secondary (leukaemia, for example) tumours may cause the testicle to enlarge and become painful. The onset is usually gradual and the pain more chronic. However, tumours may present acutely when they have been subjected to trauma. The testicle may become extremely large, although the scrotal skin is not usually erythematous. Ultrasound and full blood picture may aid in the diagnosis. Paediatric surgeons and oncologists are predominantly required in managing these patients.[11]

Irreducible inguinal hernia

Segments of intestine may on occasions descend into a hernia sac in the scrotum and become irreducible. Acute pain may be felt in the scrotum and also in the groin (see Chapter 7.11 on herniae).

Rupture of the testis

This is usually the result of trauma. The testis becomes enlarged and painful and there is associated bruising and frequently an associated hydrocele. Ultrasound examination often reveals irregularity of the testicular outline and intratesticular haematoma.[12] The patient should be referred to a surgeon for exploration and repair of the testicle.

Acute hydrocele

A patent processus vaginalis may allow intraperitoneal fluid to flow into the space around the testicle in the scrotum. Often the amount of fluid is minimal and the patient does not present acutely. Occasionally, however, intercurrent illnesses, such as gastroenteritis and upper respiratory tract infections, may result in an increase in volume of the peritoneal fluid. This leads to an increase in the amount of fluid around the testis and the patient may present to the ED with a large scrotal swelling. The testis in this situation is not painful and one can determine that the swelling does not extend into the groin. Ultrasound examination is useful in confirming the diagnosis and unnecessary surgery can be avoided.

ACUTE PROBLEMS OF THE PENIS AND FORESKIN

ESSENTIALS

1 Urinary retention may arise from phimosis or balanitis and requires urgent urinary diversion or circumcision.

2 Priapism is an acute emergency and requires urgent treatment.

Introduction

Currently, approximately 90% of young males in Australia are not circumcised. This compares to a generation ago, when the majority of males were circumcised, often in the neonatal period. As a result, problems with the foreskin are increasing and patients are often referred to the emergency department for treatment.

Parents are often unsure of the correct management of the foreskin. In most cases the foreskin should be left alone until the age of 5 or 6 and then should be retracted gently to clean the under surface of the foreskin and the glans. If the foreskin cannot be retracted easily, the use of a mild steroid ointment for a short period may correct the phimosis. If this is not successful, circumcision may be required.

Phimosis of the foreskin

In this condition the foreskin cannot be easily retracted and in the more severe cases the outflow of urine is significantly obstructed. Ballooning of the foreskin may occur with micturition when the urine flow into the foreskin space is greater than the flow exiting out of the foreskin. Urinary tract infections,[13] dysuria and possibly urinary retention may develop.[14]

A sample of urine and swabs from the foreskin should be obtained and the patient should be commenced on intravenous or oral antibiotics. In cases of urinary retention, urinary diversion may be required. For example, a suprapubic catheter may need to be inserted under general anaesthesia. Alternatively, urgent circumcision can treat the condition.[14]

In mild cases of phimosis, the application of half-strength Betnovate® ointment to the tip of the foreskin for 6 weeks has a reported success of 75–88%.[14,15]

Balanitis

This condition usually arises when phimosis of the foreskin is present and infection has occurred in the space under the foreskin. Bacteria, often enteral or cutaneous in origin, migrate into this space and as they cannot be washed away, infection results. This is frequently a subacute or chronic condition, but on occasions can be acute.

Again a sample of urine and swabs of the foreskin should be obtained and the patient should be commenced on IV or oral antibiotics. The condition usually subsides within a few days. However, in the long term, circumcision may be required.[16]

Balanitis xerotica obliterans, also called lichen sclerosus et atrophicus, is thought to be an autoimmune condition affecting the foreskin and glans. It leads to irreversible phimosis of the foreskin and presents with inability to retract the foreskin and varying degrees of urinary obstruction. It is best treated with circumcision, as studies using topical steroid treatment have failed to show any permanent improvement.[17,18]

Paraphimosis

On occasions the foreskin may be tight but the child, or parent, may have attempted to retract it and not returned it to its normal position. Oedema of the foreskin distal to the tight ring can develop and the foreskin can become painfully swollen and difficult to reduce.

The foreskin is more easily reduced the sooner that the patient is treated.[19] The patient should be given appropriate analgesia and gentle digital pressure should be used on the foreskin through saline-soaked gauze. Once some of the oedema has been dispersed the foreskin should be gently replaced in its normal position. If this is not possible the child will need to be seen by a paediatric surgeon, who may attempt the same procedure. If this again fails, the foreskin should be reduced under a general anaesthetic. Some surgeons favour circumcision whilst the child is anaesthetised so as to avoid another anaesthetic in the future.

Alternative methods described to reduce the paraphimosis are the use of hyaluronidase[20] and puncture technique[21] whereby the oedematous foreskin is punctured in several places with an 18-gauge hypodermic needle to evacuate the oedema so as to allow for easy reduction of the foreskin.

Priapism

This is an acute emergency. Low-flow priapism is due to obstruction of venous outflow from the penis. It may occur spontaneously or it can be secondary to medication, sickle cell disease or leukaemia. Uncontrolled arterial inflow, usually caused by direct trauma to the penis or perineum, results in high-flow priapism. Both types of priapism result in a painful, sustained erection. Urgent referral to a paediatric surgeon or urologist is required for immediate treatment or surgery. In the meantime, perineal compression should be attempted as it may successfully reverse high-flow priapism.[22] If this fails, colour Doppler ultrasonography of the corpora cavernosa can reveal a blood leak. Bilateral internal pudendal arteriography and embolisation can then follow.[23,24] Intracavernous injections of etilefrine can be effective in reducing priapism in children with acute sickle-cell crisis.[25] Failure to resolve the condition in a timely manner may result in permanent inability to have erections and/or penile fibrosis.[26]

References

1. Samnakay N, Cohen RJ, Orford J, et al. Androgen and oestrogen receptor status of the human appendix testis. *Pediatr Surg Int* 2003;**19**:520–4.
2. Sessions AE, Rabinowitz R, Hulbert WC, et al. Testicular torsion: Direction, degree, duration and disinformation. *J Urol* 2003;**169**:663–5.
3. Nussbaum Blask AR, Bulas D, Shalaby-Rana E, et al. Color Doppler sonography and scintigraphy of the testis: A prospective, comparative analysis in children with acute scrotal pain. *Pediatr Emerg Care* 2002;**18**:67–71.
4. Arce JD, Cortes M, Vargas JC. Sonographic diagnosis of acute spermatic cord torsion. Rotation of the cord: A key to the diagnosis. *Pediatr Radiol* 2002;**32**:485–91.
5. Dunne PJ, O'Loughlin BS. Testicular torsion: Time is the enemy. *Aust N Z J Surg* 2000;**70**:441–2 [comment].
6. Rampaul MS, Hosking SW. Testicular torsion: Most delay occurs outside the hospital. *Ann R Coll Surg Engl* 1998;**80**:169–72.
7. Rivers KK, Rivers EP, Stricker HJ, et al. The clinical utility of serologic markers in the evaluation of the acute scrotum. *Acad Emerg Med* 2000;**7**:1069–72.
8. McAndrew HF, Pemberton R, Kikiros CS, Gollow I. The incidence and investigation of acute scrotal problems in children. *Pediatr Surg Int* 2002;**18**:435–7.
9. Ng JW, Chan AY, Kong CK, Wong MK. Posterior urethral valves presenting as acute epididymo-orchitis: A case report and follow-up study. *Aust N Z J of Surg* 1996;**66**:129–30.
10. Klin B, Lotan G, Efrati Y, et al. Acute idiopathic scrotal edema in children – revisited. *J Pediatr Surg* 2002;**37**:1200–2.
11. Nichols CR. Testicular cancer. *Curr Probl Cancer* 1998;**22**:187–274.
12. Micallef M, Ahmad I, Ramesh N, et al. Ultrasound features of blunt testicular injury. *Injury* 2001;**32**:23–6.
13. Hiraoka M, Tsukahara H, Ohshima Y, Mayumi M. Meatus tightly covered by the prepuce is associated with urinary tract infection. *Pediatr Int* 2002;**44**:658–62.
14. Ashfield JE, Nickel KR, Siemens DR, et al. Treatment of phimosis with topical steroids in 194 children. *J Urol* 2003;**169**:1106–8.
15. Kikiros CS, Beasley SW, Woodward AA. The response of phimosis to local steroid application. *Pediatr Surg Int* 1993;**8**:329–33.
16. Escala JM, Rickwood AM. Balanitis. *Br J Urol* 1989;**63**:196–7.
17. Webster TM, Leonard MP. Topical steroid therapy for phimosis. *Can J Urol* 2002;**9**:1492–5.
18. Meuli M, Briner J, Hanimann B, Sacher P. Lichen sclerosus et atrophicus causing phimosis in boys: A prospective study with 5 year followup after complete circumcision. *J Urol* 1994;**152**:987–9.
19. Choe JM. Paraphimosis: Current treatment options. *Am Fam Physician* 2000;**62**:2623–8.
20. Devries CR, Miller AK, Packer MG. Reduction of paraphimosis with hyaluronidase. *Urology* 1997;**48**:464–5.
21. Fuenfer MM, Najmaldin A. Emergency reduction of paraphimosis. *Eur J Pediatr Surg* 1994;**4**:370–1.
22. Hatzichristou D, Salpiggidis G, Hatzimouratidis K, et al. Management strategy for arterial priapism: Therapeutic dilemmas. *J Urol* 2002;**168**:2074–7.
23. Volkmer BG, Nesslauer T, Kraemer SC, et al. Prepubertal high flow priapism: Incidence, diagnosis and treatment. *J Urol* 2001;**166**:1018–22.
24. Shankar KR, Babar S, Rowlands P, Jones MO. Posttraumatic high-flow priapism: Treatment with selective embolisation. *Pediatr Surg Int* 2000;**16**:454–6.
25. Gbadoe AD, Atakouma Y, Kusiaku K, Assimadi JK. Management of sickle cell priapism with etilefrine. *Arch Dis Child* 2001;**85**:52–3.
26. El-Bahnasawy MS, Dawood A, Farouk A. Low-flow priapism: Risk factors for erectile dysfunction. *BJU Int* 2002;**89**:285–90.

26.1 Acute neonatal emergencies

Paul Craven • Elly Marillier

ESSENTIALS

1 Early recognition, appropriate treatment and referral for definitive care are key to a good outcome in the sick neonate. Recognising the signs of respiratory distress in newborns and infants allows for appropriate acute management in the ED.

2 Ensuring appropriate resuscitation equipment is available for the newborn infant, with a knowledge of drug doses, is essential to appropriately manage acute cardiorespiratory arrest.

3 In the crying neonate, determine whether this presentation is part of a recurrent stereotypical pattern in an otherwise well infant, or a single acute episode. A careful history and examination will often lead to an appropriate diagnosis. Screening tests, with the exception of urine culture, have little utility. Review carefully the carer's coping skills and supports and organise appropriate follow up.

4 Recognition of peripheral versus central cyanosis in a newborn infant is essential as central cyanosis requires urgent evaluation. Respiratory and cardiac causes of cyanosis must be differentiated. Despite the majority of causes being cardiorespiratory it is important to recognise the other subtle causes of cyanosis that can affect this age group.

5 Neonatal seizures are relatively common and generally reactive in nature, and thus should not be labelled as neonatal epilepsy. Their presence is often a sign of neurological dysfunction and this should be fully investigated. The majority of neonatal seizures occur in the early neonatal period (day 1–7 of life). Neonatal seizures are often subtle; they may be missed, and are sometimes hard to differentiate from more benign movement disorders.

6 Persistent vomiting, if found in the neonate, requires full investigation. Bilious vomiting in the neonate is a surgical emergency until proven otherwise.

7 Sepsis remains the most common cause for the collapsed neonate in the emergency department.

8 In the collapsed newborn consider sepsis first then look for clues of other rarer underlying disorders if there is a poor clinical response to treatment.

9 The key to resuscitation of the newborn is adequate ventilation.

NEONATAL EMERGENCIES

Studies have indicated that shorter post-partum hospital stays have resulted in an increased attendance at the emergency department (ED) of newborn infants and those in the first month of life. The common presenting symptoms and signs were jaundice, poor feeding, breathing difficulties and irritability.

The underlying common pathologies were found to be physiological jaundice, feeding problems and suspected sepsis.

Maternal experience, social support, early postnatal discharge and perinatal instruction influenced presentation to the ED.

The infant with breathing difficulty

Respiratory emergencies are some of the commonest conditions presenting in the neonatal period. The increased work of breathing is manifested as:

- tachypnoea (RR >60 breaths per minute);
- intercostal and subcostal recession (excessive use of accessory muscles of respiration);
- flaring of the alae nares (accessory muscles of respiration);

- grunting (forced glottic closure to create positive end expiratory pressure);
- cyanosis (>5 g dL^{-1} of desaturated haemoglobin);
- apnoea (a pause in breathing of >20 seconds or a pause of less than 20 seconds associated with bradycardia);
- tracheal tug.

The causes of respiratory distress are varied and are summarised in Table 26.1.1. They can be broadly divided into primary respiratory and non-respiratory causes. Primary respiratory pathology is a direct result of upper, lower or mixed airway pathology.

This section will discuss:

- emergencies of the upper airway;
- emergencies of the lung parenchyma;
- non-pulmonary causes affecting the lung parenchyma;
- the at-risk neonate.

Upper airway obstruction

Causes

Of all cases of upper airway obstruction presenting in the neonatal period, 60% are congenital and 40% are acquired. Causes of upper airway obstruction include choanal atresia, micrognathia, macroglossia, laryngomalacia, vocal cord anomalies and tracheomalacia. There are many rare causes.

Clinical features

Stridor is the classic presenting sign of upper airway obstruction and is a rare phenomenon in the neonatal period. Stridor is an indication of partial obstruction of the large diameter airways, from either an intrinsic developmental defect or from secondary external compression and distortion. Stridor is the inspiratory noise that indicates this partial obstruction and early referral to an ear, nose and throat specialist should be considered. In addition to the stridor, infants often have an associated degree of respiratory distress, but may have a normal or hyper-expanded chest radiograph.

Investigations

These will be guided by the history and examination findings. Infants with severe stridor and respiratory distress should be urgently transported to a tertiary care centre, where intensive-care support can be continued by qualified personnel. Airway support may involve precise positioning, continuous positive airways pressure or intubation, which can prove an extremely difficult procedure in this setting. Imaging studies, including plain radiographs, computerised tomography (CT) and magnetic resonance imaging (MRI), are useful in specific clinical situations, based on the possible differential diagnosis. Other diagnostic techniques employed include barium swallow and laryngobroncho-oesophagoscopy (LBO).

Management

The management of upper airway obstruction requires the expertise of an ear, nose and throat specialist, and can range from conservative management, in laryngomalacia, ensuring adequate growth and development, to the requirement for a tracheotomy in bilateral vocal cord paralysis.

Respiratory distress attributed to lung parenchyma pathology

Causes

Respiratory distress secondary to lower respiratory tract involvement may be a significant feature of either congenital or acquired parenchymal lung disease.

Acquired conditions likely to present in the ED include pneumonia, either viral or bacterial. The commonest viral presentation is bronchiolitis secondary to respiratory syncytial virus. Other parenchymal diseases include pulmonary oedema, due to either an underlying pulmonary or cardiac anomaly.

Associated with underlying parenchymal anomalies the risks of pneumothorax are increased, once again exacerbating the respiratory distress.

Congenital anomalies that may present include cystic malformations of the lung, lobar emphysema or pleural effusions secondary to an underlying lymphatic pathology.

The causes of respiratory failure may be divided into two forms, common and uncommon:

Common

- Respiratory distress syndrome (RDS), transient tachypnoea of the newborn (TTN).
- Meconium aspiration (MAS).
- Pneumonia/sepsis.
- Drug-induced respiratory depression.
- Bronchiolitis.
- Air-leak syndrome (pneumothorax).
- Congestive heart failure.

Table 26.1.1 General causes of respiratory distress	
General causes of respiratory distress	**Specific conditions**
Respiratory disorders	Hyaline membrane disease Congenital pneumonia Meconium aspiration syndrome Transient tachypnoea of the newborn Pneumothorax Hydro/haemothorax
Upper airway abnormalities	Laryngomalacia Micrognathia Vocal cord anomalies
Cardiac anomalies	Heart failure Myocarditis Pericardial effusion Cyanotic congenital heart conditions
Structural abnormalities	Diaphragmatic hernia Congenital cystic lesions Diaphragmatic paralysis
Chest deformities	Arthrogryposis Thoracic dystrophy
Haematological causes	Anaemia
CNS lesions	Infection
Metabolic conditions	Metabolic acidosis

Uncommon

- Diaphragmatic hernia.
- Congenital airway abnormalities, such as choanal atresia.
- Pulmonary hypoplasia.
- Cystic adenomatoid malformation.
- Pulmonary haemorrhage.

Clinical features

History

In respiratory distress attributed to parenchymal involvement, a clinical history is essential to elucidate potential predisposing factors. Of the causes of parenchymal disease presenting to the ED, pneumonia and extra-pulmonary cardiac failure are the two most common causes. These can often be differentiated by clinical history.

Bacterial pneumonia in the first few hours of life may be impossible to distinguish from respiratory distress syndrome or transient tachypnoea of the newborn. Therefore, respiratory distress in newborns generally should be treated as bacterial pneumonia until proven otherwise. When associated with chorioamnionitis, it is caused most commonly by Group B streptococci (GBS) or by *Escherichia coli*. However, *Haemophilus influenzae*, *Streptococcus pneumoniae* (pneumococcus), Group D streptococci, *Listeria* and anaerobes have also been described as pathogens in this setting. Infants infected with these organisms are often preterm and have very early onset of respiratory distress. Of note, infants may also develop bacterial pneumonia transnatally in the absence of maternal chorioamnionitis. Here, the causative organism is likely to be GBS, and the onset of symptoms tends to occur 12–24 hours after birth.

Neonatal pneumonia can be either congenital or acquired. Congenital pneumonia commences before birth and the most common infecting organisms include Group B *Streptococcus* and *E. coli*. Despite the majority of infants being unwell at birth, some infants do acquire these infections after birth and present with similar signs and symptoms of respiratory distress, poor feeding, fever and apnoea. The clinical history should focus on the maternal Group B *Streptococcus* carriage in pregnancy, length of rupture of membranes, maternal antibiotic therapy during labour and maternal fever. Acquired neonatal pneumonias are

commonly viral, with respiratory syncytial virus, adenovirus and parainfluenza virus all commonly identified. A history of affected family members gives some indication of this potential.

Any infant with underlying lung pathology is at risk of air leak, and any sudden decompensation in an infant with respiratory distress should lead one to consider this diagnosis. In addition, air leak can be a spontaneous phenomenon with no identified cause.

Non-infectious causes of acquired respiratory distress include any conditions in which there is an abnormally high or low blood flow to the lungs, an increased demand for oxygen, or a decreased number of red blood cells.

The commonest non-pulmonary cause of respiratory distress seen in the ED is that of pulmonary oedema, secondary to congenital heart disease.

Congenital heart disease is one of the commonest malformations, with an incidence of 0.6%. Although 30–60% of congenital heart disease is identified antenatally, this still leaves a large percentage presenting in the postnatal period. Predischarge saturation monitoring of all newborn infants has the possibility of increasing the early identification of congenital heart disease, prior to the onset of respiratory distress, cyanosis or collapse. Cyanotic lesions generally present early but neonates with ductal-dependent systemic circulations are often well in the early neonatal period and collapse around day 4 of life. Closure of the ductus, with associated systemic collapse, is one of the commonest presentations to the ED with severe respiratory distress, secondary to associated pulmonary oedema.

Factors in the history pointing towards congenital heart disease being the cause of collapse include a family history, syndromic malformations and associated abnormalities.

In addition to predisposing factors, a history of poor feeding often predates the collapse.

Other causes of respiratory distress presenting in the ED are:

- inborn errors of metabolism, with associated acidosis, a family history, consanguinity or an abnormal smell noted from the infant;
- central nervous system anomalies;
- non-accidental injury.

Examination

Infants with disease affecting the lung parenchyma, either primary respiratory or cardiac, generally present with the classical examination findings of respiratory distress, notably: recession of the intercostal and subcostal spaces; nasal flaring; tachypnoea (>60 bpm); and expiratory grunting.

Nasal flaring is a result of the alae nasi being the first muscles to be activated during inspiration and they aim to decrease airway resistance. The recession of the inter- and subcostal spaces is a result of the compliance of the chest wall being reduced in neonates. During inspiration the pleural pressure is reduced, but in neonates with parenchymal lung disease this needs to be reduced more than normal and thus the consequences are that the compliant chest wall may cave in as a result of these more negative pressures. The recession in conjunction with the abdominal protuberance associated with diaphragmatic descent give the characteristic seesaw pattern of neonatal respiratory distress.

Infants with respiratory infections may present in a very similar manner to those with cardiac anomalies. Specific findings for infants with pneumonia may be the presence of fever or temperature instability, feed intolerance and rhinorrhoea.

If there is a suggestion of pulmonary air leak, the clinical signs are specific. There will be reduced air entry on the side of the leak, with a reduction in chest movement on that side. Percussion, although seldom used in newborn infants, should be hyper-resonant and if the air leak is under tension there may be associated displacement of the trachea and apex beat to the contralateral side.

If a primary respiratory cause cannot be identified, non-respiratory causes should be sought. Signs indicative of congenital heart disease may include weak femoral pulses, an active praecordial impulse, hepatomegaly and a cardiac murmur.

The classic cardiac lesions presenting with respiratory distress in the neonatal period include:

❶ Left to right shunting lesions (atrioventriculoseptal defects (AVSD) and ventriculoseptal defects (VSD)). Typically, large VSDs present between weeks 2 and 4 of life after the pulmonary pressures have reduced and this allows increased left to right flow with resultant pulmonary oedema. The infant will present with increasing tachypnoea, recession and poor feeding, in association with a loud cardiac murmur and crepitations audible in the chest.

❷ Duct-dependent obstructive left ventricle conditions (hypoplastic left heart, critical aortic stenosis and coarctation of the aorta). Once the ductus arteriosus closes around week 1 of life, the systemic circulation is no longer maintained. Infants present shocked, pale and with severe respiratory distress. Specifically they have weak femoral pulses and invariably a large liver.

With other causes of respiratory distress there may be features consistent with specific diagnoses. Metabolic conditions are often associated with hepatosplenomegaly, coma, hypoglycaemia and jaundice. Central nervous system (CNS) lesions may have seizures associated.

Investigations

Any infant in the first month of life with respiratory distress should be observed and monitored closely. This includes pulse rate, oxygen saturation, respiratory rate, temperature, blood pressure and capillary refill time.

The normal heart rate for a neonate in the first month of life is 120–160 bpm. Some newborn infants, however, have a resting heart rate below 90 bpm. Respiratory distress is generally associated with respiratory rate greater than 60 breaths per minute. Fever as a sign of sepsis is variable.

Plain radiographs of the chest are useful, but do not generally differentiate the various causes of respiratory distress. Sepsis and cardiac failure both demonstrate increased interstitial markings. In cardiac failure, fluid more specifically radiates into the interstitium from the hilum and in severe cases may be associated with an effusion. Again, in cardiac disease the size of the cardiac shadow may be increased. A cardiac silhouette greater than 60% of the transthoracic diameter is indicative of cardiac disease and needs to be investigated further, by means of an electrocardiogram and echocardiogram, and referral to a cardiologist.

The chest radiograph of an infant with pneumonia may show lobar or diffuse interstitial changes. Chest radiographs of infants who have bacterial pneumonia may exhibit a diffuse reticular nodular appearance but, in contrast to respiratory distress syndrome, they tend to show normal or increased lung volumes with possible focal or coarse densities. There may also be pleural effusions, particularly with GBS pneumonia. In the newborn who has bacterial pneumonia, blood cultures obtained before the initiation of antibiotics commonly grow the offending organism. Cultures of urine and cerebrospinal fluid should be obtained at the time of the blood culture if a newborn infant is systemically unwell. If the diagnosis is viral, mucus plugging, with over-aeration and hyperexpansion may be characteristic. Although tension pneumothorax should be a clinical diagnosis, the plain radiograph is good at demonstrating small pneumothoraces. An anterior pneumothorax may be subtle and easily missed by the unwary as appearing more lucent on the side of the pneumothorax in the absence of a lateral air meniscus.

Laboratory investigations, including full blood count, C-reactive protein (CRP) and blood cultures, are useful adjuncts to the diagnosis. The white cell count may show a leucocytosis with associated left shift or, more commonly, may show a consumptive picture with neutropenia and associated thrombocytopenia in the septic infant. The CRP is another non-specific marker of infection, but appears more useful in monitoring response to treatment of infection rather than in its diagnosis.

If a viral respiratory tract infection is suspected then a nasopharyngeal sample viewed with electron microscopy for respiratory viruses may reveal the common causes of bronchiolitis.

Arterial blood gas analysis or indirect transcutaneous monitoring may reveal arterial hypoxaemia and hypercarbia. The degree of hypoxaemia and acidosis will be a guide to the need for respiratory positive pressure support. In addition to diagnosing the severity of the respiratory acidosis, an arterial blood gas may also reveal a metabolic acidosis, making inborn errors of metabolism a potential differential diagnosis of the respiratory distress.

Management

A neonate with respiratory distress needs to be observed closely. Evaluation of airway, breathing and circulation are imperative, as outlined in the resuscitation guidelines devised by the International Liaison Committee on Resuscitation (ILCOR). Maintaining a neutral airway position and ensuring the airway is free of obstruction allows optimal oxygen to be delivered. Saturations should be maintained with either nasal cannulae oxygen, head box oxygen, continuous positive airways pressure or endotracheal intubation and ventilation. If working in a hospital with a Neonatal Intensive Care Unit or Paediatric Intensive Care Unit, support from personnel working in these areas can be invaluable in maintaining a patent airway.

If sepsis is suspected then intravenous antibiotics should be commenced, to cover both Gram-positive and Gram-negative bacteria and an evaluation made of the need for both fluid and inotropic support. Empiric treatment should be initiated as soon as possible with ampicillin 100 mg kg^{-1} day^{-1} divided every 12 hours (infants <1.2 kg) or every 8 hours (infants >1.2 kg) and cefotaxime 100 mg kg^{-1} day^{-1} divided every 12 hours or 150 mg kg^{-1} day^{-1} divided every 8 hours (infants >1.2 kg and >7 days old). Gentamicin is an alternative treatment, particularly when there is no evidence of meningitis. Treatment should be continued for at least 10 days if sepsis is present, although 14–21 days may be required, particularly for Gram-negative infections.

Viral infections are treated conservatively by respiratory and circulatory support as required. An unusual or unresponsive neonatal presentation of pneumonia warrants further evaluation. The maternal history may offer important clues. Neonatal pneumonia involving cytomegalovirus (CMV) or other viruses may be transmitted transplacentally. CMV pneumonia may not require treatment in the otherwise healthy infant. However, neonatal respiratory distress in the setting of perinatal exposure to herpes simplex virus, particularly if there is primary maternal genital infection, warrants treatment with aciclovir 30 mg kg^{-1} day^{-1} divided every 8 hours for 14–21 days until all cultures are negative. *Ureaplasma urealyticum* is another important organism and treatment of *Ureaplasma* infections in the newborn should include erythromycin 50 mg kg^{-1} day^{-1} divided every 6 hours.

If the cause of the respiratory distress is believed to be cardiac then once again supporting the airway, breathing and circulation is imperative. Added caution with fluid resuscitation should be considered so as not to exacerbate the cardiac failure. Use of prostaglandin E1 allows reopening of the ductus and increased systemic circulation. This is a temporising measure prior to the definitive surgery the infant may require.

Management of a pneumothorax requires either acute drainage with needle thoracocentesis, in the presence of a tension pneumothorax, or intercostal catheter insertion followed by appropriate underwater drainage. A repeat chest X-ray (CXR) to ensure adequate lung expansion is required prior to the removal of the chest drain.

The blue infant

Neonatal cyanosis is a result of deoxygenated blood in the systemic circulation. It is defined as an arterial saturation less than 90%.

History, examination and simple investigations available in the ED should be able to distinguish the cause of the cyanosis and this will predict the management of this condition.

Causes

Babies can be peripherally blue or centrally blue and this is important in differentiating the cause of the cyanosis. Peripheral cyanosis, affecting the hands and feet, known as acrocyanosis is a normal phenomenon that generally clears within 1–2 days and needs no treatment. Central cyanosis, evidenced by cyanosis of the gums and mucous membranes is generally pathological and needs urgent evaluation if presenting in the ED. Babies can be centrally cyanosed for many reasons including heart disease, lung or other breathing problems, being cold, or having seizures. Not all children who turn blue have a heart problem. A thorough history, examination and simple investigations will be able to differentiate these causes of central cyanosis.

Non-respiratory causes of cyanosis
- Cardiac defects:
  - Decreased pulmonary blood flow
  - Admixture lesions
  - Congestive heart failure (pulmonary congestion).
- Primary pulmonary hypertension of the newborn.
- Central nervous system disease:
  - Intracranial haemorrhage
  - Maternal sedative administration
  - Meningitis.
- Methaemoglobinaemia.
- Hypoglycaemia.
- Sepsis.
- Cold.

Clinical features
History
Once cyanosis has been diagnosed in an infant presenting to the ED, the most important step is to differentiate between pulmonary and cardiac causes of cyanosis.

Pulmonary causes of cyanosis include pneumonia, both bacterial and viral, pneumothorax, pleural effusions and airway anomalies. If the cause of the cyanosis is felt to be pulmonary, the infant will generally have a history of worsening respiratory distress that interferes with the infant's ability to feed successfully. The history may be indicative of an infective cause, with rhinorrhoea, fever, cough, poor feeding and worsening recession of the inter- and subcostal spaces. In addition, there may be a history of other affected family members and respiratory infections are generally more prominent in the winter months especially associated with epidemics of bronchiolitis.

Infants with cardiac causes of cyanosis may have no preceding history and generally breathe normally. A detailed antenatal history, including family history, genetic abnormalities and the results of antenatal ultrasound scans, will be important. In addition, the timing of the cyanosis may also give a clue to the diagnosis, with duct-dependent cardiac lesions generally worsening when the ductus arteriosus shuts around day 3 or 4 of life. Although congenital heart disease is generally divided into cyanotic and acyanotic, those lesions generally classified as acyanotic but duct dependent can present with severe respiratory distress and a degree of cyanosis.

In addition to congenital heart disease and pulmonary causes, an infant may present cyanosed because they have neurological depression or seizures. A history of the infant's general activity, tone and feeding patterns will be helpful. Infants with neurological depression may be hypotonic, have abnormal autonomic responses and have poor feeding with associated failure to thrive and may indeed have seizure activity.

Once again, if seizures are suspected then a detailed family history may indicate a genetic syndrome as the cause of the seizures. A thorough history of the pregnancy and delivery is also important to rule out other causes of seizures, and early checking for hypoglycaemia is essential. Considering neonatal sepsis is always imperative and a detailed history of maternal substance abuse may indicate drug withdrawal as the cause of the seizures.

Examination
Once a detailed history has been taken to elicit possible causes of cyanosis then the infant should be examined carefully.

Infants with respiratory causes for cyanosis will generally have signs of distress, namely tachypnoea, recession of the intercostal and subcostal spaces, tracheal tug, nasal flaring and expiratory grunting. As to the precise respiratory cause of this distress, septic infants often have an associated tachycardia and may have temperature instability. They may have poor capillary return and may also have associated apnoeas, a pause in breathing of greater than 20 seconds or a pause in breathing less than 20 seconds but associated with bradycardia. Infants who are septic and cyanosed may have localised respiratory infections, such as viral bronchiolitis, or may be septicaemic.

A cyanosed infant with little or no respiratory distress is more likely to have congenital heart disease. The commonest lesions presenting with cyanosis in the neonatal period are: transposition of the great arteries; total anomalous pulmonary venous return; pulmonary atresia with an intact ventricular septum; severe pulmonary stenosis; and severe tetralogy of Fallot.

Examination of a cyanosed infant with suspected cardiac disease might reveal dysmorphic features suggesting a syndromic association with congenital heart disease. Auscultation of the lung fields and praecordium may reveal evidence of pulmonary oedema and murmurs, and an abdominal examination may reveal hepatomegaly.

To differentiate an infant with non-cardiopulmonary causes for the cyanosis, the examination would need to concentrate on the neurological system of the infant. Tone, movements and reflexes will all give important information as to the neurological status. Examination for dysmorphic features and examination of the fundi and skin may add important information as to the cause of the seizures. In the neonatal period, important causes of seizures would include hypoxia, hypoglycaemia and biochemical anomalies, narcotic withdrawal and structural brain abnormalities.

Investigations

To differentiate the various causes of cyanosis in the neonatal period a full set of observations should be performed. Oxygen saturations should be performed initially in room air to serve as a baseline. Subsequent oxygen measures should be performed in 100% oxygen, achieved by means of a headbox sealed over the baby's head and neck. The so-called hyperoxia test may help to differentiate cyanotic heart disease from other causes of neonatal cyanosis. Infants with neurological or pulmonary causes of the cyanosis will demonstrate substantial increases in the arterial blood saturation, while infants with cyanotic congenital heart disease will show minimal elevation. As well as oxygen saturation changes, the difference should be confirmed with arterial blood gas analysis of arterial oxygen partial pressures. A partial pressure <100 mmHg in 100% inspired oxygen is more indicative of cardiac disease.

Once arterial oxygen saturations and blood gas analysis have been performed the infant should have a chest radiograph. Abnormalities of the lung fields may suggest a primary pulmonary cause for the cyanosis or a cardiac cause if the changes are suggestive of pulmonary oedema with increased vascular markings.

Assessing the cardiothoracic diameter and shape of the cardiac shadow may give some clues to a cardiac cause of the cyanosis. A typical boot-shaped heart is classically described in tetralogy of Fallot and an egg on a string appearance is described in transposition of the great arteries. Generally differentiating the cardiac causes of cyanosis is difficult and requires an echocardiogram. Additional investigations that may be useful

in the diagnosis of neonatal cyanosis include a full blood count to reveal polycythaemia and a raised or depressed white blood cell count, blood cultures and a nasopharyngeal aspirate.

In addition to blood gas analysis to indicate fixed or variable hypoxia, the carbon dioxide will generally be raised in respiratory pathologies contributing to the cyanosis but may be normal in cardiac disease.

An electrocardiogram (ECG) may help differentiate cardiac disease, but the gold standard investigation to help differentiate cardiac causes of cyanosis from non-cardiac causes will be an echocardiogram combined with colour Doppler flow mapping and pulsed-wave Doppler studies. The echocardiogram should be performed as a matter of urgency in such situations to allow appropriate management of congenital heart disease. Echocardiography can be easily performed by a paediatric cardiologist in the ED or the infant may need to be transferred to a specialist centre to achieve such an investigation.

If a neurological cause is suspected for the cyanosis, urgent investigation including blood sugar level monitoring is imperative. Additional biochemical investigations may include calcium, magnesium and sodium as well as specific metabolic investigations, including a urine metabolic screen and newborn screening test if inborn errors of metabolism are suspected to be causing neurological depression. If structural lesions or intra-cerebral haemorrhage is suspected, ultrasound is an easy bedside test to perform, but magnetic resonance imaging is the gold standard for CNS investigation. Additional investigations may include electroencephalogram (EEG) and urine/meconium drug screening.

Management

Any neonate that presents with cyanosis should be appropriately resuscitated as outlined in the guidelines devised by ILCOR.

Once the presence of cyanosis is determined from the physical examination of the infant, its degree of severity should be documented immediately by oximetry and confirmed by arterial blood gas and pH determinations. Arterial blood gases and pH should be determined with the patient breathing room air (if clinically stable) and following the breathing of 100% oxygen

for 5–10 minutes. If the oxygen tension rises to exceed 150 mmHg, cyanotic congenital heart disease is unlikely, although little or no change in oxygen tension strongly suggests that such a cardiac defect is the cause of the cyanosis. The gold standard for immediately ruling out non-cardiac causes of cyanosis and establishing the diagnosis of cyanotic congenital heart disease remains echocardiography. The cyanosis that results from pulmonary disease usually resolves partially, if not completely, following the administration of oxygen. Such treatment should not produce similar results in patients who have non-respiratory cyanosis. Here the cause must be determined to achieve a successful outcome.

All neonates should initially receive oxygen until a definitive diagnosis has been made. If the diagnosis is pulmonary then the addition of oxygen should resolve the cyanosis. If the respiratory distress is severe, additional support by means of positive end expiratory pressure or positive pressure ventilation may be required. If an infant requires intubation then a person skilled in this procedure should be asked to attend the ED. Following institution of airway support the infant requires intensive-care admission. Once the airway and breathing have been supported then appropriate assessment and management of the circulation is essential. In any infant with a pulmonary cause for the cyanosis, the potential for sepsis should be evaluated and treated with intravenous antibiotics.

The laboratory evaluation of most neonates who are cyanosed includes a haematocrit and haemoglobin determination, white blood cell count, differential count, blood glucose determination, and a chest radiograph. If a cardiac aetiology is likely, echocardiography is essential. In selected cases, cardiac catheterisation and angiocardiography may be necessary to define the cardiac anatomy more precisely. Electrocardiography should be performed if clinical findings suggest a tachyarrhythmia. If a CNS aetiology is suspected, appropriate scans and drug levels should be considered. The presence of methaemoglobin may be detected by placing a few drops of the patient's blood on filter paper and comparing it with normal blood. Methaemoglobin will produce a chocolate-brown colour.

Seizures that result in cyanosis should be managed according to the results of initial investigations. Hypoglycaemia should be managed with a 5 mL kg^{-1} bolus of 10% dextrose, followed by an infusion of dextrose. Hypocalcaemia should be managed with intravenous calcium and other electrolyte imbalances should be corrected before trying to control the seizure. Once treatable causes of neonatal seizures have been identified and treated then appropriate anticonvulsant therapy should be administered. Phenobarbital or phenytoin are first-line anticonvulsants used in the neonatal period.

In any infant with seizures in the first month of life, sepsis should be thoroughly investigated with both blood culture and cerebrospinal fluid (CSF) cultures for both bacteria and viruses. Treatment with antibiotics and antiviral medications should be considered if there are any risk factors, symptoms or signs of sepsis.

Of all of the above aetiologies, the most common cause of cyanosis in the neonate is a cyanotic congenital heart defect. In many such infants, pulmonary blood flow depends primarily or entirely upon the patency of the ductus arteriosus. If congenital heart disease is suspected from the hyperoxia test, chest radiograph, ECG or echocardiogram then referral should be made to a paediatric cardiologist. A discussion should take place as to whether prostaglandin E1 should be commenced to either open or maintain the patency of the ductus arteriosus and the appropriate dosage should be discussed with the accepting paediatric cardiologist. This will allow mixing of deoxygenated and oxygenated blood, increasing the oxygen saturations of the infant. A dose of 0.05–0.1 mcg kg^{-1} min^{-1} IV is generally recommended, remembering that the most serious side effects of this drug are hypoventilation and apnoea.

Once a diagnosis of congenital heart disease has been made then ongoing management by a paediatric cardiologist is essential. Transfer to a paediatric cardiology centre should be organised and the infant should be fully monitored prior to transfer, including pre- and post-ductal saturations, respiratory rate, temperature, pulse, ECG monitoring and blood pressure. Transport should be provided by a team expert in neonatal resuscitation.

The infant with possible seizures

Although the incidence of seizures is higher in the first 4 weeks of life than in any other age group, the actual incidence cannot be delineated because of the large number of subtle presentations. The seizures that do present to the ED generally do so in the early neonatal period (days 1–7) and it is essential to recognise these for two reasons:

❶ They may represent the manifestation of serious underlying disease that needs treating.

❷ If unrecognised, and thus untreated, seizures may be prolonged and possibly cause brain damage.

Seizures in the neonatal period are a result of an excessive depolarisation of neurones from many different causes. Disturbances of electrolytes (sodium, calcium, and magnesium) and an imbalance of excitatory and inhibitory amino acids have been identified as predisposing to neonatal seizure activity. It is important to identify the cause of the seizures, as many of them are easily treatable, but if missed there may be major long-term consequences.

Causes of neonatal seizures

- Hypoxia: hypoxic ischaemic encephalopathy.
- Intracranial haemorrhage: primary subarachnoid, periventricular/intraventricular, subdural.
- Electrolyte imbalance: hypoglycaemia, hypocalcaemia, hypomagnesaemia, hyponatraemia.
- Metabolic: amino acidopathies, organic acidopathies, hyperammonaemia, pyridoxine deficiency.
- Intracranial infections: bacterial and viral.
- Developmental defects: neuromigrational disorders.
- Drug withdrawal: opiates or maternal benzodiazepine abuse.
- Familial.

Clinical features

History

The clinical history will provide essential clues to the cause of the seizures. A thorough history of the pregnancy, labour and delivery should be established as well as a detailed family history of seizures.

A perinatal history of maternal fever, prolonged rupture of membranes, low vaginal swab positive for Group B *Streptococcus* and associated fetal distress may be clues to an infective cause of the seizures. In addition, a history of poor Apgar scores and poor cord blood gas results, and the need for resuscitation at birth may indicate a perinatal asphyxial event.

If a perinatal cause for the seizures is not identified in the history then a postpartum cause needs to be considered. A history of maternal substance abuse may indicate seizures secondary to neonatal abstinence syndrome and a family history of seizures is suggestive of a genetic cause for the seizures.

Poor understanding of the nutritional requirements of the newborn and excessive weight loss may indicate an electrolyte imbalance as the cause of the seizures. Hypoglycaemia and hypocalcaemia may both present with a preceding history of jitteriness.

In addition to the history of the actual cause of the seizures it is also important to get a realistic picture as to the nature of the seizures. Although most neonatal seizures are partial, they can be generalised, and there are many other presenting signs of neonatal seizure activity including: jitteriness; cyanosis; apnoea; tachycardia; lethargy; and collapse.

Examination

Any infant that has presented with seizures or potential seizures needs a thorough examination. The anterior fontanelle should be soft and non-bulging in the neonatal period. A tense fontanelle is suggestive of raised intracranial pressure. This may result from an intracranial bleed or excessive swelling secondary to neonatal meningitis. If a bleed is suspected, this may be idiopathic, secondary to a bleeding tendency or a result of non-accidental injury. If a bleeding tendency is suspected other bruising or other bleeding diatheses may be identified and the stool and urine should both be examined for the presence of blood. The head should be measured and the head circumference should be plotted on a centile chart to compare with the centile that the head circumference lay on initially. This will indicate if there is progressive hydrocephalus. Once the fontanelle has been examined the rest of the nervous system should be assessed. Tone and reflexes should be elicited to indicate any CNS involvement. The eyes should be examined for retinal haemorrhages and signs that the intracerebral injury could be deliberate. Severe hydrocephalus associated with seizures may be associated with a downward deviation of the eyes.

Considering the multitude of causes of neonatal seizures there will be many potential physical signs that can be elicited. Signs of infection, either congenital or acquired, may include a petechial rash, respiratory distress and hepatosplenomegaly, or in neonatal meningitis they may be associated with severe septic shock.

It is important to recognise that a lethargic infant may be dehydrated and suffering from the effects of an electrolyte imbalance. In addition, an infant with metabolic derangements may also present shocked, acidotic and with seizures. The metabolic derangements may have a characteristic odour that, if identified, may lead to a rapid diagnosis of the seizures.

Although there are many causes of seizures in the neonatal period, the diagnosis is only made when adequate investigations are performed. A paediatric neurologist may be involved in more intractable forms of seizure.

Investigations

Any neonate presenting to the ED with possible seizures needs prompt investigation. A first line would be to perform a full set of clinical observations, including oxygen saturations, respiratory rate, pulse rate, blood pressure temperature and ECG. Once the airway and breathing have been assessed, then a blood sugar should be performed, and serum taken for calcium, magnesium and sodium levels.

In any infant, sepsis should be high on the list of differential diagnoses and thorough investigation should be performed. This should include full blood count, blood cultures and, importantly, a lumbar puncture. The cerebrospinal fluid should be examined for evidence of both bacterial and viral infections. If viral infection is suspected then polymerase chain reaction should be performed for both enteroviruses and herpes simplex virus. Glucose and protein performed on the CSF also help guide the

differential diagnosis. If a congenital infection is possible, either the mother is non-immune or has risk factors for the possible development of rubella, cytomegalovirus or toxoplasmosis in pregnancy, then a TORCH screen should be performed.

In addition to biochemical and infective profiles, a metabolic screen should be performed on fresh urine collected from the infant, and certain inborn errors of metabolism can be eliminated by chasing the newborn screening test performed on all newborn infants between days 3 and 5 of life.

Once basic blood, urine and CSF tests have been collected, a cerebral ultrasound scan should be organised. This allows both sagittal and coronal views of the brain through the anterior and posterior fontanelles. This simple bedside test will demonstrate intracerebral haemorrhage and may demonstrate certain changes typical of congenital infections. If there is ongoing suspicion of intracerebral pathology an MRI or CT scan may be required. At this stage the infant would require admission and ongoing investigation in hospital.

Once a neonate is admitted to hospital with seizures, further investigations may involve an EEG, with video telemetry to differentiate a true seizure from other common diagnoses.

Differential diagnoses

As neonatal seizures can present with such a complex array of symptoms and signs, the list of differential diagnoses is great. Some of commoner differential diagnoses include benign neonatal sleep myoclonus, gastro-oesophageal reflux, anoxia and neonatal jitters.

Management

Any neonate presenting with a potential seizure needs urgent management. Airway, breathing and circulation should all be assessed and secured as a priority. Phenobarbitone remains the standard first-line treatment for neonatal seizures worldwide but is ineffective in many neonates. Second-line anticonvulsant regimens vary widely but usually involve the benzodiazepines (diazepam, clonazepam, lorazepam, midazolam), phenytoin, or paraldehyde.

Acute treatment

- Ensure respiratory support. Endotracheal intubation and respiratory support are often required due to the limited

respiratory reserves of the neonate. This should be considered early as the rapid correction of hypoxia aids in limiting seizure time.
- Ensure cardiac support. Fluid therapy is often required and may involve bolus replacement therapy in a shocked and acidotic infant.
- If hypoglycaemic: glucose 10% solution: 5 mL kg^{-1} IV followed by continuous infusion at 5–7 mg kg^{-1} min^{-1}.
- Other specific treatments (as indicated): calcium gluconate 5% solution 4 mL kg^{-1} IV; magnesium sulfate 50% solution 0.2 mL kg^{-1} intramuscular; pyridoxine 50–100 mg IV.
- Symptomatic treatment: phenobarbital loading dose 20 mg kg^{-1} IV; additional doses 5 mg kg^{-1} IV (10–15 minutes) to maximum of 20 mg kg^{-1}; phenytoin 20 mg kg^{-1} (1 mg kg^{-1} min^{-1}).
- Brain cooling. Newborn infants born greater than 35 weeks' gestation, who require extensive resuscitation and have poor Apgar scores and have abnormal neurological signs including seizures, may be eligible for whole body cooling. If criteria are met and temperatures are reduced to 33–34°C within 6 hours of birth, the long-term survival and survival free of significant morbidity can be significantly reduced. This MUST always be discussed with a neonatal or paediatric intensive care unit prior to commencement.

The most important determinant of prognosis is the underlying aetiology. Thus, infants who have cerebral dysgenesis have uniformly poor outcomes, and approximately 50% of those who have moderate or severe hypoxic–ischaemic encephalopathy develop sequelae. In contrast, infants who have transient metabolic derangements and are treated promptly or who have only subarachnoid haemorrhage usually have a good outcome. Intracranial infection and inborn errors of metabolism are associated with a variable prognosis.

THE VOMITING INFANT

True vomiting in babies is best divided into two broad categories: non-bilious and bilious. Bilious vomiting occurs when bile is purged along with the gastric contents. Although some small intestinal reflux into the stomach is common with all vomiting, in non-bilious vomiting, antegrade intestinal flow is preserved, and the majority of the bile drains into the more distal portions of the intestine. If an obstruction is present, non-bilious vomiting implies that the obstruction is proximal to the ampulla of Vater. Conditions leading to bilious vomiting involve either a disorder of motility or physical blockage to this antegrade flow of proximal intestinal contents distal to the ligament of Treitz.

Non-bilious vomiting

Gastro-oesophageal reflux (GOR), although not true vomiting, is frequently included in discussions of vomiting but really only occurs as a result of failed normal oesophageal function. Normally, the lower oesophageal sphincter (LES) relaxes with swallowing and propagation of oesophageal peristalsis, allowing a food bolus to enter the stomach. Its basal contraction prevents food from re-entering the oesophagus from the stomach. Transient relaxation of the LES predisposes to GOR and is the major mechanism in infants who have GOR. The LES is aided by surrounding structures, especially the crural diaphragm, and disruption of these structures, as with a hiatal hernia, contributes to the GOR in some patients. GOR also is distinguished from true vomiting by its symptoms – the emesis of GOR is effortless and generally not associated with retching or autonomic symptoms.

Both inborn errors of metabolism and endocrine disorders can cause vomiting in neonates. The physician should consider glycogen storage disease II (Pompe's disease), galactosaemia, urea cycle defects, phenylketonuria, Zellweger's disease, adrenal leukodystrophy and carnitine deficiency syndromes in the sick vomiting neonate. The inborn errors of metabolism generally present in early infancy, and the vomiting is associated with symptoms of lethargy, hypo- or hypertonia, seizures, or coma. The constellation of symptoms is similar to that seen in sepsis, necessitating a high index of suspicion in the evaluation of these patients. The presence or absence of metabolic acidosis, hypoglycaemia, hyperammonaemia,

or ketosis and a family history that includes possible consanguinity can help to determine the diagnosis.

Vomiting occurs in any neurological condition that involves increased intracranial pressure (ICP), such as hydrocephalus, congenital malformation, intracranial haemorrhage or mass lesion and infection. Additionally, babies who have seizures, autonomic disorders (Riley–Day syndrome), and conditions affecting the floor of the fourth ventricle without increased ICP frequently have their condition worsened by vomiting.

The anatomic and, thus, the generally surgical causes of non-bilious vomiting are those that affect the intestinal tract proximal to the point of bilious drainage (ampulla of Vater), which is proximal to the ligament of Treitz. These include oesophageal/gastric atresia, duplication/diverticulum/choledochal cyst, pyloric stenosis and web. Any infant who exhibits persistent non-bilious vomiting, with or without feeding, in the immediate newborn period must be suspected of having an intestinal atresia or a luminally obstructing lesion (pyloric stenosis, luminal band, web) proximal to the point of bile drainage An easy and rapid test to evaluate possible oesophageal atresia is the ability to pass a nasogastric tube easily into the stomach. After the tube has been passed, it is important to obtain a radiograph to ensure that the tube is in the stomach and not coiled in an atretic oesophagus. Any resistance to passage of the tube is an indication for evaluation by contrast radiograph for an obstruction. If an obstruction is present, naso-oesophageal tube drainage is important to prevent aspiration of pooled oesophageal secretions. Contrast studies are the standard for the diagnosis of these conditions.

Bilious vomiting

Although not absolute, anatomic conditions causing luminal obstruction distal to the ligament of Treitz usually cause bilious vomiting. Bilious vomiting is an ominous sign that mandates immediate evaluation. Conditions to be considered in the vomiting baby include intestinal atresia and stenosis, malrotation with or without volvulus and intestinal duplication. Also, malrotation with volvulus is a surgical emergency that is

diagnosed relatively easily by gastrointestinal contrast study. It is more common in older children.

Management

Any infant who is seriously ill with vomiting requires immediate resuscitation and admission to hospital. In many cases, aggressive fluid management in addition to resuscitation following ILCOR recommendations will need to be implemented without delay.

In the case of the infant with persistent non-bilious vomiting, early consultation with a paediatrician or paediatric surgeon should occur, as in many cases further evaluation may be necessary. Where an underlying metabolic or endocrine disorder was considered in the differential diagnosis, stabilisation should occur as outlined above, with particular attention to any underlying metabolic and electrolyte derangement. Early consultation with a specialist with experience in the care of these rare metabolic conditions should occur as soon as the diagnosis is entertained. Stable infants with vomiting that is not serious and who are otherwise well, such as those with GOR, can be discharged from the ED, provided that suitable follow up and family support have been organised.

For those infants with bilious vomiting, an underlying surgical disorder must be considered until proven otherwise. Early consultation with a paediatric surgeon is mandatory in every case. If the infant is seriously ill, then resuscitation should commence immediately following ILCOR recommendations, with a particular focus on maintaining circulation and fluid status in addition to correcting underlying metabolic and electrolyte derangements. After the diagnosis has been established radiographically, the gastrointestinal tract should be decompressed with a nasogastric tube, the infant kept nil by mouth and supported with intravenous fluids until definitive surgical intervention can be undertaken.

THE COLLAPSED INFANT

Occasionally, a young infant will be brought to the ED because they just don't look right to the parents. Even inexperienced parents whose first baby is just a few weeks old may notice when their child is unusually sleepy, fussy, or not eating as well as usual. To the physician in the ED, such an infant may appear quite ill, with pallor, cyanosis, or ashen in colour. The infant may be irritable or lethargic, with or without fever. In addition there may be tachypnoea or tachycardia and/or hypotension, and other signs of poor perfusion may also be apparent.

The most common entities to be considered include bacterial infection and viral syndromes. There are a number of other disorders that are uncommon, but demand diagnostic consideration because they are potentially life threatening, yet treatable (Table 26.1.2).

An infant who is critically ill in the first month of life should initially be presumed to have sepsis and empiric antibiotics commenced. As *Escherichia coli*, GBS, *Listeria*, and other anaerobes are the most likely causative organisms, a combination of ampicillin 200 mg kg^{-1} day^{-1} and gentamicin 7 mg kg^{-1} day^{-1} in divided doses is a reasonable starting point. In the case of suspected meningitis the addition of cefotaxime 200 mg kg^{-1} day^{-1} in divided doses may also be considered. This is a life-threatening situation; the airway, breathing, and circulation should be restored, vascular access obtained and supportive care commenced. The approach to the collapsed infant is presented in Figure 26.1.1.

Sepsis

Sepsis should always be considered when confronted with an ill-appearing infant. The signs and symptoms of sepsis may be quite subtle. The history may vary, and some infants may seem to be ill for several days, while others deteriorate rapidly. Any one or a combination of symptoms, such as lethargy, irritability, respiratory distress, diarrhoea, vomiting, anorexia, or fever may be a manifestation of sepsis. Fever is a very unreliable finding in the septic infant as most septic infants will be hypothermic. The septic infant is often pale, ashen, or even cyanotic, with the skin often cool and mottled owing to poor perfusion. The infant may seem lethargic, obtunded, or quite irritable. If there is marked tachycardia (heart rate approaching 200 bpm) together with tachypnoea (respiratory rate >60 breaths min^{-1}), this may herald a rapid collapse. Disseminated intravascular coagulopathy may develop, manifest as scattered petechiae or purpura. If meningitis is present

Table 26.1.2 Differential diagnosis of the collapsed infant

1. Infectious diseases
   - Bacterial sepsis
   - Meningitis
   - Urinary tract infection
   - Virus infection
   - Congenital syphilis
2. Cardiac disease
   - Congenital heart disease
   - Paroxysmal supraventricular tachycardia
   - Myocardial infarction due to anomalous coronary vessels
   - Pericarditis
   - Myocarditis
3. Endocrine disorders
   - Congenital adrenal hyperplasia
4. Metabolic disorders
   - Hyponatraemia
   - Hypernatraemia
   - Inborn errors of metabolism
   - Hypoglycaemia
   - Drug toxicity
5. Haematological disorders
   - Severe anaemia
   - Methaemoglobinaemia
6. Gastrointestinal disorders
   - Gastroenteritis with dehydration
   - Pyloric stenosis
   - Intussusception
7. Neurological disease
   - Infant botulism
   - Child-abuse intracranial bleed

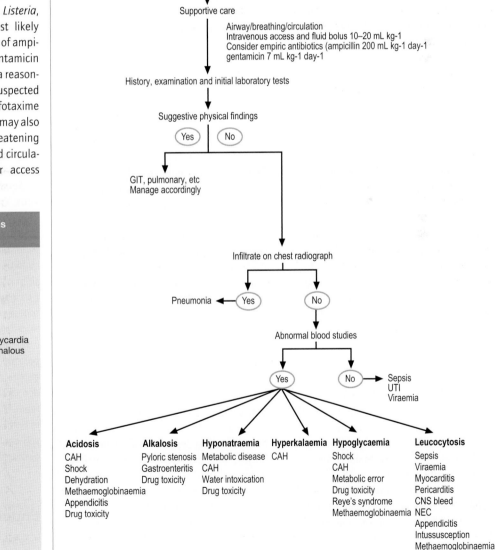

Fig. 26.1.1 Approach to the collapsing infant. Source: Adapted from Selbst SM 1985 The septic-appearing infant. Paediatr Emerg Care 3: 160–167.

there may be a bulging or tense fontanelle with a high-pitched cry. If the infection has localised elsewhere, there may be otitis media, abdominal rigidity, joint swelling or tenderness in one extremity, or possibly chest findings, such as crackles. The disease may progress rapidly, with the infant developing hypotension and/or frank shock.

A high index of suspicion is needed, as although the laboratory may be helpful in suggesting a diagnosis of sepsis, definitive cultures require time for processing. A complete blood count may reveal a leukocytosis or left shift, although this is often unreliable in infants. A coagulation profile may show evidence of disseminated intravascular coagulopathy, and blood chemistries may reveal hypoglycaemia or metabolic acidosis. Aspiration and Gram stain of urine, joint fluid, and spinal fluid, or pus from the middle ear may reveal the offending organism. Similarly, a chest X-ray may show a lobar infiltrate if pneumonia is present. A Gram stain of a petechial scraping should be considered as this will often reveal the responsible organism.

Viral infections

Overwhelming viral infections must be considered in the unwell-looking infant. Enteroviral infections in neonates commonly present as a sepsis-like illness. These infants should be investigated with both polymerase chain reaction and appropriate swabs – as directed by an infectious disease specialist. Respiratory distress will be present in all of these infants, and haemorrhagic manifestations, including gastrointestinal bleeding or bleeding into the skin, may be seen. Seizures often occur as well as icterus, splenomegaly, congestive heart failure and abdominal distension. Mortality rates for enteroviral infections in neonates are quite high. Epidemics of respiratory syncytial virus (RSV) occur in the winter, and infants may present with apnoea or respiratory distress with cyanosis. Those born prematurely, or with previous respiratory disorders, are especially susceptible to apnoea. These infants often appear septic. However, a knowledge of illness in the community and a predominance of respiratory signs may lead one to suspect RSV bronchiolitis. A rapid slide test for RSV will quickly be diagnostic. The CXR shows diffuse patchy infiltrates and possibly lobar atelectasis.

Cardiac disease

When confronted with an unwell infant, cardiac disease should be considered. An infant with a large septal defect, valvular insufficiency or stenosis, hypoplastic left heart syndrome, or coarctation of the aorta may present with congestive heart failure. The infant may arrive collapsed with clinical findings that are quite similar to those of sepsis. A chronic history of poor growth and poor feeding may suggest heart disease. The presence of a cardiac murmur is very suggestive that a structural lesion needs to be considered. The presence of a gallop rhythm, hepatomegaly, and peripheral oedema should lead to the early consideration of primary cardiac pathology. Crackles, wheezing and intercostal retractions are non-specific findings that commonly present in either heart failure or pneumonia. A CXR is the most useful investigation and will often show cardiac enlargement, pulmonary vascular engorgement or interstitial pulmonary oedema. This must be distinguished from the lobar infiltrates seen in pneumonia. An ECG may be helpful in revealing certain congenital heart lesions, in particular in hypoplastic left heart syndrome where the ECG invariably shows right axis deviation, with right atrial and ventricular enlargement. If primary cardiac pathology is considered, an early consultation with a paediatric cardiologist should occur, as an urgent echocardiogram will be essential in making the definitive diagnosis. Another important cause of the collapsed infant to consider is a tight coarctation of the aorta. In this situation the commencement of prostaglandin E1 may be life saving, stabilising the infant so that urgent transfer to a tertiary centre can take place for definitive diagnosis and operative care.

Rarely, an infant with anomalous or obstructed coronary arteries will develop a myocardial infarction and appear initially as a collapsing septic infant. Such infants present with dyspnoea, cyanosis, vomiting, pallor, and general signs of cardiac heart failure. These infants may also have cardiomegaly on CXR, and ECG changes of T-wave inversion and deep Q waves in leads I and AVL. There is a high level of urgency in transferring these infants to a tertiary centre where definitive investigation and specialist intensive care can be commenced.

An arrhythmia may cause an infant to appear quite ill. An infant with supraventricular tachycardia often presents with findings quite similar to those of a septic infant. This arrhythmia is most commonly idiopathic or may be associated with underlying heart disease drugs, fever, or infection. Infants with supraventricular tachycardia often go unrecognised at home for days, initially only exhibiting poor feeding, fussiness, and rapid breathing. If untreated, the infants will develop congestive heart failure, often presenting in a collapsed state, with a heart rate in excess of 300 bpm. The ECG will show regular atrial and ventricular beats with 1:1 conduction and the CXR may show cardiomegaly and pulmonary congestion. Management should begin with simple manoeuvres such as dunking the infant's face in a cold water/ice bath; if this is ineffective, adenosine intravenously in increments of 50 mcg kg^{-1} every 2 minutes until tachycardia resolves (maximum 4 mg). In those rare situations where there is no response to therapy, and the infant remains in heart failure, cardioversion should be considered.

Additional cardiac pathologies to be considered include myocarditis and pericarditis. Such infections are now most commonly due to *Staphylococcus aureus* and coxsackie B virus. These are often fulminant infections, and the baby with such a condition will appear critically ill. A complete physical examination may help to distinguish these conditions from other diagnoses in that signs of heart failure may be seen. Pericarditis may produce distant heart sounds together with a friction rub. Laboratory tests may be helpful, since a chest X-ray will show cardiomegaly and a suggestion of effusion if pericarditis is present. The ECG will show generalised T-wave inversion and low voltage QRS complexes, especially if pericardial fluid is present. Also, ST-T-wave abnormalities may be seen. The echocardiogram will confirm the presence or absence of a pericardial effusion.

Endocrine disorders

Infants with congenital adrenal hyperplasia may present with a history of vomiting, lethargy, or irritability. On arrival, signs of marked dehydration may be present, with tachycardia and possibly hypothermia. A history of poor feeding from birth and symptoms that have progressed over a few days may distinguish this condition from sepsis. The physical examination can establish the diagnosis in females if ambiguous genitalia are noted. Metabolic disturbance is common, with marked hyponatraemia with severe hyperkalaemia. Other non-specific laboratory findings include hypoglycaemia, acidosis, and peaked T waves or arrhythmias on the ECG. The finding of elevated urinary excretion of 17 ketosteroids confirms the diagnosis. The infant should be resuscitated as per ILCOR guidelines and initial emergency management should be discussed with a specialist so steroid replacement can be commenced as a matter of urgency. They should then be referred and transferred to a tertiary centre where management will continue with steroid replacement tailored to the infant's underlying needs.

Metabolic disorders

Metabolic disorders may result from prolonged diarrhoea or vomiting producing dehydration, electrolyte disturbances, and acid–base abnormalities, so that an infant will appear quite ill. These infants may have marked hyponatraemia, appear extremely lethargic, with slow respirations, hypothermia, and possibly seizures. Likewise, dehydrated infants with hypernatraemia may be lethargic or irritable, with muscle weakness, seizures, or coma. Those infants with persistent vomiting (classically in pyloric stenosis) may have hypochloraemic alkalosis with hypokalaemia, and they may appear weak or have cardiac dysfunction. Rare inborn errors of metabolism may produce vomiting in young infants who will then present with lethargy, seizures, or coma caused by metabolic acidosis, hyperammonaemia, or hypoglycaemia. It is thus essential to evaluate the electrolytes, acid–base status and blood sugar in young infants with significant symptoms of gastroenteritis, lethargy, or irritability and coma.

Haematological disorders

Any infant with severe anaemia or blood loss can look ill. In addition to anaemia, disorders of haemoglobin, such as

methaemoglobinaemia can produce a toxic-appearing infant. This condition was reported when the local anaesthetic agent prilocaine was used in penile blocks for circumcision, (methaemoglobinaemia is a well-known adverse effect of excessive doses of this local anaesthetic). These infants may present with cyanosis, poor feeding, vomiting, diarrhoea, lethargy, hypothermia, tachycardia, tachypnoea, hypotension and severe acidosis. They appear mottled, cyanotic, or ashen, and oxygen administration does not affect the cyanosis. The diagnosis will be confirmed by a methaemoglobin level and if elevated to 65% (normal 0–2%), the infant should be transferred to intensive care and treatment with methylene blue considered.

Gastrointestinal disorders

Gastroenteritis, even without electrolyte disturbances, can lead to severe dehydration in the infant with little reserve. Bacterial infections like *Salmonella* and *Campylobacter* and even viral agents need to be considered. A stool smear that shows polymorphonuclear leucocytes is suggestive of bacterial infection.

Pyloric stenosis is most commonly seen in male infants 4–6 weeks of age and may cause severe vomiting with significant dehydration and lethargy without fever. A careful history reveals vomiting to be the predominant feature of the illness, and there may be a positive family history for pyloric stenosis. The physical examination may reveal an abdominal mass, or 'olive', in up to 50% of cases; this strongly suggests the diagnosis of pyloric stenosis. Electrolytes typically show hypochloraemia and hypokalaemia, and alkalosis is prominent. An abdominal ultrasound gives a definitive diagnosis in the majority of cases.

While intussusception is rare in infants less than 5 months old, some young infants may present with vomiting, fever, or signs of abdominal pain (legs drawn up, irritability). The infant may appear to have spasms of pain during which he/she is quite fretful. This can be followed by apathy and listlessness. Diarrhoea is a late sign, as is the typical 'redcurrant jelly' stool. An abdominal mass may be palpated, but the diagnosis can be made using ultrasound. A plain film of the

abdomen will show evidence of small bowel obstruction.

Several other unusual but important gastrointestinal disorders have to be considered in infants. Necrotising enterocolitis occurs in premature infants in the first few weeks of life and can also occur in term infants, usually within the first 10 days of life. A history of an anoxic episode at birth, or other neonatal stresses, may be risk factors for necrotising enterocolitis. These infants are quite ill, with lethargy, irritability, and anorexia, as well as distended abdomen, bilious vomiting and bloody stools. Abdominal radiographs may be very helpful and usually show pneumatosis cystoides intestinalis because of gas in the intestinal wall. Neonatal appendicitis is a rare event, but several cases have been reported to closely mimic sepsis. The mortality for this disorder is close to 80%, and perforation obviously worsens the prognosis. Thus, rapid diagnosis is essential. The most common presenting signs include irritability, vomiting, and abdominal distension on examination. There may also be hypothermia, ashen colour, and shock as the condition progresses. There may also be oedema of the abdominal wall, localised to the right flank, and possibly erythema of the skin in that area as well. The white blood cell count may be quite elevated with a left shift, and there may be a metabolic acidosis present, as well as disseminated intravascular coagulation. Abdominal radiographs may show a paucity of gas in the right lower quadrant, evidence of free peritoneal fluid, or an abnormally thickened right abdominal wall owing to oedema. Other unusual gastrointestinal emergencies to consider include volvulus, perforation due to trauma from enemas or thermometers, and Hirschsprung's enterocolitis.

Neurological disease

The infant with botulism (*Clostridium botulinum*) may present with similar symptoms to an infant with collapse or sepsis. An infant with botulism will often be quite lethargic upon presentation to the ED, with a weak cry and possibly signs of dehydration. These infants are usually afebrile. If constipation has preceded the acute illness, botulism should be seriously considered. In Australia, the disease is most commonly associated with the ingestion of honey. The parents may note a more gradual progression of this illness. Infants with botulism are notably hypotonic, hyporeflexic, and may have increased secretions due to bulbar muscle weakness. Also, the presence of a facial droop, ophthalmoplegia, and decreased gag reflex are consistent with botulism, while they remain unusual findings for a septic infant. A stool specimen to identify toxins of *C. botulinum* may be diagnostic but requires considerable time for identification. Management is with good supportive care; an antitoxin exists but it is not readily available.

Intracranial haemorrhage secondary to non-accidental injury must be considered in the evaluation of the very ill infant. The history may or may not be helpful in establishing a diagnosis. The infant may appear gravely ill with apnoea, bradycardia, hypothermia, and bradypnoea. Careful physical examination may suggest abuse rather than any other diagnosis. The head circumference is often above the 90th percentile, the fontanelle may be full or bulging and retinal haemorrhages are found. A computer-assisted tomography scan will usually demonstrate a small posterior, interhemispheric subdural haematoma. Referral to the appropriate authority for further investigation and ongoing management is now legally mandatory and a key component of the infant's acute care.

RESUSCITATION OF THE NEWBORN INFANT

The following is based on the ILCOR recommendations for newborn infants. Resuscitation of the newborn infant presents its own set of challenges. The transition from placental gas exchange in a liquid-filled intrauterine environment to spontaneous breathing of air requires dramatic physiological changes in the infant within the first minutes to hours after birth. Up to 10% of all newborn infants may require some degree of active resuscitation at birth. In 50% of cases the need for resuscitation of the newborn infant can be predicted. However, in the ED such circumstances may arise suddenly and may occur in facilities that do not routinely provide neonatal intensive care. With adequate anticipation, it is possible to optimise the delivery setting with appropriately prepared equipment and trained personnel who are capable of functioning as a team during neonatal resuscitation.

Neonatal resuscitation can be divided into four actions: (1) basic steps, which include rapid assessment and stabilisation; (2) ventilation; (3) chest compressions; and (4) administration of medications or fluids. Tracheal intubation may be required during any of these steps. All newborn infants require rapid assessment, including examination for the presence of meconium in the amniotic fluid or on the skin; evaluation of breathing, muscle tone, and colour, and classification of gestational age as term or preterm. Newborn infants with a normal rapid assessment require only routine care (warmth, maintaining a patent airway and drying). All others receive the initial steps, including warmth, maintaining a patent airway, drying, stimulation to initiate or improve respirations, and oxygen as necessary. Subsequent evaluation and interventions are based on (1) respirations; (2) heart rate; and (3) tone. Most newborn infants require only the basic steps, but for those who require further intervention, the most crucial action is establishment of adequate ventilation. Only a very small percentage will need chest compressions and medications (<1%).

Evaluation of the newborn

Determination of the need for resuscitative efforts should begin immediately after birth and proceed throughout the resuscitation process. An initial complex of signs (meconium in the amniotic fluid or on the skin, cry or respirations, muscle tone, colour, term or preterm gestation) should be evaluated rapidly and simultaneously by visual inspection. Actions are dictated by integrated evaluation rather than by evaluation of a single vital sign, followed by action on the result, and then evaluation of the next sign (sequential action). Evaluation and intervention for the newly born are often simultaneous processes, especially when more than one trained provider is present. To enhance educational retention, this process is often taught as a sequence of distinct steps. The appropriate response to abnormal findings also depends on the time elapsed since birth and how the infant has responded to previous resuscitative interventions.

Most newborn infants will respond to the stimulation of the extrauterine environment with strong inspiratory efforts, a vigorous cry, and movement of all extremities. If these responses are intact, colour improves steadily from cyanotic or dusky to pink, and heart rate increases. The infant who responds vigorously to the extrauterine environment and who is term can remain with the mother to receive routine care (warmth, maintenance of a patent airway and drying). Indications for further assessment under a radiant warmer and possible intervention include: meconium in the amniotic fluid or on the skin, absent or weak responses, persistent cyanosis and preterm birth.

Further assessment of the newly born infant is based on (1) heart rate; (2) respiratory effort; and (3) tone. Once resuscitation has commenced oxygen saturations should also be measured continuously. After initial respiratory efforts, the newly born infant should be able to establish regular respirations sufficient to improve colour and maintain a heart rate >100 bpm. Gasping and apnoea are signs that indicate the need for assisted ventilation. Heart rate should be consistently >100 bpm in an uncompromised newly born infant. An increasing or decreasing heart rate also can provide evidence of improvement or deterioration. An uncompromised newly born infant will be able to maintain a pink colour of the mucous membranes without supplemental oxygen. Pallor may be a sign of decreased cardiac output, severe anaemia, hypovolaemia, hypothermia, or acidosis.

Basic steps

Preventing heat loss in the newborn is vital because cold stress can increase oxygen consumption and impede effective resuscitation. Placing the infant under a radiant warmer away from draughts, rapidly drying the skin, removing wet linen immediately, and wrapping the infant in warm blankets will reduce heat loss. The infant's airway is cleared by positioning of the infant in a neutral position and removal of secretions, blood, meconium or pus by suctioning if needed. If respiratory efforts are present but not producing effective tidal ventilation, often the airway is obstructed. Immediate efforts must be made to correct over-extension or flexion or to remove secretions. Aggressive pharyngeal suction can cause laryngeal spasm and vagal bradycardia and delay the onset of spontaneous breathing. When providing oropharyngeal suction, limit depth of suction to approximately 5 cm from the lips. Negative pressure of the suction apparatus should not exceed 100 mmHg (13.3 kPa or 136 cmH$_2$O). If copious secretions are present, the infant's head may be turned to the side, and suctioning may help clear the airway. Maintaining proper head position may be helpful in up to 12% of deliveries.

Clearing the airway of meconium

Approximately 12% of deliveries are complicated by the presence of meconium in the amniotic fluid. When meconium is present a significant number (20–30%) of infants will have meconium in the trachea and the need for tracheal suctioning after delivery is indicated in *depressed* infants or those apnoeic at birth. If the fluid contains meconium and the infant has depressed or absent respirations, perform direct laryngoscopy immediately after birth for suctioning of residual meconium from the hypopharynx (under direct vision) and intubation/suction of the trachea. Tracheal suctioning of the vigorous infant with meconium-stained fluid does not improve outcome. Accomplish tracheal suctioning by applying suction via a meconium aspirator to a tracheal tube as it is withdrawn from the airway. If the infant's heart rate or respiration is severely depressed, it may be necessary to institute positive-pressure ventilation despite the presence of some meconium in the airway. Babies born with meconium stained liquor who are active at birth do not require routine endotracheal suction.

Drying and maintaining a patent airway produce enough stimulation to initiate effective respirations in most newborn infants. Tactile stimulation may initiate spontaneous respirations in newly born infants who are experiencing primary apnoea. If these efforts do not result in prompt onset of effective ventilation, discontinue them because the infant is in secondary apnoea and positive-pressure ventilation will be required. If an infant remains bradycardic with a HR < 100 bpm or apnoeic, after drying and airway manoeuvres, positive pressure ventilation should be commenced. This can be commenced with air but 100% oxygen should be available if CPR is required or the newborn is ever asystolic. If positive pressure ventilation is commenced with air, an oxygen saturation probe should be attached to the newborn infant's right hand. The aim is to use blended oxygen and air to achieve saturations of 80–85% by 5 minutes and 90% by 10 minutes in a newborn term infant. If air is not available for use in a positive pressure system, resuscitation of term infants should continue in 100% oxygen. For cyanosed infants with regular respirations and a HR > 100 bpm, free-flow oxygen or blended oxygen can be delivered through a face mask and flow-inflating bag, an oxygen mask, or a hand cupped around oxygen tubing. These babies should have oxygen saturation monitors attached to achieve saturations of 80–85% by 5 minutes and 90% by 10 minutes of age. The oxygen source should deliver at least 5 L min^{-1}, and the oxygen should be held close to the face (nose) to maximise the inhaled concentration. Many self-inflating bags will not passively deliver sufficient oxygen flow (i.e. when not being squeezed). The goal of supplemental oxygen use should be normoxia. Sufficient oxygen should be administered to achieve pink colour in the mucous membranes. If cyanosis returns when supplemental oxygen is withdrawn, post-resuscitation care should include monitoring of administered oxygen concentration and arterial oxygen saturation.

Ventilation

The key to successful neonatal resuscitation is establishment of adequate ventilation. Reversal of hypoxia, acidosis, and bradycardia depends on adequate inflation of fluid-filled lungs with air or oxygen. Most newborn infants who require positive-pressure ventilation can be adequately ventilated with a bag and mask. Indications for positive-pressure ventilation include apnoea or gasping respirations, heart rate < 100 bpm, and persistent central cyanosis despite 100% oxygen. Resuscitation bags used for neonates should be no larger than 500 mL and preferably self-inflating. Newer flow driven pressure limited devices, reliant on a flow of gas to create a pressure, are also recommended and can be used in the newborn and early infant period.

Although the pressure required for establishment of air breathing is variable and unpredictable, higher inflation pressures (30–40 cmH$_2$O or higher) and longer inflation times may be required for the first several breaths than for subsequent breaths. Visible chest expansion is a more reliable sign of appropriate inflation pressures than any specific manometer reading. The assisted ventilation rate should be 40–60 breaths per minute (30 breaths per minute when chest compressions are also being delivered). Signs of adequate ventilation include bilateral expansion of the lungs, as assessed by chest wall movement and breath sounds, and improvement in heart rate and colour. If ventilation is inadequate, check the seal between mask and face, clear any airway obstruction (adjust head position, clear secretions, open the infant's mouth), and finally increase inflation pressure and check the equipment being used is not malfunctioning. Prolonged bag–mask ventilation may produce gastric inflation and this should be relieved by insertion of an orogastric tube. If such manoeuvres do not result in adequate ventilation, endotracheal intubation should follow.

After 30 seconds of adequate ventilation, spontaneous breathing and heart rate should be checked. If spontaneous respirations are present and the heart rate is ≥ 100 bpm, positive-pressure ventilation may be gradually reduced and discontinued. Gentle tactile stimulation may help maintain and improve spontaneous respirations while free-flow oxygen is administered. If spontaneous respirations are inadequate, or if heart rate remains below 100 bpm, assisted ventilation must continue with bag and mask or tracheal tube. If the heart rate is < 60 bpm, continue assisted ventilation, begin chest compressions, and consider endotracheal intubation. If chest compressions are commenced for bradycardia or asystole, 100% oxygen should also be used for the positive-pressure ventilation.

Endotracheal intubation

Endotracheal intubation may be indicated at several points during neonatal resuscitation: when tracheal suctioning for meconium is required; if bag–mask ventilation is ineffective or prolonged; when chest compressions are performed; when tracheal administration of medications is desired; or during special resuscitation circumstances, such as congenital diaphragmatic hernia or extremely low birth weight. The timing of endotracheal intubation may also depend on the skill and experience of the resuscitator. Perform endotracheal intubation orally, using a laryngoscope with a straight blade (size 0 for premature infants, size 1 for term infants). Insert the tip of the laryngoscope into the vallecula or under the epiglottis and elevate gently to reveal the vocal cords. Cricoid pressure may be helpful. Insert the tube to an appropriate depth through the vocal cords as indicated by the vocal cord guide line and check its position by the centimetre marking on the tube at the upper lip. Record and maintain this depth of insertion. Variation in head position will alter the depth of insertion and may predispose to unintentional extubation or endobronchial intubation.

After endotracheal intubation, confirm the position of the tube by the following: observing symmetrical chest-wall motion; listening for equal breath sounds, especially in the axillae, and for absence of breath sounds over the stomach; confirming the absence of gastric inflation; watching for a fog of moisture in the tube during exhalation and noting improvement in heart rate, colour, and activity of the infant. If available, the use of a carbon dioxide detecting device is extremely useful in neonatal intubation. If endotracheal intubation is unsuccessful it is possible to use a size 1 laryngeal mask airway to support breathing in infants >34 weeks gestation or more than 2 kg in weight.

Chest compressions

Asphyxia causes peripheral vasoconstriction, tissue hypoxia, acidosis, poor myocardial contractility, bradycardia, and eventually cardiac arrest. Establishment of adequate ventilation and oxygenation will restore vital signs in the vast majority of newly born infants. Initiate chest compressions if there is a heart rate <60 bpm, even if ventilation is adequate on 100% oxygen for 30 seconds. Because chest compressions may diminish the effectiveness of ventilation, do not initiate them until lung inflation and ventilation have been established. Provision of chest compressions is likely to compete with provision of effective ventilation. Coordinate compressions and ventilations to avoid simultaneous delivery. There should be a 3:1 ratio of compressions to ventilations, with 90 compressions and 30 breaths to achieve approximately 120 events per minute. Reassess the heart rate approximately every 30 seconds. Continue chest compressions until the spontaneous heart rate is ≥60 bpm.

Drugs

Drugs are rarely indicated in resuscitation of the newborn infant. Bradycardia in the newly born infant is usually the result of inadequate lung inflation or profound hypoxia, and adequate ventilation is the most important step in correcting bradycardia. Administer medications if, despite adequate ventilation with 100% oxygen and chest compressions, the heart rate remains <60 bpm. Medications and fluids are easily administered via an umbilical venous catheter or a peripherally placed intravenous catheter. The intraosseous route is less commonly needed in newborns but is useful in the emergency department in the resuscitation of infants.

Administration of adrenaline (epinephrine) is indicated when the heart rate remains <60 bpm after a minimum of 30 seconds of adequate ventilation and chest compressions. Adrenaline is particularly indicated in the presence of asystole. The recommended intravenous dose is 0.1–0.3 mL kg^{-1} of a 1:10 000 solution (0.01–0.03 mg kg^{-1}), repeated every 3–5 minutes as indicated. If endotracheal adrenaline is to be administered a higher dose is recommended of 0.5–1 mL kg^{-1} of a 1:10 000 solution (0.05–0.1 mg kg^{-1}) placed down the endotracheal tube. Higher doses have been associated with exaggerated hypertension but lower cardiac output in animals. The sequence of hypotension followed by hypertension possibly increases the risk of intracranial haemorrhage, especially in preterm infants.

Volume expanders may be necessary to resuscitate a newly born infant who is hypovolaemic. Suspect hypovolaemia in any infant who fails to respond to resuscitation. Consider volume expansion when there has been suspected blood loss or the infant appears to be in shock (pale, poor perfusion, weak pulse) and has not responded adequately to other resuscitative measures. The fluid of choice for volume expansion is an isotonic crystalloid solution such as normal saline or Ringer's lactate. Administration of O-negative red blood cells may be indicated for replacement of large-volume blood loss. The initial dose of volume expander is 10 mL kg^{-1} given by slow intravenous push over 5–10 minutes. The dose may be repeated after further clinical assessment and observation of response. Higher bolus volumes have been recommended for resuscitation of older infants. However, volume overload or complications such as intracranial haemorrhage may result from inappropriate intravascular volume expansion in asphyxiated newly born infants as well as in preterm infants.

Use of sodium bicarbonate is discouraged during brief cardiopulmonary resuscitation. If it is used during prolonged arrests unresponsive to other therapy, it should be given only after establishment of adequate ventilation and circulation. Later use of bicarbonate for treatment of persistent metabolic acidosis or hyperkalaemia should be directed by arterial blood gas levels or serum chemistries, among other evaluations. A dose of 1–2 mEq kg^{-1} of a 0.5 mEq mL^{-1} solution may be given by slow intravenous push (over at least 2 minutes) after adequate ventilation and perfusion have been established.

Naloxone hydrochloride is a narcotic antagonist without respiratory-depressant activity. It is specifically indicated for reversal of respiratory depression in a newly born infant whose mother received narcotics within 4 hours of delivery. Always establish and maintain adequate ventilation before administration of naloxone and the infant should always be transferred to a neonatal or paediatric intensive care unit for observation if naloxone has been administered. Do not administer naloxone to newly born infants whose mothers are suspected of having recently abused narcotic drugs because it may precipitate abrupt withdrawal signs in such infants. The recommended dose of naloxone is 0.1 mg kg^{-1} of a 0.4 mg mL^{-1} or 1.0 mg mL^{-1} solution given intravenously, endotracheally, or – if perfusion is adequate – intramuscularly or subcutaneously Because the duration of action of narcotics may exceed that of naloxone, continued monitoring of respiratory function is essential, and repeated naloxone doses may be necessary to prevent recurrent apnoea.

Further reading

Alexander R, Crabbe L, Sato Y, et al. Serial abuse in children who are shaken. *Am J Dis Child* 1990;**144**:58–60.

Brazelton TB. Crying in infancy. *Paediatrics* 1962;**29**:579–88.

Carey WB. The effectiveness of parent counseling in managing colic. *Paediatrics* 1994;**94**(3):333–4.

Forsyth BWC. Colic and the effect of changing formulas: A double blind, multiple-crossover study. *J Paediatr* 1989;**115**:521–6.

Holzki J, Laschat M, Stratmann C. Stridor in the neonate and infant. Implications for the paediatric anaesthetist. Prospective description of 155 patients with congenital and acquired stridor in early infancy. *Paediatr Anaestha* 1998;**8**(3):221–7.

ILCOR. International Liaison Committee on Resuscitation (ILCOR). Advisory statement: Resuscitation of the newly born infant. *Paediatrics* 1999;**103**:56.

Illingworth RS. Three month's colic. *Arch Dis Child* 1954;**145**:165–74.

Lucassen PLBJ, Assendelft WJJ, Gubbels JW, et al. Effectiveness of treatments for infantile colic: Systemic review. *Bri Med J* 1998;**316**: 1563–9.

McKenzie S. Troublesome crying in infants: Effect of advice to reduce stimulation. *Arch Dis Child* 1991;**66**: 1416–20.

Millar KR, Gloor JE, Wellington N, Joubert G. Early neonatal presentations to the paediatric ED. *Paediatr Emerg Care* 2000;**16**(3):145–50.

Poole SR. The infant with acute, unexplained, excessive crying. *Paediatrics* 1991;**88**(3):450–5.

Selbst SM. The septic-appearing infant. *Paediatr Emerg Care* 1985;**3**:160–7.

Singer JI, Rosenberg NM. A fatal case of colic. *Paediatr Emerg Care* 1992;**8**(3):171–2.

ACUTE NEONATAL PROBLEMS

TRANSPORT AND RETRIEVAL

Section editor *Ian Everitt*

27.1 Emergency medical transport and retrieval

Andrew Berry

ESSENTIALS

1 Children are different from adults and therefore can have different needs in terms of medical retrieval. Early consultation with clinicians skilled in paediatric critical care is encouraged. Their advice can assist in making a diagnosis, determining treatment and developing a transfer plan. Every hospital likely to use such a service should have a defined process for accessing it.

2 Careful stabilisation of the child 'pre-transfer' achieves the best clinical outcome. This is a combined activity of treating staff at the referring hospital and a transport team. That continuum of care is often under the supervision of remote medical experts using telephone support, conference call techniques and remote vision technology.

3 The transport network has the responsibility for the organisation of a suitable clinical escort, urgency of response and type of vehicle. Centralisation of that retrieval network ensures this occurs in a rapid and seamless manner.

4 The medical retrieval team is especially equipped and trained to handle all situations that may be encountered during patient transfer and hence are the preferred clinical escort.

5 The key to good patient outcome throughout this process remains effective communication.

6 Performance of the system should be monitored for quality purposes and system improvement. Reports should include feedback to all participants in the process.

Introduction

This chapter addresses the secondary transportation of patients; that is, inter-facility transfer. Primary transport (pre-hospital or scene transfer) is beyond the scope of the chapter. In particular, the role of 'medical retrieval' transfer is discussed. That is, where expertise normally associated with an intensive care unit (ICU) is sent from a central location to the patient and then transports the patient back to an ICU or tertiary paediatric emergency department (ED). Additionally, most medical retrieval transports of children require an emergency response because the problem is time-critical for the team expertise to reach the patient and/or the patient to reach the ICU.

It is often said that children are not small adults and in several important respects their physiology, pathophysiology and behaviour are different from adults. In patient transport, not only are these differences relevant, but the organisation of critical care services and hospital networks is also different. There is a more centralised organisation of specialist and intensive medical care for children than adults and this has implications for their transport and how transport systems are delivered.

Regionalisation

Different hospitals within a region offer differing levels of care for children. There are broadly three levels of care for children: (1) basic; (2) specialist; and (3) tertiary. In Australia and New Zealand, intensive or critical care tends to be centralised to a few tertiary hospitals. (There are 22 neonatal ICUs in Australia and six in New Zealand. There are seven full-time paediatric ICUs in Australia and one in New Zealand. Some adult units have a specialist interest in paediatric ICU as well.) This principle is based on evidence that a 'centralised' approach produces better outcomes than having a larger number of hospitals in a region each doing a small amount of critical care.[1,2] As a result:

- Most newborns likely to need critical care are delivered in tertiary perinatal centres where neonatal intensive care is available on site and from birth. Progressive improvements are being achieved in better selecting high-risk pregnancies for a more appropriate place of birth.
- Newborns with major surgical conditions or complex medical problems requiring intensive care are treated in children's hospitals.
- Infants and children requiring major surgery or intensive care are treated in children's hospitals.

Basic hospitals admit children with non-life-threatening illnesses. Regional and urban hospitals with specialist paediatric services take care of children with significant illness but not those needing intensive care. Children who need intensive care will usually require a medical retrieval team to move them safely to a tertiary hospital. Other children admitted to rural or basic hospitals with less-critical conditions may be appropriate for transfer using local clinical escorts and admission to a regional specialist hospital.

What's different about children?

This general question is addressed in other chapters. However, from a transport point of view, the type of illness or injury and the process by which a clinical diagnosis is reached are often different in children. For instance, some conditions, such as bronchiolitis, are not only largely unique to children, but manifest in quite different ways from adults. In the first few months of life, presentation with 'apnoea' along with a history of close-family upper respiratory infection suggests this diagnosis even though there may be no signs of respiratory distress or problem with gas exchange. Making this diagnosis is often possible 'over the phone' by clinicians who are experienced in paediatric critical care and offering advice from a distance. Assessing conscious state in a young child with a head injury requires knowledge of developmental milestones. A baby presenting unexpectedly at 1 week of age with 'shock' is more likely to have a congenital

heart lesion, such as left heart obstruction, than more traditional causes of shock. These and other examples require patient transfer decisions to be made by clinicians aware of these differences and skilled in eliciting information that will clarify the situation.

Referring a patient to another hospital

Referring doctor/hospital → referral doctor/hospital

Referring a patient for a higher level of care involves a dialogue between clinicians. For emergency transfers this generally involves a telephone call to a selected *referral* hospital or physician. The referrer usually makes this selection on the basis that the referral clinician has the skills and resources to deal with the problem and is geographically proximate. The ISBAR (Introduction, Situation, Background, Assessment and Recommendation)[3,4] communication technique is a useful tool to assist in this clinical conversation (Table 27.1.1).

The process of telephone triage (teletriage) requires skills of careful listening and intelligent questioning by the person taking the call. It is not learnt overnight. Clinical discussion should precede and determine the logistics of transport, not the other way around. Referral of a critical-care patient can be confounded by resource and logistic issues with the potential to prevent or impair an appropriate and constructive clinical discussion. Keep the focus of the discussion on the patient.

Table 27.1.1 ISBAR
I – Introduction. 'I am (name and role) calling from . . .. on behalf of (clinician in charge)'
S – Situation. 'I have a patient (age and weight) who is a) seriously ill, critically injured, unstable with slow/rapid deterioration, stable but I have concerns'
B – Background. 'The story is' (give information pertinent to clinical problem/age-group. May include date/time of injury/presentation, presenting signs and symptoms/medications/ recent vital signs/test results/trends in status. I've already spoken to. . . . . . (where appropriate)
A – Assessment. 'On the basis of the above, the patient's condition is. . ... They are at risk of. . .. There is a need for . . . . . .'
R – Recommendation. 'Be clear about what you are requesting, e.g. the patient needs to be intubated/in an ICU/assessed by a surgeon/ sent for urgent imaging/etc. I need your advice but at this stage do not require transfer'.

This clinical conversation is complicated by the need to decide what level of care the patient requires and whether a rural treating clinician should call a regional or a tertiary hospital. Some regional hospitals have their own retrieval capacity, allowing a child to be transported to that hospital by a non-specialist team. In some cases, a paediatric specialist may be able to travel to the referring hospital to offer on-site resuscitation, assistance and assessment in parallel with a specialist paediatric medical retrieval team responding from a distance. In some regions, highly trained paramedics or flight nurses offer a level of transport clinical escort higher than regular ambulance transport. Decisions about how these children move and whether transport should be to a regional hospital or a tertiary hospital can be difficult. Sometimes a discussion with both will help determine the best plan.

The relationships between the three levels of care are shown diagrammatically in Fig. 27.1.1.

A dialogue with one referral hospital option may recommend that the other is a more appropriate destination. Unfortunately, a series of discussions with different referral hospitals can be time-consuming and may interfere with direct patient care.

Various means have been introduced to streamline this process. In some referral hospitals, there is often a designated person available to take such calls. Occasionally, a specific telephone number in the referral hospital is advertised for that purpose. However, if that number takes the referrer down a one-way path (e.g. to a personal cellular phone), he or she may need to make other calls or await a 'call-back'. Now that hospital voice-response systems with menus designed for the public and long queues

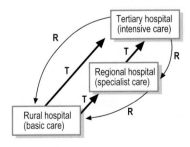

Fig. 27.1.1 The relationship between the three levels of care.

awaiting an operator have become common, simply calling the switchboard of a hospital no longer provides 'direct' access for the referring doctor.

In an ideal world the referring doctor would make just one call. After all, the clinical problem, which by definition exceeds them and/or their hospital, often requires their full attention. Only the treating doctor can place the cannula, intubate, etc. Subverting these clinical activities to make several (or many) phone calls can significantly compromise patient care and outcome. As referral hospitals become busier and/or more efficient, the availability of resources to accept the referred patient can dominate the referral process. Too often, the question of whether a 'Bed' (defined as: Space + Equipment + Nurses + Doctors + Other Resources) is available intrudes on the referral call and can interrupt the conversation with an invitation to 'try elsewhere'. Whenever the clinical referral process becomes a question of 'bed-finding', many referring doctors respond by delegating the task to others. Such staff won't necessarily have any clinical knowledge of the patient or the problem requiring transfer. Some referral hospitals have similarly delegated the process of 'bed-locating' to managers whose focus is on managing the 'bed' resource rather than entering into a clinical discussion about the patient. This combination results in lost opportunities for clinical decisions that can change the course of events independently of the transport process. For instance, an incorrect diagnosis or treatment may be recognised and corrected as the result of a clinical discussion. Having discussed the patient, an alternative referral hospital may be recommended on 'clinical' grounds. A conversation along these lines is desirable and possible, regardless of bed availability.

In regions where there are several referral hospitals serving the same referring hospitals, a single point of contact is provided for transport of a critical-care patient. In most cases, however, such 'single number' systems are designed to facilitate the logistics of transport and the clinical referral process requires a separate, additional phone call. Translated simply, this amounts to: 'find the bed and we'll arrange transport'. An integrated approach is possible, where the same number is used not only as a clinical conduit into the referral hospital 'system' but also to activate the logistics of transport.[5]

Which patients?

Selecting patients for retrieval transfer depends on the threshold for referral in each hospital; based on the role that hospital has for treating patients with problems of varying and different severity. The important point is that discussing the possibility of transfer should be part of a clinical consultation about the patient. The following list suggests conditions that should prompt that discussion with a paediatric ICU or retrieval service:

❶ Head injury (symptomatic).
❷ Altered level of consciousness (for any reason).
❸ Hypoxia despite oxygen therapy.
❹ High oxygen requirement.
❺ Respiratory failure (e.g. bronchiolitis, severe asthma, apnoea).
❻ Upper airway obstruction.
❼ Near drowning (especially with neurological depression or respiratory symptoms).
❽ Ingestion with risk of circulatory, airway or neurological compromise.
❾ Envenomation.
❿ Burns:
   - >10%
   - encircling the neck or involving the airway, face, hands, feet, perineum, or inner joint surfaces
   - associated other significant injury
   - electrical or chemical burns.
⓫ Seizures (with persisting neurological depression).
⓬ Major trauma (including spinal injury)
⓭ Metabolic disturbance, e.g.
   - diabetic ketoacidosis
   - acidaemia
   - severe biochemical abnormality.
⓮ Heart failure or arrhythmia (symptomatic).
⓯ Shock (requiring treatment with volume replacement or inotropes), e.g.
   - blood or fluid loss
   - dehydration
   - septicaemia.
⓰ Other causes of neurological depression:
   - central nervous system (CNS) infection
   - acute life-threatening episode.
⓱ Any condition with the potential for sudden cardiovascular or neurological deterioration.

Adapting such a list may be helpful in determining the local policy. **If in doubt, *consult*.**

Who will move the patient and how?

After an appropriate clinical discussion, the question of how the patient should be moved can be addressed. This can be straightforward or complex, depending on circumstances. The transfer of a patient from referring hospital to referral hospital can be accomplished in several ways. In a *patient transfer*, an escort transports the patient and then returns (in Fig. 27.1.1, T followed by R). In a *retrieval transfer*, the dispatch of a team (response) is followed by patient transport (R followed by T).

Decisions need to be made about three main topics:

❶ Clinical escort.
   a. Patient transfer:
      - ambulance officer (various levels of skill may be available)
      - nurse
      - doctor.
   b. Retrieval transfer:
      - flight nurse or flight paramedic
      - doctor (medical retrieval)
      - other.
❷ Degree of urgency.
   a. Urgent (immediate response).
   b. Emergency (specify expectation of response).
   c. Time window (before a particular time).
   d. Elective.
❸ Type of vehicle.
   a. Surface (road, boat, train, etc.).
   b. Air:
      - rotary wing
      - fixed wing.

A patient transfer is one in which the skill level of the escort is at or below that of the referring hospital. That is, the patient can be escorted by ambulance personnel (*ambulance transfer*). Alternatively, staff from the referring hospital may accompany the patient (*medical or nursing transfer*). In theory these options offer a more rapid process, although review of actual experience often shows that time benefits can be overrated. Using local resources on an ad hoc basis is often slower to mobilise than anticipated. A doctor or nurse from the referring hospital may well offer an adequate level of care but the implications for that hospital during their absence may include a significant staffing reduction for that hospital. The smaller the hospital, the greater the impact that this will have on local cover and, since distances tend to be greater for smaller hospitals, the longer this impact will last. A hospital clinician who, having cared for the patient for some time already, then leaves town escorting a patient may experience significant fatigue. There may be problems finding transport back.

On the other hand, the level of care available to the patient should not regress during the transport process. Indeed, care should increase at each stage of the patient's progress through the system. If the patient's condition is unstable, it may be better to continue treatment in the referring hospital and await the arrival of a retrieval team.

In the retrieval transfer, options for clinical escort include a flight nurse or paramedic attached to an air ambulance service. Exact team composition will vary according to local practice and the regulations governing the skills and certification required for administration of specific treatments and drugs.

Doctors participate in medical retrieval teams in Europe, South Africa and Australasia but less so in North America. Most doctors are tasked from the referral hospital but others are attached as a regional or state-wide retrieval service.

The principle of medical retrieval is to bring the required critical care skills to the patient from an ICU setting and initiate that care prior to transport. In a randomised trial, medical retrieval has been shown to offer significant benefits to preterm infants in terms of mortality and morbidity.[6] However, evidence is not so clear-cut in older age groups. Medical retrieval offers a higher level of care both during transport and, importantly, prior to travel. Patients can be stabilised prior to transport using skills and equipment not normally available in the referring hospital. This approach is preferable to hurriedly rushing from A to B with the patient in an unstable condition (the 'mercy dash') and risking en-route deterioration. To the extent that the arrival of the retrieval team in the referring hospital represents the patient's 'arrival' in intensive care, the patient should not suffer any time penalty from using the 'retrieval' rather than the 'transfer' strategy.

The exceptions are conditions requiring a procedure or an investigation that a retrieval team cannot supply. In children, the situations where this is the case are fewer than in adults. Examples include head injury requiring urgent neurosurgery, some cases of penetrating trauma, volvulus with ischaemia and transposition of the great arteries with intact septum. Some procedures may be possible in the referring hospital if those skills are part of the retrieval team. Examples include taking a surgeon (neurosurgery, ENT) or obstetrician to selected cases to perform an emergency procedure such as decompressing raised intracranial pressure or fibre-optic endoscopy for foreign body. Such options need to be planned rather than an ad hoc response.

On the other hand, there is the additional time awaiting the arrival of the 'retrieval team'. It is often tempting to say, 'we could have been there by now!' However, young children and newborns travel poorly if inadequately stabilised and the lost ground may never be regained.

Assessing the level of urgency requires assessment of how quickly skills or intervention are required in the referring hospital and also how quickly the patient needs definite care in a referral hospital. In most cases, the operational response in reaching the patient is more relevant.

Degrees of urgency

Urgent The patient is in extremis, or is deteriorating, or needs immediate, time-critical therapy.

Emergency The patient has a serious condition and the treatment required is not possible in the referring hospital.

Time window The patient needs to be at the destination by a certain time – there is a latest time by which the transfer should be concluded.

Elective The timing of transfer is discretionary – hours or days and by mutual consent.

The factors determining how quickly a team can be at the bedside include:

❶ Geographical distance.
❷ Modes of transport available.
❸ Functional distance:
  • team availability
  • vehicle availability
  • accessibility
  • number of vehicle changes.

Looking at a map to judge the time to reach the patient may be misleading. When alternative modes of transport are available, fixed wing is roughly twice the speed of helicopter and helicopter twice the speed of surface transport by road. However, the process of activating a helicopter or plane with a team on board can mean the overall response time is double or triple the flight time. The response time also includes components of travel after the flight, which may involve ground transport. The more vehicle changes that are required, the greater the overall time. Each vehicle change adds significantly to the total time. Traditionally, arbitrary distance arcs are specified to help in selecting between road, helicopter and fixed wing options. However, the cut-over from one mode of transport to another in any particular system of retrieval needs to be determined around functional distance rather than geographical distance.

No matter how fast a vehicle travels, the availability of a suitable vehicle and/or team may delay departure. Therefore deployment by road may sometimes result in a more rapid response time than by air. For a particular referring hospital, the choice of appropriate vehicle (road, helicopter or fixed wing) may differ from time to time, according to time of day and day or week.

Good data about actual response times involved in previous cases can inform the decision-making process. Such information is much more useful than simple speed versus distance graphs.

In some cases, the choice of vehicle for the patient transport phase is different from that selected for team mobilisation. If, for instance, a helicopter could not respond because of availability or weather and the retrieval was launched by road, it may be possible, and clinically appropriate, as the weather improves, to use a helicopter for the next 'leg'. When stabilisation times are significant, the use of different vehicles for the outbound and inbound legs of a retrieval may make better use of those vehicles without impairing the clinical process.

The busier a service, the more likely one mission impinges on the next. Delays awaiting a team's return from one mission should be analysed to see whether more teams should be available.

While waiting

The clinical discussion with the referral hospital should include specifics of the actual condition of the patient, their current treatment and a clearly communicated plan of management. Depending on the confidence of the referring doctor about these issues, this discussion may require more or less input from the referral doctor. Telephone advice is always central but other modalities offer additional benefits; including image (X-ray, clinical photography), remote CCTV and customised weight-specific work-plans faxed to the referring hospital. Such consultation is even more relevant when distance and the time taken to reach definitive care increases. The expertise of specialists in paediatric ICU, ED, surgery, burns, neonatology, and other paediatric disciplines, as well as toxicology and envenomation experts, is available by telephone through regional, state and national networks.

Stabilisation

Stabilisation is intended to reduce the risk of 'en route' deterioration, improve tolerance of transport and increase the safety of the process.

All patients should receive a certain amount of stabilisation prior to transport, whether their departure is imminent (as is generally the goal if a local escort is planned) or delayed until a retrieval team has arrived to transport them.

Transport medicine is not so much about how a patient is managed in a mobile setting but how to prepare for the transport process. Stabilisation involves 'packaging'

the patient so that basic physiology is controlled, with airway, breathing and circulation supported. The threshold for intervening in each of these areas is reduced for patients being moved. A successful stabilisation is one in which the risk of an unplanned intervention being necessary en route is reduced to a negligible level. Rigorous attention is required to the patency and security of the artificial airway and vascular lines. These lines and other connections to the patient, such as non-invasive monitoring probes, electrocardiogram (ECG) leads, transducers and drains, should be positioned in such a way that there is no physical force causing either traction or torsion. Despite firm fixation, these forces will cause dislodgement in transit.

Principles of medical retrieval

The 'stay and play' approach is the default for children and 'wrap and run' the exception. The 'golden hour' philosophy can be mistakenly applied to paediatric patients. It relies on battlefield experience and the principle that the outcome depends on the patient being on the operating table in less than an hour from injury. This principle evolved from management of penetrating trauma in military personnel during the Vietnam War and is rarely relevant to critically ill or injured children – particularly when they have already presented to a health facility and some or all of that 'hour' has already gone. It is tempting for rescue retrieval services, who normally deal with adults, to take this approach with children and arrive with a patient who then needs post-transport resuscitation.

Improvements in the responsiveness of retrieval teams have shortened the 'R' phase. This is gradually eroding the reflex tendency to 'wrap and run' with the patient in the hope that their condition will survive a 'mercy dash'. Such improvements are occurring through use of dedicated retrieval teams, on-site staffing and more readily available and/or faster forms of transport. Additional strategies include pre-alerting of the system during the pre-hospital phase, encouraging earlier referral by the referring hospital and more streamlined processes occurring in parallel rather than in series.

Comparing adult practice

In recent years medical retrieval services for adults have developed and are now found in both metropolitan and regional centres. It is important that paediatric clinicians have input into decisions made about any older children whom these services might plan to transport. Many older children may be appropriately moved by an adult team. Good communication between the clinical players is essential, particularly if the referring hospital calls the regional hospital that has an adult retrieval capability and it seems clear that the child is likely to need a higher level of care. In some rural emergencies, a joint response to the primary hospital by both a regional service and a specialist paediatric retrieval team may be appropriate. After such a joint response, the optimum destination for the patient can be determined (regional hospital or specialist children's hospital).

Medical retrieval teams that mostly deal with adults are often inclined to be fairly aggressive in controlling the airway. Unnecessary intubation and mechanical ventilation only complicates the post-transport management in the ICU and a little more time spent in assessment and stabilisation of, for instance, a seizure disorder may obviate this intervention.

Accompanying parents?

Parents will often wish to remain with their child. Sometimes the presence of a parent may be therapeutic if it has a calming effect on an otherwise distressed child. The child who is aware but has significant upper airway obstruction or respiratory failure is a good example. In other cases the parent may not be required to make the child's transport safe but it seems unreasonable not to make provision for a parent to travel in the ambulance or aircraft, where possible. Vehicle specifications should allow for a parent to be accommodated in paediatric medical retrievals. Should a parent be unwell themselves (e.g. a postnatal mother after an operative delivery or a parent injured in a multiple trauma case), their medical needs cannot reasonably be catered for by a medical retrieval team whose focus is on the child. Clinicians making decisions about moving these parents should judge the risks and safety of their transfer independently of the child and, if it is appropriate to move them, a suitable escort should be provided.

Prevention

The retrieval process is not an end in itself. If possible, patients should not be allowed to reach a level of clinical severity needing intensive care. Some of this involves general preventative strategies in health care and injury prevention. Those patients that do come to intensive care should, where possible, present directly to the appropriate facility. Of course, geography makes this goal unachievable in many cases. However, processes that seek to have the pre-hospital response deliver the patient to the right hospital, bypassing less-well-equipped hospitals, are becoming more sophisticated. Trends towards greater centralisation in healthcare organisation make this goal harder to achieve and the retrieval process is likely to be more frequently applied in the future. A summary of preventative strategies includes:

❶ Reduce the need.
   a. Injury prevention and immunisation programs, better interval care of recurrent severe conditions; such as asthma.
   b. Recognise the fetus at-risk of needing ICU or urgent surgery or other intervention.
   c. Plan for high-risk births to occur in a tertiary perinatal centre (major surgical and cardiac conditions).
   d. Facilitate emergency transfer of women when that will result in the birth occurring in the appropriate hospital – in particular, in preterm labour.
❷ Assist and support all participants and players (including remote, rural, regional and metropolitan hospitals) with resources, education and support to optimise the care of seriously ill or injured patients at every stage of the process.
❸ Conduct quality activities – including audit, incident monitoring, case review.

❹ Amelioration:
   a. Telemedicine – improve the referral process by adding images to enhance simple telephone conversations.
   b. Improved data interfaces between hospital systems to increase the information flow between referring hospital, retrieval team and referral hospital.

Expectations and roles

What are the expectations of those participating in the retrieval process? There are four key players:

❶ The referring clinician.
❷ The referral (receiving) clinician.
❸ The transport service.
❹ The transport clinician.

An organised and streamlined interaction between these components is required for the best results. What follows is a summary of the expectations, roles and responsibilities of each of them.

The referring clinician
- Expects to make just one phone call to initiate the process.
- Focuses on the basic principles: airway, breathing, circulation, for a child; 'warm, pink and sweet', for a newborn.
- Provides basic details of history, assessment, examination and interventions.
- Uses the ISBAR technique.
- Nominates a preferred destination, based on clinical need, proximity, family, etc.

The referral (receiving) clinician
- Offers telephone advice about management.
- Elicits appropriate additional information from the referrer.
- Assumes some responsibility for the patient and the solution of their problem.
- Accepts the transfer ('receiving') or ensures that an appropriate alternative is arranged.
- Ensures that others within the tertiary hospital are informed and involved.

- Is available to advise the referrer and/or transport team about further management.
- Reviews professional and service practice in quality activities.

The transport service
- Assesses the level of clinical care required to transport the patient.
- Selects the most appropriate (based on clinical skills) and best available (most timely) team to treat and escort the patient.
- Chooses the most appropriate transport vehicle (road or air; rotary or fixed wing) through liaison with ambulance and other vehicle providers.
- Offers a link between the referring clinician and receiving physician. This is particularly relevant when there are several potential destination units.

The transport clinician
- Participates in, or is informed about, prior clinical discussions about the patient.
- Prepares for the obvious and considers the not-so-obvious possibilities while outbound to the patient.
- Assesses the patient at 'first look' and acts according to clinical need.
- May re-triage the patient to a different level of care and/or initiate an alternative transport plan.
- Chooses between rapid-sequence and full stabilisation retrieval.
- Stabilises the patient using service-specific clinical guidelines.
- Communicates with receiving clinician(s), as appropriate.

What equipment?

Medical equipment used for patients in transport needs to be adequate to the task, robust and capable of operating at all stages of the process. It should be secured in the vehicle according to the applicable safety standards for that vehicle. A monitor or ventilator attached to an intravenous pole by friction nut or lying in the bed near the patient is not safely restrained in a moving vehicle.

Power requirements of the equipment and battery capacities should be thoroughly understood. Electrically powered devices should be able to utilise external power, where possible.

Medical oxygen and medical air should be available to supply constant flows or drive mechanical ventilators. Oxygen can be carried in aircraft or ground ambulances in compressed or liquid form. Each has its benefits but the choice depends largely on availability. Some ventilators do not require a supply of medical air.

Most modern monitors designed for transport are appropriate for children if they have suitable transducers for age for oxygen saturation monitoring, appropriate algorithms for non-invasive blood pressure measurement and selectable respiratory waveforms. Monitoring of temperature, blood pressure (nIBP and IBP), oxygen saturation, ECG and end-tidal CO_2 should be available. For the newborn, skin surface oxygen and CO_2 tension is often added.

Infusion pumps are no longer age-specific and most are capable of driving fluids at accurate low rates suitable for young children.

There are many mechanical ventilators designed for adults that are also suitable for children over the weight of about 20 kg. There are also ventilators suitable for newborns and infants up to about 5 kg. However, the patient weighing 5–20 kg presents some difficulties and a suitable transport ventilator may be hard to find.

Defibrillation equipment suitable for children should be available in the referring hospital and, in selected cases, to the team in transit. The requirement for cardioversion is quite rare in childhood and the need can *usually* be anticipated.

A portable point of care testing unit for blood gas analysis and basic chemistry is particularly useful. Even in referring hospitals with such facilities, the improved turn-around time to obtain a result may utilise the team's time far more efficiently.

Stretchers are not normally designed for young children and it is necessary to rely on paediatric immobilisation systems or restraint systems that interface between the patient and an 'adult' stretcher. Spinal immobilisation requires an age-appropriate spinal board and careful selection of cervical collars – particularly in smaller children and infants.

All equipment should be tested for electromagnetic interference and radiation. That is, susceptibility to external radiofrequency interference as well as their ability to adversely affect aircraft navigation systems. Specific items of transport equipment have been certified for use in aircraft.

The pack carried by teams should include basic and advanced life-support equipment. For inter-facility transports, some reliance on referring hospital equipment is reasonable. However, for any foreseeable need during transport itself, self-reliance is essential. On the other hand, carrying too many items or too many of a particular item can be a disadvantage. It is not possible to cater for absolutely every contingency and a 'reasonable' inventory is the product of common sense and experience.

Which vehicle?

The most frequently available transport vehicles include road ambulances, fixed-wing aircraft and helicopters. The choice of vehicle depends on the nature of the distance and the total time involved in the outward and return journeys and the requirements of the patient's illness or injury. Other considerations may include availability of airports or helipads for aircraft and weather conditions.

Remember it is not the vehicle per se that is important to the patient – it is the maximisation of available treatment, in the least time reasonably possible and movement to the tertiary centre in a careful, safe and controlled manner.

Each vehicle type has advantages and disadvantages.

Road vehicles

These are relatively slow, and are even slower if the patient cannot tolerate much movement and the driver travels cautiously to compensate. The driver can stop if required by the team, allowing the team to re-evaluate the situation and possibly perform a procedure, such as suction, intubation or chest-tube insertion.

Road vehicles are at the mercy of road congestion – even if use is made of warning devices such as lights and sirens to expedite progress.

Most road ambulance vehicles are constructed on a rigid chassis and have relatively stiff suspension. A fully configured ambulance is quite heavy, with handling and ride quality akin to a truck. For a patient with a painful injury or disease process, a road journey on anything worse than ideal road surfaces can be a very painful one. Patients with unstable cardiorespiratory status often tolerate poor road surfaces badly and need more aggressive support and/or increased sedation, analgesia or muscle relaxation to improve the situation.

Road transfers generally involve less handling, since the patient is loaded and unloaded only once. The exception is that some ambulance services conduct long-distance road trips using multiple road crews in relay.

Helicopters

These are fast and travel point to point. They generally offer a smooth trip although turbulence can have an impact on the patient as well as the team. The efficiency of a helicopter is highly dependent on whether they can offer 'door to door' service. If a road ambulance is required to provide transport between landing site and hospital, their efficiency is compromised. Even short trips by road to the helipad add substantially to the time factor. The handling of the stretcher and patient from one vehicle to another is more important that the actual road distance. Flight in poor weather may not be possible unless the aircraft and pilots are instrument flight rated. Even then, helicopters are restricted by operational limits to fuel carrying capacity, range and until recently, inability to operate in known icing conditions.

Helicopters expose the patient to the effects of altitude. Cabin pressurisation is not available. The amplitude and frequency of airframe vibration in helicopters vary according to type of blade system and the number of blades in the main rotor. Most patients seem to tolerate higher frequencies associated with multiblade aircraft better than two-bladed machines. Anecdotal experience is that newborns with persistent pulmonary hypertension actually improve as a result of these vibrations. These observations have not been tested.

Fixed-wing aircraft

These offer speed and, if pressurised, can fly higher at levels less exposed to weather and turbulence. Pressurisation systems are not designed to make patient transport easier for medical retrieval teams. They are intended to provide physiologically tolerable conditions for healthy passengers at altitudes that would not normally be comfortable. Think of it as being at the elevation of Mount Everest (8850 m, 29 035 ft) but in a cabin pressure altitude (CPA) effectively no higher than Mount Kosciusko (2228 m, 7310 ft). Healthy passengers travel reasonably comfortably at altitudes up to about 3000 m (10 000 ft) but patients should not normally be exposed to above 1200 m (4000 ft).

Patients at increased altitude can find their problems with oxygen delivery exacerbated and trapped internal fluids (gases and liquids) subject to expansion according to Boyle's law. A patient with marginal oxygenation may not tolerate a substantial altitude and trapped gases in the gut, pleural space or pericardium should be vented to atmosphere prior to flight. Otherwise, ground transport or transport by fixed-wing aircraft pressurised at or close to sea level should be used. Not all fixed-wing aircraft can pressurise the cabin to sea level equivalence – at least not without operating at a significantly lower actual altitude. Aircraft pressurisation cannot be activated on the ground, even if the airport is quite high and the patient might benefit from 'descending' to denser air. In a flight originating from an airport at a significant elevation and intending to land at sea level or at a significantly lower elevation, the pilot can dial up the destination altitude quite soon after take off. This strategy can be quite helpful in a marginal patient.

Weather factors

Both helicopters and fixed-wing aircraft are subject to weather limitations. Operated under visual flight rules (VFR), either type of aircraft can be mobilised quite quickly by day. A brief assessment of the weather is adequate and, if suitable for flight, the aircraft can be airborne within 5 to 10 minutes. The pilot navigates by visual reference to the ground and recognisable landmarks. Short-range helicopter operations are particularly suitable for this kind of operation.

At night and in poor weather, instrument flight rules (IFR) operations are generally used. A totally different approach to the planning and conduct of the flight is required. For most of the flight the pilot cannot assume that anything outside is visible and all navigation and descent to land at the destination relies on the instruments in front of him. The weather conditions at the departure point, en route and at the destination must all be assessed. Not only must the pilot be able to take off visually, but the in-flight conditions must be compatible with the aircraft's capabilities. If the expected weather conditions at the destination fall below specified minima, an alternative landing site with better weather conditions must be within range. The logical algorithms by which such assessments are made are unambiguous, quantifiable, auditable and generally not open to subjectivity. The process of IFR planning leads the pilot to give either a 'go' or 'no go' decision. The planning process might be quite complex and at least 30 minutes may be required to reach a conclusion about the flight's feasibility. A decision to go may not guarantee arrival at the intended destination. It simply says that the flight to reach that location can be attempted safely in the knowledge that landing at an alternative location (including returning to the departure point) is factored in.

As an oversimplification, modern fixed-wing aircraft are able to operate in most weather conditions. Helicopters cannot fly in cloud that is close to 0°C. (freezing point of water) or in severe turbulence. Neither type of aircraft can operate through contiguous lines of thunderstorm activity or when fog is present for take off or landing.

Communications

The process of discussing a referral and triaging the optimal transport solution relies on good communication. Earlier, reference has been made to easy access to the key personnel in the referral hospital. Subsequently, the lines of communication need to be maintained so that any change in the patient's condition or further advice sought about management can be conveyed effectively. During transport, transfer and retrieval teams should have the ability to call and be called at any phase of the process. Relaying messages through non-clinical radio operators is not sufficient. The communication devices should allow duplex (two-way simultaneous communications akin to a telephone call or face-to-face communication) for conversational dialogue between clinicians. Where conventional radios are used, a lack of familiarity with their simplex mode of operation, where a press-to-talk switch is required, can lead to information being missed because both parties talk simultaneously.

Wireless technology now makes communication more ubiquitous than ever. Cellular phones and/or satellite phones can be installed in road vehicles and aircraft used for patient transport. Performance depends on the type of technology employed and the coverage offered by the network. GSM digital phones are not designed to be used in the air and are almost useless for aeromedical work. Satellite phones require careful installation, especially in helicopters, where the aerial should not be mounted beneath the rotor hub. When installed they can be quite effective although call rates and voice delay make them less desirable than terrestrial systems. These systems are now ready to carry data as well as voice. Some services are working at creating a 'paperless' environment for the retrieval team, using electronic devices to enter patient-care information.

Medical control

Most medical retrieval teams operate under clinical policies and procedures determined in advance. Such 'off-line' control of the team's practice should be supplemented by 'on-line' control as required. That is, the team should be able to seek advice and guidance at any stage of the process by a telephone conversation in real time with a senior clinician at consultant level. It is helpful if the advice of several senior clinicians is available in a conference call whenever there are multidisciplinary management issues.

It seems ironic that once a patient is in a major institution, many levels of medical control are applied to their care. Prior to that and at the phase of their disease process when the information was leanest and the greatest uncertainty applied, the responsibility for medical care is traditionally delegated to a quite junior medical or paramedical level.

Some definitions

Common expressions

- CPA: cabin pressure altitude.
- IFR: instrument flight rules.
- VFR: visual flight rules.
- Referring: doctor or hospital with the patient needing transfer.
- Referral: doctor or hospital receiving the call and possibly accepting transfer.

Process

- Launch time: time from decision to respond to team departure
- Response time: launch time + outbound leg + circulation (time spent moving from one vehicle to the next or from the last vehicle to the bedside).
- Scene time: stabilisation time + circulation.
- Inbound leg: time travelling toward the destination hospital + circulation.
- Re-positioning leg: time taken to return from the destination to base.
- Mission time: response + scene + inbound + outbound + re-positioning.
- Restoration time: time reconfiguring equipment and restocking the kit.

Information systems

Data about patients being transported are supplied from telephone conversations in the referral process and paper records travelling with the patient or transmitted by fax. In an acute-care setting, many of the details required to assist the consultative process have yet to be committed to paper, either during pre-hospital care or in the referring hospital. Furthermore, electronic data systems developed to support pre-hospital care, EDs and neonatal nurseries are generally not designed to 'talk' with the next party in the chain. As a result, each party collects the same information and records it again. This process is inefficient and also liable to error, duplication and doubt. A challenge yet to be met is to develop a 'daisy-chain' between information systems, which allows previous information to be automatically accessible to the next 'player' in the process. From pre-hospital to referring hospital to medical retrieval team to referral hospital, each field of information should only be collected once. It should then be accessible to and shared with subsequent carers. Ultimately, this chain should link back to the referring hospital, completing a circular pathway that ensures outcome and feedback is provided to the original carers.

Quality

The search for improvement applies to patient transport as much as any other area of care. Given the multiple participants and complex and variable scenarios, a robust and thorough process of quality assurance is essential.

The medical retrieval process cannot stand alone from referring and referral hospital practice. In practice, conducting routine case debriefs, morbidity and mortality meetings and open-case presentations should include as many players as possible. To permit full participation, retrieval teams need to consider holding these activities both in referring hospitals and referral hospitals. The informal contact accompanying these quality activities breaks down barriers, increases mutual respect and facilitates telephone communication about real patients in the future.

It is also recommended that retrieval teams contribute to anonymous incident monitoring systems (AIMS). Such tools help to quantify adverse events.

Summary

- Be available.
- Teletriage intelligently.
- Respond rapidly as appropriate.
- Stabilise fully ('stay and play' rather than 'wrap and run').
- Transport carefully.
- Provide feedback to clients.
- Monitor and review practice.

References

1. Pearson GA, Shann F, Barry P, et al. Should paediatric intensive care be centralised? Trent versus Victoria. *Lancet* 1997;**349**:1213–7.
2. Lewis FR. Improved outcomes from tertiary center pediatric intensive care: A statewide comparison of tertiary and non-tertiary care facilities. *Crit Care Med* 1991;**19**(2):150–9.
3. Velji K, Ross Baker G, Fancott C, et al. Effectiveness of an adapted SBAR communication tool for a rehabilitation setting. *Healthc Q* 2008;**11**(Sp):72–9.
4. Marshall S, Harrison J, Flanagan B. The teaching of a structured tool improves the clarity and content of interprofessional clinical communication. *Qual Saf Health Care* 2009;**18**:137–40.
5. NSW Emergency Transport Service, Australia. www.nets.org.au.
6. Chance GW, Matthew JD, Gash J, et al. Neonatal transport: A controlled study of skilled assistance. Mortality and morbidity of neonates <1.5 kg birth weight. *J Pediatr* 1978;**93**(4):662–6.

27.2 Sick child in a rural hospital

Murali Narayanan • Robert Henning

ESSENTIALS

1 There are significant challenges in translating experience from the urban to rural healthcare settings including differences in the patients, illnesses and health services available.

2 The 'scoop and run' model of pre-hospital care is not appropriate in rural/remote medicine – patients must be 'packaged' as much as possible before transport.

3 Coordination between rural, central and retrieval services must be optimal.

4 Rural services should be supported through targeted training of personnel tailored to the needs of rural clinicians, easily accessible guidelines, accessible consultation services, rural clinical facilities with necessary resources and a supportive relationship with a major urban centre.

Introduction

Most emergency physicians are trained in urban centres. Their skills and knowledge are most readily applied when trained staff, equipment and hospital facilities are immediately available, and when there is ready access to specialists. This becomes an issue when the sick child presents to the emergency department in a rural hospital. Protocols and treatment plans that are appropriate to urban hospitals may be difficult to apply directly.

Challenges in the rural setting

One-third of Australians live in areas defined as rural or remote (areas outside major cities). While Aboriginal and Torres Strait Islanders (ATSI) constitute 2.5% of the total Australian population, they make up 24% of the population in remote areas and 45% of the population in very remote areas. Chronic or recurrent infection, malnutrition, lack of transport, lack of access to health care and educational deficits are all factors which contribute to poorer health status of the people living in these areas.

Income

Although the overall income differences between rich and poor may be smaller, the median household income in rural Australia is 25% lower than that in major cities, and rural families are 50% more likely to be dependent on government pensions and allowances than urban families.

Low income can lead to reluctance to consult a doctor and to reluctance of the doctor to prescribe expensive though appropriate treatments or to commit the family to expensive travel to consult specialists in urban hospitals.

Housing

The quality of housing and of home maintenance is lower in rural areas: maintenance costs are higher, and dwellings deteriorate faster in harsh environments and scarce accommodation leads to overcrowding.

Education

Lower rates of secondary school completion in rural areas than in the city affect both the child and her parents. Infant mortality is closely related to the level of education completed by the mother.

These issues apply also to children in isolated indigenous communities, where the additional problems of distance, access to health care and a relative scarcity of indigenous health workers lead to relatively late hospital presentation of severe illness.

Culture

A tradition of self-reliance and stoicism, combined with suspicion of medical services or of European society in general and varying issues with language difficulties may lead to reluctance to report illness and to delay presentation to seek medical attention. Certain cultural issues, for example not speaking the name of a deceased Aboriginal person, or the tendency of Aboriginal women to avoid eye contact with a strange man, become important considerations in the setting of paediatric emergency medicine.

The illnesses

Birth history

Low birth weight and difficult access to antenatal care in rural areas (especially in indigenous communities) can lead to severe illness in the newborn period, with consequent disability and need for hospital care.

Trauma

Age-standardised rates of serious injury in children from road trauma, interpersonal violence and self-harm increase with distance from major cities in Australia: from 50% greater in inner regional areas to 100% greater in very remote areas. Farm accidents occur frequently: 2/3 of accidental child deaths on farms occur in boys.

Farm vehicles, and especially all-terrain vehicles and four-wheel motor bikes, account for many deaths and injuries, especially to farm visitors. 35–40% of child deaths on farms are due to drowning in dams or drains, especially in children aged less than 5 years.

Infection and diet

Infective conditions, especially of the skin, respiratory and gastrointestinal systems, occur commonly in children from remote communities, where rheumatic heart disease and post-streptococcal glomerulonephritis may result.

There is lack of easy access to fresh food, fruits and vegetables in remote areas. Dietary deficiencies and substance abuse may also contribute to patterns of illness different from those found in children who present to urban hospitals.

The health services

These include community clinics staffed by nurses and/or general medical practitioners (GPs); local hospitals (staffed by nurses, remote emergency physicians and GPs) and ambulance services; regional (base) hospitals which often have paediatricians, emergency physicians, surgeons, anaesthetists and advanced radiology and pathology facilities. Finally, there are city-based patient retrieval services and tertiary hospitals with access to paediatric and neonatal intensive care facilities.

Although inner and outer regional and remote/very remote areas in Australia all have more primary care medical practitioners per 100 000 population than urban areas, this is far outweighed by the ready access of city dwellers to urban hospitals and to specialist care.

Rural general medical practitioners deal with a wide range of illness in a wide range of patients. The nature of general practice means that any single practitioner may rarely (or never) encounter any one of the critical life-threatening illnesses of childhood. This can potentially contribute to a delayed diagnosis and may lead to dilemmas in management. In many rural and remote areas, GPs may be in solo practice, so that consultation with a colleague is difficult, and many regions lack a regional paediatrician to provide timely consultation.

Regional hospitals frequently offer subspecialty clinics staffed by visiting specialists (e.g. paediatric surgery or paediatric cardiology) but these are relatively infrequent and may not coincide with the child's severe illness. The burden of diagnosis and treatment then falls on the clinician on the spot.

The resources available in rural hospitals vary: for example, pathology and radiology staff may be on-call rather than in-house after hours, and the selection of tests, scans and other investigations that are available may be limited.

Distance and difficulty of access to some rural hospitals means that the delay before arrival of a city-based retrieval team can be protracted, sometimes many hours. During this time, the rural clinician often has to manage a very ill and unstable child within the resources of the local hospital.

Caring for the critically ill child

Decisions to consider when child presents with an emergency

The 'scoop and run' model which may be appropriate in some metropolitan environments is not applicable in the remote setting. In fact, the vast distances over which these patients may need to be transported (usually by the RFDS or other state-based retrieval service) mandates that they need to be very well stabilised *prior* to transfer. It needs to be appreciated that the time taken to adequately prepare a patient for transfer from a remote setting is far in excess of the time taken for the same patient in an urban setting. Effective and ongoing communication between the treating doctor, their specialist colleagues in the tertiary emergency department or paediatric intensive care unit, and the RFDS/Retrieval Service is critical to the child's management.

Coordination of a resuscitation team prior to the child's arrival

If the staff in a remote location have prior warning of the arrival of a sick or injured child, they have the opportunity to mobilise any local resources available to them, and also to liaise with tertiary specialist colleagues and ensure that lines of communication are open for when more clinical information is available.

Potential problems to the stabilisation the child

- The reality is that should something go wrong during an air transport, it usually goes badly wrong, and is difficult to fix whilst in the air. Preparation and anticipation of the potential problems in individual cases is thus critical to minimise avoidable pitfalls, prior to patient transfer.
- Vascular access needs to be 'bullet proof' (i.e. more than one intravenous cannula, well secured, and kept patent), endotracheal tubes must be very well secured, and painful unstable injuries appropriately immobilised and pain relieved.
- Preparation of equipment, drugs: ensure there are adequate lines for potentially required infusions inserted and well secured. Plan for adequate stocks of medications, compatible fluids and disposables.
- *Local temperature issues*: for an airplane transport on a 45°C day, the temperature on the tarmac is easily 55–60°C. This may have critical implications for a neonate in a Perspex transport cot which is directly exposed to the sunlight, especially if there is a delay in boarding the craft. Equally, cold, wet and windy conditions may dramatically impact on the stability of a critically ill child.
- *Flight weather problems*: a common problem during summer in Northern Australia, air turbulence, severe electrical storms and even cyclones can have major logistical implications for the transfer of the patient. Flight plans may need to be changed, sometimes once the patient is already en route, and back-up plans need to be in place. Liaising with the highly experienced doctors and operational staff of the RFDS/ Retrieval Service is critical in such a situation.
- *Aeromedical problems:* consideration needs to be given to changes in cabin pressure, oxygenation and temperature which may affect the patient (e.g. child with a pneumothorax). The highly experienced doctors of the RFDS are an invaluable resource in this regard.

It is important to utilise the expertise of GPs and nurse practitioners, clerical staff, orderlies, RFDS staff and rural medical personnel to share the load when dealing with the multitasking required in the management of the critically ill child. Midwives are very able in caring for sick neonates. One should be mindful of the fact that it is very stressful for the healthcare practitioner dealing with a paediatric emergency in the isolated remote setting. From their perspective they should utilise all available resources to help share the load. Do not underestimate the value of the telephone as an important 'piece of resuscitation equipment' to avail resources in times of need.

Conversely, from the perspective of the receiving tertiary unit, it is important to offer ongoing advice and support, and to help plan and facilitate the transfer by liaising supportively with the transferring team (Fig. 27.2.1).

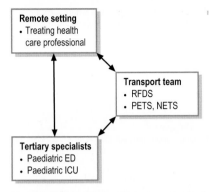

Fig. 27.2.1 The 'Communication Loop' – don't stop communicating!

What can be done to assist care in remote environments?

Personnel

The numbers of medical and nursing practitioners available in rural communities may be increased by financial and educational incentives and by imposing conditions on professional registration that require a period of rural service. These may be backed up by enhanced arrangements for in-service education, and facilitation of career paths. If these arrangements are to succeed, serious consideration must be given to spouse employment, education of children and provision of incentives such as a house and car.

Education

Regular education sessions to remote environments can be arranged through urban tertiary paediatric hospitals. These should be on-line when possible, with self-testing. They should be relevant to the needs of the local practitioner and should be followed up by face-to-face teaching sessions which are primarily hands-on, using the information given in the on-line tutorials. The hands-on teaching may consist of procedural sessions, as well as paediatric mock scenario teaching and group discussions of clinical issues which have arisen within the hospital.

This form of regular in-service teaching should be centrally coordinated, with input from the local practitioners' organisation. It must be centrally funded, with adequate time allocation in the local practitioners' calendar.

As tertiary paediatric hospitals have responsibility for medical care of children in their region, they may organise hands-on training programs (e.g. APLS courses), relevant to rural practice and located in the paediatric hospital, in which rural doctors are invited to participate.

Content of training

Illness recognition and resuscitation courses such as APLS, PALS, ATLS/EMST should be very freely available and the fees government-subsidised for nurses and doctors in rural hospitals. Follow-up training in these areas and on-line plus face-to-face courses on topics relevant to severe childhood illness should also be provided by the staff of the regional tertiary hospital.

Consultation support

A centrally organised and funded framework for provision of 24-hour, 7-day advice on all medical sub-specialties (including paediatric subspecialties) would relieve much of the uncertainty of remote rural practice and would remove many of the delays currently seen in diagnosis and management of relatively uncommon conditions.

The use of telemedicine, including teleradiology, as well as the widespread availability of point-of-care biochemical testing can narrow the uncertainty in diagnosis and allow more accurate assessment and monitoring of the response to treatment in the remote setting.

A centrally coordinated telemedicine network requires a terminal at each point of care (rural medical centre or rural hospital emergency department or paediatric ward), capable of high resolution video transmission and reception, and one or more corresponding terminals within the city paediatric hospital (and general teaching hospitals for other medical specialties). Facilities for on-line transmission of medical imaging to a centrally located radiologist are also needed.

A roster of designated subspecialty consultants with access to telemedicine facilities 24 hours per day would complete the consultation support network.

Transport

In some cases, even the above consultation system will not enable the child to be managed at the rural hospital, and specialist care at a paediatric hospital will be needed. A centrally located paediatric triage and retrieval service, staffed by nurses and doctors with training and experience in triage and paediatric retrieval (see Chapter 27.1) can transfer severely ill and unstable patients to an urban tertiary hospital.

When distances to a large city are very great, it may be more appropriate to transfer the child to a smaller base hospital closer to the child's home, if the severity of the child's illness permits.

Management protocols

These should be available for a range of severe childhood illnesses and be immediately available (e.g. on-line) in the emergency department of rural hospitals. These protocols should be up-dated regularly to keep abreast of current therapies. They should be modified to be clearly appropriate to rural hospital circumstances, although they may be adapted from those in use in the regional tertiary hospital.

These protocols should be jointly produced by tertiary hospital staff, regional paediatricians and community general practitioners, to ensure suitability for the conditions which prevail in a rural hospital. They should contain advice on when to consult, whom to consult, and how to arrange transfer to a paediatric hospital or to the paediatric ward of a regional base hospital.

Hospital facilities

Apart from telemedicine, teleradiology and point-of-care biochemistry facilities, mentioned above, the emergency department of a country hospital which only occasionally treats severely ill children needs to be equipped adequately and appropriately to deal with the child on those infrequent occasions.

A collection of appropriate resuscitation and paediatric care equipment, common to all rural hospitals, maintained by the central health authority of the state or country, devised and updated by people who are using such equipment frequently, should be supplied to each hospital. This equipment should be kept in the emergency department of the rural hospital and checked daily. When an item is used or out of date, it should be replaced promptly from the regional urban store. Such items include a paediatric range of cervical collars;

arm splints; intravenous cannulae; laryngo-scope blades; endotracheal tubes; oropharyngeal airways and laryngeal mask airways (LMAs).

Relations between rural and urban hospitals

In the interests of better coordination and of uniformly good service provision to children in rural areas, the mechanism by which facilities are extended to rural hospitals and their staff should be administered at the regional paediatric hospital. This mechanism should be sensitive to the needs of staff of rural hospitals, and responsive to their suggestions about changes.

Clearly, it is very important that tertiary hospital staff work co-operatively with practitioners in rural areas, and that members of this team are aware of each other's needs. This culture of co-operation, support and mutual respect should be part of the way in which the tertiary hospital sees its role in the health system.

Regular communication between urban and rural practitioners, aided by teaching exchanges, training visits and telemedicine consultations, can promote awareness by each party of the concerns and ideas of the other.

Further reading

Australian Institute of Health and Welfare. *Australia's health 2008*. Canberra: AIHW; 2008. Cat. no. AUS 99.

Australian Institute of Health and Welfare. *A picture of Australia's children 2009*. Canberra: AIHW; 2009. Cat. no. PHE 112.

Australian Institute of Health and Welfare. *Medical. Labour Force 2007*. National Health Labour Force Series no. 44. Canberra: AIHW; 2009.

Emergency Medicine in Rural Australia. Submission to DoHA by the Rural Doctors Association of Australia. Available from: http://www.rdaa.com.au/Uploads/Documents/Emergency%20Medicine%20in%20Rural%20Australia_20101012041618.pdf; 2007 [accessed 29.10.2010].

Fragar LJ, Stiller L, Thomas P. *Child injury on Australian farms*. Canberra: RIRDC; 2005 Rural Industries Research and Development Corporation, and Australian Centre for Agricultural Health and Safety.

Goh A Y-T, Abdel-Latif M El-A, Lum LC-S, Abu-Bakar MN. Outcome of children with different accessibility to tertiary pediatric intensive care in a developing country – a prospective cohort study. *Intens Care Med* 2003;**29**:97–102.

Marcin JP, Nesbitt TS, Kallas HJ, et al. Use of telemedicine to provide pediatric critical care inpatient consultations to underserved rural Northern California. *J Pediatr* 2004;**144**: 375–80.

Peake SL, Judd N. 2007 Supporting rural community-based critical care. *Curr Opin Crit Care* 2007;**13**:720–4.

TEACHING PAEDIATRIC EMERGENCY MEDICINE

SECTION 28

Section editor **Ian Everitt**

28.1 Availing web-based resources

Colin Parker

ESSENTIALS

1 Web resources are becoming increasingly available and integrated into every day practice.

2 Web-based products would ideally provide clinical decision support platforms, rather than being simple data repositories.

3 Users should be able to generate web material more easily via new media such as blogs, forums, wikis, social networks, podcasts and online data storage.

Accessing web-based resources

While books are still a popular medium for doctors with regard to their daily work and learning needs, the rapid progression of web-based media demands that we have a working knowledge of how to utilise this evolving technology to its maximum effect. This chapter aims to briefly explore the needs of Paediatric Emergency Medicine (PEM) staff, types of web-based solutions, and possible future trends.

Needs of paediatric emergency medicine staff

In previous times, resources for staff working in emergency departments (EDs) were scattered around notice boards, bookshelves, folders and in-trays. The technology to make these operational, educational and social resources available from a single portal is finally being utilised.

Operational materials used in everyday clinical work include work rosters, memos, notice boards, directories, as well as clinical resources. Clinical guidelines and protocols of local, national and international origin, as well as traditional textbook-style content about diseases and conditions, can be used in a traditional stand-alone way. More significantly, tools for drug doses and other clinical calculations are paving the way for interactive clinical decision support platforms, where disease management algorithms can be integrated with patient flow, investigation ordering and interpretation, and the electronic health record.

Educational materials are used to a lesser extent during everyday work and increasingly from home, the requirements varying between individuals and their learning needs. Traditionally these materials – mostly books – have been supplied by the hospital or ED library, or purchased by staff themselves for use at home. Interactive forms of learning such as lectures, tutorials and one-to-one supervision are still relevant, but can now be supplemented by newer technologies, to deliver content at a time and place convenient to the learner.

Social needs should not be overlooked, because a cohesive team environment fosters good clinical care and flow of information.

Solutions currently available on the web

Web-based resources are rapidly evolving in terms of the modes of delivery as well as format and flow of content. As books give way to CD-ROMs and software based on desktop computers, so content has moved to the internet and can be retrieved from hand-held devices such as smart-phones via wireless networks or telephone service networks. A similar evolution is happening from static html to dynamic (database-driven) content, through Web 2.0 towards the semantic web.

Traditionally, content has been provided by a limited number of authoritative sources, such as publishers of medical textbooks and journals, generally as high-quality, peer-reviewed paper publications. Many of these are reproduced on computer screens, as a paid service. While these providers will always have an important role as trustworthy sources, the trend is towards sharing more information for free, and greater use of flexible copyright licensing of intellectual property such as the Creative Commons. In the midst of this trend, content is funded either by sponsoring organisations such as governments or pharmaceutical companies, or by selling advertising on the web pages.

Web 2.0

The original internet model of web pages being published by a webmaster and distributed in a one-to-many fashion is rapidly being replaced by the web 2.0 paradigm, where content is generated by the users themselves, updated continuously and shared in an interactive way. The advantages of this wisdom of crowds approach probably outweigh the disadvantages of allowing open access for anyone to edit online content. Web 2.0 is characterised by user-generated content, in the form of metadata tags, blogs, forums, wikis, social networks, online document storage, RSS feeds, and podcasts.

Metadata, or information about data, is used to tag articles with keywords, in such a way that content from disparate sources can be browsed by clicking on the keywords associated with a particular item. This is sometimes displayed in the form of tag clouds, where commonly occurring keywords are displayed more prominently. Users can usually add metadata tags to an item, for the benefit of other users.

Blogs (web logs) started out as personal online diaries for sharing with others. The simple tools which allow non-technical users to add and update web-pages have allowed blogs to evolve into an easy way for anyone to produce their own website. Many medical blogs have thousands of subscribers who receive updates via email or Really Simple Syndication (RSS). Users can leave comments, effectively supporting online discussions.

Forums are a dedicated online space for discussion topics, usually highly specific to a defined area of interest. These discussion threads are effectively an online record of written conversation between two or more users, and their use by medical professionals,

for professional and educational matters, has been relatively limited thus far.

Wikis are web-pages that can be edited by any user, thus harnessing the power of collective knowledge, accelerating the editorial process, and keeping content current.

Social networks such as Facebook and Twitter are increasingly being used by medical professionals to broaden their social and professional networks and to share knowledge. Recognised medical experts may have tens of thousands of followers who receive the snippets of information which they choose to share.

Documents are increasingly stored on the web, in the so-called 'Cloud'. Many services allow editing and sharing of documents online, as a smarter alternative to emailing multiple versions between collaborators, and enabling easy access from any web-accessible device.

While many of us utilise the free electronic table of contents (eTOCs) services of reputable journals, often prompted by our local hospital libraries, personal experience suggests that this method of accessing information has limited usefulness. RSS is a way for information from multiple sources (feeds) to be pushed (rather than having to be actively fetched or pulled) to the user, and collated in one place, the RSS reader or feed aggregator. This allows the user to receive information in a much more efficient way than browsing journals or websites, and content can be viewed at a time and place of the clinician's choice.

Podcasts (portable broadcasts) and vodcasts (video podcasts or videocasts) are a utility which also push content to the user, in the form of audio or video content, which in the medical context usually means lectures, interviews or small-group discussions with a panel of experts. The major advantage for busy doctors and nurses is being able to enjoy these offerings while travelling, exercising, or relaxing at home.

The challenge for healthcare professionals involves assessing the quality and trustworthiness of each of these sources of information. Patients and their families may be less aware of this issue as they utilise a similar spread of information sources. We may need to offer our guidance on the content they are getting from online forums, support groups and personal blogs.

Future directions

As medicine catches up with technological advances, we can look forward to unrestricted, high-speed wireless internet access in our EDs, using hand-held and bedside devices which integrate with decision-support software and the Electronic Health Record. Information flow to patients could be facilitated by these new systems, including the electronic provision of summaries of clinical information, test results, discharge instructions, and medication lists. Educational interactive spaces incorporating RSS feeds, blogs, vodcasts, editable wikis and reference documents will probably be combined in an interactive platform where users can ask questions and discuss topics as an online community, from the comfort of home.

Hopefully, technical standards will continue to converge, allowing EDs around the country and around the world to combine their resources of hardware and data via the concept of grid computing and the deep web. By sharing unified, coordinated mega-databases of clinical data, investigation results, treatments and outcomes, we could potentially combine thousands of clinician lifetimes of individual experience into an intelligent, cohesive resource. Taking this a step further, we might eventually see internationally-coordinated administration of epidemiological data, clinical research, decision support via neural networks, and even generating new hypotheses for research via artificial intelligence systems constantly re-examining the body of clinical data.

Links

A list of useful web resources for PEM can be found at: http://lifeinthefastlane.com/resources/PEM

Further reading

http://lifeinthefastlane.com/2009/07/information-overload.
http://en.wikipedia.org/wiki/Health_2.0.
http://www.bmj.com/cgi/content/full/333/7582/1283.
http://casesblog.blogspot.com/2005/10/web-20-in-medicine.html.
http://www.slideshare.net/colinparker/emergency-medicine-web-resources. [Websites accessed 29.10.10].

28.2 Teaching paediatric emergency medicine

Colin Parker

ESSENTIALS

1 Effective communication skills and healthy attitudes are prerequisites for good paediatric emergency medicine practice, and their teaching should take precedence over teaching knowledge and skills.

2 Self preservation skills should also be taught.

3 Clinical experience is essential in gaining perspective on clinical knowledge.

4 There are unlimited methods for acquiring new knowledge; part of teaching new trainees is educating them about how to use available media and methods to best effect.

Introduction

Despite the massive explosion in the availability of information, doctors will never be replaced by computers. Paediatric emergency medicine (PEM) has elements of science, particularly with the steady growth of evidence-based medicine, but also relies heavily on the practical application of experience. Perhaps the emergent aspects of PEM, such as trauma resuscitation, have a more formulaic basis; however, clear and effective communication from the team leader is of paramount importance in a challenging resuscitation.

The bulk of PEM does not consist of emergent interventions, but rather risk stratification, and trading information with parents of children who may or may not be very unwell. Parents bring their children for reassurance, explanation, and occasionally some form of treatment. They want to feel that they have been taken seriously, and that someone cares about the well-being of their child. In short, they want to feel better after seeing the doctor.

The practice of PEM requires a set of skills, knowledge and attitudes broadly similar to those required for the practice of clinical medicine generally, but with the added requirement of having to communicate effectively under the pressures of time and emotional stress. Because doctors' attitudes are so enmeshed with ability to communicate, it is important to teach the correct attitudes before teaching skills and knowledge. Doctors with healthy attitudes will be driven to continually expand their knowledge and skills, and will seek out any available resources to improve the way they care for their patients.

Desirable attitudes in PEM

With the success of immunisation programmes and, to a lesser extent, injury prevention strategies, there seems to be a changing spectrum of illness in children presenting to emergency departments (EDs), with fewer critically unwell children, medicalisation of behavioural issues, and children with a functional component to their 'dis-ease'. In addition, the public perception of the wonders of modern medicine results in high expectations, which are sometimes difficult for clinicians to meet. The best protection is to approach with healthy attitudes:

- humility;
- caring;
- empathy and compassion;
- non-judgemental approach;
- honesty and integrity;
- advocacy and healthy paternalism;
- self-monitoring and awareness of cognitive errors in medicine.

Humility Growth in the acquisition of medical knowledge can be likened to exploring a forest: initially it is hard to see the wood for the trees; as one gets to know the landscape, one can develop an appreciation for the large valley in which the forest sits. By the third postgraduate year doctors are familiar with the whole valley. Most then travel up to the crest and realise that the valley is but a small part of the countryside, and there is in fact a vast body of knowledge which they may never know and never discover. While knowledge itself is a valuable asset, a high knowledge-to-confidence ratio is perhaps more desirable.

Caring Many communication difficulties can be overcome by having and projecting a caring attitude. With children especially, parents may not care what the doctor knows, until they know that the doctor cares. Doctors' own biases and personality differences can sometimes make this caring seem a difficult task. Projecting a caring attitude initially usually results in a positive feedback which sets the scene for genuine caring to supervene.

Empathy and compassion Doctors who are themselves parents find it easier to imagine the emotional strain of having a sick child. This tension may sometimes be expressed in fiercely protective terms by a worried parent, in the same way that patients themselves often forego the social graces when they are unwell. It is important not to take this personally, and try to imagine how the parents are feeling.

Non-judgemental approach There is a common perception among some ED staff that some children should not have been brought to the hospital because 'it's not an emergency'. They may blame the referring clinician, the parent or the patient. Everyone who brings their child to an ED has crossed some threshold of anxiety about the perceived illness, and every one of them has considered not coming to the ED. Most of them do not have significant knowledge of health-related matters. There is no place for a judgemental approach, which will not help the child or prevent a future ED visit.

Honesty and integrity   It is important to teach our colleagues humility. Doctors are often humbled by questions they cannot answer and mistakes they may have made. Appropriate teaching to junior colleagues should suggest that answers to parents should be 'I don't know but I will try to find out' and to colleagues 'that's a good idea, I forgot to check that'.

Advocacy and healthy paternalism Planning a course of action requires a collaboration between the clinician and the patient or parent. This collaboration needs to walk the fine line between patient/parent autonomy and the benefit of the unique knowledge and perspective of the health professional. In this regard, doctors need to act as advocates for the child and gently steer the collaborative decision towards one that leads to the best outcome for the patient and family.

Self-monitoring and awareness of cognitive errors   Most clinical presentations have a differential diagnosis. Healthy self-doubt and consideration of potentially bad outcomes are useful safeguards. Doctors process and synthesise available information in various ways, subject to a number of errors of cognition. These include diagnosis momentum, where doctors accept the perceptions of other clinicians and allow a diagnostic label to stick, without making an independent assessment. Or doctors may be affected by anchoring, where they decide on a particular diagnosis relatively early on in the assessment process, and reject subsequent information that does not fit. When there is some diagnostic uncertainty, the simple act of discussing the case with a colleague can often provide clarity from this cognitive fog. The main stumbling-block is the clinical maturity required to recognise feelings of uncertainty, and to act on those feelings.

Skill set for PEM

Doctors in PEM need to develop a set of practical skills, including the art of communication, clinical examination, procedural

skills, teaching and self-preservation. The most important of these is communication, a skill which is intimately entwined with attitudes and which improves with practice.

Effective communication

The groundwork for an effective consultation starts before meeting the parents. Even in busy, seemingly chaotic EDs, parents are watching and listening to those around them, especially members of staff. Individual doctors may be seen in a good light by the way they interact with staff, patients or parents, or subtle clues in the way they are introduced by their co-workers. Non-verbal aspects of communication play an important role in the initial impression; the demeanour of the doctor is probably more important than the way they are dressed, although reasonable standards in dress code assist in engendering trust.

The essential communication tasks which need to be achieved in a PEM consultation include establishing rapport, gathering information (taking a clinical history), providing information, and demonstrating the attitudes discussed previously.

An important teaching point is that gaining the trust of children starts with getting their parents or caregivers on side. The child is assessing the way their parent relates to this stranger, relying heavily on non-verbal cues to decide whether to trust the doctor. When talking to the child, an approach that illustrates the doctor's interest in them, at an age-appropriate level, is preferred. Rather than trying to playfully examine a child, time spent exclusively in play or developing rapport for the first minute or two, is time well-invested. All family members and supporting visitors should be acknowledged individually. In particular, siblings of pre-school age may become disruptive later in the consultation if they do not feel involved, and it may be helpful to give them a minor task or distraction: 'could you please hold my torch until I need it'.

History taking may be facilitated by clinical pathways, pro formas, or checklists, but diverting attention to the paperwork is a barrier to forming an effective clinical relationship. These checklists are best incorporated into practice by referring to them after the consultation, and going back to fill in the detail later; this is certainly an incentive to remember the information in future.

Several types of information may need to be provided to the patient and parents. These include imparting medical facts, explaining the natural history of a condition, describing or clarifying risk, and providing insight or perspective to the clinical situation. It may help to impart the doctor's own feelings about the clinical risk in an honest and caring way, for example, 'I'm a bit concerned about some aspects, but my feeling is that your child will be completely better in a day or two'. This often goes a long way towards managing unrealistic expectations or unreasonable demands, provided that a therapeutic relationship has been established first, such that the parents trust the doctor as someone who genuinely cares about their child.

This is perhaps the most important aspect to teach: establishing a trusting relationship built on mutual respect, by exercising the attitudes previously outlined: humility, caring, empathy, compassion, non-judgemental approach, honesty, advocacy and a healthy awareness of one's own limitations. A useful conclusion to any consultation is to invite questions. Giving the parent or patient permission to clarify any areas of concern to them provides the doctor with the opportunity to deal with any concealed dissatisfaction. It also can result in positive feedback, and reassurance that all aspects have been well explained.

Skilful clinical examination

A good physical evaluation helps to illustrate the special skills and knowledge that have been acquired by the clinician, even if these particular skills are not absolutely essential to the examination. For example, testing the tendon reflexes in a child with a minor head injury seldom changes the clinical impression, but adds value to the relationship in demonstrating thoroughness. Just as it is important to acknowledge all family members and friends at the bedside, one may need to ensure that a parent or grandparent in the waiting room is in attendance for the examination and subsequent explanation of findings. This is more time-effective than dealing with queries later.

It is important to teach that the examination of infants and toddlers should usually be more opportunistic than systematic, but also that a confident, gentle and structured examination usually inspires confidence and trust.

Mastering procedural skills

A handful of life-saving emergency procedures and a few time-important urgent practical skills need to be addressed in the training of doctors working in a paediatric emergency setting. These include basic and advanced airway and ventilation skills, intravenous and intraosseous access, and screening tests for infection such as blood cultures, lumbar puncture, and urgent urine sampling by suprapubic aspiration or urethral catheterisation.

Learning to teach

With increasing competence it is expected that most doctors will adopt the roles of supervising and teaching others. Teaching the teacher poses a new set of challenges but also brings new rewards because of the variety of learning and teaching styles amongst different individuals. The advantage to those doctors acquiring new knowledge, skills and attitudes is that they can pick and choose from a variety of teachers, and thereby develop their own style of clinical practice and teaching. Supervising colleagues involves the constant appraisal and reappraisal of clinical risk, if one considers that every clinical interaction puts three people at risk: the patient, the doctor, and the doctor in charge. Inevitably there is an element of trust, based on intuition, based on previous experiences, and based on the answers to a few pertinent questions. The safest alternative for all is for the reviewing doctor to adopt a hands-on approach and personally meet the child-parent unit, until that collegiate trust is well established and well founded.

Self-preservation

Working as a doctor in PEM is emotionally tiring, because it involves caring communication under pressure. Doctors in this environment need to be taught to be careful to avoid burnout. They should think about providing the greatest good to the greatest number of children over their professional lifetimes. A doctor who is impaired by ill-health or emotional exhaustion cannot provide good clinical care.

Strategies for avoiding burnout include learning to say no to extra work (even if it brings extra rewards), learning effective time management and prioritising tasks appropriately, physical exercise and pursuit of non-work enjoyments, and learning to build mutually supportive working relationships with colleagues. Doing meaningful work as a valued member of a supportive team is the goal to strive for.

Putting knowledge into perspective

There is no real limit to the breadth and depth of the knowledge-base of PEM. A continuous thirst for knowledge, inspired by the desirable attitudes previously mentioned, can motivate doctors in this exploration, but it is impossible for us to acquire all the medical facts, theories and controversies. The need to carry around encyclopaedic volumes of knowledge in doctors' heads is slowly diminishing as the information age starts to live up to its promise of instant availability of highly specific information. Therefore, learning how to access information, knowing where to look for high-quality, trustworthy content, and being able to critically appraise and assess the relative value of the information are becoming vitally important skills.

The value for the diagnostician in exploring a large body of knowledge such as PEM is not so much in being able to instantly recall specific facts, but rather to acquire a low-resolution background of finer forgotten details. A specific part of the clinical picture may then trigger a diagnostic thought process leading to an appropriate search.

PEM is unpredictable in terms of what challenges might come through the door at any moment, yet there are a few recurring themes which make up a large volume of the clinical work. If one excludes minor injuries and serious trauma, more than 80% of the remaining medical presentations are encompassed by six clinical scenarios: fever, breathing difficulty, vomiting with or without diarrhoea, abdominal pain, skin rash, and possible seizure. Therefore there is a relatively well-defined scope of learning for those who need to get comfortable with the majority of childhood clinical conditions presenting to an ED, and a much larger range of conditions for those who need to know more.

While experience on its own can be relatively uninformative, reflecting on experiences enables doctors to increase knowledge, and gain perspective. Thus, by seeing many patients and learning a small amount from each clinical encounter, doctors can become experienced, mature clinicians. A voluminous clinical workload without reflection, and learning without patients are both sub-optimal routes to this desired outcome.

Helping others acquire knowledge, skills and attitudes: modes of learning

A customised local solution for teaching PEM in a particular ED or institution depends on the spectrum of learners (students, nurses, doctors of varying experience and qualifications), incentives to encourage learning, and relative availability of different information resources: people, books, and other media.

The requirements of learners vary depending on whether they are nursing students, nurses of various grades, medical students, prevocational doctors, specialists-in-training from either a paediatric or an emergency medicine background, senior trainees in PEM, or consultants with different backgrounds and strengths. Learners themselves should be asked what they perceive as their general and specific goals and learning objectives.

Incentives to encourage learning include the unavoidable performance appraisal that accompanies employment as a hospital doctor, coupled with the concept of gaining a positive job reference for the next rotation. This incentive is relatively subjective, low-impact, diffuse, lacks immediate reward for good performance, and does not generally identify the acquired abilities of candidates with any degree of detail. Formal testing in the form of tests or assignments adds a dimension of anxiety and workload which may be perceived as a nuisance for both learners and teachers. For this reason, most testing is ad hoc and informal, being conducted during clinical supervision, shift handover and small-group tutorials, usually as an opportunistic, subconscious activity by a range of assessors. The traditional old-fashioned incentive of accountability for the well-being of one's patients, and the awkwardness of not knowing what to do in a given clinical situation, is perhaps being overtaken by the trend towards increasing degrees and seniority of supervision at the clinical coalface. Staff are additionally motivated to learn by their caring outlook and pride in their work. The option of a safety net should be considered, whereby there are minimum requirements of documented attendance at learning activities. Unfortunately this does not guarantee the acquisition of a minimum standard of attitudes, skills and knowledge.

Learning resources

People

The centuries-old tradition of mentorship and a clinical apprenticeship is no longer available as a one-to-one model, but this can be approximated by arranging for learners and teachers to do clinical work in the same physical space, within sight and earshot of each other. The opportunity exists in many EDs for doctors from a paediatric background to engage in a two-way exchange of ideas with those from an emergency medicine background. We learn a great deal from teaching our team-mates.

Didactic lectures are a way of sharing information with large numbers of learners, but are limited by the relative lack of interactivity, and are likely to be superseded by technological alternatives which allow the learners to choose the time and the environment most convenient for themselves. Small-group tutorials offer more interactivity, but are limited by availability of protected teaching time away from clinical duties for both learners and facilitators.

Books

Textbooks, handbooks and journals are still a convenient, reliable, low-tech learning medium. The limitations of portability, cost, and infrequent updates are still outweighed by the longstanding trusting relationship doctors have with the distributors of high-quality, peer-reviewed content from experts in their respective fields. The challenge for these distributors is to adapt their resources to newer media and models of delivery, rather than duplicate their books onto a computer screen.

Other media

Exciting new modes of learning are constantly being developed, and the current generation of learners awaits these new media with anticipation. While there is an abundance of free content available, a fair proportion of high-quality content is by paid subscription or membership. Delivery modes include audio, video, simulation with high or low-fidelity training models, dedicated software solutions, and an ever-expanding suite of web-based resources.

Audio and video reproductions of lectures, discussions, opinions and procedures may be delivered via physical media such as compact discs and digital versatile discs, or increasingly, via web technology such as streaming, mp3s, podcasts and vodcasts.

While these traditional media of text, audio and video may be individually reproduced on computers and hand-held mobile devices, the real future of web-based resources rests with combining these media into a single interactive space, managed by an active and interactive community of users. It seems likely that software solutions such as clinical decision support systems and interactive multiple choice question programs will eventually be replaced by internet-based interactive spaces or platforms combining traditional text, audio and video content with the interactivity of blogs, forums, and wikis so that users can contribute to the body of knowledge while experiencing the content in a direct and meaningful way.

Conclusions

Engaging learners in the task of acquiring the skills and knowledge for the safe and rewarding clinical practice of high-quality paediatric emergency medicine is difficult. It starts with the challenge of instilling the appropriate attitudes required to propagate these skills and knowledge in ourselves and in our colleagues.

Further reading

Groopman J. *How Doctors Think*. New York: Mariner Books, Houghton Mifflin Company; 2008.

Henry GL. Human interaction: practical ways to prevent malpractice. *Emergency Medicine Reviews and Perspectives* 2003; April 2003 (audio series).

PAEDIATRIC RESEARCH IN THE EMERGENCY DEPARTMENT

Section editor **Ian Everitt**

29.1 Research in children in the emergency department

Franz E. Babl • Meredith Borland • Andrew J. Davidson

ESSENTIALS

1 Research is essential to establish an evidence base in paediatric emergency medicine and optimise individual treatment.

2 At the core of any research project is the development of a viable research question which drives the study design.

3 A biostatistician should be involved early in the study design.

4 Agreement on key data elements and outcomes, including definitions, feasibility of collection and validity of observations must happen early in the study design.

5 Apart from a lack of subjects, the major problem in clinical research projects is poor design.

6 Good clinical research practice is important in all studies.

7 Consent and risk are key ethical issues in all studies involving children

8 Multicentre research can address the difficulty of recruiting adequate numbers of paediatric patients.

Introduction

Research is an important part of emergency medicine as it provides the scientific basis for optimal patient care. Key elements for conducting high quality, ethical research are the development of a good research question, use of an appropriate study design, adherence to good clinical research practice and an understanding of the ethical basis for research. Study design, the quality of the conduct of the study and its ethics are all intricately linked.

Increasing numbers of emergency physicians, nurses and allied health personnel are involved in research, and trainees are now required to complete research projects during training. Yet few emergency clinicians have formal research training. In addition, over the past years both national and local regulatory requirements have become more complex. Research funding is often difficult to obtain in both the emergency and paediatric setting. Hospitals and departments often have to focus on clinical care with limited resources for dedicated staff, time for research, research assistants or infrastructure for studies. Hence, there is a critical and overdue requirement for the development of paediatric emergency medicine within university academic settings, where research is highly valued and an intrinsic part of daily business.

In addition, serious outcomes and adverse events are rare in children and data collected at paediatric tertiary institutions may not be applicable to other settings. Informed consent is difficult to obtain in the emergency setting and the ethics of research in children, as a particularly vulnerable group, creates an additional degree of complexity.

However, despite these difficulties, a number of strategies can be used to overcome the perceived barriers and achieve quality research in children in the emergency department.

Research science

All research should have a sound scientific basis. Getting the science right is essential before starting any project.

Research question

The most crucial component of every project is the research question. The question defines all the other elements of the research design, including the hypothesis and objective of the project.

A good study question should be:

- original or add significantly to what is known;
- relevant and important;
- feasible, based on resources, skills, time, subject availability;
- ethical;
- plausible, that is there should be a scientific basis for the question;
- clearly defined.

Determining these factors requires clinical perspective and a detailed literature search. In clinical research the most relevant or important questions are those that actually change clinical practice.

A question can be defined in terms of the acronym PICOT:

- population (who should be in the study?);
- indicator (what is the intervention or exposure of interest?);
- comparator (what is the gold standard? comparison vs baseline vs control group?);
- outcome (what is the outcome of interest?);
- timeframe (over what time period?).

The outcome measures are often the most difficult to determine and must be clearly defined, usually with a single primary outcome to answer the study question and further secondary outcomes, which may be multiple, to expand on this question. These should be determined in advance, not after study results are in.

Literature review and level of evidence

The literature review should provide the background to the study question. Literature databases like Pubmed, Medline, Google scholar internet search engines, EMBASE and CINAHL (Cumulative Index to Nursing and Allied Health Literature) are useful but may initially be overwhelming. Helpful starting points can be standard textbooks, the Cochrane library, a search of BestBets (www.bestbets.org), BMJ Clinical Evidence (http://clinical-evidence.bmj.com) and the assistance of a medical librarian.

It is important to grade the importance of medical research evidence. There are many grading systems in use internationally. A commonly used example from National Health and Medical Research Council of Australia (NHMRC) is shown in Table 29.1.1.[1] Systematic reviews often use such a grading system as the basis for clinical management recommendations. The current standard of research evidence is the randomised clinical trial (RCT), and the highest level of evidence is meta-analysis of RCTs.

Types of studies

Studies can be grouped in a number of ways. Studies can be descriptive, analytic or interventional. Intervention studies can either assess the efficacy of the intervention (does

it work in a study?) or the effectiveness (does it work in the everyday ED situation?) (Table 29.1.2).

The ethics of medical research

Following atrocities during the Second World War, written codes of medical ethics have been developed such as the Nuremberg Code[2], the Declaration of Helsinki[3] and the Belmont Report.[4] The key principles developed in these documents still underpin most ethical guidelines.

Key principles

The key principles of research ethics include respect for persons, beneficence and justice as well as 'research merit and integrity'.

Respect for persons recognises the value of autonomy to an individual. Participants must have the power to make their own decisions, if possible. Having respect for persons requires due regard for beliefs, customs and cultural heritage of individuals as well as respecting privacy and confidentiality. Consent is the key element of respect. The consent to participate in a research project must be free and informed. Free consent implies a voluntary choice not influenced by external coercion, pressure or inducement. Informed consent implies that the participant has sufficient information and adequate understanding of

Table 29.1.1	Levels of evidence according to type of research question
Level	**Study design**
I	Evidence obtained from a systematic review of all relevant randomised controlled trials
II	Evidence obtained from at least one properly designed randomised controlled trial
III-1	Evidence obtained from well-designed pseudo-randomised controlled trials (alternate allocation or some other method)
III-2	Evidence obtained from comparative studies (including systematic reviews of such studies) with concurrent controls and allocation not randomised, cohort studies, case-control studies, or interrupted time series with a control group
III-3	Evidence obtained from comparative studies with historical control, two or more single arm studies, or interrupted time series without a parallel control group
IV	Evidence obtained from case series, either post-test or pretest/post-test

Adapted from NHMRC 1999.

Table 29.1.2 Types of studies

Study groups and question	Study type	Description	Limitations	Level of evidence
Descriptive Describes the distribution of a certain variable such as an exposure/disease/ symptom, e.g. 'How many children vomit after intranasal fentanyl?'	Case series	Case reports without control of interventions. May develop hypothesis for later prospective trials	Data often obtained retrospectively with inaccurate, incomplete or measurement bias	IV
	Cohort studies	Prospective or retrospective longer term follow up of patients. Can be observational or case-controlled	Selection bias No specific interventions performed	III-2
	Cross-sectional studies	At given time point population studied to determine prevalence (not incidence) of disease. Quick, relatively inexpensive	Causal relationship cannot be established	IV
Analytical Evaluate associations to discover cause and effect relations, e.g. 'What factors are associated with vomiting after intranasal fentanyl?'	Randomised controlled trials (RCT)	Definitive method to assess effect of intervention Allocates to intervention or control group	Difficult to conduct and large numbers may be required	II
	Case-controlled studies	Recruit disease vs non disease and assess exposure status between groups. Used for rare disease and infrequently in ED	Prone to selection bias No information on risk of disease	III-3
	Pilot study	Identifies problems with study protocol, derives mean and standard deviation for power calculations	Common euphemism for poorly planned study with inadequate numbers to detect planned outcome	
	Crossover studies	In stable disease can alternate treatments in same patients and reduces sample size	Can have high drop-out rates which significantly reduces study power	III-2
Literature review	Review	Summary of available evidence	May be incomplete due to inadequate search strategies Variable use of 'formal' critique of evidence	
	Meta-analysis	Re-analysis of previously reported trials Used to attempt to find relationships not apparent in original trials due to lack of numbers	Subject to limitations in original study design. Only 50% of published articles found in Medline search Different studies have different methodology Positive studies published more than negative studies	Depends on studies contained. If studies are level II then will be assigned level I

the proposed research, and, particularly in the paediatric context, is sufficiently mature to understand the consequences of the decision to take part in the study.

The principle of beneficence includes the concept of maximising possible benefits and minimising possible harm while avoiding unnecessary burdens. Non-therapeutic research or research where the risk of harm is possibly greater than the risk of benefit is not beneficent.

The principle of justice implies there should be no inequality in sharing the burden or risks and the benefits of research. The most obvious examples of injustice are where research benefits or risks are unevenly distributed amongst the wealthy and poor, or conducting research exclusively in minority populations to benefit non-minority populations.

Ethics of research involving children

Due to the exploitation of children prior to the Nuremberg Code there is added complexity relating to research in children. This relates to the key component of informed consent. The age at which a child develops the maturity to understand, give informed consent or accept risk for altruistic reasons is not predefined by chronological age. There is variability in this, based on complexity of the proposed intervention. It is important to note that ethical standards and criteria for study participation evolve over time, and what is acceptable now may be controversial or unacceptable in the future, just as previous standards may now be considered questionable. This is particularly so in relation to children.

Assent by the child is a requirement used in some countries (e.g. USA) from the age of approximately 7 years for studies involving children, although formal consent is still required from the legal guardians.

There are in general four recruitment scenarios for children presenting to the ED who may be enrolled in research studies:[5]

❶ Infants/toddlers without the capacity to understand or take part in discussions regarding a research project and whose parents/guardians are approached for consent.

❷ Children able to understand some relevant information and take part in limited discussion about the research, but whose consent is not required. Only parent/guardian consent is required for these children.

❸ Young people of developing maturity, able to understand the relevant information but whose relative immaturity means they remain vulnerable. The consent of these young people is required, but is not sufficient to authorise research, therefore requiring additional parent/guardian consent.

❹ Young people mature enough to understand and consent, and not vulnerable through immaturity in ways that warrant additional consent from a parent or guardian.

As children have limited capacity to consent, the degree of risk they can be exposed to needs careful consideration. In general, risk is classified in degrees, and the degree of risk acceptable depends on the importance of the study, and the likelihood of any direct benefit to the child. For example, the risk of complications from placing an intravenous cannula may be unacceptable in a child when studying a minor condition such as otitis media but acceptable in the setting of determining the effectiveness of a chemotherapy agent. In order that some important research involving children may legitimately be carried out, most jurisdictions deem that it is acceptable to have some degree of risk for the child who is unable to consent where there is no direct benefit accruing to that child, provided certain limitations are adhered to.

In addition, in the ED setting there is the added complexity relating to recruitment for a study at the time of an acute injury or illness. This makes it more difficult to fully assess the child's maturity level and understanding and to appreciate the potential for researchers to apply covert pressure to a reluctant child. Enrolment may also be curtailed by parents/guardians being unwilling or unavailable to consent during the stress of the presentation to the ED.

Ethics review process

The implementation of national guidelines and principles to individual projects is left to the discretion of committees administered locally by research institutions or hospitals. Research other than low or negligible risk research must be reviewed by a local ethics committee. Ethics committees are usually composed of representatives from clinical (doctors, nurses etc), research and community (lay people and clergy) groups. All research must be approved in writing by the sponsoring institution before it can commence. Research requiring Human Research and Ethics Committee (HREC) approval may not start until there is clear written approval from the committee.

The primary objectives of an HREC are to assess the ethical principles by which research projects in humans are proposed and conducted, protecting the welfare and rights of the research participants and to facilitate research that is or will be of benefit to the researcher's community or to humankind. HRECs may also consider all matters relating to project design, technical feasibility and any other ethical implications associated with each project. The ethics review process is not perfect and may be frustrating but a wise researcher engages with the ethics committee in a positive and helpful manner.

Many small projects can be undertaken as clinical audits and would be regarded by the community as an essential part of clinical practice, such as an analysis of the types of clinical presentations that did not wait to be seen. These projects should still be presented to the HREC, but in most institutions should undergo an expedited review, without the need for a full ethics submission and the consequent delay. In this circumstance, it is still important to plan the research project fully, as the project will not be of benefit to anyone if a researcher has not collected and analysed the data in a systematic and rigorous manner.

HREC approval is often contingent on other processes. The hospital lawyer and hospital insurer may have to sign off on high-risk projects; the trials may need registration and Therapeutic Goods Administration (TGA) notification may be required in clinical drug or device studies. A study can only be commenced once HREC approval has been obtained and only HREC approved study documents may be used during a study.

The practice and governance of research

Well-conducted clinical research is far more likely to discover the truth. There are basic professional standards in the conduct of research which must be met during this process.

Research documents

Good documentation is a key to a successful study. Documents should be kept together, be complete, dated, and secured. There should be a clear trail of all data from the point of data collection, collation into database through to publication. This trail may be scrutinised if there is any question about the veracity of a research finding. Clear documentation is also essential to reduce the chance of error and to keep the project running smoothly.

Research protocol

The key document for any study is the research protocol. It sets out why a trial should be run, acts as an operations manual and is the scientific design document for the trial. It is submitted to the HREC at the time of approval application along with the case report forms, patient information statement and consent form. The research protocol outlines in detail the research question being asked, background and rationale for the study, the design and methodology by which the question will be addressed, secondary objectives, primary and secondary outcomes, statistical considerations including sample size and power calculations. There should also be a discussion of any ethical implications of the study being undertaken. Templates for protocols can be found on the websites of a number of organisations such as the TGA.[6]

Case report forms (CRF)

The CRF is designed to record all of the required information as defined in the protocol for accurate analysis. Badly designed CRFs negatively affect the quality of data analysis and the ability of the project to answer the research question. CRFs should be designed concurrently with the protocol, preferably with input from a biostatistician and should be piloted prior to study commencement. All data collected for the study should be recorded directly, promptly, accurately and legibly.

Patient information statement and consent form

In order to gain informed consent from a potential research participant, research projects require patient information statements in plain language and consent forms that must be approved by the ethics committee prior to their use. They are intended to outline the proposed study in language lay people can understand. Good patient information statements are difficult to write and poorly written ones may cause delays in obtaining ethics approval.[7]

Study document file

The study document file should be kept in the ED administrative area and contain copies of all documentation relevant to the study in an orderly and systematic fashion. Good data handling and record keeping ensures a 'paper and electronic trail' that testifies to the accuracy of the reported data, as a study may be audited even years after it has finished.

The research team

Research is a team effort, even for a small trainee-led project. Good research practice involves having an effective team of researchers and collaborators (such as nurses, junior doctors, allied health workers) with a clear understanding of who is responsible for what and who reports to whom. Even in small studies, biostatisticians should be involved early in the design stage. They will help guide researchers to determine study design and sample size in addition to their role in database creation and data analysis.

Depending on the size and type of study, teams may include, in addition to clinicians, expert researchers, statisticians, pharmacists and/or technicians, health economists, trial coordinators, data manager, data entry staff and research nurses or assistants.

Larger studies may require several groups or committees such as a trial management group (to manage the trial on a day-to-day basis), trial steering committee, data monitoring and/or safety committee and data management committee. These committees should have regular minuted meetings.

Databases and analysis

Good data management should be carefully planned from before the first data are collected though to the analysis of data; otherwise implausible values and inconsistencies are carried through to the analysis phase, where it is very difficult to correct errors. A database is a computer software program (e.g. EpiData) where data is entered and stored in a table or file, which is called the data file. Each study patient should have a unique identifier different from the patient's hospital number to ensure confidentiality. Even for simple databases, a 'coding manual' should be created to explain variable names, describe the variables and their units, specify the number of decimals, etc. Studies are often performed over a period of time and what seems obvious at the beginning of the process may become cryptic at the analysis stage. Data must be kept securely with password protection and limited access by nominated and HREC-approved researchers, and be regularly backed up.

Reporting guidelines

The reporting of clinical trials has a recommended, standardised approach, outlined by the CONSORT Statement, an evidence based format aimed at improving the quality and integrity of reporting for RCTs. CONSORT consists of a checklist and flow diagram for reporting a RCT.[8] The flow diagram provides readers with a clear picture of the progress of all participants in the trial, from the time they are randomised until the end of their involvement. Both documents are also very helpful at the design stage of the trial and ensure that the research protocol is comprehensive and logical.

There are also a number of reporting guidelines for other types of studies. Information about reporting guidelines, including key checklists and flow diagrams, is listed at the EQUATOR website.[9]

Key regulatory documents

The National Statement on Ethical Conduct in Human Research[5]

The peak medical research bodies in Australia (NHMRC, Australian Research Council (ARC) and the Australian Vice Chancellors' Committee (AVCC)) produce this joint statement which is Australia's primary source of guidance promoting ethically sound review and conduct of human research with national standards to guide institutions, researchers and HRECs.

International Conference on Harmonisation of Good Clinical Practice guidelines (ICH-GCP)[10]

This is an international document accepted in Australia. It was developed through a drive to regulate requirements for a single market for pharmaceuticals. ICH-GCP is also known as GCP or GCRP (good clinical research practice). It is an overarching ethical and quality standard for the design, conduct, performance, recording, analysis, monitoring, auditing and reporting of clinical research. It also includes protection of human rights as a subject in clinical trial.

Australian Code for the Responsible Conduct of Research[11]

Having been jointly authored by ARC, AVCC, and NHMRC, this code is designed to guide institutions and researchers in how to achieve and maintain responsible research practice.

All research in Australia must abide by the National Statement. The National Statement requires that research is conducted in accordance with the Australian Code of Conduct. However, this document does not provide an exhaustive description of how to conduct research. The TGA has published a more detailed document describing how research should be performed in Australia which in turn requires that researchers follow relevant sections of the ICH GCP.[10]

The aim of these documents is not only to increase the scientific quality and hence the veracity of findings but also to ensure research is conducted in an ethically responsible manner and that the findings are verifiable. Being compliant with these documents assures the public that the data and reported results are credible and accurate and that the rights, integrity and confidentiality of human research subjects have been protected.

Project registration

Since July 2005 all clinical trials must be registered on a Clinical Trials Register before the enrolment of the first participant. The guidelines of the International Committee of Medical Journal Editors (ICMJE) state that any trial must be registered in order to be published in any of their comprehensive list of journals.[12] The purpose of trial registration is a greater efficiency by reducing unnecessary duplication of research effort, better compliance, and a greater assurance that all clinical trials reports are reported, including those with negative results. There are several clinical trial registers worldwide including the Australian and New Zealand Clinical Trial Registry (ANZCTR).[13]

Privacy and confidentiality

Clinical research almost invariably involves the use of personal information. Patients provide information with the expectation that it will be treated confidentially and the unauthorised disclosure of such information may be a risk to the subject which should be considered in any research project. Similar to medical records in general, patient privacy laws apply to research records.

Multicentre research

Some of the difficulties in emergency research in children, such as the low frequency of major outcomes or limited applicability of findings, can be overcome by co-operating with other institutions. This recognition has led to a number of co-operative research networks, initially in North America (Pediatric Emergency Research Canada (PERC) and Pediatric Emergency Care Applied Research Network (PECARN)), in Australia and New Zealand (Paediatric Research in Emergency Departments International Collaborative (PREDICT)) and now also in Europe (Research in European Paediatric Emergency Departments (REPEDS)). These networks have increased the profile of paediatric emergency medicine, illustrated the similarities and differences in practice across geographical areas and are increasing the evidence base for interventions.[14]

Funding research

Finding funding for research is a challenge. In Australia the major large sources are ARC and NHMRC grants, with smaller disease- and specialty-specific competitive funding bodies such as Diabetes Australia Research Trust, National Heart Foundation, and so on. Obtaining such funding requires a robust research question and study design, and a strong track record. Evidence of seed funding and pilot data is also useful. Seed funding may come from professional societies, research institutions and private practice funds. Infrastructure support may come from the hospitals, universities or research institutes. Philanthropic funds are also available, though these are increasingly competitive. Collaboration with other successful groups and researchers is another key to funding success.

Controversies and future directions

❶ Trainees are expected to undertake research during their training. Due to time constraints this encourages low level studies and biases against RCTs or Systematic Reviews. Supervisors should offer research training for trainees.

❷ Most public hospital departments are poorly resourced both financially and with research-specific personnel to undertake research in emergencies in children. There is a pressing need for the development of university departments of paediatric emergency medicine.

❸ The development of cross linkages through research networks such as PREDICT has helped build capacity in emergency departments. It has also provided increased exposure of paediatric emergency research to funding agencies which may be the basis for developing high level research studies with dissemination of both research projects and their results into more emergency departments.

❹ Expansion of cross-linkages between international research networks is being developed and should further enhance the dissemination of evidence based emergency medicine.

References

1. National Health and Medical Research Council of Australia. *Levels of Evidence Guidelines.* Available from: http://www.nhmrc.gov.au/guidelines/consult/consultations/add_levels_grades_dev_guidelines2.htm [accessed 29.10.10].
2. National Institutes of Health. Office of Human Subjects Research. *Regulations and Ethical Guidelines.* Available from:http://ohsr.od.nih.gov/guidelines/nuremberg.html [accessed 29.10.10].
3. World Medical Association Declaration of Helsinki. *Ethical Principles of Medical Research involving Human Subjects.* Available from:http://www.wma.net/en/30publications/10policies/b3/index.html [accessed 29.10.10].
4. National Institutes of Health. Office of Human Subjects Research. *Regulations and Ethical Guidelines.* Available from:http://ohsr.od.nih.gov/guidelines/belmont.html [accessed 29.10.10].
5. National Health and Medical Research Council. Australian Research Council. Australian Vice Chancellors' Committee. *National Statement on Ethical Conduct in Human Research.* Available from:http://www.nhmrc.gov.au/PUBLICATIONS/ethics/2007_humans/contents.htm [accessed 29.10.10].
6. Therapeutics Goods Administration. Available from:www.tga.gov.au/docs/pdf/euguide/ich/ich13595.pdf [accessed 29.10.10].
7. Green JB, Duncan RE, Barnes GL, Oberklaid F. Putting the 'informed' into 'consent': a matter of plain language. *J Paediatr Child Health* 2003;**39**(9):700–3.
8. CONSORT group. *The CONSORT Statement.* Available from:http://www.consort-statement.org/consort-statement/ [accessed 29.10.10].
9. EQUATOR Network. *Introduction to reporting guidelines.* Available from: http://www.equator-network.org/resource-centre/library-of-health-research-reporting/reporting-guidelines/ [accessed 20.10.10].
10. *International Conference on Harmonisation of Technical Requirements for Registration of Pharmaceuticals for Human Use.' ICH Guidelines.* Available from:http://www.ich.org/cache/compo/276-254-1.html [accessed 29.10.10].
11. National Health and Medical Research Council. Australian Research Council. Australian Vice Chancellors' Committee. *Australian Code for the Responsible Conduct of Research.* 2007. Available from: http://www.nhmrc.gov.au/_files_nhmrc/file/publications/synopses/r39.pdf [accessed 29.10.10].
12. International Committee of Medical Journal Editors. *Uniform Requirements for Manuscripts Submitted to Biomedical Journals: Publishing and Editorial Issues Related to Publication in Biomedical Journals: Obligation to Register Clinical Trials.* Available from:http://www.icmje.org/publishing_10register.html [accessed 29.10.10].
13. *Australian and New Zealand Clinical Trials Registry.* Available from:www.anzctr.org.au; [accessed 20.10.10].
14. Kuppermann N, Holmes JF, Dayan PS, et al. Identification of children at very low risk of clinically-important brain injuries after head trauma: a prospective cohort study. *Lancet* 2009;**374**(9696):1160–70.

ADOLESCENT MEDICINE IN THE EMERGENCY DEPARTMENT

SECTION

30

Section editor **Ian Everitt**

30.1 Adolescent medicine in the emergency department

Katherine Barton • Donald Payne

ESSENTIALS

1 Establishing rapport is essential for a successful adolescent health consultation.

2 Interviewing adolescents in a quiet, more private setting, removed from the main ED, is a great advantage.

3 It is important to see adolescents on their own.

4 Using the HEADSS framework as an *aide-mémoire* will help exploration of relevant psychosocial issues.

5 Explanation of confidentiality is essential.

6 Discussion should be professional and in language the young person is able to understand.

Introduction

Many health professionals find working with adolescents challenging. Communication can be difficult, the priorities of adolescents are different to those of adults and issues of consent, confidentiality and privacy take on particular significance.[1] Adolescents also take time, which is not always readily available in the emergency department (ED). The perceived discomfort that some professionals experience working with adolescents usually reflects a lack of training in this area.[2] However, as with any area of medicine, specific training can lead to an increase in clinicians' competence and confidence in dealing with adolescents.[3] Keys to working effectively with this group include developing confidence in talking to adolescents and understanding the concept of adolescent development.

Although different age ranges have been proposed, it is more appropriate to think of adolescence as a process – during which an individual moves from being a dependent child to an independent adult.[4] The developmental changes that occur during adolescence include the obvious physical changes of growth and puberty as well as the less well-recognised cognitive and social changes. A key task of adolescence is for individuals to establish their own identity and self-image. This involves developing independence from parents, forming relationships outside the family, challenging authority and experimenting with different behaviours, some of which can pose a health risk. Health professionals working with adolescents need to acknowledge this process and be aware of the impact of emerging adolescent behaviours on health outcomes, as well as the effect of illness on normal adolescent development.[4,5]

Adolescent health problems in the ED

Whether the setting is an adult, mixed or paediatric ED, all emergency doctors are likely to see adolescents in their daily practice. The leading causes of death among adolescents and young adults are motor vehicle accidents and suicide.[6] The most common causes of morbidity include injuries (both intentional and non-intentional), mental health problems, drug and alcohol misuse and sexual health problems (Table 30.1.1). In addition, the number of adolescents and young adults growing up with chronic diseases of childhood is increasing as a result of improved treatment of these conditions. Many presentations to ED for primary physical problems are linked with psychosocial issues or with health risk behaviours, such as drug and alcohol use, unsafe sex and physical risk-taking. Clinicians working in ED must therefore be aware of these underlying risk factors and feel confident in being able to discuss them and liaise with local adolescent resources as needed.

The approach to the adolescent in the ED

Establishing rapport

Establishing rapport is essential for a successful adolescent health consultation. Empathy, trust and respect are important keys in any doctor–patient relationship, but especially so for adolescents. Establishing rapport in ED can be challenging, but not impossible. Adolescents may present to an adult department, where they could find themselves surrounded by much older patients, or to a paediatric department, full of infants, toddlers and understandably anxious parents. The setting may therefore have a significant impact on the consultation. The

---

Table 30.1.1 Health issues for adolescents presenting to medical care

Accidents and injuries: motor vehicle accidents, bicycle and pedestrian accidents, work related injuries, falls, assaults, poisonings
Mental health issues: anxiety, depression, self harm, suicide attempts, psychosis, personality disorders, eating disorders
Drug related: alcohol, illicit drug use
Infectious diseases: e.g. influenza, meningococcal infection, pneumonia
Chronic disease: asthma, cystic fibrosis, diabetes mellitus, inflammatory bowel disease, chronic pain/fatigue syndromes, allergies
Sexual health: pregnancy, sexually transmitted infections

Source: Australian Institute of Health and Welfare (AIHW) 2007. Young Australians – Their Health and Well Being 2007. Cat. No. PHE 87. Canberra. www.aihw.gov.au.

---

ability to see adolescents in a quiet, more private setting, removed from the main business of the ED, is a great advantage.

Seeing adolescents alone

It is important to see adolescents on their own, separate from parents, for at least part of the consultation. This helps to establish rapport and trust and optimises the chances that the young person will talk openly about relevant issues. Adolescents often contribute little to the history when parents are present. However, on their own, they are much more likely to open up. Parents may find it difficult to separate from the adolescent for the health consultation. This process is helped by explaining that it is routine practice to see adolescents on their own and emphasising the importance of the young person beginning to take responsibility for their own health. Spending time with parents on their own afterwards (after discussing with the young person what you will tell them) may alleviate their anxieties.

Unless the urgency of the situation dictates otherwise, it is helpful to begin the consultation by asking adolescents one or two general questions (e.g. what school do you go to? where do you live? who else is at home?) rather than immediately focusing on the medical presentation. This helps to put them at ease and shows that you see them as a person first who happens to have a medical problem.

Using the HEADSS framework

Table 30.1.2 shows the HEADSS framework, used widely around the world, which acts as a helpful guide for clinicians to use when interviewing adolescents.[7] HEADSS begins with relatively unthreatening questions about home, school and activities. These have the dual purpose of gathering information and allowing time to develop rapport. However, difficulties in these areas (e.g. prolonged school absence, no hobbies or interests) may be a reflection of problems in other areas. As mentioned earlier, mental health problems, such as anxiety or depression, and health risk behaviours such as smoking, alcohol and other drug use are common in adolescents and should always be considered.

Doctors may find it difficult to communicate with adolescents with regards to health risk behaviours. It is important to remain

---

Table 30.1.2 HEADSS

H Home
Where do you live? Who lives with you?
How do you get on with the people you live with?
Who would you talk to if you had a problem?
E Education (or employment)
Which school do you go to? Which year are you in?
Which subjects do you enjoy? What are you good at?
Who do you spend time with at school? What are the teachers like?
A Activities
What do you enjoy doing outside of school?
Are you in any clubs or sports teams?
Who do you meet up with at weekends?
D Drugs
Do your friends smoke cigarettes or drink alcohol? How about you?
How much do you smoke/drink? Every day? At weekends?
Have you ever tried marijuana or other drugs?
S Sexuality
Do any of your friends have girlfriends/boyfriends? How about you?
Have you ever had sex? Do you use condoms/the pill?
S Suicide
How would you describe your mood? Do you ever get really down?
Some people who feel really down often feel like hurting themselves or even killing themselves. Have you ever felt like that?
Have you ever tried to hurt yourself?

---

empathic and non-judgemental but to convey concern about risk taking and its potentially harmful consequences. It is also important to frame discussions about treatment options in language which the young person is likely to understand.[4] Tailoring your approach depending on the developmental stage of the adolescent allows you to take a thorough history more easily. For example, younger adolescents (with more concrete thinking) respond best to simple, closed questions. Older adolescents understand more abstract concepts and can more easily answer open-ended questions and contemplate the future. This becomes important when discussing adherence to treatment and health risk behaviours. Younger adolescents are only able to comprehend short-term consequences, whereas older adolescents can foresee the longer-term implications of their behaviour. At times, adolescent patients will be difficult to engage. This is especially so considering that many presentations to ED will be in relation to sensitive issues such as psychosocial problems or substance abuse. It is often a situation of high stress for both the young person and their family. Acknowledging this and demonstrating patience is important.

Confidentiality

One of the barriers to adolescents seeking medical care is a perceived lack of confidentiality. Establishing confidentiality is thus essential at the beginning of the adolescent consultation. It is important to explain that, whilst you may discuss aspects of their case with colleagues and write in patient notes, you will not discuss things with their parents without their permission. It is also essential to explain the limitations of confidentiality. The disclosure of any activity that puts the patient at serious risk of significant harm (such as suicidal thoughts or physical/sexual abuse) cannot remain confidential. Neither can the disclosure of activities that put others at risk. Clearly, establishing confidentiality at the beginning of a consultation fosters an honest and open communication between the doctor and the young person. Adolescents who are assured of some degree of confidentiality are more likely to speak frankly.[8] In practice, this increases the chances of being able to address a range of health-related issues, such as treatment adherence, mood and drug and alcohol use, thus opening up the possibility of providing effective health care.

The mature minor principle

The legal age for consent to treatment varies between states within Australia.[5] However, when working with adolescents, regardless of their age, the mature minor principle can always be employed.[9] This states that a young person can consent to treatment without parental knowledge if they are considered to be competent to do so by their treating clinician. The clinician must be confident that the young person understands the proposed treatment, its benefits and risks and is able to make an informed decision. An adolescent's competence to consent to treatment will clearly depend on the complexity of the treatment proposed. In practice it is best to try to encourage adolescents to involve their parents, or another adult whom they trust, in any treatment decision. However, sometimes adolescents will choose not to involve their parents. In these circumstances it is sensible for clinicians to consult with another colleague rather than taking sole responsibility for difficult decisions. Clinicians have a duty of care to provide the best

treatment for their patients at the time of presentation. In addition, for adolescents, it is particularly important that their experience of health services is a positive one, thereby optimising the chances that they will feel confident to access appropriate health services in the future.

Psychosocial screening

Adolescence is a critical time when health behaviours are established, and doctors can have an important role in reinforcing positive health behaviours. Presentations to ED should be seen as an opportunity for health promotion, especially considering many young people do not have a local general practitioner.[6] Although more pertaining to a physician consultation in an outpatient clinic setting, psychosocial screening (HEADSS) can be a very useful tool in the ED consultation. Due to the fact that many young people present with mental health issues, it is important to assess the psychosocial factors that may be contributing to the current presentation. This is especially important when young people present to the emergency department with mental health issues, alcohol and drug issues and chronic unexplained problems such as pain and fatigue. It is helpful to summarise in advance the types of questions you plan to ask and to explain their relevance to health outcomes. Normalising the process by explaining that you ask all adolescents these same questions can help make the young person feel more at ease. Beginning with an explanation about confidentiality is essential.[5] Sensitive questions can be more easily asked using a third person approach, such as 'Do any of your friends use marijuana?' before progressing to asking about the patient themselves.

Physical examination

The examination of the adolescent patient is essentially the same as the examination of an adult patient, from general inspection and observations to a systematic approach to each of the major systems. However, clinicians must be sensitive to the developmental stage of the young person. Priority should be placed on *privacy*, and making the young person feel comfortable. Simply explaining what you are about to do can ease embarrassment. It is sensible to try to find a chaperone to be present during an examination.

Accurate staging of puberty may be required in certain cases. At the end of the examination, the findings should be explained in language the young person is able to understand. If the examination is normal, a simple explanation of this fact will be very reassuring for a young person.[4]

Linking adolescents with community follow up

Given that mental health problems, health risk behaviours and sexual health problems are common among adolescents and young adults presenting to ED, it is useful for clinicians to have access to information about youth-friendly services available in the local community. These include sexual health clinics, drug and alcohol centres, mental health services and drop-in centres. Some may require a referral, others may accept self-referrals. Clinicians should be able to provide adolescents with written information and website addresses. Education should also be considered. If appropriate (e.g. those with prolonged school absence), an attempt should be made to link adolescents with hospital school services, where they exist.[10]

Summary

Adolescents require clinicians to have a different approach compared to paediatric or adult patients. Priorities should include privacy, confidentiality and adequate time spent with the young person. The reasons for presenting to ED are often complex. Performing a psychosocial screen can be very rewarding. Many young people have no general practitioner and therefore ED visits should be seen as an opportunity for preventive health screening, in addition to acute management. Training in adolescent health for all staff working in ED will be of benefit to both patients and staff.

Controversies and future directions

Where should adolescents and young adults be seen?

There is no consistent policy between different hospitals regarding the upper age limit for attendance at a paediatric ED. Some departments will not treat adolescents once they reach the age of 14, while others continue to see young adults into their early 20s. Regardless of the age of the patient, it is important that each ED has the staff and facilities to provide developmentally appropriate care for adolescents and young adults.

Facilities for managing aggressive, intoxicated or distressed adolescents.

ED staff need to be able to manage these patients with access to appropriate facilities, such as secure, safe rooms that are equipped to allow adolescents to recover without the risk of harming themselves or others. ED staff require specific training to ensure that they are both competent and confident in managing these patients.

Opportunistic health screening

Attendance at ED can highlight the presence of underlying health problems (e.g. anxiety, depression) or health-risk behaviours (e.g. alcohol or other drug use; unprotected sex). Attempting to address these issues is not straightforward and may be considered to be an inappropriate use of health professionals' time in ED. However, addressing these issues has the potential to prevent subsequent problems and re-attendance at ED.

References

1. Payne D, Martin C, Viner R, Skinner R. Adolescent medicine in paediatric practice. *Arch Dis Child* 2005;**90**:1133–7.
2. McDonagh JE, Southwood TR, Shaw KL. Unmet education and training needs of rheumatology health professionals in adolescent health and transitional care. *Rheumatology* 2004;**43**:737–43.
3. Sanci LA, Coffey CM, Veit FC, et al. Evaluation of the effectiveness of an educational intervention for general practitioners in adolescent health care: randomised controlled trial. *Br Med J* 2000;**320**:224–230.
4. Christie D, Viner R. Adolescent development. *Br Med J* 2005;**330**:301–4.
5. *Adolescent Health GP Resource Kit.* 2nd ed. Available from:http://www.caah.chw.edu.au/resources/#03 [accessed 29.10.10].
6. Australian Institute of Health and Welfare (AIHW). *Young Australians – their health and wellbeing 2007.* 2007 Available from:www.aihw.gov.au/publications/index.cfm/title/10451 [accessed 29.10.10].
7. Goldenring JM, Cohen E. Getting into adolescent heads. *Contemp Pediatr* 1988;(July):75–90.
8. Ford CA, Millstein SG, Halpern-Felsher BL, et al. Influence of physician confidentiality assurances on adolescents' willingness to disclose information and seek future health care. A randomized controlled trial. *JAMA* 1997;**278**:1029–34.
9. Sanci LA, Sawyer SM, Kang MS, et al. Confidential health care for adolescents: reconciling clinical evidence with family values. *Med J Aust* 2005;**183**:410–4.
10. *Hospital School Services.* Available from: www.hospitalschoolservices.wa.edu.au [accessed 29.10.10].

Index